VARCAROLIS'

Foundations of Psychiatric Mental Health Nursing

A CLINICAL APPROACH

VARCAROLIS'

Foundations of Psychiatric Mental Health Nursing

A CLINICAL APPROACH

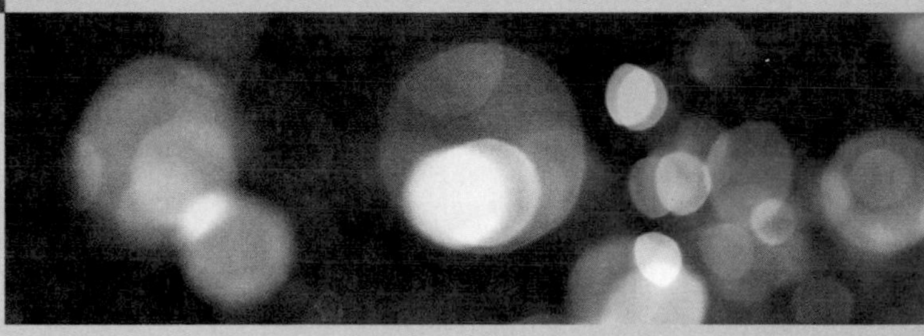

SEVENTH EDITION

Margaret Jordan Halter, PhD, PMHCNS

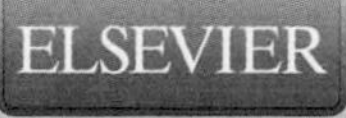

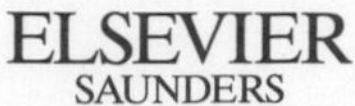

ELSEVIER
SAUNDERS

3251 Riverport Lane
St. Louis, Missouri 63043

VARCAROLIS' FOUNDATIONS OF PSYCHIATRIC MENTAL HEALTH NURSING: A CLINICAL APPROACH

ISBN: 978-1-4557-5358-1

Notices

Knowledge and best practice in this field are constantly changing. As new research and experience broaden our understanding, changes in research methods, professional practices, or medical treatment may become necessary.

Practitioners and researchers must always rely on their own experience and knowledge in evaluating and using any information, methods, compounds, or experiments described herein. In using such information or methods they should be mindful of their own safety and the safety of others, including parties for whom they have a professional responsibility.

With respect to any drug or pharmaceutical products identified, readers are advised to check the most current information provided (i) on procedures featured or (ii) by the manufacturer of each product to be administered, to verify the recommended dose or formula, the method and duration of administration, and contraindications. It is the responsibility of practitioners, relying on their own experience and knowledge of their patients, to make diagnoses, to determine dosages and the best treatment for each individual patient, and to take all appropriate safety precautions.

To the fullest extent of the law, neither the Publisher nor the authors, contributors, or editors assume any liability for any injury and/or damage to persons or property as a matter of products liability, negligence or otherwise, or from any use or operation of any methods, products, instructions, or ideas contained in the material herein.

Library of Congress Cataloging-in-Publication Data

Varcarolis' foundations of psychiatric mental health nursing : a clinical approach. — 7th ed. / [edited by] Margaret Jordan Halter.
p. ; cm.
Foundations of psychiatric mental health nursing
Rev. ed. of: Foundations of psychiatric mental health nursing / [edited by] Elizabeth M. Varcarolis, Margaret Jordan Halter. 6th ed. c2010.
Includes bibliographical references and index.
ISBN 978-1-4557-5358-1 (pbk. : alk. paper)
I. Halter, Margaret J. (Margaret Jordan) II. Varcarolis, Elizabeth M. III. Foundations of psychiatric mental health nursing. IV. Title: Foundations of psychiatric mental health nursing.
[DNLM: 1. Mental Disorders—nursing. 2. Psychiatric Nursing. WY 160]
RC440
616.89'0231—dc23

2013012893

Senior Content Strategist: Yvonne Alexopoulos
Senior Content Development Specialist: Lisa P. Newton
Publishing Services Manager: Jeff Patterson
Senior Project Manager: Clay S. Broeker
Design Direction: Karen Pauls

Printed in the United States of America

Last digit is the print number: 9 8 7 6 5 4 3 2 1

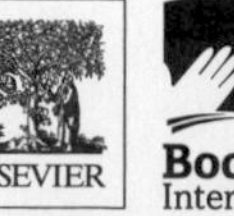

In honor of my grandmother, Edith (1882-1927), who lost her life to depression before hope of recovery existed.

1-in-128 odds for 7 female births in a row . . . to our dear daughters, Elissa, Emily, and Monica, and their daughters, Kiran, Leela, Vivienne, and Violette. My husband, Paul, is a loved man indeed!

And finally, to my twin sister, Anne. What a bonus in life.

ACKNOWLEDGMENTS

My ancestors were storytellers. Boxes of diaries, articles, newspaper clippings, and books in an unused closet detail many of their moves and thoughts. The family tree includes a newspaper editor, a historian, a poet, and a nonfiction writer. One great aunt, Ella Chalfant, published a book titled *A Goodly Heritage* in 1955 and was likely an early feminist. Her book centered on inheritance laws in the 1800s and featured copies of wills that demonstrated the disenfranchisement of women (e.g., a husband needed to leave a wife's clothing to her on his death). As a registered nurse, I did have the opportunity to write some stories (in the form of nurses notes); as a tenure-track faculty member, I was required to write some stories (in the form of presentations and publications).

A 2004 phone call finally put me on the path to more fully join these relatives in their vocation. I was in my office when the phone rang. A pleasant voice with a slight New York accent says, "Peggy? Hi, this is Betsy Varcarolis." I knew the name at once. She went on, "The reason I'm calling is that I very much enjoyed your article, "Stigma and help seeking related to depression: A study of nursing students." I would like to feature it as an Evidence-Based Practice box in the fifth edition of my book." I was thrilled—what an honor!

This was the beginning. After that call, my work progressed from chapter reviewer to chapter writer to textbook editor. I accomplished these milestones as an apprentice of Elizabeth Varcarolis, the genius who conceived and published the first edition of *Foundations of Psychiatric Mental Health Nursing* in 1990 and went on to make this textbook a leader in the specialty of psychiatric nursing. Betsy has the rare gift of making the complex understandable and of making impersonal learning a joint process in which the experts talk with the students rather than just providing information.

In this seventh edition of the book, Elizabeth Varcarolis is honored with her name being added to the title. My sincere thanks and gratitude go out to Betsy for what she has done for my life goals, the profession, countless students, and recipients of psychiatric mental health care. I wish for her all the best as she enjoys retirement with her husband, Paul.

My heartfelt appreciation also goes out to the talented group of writers who contributed to the seventh edition. This was an especially challenging version since the publication year was the same as for the *Diagnostic and Statistical Manual's* fifth edition. Clinical chapters were rearranged, and content was added and deleted. My particular thanks go to those contributors who created new chapters and incorporated new content.

I have a talented pool of veteran writers, and their knowledge and passion continue to influence psychiatric nursing in this edition. I have also welcomed a new cohort of writers whose expertise was both recognized and sought. It has truly been a joy working with each of you. Thanks for the countless hours you spent researching, writing, and rewriting!

A huge debt of gratitude goes to the many educators and clinicians who reviewed the manuscript and offered valuable suggestions, ideas, opinions, and criticisms. All comments were appreciated and helped refine and strengthen the individual chapters.

Throughout this project, a number of people at Elsevier provided superb support. Sincere thanks go to Clay Broeker, my gracious project manager, and to Karen Pauls, a talented and creative designer. Special gratitude goes to the team who got this project off the ground and kept it airborne for nearly 2 years. Yvonne Alexopoulos, senior content strategist, kept me on a straight path; Lisa Newton, senior content development specialist, was my ever-optimistic team member who celebrated each milestone; and Kit Blanke (Mr. Kit Blanke), content coordinator, helped keep me organized and up to speed on technological advances. My sincere thanks go out to the whole Elsevier team.

Peggy Halter

CONTRIBUTORS

Lois Angelo, APRN, BC
Assistant Professor of Nursing
Massachusetts College of Pharmacy and Health Sciences
Boston, Massachusetts
Chapter 17: Somatic Symptom Disorders

Carolyn Baird, DNP, MBA, RN-BC, CARN-AP, ICCDPD
Co-Occurring Disorders Therapist
Counseling and Trauma Services
Canonsburg, Pennsylvania
Chapter 22: Substance-Related and Addictive Disorders

Leslie A. Briscoe, PMHNP-BC
Psychiatric Nurse Practitioner
U.S. Department of Veterans Affairs
Cleveland, Ohio
Chapter 30: Psychosocial Needs of the Older Adult

Penny S. Brooke, APRN, MS, JD
Professor Emeritus
University of Utah,
Salt Lake City, Utah
Chapter 6: Legal and Ethical Guidelines for Safe Practice

Claudia A. Cihlar, PhD, PMHCNS-BC
Coordinator of Behavioral Health Services
Center for Psychiatry
Akron General Medical Center
Akron, Ohio
Chapter 24: Personality Disorders

Alison M. Colbert, PhD, APRN, BC
Assistant Professor
Duquesne University
Pittsburgh, Pennsylvania
Chapter 32: Forensic Psychiatric Nursing

Laura Cox Dzurec, PhD, PMHCNS, BC
Dean, College of Nursing
Kent State University
Chapter 34: Family Interventions
Chapter 35: Integrative Care

Carissa R. Enright, RN, MSN, PMHNP-BC
Associate Clinical Professor
Texas Woman's University
Psychiatric Consult Liaison
Presbyterian Hospital of Dallas
Dallas, Texas
Chapter 18: Feeding, Eating, and Elimination Disorders

Jodie Flynn, MSN, RN, SANE-A, SANE-P, D-ABMDI
Undergraduate Program Coordinator
Dwight Schar College of Nursing and Health Sciences
Ashland University
Mansfield, Ohio
Chapter 29: Sexual Assault

Kimberly Gregg, PhD(c), MS, PMHCNS-BC
Psychiatric Mental Health Clinical Nurse Specialist
Hennepin County Medical Center
Minneapolis, Minnesota
Clinical Assistant Professor, University of North Dakota
Grand Forks, North Dakota
Chapter 5: Cultural Implications for Psychiatric Mental Health Nursing

Faye J. Grund, PhD(c), APRN, PMHNP-BC
Interim Dean
Dwight Schar College of Nursing and Health Sciences
Ashland University
Mansfield, Ohio
Chapter 25: Suicide and Non-Suicidal Self-Injury

Mary A. Gutierrez, PharmD, BCPP
Professor of Clinical Pharmacy and Psychiatry
Department of Pharmacotherapy and Outcomes Science
Loma Linda University School of Pharmacy
Loma Linda, California
Chapter 3: Biological Basis for Understanding Psychiatric Disorders and Treatments

Monica J. Halter, APRN, PMHNP-BC
Psychiatric Nurse Practitioner
Psychological and Behavioral Consultants
Cleveland, Ohio
Chapter 4: Settings for Psychiatric Care

Edward A. Herzog, RN, BSN, MSN, CNS
Lecturer
College of Nursing
Kent State University
Kent, Ohio
Chapter 12: Schizophrenia and Schizophrenia Spectrum Disorders
Chapter 31: Serious Mental Illness

Diane K. Kjervik, JD, RN, FAAN
Professor Emeritus
School of Nursing
University of North Carolina at Chapel Hill
Chapel Hill, North Carolina
Chapter 6: Legal and Ethical Guidelines for Safe Practice

Mallie Kozy, PhD, PMHCNS-BC
Associate Professor, Chair
Undergraduate Nursing Studies, College of Nursing
Lourdes University
Sylvania, Ohio
Chapter 14: Depressive Disorders

Jerika T. Lam, PharmD, AAHIVE
Assistant Director
Inpatient Pharmacy Department
Kaiser Moreno Valley Hospital
Moreno Valley, California
Chapter 3: Biological Basis for Understanding Psychiatric Disorders and Treatments

Lorann Murphy, MSN, PMHCNS-BC
Clinical Nurse Specialist
Lutheran Hospital
Cleveland, Ohio
Chapter 27: Anger, Aggression, and Violence

Cindy Parsons, DNP, ARNP, PMHNP-BC, FAANP
Associate Professor of Nursing
University of Tampa
Tampa, Florida
Chapter 11: Childhood and Neurodevelopmental Disorders

Donna Rolin-Kenny, PhD, APRN, PMHCNS-BC
Assistant Professor, School of Nursing
University of Texas at Austin
Austin, Texas
Chapter 33: Therapeutic Groups

Judi Sateren, MS, RN
Associate Professor Emerita
St. Olaf College
Northfield, Minnesota
Chapter 28: Child, Older Adult, and Intimate Partner Violence

Mary Ann Schaepper, MD, MEd
Director of Psychiatry Residency Training
Loma Linda University Medical Center
Associate Professor of Psychiatry
Loma Linda University School of Medicine
Loma Linda, California
Chapter 3: Biological Basis for Understanding Psychiatric Disorders and Treatments

L. Kathleen Sekula, PhD, APRN, FAAN
Associate Professor and Director
Forensic Graduate Nursing Programs
Duquesne University
Pittsburgh, Pennsylvania
Chapter 32: Forensic Psychiatric Nursing

Jane Stein-Parbury, RN, BSN, MEd, PhD, FRCNA
Professor of Mental Health Nursing
Faculty of Health, University of Technology
Director
Area Professorial Mental Health Nursing Unit
South East Sydney Local Health District
Sydney, Australia
Chapter 23: Neurocognitive Disorders

Christine Tebaldi, MS, PMHNP-BC
Director of Psychiatric Emergency and Consultative Services
Community Hospital Programs
McLean Hospital
Belmont, Massachusetts
Chapter 4: Settings for Psychiatric Care

Margaret Trussler, MS, APRN-BC
Sleep Health Centers
Boston, Massachusetts
Clinical Faculty
University of Massachusetts
Worcester, Massachusetts
Chapter 19: Sleep-Wake Disorders

Elizabeth M. Varcarolis, RN, MA
Professor Emeritus and former Deputy Chairperson
Department of Nursing
Borough of Manhattan Community College
Associate Fellow
Albert Ellis Institute for Rational Emotional Behavioral Therapy (REBT)
New York, New York
Chapter 7: The Nursing Process and Standards of Care for Psychiatric Mental Health Nursing
Chapter 8: Therapeutic Relationships
Chapter 9: Communication and the Clinical Interview
Chapter 10: Understanding and Managing Responses to Stress
Chapter 16: Anxiety and Obsessive-Compulsive Related Disorders

Kathleen Wheeler, PhD, APRN-BC, PMHCNS, PMHNP, FAAN
Professor
Fairfield University School of Nursing
Fairfield, Connecticut
Chapter 16: Trauma, Stressor-Related, and Dissociative Disorders

Rick Zoucha, PhD, APRN-BC, CTN-A
Associate Professor, School of Nursing
Duquesne University
Pittsburgh, Pennsylvania
Chapter 5: Cultural Implications for Psychiatric Mental Health Nursing

Ancillary Writers

Teresa S. Burckhalter, MSN, RN, BC
Nursing Instructor
Technical College of the Lowcountry
Beaufort, South Carolina
Test Bank

Patricia Clayburn, MSN, RN
Professional Instructor
Dwight Schar College of Nursing
Ashland University
Ashland, Ohio
Chapter Review Questions

Marie Messier, MSN, RN
Associate Professor of Nursing
Germanna Community College
Locust Grove, Virginia
Case Studies/Nursing Care Plans

Kathleen Slyh, RN, MSN
Nursing Instructor
Technical College of the Lowcountry
Beaufort, South Carolina
PowerPoint Presentations

Linda Turchin, RN, MSN, CNE
Assistant Professor of Nursing
Fairmont State University
Fairmont, West Virginia
Test Bank Reviewer
Pre-Tests/Post-Tests

Linda Wendling, MS, MFA
Learning Theory Consultant
University of Missouri—St. Louis
St. Louis, Missouri
TEACH for Nurses

REVIEWERS

Irma Aguilar, RN, PhD
Associate Professor
Tarrant County College District
Fort Worth, Texas

Claudia Chiesa, PhD, RPh
Staff Pharmacist
Catalina Pharmacy Management Services
Tucson, Arizona

Phyllis M. Jacobs, RN, MSN
Assistant Professor
Wichita State University
Wichita, Kansas

Susan Justice, MSN, RN, CNS
Clinical Instructor
Psychiatric Nursing Lead Faculty
University of Texas College of Nursing
Arlington, Texas

Marti Rickel, RN, MSN
Instructor
North Seattle Community College
Seattle, Washington

Donna Rolin-Kenny, PhD, APRN, PMHCNS-BC,
Assistant Professor, School of Nursing
University of Texas at Austin
Austin, Texas

Judge Elinore Marsh Stormer
Summit County Probate Court
Akron, Ohio

Sheila R. Webster, MA, RN, PMHCNS-BC
Lecturer
Kent State University
Kent, Ohio

TO THE INSTRUCTOR

The role of the health care provider continues to become more challenging as our health care system is compromised by increasing federal cuts, lack of trained personnel, and the dictates of health maintenance organizations (HMOs) and behavioral health maintenance organizations (BHMOs). We nurses and our patients are from increasingly diverse cultural and religious backgrounds, bringing with us a wide spectrum of beliefs and practices. An in-depth consideration and understanding of cultural, religious/spiritual, and social practices is paramount in the administration of appropriate and effective nursing care and is emphasized throughout this text.

We are living in an age of fast-paced research in neurobiology, genetics, and psychopharmacology, as well as research to find the most effective evidence-based approaches for patients and their families. Legal issues and ethical dilemmas faced by the health care system are magnified accordingly. Given these myriad challenges, knowing how best to teach our students and serve our patients can seem overwhelming. With contributions from several knowledgeable and experienced nurse educators, our goal is to bring to you the most current and comprehensive trends and evidence-based practices in psychiatric mental health nursing.

CONTENT NEW TO THIS EDITION

The following topics are at the forefront of nursing practice and psychiatric-mental health care and are considered in detail in this seventh edition:

- Clinical disorders that are consistent with the *DSM-5* are presented along with corresponding nursing care.
- New and recombined *DSM-5* disorders are presented, including hoarding disorder, disruptive mood dysregulation disorder, premenstrual dysphoric disorder, binge eating disorder, and autism spectrum disorder.
- Quality and Safety Education for Nurses (QSEN) content—patient-centered care, teamwork and collaboration, evidence-based practice, quality improvement, safety, and informatics—are integrated naturally in the application of the nursing process.
- The social influence of mental health care and the importance of legislation are stressed throughout and are highlighted in Health Policy boxes.
- A complete update has been made on the biological basis for understanding psychiatric disorders and treatments (Chapter 3).
- Settings for psychiatric care are presented along a continuum of acuity and take into account the changing needs of individuals seeking and/or requiring psychiatric services (Chapter 4).
- Trauma, stressor-related, and dissociative disorders are given increased attention in a separate chapter to reflect the increasing recognition of these problems (Chapter 16).
- Screenings and severity ratings are introduced in Chapter 1 and included throughout most clinical chapters
- Chapter 19 provides an in-depth look at both normal sleep and also the cross-cutting problem of altered sleep that accompanies and/or exacerbates psychiatric disorders.
- A separate chapter focuses on impulse control disorders (Chapter 20).
- The terms *substance abuse* with *substance dependence* have been consolidated into the single problem of substance use disorder (Chapter 22)

Refer to the To the Student section of this introduction on pages xv-xvi for examples of thoroughly updated **familiar features with a fresh perspective,** including Evidence-Based Practice boxes, Considering Culture boxes, Health Policy boxes, Key Points to Remember, Assessment Guidelines, and Vignettes, among others.

ORGANIZATION OF THE TEXT

Chapters are grouped in units to emphasize the clinical perspective and facilitate location of information. The order of the clinical chapters approximates those found in the *DSM-5*. All clinical chapters are organized in a clear, logical, and consistent format with the nursing process as the strong, visible framework. The basic outline for clinical chapters is:

- **Clinical Picture:** Identifies disorders that fall under the umbrella of the general chapter name. This section presents an overview of the disorder(s) and includes strong source material.
- **Epidemiology:** Helps the student to understand the extent of the problem and characteristics of those who would more likely be affected. This section provides information related to prevalence, lifetime incidence, age of onset, and gender differences.
- **Comorbidity:** Describes the most common conditions that are associated with the psychiatric disorder. Knowing that comorbid disorders are often part of the clinical picture of specific disorders helps students as well as clinicians understand how to better assess and treat their patients.
- **Etiology:** Provides current views of causation along with formerly held theories. It is based on the biopsychosocial triad and includes biological, psychological, and environmental factors.
- **Assessment:**
  - **General Assessment:** Appropriate assessment for a specific disorder, including assessment tools and rating scales. The rating scales included help to highlight important areas in the assessment of a variety of behaviors or mental conditions. Because many of the answers are subjective in nature, experienced clinicians use these tools as a guide when planning care, in addition to their knowledge of their patients.

- **Self-Assessment:** Discusses the nurse's thoughts and feelings that may need to be addressed to enhance self-growth and provide the best possible and most appropriate care to the patient.
- **Assessment Guidelines:** Provides a summary of specific areas to assess by disorder.

- **Diagnosis:** NANDA International–approved nursing diagnoses are used in all nursing process sections.
- **Outcomes Identification:** *NIC* classifications for interventions and *NOC* classifications for outcomes are introduced in Chapter 8 and used throughout the text when appropriate.
- **Planning**
- **Implementation:** Interventions follow the Standards of Practice and Professional Performance set by *Psychiatric-Mental Health Nursing: Scope and Standards of Practice* (2007), developed collaboratively by the American Nurses Association, American Psychiatric Nurses Association, and International Society of Psychiatric–Mental Health Nurses. These standards are incorporated throughout the chapters and are listed on the inside back cover for easy reference.
- **Evaluation**

TEACHING AND LEARNING RESOURCES

For Instructors

Instructor Resources on Evolve, available at http://evolve.elsevier.com/Varcarolis, provide a wealth of material to help you make your psychiatric nursing instruction a success. In addition to all of the Student Resources, the following are provided for Faculty:

- **TEACH for Nurses Lesson Plans,** based on textbook chapter Learning Objectives, serve as ready-made, modifiable lesson plans and a complete roadmap to link all parts of the educational package. These concise and straightforward lesson plans can be modified or combined to meet your particular scheduling and teaching needs.
- **PowerPoint Presentations** are organized by chapter, with approximately 750 slides for in-class lectures. These are detailed and include customizable text and image lecture slides to enhance learning in the classroom or in Web-based course modules. If you share them with students, they can use the note feature to help them with your lectures.
- **Audience Response Questions for i>clicker and other systems** are provided with two to five multiple-answer questions per chapter to stimulate class discussion and assess student understanding of key concepts.
- The **Test Bank** has more than 1800 test items, complete with the correct answer, rationale, cognitive level of each question, corresponding step of the nursing process, appropriate NCLEX Client Needs label, and text page reference(s).
- A **DSM-5 Webinar** explaining the changes in structure and disorders is available for reference.

For Students

Student Resources on Evolve, available at http://evolve.elsevier.com/Varcarolis, provide a wealth of valuable learning resources. The Evolve Resources page near the front of the book gives login instructions and a description of each resource.

- The **Answer Key to Chapter Review Questions** provides answers and rationales for the Chapter Review questions at the end of each chapter.
- The **Answer Key to Critical Thinking Guidelines** provides possible outcomes for the Critical Thinking questions at the end of each chapter.
- **Case Studies and Nursing Care Plans** provide detailed case studies and care plans for specific psychiatric disorders to supplement those found in the textbook.
- **NCLEX® Review Questions,** provided for each chapter, will help you prepare for course examinations and for your RN licensure examination.
- **Pre-Tests and Post-Tests** provide interactive self-assessments for each chapter of the textbook, including instant scoring and feedback at the click of a button.

We are grateful to educators who send suggestions and provide feedback and hope this seventh edition continues to help students learn and appreciate the scope of psychiatric mental health nursing practice.

Peggy Halter

TO THE STUDENT

Psychiatric mental health nursing challenges us to understand the complexities of human behavior. In the chapters that follow, you will learn about people with psychiatric disorders and how to provide them with quality nursing care. As you read, keep in mind these special features.

READING AND REVIEW TOOLS

❶ **Key Terms and Concepts** and ❷ **Objectives** introduce the chapter topics and provide a concise overview of the material discussed.

Key Points to Remember listed at the end of each chapter reinforce essential information.

Critical Thinking activities at the end of each chapter are scenario-based critical thinking problems for practice in applying what you have learned. **Answer Guidelines** can be found on the Evolve website.

Multiple-choice **Chapter Review** questions at the end of each chapter help you review the chapter material and study for exams. **Answers** with **rationales** and textbook **page references** are located on the Evolve website.

ADDITIONAL LEARNING RESOURCES

Your ❸ **Evolve Resources** at **http://evolve.elsevier.com/Varcarolis** offer more helpful study aids, such as additional Case Studies and Nursing Care Plans.

CHAPTER FEATURES

❹ **Vignettes** describe the unique circumstances surrounding individual patients with psychiatric disorders.

❺ **Self-Assessment** sections discuss a nurse's thoughts and feelings that may need to be addressed to enhance self-growth and provide the best possible and most appropriate care to the patient.

❻ **Assessment Guidelines** in the clinical chapters provide summary points for patient assessment.

❼ **Evidence-Based Practice** boxes demonstrate how current research findings affect psychiatric mental health nursing practice and standards of care.

❽ **Guidelines for Communication** boxes provide tips for communicating therapeutically with patients and their families.

Considering Culture boxes reinforce the importance of providing culturally competent care.

Drug Treatment tables present the latest information on medications used to treat psychiatric disorders.

❾ **Patient and Family Teaching** boxes underscore the nurse's role in helping patients and families understand psychiatric disorders, treatments, complications, and medication side effects, among other important issues.

Case Studies and Nursing Care Plans present individualized histories of patients with specific psychiatric disorders following the steps of the nursing process. Interventions with rationales and evaluation statements are presented for each patient goal.

CHAPTER 16

Trauma, Stressor-Related, and Dissociative Disorders

Kathleen Wheeler

3 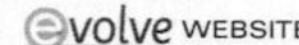 WEBSITE

Visit the Evolve website for a pretest on the content in this chapter.
http://evolve.elsevier.com/Varcarolis

Pre-Test interactive review

2 **OBJECTIVES**

1. Describe clinical manifestations of each disorder covered under the general umbrella of trauma-related and dissociative disorders.
2. Describe the symptoms, epidemiology, comorbidity, and etiology of trauma-related disorders in children.
3. Discuss at least five of the neurobiological changes that occur with trauma.
4. Apply the nursing process to the care of children who are experiencing trauma-related disorders.
5. Differentiate between the symptoms of posttraumatic stress, acute stress, and adjustment disorders in adults.
6. Describe the symptoms, epidemiology, comorbidity, and etiology of trauma-related disorders in adults.
7. Discuss how to deal with common reactions the nurse may experience while working with a patient who has suffered trauma.
8. Apply the nursing process to trauma-related disorders in adults.
9. Develop a teaching plan for a patient who suffers from posttraumatic stress disorder.
10. Identify dissociative disorders, including depersonalization/derealization disorder, dissociative amnesia, and dissociative identity disorder
11. Create a nursing care plan incorporating evidence-based interventions for symptoms of dissociation, including flashbacks, amnesia, and impaired self-care.
12. Role-play intervening with a patient who is experiencing a flashback.

1 **KEY TERMS AND CONCEPTS**

acute stress disorder
adjustment disorder
alternate personality (alter)
debriefing
depersonalization
derealization
disinhibited social engagement disorder
dissociation
dissociative amnesia
dissociative fugue
dissociative identity disorder
eye movement desensitization and reprocessing
flashbacks
hypervigilance
neuroplasticity
posttraumatic stress disorder (PTSD)
reactive attachment disorder
resilience
trauma-informed care
window of tolerance

304

---

466 UNIT IV Psychobiological Disorders

profound lack of empathy, also known as callousness. This callousness results in a lack of concern about the feelings of others, the absence of remorse or guilt except when facing punishment, and a disregard for meeting school, family, and other obligations.

These individuals tend to exhibit a shallow, unexpressive, and superficial affect; however, they may also be adept at portraying themselves as concerned and caring if these attributes help them to manipulate and exploit others. A person with antisocial personality disorder may be able to act witty and charming and be good at flattery and manipulating the emotions of others.

EPIDEMIOLOGY

Antisocial personality disorder is the most researched personality disorder, probably due to its marked impact on society in the form of criminal activity. The prevalence of antisocial personality disorder is about 1.1% in community studies (Skodol et al., 2011). While the disorder is much more common in men (3% versus 1%), women may be underdiagnosed due to the traditional close association of this disorder with males.

ETIOLOGY

Biological Factors

Antisocial personality disorder is genetically linked, and twin studies indicate a predisposition to this disorder. Kendler and colleagues (2012) note that the main two dimensions of genetic risk include the trait of aggressive-disregard (violent tendencies without concern for others) and the trait of disinhibition (lack of concern for consequences).

An alteration in serotonin transmission has also been implicated with the aggression and impulsivity that frequently accompany this disorder. Levels of a metabolite of serotonin, 5-hydroxyindoleacetic acid, can be measured in urine and cerebrospinal fluid. It has been found to be lower in individuals with antisocial personality disorder. Lower levels of serotonin along with dopamine hyperfunction may contribute to aggression, disinhibition, and comorbid substance abuse (Seo et al., 2008).

Environmental Factors

It is likely that a genetic predisposition for characteristics of antisocial personality disorder such as a lack of empathy may be set into motion by a childhood environment of inconsistent parenting and discipline, significant abuse, and extreme neglect. Children reflect parental attitudes and behaviors in the absence of more prosocial influences. Virtually all individuals who eventually develop this disorder have a history of impulse control and conduct problems as children and adolescents. Chapter 21 describes impulse control and conduct disorders in greater detail.

Cultural Factors

Assigning a diagnosis of personality disorder cannot be entirely separated from the cultural context of both the individual and the person diagnosing. Cultural bias, including race, ethnicity, ageism, religion, and gender expectations may unintentionally enter into the categorization. Some studies have found a higher prevalence rate of antisocial personality disorder in African Americans and in persons with co-occurring substance dependence (McGilloway et al, 2010).

VIGNETTE 4

Richard is a 25-year-old divorced cab driver who is referred to the hospital by the court for competency evaluation after an assault charge. He told the arresting officer that he has bipolar disorder. He has a history of substance abuse and multiple arrests for disorderly conduct or assault. During his intake interview, he is polite and even flirtatious with the female registered nurse. He insists that he is not responsible for his behavior because he is manic. The only symptom he describes is irritability. Richard points out that he cannot tolerate any psychotropic medications because of the side effects. He also notes that he has dropped out of three clinics after several visits because "the staff don't understand me."

APPLICATION OF THE NURSING PROCESS

ASSESSMENT

People with antisocial personality disorder do not enter the health care system for treatment of this disorder unless they have been court-ordered to do so. Psychiatric admissions may be initiated for anxiety and depression. Entering treatment may also be a way to avoid or address legal, financial, occupational, or other circumstances. Health care workers also encounter people with this disorder based on the physical consequences of high-risk behaviors, such as acute injury and substance use. Keep in mind that questions asked during the assessment phase may not always result in accurate responses since the patient may become defensive or simply not tell the truth.

Self-Assessment 5

You may respond to a person with antisocial personality disorder in a variety of ways. Because these individuals have the capacity to be charming, you may want to defend the person as someone who is being unfairly treated and misunderstood. These feelings should be explored with your faculty or other experienced personnel. Conversely, if you are aware that your patient has a history of criminal acts, you may feel disdain or personally threatened. Again, share your concerns with people who are experienced in caring for this population. Awareness and monitoring of one's own stress responses to patient behaviors facilitate more effective and therapeutic intervention, regardless of the specific approach to their care.

ASSESSMENT GUIDELINES 6

Antisocial Personality Disorder

1. Assess current life stressors.
2. Assess for suicidal, violent, and/or homicidal thoughts.
3. Assess anxiety, aggression, and anger levels.
4. Assess motivation for maintaining control.
5. Assess for substance misuse (past and present).

CHAPTER 16 Trauma, Stressor-Related, and Dissociative Disorders 307

7 **EVIDENCE-BASED PRACTICE**

Traumatic Stress Responses among Nurses

Buurman, B. M., Mank, A.P.M., Beijer, H.J.M., & Olff, M. (2011). Coping with serious events at work: A study of traumatic stress among nurses. *Journal of the American Psychiatric Nurses Association, 17,* 321-329.

Problem

Nurses frequently encounter traumatic events and experience chronic stress in the workplace that can lead to PTSD and burnout. Events that are traumatic include aggression among themselves as well as witnessing the pain, suffering, and death of others. These serious events involve helplessness, fear, or horror that can lead to PTSD while chronic interpersonal stressors at work often lead to burnout.

Purpose of Study

The purpose of this study was to describe the nature and number of serious events nurses encounter and their coping and reactions and to investigate which factors were related to traumatic stress after a serious event.

Methods

Nurses ($n = 69$) at a large university hospital in Amsterdam were asked to complete two questionnaires, the Utrecht Coping List and the List of Serious Events and Traumatic Stress in Nursing.

Key Findings

- 98% of nurses reported traumatic stress with a mean of 8 serious events experienced in the past 5 years.
- Active coping decreased the risk of experiencing traumatic stress while comforting cognition and social support increased the likelihood of appraising a serious event as traumatic.

Implications for Nursing Practice

Many nurses experience traumatic stress. Nurses need additional help particularly after events that threaten their physical integrity. More experienced nurses had more reactions after patients' deaths, perhaps because of cumulative trauma. Thus, experienced nurses are particularly vulnerable for developing PTSD and burnout. Interventions should be initiated consistently after traumatic events, and future research is warranted in order to determine what interventions are most effective in preventing PTSD and burnout.

anxious state. This theory provides an explanation of why many people with PTSD also suffer from depression.

Psychological Factors

Attachment Theory

A psychological theory that has important implications for trauma-related disorders is that of attachment theory. This theory describes the importance and dynamics of the early relationship between the infant and the caretaker based on the early work of Bowlby (1988). Attachment patterns or schemas are formed early in life through interaction and experiences with caregivers, and this relationship is embedded in implicit emotional and somatic memories. Research has demonstrated that these templates or patterns of attachment persist into adulthood. These schemas were studied and classified for young children and include secure, avoidant, ambivalent, and disorganized attachment styles (Ainsworth, 1967).

Environmental Factors

To a greater degree than adults, children are dependent on others. It is this dependency in tandem with the neuroplasticity (malleability) of the developing brain that can increase vulnerability to adverse life experiences. External factors in the environment can either support or put stress on children and adolescents and shape development. Young persons are vulnerable in an environment in which systems (e.g., schools, court systems) and adults (e.g., parents, counselors) have power and control. Parents model behavior and provide the child with a view of the world. If parents are abusive, rejecting, or overly controlling, the child may suffer detrimental effects during the period of development when the trauma occurs. Most children, however, who suffer a traumatic and stressful event do develop normally.

Poverty, parental substance abuse, and exposure to violence have received increasing attention and place minority children at greater risk for trauma and stress. Pervasive and persistent economic, social, and ethnic disparities are called the "millennial morbidities" (Shonkoff & Garner, 2012). A review of 58 studies found that racial and ethnic disparities in children's health are worsening (Flores, 2010). Differences in cultural expectations, presence of stresses, and lack of support by the dominant culture may have profound effects and increase the risk of mental, emotional, and academic problems. Family stability may provide cushioning effects in the face of poverty and adversity. Working with children and adolescents from diverse backgrounds requires an increased awareness of one's own biases and of the patient's needs.

The term resilience refers to positive adaptation, or the ability to maintain or regain mental health despite adversity. Studies have shown that factors that enhance resilience include the presence of supportive relationships and attachments as well as the avoidance of frequent and prolonged stress (Herrman et al., 2011). Children brought up in a chaotic or non-nurturing environment suffer neurological consequences that are long-lasting and difficult to remediate (Shonkoff & Garner, 2012). Toxic stress and adverse childhood experiences have been found to result in lifelong consequences for both psychological and physical health (Shonkoff, 2010). Trauma in early childhood also plays a role in the intergenerational transmission of disparities in health outcomes. The nurse's role is to identify and foster qualities to keep at-risk children from developing emotional problems.

Attachment at its most basic level ensures survival of the species. Lack of attachment is counter to such a basic drive. Tizard (1977) conducted one of the best-known early studies related to attachment disorder. Children in this study were abandoned by their parents and lived in an institutional setting. They were provided with play areas, books, and basic needs. What they were not provided with was an adequate ratio of caregivers to children, and caregivers were instructed not to form attachments with the children. After 4 years, eight of the 26 children managed to somehow form attachment with caregivers, eight of the children became emotionally unresponsive, and 10 of the children became indiscriminately

---

CHAPTER 12 Schizophrenia and Schizophrenia Spectrum Disorders 213

BOX 12-4 GUIDELINES FOR COMMUNICATION WITH PATIENTS EXPERIENCING DELUSIONS 8

- To build trust, be open, honest, genuine, and reliable.
- Respond to suspicion in a matter-of-fact, empathic, supportive, and calm manner.
- Ask the patient to describe his beliefs. Example: "Tell me more about someone trying to hurt you."
- Avoid debating the delusional content, but interject doubt where appropriate. Example: "It seems as if it would be hard for a girl that small to hurt you."
- Validate if part of the delusion is real. Example: "Yes, there was a man at the nurse's station, but I did not hear him talk about you."
- Focus on the feelings or theme that underlie or flow from the delusions. Example: "You seem to wish you could be more powerful" or "It must feel frightening to believe others want to hurt you."
- Once trust has been established, acknowledge that, while the belief seems very real to the patient, illnesses can sometimes make things seem true even though they aren't. Introducing this obliquely can make it less confrontational: "I wonder if that might be what is happening here, because what seems true to you does not seem true to others."
- Once the patient has begun to question the delusion and/or understand the concept of delusions, label subsequent delusions to help the patient recognize them as well.
- Do not dwell excessively on the delusion. Instead, refocus onto reality-based topics. If the patient obsesses about delusions, set limits on the amount of time you will talk about them, and explain your reason.
- Observe for events that trigger delusions. If possible, help the patient find ways to avoid such triggers or reduce associated anxiety.
- Promote improved reality testing by guiding the patient to question his beliefs: "I wonder if there might be any other explanation why others might be avoiding you? Instead of hating you, might they simply be busy?"

Data from Farhall, J., Greenwood, K. M., & Jackson, H. J. (2007). Coping with hallucinated voices in schizophrenia: A review of self-initiated strategies and therapeutic interventions. *Clinical Psychology Review, 27,* 476-493.

BOX 12-5 PATIENT AND FAMILY TEACHING: SCHIZOPHRENIA 9

Further information can be found in the Substance Abuse and Mental Health Services Administration (SAMHSA) pamphlet *Developing A Recovery And Wellness Lifestyle: A Self-Help Guide,* available at http://mentalhealth.samhsa.gov/publications/allpubs/SMA-3718 or via the Wellness Recovery Action Plan (WRAP) website (M. A. Copeland and staff): www.mentalhealthrecovery.com

1. Learn all you can about the illness.
   - Attend educational and support groups.
   - Join the National Alliance on Mental Illness (NAMI).
   - Read books about mental illness such as *Surviving Schizophrenia: A Manual for Families, Patients, and Providers* by E. Fuller Torrey.
   - Access trusted websites such as the National Institute of Mental Health (www.nimh.nih.gov).
2. Develop a relapse prevention plan.
   - Know the early warning signs of relapse (e.g., avoiding others, trouble sleeping, troubling thoughts).
   - Make a list of whom to call, what to do, and where to go if signs of relapse appear. Keep it with you.
   - Relapse is part of the illness, not a sign of failure.
3. Participate in family, group, and individual therapy.
4. Learn new ways to act and coping skills to help handle family, work, and social stress. Get information from your nurse, case manager, doctor, NAMI, community mental health groups, or a hospital. Everyone needs a place to talk about fears and losses and to learn new ways of coping.
5. Have a plan, on paper, of what to do to cope with stressful times.
6. Adhere to treatment. People who adhere to treatment that works for them are more likely to get better and stay better.
   - Engaging in struggles over adherence does not help, but tying adherence to the patient's own goals does. ("Staying in treatment will help you keep your job and avoid trouble with the police.")
   - Share concerns about troubling side effects or concerns (e.g., sexual problems, weight gain, "feeling funny") with your nurse, case manager, doctor, or social worker; most side effects can be helped.
   - Keeping side effects a secret or stopping medication can prevent you from having the life you want.
7. Avoid alcohol and/or drugs; they can act on the brain and cause a relapse.
8. Keep in touch with supportive people.
9. Keep healthy and stay in balance.
   - Taking care of one's diet, health, and hygiene helps prevent medical illnesses.
   - Maintain a regular sleep pattern.
   - Keep active (hobbies, friends, groups, sports, job, special interests).
   - Nurture yourself, and practice stress-reduction activities daily.

Data from *Beyond symptom control: Moving towards positive patient outcomes.* Paper presented at the American Psychiatric Association 55th Institute on Psychiatric Services, October 29 to November 2, 2003, Boston, MA. Retrieved from www.medscape.com/viewprogram/2835_pnt. Further information can be found in the Substance Abuse and Mental Health Services Administration (SAMHSA) pamphlet *Developing a recovery and wellness lifestyle: A self-help guide,* available at http://mentalhealth.samhsa.gov/publications/allpubs/SMA-3718, or via the Wellness Recovery Action Plan (WRAP) website (M. A. Copeland and staff) at www.mentalhealthrecovery.com.

CONTENTS

UNIT I FOUNDATIONS IN THEORY

UNIT II FOUNDATIONS FOR PRACTICE

UNIT IV PSYCHOBIOLOGICAL DISORDERS

UNIT V TRAUMA INTERVENTIONS

CHAPTER

1

Mental Health and Mental Illness

Margaret Jordan Halter

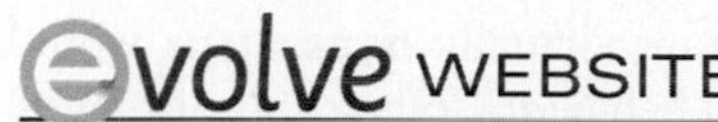

Visit the Evolve website for a pretest on the content in this chapter: http://evolve.elsevier.com/Varcarolis

Pre-Test interactive review

OBJECTIVES

1. Describe the continuum of mental health and mental illness.
2. Explore the role of resilience in the prevention of and recovery from mental illness and consider resilience in response to stress.
3. Identify how culture influences the view of mental illnesses and behaviors associated with them.
4. Discuss the nature/nurture origins of psychiatric disorders.
5. Summarize the social influences of mental health care in the United States.
6. Explain how epidemiological studies can improve medical and nursing care.
7. Identify how the *Diagnostic and Statistical Manual, fifth edition (DSM-5)* is used for diagnosing psychiatric conditions.
8. Describe the specialty of psychiatric mental health nursing and list three phenomena of concern.
9. Compare and contrast a *DSM-5* medical diagnosis with a nursing diagnosis.
10. Discuss future challenges and opportunities for mental health care in the United States.
11. Describe direct and indirect advocacy opportunities for psychiatric mental health nurses.

KEY TERMS AND CONCEPTS

advanced practice registered nurse–psychiatric mental health (APRN-PMH)
basic level registered nurse
clinical epidemiology
comorbid condition
cultural competence
Diagnostic and Statistical Manual of Mental Disorders, fifth edition (DSM-5)
diathesis-stress model
electronic health care
epidemiology
incidence
mental health
mental health continuum
mental illness
Nursing Interventions Classification (NIC)
Nursing Outcomes Classification (NOC)
phenomena of concern
prevalence
psychiatric mental health nursing
psychiatry's definition of mental health
recovery
registered nurse–psychiatric mental health (RN-PMH)
resilience
stigma

If you are a fan of vintage films, you may have witnessed a scene similar to this: A doctor, wearing a lab coat and an expression of deep concern, enters a hospital waiting room and delivers the bad news to an obviously distraught gentleman who is seated there. The doctor says "I'm afraid your wife has suffered a nervous breakdown," and from that point on, the woman's condition is only vaguely described. The husband dutifully visits her at a gated asylum, where the staff regard him with sad expressions. He may find his wife confined to her bed, or standing by the window and staring vacantly into the middle distance, or sitting motionless in the hospital garden. The viewer can only speculate about the nature of the problem but may assume she has had an emotional collapse.

CONTINUUM OF MENTAL HEALTH AND MENTAL ILLNESS

We have come a long way in acknowledging psychiatric disorders and increasing our understanding of them since the days of "nervous breakdowns." In fact, the World Health Organization (WHO) (2010) maintains that a person cannot be considered healthy without taking into account mental health as well as physical health.

The WHO defines **mental health** as a state of well-being in which each individual is able to realize his or her own potential, cope with the normal stresses of life, work productively, and make a contribution to the community. Mental health provides people with the capacity for rational thinking, communication skills, learning, emotional growth, resilience, and self-esteem (U.S. Department of Health and Human Services [USDHHS], 1999). Some of the attributes of mentally healthy people are presented in Figure 1-1.

Psychiatry's definition of mental health evolves over time. It is a definition shaped by the prevailing culture and societal values, and it reflects changes in cultural norms, society's expectations, political climates, and even reimbursement criteria by third-party payers. In the past, the term *mental illness* was applied to behaviors considered "strange" and "different"—behaviors that occurred infrequently and deviated from an established norm. Such criteria are inadequate because they suggest that mental health is based on conformity, and if such definitions were used, nonconformists and independent thinkers like Abraham Lincoln, Mahatma Gandhi, and Socrates would be judged mentally ill. Although the sacrifices of a Mother Teresa or the dedication of Martin Luther King Jr. are uncommon, virtually none of us would consider these much-admired behaviors to be signs of mental illness.

Mental illness refers to all mental disorders with definable diagnoses. These disorders are manifested in significant dysfunction that may be related to developmental, biological, or psychological disturbances in mental functioning. (APA, 2013). The cognition may be impaired—as in Alzheimer's disease; emotions may be affected—as in major depression; and behavioral alterations may be apparent—as in schizophrenia; or the

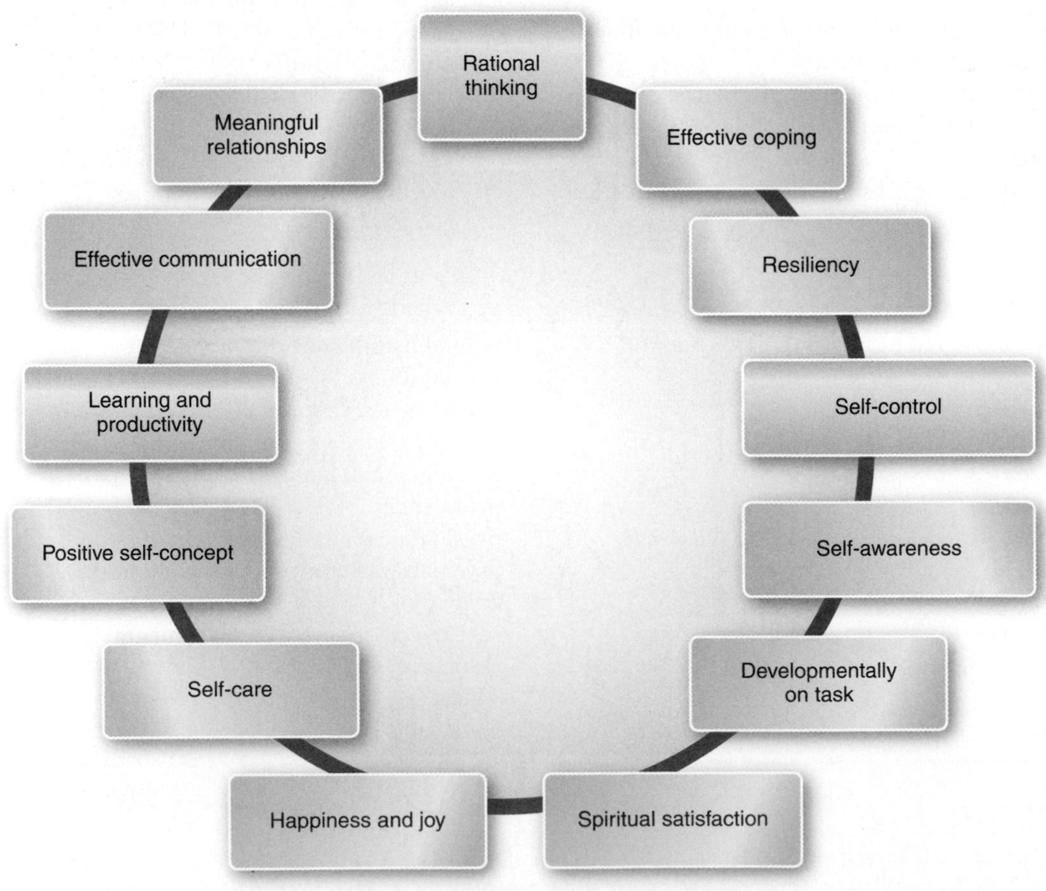

FIG 1-1 Some attributes of mental health.

patient may display some combination of the three. Behavior that deviates from socially accepted norms does not indicate a mental illness unless there is significant disturbance in mental functioning.

You may be wondering if there is some middle ground between mental health and mental illness. After all, it is a rare person who does not have doubts as to his or her sanity at one time or another. The answer is that there is a definite middle ground; in fact, mental health and mental illness can be conceptualized as points along a **mental health continuum** (Figure 1-2).

Well-being is characterized by adequate to high-level functioning in response to routine stress and resultant anxiety or distress. Nearly all of us experience emotional problems or concerns or occasions when we are not at our best. We may feel lousy temporarily, but signs and symptoms are not of sufficient duration or intensity to warrant a psychiatric diagnosis. We may spend a day or two in a gray cloud of self-doubt and recrimination over a failed exam, a sleepless night filled with worry and obsession about normally trivial concerns, or months of genuine sadness and mourning after the death of a loved one. During those times, we are fully or vaguely aware that we are not functioning optimally; however, time, exercise, a balanced diet, rest, interaction with others, mental reframing, or even early intervention and treatment may alleviate these problems or concerns. It is not until we experience marked distress or suffer from impairment or inability to function in our everyday lives that the line is crossed into mental illness.

People who have experienced mental illness can testify to the existence of changes in functioning. The following comments of a 40-year-old woman illustrate the continuum between illness and health as her condition ranged from (1) deep depression to (2) mania to (3) health:

1. It was horror and hell. I was at the bottom of the deepest and darkest pit there ever was. I was worthless and unforgivable. I was as good as—no, worse than—dead.
2. I was incredibly alive. I could sense and feel everything. I was sure I could do anything, accomplish any task, create whatever I wanted, if only other people wouldn't get in my way.
3. Yes, I am sometimes sad and sometimes happy and excited, but nothing as extreme as before. I am much calmer. I realize now that, when I was manic, it was a pressure-cooker feeling. When I am happy now, or loving, it is more peaceful and real. I have to admit that I sometimes miss the intensity—the sense of power and creativity—of those manic times. I never miss anything about the depressed times, but of course the power and the creativity never bore fruit. Now I do get things done, some of the time, like most people. And people treat me much better now. I guess I must seem more real to them. I certainly seem more real to me (Altrocchi, 1980).

Contributing Factors

Many factors can affect the severity and progression of a mental illness as well as the mental health of a person who does not have a mental illness (Figure 1-3). If possible, these influences need to be evaluated and factored into an individual's plan of care. In fact, the ***Diagnostic and Statistical Manual of Mental Disorders, fifth edition (DSM-5)***, a 1.5-inch-thick manual that classifies 157 separate disorders, states that there is evidence suggesting that the symptoms and causes of a number of disorders are influenced by cultural and ethnic factors (APA, 2013). The *DSM-5* is discussed in further detail later in this chapter.

Resilience

Researchers, clinicians, and consumers are all interested in actively facilitating mental health and reducing mental illness. A characteristic of mental health, increasingly being promoted and essential to the recovery process, is **resilience**. Resilience is closely associated with the process of adapting and helps people facing tragedies, loss, trauma, and severe stress. It is the ability and capacity for people to secure the resources they need to support their well-being, such as children of poverty and abuse seeking out trusted adults who provide them with the psychological and physical resources that allow them to excel. This social support actually brings about chemical changes in the body through the release of oxytocin, which mutes the destructive stress-related chemicals (Southwick & Charney, 2012).

Disasters, such as the attack on the World Trade towers in 2001 and the devastation of Hurricane Sandy in 2012, in which people pulled together to help one another and carried on despite

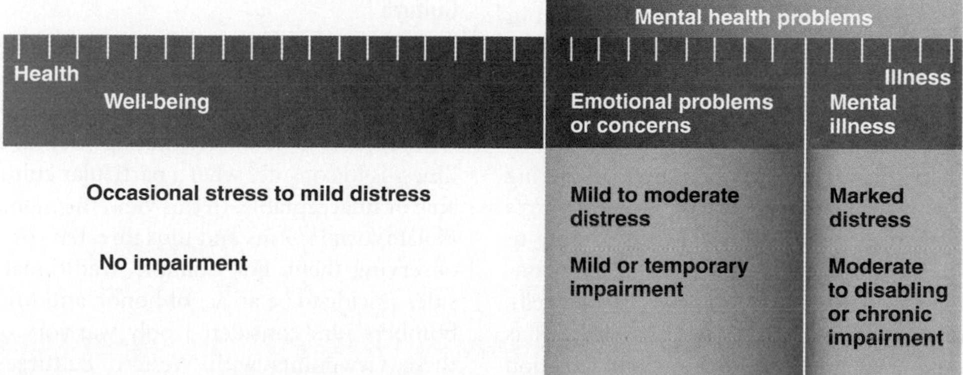

FIG 1-2 Mental Health–Mental Illness Continuum. (From University of Michigan, "Understanding U." [2007]. What is mental health? Retrieved from http://www.hr.umich.edu/mhealthy/programs/mental_emotional/understandingu/learn/mental_health.html.)

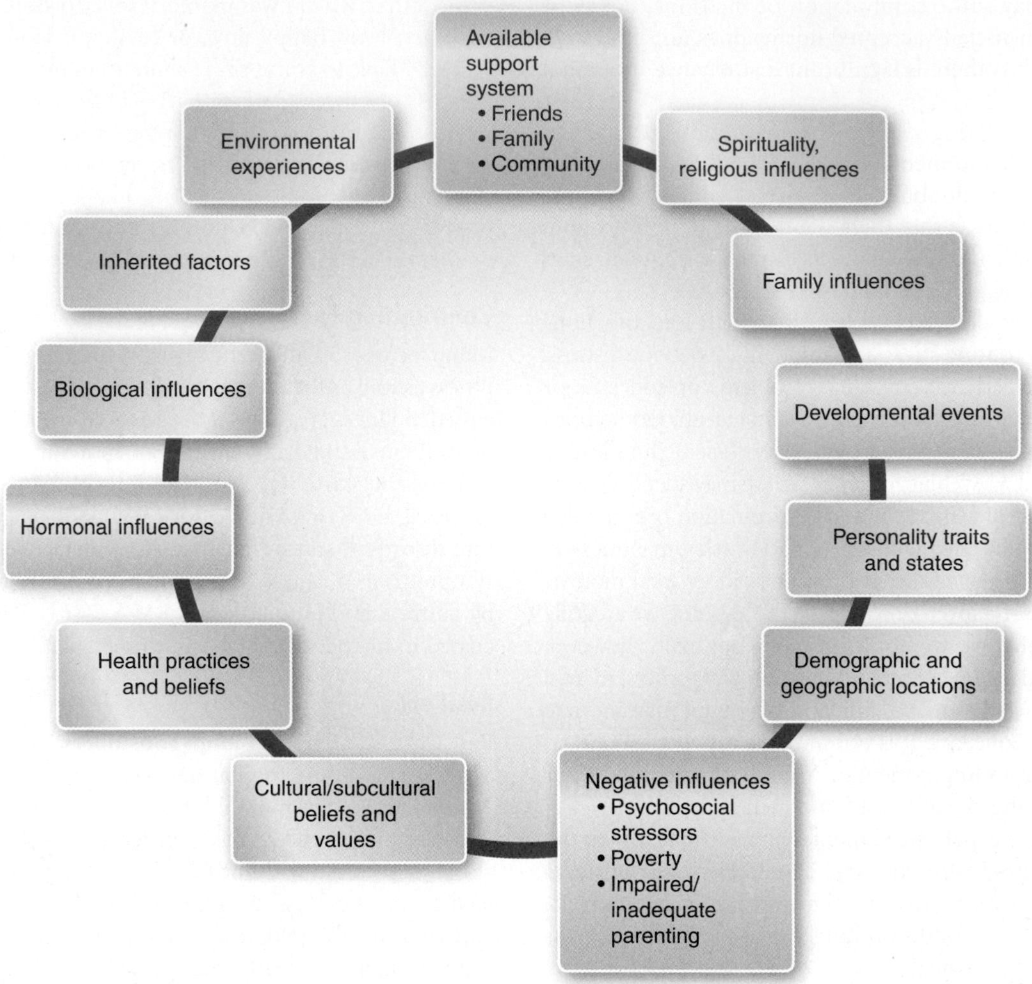

FIG 1-3 Influences that can have an impact on an individual's mental health.

horrendous loss, illustrate resilience. Being resilient does not mean being unaffected by stressors; it means recognizing the feelings, readily dealing with them, and learning from the experience rather than falling victim to negative emotions.

Accessing and developing this trait assists people in bouncing back from painful experiences and difficult events; it is characterized by optimism, a sense of mastery, and competence (Southwick & Charney, 2012). It is not an unusual quality; it is possessed by regular, everyday people and can be enhanced in almost everyone. One of the most important qualities is the ability to identify the problems and challenges, accepting those things that cannot be changed and then focusing on what can be overcome.

Research demonstrates that early experiences in mastering difficult or stressful situations enhance the prefrontal cortex's resiliency in coping with difficult situations later. According to Amat and colleagues (2006), when rats were exposed to uncontrollable stresses, their brains turned off mood-regulating cells, and they developed a syndrome much like major depression. Rats that were first given the chance to control a stressful situation were better able to respond to subsequent stress for up to a week following the success. In fact, when the successful rats were faced with uncontrollable stress, their brain cells responded as if they were in control.

People who are resilient are effective at regulating their emotions and not falling victim to negative, self-defeating thoughts. You can get an idea of how good you are at regulating your emotions by taking the Resilience Factor Test in Box 1-1.

Culture

There is no standard measure for mental health, in part because it is culturally defined and is based on interpretations of effective functioning according to societal norms (WHO, 2007). One approach in differentiating mental health from mental illness is to consider what a particular culture regards as acceptable or unacceptable. In this view, the mentally ill are those who violate social norms and thus threaten (or make anxious) those observing them. For example, traditional Japanese may consider suicide to be an act of honor, and Middle Eastern "suicide bombers" are considered holy warriors or martyrs. Contrast these viewpoints with Western culture, where people who attempt or complete suicides are nearly always considered mentally ill.

BOX 1-1 THE RESILIENCE FACTOR TEST

Use the following scale to rate each item listed below:
1 = Not true of me
2 = Sometimes true
3 = Moderately true
4 = Usually true
5 = Very true

1. Even if I plan ahead for a discussion with my spouse, my boss, or my child, I still find myself acting emotionally.
2. I am unable to harness positive emotions to help me focus on a task.
3. I can control the way I feel when adversity strikes.
4. I get carried away by my feelings.
5. I am good at identifying what I am thinking and how it affects my mood.
6. If someone does something that upsets me, I am able to wait until an appropriate time when I have calmed down to discuss it.
7. My emotions affect my ability to focus on what I need to get done at home, school, or work.
8. When I discuss a hot topic with a colleague or family member, I am able to keep my emotions in check.

ADD YOUR SCORE ON THE FOLLOWING ITEMS:	ADD YOUR SCORE ON THE FOLLOWING ITEMS:
3 _____	1 _____
5 _____	2 _____
6 _____	4 _____
8 _____	7 _____
Positive total = _____	Negative total = _____

Positive total minus negative total = _____

A score higher than 13 is rated as above average in emotional regulation.

A score between 6 and 13 is inconclusive.

A score lower than 6 is rated as below average in emotional regulation.

If your emotional regulation is below average, you may need to master some calming skills. Here are a few tips:

- When anxiety strikes, your breathing may become shallow and quick. You can help control the anxiety by controlling your breathing. Inhale slowly through your nose, breathing deeply from your belly, not your chest.
- Stress will make your body tight and stiff. Again, you can counter the effects of stress on the body and brain if you relax your muscles.
- Try positive imagery; create an image that is relaxing, such as visualizing yourself on a secluded beach.
- Resilience is within your reach.

From *The resilience factor: 7 essential skills for overcoming life's obstacles* by Karen Reivich, PhD and Andrew Shatte, PhD. Copyright © 2002 by Karen Reivich and Andrew Shatte. Used by permission of Broadway Books, a division of Random House, Inc. Any third party use of this material, outside of this publication, is prohibited. Interested parties must apply directly to Random House, Inc. for permission.

Throughout history, people have interpreted health or sickness according to their own current views. A striking example of how cultural change influences the interpretation of mental illness is an old definition of *hysteria*. According to Webster's Dictionary (Porter, 1913), hysteria was "A nervous affection, occurring almost exclusively in women, in which the emotional and reflex excitability is exaggerated, and the will power correspondingly diminished, so that the patient loses control over the emotions, becomes the victim of imaginary sensations, and often falls into paroxysm or fits." Treatment for this condition, thought to be the result of sexual deprivation, often involved sexual outlets for afflicted women. According to some authors, this diagnosis fell into disuse as women's rights improved, the family atmosphere became less restrictive, and societal tolerance of sexual practices increased.

Cultures differ in not only their views regarding mental illness but also the types of behavior categorized as mental illness. Culture-bound syndromes seem to occur in specific sociocultural contexts and are easily recognized by people in those cultures (Stern et al., 2010). For example, one syndrome recognized in parts of Southeast Asia is running amok, in which a person (usually a male) runs around engaging in almost indiscriminate violent behavior. Pibloktoq, an uncontrollable desire to tear off one's clothing and expose oneself to severe winter weather, is a recognized psychological disorder in parts of Greenland, Alaska, and the Arctic regions of Canada. In the United States, anorexia nervosa (see Chapter 18) is recognized as a psychobiological disorder that entails voluntary starvation. The disorder is well known in Europe, North America, and Australia but unheard of in many other parts of the world.

What is to be made of the fact that certain disorders occur in some cultures but are absent in others? One interpretation is that the conditions necessary for causing a particular disorder occur in some places but are absent in other places. Another interpretation is that people learn certain kinds of abnormal behavior by imitation; however, the fact that some disorders may be culturally determined does not prove that all mental illnesses are so determined. The best evidence suggests that schizophrenia (see Chapter 12) and bipolar disorders (see Chapter 13) are found throughout the world. The symptom patterns of schizophrenia have been observed in Western culture and among indigenous Greenlanders and West African villagers.

Perceptions of Mental Health and Mental Illness

Mental Illness Versus Physical Illness

People commonly make a distinction between mental illnesses and physical illnesses. It is an odd distinction, considering that *mental* refers to the brain, the most complex and sophisticated part of the body, the organ responsible for the higher thought processes that set us apart from other creatures. Surely the workings of the brain—the synaptic connections, the areas of functioning, the spinal innervations and connections—are *physical*. One problem with this distinction is that it implies that psychiatric disorders are "all in the head" and therefore under personal control and indistinguishable from a choice to indulge in bad behavior. Although some physical disorders, such as a broken arm from skiing or lung cancer from smoking, are blamed on the victim, the majority of physical illnesses are considered to be beyond personal responsibility.

Perhaps the origin of this distinction between mental and physical illness lies in the religious and philosophical tradition of explaining the unexplainable by assigning a mystical or spiritual origin to cognitive processes and emotional activities. Despite many advances in understanding, mental illnesses continue to be viewed differently from illnesses that originate in other parts of the body.

Consider that people with epilepsy were once thought to be possessed by demons, under the attack of gods, or cursed; they were subjected to horrible "cures" and treatments. Today, most people would say that epilepsy is a disorder of the mind and not under personal control because we can *see* epilepsy on brain scans as areas of overactivity and excitability. There are no specific biological tests to diagnose most psychiatric disorders—no cranium culture for depression and no MRI for obsessive-compulsive disorder (OCD); however, researchers are convinced that the root of most mental disorders lies in intercellular abnormalities, and we can now see clear signs of altered brain function in several mental disorders, including schizophrenia, OCD, stress disorders, and depression.

Nature Versus Nurture

For students, one of the most intriguing aspects of learning about mental illnesses is understanding their origins. Although for centuries people believed that extremely unusual behaviors were due to demonic forces, in the late 1800s, the mental health pendulum swung briefly to a biological focus with the "germ theory of diseases." Germ theory explained mental illness in the same way other illnesses were being described—that is, they were caused by a specific agent in the environment (Morgan, McKenzie, & Fearon, 2008). This theory was abandoned rather quickly since clinicians and researchers could not identify single causative factors for mental illnesses; there was no "mania germ" that could be viewed under a microscope and subsequently treated.

Although ineffective biological treatments for mental illness continued to be explored, psychological theories dominated and focused on the science of the mind and behavior over the next half century. These theories explained the origin of mental illness as faulty psychological processes that could be corrected by increasing personal insight and understanding. For example, a patient experiencing depression and apathy might be assisted to explore feelings left over from childhood, when overly protective parents harshly discouraged his attempts at independence.

This psychological focus was challenged in 1952 when chlorpromazine (Thorazine) was found to have a calming effect on agitated, out-of-control patients. Imagine what this must have been like for clinicians who had resorted to every biological treatment imaginable, including wet wraps, insulin shock therapy, and psychosurgery (in which holes were drilled in the head of a patient and probes inserted in the brain) in a futile attempt to change behavior. Many began to believe that if psychiatric problems respond to medications that alter intercellular components, a disruption of intercellular components must already be present. At this point, the pendulum made steady and sure progress toward a biological explanation of psychiatric problems and disorders.

Currently, the **diathesis-stress model**—in which diathesis represents biological predisposition and stress represents environmental stress or trauma—is the most accepted explanation for mental illness. This nature-*plus*-nurture argument asserts that most psychiatric disorders result from a combination of genetic vulnerability and negative environmental stressors. While one person may develop major depression largely as the result of an inherited and biological vulnerability that alters brain chemistry, another person with little vulnerability may develop depression from changes in brain chemistry caused by the insults of a stressful environment.

Social Influences on Mental Health Care

Consumer Movement and Mental Health Recovery

In the latter part of the 20th century, tremendous energy was expended on putting the notion of equality into widespread practice in the United States. Treating people fairly and extinguishing labels became a cultural focus. In regard to mental illness, decades of institutionalization had created political and social concerns that gave rise to a mental health movement similar to women's rights movements, civil rights movements, disabilities rights movements, and gay rights movements. Groups of people with mental illnesses—or mental health consumers—began to advocate for their rights and the rights of others with mental illness and to fight stigma, discrimination, and forced treatment.

In 1979, people with mental illnesses and their families formed a nationwide advocacy group, the National Alliance on Mental Illness (NAMI). In the 1980s, individuals in the consumer movement organized by NAMI began to resist the traditional arrangement of mental health care providers who dictated care and treatment without input from the patient. This "paternalistic" relationship was not just demoralizing; it also implied that patients were not competent to make their own decisions. Consumers rebelled and demanded increased involvement in decisions concerning their treatment.

The consumer movement also promoted the notion of **recovery**, a new and an old idea in mental health. On one hand, it represents a concept that has been around a long time: that some people—even those with the most serious illnesses, such as schizophrenia—recover. One such recovery was depicted in the movie "A Beautiful Mind," wherein a brilliant mathematician, John Nash, seems to have emerged from a continuous cycle of devastating psychotic relapses to a state of stabilization and recovery (Howard, 2001). On the other hand, a newer conceptualization of recovery evolved into a consumer-focused process "in which people are able to live, work, learn, and participate fully in their communities" (U.S. Department of Health and Human Services, 2003).

According to the Substance Abuse and Mental Health Services Administration (SAMHSA) (2011), recovery is defined as "a process of change through which individuals improve their health and wellness, live a self-directed life, and strive to reach their full potential." The focus is on the consumer and what he or she can do. An example of recovery follows:

VIGNETTE

Jeff was diagnosed with schizophrenia when he began to hear voices as a college student. He dropped out of school and had a series of hospitalizations, outpatient treatments, and ultimately nonadherence to the plan of care. He was put on Social Security Disability and never worked again after he lost his part-time job at a factory. For 20 years, Jeff has been told what medication to take, where to live, and what to do.

At the community health center where he receives services he met Linda, who was involved with a recovery support group. She told him about it and gave him a pamphlet with a list of the 10 guiding principles of recovery, which were:

Self-directed: Consumers lead, control, exercise choice over, and determine their own path of recovery.

Individual- and person-centered: Recovery is based on unique strengths and resiliencies, as well as needs, preferences, experiences (including past trauma), and cultural backgrounds.

Empowering: Consumers have the authority to choose from a range of options, participate in all decisions that will affect their lives, and be educated and supported in so doing.

Holistic: Recovery encompasses an individual's whole life, including mind, body, spirit, and community.

Nonlinear: Recovery is based on continual growth, occasional setbacks, and learning from experience.

Strengths-based: Recovery is focused on valuing and building on the multiple capacities, resiliencies, talents, coping abilities, and inherent worth of individuals.

Peer-supported: Consumers encourage and engage each other in recovery and provide a sense of belonging, supportive relationships, valued roles, and community.

Respect: Community, systems, and societal acceptance and appreciation of consumers—including protecting their rights and eliminating discrimination and stigma—are crucial in achieving recovery.

Responsibility: Consumers have a personal responsibility for their own self-care and recovery, for understanding and giving meaning to their experiences, and for identifying coping strategies and healing processes to promote their own wellness.

Hope: Recovery provides the essential motivating message of a better future: that people can and do overcome the barriers and obstacles that confront them. Hope is the catalyst of the recovery process.

Jeff's involvement in a recovery support group has changed his view of himself, and he has taken the lead role in his own recovery: "See, nobody knows your body better than you do, and some, maybe some mental health providers or doctors, think, 'Hey, I am the professional, and you're the person seeing me. I know what's best for you.' But technically, it isn't true. They only provide you with the tools to get better. They can't crawl inside you and see how you are."

After 20 years, Jeff asked for and received newer, more effective medications. He has moved into his own apartment and returned to college with a focus on information technology. He has his high and low days but maintains goals, hope, and a purpose for his life. Jeff attends regular recovery support groups, has taken up bicycling, and is purchasing a condominium along with his new wife.

Decade of the Brain

In 1990, President George H.W. Bush designated the last decade of the 1900s as the Decade of the Brain. The overriding goal of this designation was to make legislators and the public aware of the advances that had been made in neuroscience and brain research. This U.S. initiative stimulated a worldwide growth of scientific research. Among the advances and progress made during the Decade of the Brain were the following:

- Understanding the genetic basis of embryonic and fetal neural development
- Mapping genes involved in neurological illnesses, including mutations associated with Parkinson's disease, Alzheimer's disease, and epilepsy
- Discovering that the brain uses a relatively small number of neurotransmitters but has a vast assortment of neurotransmitter receptors
- Uncovering the role of cytokines (proteins involved in the immune response) in such brain disorders as depression
- Refining neuroimaging techniques, such as positron emission tomography (PET) scans, magnetic resonance imaging (MRI), magnetoencephalography, and event-related electroencephalography (EEG), has improved our understanding of normal brain functioning as well as areas of difference in pathological states
- Bringing together computer modeling and laboratory research, which resulted in the new discipline of computational neuroscience.

Surgeon General's Report on Mental Health

The first Surgeon General's report on the topic of mental health was published in 1999 (USDHHS, 1999). This landmark document was based on an extensive review of the scientific literature in consultation with mental health providers and consumers. The two most important messages from this report were that (1) mental health is fundamental to overall health, and (2) there are effective treatments for mental health. The report is reader-friendly and a good introduction to mental health and illness. You can review the report at http://www.surgeongeneral.gov/library/mentalhealth/home.html.

Human Genome Project

The Human Genome Project was a 13-year project that lasted from 1990–2003 and was completed on the 50th anniversary of the discovery of the DNA double helix. The project has strengthened biological and genetic explanations for psychiatric conditions (Cohen, 2000). The goals of the project (U.S. Department of Energy, 2008) were to do the following:

- **Identify** the approximately 20,000 to 25,000 genes in human DNA.
- **Determine** the sequences of the 3 billion chemical base pairs that make up human DNA.
- **Store** this information in databases.
- **Improve** tools for data analysis.
- **Address** the ethical, legal, and social issues that may arise from the project.

Although researchers have begun to identify strong genetic links to mental illness (as you will see in the chapters on clinical disorders), it will be some time before we understand the exact nature of genetic influences on mental illness. What we do know is that most psychiatric disorders are the result of multiple mutated or defective genes, each of which in combination may contribute to the disorder.

President's New Freedom Commission on Mental Health

In 2003, the President's New Freedom Commission on Mental Health chaired by Michael F. Hogan, the director of Ohio's Department of Mental Health, released its recommendations for mental health care in America. This was the first commission since First Lady Rosalyn Carter's (wife of President Jimmy Carter) in 1978. The report noted that the system of delivering mental health care in America was "in a shambles." It called for a streamlined system with a less fragmented delivery of care. It advocated early diagnosis and treatment, a new expectation for principles of recovery, and increased assistance in helping people find housing and work. Box 1-2 describes the goals necessary for such a transformation of mental health care in the United States.

Institute of Medicine

The "Improving the Quality of Health Care for Mental and Substance-Use Conditions: Quality Chasm Series" was released in 2005 by the Institute of Medicine (IOM). It highlighted effective treatments for mental illness and addressed the huge gap between the best care and the worst. It focused on such issues as the problem of coerced (forced) treatment, a system that treats mental health issues separately from physical health problems, and lack of quality control. The report encouraged health care workers to focus on safe, effective, patient-centered, timely, efficient, and equitable care.

Another important and related publication issued by the Institute of Medicine in 2011 is "The Future of Nursing: Focus on Education." This report contends that the old way of training nurses is not adequate for the 21st century's complex requirements. It calls for highly educated nurses who are prepared to care for an aging and diverse population with an increasing incidence of chronic disease. They recommended that nurses be trained in leadership, health policy, system improvement, research, and teamwork.

Recommendations from both documents were addressed by a group called Quality and Safety Education for Nurses (QSEN; pronounced *Q-sen*) and were funded by the Robert Wood Johnson Foundation. They have developed a structure to support the education of future nurses who possess the knowledge, skills, and attitudes to continuously improve the safety and quality of healthcare. Consider this tragic story:

> *Betsy Lehman was a health reporter for the Boston Globe and was married to a cancer researcher. She herself was diagnosed with cancer and was mistakenly prescribed an extremely high and wrong dose of an anti-cancer drug. Ms. Lehman sensed something was wrong and appealed to the health care providers, who did not respond. The day before she died, she begged others to help because the professionals were not listening (Robert Wood Johnson, 2011).*

How could her death have been prevented? Consider the key areas of care promoted by QSEN and how they could have prevented Ms. Lehman's death:

1. **Patient-centered care:** Care should be given in an atmosphere of respect and responsiveness, and the patient's values (rather than our own), preferences, and needs should guide care.
2. **Teamwork and collaboration:** Nurses and interprofessional teams need to maintain open communication, respect, and shared decision making.
3. **Evidence-based practice:** Optimal health care is the result of integrating the best current evidence while considering the patient/family values and preferences.
4. **Quality improvement:** Nurses should be involved in monitoring the outcomes of the care that they give. They should also be care designers and test changes that will result in quality improvement.
5. **Safety:** The care provided should not add further injury (e.g., nosocomial infections). Harm to patients and providers is minimized through both system effectiveness and individual performance.
6. **Informatics:** Information and technology is used to communicate, manage knowledge, mitigate error, and support decision making.

BOX 1-2 GOALS FOR A TRANSFORMED MENTAL HEALTH SYSTEM IN THE UNITED STATES

Goal 1
Americans understand that mental health is essential to overall health.

Goal 2
Mental health care is consumer- and family-driven.

Goal 3
Disparities in mental health services are eliminated.

Goal 4
Early mental health screening, assessment, and referral to services are common practice.

Goal 5
Excellent mental health care is delivered, and research is accelerated.

Goal 6
Technology is used to access mental health care and information.

Data from U.S. Department of Health and Human Services, President's New Freedom Commission on Mental Health. (2003). *Achieving the promise: Transforming mental health care in America.* USDHHS Publication No. SMA-03-3832. Retrieved from http://www.mentalhealthcommission.gov/reports/finalreport/fullreport-02.htm.

Legislation and Funding Mental Health

Imagine insurance companies singling out a group of disorders such as cardiac disease. Imagine people with cardiac disease being assigned higher co-pays and specifying the number of times patients could be reimbursed for treatment for the entire course of their lives. People would be outraged by such discrimination. Yet this is exactly what has happened with psychiatric disorders.

Here are the problems: Some insurance companies did not cover mental health care at all, identified yearly or lifetime limits on mental health coverage, limited the number of hospital days or outpatient treatment sessions, or assigned higher copayments or deductibles for those in need of psychiatric services. While this saved money for insurers, costs were shifted to taxpayers, and many people gave up and suffered needlessly. Advocates fought to remedy reimbursement inequities for years. In response to this problem, the Mental Health Parity Act of 1996 was signed into law. *Parity* simply refers to equivalence, and this legislation required insurers that provide mental health coverage to offer annual and lifetime benefits at the same level provided for medical/surgical coverage. Unfortunately, by the year 2000, the Government Accounting Office found that although 86% of health plans complied with the 1996 law, 87% of those plans actually imposed new limits on mental health coverage.

The Wellstone-Domenici Parity Act built on the 1996 legislation. It was enacted into law on October 3, 2008, for group health plans with more than 50 employees. While mental health and addictions coverage was still not mandated under any plan, the new law required that any plan providing mental health coverage must do so in the same manner as medical/surgical coverage. Equal coverage includes deductibles, copayments, coinsurance, and out-of-pocket expenses as well as treatment limitations (e.g., frequency of treatment and number/frequency of visits).

This parity legislation happened right before the passage of the Patient Protection and Affordable Care Act of 2010 (ACA). The ACA has been described as the most significant health care legislation since the creation of Medicare and Medicaid in 1965. A huge and comprehensive law, the ACA has several major goals. First, it provides coverage for most Americans who are uninsured through a combination of expanded Medicaid eligibility (for the very poor), creation of Health Insurance Exchanges in the states (to serve as a broker to help uninsured consumers choose among various plans), and the so-called "insurance mandate," a requirement that people without coverage obtain it.

A second goal of the ACA is to improve the quality of health care by moving away from payment based on the number of services provided and instead rewarding providers for care that keeps people healthy These reforms resonate with nurses who are experts in health promotion and in holistic care, which considers the significance of mental health as a component of overall health. ACA provided for $30 million to train 600 nurse practitioners to provide comprehensive primary care.

Wellness-oriented care was also emphasized by the ACA's support for primary care practices in Patient Centered Medical/Health Homes. It also promoted nurse practitioner-led clinics by providing $15 million for 10 nurse-managed health clinics. Such programs will place a greater emphasis on mental health care integrated into primary care, and these approaches lean heavily on psychiatric nurses as part of the primary care team.

EPIDEMIOLOGY OF MENTAL DISORDERS

Epidemiology, as it applies to psychiatric mental health, is the quantitative study of the distribution of mental disorders in human populations. Once the distribution of mental disorders has been determined quantitatively, epidemiologists can identify high-risk groups and high-risk factors associated with illness onset, duration, and recurrence. The further study of risk factors for mental illness may then lead to important clues about the etiology of various mental disorders.

Annually an estimated 26.2% of Americans aged 18 and older—about one in four adults—suffer from a diagnosable mental disorder (Kessler et al., 2005). When this percentage is applied to the 2012 U.S. Census residential population estimate, the figure translates into 82 million people. In addition, neuropsychiatric disorders are the leading category of disease, with twice the disability as the next category, cardiovascular diseases. More than a third of this disability is due to depression. Many individuals have more than one mental disorder at a time; this co-occurrence is known as having a **comorbid condition**.

Two different but related words used in epidemiology are **incidence** and **prevalence**. *Incidence* refers to the number of new cases of mental disorders in a healthy population within a given period of time—for example, the number of Atlanta adolescents who were newly diagnosed with major depression between 2000 and 2001. This is usually annual. *Prevalence* describes the *total number of cases*, new and existing, in a given population during a specific period of time, regardless of when they became ill (e.g., the number of adolescents who screen positive for major depression in New York City schools between 2000 and 2010).

A disease with a short duration, such as the common cold, tends to have a high incidence (many new cases in a given year), and a low prevalence (not many people suffering from a cold at any given time). Conversely, a chronic disease such as diabetes will have a low incidence because the person will be dropped from the list of new cases after the first year (or whatever time increment is being used).

Lifetime risk data, or the risk that one will develop a disease in the course of a lifetime, will be higher than both incidence and prevalence. According to Kessler, Berglund, and colleagues (2005), 46.4% of all Americans will meet criteria for a psychiatric disorder in a lifetime. Table 1-1 shows the prevalence of some psychiatric disorders in the United States.

Originally, epidemiology meant the study of epidemics. **Clinical epidemiology** is a broad field that examines health and illness at the population level. Studies use traditional epidemiological methods and are conducted in groups usually defined by the illness or symptoms or by the diagnostic procedures or treatments given for the illness or symptoms. Clinical epidemiology includes the following:

- Studies of the natural history, or what happens if there is no treatment and the problem is left to run its course, of an illness
- Studies of diagnostic screening tests
- Observational and experimental studies of interventions used to treat people with the illness or symptoms

TABLE 1-1 TWELVE-MONTH PREVALENCE OF PSYCHIATRIC DISORDERS IN THE UNITED STATES

DISORDER	PREVALENCE OVER 12 MONTHS (%)	12 MONTH % RECEIVING TREATMENT	COMMENTS
Schizophrenia	1.1	45.8	Affects men and women equally
Major depressive disorder	6.7	51.7	Leading cause of disability in United States and established economies worldwide Nearly twice as many women (6.5%) as men (3.3%) suffer from major depressive disorder every year
Bipolar disorder	2.6	48.8	Affects men and women equally
Generalized anxiety disorder	3.1	43.2	Can begin across life cycle; risk is highest between childhood and middle age
Panic disorder	2.7	59.1	Typically develops in adolescence or early adulthood About 1 in 3 people with panic disorder develop agoraphobia
Obsessive-compulsive disorder	1	No data	First symptoms begin in childhood or adolescence
Posttraumatic stress disorder (PTSD)	3.5	49.9	Can develop at any time About 30% of Vietnam veterans experienced PTSD after the war; percentage high among first responders to 9/11/01 U.S. terrorist attacks
Social phobia	6.8	40.1	Typically begins in childhood or adolescence
Agoraphobia	.08	45.8	Begins in young adulthood
Specific phobia	8.7	32.4	Begins in childhood
Any personality disorder	9.1	No data	Antisocial personality disorder more common in men
Alzheimer's disease	10 (65+) 50 (85 years+)		Rare, inherited forms can strike in the 30s-40s

Data from National Institute of Mental Health. (2008). *Statistics*. Retrieved from http://www.nimh.nih.gov/statistics/index.shtml.

Results of epidemiological studies are routinely included in the *DSM-5* to describe the frequency of mental disorders. Analysis of such studies can reveal the frequency with which psychological symptoms appear together with physical illness. For example, epidemiological studies demonstrate that depression is a significant risk factor for death in people with cardiovascular disease and premature death in people with breast cancer.

Classification of Mental Disorders

Nursing care, as opposed to medical care, is care based on responses to illness. Nurses do not treat major depression per se; they treat the problems associated with depression, such as insomnia or hopelessness and provide effective nursing care using the nursing process as a guide. If human beings have biological, psychological, social, and spiritual components and needs, then holistic nursing allows nurses to assess and plan for the whole individual. Nurses, physicians, and other health care providers are part of a multidisciplinary team that, when well-coordinated, can provide optimal care for the biological, psychological, social, and spiritual needs of patients.

To carry out their diverse professional responsibilities, educators, clinicians, and researchers need clear and accurate guidelines for identifying and categorizing mental illness. For clinicians in particular, such guidelines help in planning and evaluating their patients' treatment. A necessary element for categorization is agreement regarding which behaviors constitute a mental illness. At present, there are two major classification systems used in the United States: the *Diagnostic and Statistical Manual, fifth edition (DSM-5)* and the *International Classification of Disease, Ninth Revision, Clinical Modification (ICD-9-CM)* (WHO, 2007). Both are important in terms of planning for patient care and determining reimbursement for services rendered, and this text will discuss both. More attention will be devoted to the *DSM-5* because it is the dominant mode of understanding and diagnosing mental illness in the United States and the framework for describing psychiatric disorders in this text.

The *DSM-5*

The *Diagnostic and Statistical Manual (DSM)* is a publication of the American Psychiatric Association (APA). It is the official guideline for diagnosing psychiatric disorders. First published in 1952, the 2013 edition describes criteria for 157 disorders. The development of the *DSM-5* was influenced by clinical field trials conducted by psychiatrists, advanced practice psychiatric-mental health nurses, psychologists, licensed clinical social workers, licensed counselors, and licensed marriage and family therapists. It identifies disorders based on criteria in clin ical settings such as inpatient, outpatient, partial hospitalization, consultation-liaison, clinics, private practice, primary care, and community populations. The *DSM* also serves as a tool for collecting epidemiological statistics about the diagnosis of psychiatric disorders.

A common misconception is that a classification of mental disorders classifies *people*, when the *DSM* actually classifies *disorders*. For this reason, the *DSM* and this textbook avoid the use of expressions such as "a schizophrenic" or "an alcoholic." Viewing the person as a person and not an illness requires more accurate terms such as "an individual with schizophrenia" or "my patient has major depression."

Since the third edition of the *DSM* appeared in 1980, the criteria for classification of mental disorders have been sufficiently detailed for clinical, teaching, and research purposes. As an example, Box 1-3 shows the specific criteria provided in the most current edition, *DSM-5*, for the diagnosis of generalized anxiety disorder. Box 1-4 contains a tool to rate the severity of symptoms in this disorder.

The *DSM-5* Organizational Structure

The *DSM-5* (APA, 2013) organizes diagnoses for psychiatric disorders on a developmental hierarchy. This hierarchy means that disorders that are usually seen in infancy, childhood, and adolescence are listed in the first chapter, Neurodevelopmental Disorders, and disorders that occur later in life, such as the Neurocognitive Disorders, are further down on the list. Also, within each chapter specific disorders are listed based on when they typically occur, from youngest to oldest. Diagnostic groups that are related to one another have been closely situated. Examples of this strategic placement include Schizophrenia Spectrum Disorders next to Bipolar Related Disorders and Feeding and Eating Disorders next to Elimination Disorders.

1. Neurodevelopmental Disorders
2. Schizophrenia Spectrum Disorders
3. Bipolar and Related Disorders
4. Depressive Disorders
5. Anxiety Disorders
6. Obsessive-Compulsive Disorders
7. Trauma and Stressor-Related Disorders
8. Dissociative Disorders
9. Somatic Symptom Disorders
10. Feeding and Eating Disorders
11. Elimination Disorders
12. Sleep-Wake Disorders
13. Sexual Dysfunctions
14. Gender Dysphoria
15. Disruptive, Impulse Control, and Conduct Disorders
16. Substance Related and Addictive Disorders
17. Neurocognitive Disorders
18. Personality Disorders
19. Paraphilic Disorders
20. Other Disorders

The previous version, the *DSM-IV-TR*, included a five-axis system whereby Axis I was the psychiatric diagnosis, Axis II was reserved for personality disorders, Axis III identified general medical conditions, Axis IV was environmental stressors, and Axis V provided a tool that measured global functioning with a specific number from 0 to 100. The latest version collapses the first three categories into a single axis. Environmental stressors and concerns are addressed by specific codes. The APA recommends a tool such as the 36-item World Health Organization Disability Assessment Schedule (WHODAS) to measure global functioning; it is available at http://www.who.int/classifications/icf/whodasii/en/.

BOX 1-3 *DSM-5* CRITERIA FOR GENERALIZED ANXIETY DISORDER

A. Excessive anxiety and worry (apprehensive expectation), occurring more days than not for at least 6 months, about a number of events or activities (such as work or school performance).
B. The individual finds it difficult to control the worry.
C. The anxiety and worry are associated with three (or more) of the following six symptoms (with at least some symptoms having been present for more days than not for the past 6 months): (**Note:** Only one item is required in children.)
   1. Restlessness or feeling keyed up or on edge
   2. Being easily fatigued.
   3. Difficulty concentrating or mind going blank.
   4. Irritability.
   5. Muscle tension
   6. Sleep disturbance (difficulty falling or staying asleep, or restless, unsatisfying sleep).
D. The anxiety, worry, or physical symptoms cause clinically significant distress or impairment in social, occupational, or other important areas of functioning.
E. The disturbance is not attributable to the physiological effects of a substance (e.g., a drug of abuse, a medication) or another medical condition (e.g., hyperthyroidism).
F. The disturbance is not better explained by another mental disorder (e.g., anxiety or worry about having panic attacks in panic disorder, negative evaluation in social anxiety disorder [social phobia], contamination or other obsessions in obsessive-compulsive disorder, separation from attachment figures in separation anxiety disorder, reminders of traumatic events in posttraumatic stress disorder, gaining weight in anorexia nervosa, physical complaints in somatic symptom disorder, perceived appearance flaws in body dysmorphic disorder, having a serious illness in illness anxiety disorder, or the content of delusional beliefs in schizophrenia or delusional disorder).

From American Psychiatric Association. (2013). *Diagnostic and statistical manual of disorders* (5th ed.). Washington, DC: Author.

BOX 1-4 PROMIS TOOL FOR ANXIETY (SHORT FORM)

Please respond to each question or statement by marking one box per row. In the past 7 days . . .

		NEVER	RARELY	SOMETIMES	OFTEN	ALWAYS
EDANX01 1	I felt fearful	☐ 1	☐ 2	☐ 3	☐ 4	☐ 5
EDANX40 2	I found it hard to focus on anything other than my anxiety	☐ 1	☐ 2	☐ 3	☐ 4	☐ 5
EDANX41 3	My worries overwhelmed me	☐ 1	☐ 2	☐ 3	☐ 4	☐ 5
EDANX53 4	I felt uneasy	☐ 1	☐ 2	☐ 3	☐ 4	☐ 5
EDANX46 5	I felt nervous	☐ 1	☐ 2	☐ 3	☐ 4	☐ 5
EDANX07 6	I felt like I needed help for my anxiety	☐ 1	☐ 2	☐ 3	☐ 4	☐ 5
EDANX05 7	I felt anxious	☐ 1	☐ 2	☐ 3	☐ 4	☐ 5
EDANX54 8	I felt tense	☐ 1	☐ 2	☐ 3	☐ 4	☐ 5

National Institutes of Health. (2012). *PROMIS item bank v1.0—Emotional distress—Anxiety—Short form 8a.* Retrieved from https://www.assessmentcenter.net/PromisForms.aspx.

The *ICD-9-CM*

In an increasingly global society, it is important to view the United States' diagnosis and treatment of mental illness as part of a bigger picture. An international standard for diagnostic classification for all diseases is the *International Classification of Diseases, Ninth Revision, Clinical Modification* (*ICD-9-CM*) (WHO, 2011). The United States has adapted this resource to its system with a "clinical modification," hence its title of *ICD-9-CM*. Clinical descriptions of mental and behavioral disorders are divided into two broad classifications with subclassifications:

Psychosis
- Organic psychotic conditions
- Other psychoses

Neurotic disorders, personality disorders, and other nonpsychotic disorders
- Neurotic disorders
- Personality disorders
- Psychosexual disorders
- Psychoactive disorders
- Other adult onset disorders
- Mental disorders diagnosed in childhood

The United States Centers for Medicare and Medicaid Services mandated a switch to the newer version of this system, the *ICD-10*, effective October 2014. This version contains 68,000 codes as compared to the 13,000 in the *ICD-9*. Efforts were made by the American Psychiatric Association to make the DSM-5 correspond more closely with this system. Clinical descriptions of mental and behavior disorders are divided into 11 disease classifications:

1. Organic—including symptomatic—mental disorders
2. Mental and behavioral disorders due to psychoactive substance use
3. Schizophrenia, schizotypal, and delusional disorders
4. Mood (affective) disorders
5. Neurotic, stress-related, and somatoform disorders
6. Behavioral syndromes associated with physiological disturbances and physical factors
7. Disorders of adult personality and behavior
8. Mental retardation
9. Disorders of psychological development
10. Behavioral and emotional disorders with onset usually occurring in childhood and adolescence
11. Unspecified mental disorder

PSYCHIATRIC MENTAL HEALTH NURSING

In all clinical settings, nurses work with people who are going through crises, including physical, psychological, mental, and spiritual distress. You will encounter patients who are experiencing feelings of hopelessness, helplessness, anxiety, anger, low self-esteem, or confusion. You will meet people who are withdrawn, suspicious, elated, depressed, hostile, manipulative, suicidal, intoxicated, or withdrawing from a substance. Most of you have already come across people who are going through difficult times in their lives. While you may have handled these situations well, there may have been times when you wished you had additional skills and knowledge. Basic psychosocial nursing concepts will become central to your practice of nursing and increase your competency as a practitioner in all clinical settings. Whatever setting you choose to work in, you will have the opportunity to improve the lives of people who are experiencing mental illness as an additional challenge to their health care needs.

Your experience in the psychiatric nursing rotation will greatly increase your insight into the experiences of others and may help you gain insight into yourself. This part of your nursing education will provide essential information about psychiatric disorders and the opportunity to learn new skills for dealing with a variety of challenging behaviors. The remaining sections of this chapter present a brief overview of what psychiatric nurses do, their scope of practice, and the challenges and evolving roles for the future health care environment.

What Is Psychiatric Mental Health Nursing?

Psychiatric mental health nursing, a core mental health profession, employs a purposeful use of self as its art and a wide range of nursing, psychosocial, and neurobiological theories and research evidence as its science (American Nurses Association [ANA], 2007). Psychiatric mental health nurses work with people throughout the life span: children, adolescents, adults, and the elderly. Psychiatric mental health nurses assist healthy people who are in crisis or who are experiencing life problems as well as those with long-term mental illness. Their patients may include people with dual diagnoses (a mental disorder and a coexisting substance disorder), homeless persons and families, forensic patients (people in jail), individuals who have survived abusive situations, and people in crisis. Psychiatric mental health nurses work with individuals, couples, families, and groups in every nursing setting. They work with patients in hospitals, in their homes, in halfway houses, in shelters, in clinics, in storefronts, on the street—virtually everywhere.

The *Psychiatric-Mental Health Nursing: Scope and Standards of Practice* defines the specific activities of the psychiatric mental health nurse. This publication—jointly written in 2007 by the American Nurses Association (ANA), the American Psychiatric Nurses Association (APNA), and the International Society of Psychiatric-Mental Health Nurses (ISPN)—defines the focus of **psychiatric mental health nursing** as "promoting mental health through the assessment, diagnosis, and treatment of human responses to mental health problems and psychiatric disorders" (p. 14). The psychiatric mental health nurse uses the same nursing process you have already learned to assess and diagnose patients' illnesses, identify outcomes, and plan, implement, and evaluate nursing care. Box 1-5 describes **phenomena of concern** for psychiatric mental health nurses.

Classification of Nursing Diagnoses, Outcomes, and Interventions

To provide the most appropriate and scientifically sound care, the psychiatric mental health nurse uses standardized classification systems developed by professional nursing groups. The *Nursing Diagnoses: Definitions and Classification 2012-2014* of the North American Nursing Diagnosis Association International (NANDA-I) (Herdman, 2012) provides 216 standardized diagnoses, more than 40% of which are related to psychosocial/psychiatric nursing care. These diagnoses provide a common language to aid in the selection of nursing interventions and ultimately lead to outcome achievement.

BOX 1-5 PHENOMENA OF CONCERN FOR PSYCHIATRIC-MENTAL HEALTH NURSES

Phenomena of concern for psychiatric-mental health nurses include:

- Promotion of optimal mental and physical health and well-being and prevention of mental illness.
- Impaired ability to function related to psychiatric, emotional, and physiological distress.
- Alterations in thinking, perceiving, and communicating due to psychiatric disorders or mental health problems.
- Behaviors and mental states that indicate potential danger to self or others.
- Emotional stress related to illness, pain, disability, and loss.
- Symptom management, side effects, or toxicities associated with self-administered drugs, psychopharmacological intervention, and other treatment modalities.
- The barriers to treatment efficacy and recovery posed by alcohol and substance abuse and dependence.
- Self-concept and body image changes, developmental issues, life process changes, and end-of-life issues.
- Physical symptoms that occur along with altered psychological status.
- Psychological symptoms that occur along with altered physiological status.
- Interpersonal, organizational, sociocultural, spiritual, or environmental circumstances or events that have an effect on the mental and emotional well-being of the individual and family or community.
- Elements of recovery, including the ability to maintain housing, employment, and social support, that help individuals re-engage in seeking meaningful lives.
- Societal factors such as violence, poverty, and substance abuse.

From American Psychiatric Nurses Association, International Society of Psychiatric-Mental Health Nurses, & American Nurses Association. (2007). *Psychiatric-mental health nursing: Scope and standards of practice.* Silver Spring, MD: NurseBooks.org.

DSM-5 and NANDA-I–Approved Nursing Diagnoses

Psychiatric mental health nursing includes the diagnosis and treatment of human responses to actual or potential mental health problems. A nursing diagnosis "is a clinical judgment about individual, family, or community responses to actual or potential health problems and life processes" (Herdman, 2012, p. 515). While the *DSM-5* is used to diagnose a psychiatric disorder, a well-defined nursing diagnosis provides the framework for identifying appropriate nursing interventions for dealing with the patient's reaction to the disorder. Those reactions might include confusion, low self-esteem, impaired ability to function in job or family situations, and so on.

The last page of this text (opposite the inside back cover) lists NANDA-I–approved nursing diagnoses, and the individual clinical chapters (11 through 24) offer suggestions for potential nursing diagnoses for the behaviors and phenomena often encountered in association with specific disorders. A more thorough discussion of nursing diagnoses in psychosocial nursing can be found in Chapter 7.

Nursing Outcomes Classification (NOC)

The *Nursing Outcomes Classification (NOC)* is a comprehensive source of standardized outcomes, definitions of these outcomes, and measuring scales that help to determine the outcome of nursing interventions (Moorhead et al., 2013). Outcomes are organized into seven domains: functional health, physiologic health, psychosocial health, health knowledge and behavior, perceived health, family health, and community health. The psychosocial health domain includes four classes: psychological well-being, psychosocial adaptation, self-control, and social interaction.

Nursing Interventions Classification (NIC)

The *Nursing Interventions Classification (NIC)* is another tool used to standardize, define, and measure nursing care. Bulechek, Butcher, Dochterman, and Wagner (2013) define a nursing intervention as "any treatment, based upon clinical judgment and knowledge, that a nurse performs to enhance patient/client outcomes" (p. xxi), including direct and indirect care through a series of nursing activities. There are seven domains: basic physiological, complex physiological, behavioral, safety, family, health system, and community. Two domains relate specifically to psychiatric nursing: behavioral, including communication, coping, and education, and safety, covering crisis and risk management.

Levels of Psychiatric Mental Health Clinical Nursing Practice

Psychiatric mental health nurses are registered nurses educated in nursing and licensed to practice in their individual states. Psychiatric nurses are qualified to practice at two levels, basic and advanced, depending on educational preparation. Table 1-2 describes basic and advanced psychiatric nursing interventions.

Basic Level

Basic level registered nurses are professionals who have completed a nursing program, passed the state licensure examination, and are qualified to work in most any general or specialty area. The registered nurse–psychiatric mental health (RN-PMH) is a nursing graduate who possesses a diploma, an associate degree, or a baccalaureate degree and chooses to work in the specialty of psychiatric mental health nursing. At the basic level, nurses work in various supervised settings and perform multiple roles such as staff nurse, case manager, home care nurse, and so on.

After 2 years of full-time work as a registered nurse, 2000 clinical hours in a psychiatric setting, and 30 hours of continuing education in psychiatric nursing, a baccalaureate-prepared nurse may take a certification examination administered by the American Nurses Credentialing Center (the credentialing arm of the American Nurses Association) to demonstrate clinical competence in psychiatric mental health nursing. After passing the examination, a board-certified credential is added to the RN title resulting in RN-BC. Certification gives nurses a sense of mastery and accomplishment, identifies them as competent clinicians, and satisfies a requirement for reimbursement by employers in some states.

Advanced Practice

The psychiatric clinical nurse specialist was one of the first advanced practice roles to be developed in the United States in the 1950s. These nurse specialists were trained to provide individual therapy and group therapy in state psychiatric hospitals and to provide training for other staff. Eventually they, along with psychiatric nurse practitioners who were introduced in the mid-1960s, gained diagnostic privileges, prescriptive authority, and permission to engage in psychotherapy.

TABLE 1-2 BASIC LEVEL AND ADVANCED PRACTICE PSYCHIATRIC MENTAL HEALTH NURSING INTERVENTIONS

BASIC LEVEL INTERVENTION	DESCRIPTION
Coordination of care	Coordinates implementation of the nursing care plan and documents coordination of care.
Health teaching and health maintenance	Individualized anticipatory guidance to prevent or reduce mental illness or enhance mental health (e.g., community screenings, parenting classes, stress management)
Milieu therapy	Provides, structures, and maintains a safe and therapeutic environment in collaboration with patients, families, and other health care clinicians
Pharmacological, biological, and integrative therapies	Applies current knowledge to assessing patient's response to medication, provides medication teaching, and communicates observations to other members of the health care team
ADVANCED PRACTICE INTERVENTION	**DESCRIPTION**
All of the above plus:	
Medication prescription and treatment	Prescription of psychotropic medications, with appropriate use of diagnostic tests; hospital admitting privileges
Psychotherapy	Individual, couple, group, or family therapy, using evidence-based therapeutic frameworks and the nurse-patient relationship
Consultation	Sharing of clinical expertise with nurses or those in other disciplines to enhance their treatment of patients or address systems issues

Data from American Psychiatric Nurses Association, International Society of Psychiatric-Mental Health Nurses, & American Nurses Association. (2007). *Psychiatric-mental health nursing: Scope and standards of practice.* Silver Spring, MD: NurseBooks.org.

Currently, the **advanced practice registered nurse–psychiatric mental health (APRN-PMH)** is a licensed registered nurse with a Master of Science in Nursing (MSN) or Doctor of Nursing Practice (DNP) in psychiatric nursing. This DNP is not to be confused with a doctoral degree in nursing (PhD), which is a research degree, whereas the DNP is a practice doctorate that prepares advanced practice nurses. The APRN-PMH may function autonomously depending on the state and is eligible for specialty privileges. Some advanced practice nurses continue their education to the doctoral (PhD) level.

Unlike other specialty areas, there is no significant difference between a psychiatric nurse practitioner (NP) and a clinical nurse specialist (CNS) as long as the CNS has achieved prescriptive authority. Certification is required and is obtained through the American Nurses Credentialing Center. Four examinations are currently available, including two for psychiatric NPs and two for CNSs:

1. Psychiatric–Mental Health Nurse Practitioner (across the life span)–Board Certified (PMHNP-BC)
2. Adult Psychiatric & Mental Health Nurse Practitioner (PMHNP-BC)*
3. Adult Psychiatric & Mental Health Clinical Nurse Specialist (PMHCNS-BC)*
4. Child/Adolescent Psychiatric & Mental Health Clinical Nurse Specialist (PMHCNS-BC)*

FUTURE CHALLENGES AND ROLES FOR PSYCHIATRIC MENTAL HEALTH NURSES

Significant trends that will affect the future of psychiatric nursing in the United States include educational challenges, an aging population, increasing cultural diversity, and expanding technology.

Educational Challenges

Psychiatric mental health nurses at both the basic and advanced practice level continue to be in demand. As with any specialty area in hospital settings, psychiatric nurses are caring for more acutely ill patients. In the 1980s, it was common for patients who were depressed and suicidal to have insurance coverage for about 2 weeks. Now patients are lucky to be covered for 3 days, if they are covered at all. This means that nurses need to be more skilled and be prepared to discharge patients for whom the benefit of their care will not always be evident.

Challenges in educating students who possess the skills to eventually become psychiatric mental health nurses are related to this level of acute care and also to dwindling inpatient populations. Clinical rotations in general medical centers are becoming less available, and faculty are fortunate to secure rotations in state psychiatric hospitals and veterans administration facilities. Community psychiatric settings also provide students with valuable experience, but the logistics of placing and supervising students in multiple sites has required creativity on the part of nursing educators. Some schools have established integrated rotations that allow students to work outside the psychiatric setting with patients who have mental health issues—for example, caring for a depressed person on an orthopedic floor.

Nurse-led health homes and clinics are becoming increasingly common. Community nursing centers that can secure funding serve low-income and uninsured people. In this model, psychiatric mental health nurses work with primary care nurses to provide comprehensive care, usually funded by scarce grants from academic centers. These centers use a nontraditional approach of combining primary care and health promotion interventions. Advanced practice psychiatric nurses have also been extremely successful in setting up private practices where they provide both psychotherapy and medication management.

An Aging Population

As the number of older adults grows, the prevalence of Alzheimer's disease and other dementias requiring skilled nursing care in inpatient settings is likely to increase. Healthier older adults will need more services at home, in retirement communities, or in assisted living facilities. For more information on the needs of older adults, refer to Chapters 23, 28, and 30.

Cultural Diversity

Cultural diversity is steadily increasing in the United States. The United States Census Bureau (2012) notes that for the first time in our history a majority (50.4%) of children less than 1 year of age were minorities as of July 1, 2011. Percentages of Hispanics (who may be of any race) are projected to nearly double in numbers during those years, from 16% of the population to over 30%. Psychiatric mental health nurses will need to increase their **cultural competence**; that is, their sensitivity to different cultural views regarding health, illness, and response to treatment.

Science, Technology, and Electronic Health Care

Genetic mapping from the Human Genome Project has resulted in a steady stream of research discoveries concerning genetic markers implicated in a variety of psychiatric illnesses. This information could be helpful in identifying at-risk individuals and in targeting medications specific to certain genetic variants and profiles; however, the legal and ethical implications of responsibly using this technology are staggering. For example:

- Would you want to know you were at risk for a psychiatric illness such as bipolar disorder?
- Who should have access to this information—your primary care provider, insurer, future spouse, a lawyer in a child-custody battle?
- Who will regulate genetic testing centers to protect privacy and prevent 21st-century problems such as identity theft and fraud?

Despite these concerns, the next decade holds great promise in the diagnosis and treatment of psychiatric disorders, and nurses

*In 2014, all but the Psychiatric & Mental Health Nurse Practitioner credentialing exams will be retired. Nurses who are already certified with these credentials can renew their certification using professional development activities and clinical practice hours to maintain their certified status as long as their certification does not lapse.

will be central as educators and caregivers. Scientific advances through research and technology are certain to shape psychiatric mental health nursing practice. Magnetic resonance imaging research, in addition to comparing healthy people to people diagnosed with mental illness, is now focusing on development of preclinical profiles of children and adolescents. The hope of this type of research is to identify people at risk for developing mental illness, which allows earlier interventions to try to decrease impairment.

Electronic health care services provided from a distance are gaining wide acceptance. In the early days of the Internet, consumers were cautioned against the questionable wisdom of seeking advice through an unregulated medium; however, the Internet has transformed the way we approach health care needs and allows people to be their own advocates.

The APA (2008) promotes telepsychiatry through audio and visual media as an effective way to reach underserved populations and those who are homebound. This allows for assessment and diagnosis, medication management, and even group therapy. Psychiatric nurses may become more active in developing websites for mental health education, screening, or support, especially to reach geographically isolated areas. Many health agencies hire nurses to staff help lines or hotlines, and as the provision of these cost-effective services increase, so will the need for bilingual resources.

ADVOCACY AND LEGISLATIVE INVOLVEMENT

The role of the psychiatric mental health nurse as patient advocate continues to evolve. Through direct care and indirect action nurses advocate for the psychiatric patient. As a patient advocate, the nurse reports incidents of abuse or neglect to the appropriate authorities for immediate action. The nurse also upholds patient confidentiality, which has become more of a challenge as the use of electronic medical records increases. Another form of nursing advocacy is supporting the patient's right to make decisions regarding treatment. Within managed care, situations in which the patient disagrees with the treatment approved continue to arise.

On an indirect level, the nurse may choose to be active in consumer mental health groups (such as NAMI) and state and local mental health associations to reduce the **stigma** of mental illness and to support consumers of mental health care. The nurse can also be vigilant about reviewing local and national legislation affecting health care to identify potential detrimental effects on the mentally ill. Especially during times of fiscal crisis, lawmakers are inclined to decrease or eliminate funding for vulnerable populations who do not have a strong political voice.

The American Psychiatric Nurses Association (2008) is investing increased energy into monitoring legislative, regulatory, and policy matters affecting psychiatric nursing and mental health in order to positively affect the care of people with psychiatric disorders. As the 24-hours-a-day, 7-days-a-week caregivers and members of the largest group of health care professionals, nurses are in the enviable position of being expert advocates for individuals with mental illness and having the potential to exert tremendous influence on legislation.

When commissions and task forces are developed, however, nurses are not usually the first group to be considered to provide input and expertise for national, state, and local decision makers. In fact, nursing presence is often absent at the policymaking table. Consider the President's New Freedom Commission for Mental Health (2003), which included psychiatrists (medical doctors), psychologists (PhDs), academics, and policymakers—but no nurses. It is difficult to understand how the largest contingent of mental health care providers in the United States could be excluded from a group that would determine the future of mental health care.

It is in the best interest of consumers of mental health care that all members of the collaborative health care team, including nurses, be involved in decisions and legislation that will affect their care. Current political issues that need monitoring and support include mental health parity, discriminatory media portrayal, standardized language and practices, and advanced practice issues, such as prescriptive authority over Schedule II drugs and government and insurance reimbursement for nursing care.

KEY POINTS TO REMEMBER

- Mental health and illness are not either/or propositions but endpoints on a continuum.
- The study of epidemiology can help identify high-risk groups and behaviors. In turn, this can lead to a better understanding of the causes of some disorders. Prevalence rates help us identify the proportion of a population experiencing a specific mental disorder at a given time.
- Recognizing that mental disorders are biologically based with environmental mediation, it is easier to see how they can be classified as medical disorders.
- The *DSM-5* provides criteria for psychiatric disorders and a basis for the development of comprehensive and appropriate interventions.
- Culture influences behavior, and symptoms may reflect a person's cultural patterns or beliefs. Symptoms must be understood in terms of a person's cultural background.
- Psychiatric mental health nurses work with a broad population of patients in diverse settings to promote optimal mental health.
- Standardized nursing classification systems (*NANDA-I, NOC, NIC*) are used to form and communicate patient problems, outcomes, and interventions specific to nursing care.
- Psychiatric mental health nurses function at a basic or advanced level of practice with clearly defined roles.
- Due to social, cultural, scientific, and political factors, the future holds many challenges and possibilities for the psychiatric mental health nurse.

CRITICAL THINKING

1. Brian, a college sophomore with a grade-point average of 3.4, is brought to the emergency department after a suicide attempt. He has been extremely depressed since the death of his girlfriend 5 months previously when the car he was driving crashed. His parents are devastated, and they believe that taking one's own life prevents a person from going to heaven.

   Brian has epilepsy and has had more seizures since the auto accident. He says he should be punished for his carelessness and does not care what happens to him. He has stopped going to classes and no longer shows up for his part-time job of tutoring young children in reading.

   a. What might be a possible *DSM-5* (medical) diagnosis?
   b. What are some factors that you should assess regarding aspects of Brian's overall health and other influences that can affect mental health?
   c. If an antidepressant medication could help Brian's depression, explain why this alone would not meet his multiple needs. What issues do you think have to be addressed if Brian is to receive a holistic approach to care?
   d. Formulate two potential nursing diagnoses for Brian.
   e. Would Brian's parents' religious beliefs factor into your plan of care? If so, how?
2. In a small group, share experiences you have had with others from unfamiliar cultural, ethnic, religious, or racial backgrounds, and identify two positive learning experiences from these encounters.
3. Would you feel comfortable referring a family member to a mental health clinician? What factors influence your feelings?
4. How could basic and advanced practice psychiatric mental health nurses work together to provide the highest quality of care?
5. Would you consider joining a professional group or advocacy group that promotes mental health? Why or why not?

CHAPTER REVIEW

1. Which statement about mental illness is true?
   a. Mental illness is a matter of individual nonconformity with societal norms.
   b. Mental illness is present when individual irrational and illogical behavior occurs.
   c. Mental illness changes with culture, time in history, political systems, and the groups defining it.
   d. Mental illness is evaluated solely by considering individual control over behavior and appraisal of reality.
2. A nursing student new to psychiatric mental health nursing asks a peer what resources he can use to figure out which symptoms are present in a specific psychiatric disorder. The best answer would be:
   a. *Nursing Interventions Classification (NIC)*
   b. *Nursing Outcomes Classification (NOC)*
   c. NANDA-I nursing diagnoses
   d. *DSM-5*
3. Epidemiological studies contribute to improvements in care for individuals with mental disorders by:
   a. Providing information about effective nursing techniques.
   b. Identifying risk factors that contribute to the development of a disorder.
   c. Identifying who in the general population will develop a specific disorder.
   d. Identifying which individuals will respond favorably to a specific treatment.
4. Which statement best describes a major difference between a *DSM-5* diagnosis and a nursing diagnosis?
   a. There is no functional difference between the two; both serve to identify a human deviance.
   b. The *DSM-5* diagnosis disregards culture, whereas the nursing diagnosis takes culture into account.
   c. The *DSM-5* is associated with present symptoms, whereas a nursing diagnosis considers past, present, and potential responses to actual mental health problems.
   d. The *DSM-5* diagnosis impacts the choice of medical treatment, whereas the nursing diagnosis offers a framework for identifying multidisciplinary interventions.
5. The intervention that can be practiced by an advanced practice registered nurse in psychiatric mental health but cannot be practiced by a basic level registered nurse is:
   a. Advocacy
   b. Psychotherapy
   c. Coordination of care
   d. Community-based care

Answers to Chapter Review
1. c; 2. d; 3. c; 4. c; 5. b.

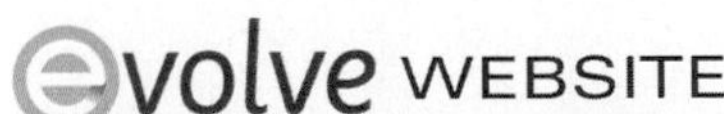

Visit the Evolve website for a posttest on the content in this chapter: http://evolve.elsevier.com/Varcarolis

Post-Test interactive review

REFERENCES

Altrocchi, J. (1980). *Abnormal behavior*. New York: Harcourt Brace Jovanovich.

Amat, J., Paul, E., Zarza, C., Watkins, L. R., & Maier, S. F. (2006). Previous experience with behavioral control over stress blocks the behavioral and dorsal raphe activating effects of later uncontrollable stress: Role of the ventral medial prefrontal cortex. *Journal of Neuroscience, 26*(51), 13,264–13,272.

American Psychiatric Nurses Association. (2008). *Institute for mental health advocacy*. Retrieved from http://www.apna.org/i4a/pages/index.cfm?pageid=3637.

American Psychiatric Nurses Association, International Society of Psychiatric-Mental Health Nurses, & American Nurses Association. (2007). *Psychiatric-mental health nursing: Scope and standards of practice*. Silver Spring, MD: NurseBooks.org.

American Psychiatric Association. (2013). *Diagnostic and statistical manual of mental disorders* (5th ed.). Washington, DC: Author.

Bulechek, G. M., Butcher, H. K., Dochterman, J. M., & Wagner, C. (2013). *Nursing interventions classification (NIC)* (6th ed.). St. Louis: Mosby.

Cohen, J. I. (2000). Stress and mental health: A biobehavioral perspective. *Issues in Mental Health Nursing, 21,* 185–202.

Herdman, T. H. (Ed.). (2012). *NANDA international nursing diagnoses: Definitions and classification, 2012–2014*. Oxford, UK: Wiley-Blackwell.

Howard, R. (Director). (2001). *A beautiful mind* [film]. Los Angeles: Universal Pictures.

Institute of Medicine. (2011). *The future of nursing: focus on education*. Retrieved from http://www.iom.edu/Reports/2010/The-Future-of-Nursing-Leading-Change-Advancing-Health/Report-Brief-Education.aspx.

Institute of Medicine. (2006). *Improving the quality of health care for mental and substance-use conditions: Quality chasm series*. Washington, DC: National Academies Press.

Kessler, R. C., Berglund, P., Demler, O., Jin, R., & Walters, E. E. (2005). Lifetime prevalence and age-of-onset distributions of DSM-IV disorders in the national comorbidity survey replication. *Archives of General Psychiatry, 62,* 593–602.

Kessler, R. C., Chiu, W. T., Demler, O., & Walters, E. E. (2005). Prevalence, severity, and comorbidity of twelve-month DSM-IV disorders in the National Comorbidity Survey Replication (NCS-R). *Archives of General Psychiatry, 62*(6), 617–27.

Moorhead, S., Johnson, M., Maas, M. L., & Swanson, E. (2013). *Nursing outcomes classification (NOC)* (5th ed.). St Louis: Mosby.

Morgan, C., McKenzie, K., & Fearon, P. (2008). *Society and psychosis*. London, UK: Cambridge.

Porter, N. (Ed.), (1913). *Webster's revised unabridged dictionary*. Boston, MA: Merriam.

Robert Wood Johnson Foundation. (2011). *QSEN branches out*. Retrieved from http://www.rwjf.org/humancapital/product.jsp?id=72552.

Southwick, S. M., & Charney, D. S. (2012). The science of resilience: Implications for the prevention and treatment of depression. *Science, 338*(6103), 79–82. doi:10.1126/science.1222942.

Stern, T. A., Fricchione, G. L., Cassem, N. H., Jellinek, M. S., & Rosenbaum, J. F. (2010). *Massachusetts General Hospital handbook of general hospital psychiatry* (6th ed.). Philadelphia, PA: Saunders.

Substance Abuse and Mental Health Services Administration. (2011). *SAMHSA announces a working definition of "recovery" from mental disorders and substance use disorders*. Retrieved from http://www.samhsa.gov/newsroom/advisories/1112223420.aspx.

United States Census Bureau. (2012). *Most children younger than one are minorities, Census Bureau reports*. Retrieved from http://www.census.gov/newsroom/releases/archives/population/cb12-90.html.

United States Department of Energy. (2008). *The human genome project information*. Retrieved from http://www.ornl.gov/sci/techresources/Human_Genome/home.shtml.

United States Department of Health and Human Services, Health Resources and Services Administration. (2004). *The registered nurse population: Findings from the 2004 national sample survey of registered nurses*. Retrieved from http://bhpr.hrsa.gov/healthworkforce/rnsurvey04/.

United States Department of Health and Human Services, U.S. Public Health Service. (1999). *Mental health: a report of the Surgeon General*. Washington, DC: U.S. Government Printing Office.

World Health Organization. (2010). *Mental health: Strengthening Our response*. Retrieved from http://www.who.int/mediacentre/factsheets/fs220/en/.

World Health Organization. (2007). ICD-10: International statistical classification of diseases and related health problems (10th rev. ed.). New York, NY: Author.

CHAPTER

2

Relevant Theories and Therapies for Nursing Practice

Margaret Jordan Halter

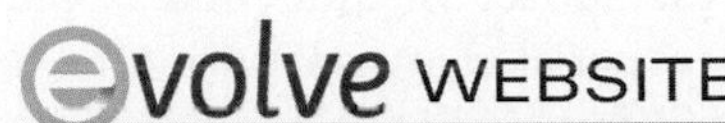

Visit the Evolve website for a pretest on the content in this chapter: http://evolve.elsevier.com/Varcarolis

Pre-Test interactive review

OBJECTIVES

1. Evaluate the premises behind the various therapeutic models discussed in this chapter.
2. Describe the evolution of therapies for psychiatric disorders.
3. Identify ways each theorist contributes to the nurse's ability to assess a patient's behaviors.
4. Provide responses to the following based on clinical experience:
   a. An example of how a patient's irrational beliefs influenced behavior.
   b. An example of countertransference in your relationship with a patient.
   c. An example of the use of behavior modification with a patient.
5. Identify Peplau's framework for the nurse-patient relationship.
6. Choose the therapeutic model that would be most useful for a particular patient or patient problem.

KEY TERMS AND CONCEPTS

automatic thoughts
behavior therapy
biofeedback
classical conditioning
cognitive-behavioral therapy (CBT)
cognitive distortions
conditioning
conscious
countertransference
defense mechanisms
ego
extinction
id
interpersonal psychotherapy
milieu therapy
negative reinforcement
operant conditioning
positive reinforcement
preconscious
psychodynamic therapy
punishment
reinforcement
superego
systematic desensitization
transference
unconscious

Every professional discipline, from math and science to philosophy and psychology, bases its work and beliefs on theories. Most of these theories can best be described as explanations, hypotheses, or hunches, rather than testable facts. For students, the word *theory* may conjure up some dry, conceptual images, vaguely recalling the physicists' theory of relativity or the geologists' plate tectonics. Compared to most other theories, however, psychological theories are filled with familiar concepts since terms from psychological theories have filtered their way into parts of mainstream thinking and speech. Advertisements use the behaviorist ploy of linking a gorgeous, seductive woman to the family-style utilitarian minivan. And who has not attributed language mistakes to subconscious motivation? As the fictional king greets his queen: "Good morning, my beheaded . . . I mean my beloved!" we comprehend the Freudian slip.

Dealing with other people is one of the most universally anxiety-provoking activities, and psychological theories provide plausible explanations for perplexing behavior. Maybe the guy at the front desk who never greets you in the morning does not really despise you; maybe he has an inferiority complex because his mother was cold and his father was absent from the home. In much the same way, patient stories are complex and always unique. It is useful to have a broad base of knowledge about personality development, human needs, the ingredients of mental health, contributing factors to mental illness, and the importance of relationships.

This chapter will provide you with snapshots of some of the most influential psychological theories. It will also provide an overview of the treatment, or therapy, they inspired and the contributions they have made to the practice of psychiatric mental health nursing. The theoretical journey begins with a look at Sigmund Freud, often referred to as the "father of psychoanalysis, and it moves on to Erik Erikson and Harry Stack Sullivan, who initially were devotees of Freud but later found Freudian theory lacking and took a divergent path. The chapter then focuses on the theory of the "mother of psychiatric nursing," Hildegard Peplau. Abraham Maslow, a representative theorist from the humanistic approach to psychiatry, follows her work. Ivan Pavlov, John B. Watson, and B. F. Skinner represent the behaviorist approach. The final leg of this trip explores two dominant approaches to treating psychiatric illness: cognitive-behavioral therapy and biological therapies. Each of these theoretical approaches and therapies is evaluated for relevance to psychiatric mental health nursing. Let's begin our expedition!

PSYCHOANALYTIC THEORIES AND THERAPIES

Sigmund Freud's Psychoanalytic Theory

Sigmund Freud (1856-1939), an Austrian neurologist, revolutionized thinking about mental health disorders with his groundbreaking theory of personality structure, levels of awareness, anxiety, the role of defense mechanisms, and the stages of psychosexual development. Originally, he was searching for biological treatments for psychological disturbances and even experimented with using cocaine as medication. He soon abandoned the physiological approach and focused on psychological treatments. Freud came to believe that the vast majority of mental disorders were due to unresolved issues that originated in childhood. He arrived at this conclusion through his experiences treating people with hysteria, individuals who were suffering physical symptoms despite the absence of an apparent physiological cause.

As part his treatment, Freud initially used hypnosis, but this provided mixed therapeutic results. He then changed his approach to talk therapy, known as the *cathartic method*. Today, we refer to catharsis as "getting things off our chests." Talk therapy evolved to include "free association," which requires full and honest disclosure of thoughts and feelings as they come to mind. Dream analysis became an essential part of his therapy since Freud believed that urges and impulses of the unconscious mind were symbolically played out in dreams. Freud (1961, 1969) concluded that talking about difficult emotional issues had the potential to heal the wounds causing mental illness. Viewing the success of these therapeutic approaches led Freud to construct his psychoanalytic theory.

Levels of Awareness

Through the use of talk therapy and free association, Freud came to the conclusion that there were three levels of psychological awareness in operation. He offered a topographic theory of how the mind functions, a description of the landscape of the mind. He used the image of an iceberg to describe these levels of awareness (Figure 2-1).

Conscious. Freud described the conscious part of the mind as the tip of the iceberg. It contains all the material a person is aware of at any one time, including perceptions, memories, thoughts, fantasies, and feelings.

Preconscious. Just below the surface of awareness is the preconscious, which contains material that can be retrieved rather easily through conscious effort.

Unconscious. The unconscious includes all repressed memories, passions, and unacceptable urges lying deep below the surface. It is believed that the memories and emotions associated with trauma are often "placed" in the unconscious because the individual finds it too painful to deal with them. The unconscious exerts a powerful yet unseen effect on the conscious thoughts and feelings of the individual. The individual is usually unable to retrieve unconscious material without the assistance of a trained therapist; however, with this assistance, unconscious material can be brought into conscious awareness.

Personality Structure

Freud (1960) delineated three major and distinct but interactive systems of the personality: the id, the ego, and the superego.

Id. At birth we are all id. The id is the source of all drives, instincts, reflexes, needs, genetic inheritance, and capacity to respond, as well as all the wishes that motivate us. The id cannot tolerate frustration and seeks to discharge tension and return to a more comfortable level of energy. The id lacks the ability to problem solve; it is not logical and operates according to the pleasure principle. The only needs that count are its own. A hungry, screaming infant is the perfect example of id.

Ego. Within the first few years of life as the child begins to interact with others, the ego develops. The ego is the problem solver and reality tester. It is able to differentiate subjective experiences, memory images, and objective reality and attempts to negotiate with the outside world. The ego follows the reality

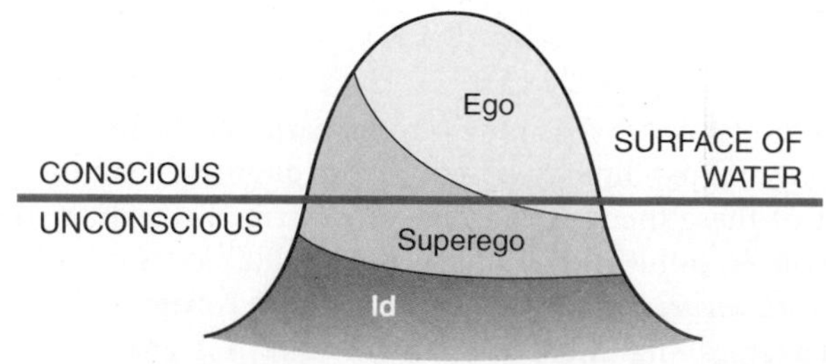

FIG 2-1 The mind as an iceberg.

principle, which says to the id, "You have to delay gratification for right now," and then sets a course of action. For example, a hungry man feels tension arising from the id that wants to be fed. His ego allows him not only to think about his hunger but to plan where he can eat and to seek that destination. This process is known as reality testing because the individual is factoring in reality to implement a plan to decrease tension.

Superego. The superego, the last portion of the personality to develop, represents the moral component of personality. The superego consists of the conscience (all the "should nots" internalized from parents) and the ego ideal (all the "shoulds" internalized from parents). The superego represents the ideal rather than the real; it seeks perfection, as opposed to seeking pleasure or engaging reason.

In a mature and well-adjusted individual, the three systems of the personality—the id, the ego, and the superego—work together as a team under the administrative leadership of the ego. If the id is too powerful, the person will lack control over impulses; if the superego is too powerful, the person may be self-critical and suffer from feelings of inferiority.

Defense Mechanisms and Anxiety

Freud (1969) believed that anxiety is an inevitable part of living. The environment in which we live presents dangers and insecurities, threats and satisfactions. It can produce pain and increase tension or produce pleasure and decrease tension. The ego develops defenses, or defense mechanisms, to ward off anxiety by preventing conscious awareness of threatening feelings.

Defense mechanisms share two common features: (1) they all (except suppression) operate on an unconscious level and (2) they deny, falsify, or distort reality to make it less threatening. Although we cannot survive without defense mechanisms, it is possible for our defense mechanisms to distort reality to such a degree that we experience difficulty with healthy adjustment and personal growth. Chapter 12 offers further discussions of defense mechanisms.

Psychosexual Stages of Development

Freud believed that human development proceeds through five stages from infancy to adulthood. His main focus, however, was on events that occur during the first 5 years of life. From Freud's perspective, experiences during the early stages determined an individual's lifetime adjustment patterns and personality traits. In fact, Freud thought that personality was formed by the time the child entered school and that subsequent growth consisted of elaborating on this basic structure. Freud's psychosexual stages of development are presented in Table 2-1.

Implications for Psychiatric Mental Health Nursing

Freud's theory has relevance to psychiatric mental health nursing practice at many junctures. First, the theory offers a comprehensive explanation of complex human processes and suggests that the formation of a patient's personality is strongly influenced by childhood experiences. Freud's theory of the unconscious mind is particularly valuable as a baseline for considering the complexity of human behavior. By considering conscious and unconscious influences, a nurse can identify and begin to think about the root causes of patient suffering. Freud emphasized the importance of individual talk sessions characterized by attentive listening, with a focus on underlying themes as an important tool of healing in psychiatric care.

Classical Psychoanalysis

Classical psychoanalysis, as developed by Sigmund Freud, is seldom used today. Freud's premise that all mental illness is caused by early intrapsychic conflict is no longer widely thought to be valid, and such therapy requires an unrealistically lengthy period of treatment (i.e., three to five times a week for nearly six years), making it prohibitively expensive and not insured for most. There are two concepts from classic psychoanalysis that are important for nurses to know: transference and countertransference (Freud, 1969).

Transference refers to feelings that the patient has toward health care workers that were originally held toward significant others in his or her life. When transference occurs, these feelings become available for exploration with the patient. Such exploration helps the patient to better understand certain feelings and behaviors. Countertransference refers to unconscious feelings that the health care worker has toward the patient. For instance, if the patient reminds you of someone you do not like, you may unconsciously react as if the patient were that individual. Countertransference underscores the importance of maintaining self-awareness and seeking supervisory guidance as therapeutic relationships progress. Chapter 10 talks more about countertransference and the nurse-patient relationship.

Psychodynamic Therapy

Psychodynamic therapy follows the psychoanalytic model by using many of the tools of psychoanalysis, such as free association, dream analysis, transference, and countertransference; however, the therapist has increased involvement and interacts with the patient more freely than in traditional psychoanalysis. The therapy is oriented more to the here and now and makes less of an attempt to reconstruct the developmental origins of conflicts (Dewan, Steenbarger, & Greenberg, 2011). Psychodynamic therapy tends to last longer than other common therapeutic modalities and may extend for more than 20 sessions, which insurance companies often reject.

The best candidates for psychodynamic therapy are relatively healthy and well-functioning individuals, sometimes referred to as the "worried well," who have a clearly circumscribed area of difficulty and are intelligent, psychologically minded, and well motivated for change. Patients with psychosis, severe depression, borderline personality disorders, and severe character disorders are not appropriate candidates for this type of treatment. Supportive therapies, which are within the scope of practice of the basic level psychiatric nurse, are useful for these patients. A variety of supportive therapies are described in chapters concerning specific disorders (Chapters 11 to 24).

At the start of treatment, the patient and therapist agree on what the focus will be and concentrate their work on that focus. Sessions are held weekly, and the total number of sessions to be held is determined at the outset of therapy. There is a rapid, back-and-forth pattern between patient and therapist, with both

TABLE 2-1 FREUD'S PSYCHOSEXUAL STAGES OF DEVELOPMENT

STAGE (AGE)	SOURCE OF SATISFACTION	PRIMARY CONFLICT	TASKS	DESIRED OUTCOMES	OTHER POSSIBLE PERSONALITY TRAITS
Oral (0-1 yr)	Mouth (sucking, biting, chewing)	Weaning	Mastery of gratification of oral needs; beginning of ego development (4-5 mo)	Development of trust in the environment, with the realization that needs can be met	Fixation at the oral stage is associated with passivity, gullibility, and dependence; the use of sarcasm; may develop orally focused habits (e.g., smoking, nail-biting).
Anal (1-3 yr)	Anal region (expulsion and retention of feces)	Toilet training	Beginning of development of a sense of control over instinctual drives; ability to delay immediate gratification to gain a future goal	Control over impulses	Fixation at the anal stage is associated with anal retentiveness (stinginess, rigid thought patterns, obsessive-compulsive disorder) or anal-expulsive character (messiness, destructiveness, cruelty).
Phallic (oedipal) (3-6 yr)	Genitals (masturbation)	Oedipus and Electra	Sexual identity with parent of same sex; beginning of superego development	Identification with parent of the same sex	Fixation may result in reckless, self-assured, and narcissistic, person. Lack of resolution may result in inability to love and difficulties with sexual identity.
Latency (6-12 yr)	—	—	Growth of ego functions (social, intellectual, mechanical) and the ability to care about and relate to others outside the home (peers of the same sex)	The development of skills needed to cope with the environment	Fixations can result in difficulty identifying with others and in developing social skills, leading to a sense of inadequacy and inferiority.
Genital (12 yr and beyond)	Genitals (sexual intercourse)	—	Development of satisfying sexual and emotional relationship; emancipation from parents—planning of life goals and development of a sense of personal identity	The ability to be creative and find pleasure in love and work	Inability to negotiate this stage may derail emotional and financial independence, may impair personal identity and future goals, and disrupt ability to form satisfying intimate relationships.

Data from Gleitman, H. (1981). *Psychology.* New York, NY: W. W. Norton.

participating actively. The therapist intervenes constantly to keep the therapy on track, either by redirecting the patient's attention or by interpreting deviations from the focus to the patient.

Brief therapies share the following common elements:

- The central focus is established early, usually during the first session or two.
- Clear expectations are established for time-limited therapy with improvement demonstrated within a small number of sessions.
- Goals are concrete, and there is one major focus on improving the patient's worst symptoms, improving coping skills, and helping the patient understand what is going on in his or her life.
- Interpretations are directed toward present-life circumstances and patient behavior rather than toward the historical significance of feelings.
- There is a general understanding that psychotherapy does not cure but that it can help troubled individuals learn to better deal with life's inevitable stressors.

Erik Erikson's Ego Theory

Erik Erikson (1902-1994), an American psychoanalyst, was also a follower of Freud; however, Erikson (1963) believed that Freudian theory was restrictive and negative in its approach. He also stressed that an individual's development is influenced by more than the limited mother-child-father triangle and that culture and society exert significant influence on personality. According to Erikson, personality was not set in stone at age 5, as Freud suggested, but continued to develop throughout the life span.

Erikson described development as occurring in eight predetermined and consecutive life stages (psychosocial crises), each of which consists of two possible outcomes (e.g., industry vs. inferiority). The successful or unsuccessful completion of each stage will affect the individual's progression to the next (Table 2-2). For example, Erikson's crisis of industry versus inferiority occurs from the ages of 7 to 12. During this stage, the child's task is to gain a sense of personal abilities and competence and to expand relationships

TABLE 2-2 ERIKSON'S EIGHT STAGES OF DEVELOPMENT

APPROXIMATE AGE	DEVELOPMENTAL TASK	PSYCHOSOCIAL CRISIS	SUCCESSFUL RESOLUTION OF CRISIS	UNSUCCESSFUL RESOLUTION OF CRISIS
Infancy (0-1½ yr)	Forming attachment to mother, which lays foundations for later trust in others	Trust vs. mistrust	Sound basis for relating to other people; trust in people; faith and hope about environment and future "If he's late in picking me up, there must be a good reason."	General difficulties relating to people effectively; suspicion; trust-fear conflict; fear of future "I can't trust anyone; no one has ever been there when I needed them."
Early childhood (1½-3 yr)	Gaining some basic control of self and environment (e.g., toilet training, exploration)	Autonomy vs. shame and doubt	Sense of self-control and adequacy; will power "I'm sure that with the proper diet and exercise program, I can achieve my target weight."	Independence/fear conflict; severe feelings of self-doubt "I could never lose the weight they want me to, so why even try?"
Preschool (3-6 yr)	Becoming purposeful and directive	Initiative vs. guilt	Ability to initiate one's own activities; sense of purpose "I like to help mommy set the table for dinner."	Aggression/fear conflict; sense of inadequacy or guilt "I wanted the candy, so I took it."
School age (6-12 yr)	Developing social, physical, and school skills	Industry vs. inferiority	Competence; ability to work "I'm getting really good at swimming since I've been taking lessons."	Sense of inferiority; difficulty learning and working "I can't read as well as the others in my class; I'm just dumb."
Adolescence (12-20 yr)	Making transition from childhood to adulthood; developing sense of identity	Identity vs. role confusion	Sense of personal identity; fidelity "I'm going to go to college to be an engineer; I hope to get married before I am 30."	Confusion about who one is; weak sense of self "I belong to the gang because without them, I'm nothing."
Early adulthood (20-35 yr)	Establishing intimate bonds of love and friendship	Intimacy vs. isolation	Ability to love deeply and commit oneself "My husband has been my best friend for 25 years."	Emotional isolation; egocentricity "There's no one out there for me."
Middle adulthood (35-65 yr)	Fulfilling life goals that involve family, career, and society; developing concerns that embrace future generations	Generativity vs. self-absorption	Ability to give and to care for others "I'm joining the political action committee to help people get the health care they need."	Self-absorption; inability to grow as a person "After I work all day, I just want to watch television and don't want to be around people."
Later years (65 yr to death)	Looking back over one's life and accepting its meaning	Integrity vs. despair	Sense of integrity and fulfillment; willingness to face death; wisdom "I've led a happy, productive life, and I still have plenty to give."	Dissatisfaction with life; denial of or despair over prospect of death "What a waste my life has been; I'm going to die alone."

Data from Erikson, E. H. (1963). *Childhood and society.* New York, NY: W. W. Norton; Altrocchi, J. (1980). *Abnormal psychology* (p. 196). New York, NY: Harcourt Brace Jovanovich.

beyond the immediate family to include peers. The attainment of this task (industry) brings with it the virtue of confidence. The child who fails to navigate this stage successfully is unable to master age-appropriate tasks, cannot make a connection with peers, and will feel like a failure (inferiority).

Implications for Psychiatric Mental Health Nursing

Erikson's developmental model is an essential component of patient assessment. Analysis of behavior patterns using Erikson's framework can identify age-appropriate or arrested development of normal interpersonal skills. A developmental framework helps the nurse know what types of interventions are most likely to be effective. For example, children in Erikson's initiative-versus-guilt stage of development respond best if they actively participate and ask questions. Older adults respond to a life-review strategy that focuses on the integrity of their life as a tapestry of experience. In the therapeutic encounter, individual responsibility and the capacity for improving one's functioning are addressed. Treatment approaches and interventions can be tailored to the patient's developmental level.

INTERPERSONAL THEORIES AND THERAPIES

Harry Stack Sullivan's Interpersonal Theory

Harry Stack Sullivan (1892-1949), an American-born psychiatrist, initially approached patients from a Freudian framework, but he became frustrated by dealing with what he considered unseen and private mental processes within the individual. He turned his attention to interpersonal processes that could be observed in a social framework. Sullivan (1953) defined *personality* as behavior that can be observed within interpersonal relationships. This premise led to the development of his interpersonal theory.

According to Sullivan, the purpose of all behavior is to get needs met through interpersonal interactions and to decrease or avoid anxiety. He defined *anxiety* as any painful feeling or emotion that arises from social insecurity or prevents biological needs from being satisfied. Sullivan coined the term *security operations* to describe measures the individual employs to reduce anxiety and enhance security. Collectively, all of the security operations an individual uses to defend against anxiety and ensure self-esteem make up the *self-system*.

There are many parallels between Sullivan's notion of security operations and Freud's concept of defense mechanisms. Both are processes of which we are unaware, and both are ways in which we reduce anxiety. Freud's defense mechanism of repression, however, is an intrapsychic activity, whereas Sullivan's security operations are interpersonal relationship activities that can be observed.

Implications for Psychiatric Mental Health Nursing

Sullivan's theory is the foundation for Hildegard Peplau's nursing theory of interpersonal relationships examined later in this chapter. Sullivan believed that therapy should educate patients and assist them in gaining personal insight. Sullivan first used the term *participant observer*, which underscores that professional helpers cannot be isolated from the therapeutic situation if they are to be effective. Sullivan would insist that the nurse interact with the patient as an authentic human being. Mutuality, respect for the patient, unconditional acceptance, and empathy, which are considered essential aspects of modern therapeutic relationships, were important aspects of Sullivan's theory of interpersonal therapy.

Sullivan also demonstrated that a psychotherapeutic environment characterized by an accepting atmosphere that provided numerous opportunities for practicing interpersonal skills and developing relationships is an invaluable treatment tool. Group psychotherapy, family therapy, and educational and skill training programs, as well as unstructured periods, can be incorporated into the design of a psychotherapeutic environment to facilitate healthy interactions. This method is used today in virtually all residential and day hospital settings.

Interpersonal Psychotherapy

Interpersonal psychotherapy is an effective short-term therapy derived from the school of psychiatry that originated with Adolph Meyer and Harry Stack Sullivan. The assumption is that psychiatric disorders are influenced by interpersonal interactions and the social context. The goal of interpersonal psychotherapy is to reduce or eliminate psychiatric symptoms (particularly depression) by improving interpersonal functioning and satisfaction with social relationships (Dewan, Steenbarger, & Greenberger, 2011). Interpersonal psychotherapy has proved successful in the treatment of depression. Treatment is predicated on the notion that disturbances in important interpersonal relationships (or a deficit in one's capacity to form those relationships) can play a role in initiating or maintaining clinical depression. In interpersonal psychotherapy, the therapist identifies the nature of the problem to be resolved and then selects strategies consistent with that problem area. Four types of problem areas have been identified (Hollon & Engelhardt, 1997):

1. **Grief:** Complicated bereavement following the death or loss of a loved one
2. **Role disputes:** Conflicts with a significant other
3. **Role transition:** Problematic change in life status or social or vocational role
4. **Interpersonal deficit:** An inability to initiate or sustain close relationships

Hildegard Peplau's Theory of Interpersonal Relationships in Nursing

Hildegard Peplau (1909-1999) (Figure 2-2), influenced by the work of Sullivan and learning theory, developed the first systematic theoretical framework for psychiatric nursing in her groundbreaking book *Interpersonal Relations in Nursing* (1952). Peplau not only established the foundation for the professional practice of psychiatric nursing but also continued to enrich psychiatric nursing theory and work for the advancement of nursing practice throughout her career.

Peplau was the first nurse to identify psychiatric mental health nursing both as an essential element of general nursing and as a specialty area that embraces specific governing principles. She was also the first nurse theorist to describe the nurse-patient relationship as the foundation of nursing practice (Forchuk, 1991). In shifting the focus from what nurses do *to* patients to what nurses do *with* patients, Peplau (1989) engineered a major paradigm shift from a model focused on medical treatments to an interpersonal relational model of nursing practice.

She viewed nursing as an educative instrument designed to help individuals and communities use their capacities in living more productively (Peplau, 1987). Her theory is mainly concerned with the processes by which the nurse helps patients make positive changes in their health care status and well-being. She believed that illness offered a unique opportunity for experiential learning, personal growth, and improved coping strategies and that psychiatric nurses play a unique role in facilitating this growth (Peplau, 1982a, 1982b).

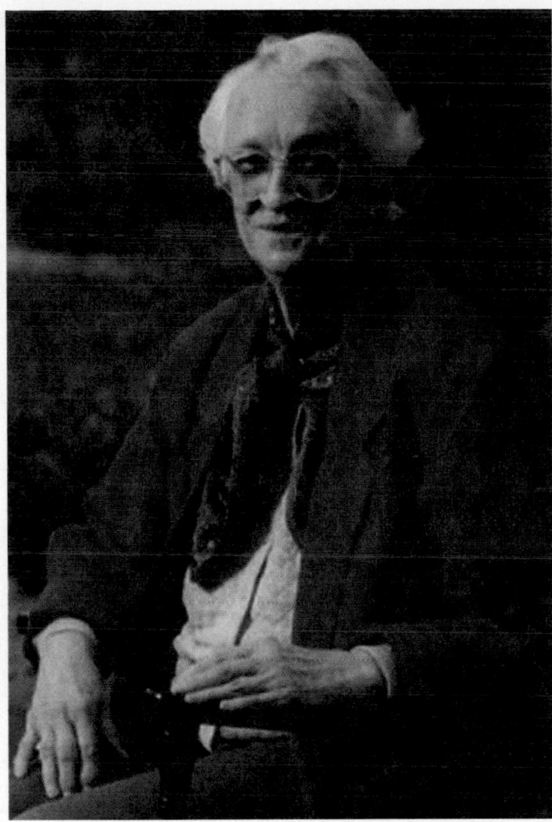

FIG 2-2 Hildegard Peplau.

Peplau identified stages of the nurse-patient relationship (Chapter 9) and also used the technique of process recording to help her students hone their communication and relationship skills (see Table 10-4). The skills of the psychiatric nurse include observation, interpretation, and intervention. The nurse observes and listens to the patient, developing impressions about the meaning of the patient's situation. By employing this process, the nurse is able to view the patient as a unique individual. The nurse's inferences are then validated with the patient for accuracy.

Peplau proposed an approach in which nurses are both participants and observers in therapeutic conversations. She believed it was essential for nurses to observe the behavior not only of the patient but also of themselves. This self-awareness on the part of the nurse is essential in keeping the focus on the patient and in keeping the social and personal needs of the nurse out of the nurse-patient conversation.

Peplau spent a lifetime illuminating the science and art of professional nursing practice, and her work has had a profound effect on the nursing profession, nursing science, and the clinical practice of psychiatric nursing (Haber, 2000). The *art* component of nursing consists of the care, compassion, and advocacy nurses provide to enhance patient comfort and well-being. The *science* component of nursing involves the application of knowledge to understand a broad range of human problems and psychosocial phenomena, intervening to relieve patients' suffering and promote growth (Haber, 2000). In her works, Peplau (1995) constantly reminds nurses to "care for the person as well as the illness" and to "think exclusively of patients as persons."

Implications for Psychiatric Mental Health Nursing

Perhaps Peplau's most universal contribution to the everyday practice of psychiatric mental health nursing is her application of Sullivan's theory of anxiety to nursing practice. She described the effects of different levels of anxiety (mild, moderate, severe, and panic) on perception and learning. She promoted interventions to lower anxiety, with the aim of improving patients' abilities to think and function at more satisfactory levels. More on the application of Peplau's theory of anxiety and interventions is presented in Chapter 12.

Table 2-3 lists additional nursing theorists and summarizes their major contributions and the impact of these contributions on psychiatric mental health nursing.

TABLE 2-3 ADDITIONAL THEORISTS WHOSE CONTRIBUTIONS INFLUENCE PSYCHIATRIC MENTAL HEALTH NURSING

THEORIST	SCHOOL OF THOUGHT	MAJOR CONTRIBUTIONS	RELEVANCE TO PSYCHIATRIC MENTAL HEALTH NURSING
Carl Rogers	Humanism	Developed a person-centered model of psychotherapy. Emphasized the concepts of: Congruence—authenticity of the therapist in dealings with the patient. Unconditional acceptance and positive regard—climate in the therapeutic relationship that facilitates change. Empathetic understanding—therapist's ability to apprehend the feelings and experiences of the patient as if these things were happening to the therapist.	Encourages nurses to view each patient as unique. Emphasizes attitudes of unconditional positive regard, empathetic understanding, and genuineness that are essential to the nurse-patient relationship. *Example:* The nurse asks the patient, "What can I do to help you regain control over your anxiety?"
Jean Piaget	Cognitive development	Identified stages of cognitive development, including sensorimotor (0-2 yr); preoperational (2-7 yr); concrete operational (7-11 yr); and formal operational (11 yr-adulthood). These describe how cognitive development proceeds from reflex activity to application of logical solutions to all types of problems.	Provides a broad base for cognitive interventions, especially with patients with negative self-views. *Example:* The nurse shows an 8-year-old all the equipment needed to start an IV when discussing the fact that he will need one prior to surgery.

Continued

TABLE 2-3 ADDITIONAL THEORISTS WHOSE CONTRIBUTIONS INFLUENCE PSYCHIATRIC MENTAL HEALTH NURSING—cont'd

THEORIST	SCHOOL OF THOUGHT	MAJOR CONTRIBUTIONS	RELEVANCE TO PSYCHIATRIC MENTAL HEALTH NURSING
Lawrence Kohlberg	Moral development	Posited a six-stage theory of moral development.	Provides nurses with a framework for evaluating moral decisions.
Albert Ellis	Existentialism	Developed approach of rational emotive behavioral therapy that is active and cognitively oriented; confrontation used to force patients to assume responsibility for behavior; patients are encouraged to accept themselves as they are and are taught to take risks and try out new behaviors.	Encourages nurses to focus on "here-and-now" issues and to help the patient live fully in the present and look forward to the future. *Example:* The nurse encourages the patient to vacation with her family even though she will be wheelchair-bound until her leg fracture heals
Albert Bandura	Social learning theory	Responsible for concepts of modeling and self-efficacy: person's belief or expectation that he or she has the capacity to effect a desired outcome through his or her own efforts.	Includes cognitive functioning with environmental factors, which provides nurses with a comprehensive view of how people learn. *Example:* The nurse helps the teenage patient identify three negative outcomes of tobacco use
Viktor Frankl	Existentialism	Developed "logotherapy," a form of support offered to help people find their sense of self-respect. Logotherapy is a future-oriented therapy focused on one's need to find meaning and value in living as one's most important life task.	Focuses nurse beyond mere behaviors to understanding the meaning of these behaviors to the patient's sense of life meaning. *Example:* The nurse listens attentively as the patient describes what it's been like since her daughter died.

Data from Bandura, A. (1977). *Social learning theory.* Englewood Cliffs, NJ: Prentice-Hall; Bernard, M. E., & Wolfe, J. L. (Eds.). (1993). *The RET resource book for practitioners.* New York, NY: Institute for Rational-Emotive Therapy; Ellis, A. (1989). *Inside rational emotive therapy.* San Diego, CA: Academic Press; Frankl, V. (1969). *The will to meaning.* Cleveland, OH: New American Library; Kohlberg, L. (1986). A current statement on some theoretical issues. In S. Modgil & C. Modgil (Eds.), *Lawrence Kohlberg.* Philadelphia, PA: Palmer; Rogers, C. R. (1961). *On becoming a person.* Boston, MA: Houghton Mifflin.

BEHAVIOR THEORIES AND THERAPIES

Behavior theories also developed as a protest response to Freud's assumption that a person's destiny was carved in stone at a very early age. Behaviorists have no concern with inner conflicts but argue that personality simply consists of learned behaviors. Consequently, personality becomes synonymous with behavior—if behavior changes, so does the personality.

The development of behavior models began in the 19th century as a result of Ivan Pavlov's laboratory work with dogs. It continued into the 20th century with John B. Watson's application of these models to shape behavior and B. F. Skinner's research on rat behavior. These behavior theorists developed systematic learning principles that could be applied to humans. Behavior models emphasize the ways in which observable behavior responses are learned and can be modified in a particular environment. Pavlov's, Watson's, and Skinner's models focus on the belief that behavior can be influenced through a process referred to as conditioning. **Conditioning** involves pairing a behavior with a condition that reinforces or diminishes the behavior's occurrence.

Ivan Pavlov's Classical Conditioning Theory

Ivan Pavlov (1849-1936) was a Russian physiologist. He won a Nobel Prize for his outstanding contributions to the physiology of digestion, which he studied through his well-known experiments with dogs. In incidental observation of the dogs, Pavlov noticed that the dogs were able to anticipate when food would be forthcoming and would begin to salivate even before actually tasting the meat. Pavlov labeled this process psychic secretion. He hypothesized that the psychic component was a learned association between two events: the presence of the experimental apparatus and the serving of meat.

Pavlov formalized his observations of behaviors in dogs in a theory of **classical conditioning**. Pavlov (1928) found that when a neutral stimulus (a bell) was repeatedly paired with another stimulus (food that triggered salivation), eventually the sound of the bell alone could elicit salivation in the dogs. An example of this response in humans would be an individual who became very ill as a child after eating spoiled coleslaw at a picnic and later in life feels nauseated whenever he smells coleslaw. It is important to recognize that classical conditioned responses are *involuntary*—not under conscious personal control—and are not spontaneous choices.

John B. Watson's Behaviorism Theory

John B. Watson (1878-1958) was an American psychologist who rejected the unconscious motivation of psychoanalysis as being too subjective. He developed the school of thought referred to as *behaviorism*, which he believed was more objective or measurable. Watson contended that personality traits and responses—adaptive and maladaptive—were socially learned through classical conditioning. In a famous (but terrible) experiment, Watson stood behind Little Albert, a 9-month-old who liked animals, and made a loud noise with a hammer every time the infant reached for a white rat. After this experiment, Little Albert became terrified at the sight of white fur or hair, even in the absence of a loud noise. Watson concluded that controlling the environment could mold behavior and that anyone could be trained to be anything, from a beggar man to a merchant.

B.F. Skinner's Operant Conditioning Theory

B.F. Skinner (1904-1990) represented the second wave of behavioral theorists. Skinner (1987) researched operant conditioning, in which *voluntary* behaviors are learned through consequences, and behavioral responses are elicited through reinforcement, which causes a behavior to occur *more* frequently. A consequence can be a positive reinforcement, such as receiving a reward (getting a 3.8 GPA after studying hard all semester), or a negative reinforcement, such as the removal of an objectionable or aversive stimulus (walking freely through a park once the vicious dog is picked up by the dogcatcher).

Other techniques can cause behaviors to occur *less* frequently. One technique is an unpleasant consequence, or punishment. Driving too fast may result in a speeding ticket, which—in mature and healthy individuals—decreases the chances that speeding will occur. Absence of reinforcement, or extinction, also decreases behavior by withholding a reward that has become habitual. If a person tells a joke and no one laughs, for example, the person is less apt to tell jokes because his joke-telling behavior is not being reinforced. Teachers employ this strategy in the classroom when they ignore acting-out behavior that had previously been rewarded by more attention.

Figure 2-3 illustrates the differences between classical conditioning (in which an involuntary reaction is caused by a stimulus) and operant conditioning (in which voluntary behavior is learned through reinforcement).

Implications for Psychiatric Mental Health Nursing

Skinner's behavioral model provides a concrete method for modifying or replacing behaviors. Behavior management and modification programs based on his principles have proven to be successful in altering targeted behaviors. *Programmed learning* and *token economies* represent extensions of Skinner's thoughts on learning. Behavioral methods are particularly effective with children, adolescents, and individuals with many forms of chronic mental illness.

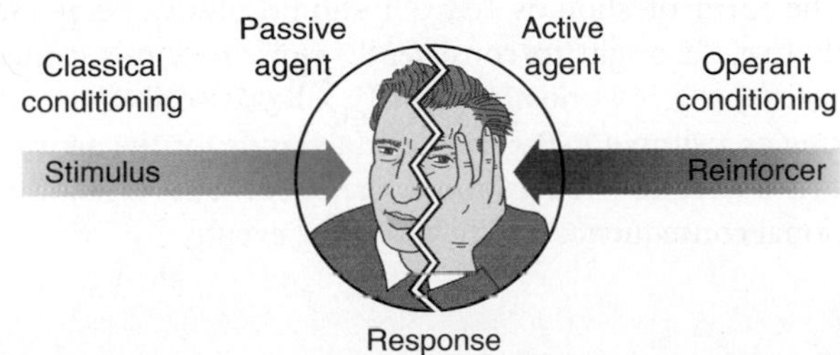

FIG 2-3 Classical versus operant conditioning. (From Carson, V. B. [2000]. *Mental health nursing: The nurse-patient journey* [2nd ed., p. 121]. Philadelphia, PA: Saunders.)

Behavior Therapy

Behavior therapy is based on the assumption that changes in maladaptive behavior can occur without insight into the underlying cause. This approach works best when it is directed at specific problems and the goals are well defined. Behavior therapy is effective in treating people with phobias, alcoholism, schizophrenia, and many other conditions. Four types of behavior therapy are discussed here: modeling, operant conditioning, systematic desensitization, and aversion therapy.

Modeling

In modeling, the therapist provides a role model for specific identified behaviors, and the patient learns through imitation. The therapist may do the modeling, provide another person to model the behaviors, or present a video for the purpose. Bandura, Blahard, and Ritter (1969) were able to help people reduce their phobias about nonpoisonous snakes by having them first view close-ups of filmed encounters between people and snakes that resulted in successful outcomes and then view live encounters between people and snakes that also had successful outcomes. In a similar fashion, some behavior therapists use role-playing in the consulting room. They demonstrate patterns of behavior that might prove more effective than those usually engaged in and then have the patients practice these new behaviors. For example, a student who does not know how to ask a professor for an extension on a term paper would watch the therapist portray a potentially effective way of making the request. The clinician would then help the student practice the new skill in a similar role-playing situation.

Operant Conditioning

Operant conditioning is the basis for behavior modification and uses positive reinforcement to increase desired behaviors. For example, when desired goals are achieved or behaviors are performed, patients might be rewarded with tokens. These tokens can be exchanged for food, small luxuries, or privileges. This reward system is known as a *token economy*.

Operant conditioning has been useful in improving the verbal behaviors of mute, autistic, and developmentally disabled children. In patients with severe and persistent mental illness, behavior modification has helped increase levels of self-care, social behavior, group participation, and more. You may find this a useful technique as you proceed through your clinical rotations.

A familiar case in point of positive reinforcement is the mother who takes her preschooler along to the grocery store, and the child starts acting out, demanding candy, nagging, crying, and yelling. Here are examples of three ways the child's behavior can be reinforced:

ACTION	RESULT
1. The mother gives the child the candy.	The child continues to use this behavior. This is positive reinforcement of negative behavior.
2. The mother scolds the child.	Acting out may continue, because the child gets what he really wants—attention. This positively rewards negative behavior.
3. The mother ignores the acting out but gives attention to the child when he is acting appropriately.	The child gets a positive reward for appropriate behavior.

Systematic Desensitization

Systematic desensitization is another form of behavior modification therapy that involves the development of behavior tasks customized to the patient's specific fears; these tasks are presented to the patient while using learned relaxation techniques. The process involves four steps:

1. The patient's fear is broken down into its components by exploring the particular stimulus cues to which the patient reacts. For example, certain situations may precipitate a phobic reaction, whereas others do not. Crowds at parties may be problematic, whereas similar numbers of people in other settings do not cause the same distress.
2. The patient is incrementally exposed to the fear. For example, a patient who has a fear of flying is introduced to short periods of visual presentations of flying—first with still pictures, then with videos, and finally in a busy airport. The situations are confronted while the patient is in a relaxed state. Gradually, over a period of time, exposure is increased until anxiety about or fear of the object or situation has ceased.
3. The patient is instructed in how to design a hierarchy of fears. For fear of flying, a patient might develop a set of statements representing the stages of a flight, order the statements from the most fearful to the least fearful, and use relaxation techniques to reach a state of relaxation as they progress through the list.
4. The patient practices these techniques every day.

Aversion Therapy

Today, aversion therapy (which is akin to punishment) is used widely to treat behaviors such as alcoholism, sexual deviation, shoplifting, hallucinations, violent and aggressive behavior, and self-mutilation. Aversion therapy is sometimes the treatment of choice when other less drastic measures have failed to produce the desired effects. The following are three paradigms for using aversive techniques:

1. Pairing of a maladaptive behavior with a noxious stimulus (e.g., pairing the sight and smell of alcohol with electric shock), so that anxiety or fear becomes associated with the once-pleasurable stimulus
2. Punishment (e.g., punishment applied after the patient has had an alcoholic drink)
3. Avoidance training (e.g., patient avoids punishment by pushing a glass of alcohol away within a certain time limit)

Simple examples of extinguishing undesirable behavior through aversion therapy include painting foul-tasting substances on the fingernails of nail biters or the thumbs of thumb suckers. Other examples of aversive stimuli are chemicals that induce nausea and vomiting, noxious odors, unpleasant verbal stimuli (e.g., descriptions of disturbing scenes), costs or fines in a token economy, and denial of positive reinforcement (e.g., isolation).

Before initiating any aversive protocol, the therapist, treatment team, or society *must* answer the following questions:

- Is this therapy in the best interest of the patient?
- Does its use violate the patient's rights?
- Is it in the best interest of society?

If aversion therapy is chosen as the most appropriate treatment, ongoing supervision, support, and evaluation of those administering it must occur.

Biofeedback

Biofeedback is also a form of behavior therapy and is successfully used today, especially for controlling the body's physiological response to stress and anxiety. Biofeedback is discussed in detail in Chapter 12.

COGNITIVE THEORIES AND THERAPIES

While behaviorists focused on increasing, decreasing, or eliminating measurable behaviors, little attention was paid to the thoughts, or cognitions, that were involved in these behaviors. Rather than thinking of people as passive recipients of environmental conditioning, cognitive theorists proposed that there is a dynamic interplay between individuals and the environment. These theorists believe that thoughts come before feelings and actions, and thoughts about the world and our place in it are based on our own unique perspectives, which may or may not be based on reality. Two of the most influential theorists and their therapies are presented here.

Rational-Emotive Behavior Therapy

Rational-Emotive Behavior Therapy (REBT) was developed by Albert Ellis (1913-2007) in 1955. The aim of REBT is to eradicate core irrational beliefs by helping people recognize thoughts that are not accurate, sensible, or useful. These thoughts tend to take the form of shoulds (e.g., "I should always be polite"), oughts (e.g., "I ought to consistently win my tennis games"), and musts (e.g., "I must be thin"). Ellis described negative thinking as a simple A-B-C process. *A* stands for the activating event, *B* stands for beliefs about the event, and *C* stands for emotional consequence as a result of the event.

A	→	B	→	C
Activating Event		Beliefs		Emotional Consequence

Perception influences all thoughts, which in turn influence our behaviors. It often boils down to the simple notion of perceiving the glass as half full or half empty. For example, imagine you have just received an invitation to a birthday party (activating event). You think, "I hate parties. Now I have to hang out with people who don't like me, instead of watching my favorite television shows. They probably just invited me to get a gift" (beliefs). You will probably be miserable (emotional consequence) if you go. On the other hand, you may think, "I love parties! This will be a great chance to meet new people, and it will be fun to shop for the perfect gift" (beliefs). You could have a delightful time (emotional consequence).

Although Ellis (Figure 2-4) admits that the role of past experiences is instrumental in current beliefs, the focus of rational-emotive behavior therapy is on present attitudes, painful feelings, and dysfunctional behaviors. If our beliefs are negative and self-deprecating, we are more susceptible to depression and anxiety. Ellis noted that while we cannot change the past, we can change the way we are now. He was pragmatic in his approach to mental illness and colorful in his therapeutic advice. "It's too [darn] bad you panic, but you don't die from it! Get them over the panic about panic, you may find the panic disappears" (Ellis, 2000).

Cognitive-Behavioral Therapy

Aaron T. Beck (see Figure 2-4), another adherent of Sigmund Freud's tenets, was originally trained in psychoanalysis but is regarded as a Neo-Freudian. When he attempted to study depression from a psychoanalytic perspective, he became convinced that people with depression generally had stereotypical patterns of negative and self-critical thinking that seemed to distort their ability to think and process information. **Cognitive-behavioral therapy (CBT)** is based on both cognitive psychology and behavioral theory. It is a commonly employed, effective, and well-researched therapeutic tool.

Beck's method (Beck, 1979), the basis for CBT, is an active, directive, time-limited, structured approach used to treat a variety of psychiatric disorders (e.g., depression, anxiety, phobias, and pain problems). It is based on the underlying theoretical principle that feelings and behaviors are largely determined by the way people think about the world and their place in it (Beck, 1967, 1976). Their cognitions (verbal or pictorial events in their streams of consciousness) are based on attitudes or assumptions developed from previous experiences. These cognitions may be fairly accurate, or they may be distorted.

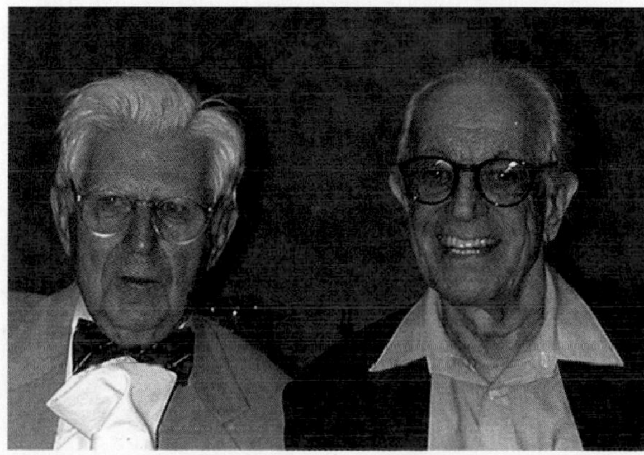

FIG 2-4 Aaron Beck and Albert Ellis. (Courtesy of Fenichel, 2000.)

According to Beck, people have *schemas*, or unique assumptions about themselves, others, and the world in general. For example, if a person has the schema "The only person I can trust is myself," he or she will have expectations that everyone else has questionable motives, will lie, and will eventually hurt him or her. Other negative schemas include incompetence, abandonment, evilness, and vulnerability. People are typically not aware of such cognitive biases, but recognizing them as beliefs and attitudes based on distortions and misconceptions will help make it apparent when dysfunctional schemas underlie our thinking.

Rapid, unthinking responses based on schemas are known as **automatic thoughts**. These responses are particularly intense and frequent in psychiatric disorders such as depression and anxiety. Often automatic thoughts, or **cognitive distortions**, are irrational and lead to false assumptions and misinterpretations. For example, if a person interprets all experiences in terms of whether he or she is competent and adequate, thinking may be dominated by the cognitive distortion, "Unless I do everything perfectly, I'm a failure." Consequently, the person reacts to situations in terms of adequacy, even when these situations are unrelated to whether he or she is personally competent. Table 2-4 describes common cognitive distortions.

The therapeutic techniques of the cognitive therapist are designed to identify, reality test, and correct distorted conceptualizations and the dysfunctional beliefs underlying them. In other words, the cognitive therapist helps patients change the way they think and thereby reduce symptoms. Patients are taught to challenge their own negative thinking and substitute it with positive, rational thoughts. They are taught to recognize when thinking is based on distortions and misconceptions. Homework assignments play an important role in CBT. A particularly useful technique is the use of a four-column format to record the precipitating event or situation, the resulting automatic thought, the proceeding feeling(s) and behavior(s), and finally, a challenge to the negative thoughts, based on rational evidence and thinking. The following is an example of the type of analysis done by a patient receiving CBT.

A 24-year-old nurse recently discharged from the hospital for severe depression presented this record (Beck, 1979):

EVENT	FEELING	COGNITIONS	OTHER POSSIBLE INTERPRETATIONS
While at a party, Cory asked me, "How is it going?" a few days after I was discharged from the hospital.	Anxious	Cory thinks I am crazy. I must really look bad for him to be concerned.	He really cares about me. He noticed that I look better than before I went into the hospital and wants to know if I feel better too.

TABLE 2-4 SELECTED NURSING THEORISTS, THEIR MAJOR CONTRIBUTIONS, AND THEIR IMPACT ON PSYCHIATRIC MENTAL HEALTH NURSING

NURSING THEORIST	FOCUS OF THEORY	CONTRIBUTION TO PSYCHIATRIC MENTAL HEALTH NURSING
Patricia Benner	"Caring" as foundation for nursing	Benner encourages nurses to provide caring and comforting interventions. She emphasizes the importance of the nurse-patient relationship and the importance of teaching and coaching the patient and bearing witness to suffering as the patient deals with illness.
Dorothea Orem	Goal of self-care as integral to the practice of nursing	Orem emphasizes the role of the nurse in promoting self-care activities of the patient; this has relevance to the seriously and persistently mentally ill patient.
Sister Callista Roy	Continual need for people to adapt physically, psychologically, and socially	Roy emphasizes the role of nursing in assisting patients to adapt so that they can cope more effectively with changes.
Betty Neuman	Impact of internal and external stressors on the equilibrium of the system	Neuman emphasizes the role of nursing in assisting patients to discover and use stress-reducing strategies.
Joyce Travelbee	Meaning in the nurse-patient relationship and the importance of communication	Travelbee emphasizes the role of nursing in affirming the suffering of the patient and in being able to alleviate that suffering through communication skills used appropriately through the stages of the nurse-patient relationship.

Data from Benner, P., & Wrubel, J. (1989). *The primacy of caring: Stress and coping in health and illness.* Menlo Park, CA: Addison-Wesley; Leddy, S., & Pepper, J. M. (1993). *Conceptual bases of professional nursing* (3rd ed., pp. 174-175). Philadelphia, PA: Lippincott; Neuman, B., & Young, R. (1972). A model for teaching total-person approach to patient problems. *Nursing Research, 21*, 264-269; Orem, D. E. (1995). *Nursing: Concepts of practice* (5th ed.). New York, NY: McGraw-Hill; Roy, C., & Andrews, H. A. (1991). *The Roy adaptation model: The definitive statement.* Norwalk, CT: Appleton & Lange; Travelbee, J. (1961). *Intervention in psychiatric nursing.* Philadelphia, PA: F. A. Davis.

Table 2-5 compares and contrasts psychodynamic, interpersonal, cognitive-behavioral, and behavioral therapies.

Implications for Psychiatric Mental Health Nursing

Recognizing the interplay between events, negative thinking, and negative responses can be beneficial from both a patient-care standpoint and a personal one. As a supportive therapeutic measure, helping the patient identify negative thought patterns is a worthwhile intervention. Workbooks are available to aid in the process of identifying cognitive distortions.

The cognitive approach can also help nurses understand their own responses to a variety of difficult situations. One example might be the anxiety that some students feel regarding the psychiatric nursing clinical rotation. Students may overgeneralize ("All psychiatric patients are dangerous.") or personalize ("My patient doesn't seem to be better; I'm

TABLE 2-5 COMMON COGNITIVE DISTORTIONS

DISTORTION	DEFINITION	EXAMPLE
All-or-nothing thinking	Thinking in black and white, reducing complex outcomes into absolutes	Although Lindsey earned the second highest score in the state's cheerleading competition, she consistently referred to herself as "a loser."
Overgeneralization	Using a bad outcome (or a few bad outcomes) as evidence that nothing will ever go right again	Andrew had a minor traffic accident. He is reluctant to drive and says, "I shouldn't be allowed on the road."
Labeling	A form of generalization in which a characteristic or event becomes definitive and results in an overly harsh label for self or others	"Because I failed the advanced statistics exam, I am a failure. I might as well give up. I may as well quit and look for an easier major."
Mental filter	Focusing on a negative detail or bad event and allowing it to taint everything else	Anne's boss evaluated her work as exemplary and gave her a few suggestions for improvement. She obsessed about the suggestions and ignored the rest.
Disqualifying the positive	Maintaining a negative view by rejecting information that supports a positive view as being irrelevant, inaccurate, or accidental	"I've just been offered the job I thought I always wanted. There must have been no other applicants."
Jumping to conclusions	Making a negative interpretation despite the fact that there is little or no supporting evidence	"My fiancé, Juan, didn't call me for 3 hours, which just proves he doesn't love me anymore."

TABLE 2-5 COMMON COGNITIVE DISTORTIONS—cont'd

DISTORTION	DEFINITION	EXAMPLE
a. Mind-reading	Inferring negative thoughts, responses, and motives of others	Isabel is giving a presentation and a man in the audience is sleeping. She panics, "I must be boring."
b. Fortune-telling error	Anticipating that things will turn out badly as an established fact	"I'll ask her out, but I know she won't have a good time."
Magnification or minimization	Exaggerating the importance of something (such as a personal failure or the success of others) or reducing the importance of something (such as a personal success or the failure of others)	"I'm alone on a Saturday night because no one likes me. When other people are alone, it's because they want to be."
a. Catastrophizing	Catastrophizing is an extreme form of magnification in which the very worst is assumed to be a probable outcome.	"If I don't make a good impression on the boss at the company picnic, she will fire me."
Emotional reasoning	Drawing a conclusion based on an emotional state	"I'm nervous about the exam. I must not be prepared. If I were, I wouldn't be afraid."
"Should" and "must" statements	Rigid self-directives that presume an unrealistic amount of control over external events	Renee believes that a patient with diabetes has high blood sugar today because she's not a very good nurse and that her patients should always get better.
Personalization	Assuming responsibility for an external event or situation that was likely outside personal control.	"I'm sorry your party wasn't more fun. It's probably because I was there."

Modified from Burns, D.D. (1989). *The feeling good handbook.* New York, NY: William Morrow.

probably not doing him any good.") the situation. The key to effectively using this approach in clinical situations is to challenge the negative thoughts not based on facts and then replace them with more realistic appraisals.

HUMANISTIC THEORIES

In the 1950s, humanistic theories arose as a protest against both the behavioral and psychoanalytic schools, which were thought to be pessimistic, deterministic, and dehumanizing. Humanistic theories focus on human potential and free will to choose life patterns that are supportive of personal growth. Humanistic frameworks emphasize a person's capacity for self-actualization. This approach focuses on understanding the patient's perspective as she or he subjectively experiences it. There are a number of humanistic theorists, and this text will explore Abraham Maslow and his theory of self-actualization.

Abraham Maslow's Humanistic Psychology Theory

Abraham Maslow (1908-1970), considered the father of humanistic psychology, introduced the concept of a "self-actualized personality" associated with high productivity and enjoyment of life (Maslow, 1963, 1968). He criticized psychology for focusing too intently on humanity's frailties and not enough on its strengths. Maslow contended that the focus of psychology must go beyond experiences of hate, pain, misery, guilt, and conflict to include love, compassion, happiness, exhilaration, and well-being.

Hierarchy of Needs

Maslow conceptualized human motivation as a hierarchy of dynamic processes or needs that are critical for the development of all humans. Central to his theory is the assumption that humans are active rather than passive participants in life, striving for self-actualization. Maslow (1968) focused on human need fulfillment, which he categorized into six incremental stages, beginning with physiological survival needs and ending with self-transcendent needs (Figure 2-5). The hierarchy of needs is conceptualized as a pyramid, with the strongest, most fundamental needs placed on the lower levels. The higher levels—the more distinctly human needs—occupy the top sections of the pyramid. When lower-level needs are met, higher needs are able to emerge.

- **Physiological needs:** The most basic needs are the physiological drives—needing food, oxygen, water, sleep, sex, and a constant body temperature. If all needs were deprived, this level would take priority over the rest.
- **Safety needs:** Once physiological needs are met, safety needs emerge. They include security; protection; freedom from fear, anxiety, and chaos; and the need for law, order, and limits. Adults in a stable society usually feel safe, but they may feel threatened by debt, job insecurity, or lack of insurance. It is during times of crisis, such as war, disasters, assaults, and social breakdown, when safety needs take precedence. Children, who are more vulnerable and dependent, respond far more readily and intensely to safety threats.
- **Belonging and love needs:** People have a need for intimate relationships, love, affection, and belonging and will seek to overcome feelings of loneliness and alienation. Maslow stresses the importance of having a family and a home and being part of identifiable groups.
- **Esteem needs:** People need to have a high self-regard and have it reflected to them from others. If self-esteem needs are met, they feel confident, valued, and valuable. When self-esteem is compromised, they feel inferior, worthless, and helpless.
- **Self-actualization:** Human beings are preset to strive to be everything they are capable of becoming. Maslow said,

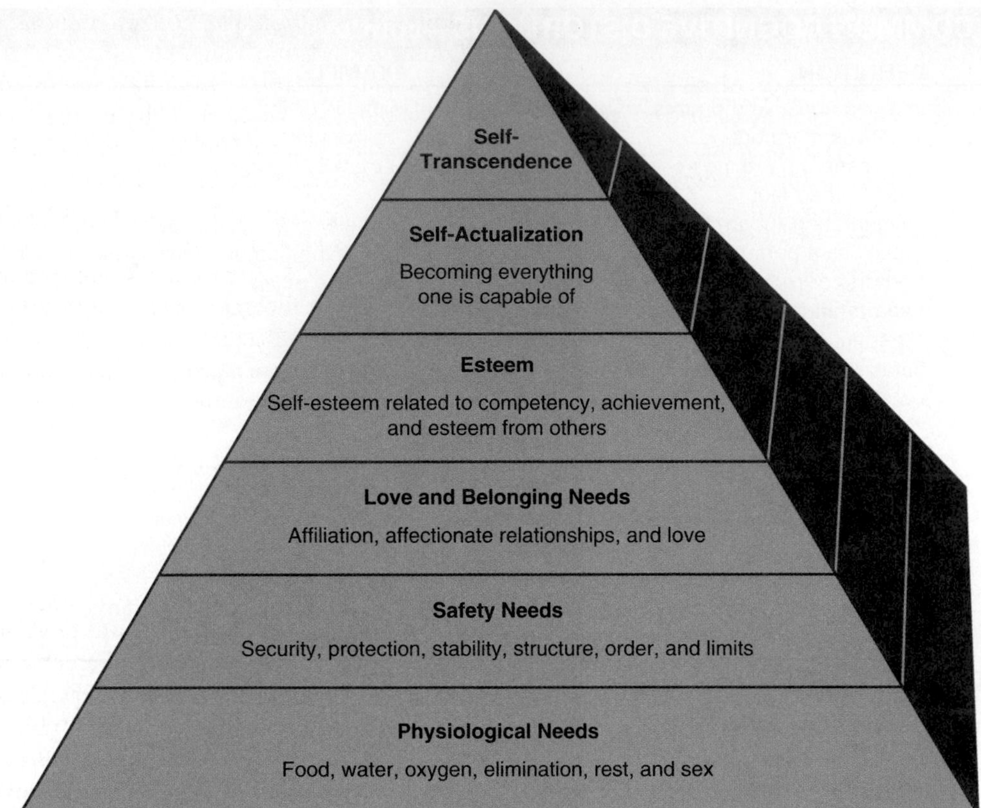

FIG 2-5 Maslow's hierarchy of needs. (Adapted from Maslow, A. H. [1972]. *The farther reaches of human nature*. New York, NY: Viking.)

"What a man *can* be, he *must* be." What people are capable of becoming is highly individual—an artist must paint, a writer must write, and a healer must heal. The drive to satisfy this need is felt as a sort of restlessness, a sense that something is missing. It is up to each person to choose a path that will bring about inner peace and fulfillment.

Although Maslow's early work included only five levels of needs, he later took into account two additional factors: (1) cognitive needs (the desire to know and understand) and (2) aesthetic needs (Maslow, 1970). He describes the acquisition of knowledge (our first priority) and the need to understand (our second priority) as being hard-wired and essential; he identified the aesthetic need for beauty and symmetry as universal. How else, after all, do we explain the impulse to straighten a crooked picture?

Maslow based his theory on the results of clinical investigations of people who represented self-actualized individuals who moved in the direction of achieving and reaching their highest potentials. Among those Maslow chose to investigate were historical figures such as Abraham Lincoln, Thomas Jefferson, Harriet Tubman, Walt Whitman, Ludwig van Beethoven, William James, and Franklin D. Roosevelt, as well as others such as Albert Einstein, Eleanor Roosevelt, and Albert Schweitzer, who were living at the time they were studied. This investigation led Maslow (1963, 1970) to identify some basic personality characteristics that distinguish self-actualizing people from those who might be called "ordinary" (Box 2-1).

BOX 2-1 SOME CHARACTERISTICS OF SELF-ACTUALIZED PERSONS

- Accurate perception of reality. Not defensive in their perceptions of the world.
- Acceptance of themselves, others, and nature.
- Spontaneity, simplicity, and naturalness. Self-actualized individuals (SAs) do not live programmed lives.
- Problem-centered rather than self-centered orientation. Possibly the most important characteristic. SAs have a sense of a mission to which they dedicate their lives.
- Pleasure in being alone and in ability to reflect on events.
- Active social interest.
- Freshness of appreciation. SAs don't take life for granted.
- Mystical or peak experiences. A peak experience is a moment of intense ecstasy, similar to a religious or mystical experience, during which the self is transcended.
- SAs may become so involved in what they are doing that they lose all sense of time and awareness of self (*flow experience*).
- Lighthearted sense of humor that indicates "we're in it together" and lacks sarcasm or hostility.
- Fairness and respect for people of different races, ethnicities, religions, and political views.
- Creativity, especially in managing their lives.
- Resistance to conformity (enculturation). SAs are autonomous, independent, and self-sufficient.

From Maslow, A. H. (1970). *Motivation and personality*. New York, NY: Harper & Row.

Implications for Psychiatric Mental Health Nursing

The value of Maslow's model in nursing practice is twofold. First, an emphasis on human potential and the patient's strengths is key to successful nurse-patient relationships. Second, the model helps establish what is most important in the sequencing of nursing actions in the nurse-patient relationship. For example, to collect any but the most essential information when a patient is struggling with drug withdrawal is inappropriate. Following Maslow's model as a way of prioritizing actions, the nurse meets the patient's physiological need for stable vital signs and pain relief before collecting general information for a nursing database.

BIOLOGICAL THEORIES AND THERAPIES

The Advent of Psychopharmacology

In 1950, a French drug firm synthesized chlorpromazine—a powerful antipsychotic medication—and psychiatry experienced a revolution. The advent of psychopharmacology presented a direct challenge to psychodynamic approaches to mental illness. The dramatic experience of observing patients freed from the bondage of psychosis and mania by powerful drugs such as chlorpromazine and lithium left witnesses convinced of the critical role of the brain in psychiatric illness. When President George H.W. Bush declared the 1990s the Decade of the Brain, vast amounts of research monies and effort were directed at study of the structure and functions of the brain.

Since the discovery of chlorpromazine, many other medications have proven effective in controlling psychosis, mania, depression, and anxiety. These medications greatly reduce the need for hospitalization and dramatically improve the lives of people suffering from serious psychiatric difficulties. Today, psychoactive medications exert differential effects on different neurotransmitters and help restore brain function, allowing patients with mental illness to continue living productive lives with greater satisfaction and far less emotional pain.

The Biological Model

A biological model of mental illness focuses on neurological, chemical, biological, and genetic issues and seeks to understand how the body and brain interact to create emotions, memories, and perceptual experiences. A biological perspective views abnormal behavior as part of a disease process or a defect and seeks to stop or alter it. The biological model locates the illness or disease in the body—usually in the limbic system of the brain and the synapse receptor sites of the central nervous system—and targets the site of the illness using physical interventions such as drugs, diet, or surgery.

The recognition that psychiatric illnesses are as physical in origin as diabetes and coronary heart disease serves to decrease the stigma surrounding them. Just as someone with diabetes or heart disease cannot be held responsible for their illness, patients with schizophrenia or bipolar affective disorder are no more to blame.

Implications for Psychiatric Mental Health Nursing

Historically, psychiatric mental health nurses always have attended to the physical needs of psychiatric patients. Nurses administer medications; monitor sleep, activity, nutrition, hydration, elimination, and other functions; and prepare patients for somatic therapies, such as electroconvulsive therapy. They have continued to do so with the advancement of the biological model, which has not altered the basic nursing strategies: focusing on the qualities of a therapeutic relationship, understanding the patient's perspective, and communicating in a way that facilitates the patient's recovery.

One of the risks in adopting a biological model to the exclusion of all other theoretical perspectives is that such a theory ignores the myriad other influences, including social, environmental, cultural, economic, spiritual, and educational factors that play a role in the development and treatment of mental illness.

ADDITIONAL THERAPIES

Milieu Therapy

In 1948, Bruno Bettelheim coined the term **milieu therapy** to describe his use of the total environment to treat disturbed children. Bettelheim created a comfortable, secure environment (or milieu) in which psychotic children were helped to form a new world. Staff members were trained to provide 24-hour support and understanding for each child on an individual basis. In 1953, Maxwell Jones in Great Britain wrote the book *The Therapeutic Community.* This book both laid the groundwork for the milieu therapy movement in the United States and defined the nurse's role in this therapy.

Milieu is sometimes a difficult concept to grasp. It is an all-inclusive term that recognizes the people (the patients and staff), the setting, the structure, and the emotional climate as all-important to healing. Milieu therapy takes naturally occurring events in the environment and uses them as rich learning opportunities for patients. There are certain basic characteristics of milieu therapy, regardless of whether the setting involves treatment of psychotic children, patients in a psychiatric hospital, drug abusers in a residential treatment center, or psychiatric patients in a day hospital. Milieu therapy, or a therapeutic community, has as its locus a living, learning, or working environment. Such therapy may be based on any number of therapeutic modalities, from structured behavior therapy to spontaneous, humanistic-oriented approaches.

Implications for Psychiatric Mental Health Nursing

Milieu therapy is a basic intervention in nursing practice. Nurses are constantly involved in the assessment and provision of safe and effective milieus for their patients. Common examples include providing a safe environment for the suicidal patient or a patient with a cognitive disorder (e.g., Alzheimer's disease), referring abused women to safe houses, and advocating for children suspected of being abused in their home environments.

CONCLUSION

In this chapter you were introduced to some of the historically significant theories and therapies, therapies that are widely used today, and the theoretical implications for nursing care. Table 2-6 lists additional theorists whose contributions influence psychiatric mental health nursing.

TABLE 2-6 **COMPARISON OF PSYCHOANALYTIC, INTERPERSONAL, COGNITIVE-BEHAVIORAL, AND BEHAVIORAL THERAPIES**

	PSYCHODYNAMIC THERAPY	INTERPERSONAL THERAPY	COGNITIVE-BEHAVIORAL THERAPY	BEHAVIOR THERAPY
Treatment focus	Unresolved past relationships and core conflicts	Current interpersonal relationships and social supports	Thoughts and cognitions	Learned maladaptive behavior
Therapist role	Significant other Transference object	Problem solver	Active, directive, challenging	Active, directive teacher
Primary disorders treated	Anxiety Depression Personality disorders	Depression	Depression Anxiety/panic Eating disorders	Posttraumatic stress disorder Obsessive compulsive disorder Panic disorder
Length of therapy	20 + sessions	Short term (12-20 sessions)	Short term (5-20 sessions)	Varies, typically fewer than 10 sessions
Technique	Therapeutic alliance Free association Understanding transference Challenging defense mechanisms	Facilitate new patterns of communication and expectations for relationships	Evaluating thoughts and behaviors Modifying dysfunctional thoughts and behaviors	Relaxation Thought stopping Self-reassurance Seeking social support

Data from Dewan, M. J., Steenbarger, B. N., & Greenberg, R. P. (2011). Brief psychotherapies. In R. E. Hales, S. C. Yudofsky, & G. O. Gabbard (Eds.), *Essentials of psychiatry* (3rd ed., pp. 525-539). Arlington, VA: American Psychiatric Publishing.

There are literally hundreds of therapies in use today. The Substance Abuse and Mental Health Services Administration (SAMHSA) maintains a National Registry of Evidence-based Practices and Programs. New therapies are entered into the database all the time. Examples of therapies that were added in 2012 include College Drinkers Check-Up, Dynamic Deconstructive Psychotherapy, and Mindfulness Based Stress Reduction. The registry can be accessed at http://www.nrepp.samhsa.gov/ViewAll.aspx

You will be introduced to other therapeutic approaches later in the book. Crisis intervention (Chapter 25) is an approach you will find useful, not only in psychiatric mental health nursing but also in other nursing specialties. Group therapy (Chapter 33) and family interventions (Chapter 34), which are appropriate for the basic level practitioner, will also be discussed.

KEY POINTS TO REMEMBER

- Sigmund Freud advanced the first theory of personality development.
- Freud articulated levels of awareness (unconscious, preconscious, conscious) and demonstrated the influence of our unconscious behavior on everyday life, as evidenced by the use of defense mechanisms.
- Freud identified three psychological processes of personality (id, ego, superego) and described how they operate and develop.
- Freud articulated one of the first modern developmental theories of personality, based on five psychosexual stages.
- Various psychoanalytic therapies have been used over the years. Currently, a short-term, time-limited version of psychotherapy is common.
- Erik Erikson expanded on Freud's developmental stages to include middle age through old age. Erikson called his stages *psychosocial stages* and emphasized the social aspect of personality development.
- Harry Stack Sullivan proposed the interpersonal theory of personality development, which focuses on interpersonal processes that can be observed in a social framework.
- Hildegard Peplau, a nursing theorist, developed an interpersonal theoretical framework that has become the foundation of psychiatric mental health nursing practice.
- Abraham Maslow, the founder of humanistic psychology, offered the theory of self-actualization and human motivation that is basic to all nursing education today.
- Cognitive-behavioral therapy is the most commonly used, accepted, and empirically validated psychotherapeutic approach.
- A biological model of mental illness and treatment dominates care for psychiatric disorders.
- Milieu therapy is a philosophy of care in which all parts of the environment are considered to be therapeutic opportunities for growth and healing. The milieu includes the people (patients and staff), setting, structure, and emotional climate.

CRITICAL THINKING

1. Consider how the theorists and theories discussed in this chapter have had an impact on your practice of nursing:
   a. How do Freud's concepts of the conscious, preconscious, and unconscious affect your understanding of patients' behaviors?
   b. Do you believe Erikson's psychosocial stages represent a sound basis for identifying disruptions in stages of development in your patients? Support your position with a clinical example.
   c. What are the implications of Sullivan's focus on the importance of interpersonal relationships for your interactions with patients?
   d. Peplau believed that nurses must exercise self-awareness within the nurse-patient relationship. Describe situations in your student experience in which this self-awareness played a vital role in your relationships with patients.
   e. Identify someone you believe to be self-actualized. What characteristics does this person have that support your assessment? How do you make use of Maslow's hierarchy of needs in your nursing practice?
   f. What do you think about the behaviorist point of view that to change behaviors is to change personality?
2. Which of the therapies described in this chapter do you think can be the most helpful to you in your nursing practice? What are your reasons for this choice?

CHAPTER REVIEW

1. Which contribution to modern psychiatric mental health nursing practice was made by Freud?
   a. The theory of personality structure and levels of awareness
   b. The concept of a "self-actualized personality"
   c. The thesis that culture and society exert significant influence on personality
   d. Provision of a developmental model that includes the entire life span
2. The theory of interpersonal relationships developed by Hildegard Peplau is based on the foundation provided by which early theorist?
   a. Freud
   b. Piaget
   c. Sullivan
   d. Maslow
3. The concepts at the heart of Sullivan's theory of personality are:
   a. needs and anxiety.
   b. basic needs and meta-needs.
   c. schemas, assimilation, and accommodation.
   d. developmental tasks and psychosocial crises.
4. The premise that an individual's behavior and affect are largely determined by his or her attitudes and assumptions about the world underlies:
   a. modeling.
   b. milieu therapy.
   c. cognitive-behavioral therapy.
   d. psychoanalytic psychotherapy.
5. Providing a safe environment for patients with impaired cognition, planning unit activities to stimulate thinking, and including patients and staff in unit meetings are all part of:
   a. milieu therapy.
   b. cognitive-behavioral therapy.
   c. behavior therapy.
   d interpersonal psychotherapy.

Answers to Chapter Review
1. a; 2. c; 3. a; 4. c; 5. a.

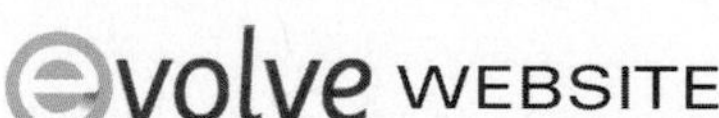

WEBSITE

Visit the Evolve website for a posttest on the content in this chapter: http://evolve.elsevier.com/Varcarolis

Post-Test interactive review

REFERENCES

Beck, A. T. (1967). *Depression: Clinical, experimental and theoretical aspects.* New York: Harper & Row.

Beck, A. T., Rush, A. J., Shaw, B. F., & Emery, G. (1979). *Cognitive therapy of depression.* New York: Guilford Press.

Bulechek, G. M., Butcher, H.K., Dochterman, J. M., & Wagner, C. (2013). *Nursing interventions classification (NIC)* (6th ed.). St. Louis: Mosby.

Dewan, M. J., Steenbarger, B. N., & Greenberg, R. P. (2011). Brief psychotherapy. In R. E. Hales, S. C. Yudofsky, & G. O. Gabbard (Eds.), *Essentials of psychiatry* (pp. 525–540). Arlington, VA: American Psychiatric Publishing.

Ellis, A. (2000, August). *On therapy: A dialogue with Aaron T. Beck and Albert Ellis.* Discussion at the American Psychological Association's 108th Convention, Washington, DC.

Erikson, E. H. (1963). *Childhood and society.* New York: W. W. Norton.

Forchuk, C. (1991). A comparison of the works of Peplau and Orlando. *Archives of Psychiatric Nursing, 5*(1), 38–45.

Freud, S. (1960). *The ego and the id* (J. Strachey, trans.). New York , NY: W. W. Norton (Original work published in 1923).

Freud, S. (1961). *The interpretation of dreams* (J. Strachey, ed. & trans.). New York: Scientific Editions (original work published in 1899).

Freud, S. (1969). *An outline of psychoanalysis* (J. Strachey, trans.). New York: W. W. Norton (original work published in 1940).

Haber, J. (2000). Hildegard E. Peplau: The psychiatric nursing legacy of a legend. *Journal of the American Psychiatric Nurses Association, 6*(2), 56–62.

Herdman, T. H. (Ed.), (2012) *NANDA international nursing diagnoses: Definitions and classification, 2012-2014.* Oxford, UK: Wiley-Blackwell.

Hollon, S. D., & Engelhardt, N. (1997). Review of psychosocial treatment of mood disorders. In D. L. Dunner (Ed.), *Current psychiatric therapy II* (pp. 296–301). Philadelphia: Saunders.

Jones, M. (1953). *The therapeutic community.* New York: Basic Books.

Maslow, A. H. (1963). Self-actualizing people. In G. B. Levitas (Ed.), *The world of psychology* (vol. 2, pp. 527–556). New York: Braziller.

Maslow, A. H. (1968). *Toward a psychology of being.* Princeton, NJ: Van Nostrand.

Maslow, A. H. (1970). *Motivation and personality* (2nd ed.). New York, NY: Harper & Row.

Moorhead, S., Johnson, M., Maas, M. L., & Swanson, E. (2013). *Nursing outcomes classification (NOC)* (5th ed.). St Louis: Mosby.

Pavlov, I. (1928). *Lectures on conditioned reflexes* (W. H. Grant, trans.). New York: International Publishers.

Peplau, H. E. (1952). *Interpersonal relations in nursing: A conceptual frame of reference for psychodynamic nursing.* New York, NY: Putnam.

Peplau, H. E. (1982a). Therapeutic concepts. In S. A. Smoyak & S. Rouslin (Eds.), *A collection of classics in psychiatric nursing literature* (pp. 91–108). Thorofare, NJ: Slack.

Peplau, H. E. (1982b). Interpersonal techniques: the crux of psychiatric nursing. In S. A. Smoyak & S. Rouslin (Eds.), *A collection of classics in psychiatric nursing literature* (pp. 276–281). Thorofare, NJ: Slack.

Peplau, H. E. (1987). Interpersonal constructs for nursing practice. *Nursing Education Today, 7,* 201–208.

Peplau, H. E. (1989). Future directions in psychiatric nursing from the perspective of history. *Journal of Psychosocial Nursing, 27*(2), 18–28.

Peplau, H. E. (1995). Another look at schizophrenia from a nursing standpoint. In C. A. Anderson (Ed.), *Psychiatric nursing 1946-94: The state of the art* (pp. 3–8). St. Louis: Mosby.

Skinner, B. F. (1987). Whatever happened to psychology as the science of behavior? *American Psychologist, 42,* 780–786.

Substance Abuse and Mental Health Services Administration. (2012). *National Registry of Evidence-Based Practices and Programs.* Retrieved from http://www.nrepp.samhsa.gov/ViewAll.aspx.

Sullivan, H. S. (1953). *The interpersonal theory of psychiatry.* New York, NY: W. W. Norton.

Watson, J. B. (1919). *Psychology from the standpoint of a behaviorist.* Philadelphia, PA: Lippincott.

CHAPTER

3

Biological Basis for Understanding Psychiatric Disorders and Treatments

Mary A. Gutierrez, Jerika T. Lam, and Mary Ann Schaepper

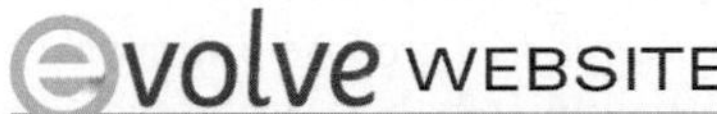

Visit the Evolve website for a pretest on the content in this chapter: http://evolve.elsevier.com/Varcarolis

Pre-Test interactive review

OBJECTIVES

1. Discuss major functions of the brain and how psychotropic drugs can alter these functions.
2. Identify how specific brain functions are altered in certain mental disorders (e.g., depression, anxiety, schizophrenia).
3. Describe how a neurotransmitter functions as a chemical messenger.
4. Describe how the use of imaging techniques can be helpful for understanding mental illness.
5. Develop a teaching plan that includes side effects from dopamine blockage (e.g., antipsychotic drugs) such as motor abnormalities.
6. Describe the result of blockage of the muscarinic receptors and the α_1 receptors by the standard neuroleptic drugs.
7. Identify the main neurotransmitters that are affected by the following psychotropic drugs and their subgroups:
   Antianxiety and hypnotic drugs
   Antidepressant drugs
   Mood stabilizers
   Antipsychotic drugs
   Psychostimulants
   Anticholinesterase inhibitors
8. Identify special dietary and drug restrictions in a teaching plan for a patient taking a monoamine oxidase inhibitor.
9. Identify specific cautions you might incorporate into your medication teaching plan with regard to the following:
   Herbal treatments
   Genetic pharmacology (i.e., variations in effects and therapeutic actions of medications among different ethnic groups)

KEY TERMS AND CONCEPTS

antagonists
antianxiety (anxiolytic) drugs
anticholinesterase inhibitors
atypical antipsychotics
circadian rhythms
conventional antipsychotics
hypnotic
limbic system
lithium
monoamine oxidase inhibitors (MAOIs)
mood stabilizers
neurons
neurotransmitter
pharmacodynamics
pharmacokinetics
receptors
reticular activating system (RAS)
reuptake
selective serotonin reuptake inhibitors (SSRIs)
synapse
therapeutic index
tricyclic antidepressants (TCAs)

Although the origin of a psychiatric illness may be related to a number of factors, such as genetics, neurodevelopmental factors, drugs, infection, and bad experiences, there is ultimately a physiological alteration in brain function that accounts for the disturbances in the patient's behavior and mental experiences. These physiological alterations are the targets of the psychotropic (Greek for *psyche,* or mind, + *trepein,* to turn) drugs used to treat mental disease. From a holistic point of view, mental disorders have psychobiological components that support the efficacy of treating these disorders both pharmacologically and with appropriate psychotherapy, or "talk" therapy that provides social and psychological support and actually alters brain function (Karlsson, 2011).

The treatment of mental illness with psychotropic drugs extends back more than half a century, yet a full understanding of how these drugs improve the symptoms of these illnesses continues to elude investigators. Early biological theories associated a single neurotransmitter with a specific disorder. The dopamine theory of schizophrenia and the monoamine theory of depression are now viewed as overly simplistic because a large number of other neurotransmitters, hormones, and co-regulators are now thought to play important and complex roles. The focus of research on neurotransmitters is now on how they are released from presynaptic cells and then act on postsynaptic cells and on how psychotropic drugs interact with these substances to make changes in brain functioning.

Recent discoveries have influenced the direction of research and treatment. While scientists have long known about basic receptors for neurotransmitters, many subtypes of receptors for the various neurotransmitters have been discovered in recent years.

The overall purpose of this chapter is to relate psychiatric disturbances and the psychotropic drugs used to treat them to normal brain structure and function. First, this chapter looks at the normal functions of the brain and how these functions are carried out from an anatomical and physiological perspective. Then, it reviews current theories of the psychobiological basis of various types of emotional and physiological dysfunctions. Finally, the chapter reviews the major drugs used to treat mental disorders, explains how they work, and identifies how both the beneficial and the problematic effects of psychiatric drugs relate to their interaction with various neurotransmitter-receptor systems.

Despite new information about the complex brain functions and neurotransmitters, there is still much to be clarified in understanding the complex ways in which the brain carries out its normal functions, is altered during disease, and is improved upon by pharmacological intervention. After reading this chapter, you should have a neurobiological framework into which you can place existing, as well as future, information about mental illnesses and their treatments. Additional, detailed information regarding adverse and toxic effects, dosage, nursing implications, and teaching tools is presented in the appropriate clinical chapters (Chapters 11-24).

STRUCTURE AND FUNCTION OF THE BRAIN

Functions and Activities of the Brain

Regulating behavior and carrying out mental processes are important, but far from the only, responsibilities of the brain. Box 3-1 summarizes some of the major functions and activities of the brain. Because all of these brain functions are carried out by similar mechanisms (interactions of neurons) often in similar locations, it is not surprising that mental disturbances are often associated with alterations in other brain functions and that the drugs used to treat mental disturbances can also interfere with other activities of the brain.

Maintenance of Homeostasis

The brain serves as the coordinator and director of the body's response to both internal and external changes. Appropriate responses require a constant monitoring of the environment, interpretation and integration of the incoming information, and control over the appropriate organs of response. The goal of these responses is to maintain homeostasis and thus to maintain life.

Information about the external world is relayed from various sense organs to the brain by the peripheral nerves. This information, which is at first received as a gross sensation, such as light, sound, or touch, must ultimately be interpreted as a key, a train whistle, or a hand on the back, respectively. Interestingly, a component of major psychiatric disturbance (e.g., schizophrenia) is an alteration of sensory experience; thus, the patient may experience a sensation that does not originate in the external world. For example, people with schizophrenia may hear voices talking to them (i.e., auditory hallucination).

The brain not only monitors the external world but also keeps a close watch on the internal functions; thus, the brain continuously receives information about blood pressure, body temperature, blood gases, and the chemical composition of the body fluids so that it can direct the appropriate responses required to maintain homeostasis.

To respond to external changes, the brain has control over the skeletal muscles. This control involves the ability to initiate contraction (i.e., to contract the biceps and flex the arm) but also to fine-tune and coordinate contraction so that a person can, for example, guide the fingers to the correct keys on a piano. Unfortunately, both psychiatric disease and the treatment of psychiatric disease with psychotropic drugs are often associated with disturbance of movement.

It is important to remember that the skeletal muscles controlled by the brain include the diaphragm, which is essential for

BOX 3-1 FUNCTIONS OF THE BRAIN

- Monitor changes in the external world.
- Monitor the composition of body fluids.
- Regulate the contractions of the skeletal muscles.
- Regulate the internal organs.
- Initiate and regulate the basic drives: hunger, thirst, sex, aggressive self-protection.
- Mediate conscious sensation.
- Store and retrieve memories.
- Regulate mood (affect) and emotions.
- Think and perform intellectual functions.
- Regulate the sleep cycle.
- Produce and interpret language.
- Process visual and auditory data.

breathing, and the muscles of the throat, tongue, and mouth, which are essential for speech; thus, drugs that affect brain function can stimulate or depress respiration or lead to slurred speech.

Adjustments to changes within the body require that the brain exert control over the various internal organs. For example, if blood pressure drops, the brain must direct the heart to pump more blood and the smooth muscles of the arterioles to constrict. This increase in cardiac output and vasoconstriction allows the body to return blood pressure to its normal level.

Regulation of the Autonomic Nervous System and Hormones

The autonomic nervous system and the endocrine system serve as the communication links between the brain and the cardiac muscle, smooth muscle, and glands of which the internal organs are composed (Figure 3-1). If the brain needs to stimulate the heart, it must activate the sympathetic nerves to the sinoatrial node and the ventricular myocardium. If the brain needs to bring about vasoconstriction, it must activate the sympathetic nerves to the smooth muscles of the arterioles.

The linkage between the brain and the internal organs that allows for the maintenance of homeostasis may also serve to translate mental disturbances, such as anxiety, into alterations of internal function. For example, anxiety can activate the sympathetic nervous system, leading to symptoms such as increased heart rate and blood pressure, shortness of breath, and sweating.

The brain also exerts influence over the internal organs by regulating hormonal secretions of the pituitary gland, which in turn regulates other glands. A specific area of the brain, the hypothalamus, secretes hormones called releasing factors. These hormones act on the pituitary gland to stimulate or inhibit the synthesis and release of pituitary hormones. Once in the general circulation they influence various internal activities. An example of this linkage is the release of gonadotropin-releasing hormone by the hypothalamus at the time of puberty. This hormone stimulates the release of two gonadotropins—follicle-stimulating hormone and luteinizing hormone—by the pituitary gland, which consequently activates the ovaries or testes. This linkage may explain why anxiety or depression in some women may lead to disturbances of the menstrual cycle.

The relationship between the brain, the pituitary gland, and the adrenal glands is particularly important in normal and abnormal mental function. Specifically, the hypothalamus secretes corticotropin-releasing hormone (CRH), which stimulates the pituitary to release corticotropin, which in turn stimulates the cortex of each adrenal gland to secrete the hormone cortisol. This system is activated as part of the normal response to a variety of mental and physical stresses. Among many other actions, all three hormones—CRH, corticotropin, and cortisol—influence the functions of the nerve cells of the brain. There is considerable evidence that this system is overactive in anxiety and that the normal negative feedback mechanism that is supposed to bring the hormone levels back down does not respond properly.

Control of Biological Drives and Behavior

To understand the neurobiological basis of mental disease and its treatment, it is helpful to distinguish between the various

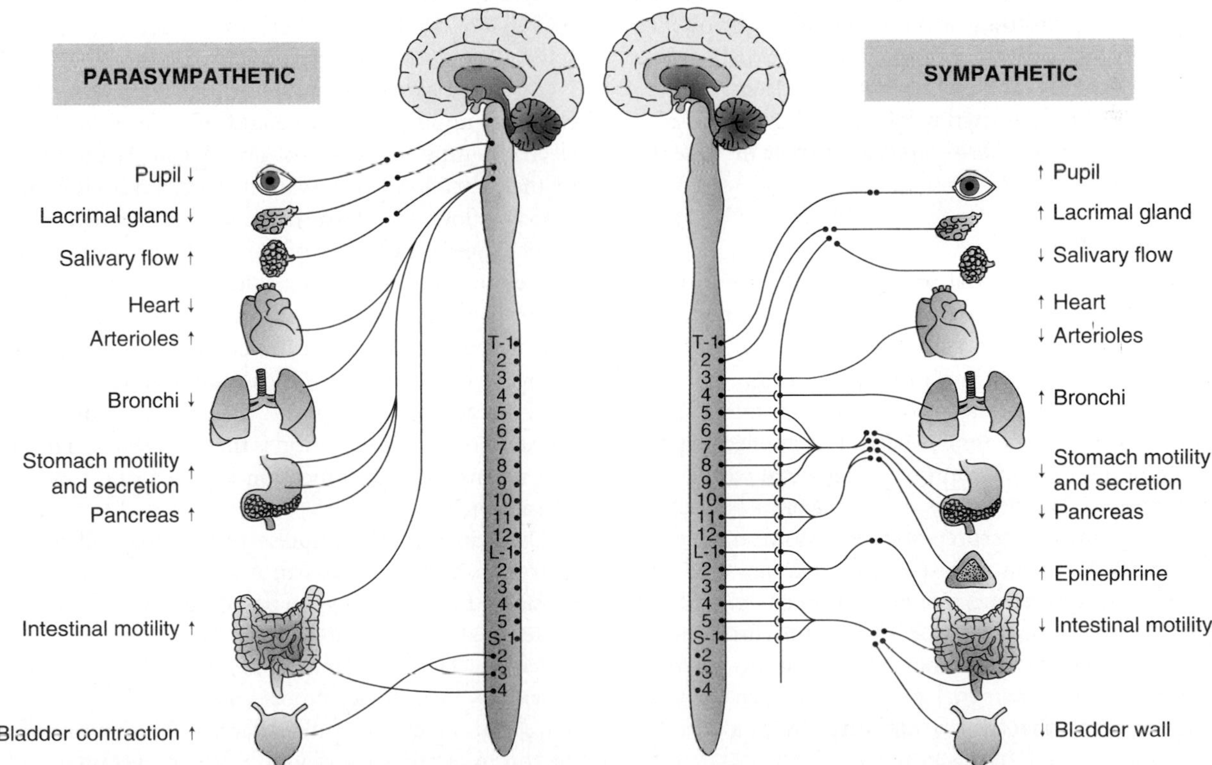

FIG 3-1 The autonomic nervous system has two divisions: the sympathetic and parasympathetic. The sympathetic division is dominant in stress situations, such as those involving fear and anger (known as the fight-or-flight response).

types of brain activity that serve as the basis of mental experience and behavior. An understanding of these activities shows where to look for disturbed function and what to hope for in treatment. The brain, for example, is responsible for the basic drives, such as sex and hunger, that play a strong role in molding behavior. Disturbances of these drives (e.g., overeating or undereating, loss of sexual interest) can be an indication of an underlying psychiatric disorder such as depression.

Cycle of Sleep and Wakefulness. The entire cycle of sleep and wakefulness, as well as the intensity of alertness while the person is awake, is regulated and coordinated by various regions of the brain. Although we do not fully understand the true homeostatic function of sleep, we know that it is essential for both physiological and psychological well-being. Assessment of sleep patterns is part of what is required to determine a psychiatric diagnosis.

Unfortunately, many of the drugs used to treat psychiatric problems interfere with the normal regulation of sleep and alertness. Drugs with a sedative-hypnotic effect can blunt the degree to which a person feels alert and focused and can cause drowsiness. The sedative-hypnotic effect requires caution in using these drugs while engaging in activities that require a great deal of attention, such as driving a car or operating machinery. One way of minimizing the danger is to take drugs at night just before bedtime.

Circadian Rhythms. The cycle of sleep and wakefulness is only one aspect of circadian rhythms, the fluctuation of various physiological and behavioral parameters over a 24-hour cycle. Other variations include changes in body temperature, secretion of hormones such as corticotropin and cortisol, and secretion of neurotransmitters such as norepinephrine and serotonin. Both norepinephrine and serotonin are thought to be involved in mood; thus, daily fluctuations of mood may be partially related to circadian variations in these neurotransmitters. There is evidence that the circadian rhythm of neurotransmitter secretion is altered in psychiatric disorders, particularly in those that involve mood.

Conscious Mental Activity

All aspects of conscious mental experience and sense of self originate from the neurophysiological activity of the brain. Conscious mental activity can be a basic, meandering stream of consciousness that can flow from thoughts of future responsibilities, memories, fantasies, and so on. Conscious mental activity can also be much more complex when it is applied to problem solving and the interpretation of the external world. Both the basic stream of consciousness and the complex problem solving and environment interpretation can become distorted in psychiatric illness. A person with schizophrenia may have chaotic and incoherent speech and thought patterns (e.g., a jumble of unrelated words known as word salad and unconnected phrases and topics known as looseness of association) and delusional interpretations of personal interactions, such as beliefs about people or events that are not supported by data or reality.

Memory

An extremely important component of mental activity is memory, the ability to retain and recall past experiences. From both an anatomical and a physiological perspective, there is thought to be a major difference in the processing of short- and long-term memory. This can be seen dramatically in some forms of cognitive mental disorders such as dementia, in which a person has no recall of the events of the previous few minutes but may have vivid recall of events that occurred decades earlier.

Social Skills

An important, and often neglected, aspect of brain functioning involves the social skills that make interpersonal relationships possible. In almost all types of mental illness, from mild anxiety to severe schizophrenia, difficulties in interpersonal relationships are important parts of the disorder, and improvements in these relationships are important gauges of progress. The connection between brain activity and social behavior is an area of intense research and is thought to be a combination of genetic makeup combined with individual experience. There is evidence that positive reward-based experiential learning and negative avoidance learning may involve different areas of the brain.

Cellular Composition of the Brain

The brain is composed of approximately 100 billion neurons, nerve cells that conduct electrical impulses, as well as other types of cells that surround the neurons. Most functions of the brain, from regulation of blood pressure to the conscious sense of self, are thought to result from the actions of individual neurons and the interconnections between them. Although neurons come in a great variety of shapes and sizes, all carry out the same three types of physiological actions: (1) respond to stimuli, (2) conduct electrical impulses, and (3) release chemicals called neurotransmitters.

An essential feature of neurons is their ability to conduct an electrical impulse from one end of the cell to the other. This electrical impulse consists of a change in membrane permeability that first allows the inward flow of sodium ions and then the outward flow of potassium ions. The inward flow of sodium ions changes the polarity of the membrane from positive on the outside to positive on the inside. Movement of potassium ions out of the cell returns the positive charge to the outside of the cell. Because these electrical charges are self-propagating, a change at one end of the cell is conducted along the membrane until it reaches the other end (Figure 3-2). The functional significance of this propagation is that the electrical impulse serves as a means of communication between one part of the body and another.

Once an electrical impulse reaches the end of a neuron, a neurotransmitter is released. A neurotransmitter is a chemical substance that functions as a neuromessenger. Neurotransmitters are released from the axon terminal at the presynaptic neuron on excitation. This neurotransmitter then diffuses across a space, or synapse, to an adjacent postsynaptic neuron, where it attaches to receptors on the neuron's surface. It is this interaction from one neuron to another, by way of a neurotransmitter and receptor, that allows the activity of one neuron to influence the activity of other neurons. Depending on the chemical structure of the neurotransmitter and the specific type of receptor to which it

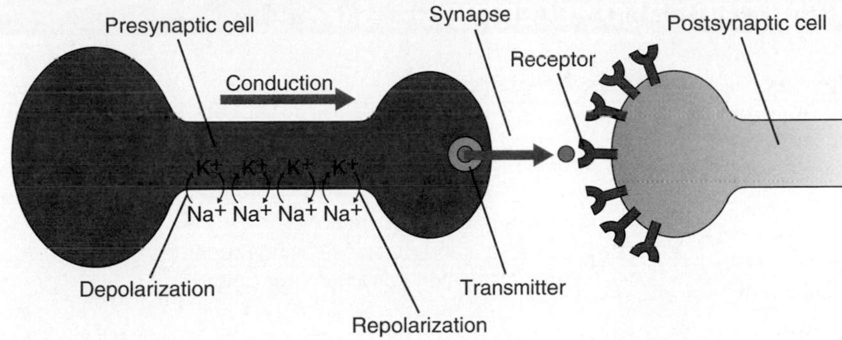

FIG 3-2 Activities of neurons. Conduction along a neuron involves the inward movement of sodium ions (Na^+) followed by the outward movement of potassium ions (K^+). When the current reaches the end of the cell, a neurotransmitter is released. The neurotransmitter crosses the synapse and attaches to a receptor on the postsynaptic cell. The attachment of neurotransmitter to receptor either stimulates or inhibits the postsynaptic cell.

attaches, the postsynaptic cell will be rendered either more or less likely to initiate an electrical impulse. It is the interaction between neurotransmitter and receptor that is a major target of the drugs used to treat psychiatric disease. Table 3-1 lists important neurotransmitters and the types of receptors to which they attach. Also listed are the mental disorders associated with an increase or decrease in these neurotransmitters.

After attaching to a receptor and exerting its influence on the postsynaptic cell, the neurotransmitter separates from the receptor and is destroyed. The process of neurotransmitter destruction is described in Box 3-2. There are two basic mechanisms by which neurotransmitters are destroyed. Some neurotransmitters (e.g., acetylcholine) are destroyed by specific enzymes at the postsynaptic cell. The enzyme that destroys acetylcholine is called acetylcholinesterase (most enzymes start with the name of the neurotransmitter they destroy and end with the suffix –ase). Other neurotransmitters (e.g., norepinephrine) are taken back into the presynaptic cell from which they were originally released by a process called cellular **reuptake** and are either reused or destroyed by intracellular enzymes. In the case of the monoamine neurotransmitters (e.g., norepinephrine, dopamine, serotonin), the destructive enzyme is called monoamine oxidase (MAO).

Some neurotransmitters regulate concentration at the postsynaptic receptors by exerting their own feedback inhibition of their own release. This is accomplished by the attachment of neurotransmitters to presynaptic receptors at the synapse, which act to inhibit the further release of neurotransmitters.

TABLE 3-1 TRANSMITTERS AND RECEPTORS

TRANSMITTERS	RECEPTORS	EFFECTS/COMMENTS	ASSOCIATION WITH MENTAL HEALTH
Monoamines			
Dopamine (DA)	D_1, D_2, D_3, D_4, D_5	• Involved in fine muscle movement • Involved in integration of emotions and thoughts • Involved in decision making • Stimulates hypothalamus to release hormones (sex, thyroid, adrenal)	*Decrease:* • Parkinson's disease • Depression *Increase:* • Schizophrenia • Mania
Norepinephrine (NE) (noradrenaline)	α_1, α_2, β_1, β_2	• Level in brain affects mood • Attention and arousal • Stimulates sympathetic branch of autonomic nervous system for "fight or flight" in response to stress	*Decrease:* • Depression *Increase:* • Mania • Anxiety states • Schizophrenia
Serotonin (5-HT)	5-HT_1, 5-HT_2, 5-HT_3, 5-HT_4	• Plays a role in sleep regulation, hunger, mood states, and pain perception • Hormonal activity • Plays a role in aggression and sexual behavior	*Decrease:* • Depression *Increase:* • Anxiety states
Histamine	H_1, H_2	• Involved in alertness • Involved in inflammatory response • Stimulates gastric secretion	*Decrease:* • Sedation • Weight gain

Continued

TABLE 3-1 TRANSMITTERS AND RECEPTORS—cont'd

TRANSMITTERS	RECEPTORS	EFFECTS/COMMENTS	ASSOCIATION WITH MENTAL HEALTH
Amino Acids			
γaminobutyric acid (GABA)	$GABA_A$, $GABA_B$	• Plays a role in inhibition; reduces aggression, excitation, and anxiety • May play a role in pain perception • Has anticonvulsant and muscle-relaxing properties • May impair cognition and psychomotor functioning	*Decrease:* • Anxiety disorders • Schizophrenia • Mania • Huntington's disease *Increase:* • Reduction of anxiety
Glutamate	NMDA, AMPA	• Is excitatory • AMPA plays a role in learning and memory	*Decrease (NMDA):* • Psychosis *Increase (NMDA):* • Prolonged increased state can be neurotoxic • Neurodegeneration in Alzheimer's disease *Increase (AMPA):* • Improvement of cognitive performance in behavioral tasks
Cholinergics			
Acetylcholine (ACh)	Nicotinic, muscarinic (M_1, M_2, M_3)	• Plays a role in learning, memory • Regulates mood: mania, sexual aggression • Affects sexual and aggressive behavior • Stimulates parasympathetic nervous system	*Decrease:* • Alzheimer's disease • Huntington's disease • Parkinson's disease *Increase:* • Depression
Peptides (Neuromodulators)			
Substance P (SP)	SP	• Centrally active SP antagonist has antidepressant and anti-anxiety effects in depression • Promotes and reinforces memory • Enhances sensitivity to pain receptors to activate	• Involved in regulation of mood and anxiety • Role in pain management
Somatostatin (SRIF)	SRIF	Altered levels associated with cognitive disease	*Decrease:* Alzheimer's disease Decreased levels of SRIF found in spinal fluid of some depressed patients *Increase:* Huntington's disease
Neurotensin (NT)	NT	Endogenous antipsychotic-like properties	Decreased levels found in spinal fluid of patients with schizophrenia

AMPA, α-Amino-3-hydroxy-5-methyl-4-isoxazolepropionic acid; *NMDA,* N-methyl-d-aspartate.

A neuron may release a specific neurotransmitter that stimulates or inhibits a postsynaptic membrane receptor. Negative feedback on a presynaptic receptor should maintain a normal balance of neurotransmitters; however, researchers have also found that neurons may release more than one chemical at the same time. Larger molecules, neuropeptides, may bring about long-term changes in the postsynaptic cells by joining neurotransmitters such as norepinephrine or acetylcholine. The result of these changes is an alteration of basic cell functions or genetic expression and may lead to modifications of cell shape and responsiveness to stimuli. Ultimately, this means that the action of one neuron on another affects not only the immediate response of that neuron but also its sensitivity to future influence. The long-term implications of this for neural development, normal and abnormal mental health, and the treatment of psychiatric disease are being investigated.

Communication in nerve cells goes from presynaptic to postsynaptic; however, researchers have found that the communication between neurons at a synapse does not just go in one direction. Influencing the growth, shape, and activity of

BOX 3-2 DESTRUCTION OF NEUROTRANSMITTERS

A full explanation of the various ways in which psychotropic drugs alter neuronal activity requires a brief review of the manner in which neurotransmitters are destroyed after attaching to the receptors. To avoid continuous and prolonged action on the postsynaptic cell, the neurotransmitter is released shortly after attaching to the postsynaptic receptor. Once released, the neurotransmitter is destroyed in one of two ways.

One way is the immediate inactivation of the neurotransmitter at the postsynaptic membrane. An example of this method of destruction is the action of the enzyme acetylcholinesterase on the neurotransmitter acetylcholine. Acetylcholinesterase is present at the postsynaptic membrane and destroys acetylcholine shortly after it attaches to nicotinic or muscarinic receptors on the postsynaptic cell.

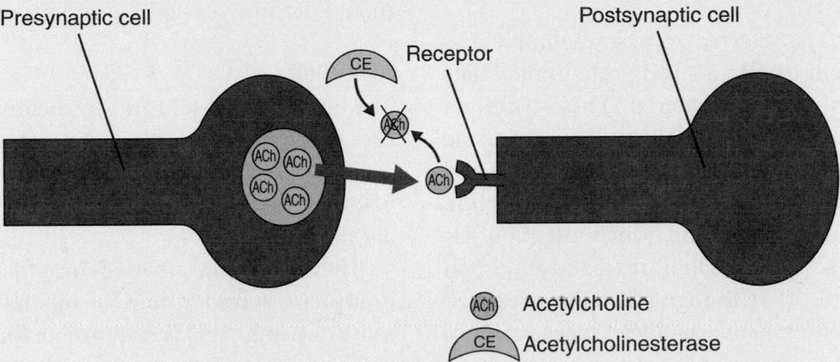

A *second* method of neurotransmitter inactivation is a little more complex. After interacting with the postsynaptic receptor, the neurotransmitter is released and taken back into the presynaptic cell, the cell from which it was released. This process, referred to as the reuptake of neurotransmitter, is a common target for drug action. Once inside the presynaptic cell, the neurotransmitter is either recycled or inactivated by an enzyme within the cell. The monoamine neurotransmitters norepinephrine, dopamine, and serotonin are all inactivated in this manner by the enzyme monoamine oxidase.

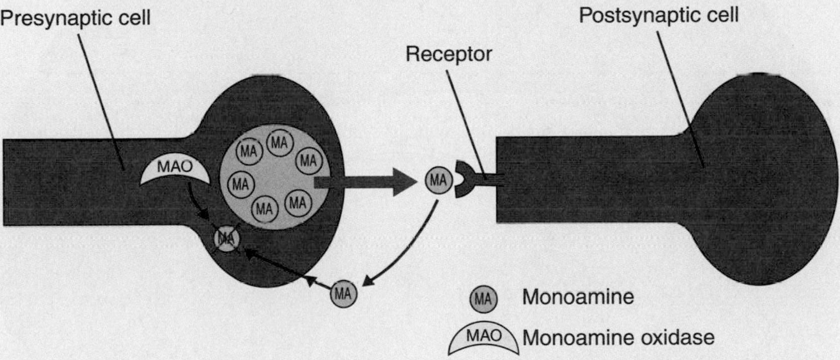

Looking at this second method, you might naturally ask what prevents the enzyme from destroying the neurotransmitter before its release. The answer is that before release the neurotransmitter is stored within a membrane and is protected. After release and reuptake, the neurotransmitter is either destroyed by the enzyme or reenters the membrane to be used again.

presynaptic cells are protein and simple gases, such as carbon monoxide and nitrous oxide, called neurotrophic factors. These factors are thought to be particularly important during the development of the fetal brain, guiding the growing brain to form the proper neuronal connections. It is apparent that the brain retains anatomical plasticity throughout life and that internal and external influences can alter the synaptic network of the brain. Altered genetic expression or environmental trauma can change these factors and result in negative and positive consequences on mental function and psychiatric disease.

Other chemicals, such as steroid hormones, brought to the neurons by the blood can influence the development and responsiveness of neurons. Estrogen, testosterone, and cortisol can bind to neurons, where they can cause short- and long-term changes in neuronal activity. A clear example of this is evident in the psychosis that can result from the hypersecretion of cortisol in Cushing's disease or from the use of prednisone in high doses to treat chronic inflammatory disease.

Organization of the Brain

Brainstem

The central core of the brainstem regulates the internal organs and is responsible for such vital functions as the regulation of blood gases and the maintenance of blood pressure. The hypothalamus, a small area in the ventral superior portion of the brainstem, plays a vital role in such basic drives as hunger, thirst, and sex. It also serves as a crucial psychosomatic link between higher brain activities, such as thought and emotion, and the functioning of the internal organs. The brainstem also serves as an initial processing center for sensory information that is then sent on to the cerebral cortex. Through projections of the reticular activating system (RAS), the brainstem regulates the entire cycle of sleep and wakefulness and the ability of the cerebrum to carry out conscious mental activity.

Other ascending pathways, referred to as mesolimbic and mesocortical pathways, seem to play a strong role in modulating the emotional value of sensory material. These pathways project to those areas of the cerebrum collectively known as the limbic system, which plays a crucial role in emotional status and psychological function. They use norepinephrine, serotonin, and dopamine as their neurotransmitters. Much attention has been paid to the role of these pathways in normal and abnormal mental activity. For example, it is thought that the release of dopamine from the ventral tegmental pathway plays a role in psychological reward and drug addiction. The neurotransmitters released by these neurons are major targets of the drugs used to treat psychiatric disease.

Cerebellum

Located behind the brainstem, the cerebellum (Figure 3-3) is primarily involved in the regulation of skeletal muscle coordination and contraction and the maintenance of equilibrium. It plays a crucial role in coordinating contractions so that movement is accomplished in a smooth and directed manner.

Cerebrum

The human brainstem and cerebellum are similar in both structure and function to these same structures in other mammals. The development of a much larger and more elaborate cerebrum is what distinguishes human beings from the rest of the animal kingdom.

The cerebrum, situated on top of and surrounding the brainstem, is responsible for mental activities and a conscious sense of being. This is responsible for our conscious perception

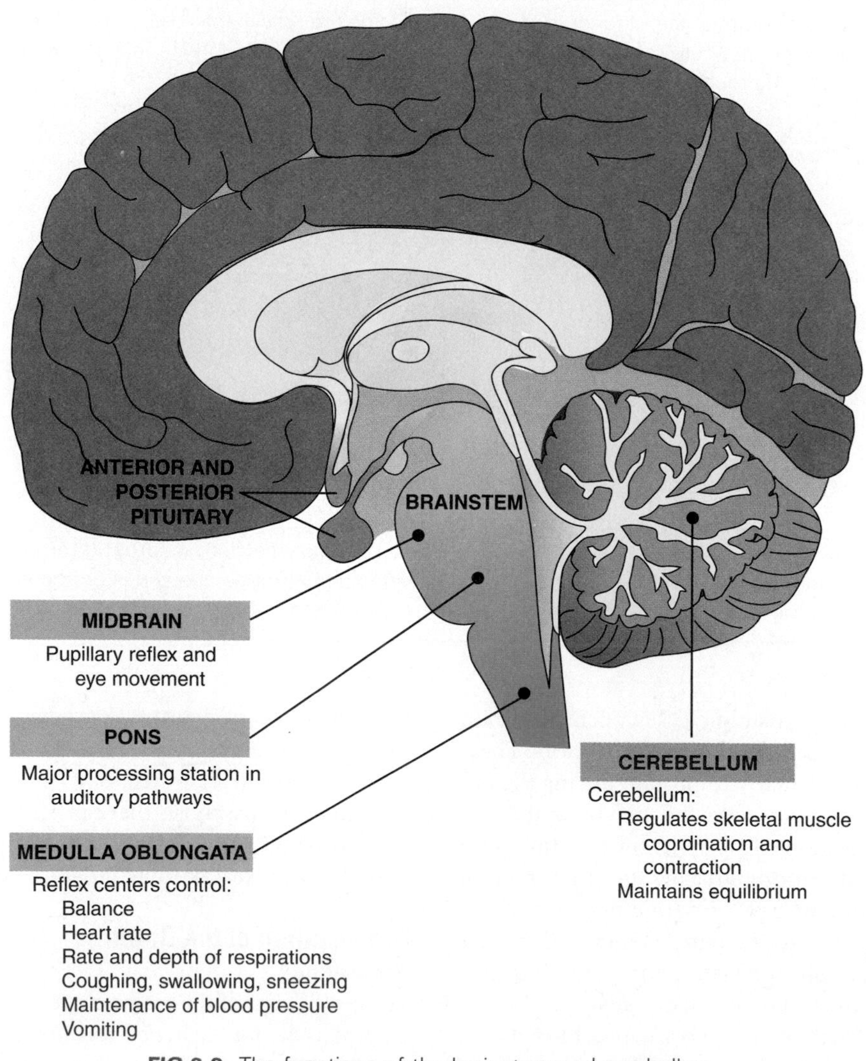

FIG 3-3 The functions of the brainstem and cerebellum.

of the external world and our own body, emotional status, memory, and control of skeletal muscles that allow willful direction of movement. The cerebrum is also responsible for language and the ability to communicate.

The cerebrum consists of surface, the cerebral cortex, and deep areas of integrating gray matter that include the basal ganglia, amygdala, and hippocampus. Tracts of white matter link these areas with each other and the rest of the nervous system. The cerebral cortex, which forms the outer layer of the brain, is responsible for conscious sensation and the initiation of movement. Certain areas of the cortex are responsible for specific sensations. For example, the sensation of touch resides in the parietal cortex, sounds are based in the temporal cortex, and vision is housed in the occipital cortex. Likewise, a specific area of the frontal cortex controls the initiation of skeletal muscle contraction. Of course, all areas of the cortex are interconnected so that an appropriate picture of the world can be formed and, if necessary, linked to a proper response (Figure 3-4).

Both sensory and motor aspects of language reside in specialized areas of the cerebral cortex. Sensory language functions

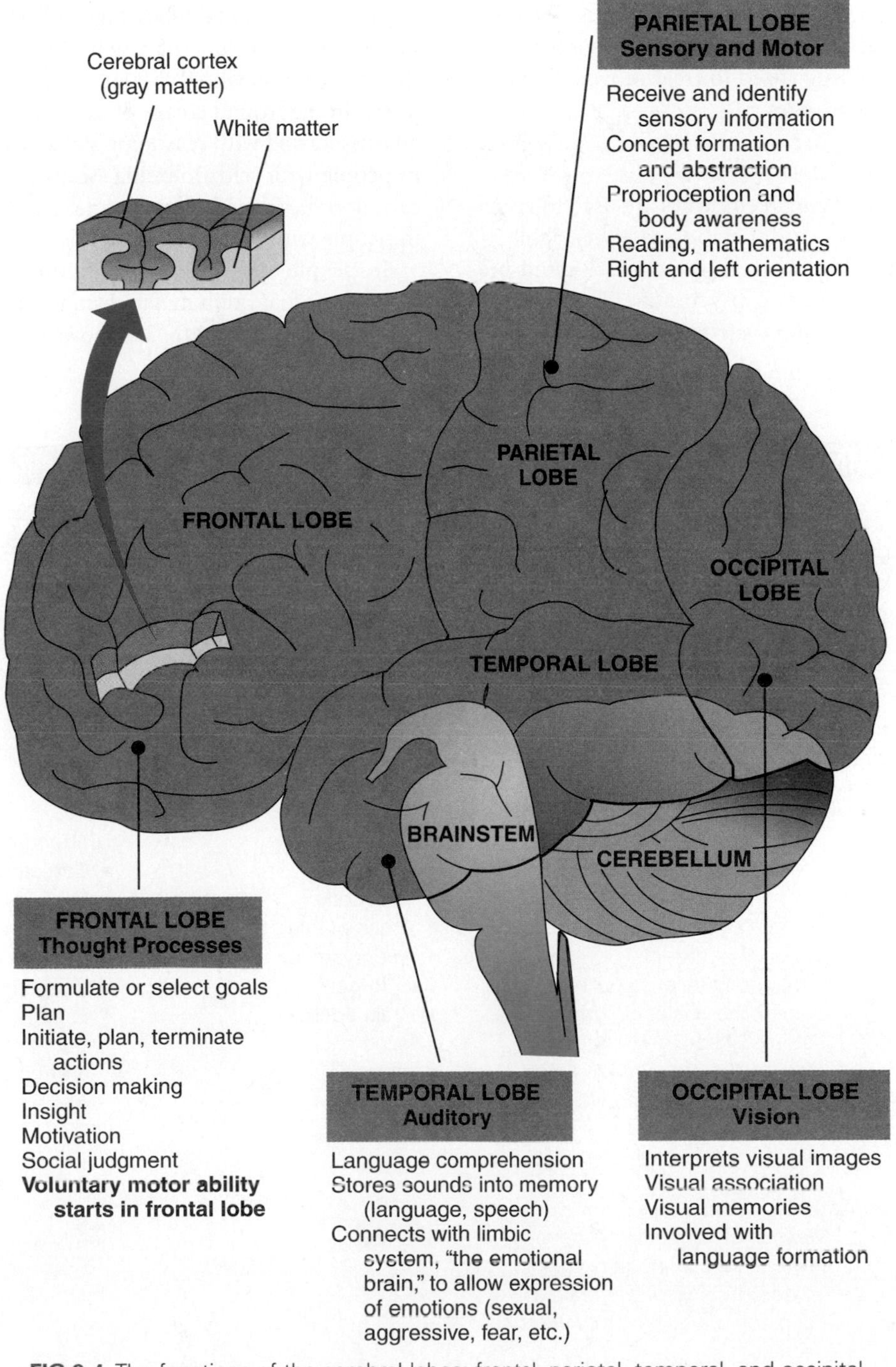

FIG 3-4 The functions of the cerebral lobes: frontal, parietal, temporal, and occipital.

include the ability to read, understand spoken language, and know the names of objects perceived by the senses. Motor functions involve the physical ability to use muscles properly for speech and writing. In both neurological and psychological dysfunction, the use of language may become compromised or distorted. The change in language ability may be a factor in determining a diagnosis.

Underneath the cerebral cortex there are pockets of integrating gray matter deep within the cerebrum. Some of these, the basal ganglia, are involved in the regulation of movement. Others, the amygdala and hippocampus, are involved in emotions, learning, memory, and basic drives. Significantly, there is an overlap of these areas both anatomically and in the types of neurotransmitters employed. One important consequence is that drugs used to treat emotional disturbances may cause movement disorders, and drugs used to treat movement disorders may cause emotional changes.

Visualizing the Brain

A variety of noninvasive imaging techniques are used to visualize brain structure, functions, and metabolic activity. Table 3-2 identifies some common brain imaging techniques and preliminary findings as they relate to psychiatry. There are two types of neuroimaging techniques: structural and functional. Structural imaging techniques (e.g., computed tomography [CT] and magnetic resonance imaging [MRI]) provide overall images of the brain and layers of the brain. Functional imaging techniques (e.g., positron emission tomography [PET] and single photon emission computed tomography [SPECT]) reveal physiological activity in the brain, as described in Table 3-2.

PET scans are particularly useful in identifying physiological and biochemical changes as they occur in living tissue. Usually, a radioactive "tag" is used to trace compounds such as glucose in the brain. Glucose use is related to functional activity in certain areas of the brain. For example, in unmedicated patients with schizophrenia, PET scans may show a decreased use of glucose in the frontal lobes. Figure 3-5 shows lower brain activity in the frontal lobe of a twin diagnosed with schizophrenia than in the twin who does not share the diagnosis. The area affected in the frontal cortex of the twin with schizophrenia is an area associated with reasoning skills, which are greatly impaired in people with schizophrenia. Scans such as these suggest a location in the frontal cortex as the site of functional impairment in people with schizophrenia.

In people with obsessive-compulsive disorder (OCD), PET scans show that brain metabolism is increased in certain areas of the frontal cortex. Figure 3-6 shows increased brain metabolism

TABLE 3-2 COMMON BRAIN IMAGING TECHNIQUES

TECHNIQUE	DESCRIPTION	USES	PSYCHIATRIC RELEVANCE AND PRELIMINARY FINDINGS
Electrical: Recording Electrical Signals from the Brain			
Electroencephalograph (EEG)	A recording of electrical signals from the brain made by hooking up electrodes to the subject's scalp.	Can show the state a person is in — asleep, awake, anesthetized — because the characteristic patterns of current differ for each of these states.	Provides support from a wide range of sources that brain abnormalities exist; may lead to further testing.
Structural: Show Gross Anatomical Details of Brain Structures			
Computerized axial tomography (CT)	A series of x-ray images is taken of the brain and a computer analysis produces "slices" providing a precise 3D-like reconstruction of each segment.	Can detect: • Lesions • Abrasions • Areas of infarct • Aneurysm	Schizophrenia • Cortical atrophy • Third ventricle enlargement • Cognitive disorders • Abnormalities
Magnetic resonance imaging (MRI)	A magnetic field is applied to the brain. The nuclei of hydrogen atoms absorb and emit radio waves that are analyzed by computer, which provides 3D visualization of the brain's structure in sectional images.	Can detect: • Brain edema • Ischemia • Infection • Neoplasm • Trauma	Schizophrenia • Enlarged ventricles • Reduction in temporal lobe and prefrontal lobe
Functional: Show Some Activity of the Brain			
Functional magnetic resonance imaging (fMRI)	Measures brain activity indirectly by changes in blood oxygen in different parts of the brain as subjects participate in various activities.	See MRI	See MRI

TABLE 3-2 **COMMON BRAIN IMAGING TECHNIQUES—cont'd**

TECHNIQUE	DESCRIPTION	USES	PSYCHIATRIC RELEVANCE AND PRELIMINARY FINDINGS
Positron-emission tomography (PET)	Radioactive substance (tracer) is injected, travels to the brain, and shows up as bright spots on the scan. Data collected by the detectors are relayed to a computer, which produces images of the activity and 3D visualization of the CNS.	Can detect: • Oxygen utilization • Glucose metabolism • Blood flow • Neurotransmitter-receptor interaction	Schizophrenia • Increased D_2, D_3 receptors in caudate nucleus • Abnormalities in limbic system • Mood disorder • Abnormalities in temporal lobes • Adult ADHD • Decreased utilization of glucose
Single photon emission computed tomography (SPECT)	Similar to PET but uses radionuclides that emit γ-radiation (photons). Measures various aspects of brain functioning and provides images of multiple layers of the CNS (as does PET).	Can detect: • Circulation of cerebrospinal fluid • Similar functions to PET	See PET

ADHD, Attention deficit hyperactivity disorder; *CNS,* central nervous system; *3D,* three-dimensional.

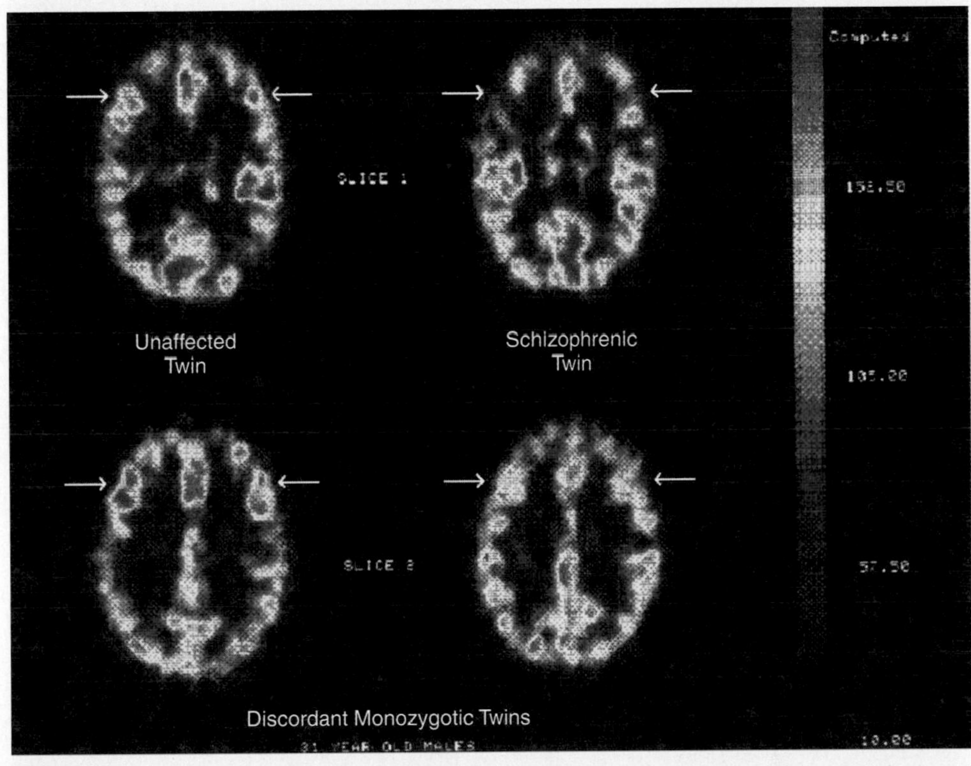

FIG 3-5 Positron emission tomographic (PET) scans of blood flow in identical twins, one of whom has schizophrenia, illustrate that individuals with this illness have reduced brain activity in the frontal lobes when asked to perform a reasoning task that requires activation of this area. Patients with schizophrenia also perform poorly on the task. This suggests a site of functional impairments in schizophrenia (From Karen Berman, MD, courtesy of National Institute of Mental Health, Clinical Brain Disorders Branch.)

in an individual with OCD compared with someone who does not have OCD, suggesting altered brain function in people with OCD.

PET scans of individuals with depression show decreased brain activity in the prefrontal cortex. Figure 3-7 shows the results of a PET scan taken after a form of radioactively tagged glucose was used as a tracer to visualize brain activity. The patient with depression shows reduced brain activity compared with someone who does not have depression. Figure 3-8 shows three views of a PET scan of the brain of a patient with Alzheimer's disease.

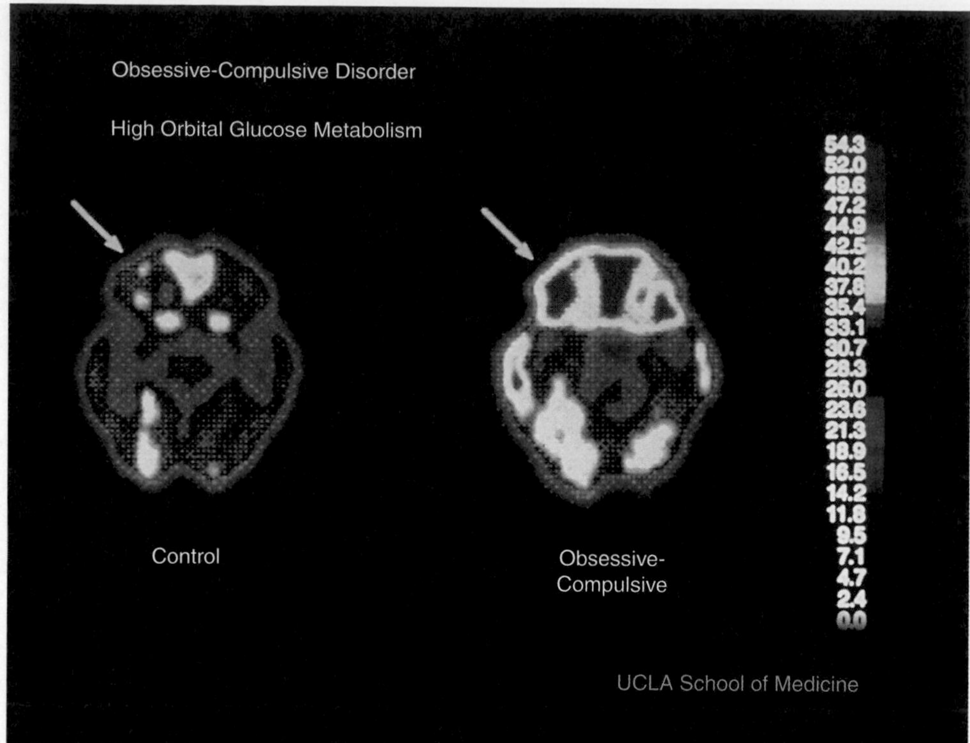

FIG 3-6 Positron emission tomographic (PET) scans show increased brain metabolism *(brighter colors)*, particularly in the frontal cortex, in a patient with obsessive-compulsive disorder (OCD), compared with a control. This suggests altered brain function in OCD. (From Lewis Baxter, MD, University of Alabama, courtesy of National Institute of Mental Health.)

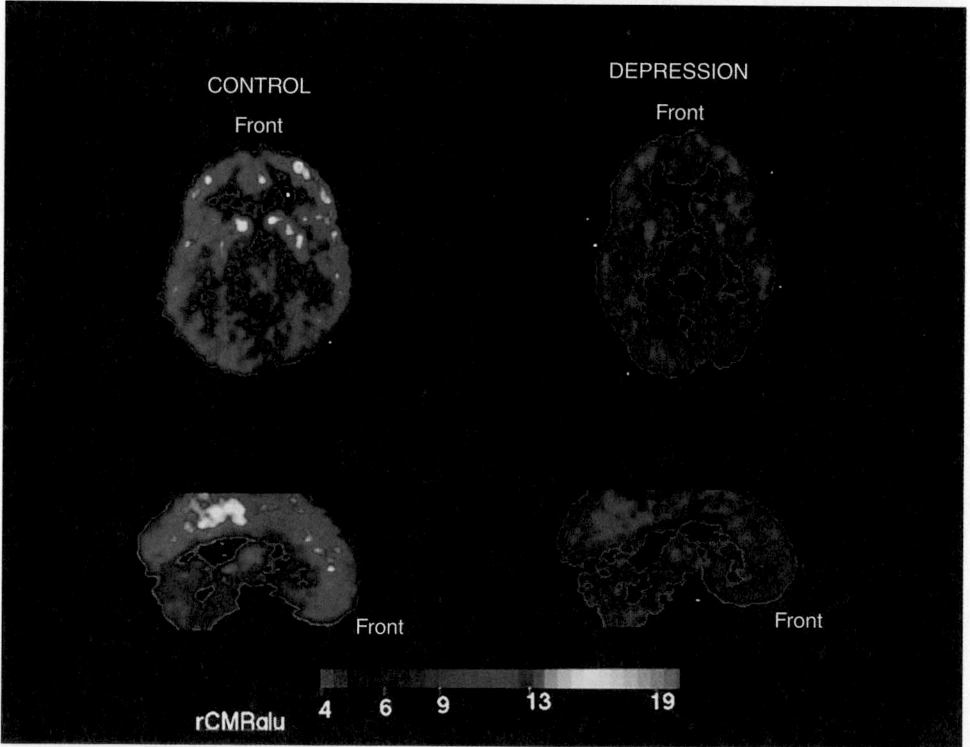

FIG 3-7 Positron emission tomographic (PET) scans of a patient with depression *(right)* and a person without depression *(left)* reveal reduced brain activity *(darker colors)* in depression, especially in the prefrontal cortex. A form of radioactively tagged glucose was used as a tracer to visualize levels of brain activity. (From Mark George, MD, courtesy of National Institute of Mental Health, Biological Psychiatry Branch.)

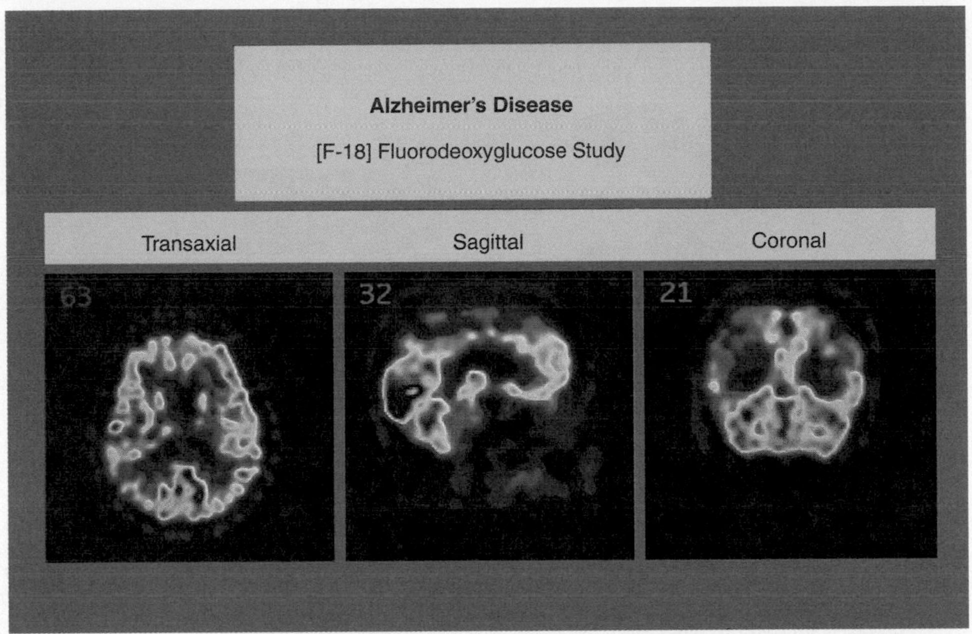

FIG 3-8 Positron emission tomographic (PET) scan of a patient with Alzheimer's disease demonstrates a classic pattern for areas of hypometabolism in the temporal and parietal regions of the brain. Areas of reduced metabolism *(dark blue and black regions)* are very noticeable in the sagittal and coronal views. (Courtesy of PET Imaging Center, Department of Radiology, University of Iowa Hospitals and Clinics, Iowa City.)

Modern imaging techniques have become important tools in assessing molecular changes in mental disease and marking the receptor sites of drug action. From a psychiatric perspective, it is important to understand where in the brain the various components of psychological activity take place and what types of neurotransmitters and receptors underlie this activity physiologically. Our understanding of both of these questions is far from complete; however, it is thought that the limbic system—a group of structures that includes parts of the frontal cortex, the basal ganglia, and the brainstem—is a major locus of psychological activity.

Within these areas, the monoamine neurotransmitters (norepinephrine, dopamine, and serotonin), the amino acid neurotransmitters (glutamate and γ-aminobutyric acid [GABA]), and the neuropeptides (corticotropin releasing hormone [CRH] and endorphin), as well as acetylcholine, play a major role. Alterations in these areas are thought to form the basis of psychiatric disease and are the target for pharmacological treatment.

Disturbances of Mental Function

Most origins of mental dysfunction are unknown, but known causes are drugs (e.g., lysergic acid diethylamide [LSD]), long-term use of high daily doses of prednisone, excess levels of hormones (e.g., thyroxine, cortisol), infection (e.g., encephalitis, acquired immunodeficiency syndrome [AIDS]), and physical trauma. Even when the cause is known, the link between the causative factor and the mental dysfunction is far from understood.

There is often a genetic predisposition for psychiatric disorders. The incidence of both thought and mood disorders are higher in relatives of people with these diseases than in the general population. Identical twins provide a measure of how strongly inheritance is implicated through a concept known as concordance rate. Concordance refers to how often one twin will be affected by the same illness as the other twin; there is a strong concordance among identical twins even when they are raised apart. A 100% concordance rate would mean that if one twin has a disorder, the other one would also have it, which would be the case for strictly inherited disorders. For schizophrenia, the concordance rate is 50%, meaning that inheritance is half of the equation and that other factors are involved.

Researchers ultimately want to be able to understand mental dysfunction in terms of altered activity of neurons in specific areas of the brain; the hope is that such an understanding will lead to better treatments and possible prevention of mental disorders. Current interest is focused on certain neurotransmitters and their receptors, particularly in the limbic system, which links the frontal cortex, basal ganglia, and upper brainstem. As mentioned earlier, the neurotransmitters that have been most consistently linked to mental activity are norepinephrine, dopamine, serotonin, GABA, and glutamate.

Although the underlying physiology is complex, it is thought that a deficiency of norepinephrine or serotonin, or both, may serve as the biological basis of depression. Figure 3-9 shows that an insufficient degree of transmission may be due to a deficient release of neurotransmitters by the presynaptic cell or to a loss of the ability of postsynaptic receptors to respond to the neurotransmitters. Changes in neurotransmitter release and receptor response can be both a cause and a consequence of intracellular changes in the neurons involved. Thought disorders such as schizophrenia are associated physiologically with excess transmission of the neurotransmitter dopamine, among other changes. As illustrated in Figure 3-10, this may be due to either

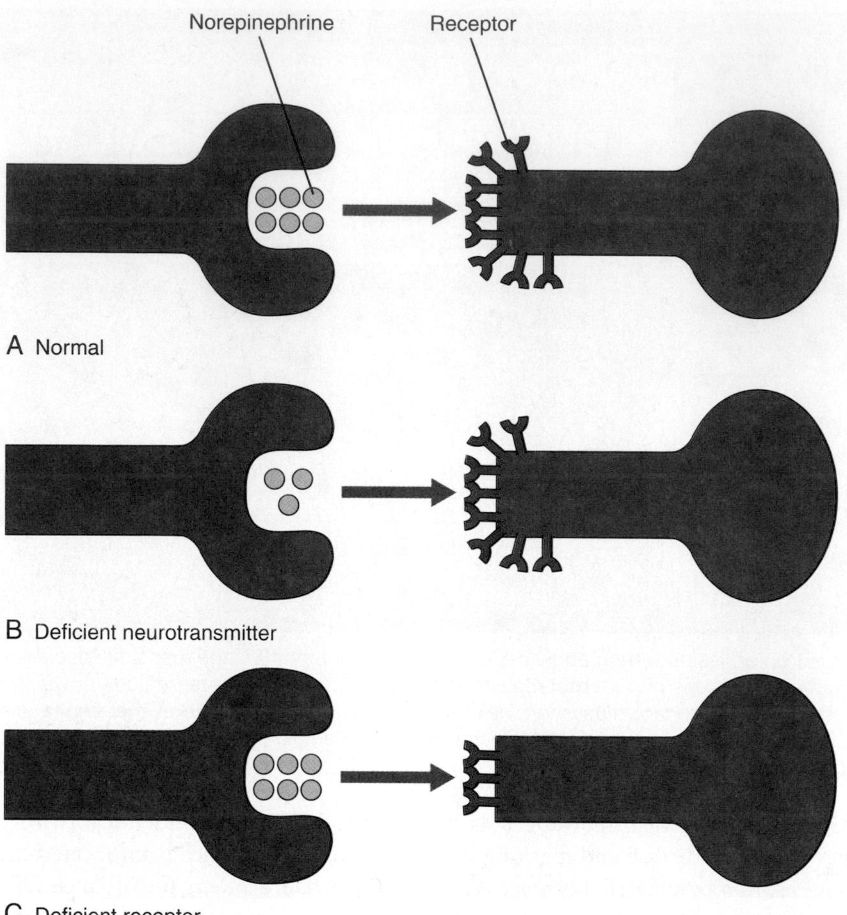

FIG 3-9 Normal transmission of neurotransmitters *(A)*. Deficiency in transmission may be due to deficient release of neurotransmitter, as shown in *B,* or to a reduction in receptors, as shown in *C*.

an excess release of neurotransmitter or an increase in receptor responsiveness.

Glutamate may have a direct influence on the activity of dopamine-releasing cells. A recent study showed preliminary in vivo evidence of the relationship between hippocampal glutamatergic and striatal dopaminergic function being abnormal in people at high risk of psychosis (Stone, 2010).

The neurotransmitter γ-aminobutyric acid (GABA) seems to play a role in modulating neuronal excitability and anxiety. Not surprisingly, many **antianxiety (anxiolytic) drugs** act by increasing the effectiveness of this neurotransmitter. This is accomplished primarily by increasing receptor responsiveness.

It is important to keep in mind that the various areas of the brain are interconnected structurally and functionally by a vast network of neurons. This network serves to integrate the many and varied activities of the brain. A limited number of neurotransmitters are used in the brain, and thus a particular neurotransmitter is often used by different neurons to carry out quite different activities. For example, dopamine is used by neurons involved in not only thought processes but also the regulation of movement. As a result, alterations in neurotransmitter activity, due to a mental disturbance or to the drugs used to treat the disturbance, can affect more than one area of brain activity. Alterations in mental status, whether arising from disease or from medication, are often accompanied by changes in basic drives, sleep patterns, body movement, and autonomic functions.

MECHANISMS OF ACTION OF PSYCHOTROPIC DRUGS

When studying drugs, it is important to keep in mind the concepts of pharmacodynamics and pharmacokinetics. **Pharmacodynamics** refers to the biochemical and physiological effects of drugs on the body, which include the mechanisms of drug action and its effect. The term **pharmacokinetics** refers to the actions of the person on the drug. How is the drug absorbed into the blood? How is it transformed in the liver? How is it distributed in the body? How is it excreted by the kidney? Pharmacokinetics determines the blood level of a drug and is used to guide the dosage schedule. It is also used to determine the type and amount of drug used in cases of liver and kidney disease.

The processes of pharmacokinetics and pharmacodynamics play an extensive role in how genetic factors give rise to interindividual and cross-ethnic variations in drug response. The Considering Culture box discusses how the area of pharmacogenetics may influence the way health care providers tailor their prescriptions for patients.

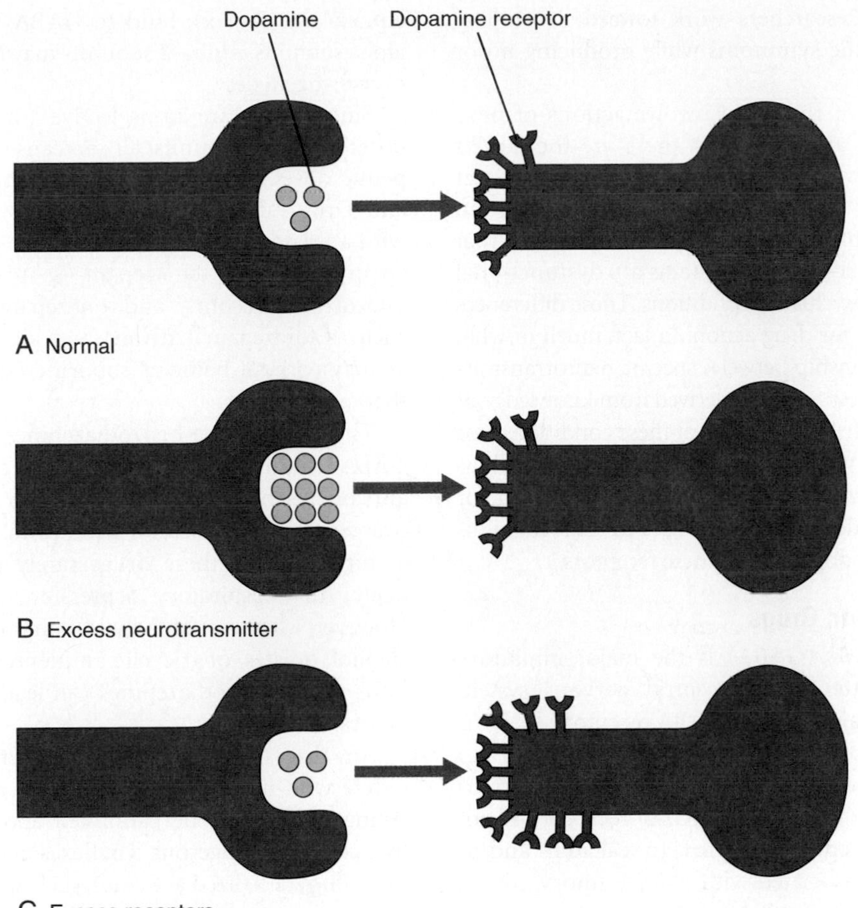

FIG 3-10 Causes of excess transmission of neurotransmitters. Excess transmission may be due to excess release of neurotransmitter, as shown in *B*, or to excess responsiveness of receptors, as shown in *C*.

CONSIDERING CULTURE

Pharmacogenetics

Pharmacogenetics explains how genetic variation leads to altered drug responses in different individuals and ethnic groups. Variation of drug metabolism via the CYP450 enzymes leads to significant differences in psychotropic drug concentrations. People who metabolize drugs poorly will experience more adverse drug reactions; people who metabolize drugs extensively may have less of a therapeutic response to treatment.

Three CYP450 enzymes are responsible for metabolizing all the currently available selective serotonin reuptake inhibitors (SSRIs) such as Prozac. Poor metabolism of one of these enzymes, CYP450 2D6, occurs in about 15% of Caucasians. Poor metabolism of another of these enzymes, CYP450 2C19, occurs in about 20% of Asian subgroups.

Although an immense amount of progress has been made to unravel the complex pharmacogenetics that influence a patient's treatment responses, considerable scientific and clinical work remains to be completed. There are still challenges to achieving the goals of personalized treatments in psychiatry. For patients with treatment failure or excessive adverse drug reactions, there are FDA-approved CYP450 genotyping tests available to determine if patients are poor, extensive, or rapid metabolizers.

Zandi, P.P., & Judy, J.T. (2010). The promise and reality of pharmacogenetics in psychiatry. *The Psychiatric Clinics of North America, 33,* 181-224.

Many drugs are transformed by the liver into active metabolites—chemicals that also have pharmacological actions. This knowledge is used by researchers in designing new drugs that make use of the body's own mechanisms to activate a chemical for pharmacological use.

An ideal psychiatric drug would relieve the mental disturbance of the patient without inducing additional cerebral (mental) or somatic (physical) effects. Unfortunately, in psychopharmacology—as in most areas of pharmacology—there are no drugs that are both fully effective and free of undesired side effects. Researchers work toward developing medications that target the symptoms while producing no or few side effects.

Because all activities of the brain involve actions of neurons, neurotransmitters, and receptors, these are the targets of pharmacological intervention. Most psychotropic drugs act by either increasing or decreasing the activity of certain neurotransmitter-receptor systems. It is generally agreed that different neurotransmitter-receptor systems are dysfunctional in persons with different psychiatric conditions. These differences offer more specific targets for drug action. In fact, much of what is known about the relationship between specific neurotransmitters and specific disturbances has been derived from knowledge of the pharmacology of the drugs used to treat these conditions. For example, most agents that were effective in reducing the delusions and hallucinations of schizophrenia blocked the D_2 receptors for dopamine. It was concluded that delusions and hallucinations result from overactivity of dopamine at these receptors.

Antianxiety and Hypnotic Drugs

Gamma-aminobutyric acid (GABA) is the major inhibitory (calming) neurotransmitter in the central nervous system (CNS). There are three major types of GABA receptors: $GABA_A$, $GABA_B$, and $GABA_C$ receptors. The various subtypes of $GABA_A$ receptors are the targets of benzodiazepines (BZDs), barbiturates, and alcohol. While the role of $GABA_C$ receptors is not defined, the $GABA_B$ receptors coupled to calcium and/or potassium channels are associated with pain, memory, mood, and other CNS functions. Drugs that enhance $GABA_A$ receptors exert a sedative-hypnotic action on brain function. The most commonly used anti-anxiety agents are the benzodiazepines.

Benzodiazepines

Benzodiazepines (BZDs) potentiate, or promote the activity of GABA by binding to a specific receptor on the $GABA_A$ receptor complex. This binding results in an increased frequency of chloride channel opening causing membrane hyperpolarization, which inhibits cellular excitation. If cellular excitation is decreased, the result is a calming effect. Figure 3-11 shows that BZDs, such as diazepam (Valium), clonazepam (Klonopin), and alprazolam (Xanax), bind to $GABA_A$ receptors with different alpha subunits. Alpha-2 subunits may be the most important for decreasing anxiety.

Since BZDs are nonselective for $GABA_A$ receptors with different alpha subunits, all can cause sedation at higher therapeutic doses. There are five BZDs approved by the U.S. Food and Drug Administration (FDA) for treatment of insomnia with a predominantly **hypnotic** (sleep-inducing) effect : flurazepam (Dalmane), temazepam (Restoril), triazolam (Halcion), estazolam (Prosom), and quazepam (Doral). Other BZDs, such as lorazepam (Ativan) and alprazolam (Xanax), reduce anxiety without being as soporific (sleep producing) at lower therapeutic doses.

The fact that the benzodiazepines potentiate the ability of GABA to inhibit neurons probably accounts for their efficacy as anticonvulsants and for their ability to reduce the neuronal overexcitement of alcohol withdrawal. When used alone, even at high dosages, these drugs rarely inhibit the brain to the degree that respiratory depression, coma, and death result. However, when combined with other CNS depressants, such as alcohol, opiates, or tricyclic antidepressants, the inhibitory actions of the benzodiazepines can lead to life-threatening CNS depression.

Any drug that inhibits electrical activity in the brain can interfere with motor ability, attention, and judgment. A patient taking BZDs must be cautioned about engaging in activities that could be dangerous if reflexes and attention are impaired, including specialized activities, such as working in construction, and more common activities, such as driving a car. In older adults, the use of BZDs may contribute to falls and broken bones. Ataxia is a common side effect secondary to the abundance of GABA receptors in the cerebellum.

Short-Acting Sedative-Hypnotic Sleep Agents

A newer class of hypnotics, termed the "Z-drugs," includes zolpidem (Ambien), zaleplon (Sonata), and eszopiclone (Lunesta). They have sedative effects without the anti-anxiety, anticonvulsant, or muscle relaxant effects of BZDs, and they demonstrate selectivity for $GABA_A$ receptors containing alpha-1 subunits. The drugs' affinity to α-1 subunits has the potential for amnestic

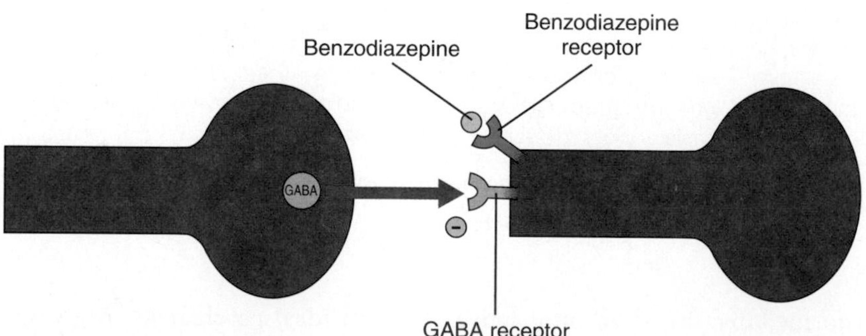

FIG 3-11 Action of the benzodiazepines. Drugs in this group attach to receptors adjacent to the receptors for the neurotransmitter γ-aminobutyric acid (GABA). Drug attachment to these receptors results in a strengthening of the inhibitory effects of GABA. In the absence of GABA there is no inhibitory effect of benzodiazepines.

and ataxic side effects, and the onset of action is faster than that of most BZDs. It is important to inform patients taking non-benzodiazepine hypnotic agents about the quick onset and to take them when they are ready to go to sleep.

Most of these drugs have short half-lives, which determine the duration of action. Eszopiclone has the longest duration of action (an average of 7-8 hours of sleep per therapeutic dose), while the other two are much shorter. Eszopiclone also has a unique side effect of an unpleasant taste upon awakening. Although tolerance and dependence are reportedly less than with BZDs, all of the BZDs and Z-hypnotics are categorized as schedule C-IV by the U.S. Drug Enforcement Administration (DEA).

Melatonin Receptor Agonists

Melatonin is a hormone that is only excreted at night as part of the normal circadian rhythm. Ramelteon (Rozerem) is a melatonin (MT) receptor agonist and acts much the same way as endogenous (i.e., naturally occurring) melatonin. It has a high selectivity and potency at the MT1 receptor site—which is thought to regulate sleepiness—and at the MT2 receptor site—which is thought to regulate circadian rhythms. This is one of two hypnotic medications approved for the treatment of insomnia that is not classified as a scheduled substance, or one having abuse potential, by the DEA. Side effects include headache and dizziness. Long-term use of ramelteon above therapeutic doses can lead to increased prolactin and associated side effects (e.g., sexual dysfunction).

Doxepin

Doxepin (Silenor) is the low-dose formulation (3 mg and 6 mg tablets) of the antidepressant doxepin. Silenor is labeled for the treatment of insomnia characterized by difficulty in maintaining sleep (Patel, 2011). Mechanism of action for its sedative effect is most likely from histamine-1 blockade. Patients with severe urinary retention or on MAOIs should avoid this medication. The use of other CNS depressants and sedating antihistamines should also be avoided. Silenor was mainly studied in the geriatric population, where it showed an improvement in total sleep duration with no significant decrease in time of sleep onset.

Buspirone

Buspirone (BuSpar) is a drug that reduces anxiety without having strong sedative-hypnotic properties. Because this agent does not leave the patient sleepy or sluggish, it is often much better tolerated than the benzodiazepines. It is not a CNS depressant and, thus, does not have as great a danger of interaction with other CNS depressants, such as alcohol. Also, there is not the potential for addiction that exists with benzodiazepines.

Although the mechanism of action of buspirone is not clearly understood, one possibility is illustrated in Figure 3-12. Buspirone seems to act as a partial serotonin agonist at the 5-HT_{1A} and 5-HT2 receptors; it also has a moderate affinity for D2 receptors, and effects include dizziness and insomnia.

Refer to Chapter 15 on anxiety disorders for a discussion of the adverse reactions, dosages, nursing implications, and patient and family teaching for the anti-anxiety drugs. Refer to Chapter 19 on sleep disorders for a more detailed discussion on medication to promote sleep.

Treating Anxiety Disorders with Antidepressants

The symptoms, neurotransmitters, and circuits associated with anxiety disorders overlap extensively with those of depressive disorders (refer to Chapters 14 and 15), and many antidepressants have proven to be effective treatments for anxiety disorders. Selective serotonin reuptake inhibitors (SSRIs) are often used to treat obsessive-compulsive disorder (OCD), social anxiety disorder (SAD), generalized anxiety disorder (GAD), and panic disorder (PD). Venlafaxine (Effexor XR), is used to treat GAD, SAD, and PD. Duloxetine (Cymbalta) has FDA approval for GAD.

Antidepressant Drugs

Our understanding of the neurophysiological basis of mood disorders is far from complete; however, a great deal of evidence

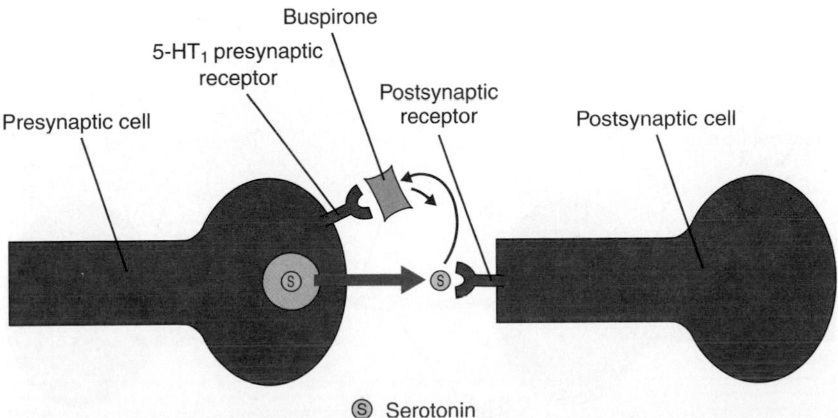

FIG 3-12 Action of buspirone. A proposed mechanism of action of buspirone is that it blocks feedback inhibition by serotonin. This leads to increased release of serotonin by the presynaptic cell. *5-HT1,* Serotonin.

seems to indicate that the neurotransmitters norepinephrine and serotonin play a major role in regulating mood. It is thought that a transmission deficiency of one or both of these monoamines within the limbic system underlies depression. One piece of evidence is that all of the drugs that show efficacy in the treatment of depression increase the synaptic level of one or both of these neurotransmitters. Figure 3-13 identifies the side effects of specific neurotransmitters being blocked or activated. Figure 3-14 illustrates the normal release, reuptake, and destruction of the monoamine neurotransmitters. A grasp of this underlying physiology is essential for understanding the mechanisms by which the antidepressant drugs are thought to act.

Three hypotheses of antidepressants' mechanism of action:

1. The *monoamine hypothesis of depression* suggests that there is a deficiency in one or more of the three neurotransmitters: serotonin, norepinephrine, or dopamine. The theory is that increasing these neurotransmitters alleviates depression.
2. The *monoamine receptor hypothesis of depression* suggests that low levels of neurotransmitters cause postsynaptic receptors to be up-regulated (increased in sensitivity or number). Increasing neurotransmitters by antidepressants results in down-regulation (desensitization) of key neurotransmitter receptors (Stahl, 2008). Delayed length of time for down-regulation may answer the question of why it takes so long

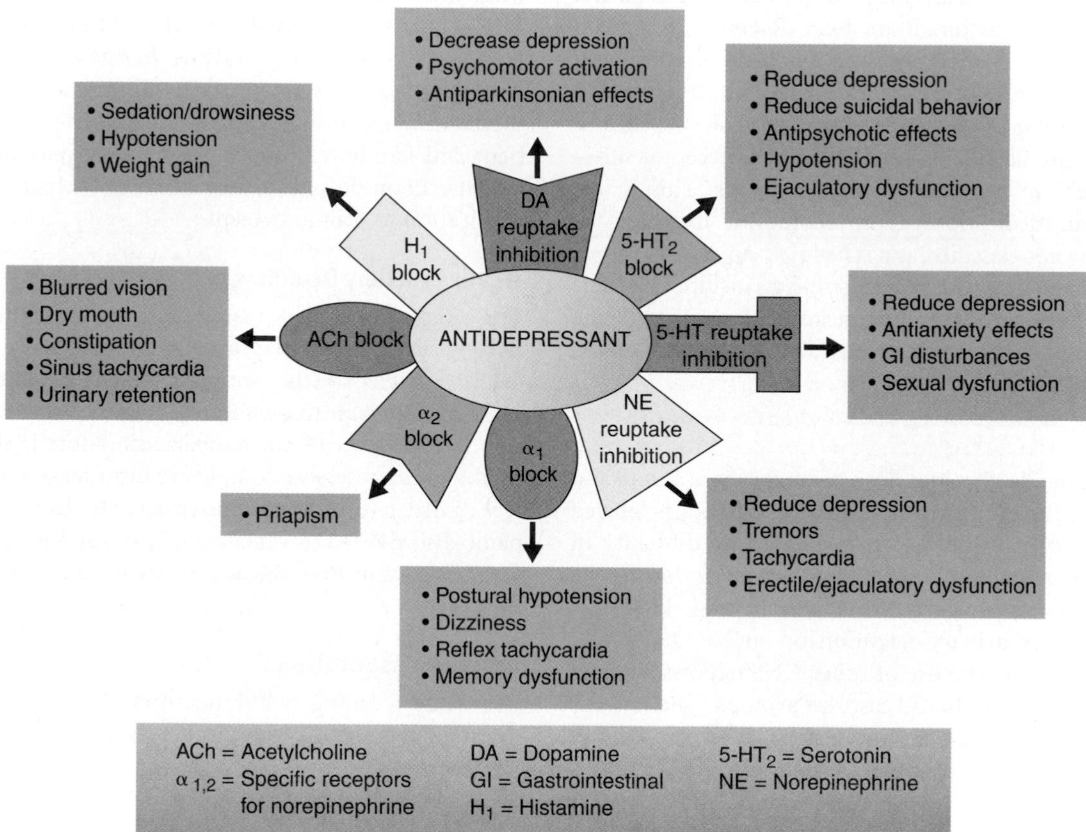

FIG 3-13 Possible effects of receptor binding of the antidepressant medications.

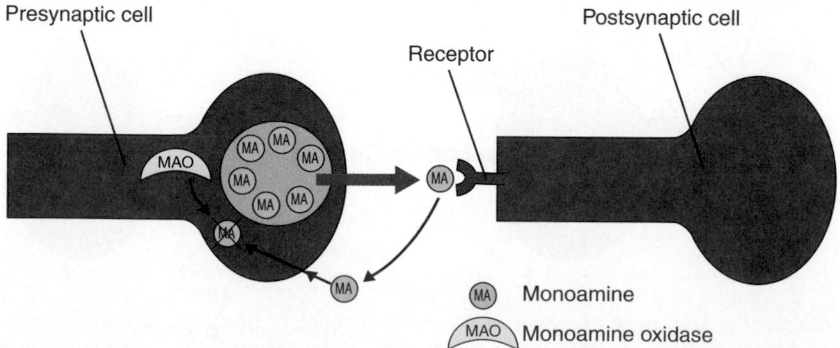

FIG 3-14 Normal release, reuptake, and destruction of the monoamine neurotransmitters.

for antidepressants to work, especially if they rapidly increase neurotransmitters.

3. Another hypothesis for the mechanism of antidepressant drugs is that with prolonged use they increase production of neurotrophic factors.These factors regulate the survival of neurons and enhance the sprouting of axons to form new synaptic connections (Stahl, 2008).

Tricyclic Antidepressants

Tricyclic antidepressants (TCAs) and heterocyclic antidepressants were widely used prior to the development of SSRIs. They are no longer first-line medications since they have more side effects, take longer to reach an optimal dose, and are far more lethal in overdose. The tricyclic antidepressants are thought to act primarily by blocking the reuptake of norepinephrine for the secondary amines (e.g., nortriptyline [Pamelor]) and both norepinephrine and serotonin for the tertiary amines (e.g., amitriptyline [Elavil], imipramine [Tofranil]). As shown in Figure 3-15, this blockage prevents norepinephrine from coming into contact with its degrading enzyme, MAO, and thus increases the level of norepinephrine at the synapse. Similarly, the tertiary tricyclic antidepressants block the reuptake and destruction of serotonin and increase the synaptic level of this neurotransmitter. Visit the Evolve website for a more thorough discussion of how tricyclic antidepressants work.

To varying degrees, many of the tricyclic drugs also block the muscarinic receptors that normally bind acetylcholine. As discussed in the previous section, this blockage leads to typical anticholinergic effects, such as blurred vision, dry mouth, tachycardia, urinary retention, and constipation. These adverse effects can be troubling to patients and limit their adherence to the regimen.

Depending on the individual drug, these agents can also block H1 receptors in the brain. Blockage of these receptors by any drug causes sedation and drowsiness, an unwelcome symptom in daily use (see Figure 3-13). Persons taking tricyclic antidepressants often have adherence issues because of their adverse reactions. Tricyclic antidepressant overdose can be fatal secondary to cardiac conduction disturbances from excessive sodium channel blockade.

Selective Serotonin Reuptake Inhibitors

As the name implies, the selective serotonin reuptake inhibitors (SSRIs), such as fluoxetine (Prozac), sertraline (Zoloft), paroxetine (Paxil), citalopram (Celexa), escitalopram (Lexapro), and fluvoxamine (Luvox), preferentially block the reuptake and the degradation of serotonin, but they each have different effects on neurotransmitters.

Fluoxetine is a 5-HT_{2C} antagonist, which can lead to the anorexic and antibulimic effects of fluoxetine at higher doses. Both sertraline and fluvoxamine have σ-1 receptor binding property. Sigma-1 action is not well understood but may contribute to antianxiety and antipsychotic actions.

Paroxetine is the most anticholinergic among the SSRIs due to its muscarinic-1 antagonist property. Although it is less anticholinergic than the tricyclic antidepressants, paroxetine may not be the best choice for patients with contraindications with anticholinergic agents (e.g., narrow angle glaucoma). Citalopram has R- and S-enantiomers. At lower doses, the R-isomer may inhibit the increased 5-HT effects of the S-isomer leading to inconsistent efficacy. Escitalopram has the S-enantiomer only without the R-enantiomer, which explains its more predictable efficacy at lower doses (Stahl, 2008).

SSRIs, as a group, have less ability to block the muscarinic and histamine$_1$ (H_1) receptors than do the tricyclic antidepressants. As a result of their more selective action, they seem to show comparable efficacy without eliciting the anticholinergic and sedating side effects that limit patient compliance. However, SSRIs have other side effects resulting from stimulation of different 5-HT receptors. Stimulation of the 5-HT_{2A} and 5-HT_{2C} receptors in the spinal cord may inhibit the spinal reflexes of orgasm, while stimulation of the 5-HT_{2A} receptors in the mesocortical area may decrease dopamine activity in this area, leading to apathy and low libido. Stimulation of the 5-HT_3 receptors in the hypothalamus or brainstem may cause nausea or vomiting, while gastrointestional (GI) side effects are secondary to the 5-HT_3 and/or 5-HT_4 receptors in the GI tract (Stahl, 2008) (Figure 3-16). Visit the Evolve website for a more detailed explanation of how the SSRIs work.

Serotonin-Norepinephrine Reuptake Inhibitors

Serotonin-norepinephrine reuptake inhibitors (SNRIs) medications increase both serotonin and norepinephrine. Venlafaxine (Effexor) is more of a serotonergic agent at lower therapeutic doses, and norepinephrine reuptake blockade occurs at higher doses, leading to the dual SNRI action. Hypertension may be

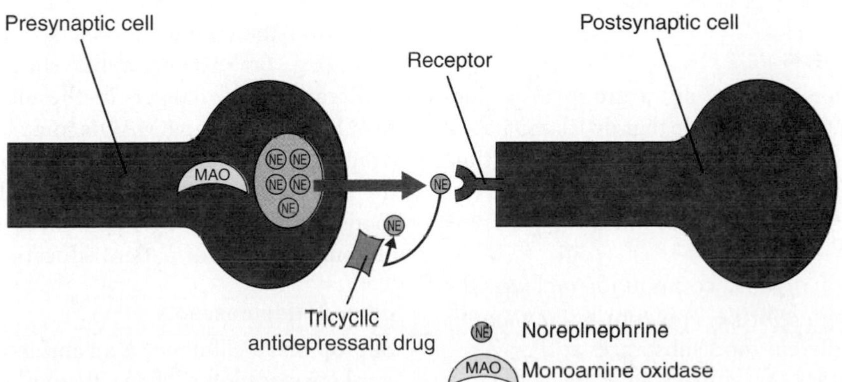

FIG 3-15 How the tricyclic antidepressants block the reuptake of norepinephrine.

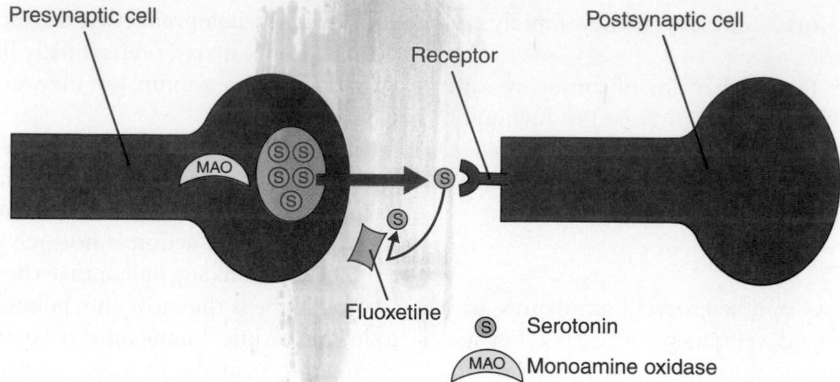

FIG 3-16 How the selective serotonin reuptake inhibitors (SSRIs) work.

induced in about 5% of patients is a dose-dependent effect based on norepinephrine reuptake blockade. Doses higher than 150 mg/day can increase diastolic blood pressure about 7-10 mm Hg.

Desvenlafaxine (Pristiq) is a metabolite of venlafaxine. When normal metabolizers take venlafaxine, the majority of the benefit comes from venlafaxine being metabolized into desvenlafaxine. Therefore, the mechanism of actions and effects of the two antidepressants are very similar.

Duloxetine (Cymbalta) is an SNRI indicated for both depression and GAD as well as diabetic peripheral neuropathy and fibromyalgia. Like the tricyclic antidepressants, many of the SNRIs also have therapeutic effects on neuropathic pain. The common underlying mechanism of neuropathic pain is nerve injury or dysfunction. The mechanism by which tricyclic antidepressants and SNRIs reduce neuropathic pain is activating the descending norepinephrine and 5-HT pathways to the spinal cord, thereby limiting pain signals ascending to the brain.

Serotonin-Norepinephrine Disinhibitors

The class of drugs described as serotonin-norepinephrine disinhibitors (SNDIs) is represented by only one drug, mirtazapine (Remeron), which increases norepinephrine and serotonin transmission by antagonizing (blocking) presynaptic alpha-2 noradrenergic receptors. Mirtazapine offers both antianxiety and antidepressant effects with minimal sexual dysfunction and improved sleep. This antidepressant is particularly suited for the patient with nausea because it is an antiemetic. The most common side effects are sedation and weight gain secondary to potent H_1 blockade and 5-HT_{2C} blockade (Stahl, 2008).

Monoamine Oxidase Inhibitors

Monoamine oxidase inhibitors (MAOIs) are a group of antidepressant drugs that illustrate the principle that drugs can have a desired and beneficial effect in the brain while at the same time having possibly dangerous effects elsewhere in the body. To understand the action of these drugs, keep in mind the following definitions:

- Monoamines: a type of organic compound; includes the neurotransmitters norepinephrine, epinephrine, dopamine, serotonin, and many different food substances and drugs
- Monoamine oxidase (MAO): an enzyme that destroys monoamines
- Monoamine oxidase inhibitors (MAOIs): drugs that prevent the destruction of monoamines by inhibiting the action of MAO

Monoamine neurotransmitters, as well as any monoamine food substance or drugs, are degraded (destroyed) by the enzyme MAO, which is located in neurons and in the liver. Antidepressant drugs such as isocarboxazid (Marplan), phenelzine (Nardil), selegiline (EMSAM), and tranylcypromine (Parnate), are MAOIs. They act by inhibiting the enzyme and interfering with the destruction of the monoamine neurotransmitters, thereby leaving more of them available. This in turn increases the synaptic level of the neurotransmitters and makes possible the antidepressant effects of these drugs (Figure 3-17). Visit the Evolve website for a more comprehensive explanation of how MAOIs work.

The problem with inhibiting MAO is that this enzyme is also used by the liver to degrade monoamine substances that enter the body through food. One monoamine, tyramine, is present in many food substances, such as aged cheeses, pickled or smoked fish, and wine. If the liver cannot break down the tyramine from these substances, it can produce significant vasoconstriction resulting in an elevation in blood pressure and the threat of hypertension.

In addition to food, a substantial number of drugs, such as other antidepressants and sympathomimetic drugs, are chemically monoamines. Dosages of these drugs are affected by the rate at which MAO destroys them in the liver. In a patient taking drugs to inhibit MAO, the blood level of monoamine drugs can reach high levels and cause serious toxicity. Thus, MAOIs are contraindicated with concurrent use of any other antidepressants and sympathomimetic drugs. Concurrent use with some over-the-counter products with sympathomimetic properties (e.g., oral decongestants) should be avoided.

Because of the dangers that result from inhibition of hepatic MAO, patients taking MAOIs must be given a list of foods and drugs that need to be avoided. Chapter 14 discusses the treatment of depression and contains a list of foods to avoid and foods to be taken in moderation, along with nursing measures and instructions for patient education.

Other Antidepressants

Bupropion (Wellbutrin) is an antidepressant that is also used for smoking cessation (Zyban). It seems to act as a norepinephrine-dopamine reuptake inhibitor and also inhibits nicotinic

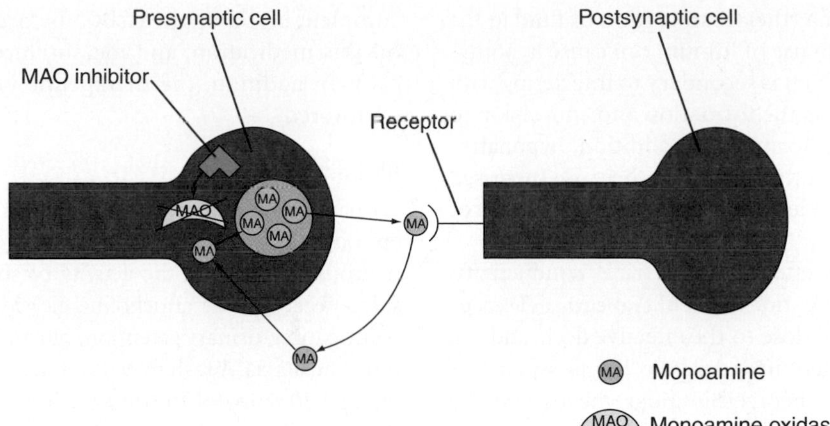

FIG 3-17 Blocking of monoamine oxidase (MAO) by inhibiting agents (MAOIs), which prevents the breakdown of monoamine by MAO.

acetylcholine receptors to reduce the addictive action of nicotine. With no 5HT activities, it does not cause sexual side effects. Side effects include insomnia, tremor, anorexia, and weight loss. It is contraindicated in patients with a seizure disorder, in patients with a current or prior diagnosis of bulimia or anorexia nervosa, and in patients undergoing abrupt discontinuation of alcohol or sedatives (including benzodiazepines) due to the potential of seizures.

Vilazodone (Viibryd) is a newer antidepressant, approved by the FDA in January 2011. The mechanism of action includes enhancing the release of serotonin by inhibiting the serotonin transporter (similar to SSRIs) and by stimulating serotonin (5-HT_{1A}) receptors via partial agonism (similar to the anxiolytic medication buspirone). With this dual activity, vilazodone is considered to be a serotonin partial agonist–reuptake inhibitor (SPARI). Commonly observed adverse reactions during clinical trials included diarrhea, nausea, insomnia, and vomiting. This antidepressant should be taken with food for better bioavailability, and nighttime doses should be avoided due to insomnia.

Antidepressants that can cause insomnia should be noted since patients may have drug-induced insomnia. Medications prescribed BID dosing are often interpreted by patients as taking the medication in the morning and at night, which can cause insomnia (e.g., bupropion BID). When the prescription is for QD administration (e.g.., vilazodone QD), without specifying taking it at morning or night, patients may choose the administration time that is most convenient for them without knowing the possible drug-induced insomnia.

Trazodone was not used for antidepressant treatment for many years, but was often given, along with another agent, for the treatment of insomnia, as sedation is one of the common side effects. In 2010 a trademarked version, Oleptro, was FDA-approved as an extended-release drug indicated for the use of major depressive disorder in adults. Its antidepressant effects are due to its action as a 5-HT reuptake inhibitor and 5-$HT_{2A/2C}$ antagonist. The common side effects are sedation and orthostatic hypotension. Its sedative effect is from potent H_1 blockade, and orthostasis is from α-1 blockade.

Mood Stabilizers

Lithium

Although the efficacy of **lithium** (Eskalith, Lithobid) as a **mood stabilizer** in patients with bipolar (manic-depressive) disorder has been established for many years, its mechanism of action is still far from understood. As a positively charged ion, similar in structure to sodium and potassium, lithium may well act by affecting electrical conductivity in neurons.

As discussed earlier, an electrical impulse consists of the inward, depolarizing flow of sodium followed by an outward, repolarizing flow of potassium. These electrical charges are propagated along the neuron so that, if they are initiated at one end of the neuron, they will pass to the other end. Once they reach the end of a neuron, a neurotransmitter is released.

It may be that an overexcitement of neurons in the brain underlies bipolar disorder and that lithium interacts in some complex way with sodium and potassium at the cell membrane to stabilize electrical activity. Also, lithium may reduce excitatory neurotransmitter glutamate and exert an antimanic effect. The other mechanisms by which lithium work to regulate mood include the noncompetitive inhibition of the enzyme inositol monophosphatase. Inhibition of 5-HT autoreceptors by lithium is more related to lithium's antidepressant effects rather than its antimanic effects.

While we do not know exactly how lithium works, we are certain that its influence on electrical conductivity results in adverse effects and toxicity. By altering electrical conductivity, lithium represents a potential threat to all body functions that are regulated by electrical currents. Foremost among these functions is cardiac contraction; lithium can induce, although not commonly, sinus bradycardia. Extreme alteration of cerebral conductivity with overdose can lead to convulsions. Alteration in nerve and muscle conduction can commonly lead to tremor at therapeutic doses or more extreme motor dysfunction with overdose.

Sodium and potassium play a strong role in regulating fluid balance, and the distribution of fluid in various body compartments explains the disturbances in fluid balance that can be caused by lithium. These include polyuria (the output of large volumes of urine) and edema (the accumulation of fluid in the interstitial space). Long-term use of lithium can cause hypothyroidism in some patients, which is secondary to interfering with the iodine molecules affecting the formation and conversion to its active form (T3) thyroid hormone. In addition, hyponatremia can increase the risk of lithium toxicity because increased renal reabsorption of sodium leads to increased reabsorption of lithium as well.

Primarily because of its effects on electrical conductivity, lithium has a low therapeutic index. The **therapeutic index** represents the ratio of the lethal dose to the effective dose, and is a measure of overall drug safety in regards to the possibility of overdose or toxicity. A low therapeutic index means that the blood level of a drug that can cause death is not far above the blood level required for drug effectiveness. Blood level of lithium needs to be monitored on a regular basis to be sure that the drug is not accumulating and rising to dangerous levels. Table 3-3 lists some of the adverse effects of lithium. Chapter 13 considers lithium treatment in more depth and discusses specific dosage-related adverse and toxic effects, nursing implications, and the patient teaching plan.

Anticonvulsant Drugs

Valproate (available as divalproex sodium [Depakote] and valproic acid [Depakene]), carbamazepine (Tegretol), and lamotrigine (Lamictal) have demonstrated efficacy in the treatment of bipolar disorders (APA, 2008). Their anticonvulsant properties derive from the alteration of electrical conductivity in membranes; in particular, they reduce the firing rate of very-high-frequency neurons in the brain. It is possible that this membrane-stabilizing effect accounts for the ability of these drugs to reduce the mood swings that occur in patients with bipolar disorders. Other proposed mechanisms as mood stabilizers are glutamate antagonists and GABA agonist.

Valproate

Valproate (Depakote and Depakene) is structurally different from other anticonvulsants and psychiatric drugs that show efficacy in the treatment of bipolar disorder. Divalproex is recommended for mixed episodes and has been found useful for rapid cycling. Common side effects include tremor, weight gain, and sedation. Occasional serious side effects are thrombocytopenia, pancreatitis, hepatic failure, and birth defects. Baseline levels are measured for liver function indicators and complete blood count (CBC) before an individual is started on this medication, and measurements are repeated periodically. In addition, the therapeutic blood level of the drug is monitored.

Carbamazepine

Carbamazepine (Tegretol) is useful in preventing mania during episodes of acute mania. It reduces the firing rate of overexcited neurons by reducing the activity of sodium channels. Common side effects include anticholinergic side effects (e.g., dry mouth, constipation, urinary retention, blurred vision), orthostasis, sedation, and ataxia. A rash may occur in about 10% of patients during the first 20 weeks of treatment. This potentially serious side effect should be reported immediately to the care provide because it could progress to a life-threatening exfoliative dermatitis or Stevens-Johnson syndrome (Martinez, Marangell, & Martinez, 2011). Recommended baseline laboratory work includes liver function tests, CBC, electrocardiogram, and electrolyte levels. Blood levels are monitored to avoid toxicity (> 12 mcg/mL), but there are no established therapeutic blood levels for carbamazepine in the treatment of bipolar disorder.

Lamotrigine

Lamotrigine (Lamictal) is approved by the FDA for maintenance therapy of bipolar disorder, but it is not effective in acute mania. Lamotrigine works well in treating the depression of bipolar disorder with less incidence of switching the patient into mania than antidepressants. It modulates the release of glutamate and aspartate. Patients should promptly report any rashes, which could be a sign of life-threatening Stevens-Johnson syndrome. This can be minimized by slow titration to therapeutic doses.

Other Anticonvulsants

Other anticonvulsants used as mood stabilizers are gabapentin (Neurontin), topiramate (Topamax), and oxcarbazepine (Trileptal). None of them has FDA approval as a mood stabilizer, and studies to support their use as primary treatments for bipolar disorder are lacking. Antipsychotic medications and antianxiety medications, such as clonazepam (Klonopin) are used for their calming effects during mania. Refer to Chapter 13 for a more detailed discussion of these medications.

Antipsychotic Drugs

First-Generation Antipsychotics

The first generation of antipsychotic drugs is also referred to as **conventional antipsychotics**, *typical antipsychotics*, and *standard antipsychotics*. These drugs are strong **antagonists** (blocking the action) of the D_2 receptors for dopamine. By binding to these receptors and blocking the attachment of dopamine, they reduce dopaminergic transmission. It has been postulated that an overactivity of the dopamine system in certain areas of the mesolimbic system may be responsible for at least some of the symptoms of schizophrenia; thus, blockage of dopamine may reduce these symptoms. This is thought to be particularly true of the "positive" symptoms of schizophrenia, such as delusions (e.g., paranoid and grandiose ideas) and hallucinations

TABLE 3-3 ADVERSE EFFECTS OF LITHIUM

SYSTEM	ADVERSE EFFECTS
Nervous and muscular	Tremor, ataxia, confusion, convulsions
Digestive	Nausea, vomiting, diarrhea
Cardiac	Arrhythmias
Fluid and electrolyte	Polyuria, polydipsia, edema
Endocrine	Goiter and hypothyroidism

(e.g., hearing or seeing things not present in reality). Refer to Chapter 12 for a more detailed discussion of schizophrenia and its symptoms.

These drugs are also antagonists—to varying degrees—of the muscarinic receptors for acetylcholine, α_1 receptors for norepinephrine, and histamine$_1$ (H_1) receptors for histamine. Although it is unclear if this antagonism plays a role in the beneficial effects of the drugs, it is certain that antagonism is responsible for some of their major side effects (refer to Chapter 12).

Figure 3-18 illustrates the proposed mechanism of action of the first generation antipsychotics, which include the phenothiazines, thioxanthenes, butyrophenones, and pharmacologically related agents. As summarized in Figure 3-19, many of the untoward side effects of these drugs can be understood as a logical extension of their receptor-blocking activity. Because dopamine (D_2) in the basal ganglia plays a major role in the regulation of movement, it is not surprising that dopamine blockage can lead to motor abnormalities (extrapyramidal side effects), such as parkinsonism, akinesia, akathisia, dyskinesia, and tardive dyskinesia.

Nurses and physicians often monitor patients for evidence of involuntary movements after administration of the first generation antipsychotic agents. One popular scale is called the Abnormal Involuntary Movement Scale (AIMS). Refer to Chapter 12 for an example AIMS and a discussion of the clinical use of antipsychotic drugs, side effects, specific nursing interventions, and patient teaching strategies.

An important physiological function of dopamine is that it acts as the hypothalamic factor that inhibits the release of prolactin from the anterior pituitary gland; thus, blockage of dopamine transmission can lead to increased pituitary secretion of prolactin. In women, this hyperprolactinemia can result in amenorrhea (absence of the menses) or galactorrhea (breast milk flow), and in men, it can lead to gynecomastia (development of the male mammary glands).

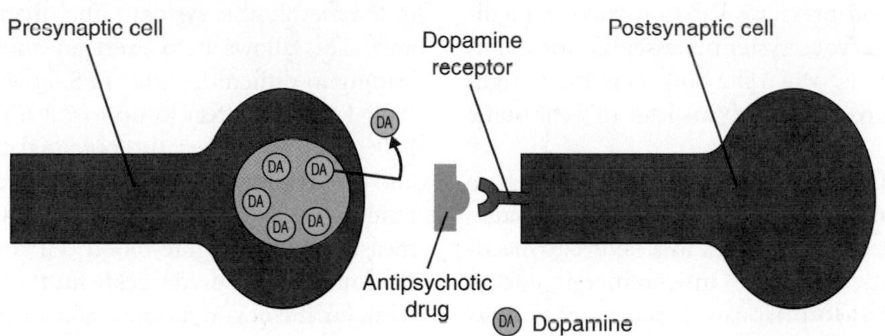

FIG 3-18 How the first generation antipsychotics block dopamine receptors.

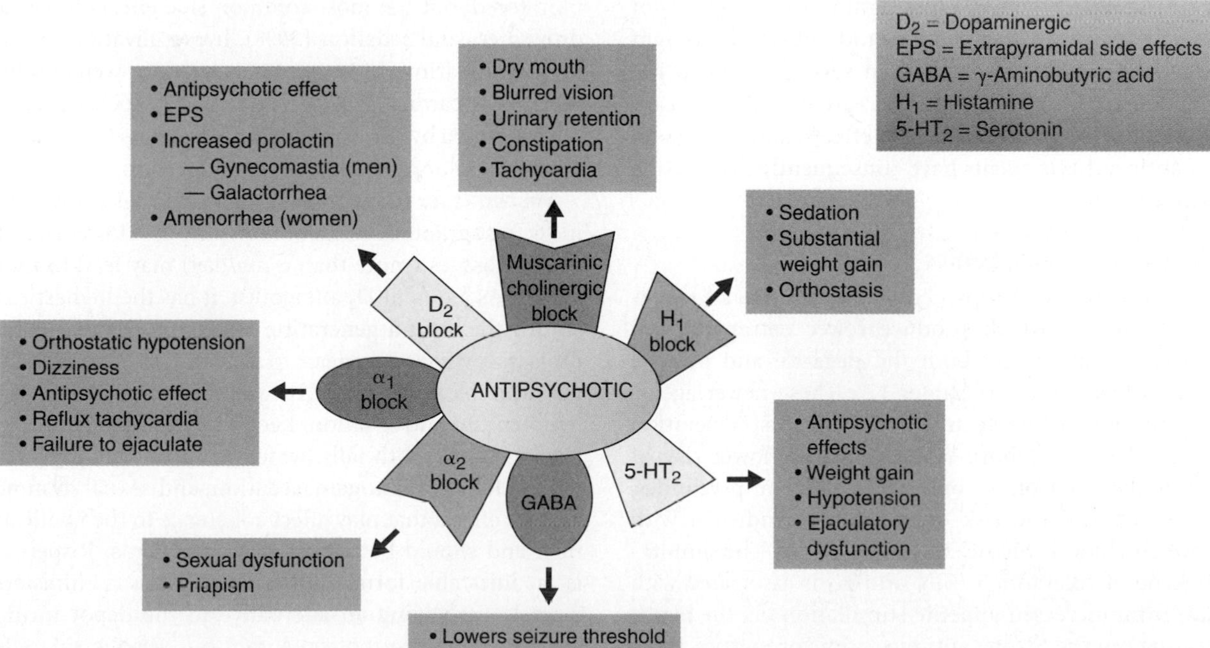

FIG 3-19 Adverse effects of receptor blockage of antipsychotic agents. (From Varcarolis, E. [2004]. *Manual of psychiatric nursing care plans* [2nd ed.]. St. Louis, MO: Elsevier.)

Acetylcholine is the neurotransmitter released by the postganglionic neurons of the parasympathetic nervous system. Through its attachment to muscarinic receptors on internal organs, it serves to help regulate internal function. Blockage of the muscarinic receptors by phenothiazines and a wide variety of other psychiatric drugs can lead to a constellation of untoward effects, which are predictable based on knowledge of the normal physiology of the parasympathetic nervous system. These side effects usually involve blurred vision, dry mouth, constipation, and urinary hesitancy. These drugs can also impair memory since acetylcholine is important for memory function.

In addition to blocking dopamine and muscarinic receptors, many of the first-generation antipsychotic drugs act as antagonists at the α_1 receptors for norepinephrine. These receptors are found on smooth muscle cells that contract in response to norepinephrine from sympathetic nerves. For example, the ability of sympathetic nerves to constrict blood vessels is dependent on the attachment of norepinephrine to α_1 receptors; thus, blockage of these receptors can bring about vasodilatation and a consequent drop in blood pressure. Vasoconstriction mediated by the sympathetic nervous system is essential for maintaining normal blood pressure when the body is in the upright position; blockage of the α_1 receptors can lead to orthostatic hypotension.

The α_1 receptors are also found on the vas deferens and are responsible for the propulsive contractions leading to ejaculation. Blockage of these receptors can lead to a failure to ejaculate. Potent α_1 antagonists with little anticholinergic effects, such as trazodone, can lead to priapism, a painful prolonged erection that is caused by the inability for detumesence (subsidence of erection).

Finally, many of these first generation antipsychotic agents, as well as a variety of other psychiatric drugs, block the H_1 receptors for histamine. The two most significant side effects of blocking these receptors are sedation and substantial weight gain. The sedation may be beneficial in severely agitated patients. Nonadherence to the medication regimen is a significant issue because of these troublesome side effects, and the second generation antipsychotic agents have consequently become the drugs of choice.

Second-Generation Antipsychotics

The second generation of antipsychotic drugs is also known as atypical antipsychotics, which produce fewer extrapyramidal side effects (EPS) and target both the negative and positive symptoms of schizophrenia (Chapter 12). These newer agents are often chosen as first-line treatments over the first-generation antipsychotics described above because of their lower risk of EPS. Most of the available second-generation antipsychotics, however, can increase the risk of metabolic syndrome with increased weight, blood glucose, and triglycerides. The simultaneous blockade of receptors 5-HT_{2C} and H_1 is associated with weight gain from increased appetite stimulation via the hypothalamic eating centers. Strong antimuscarinic properties at the M3 receptor on the pancreatic beta cells can cause insulin resistance leading to hyperglycemia. The receptor responsible for elevated triglycerides is currently unknown (Stahl, 2008). Clozapine and olanzapine have the highest risk of causing metabolic syndrome while aripiprazole and ziprasidone have the lowest risk.

The second generation antipsychotics are predominantly D_2 (dopamine) and 5-HT_{2A} (serotonin) antagonists (blockers). The blockade at the mesolimbic dopamine pathway decreases psychosis, similar to the mechanism by which the first-generation antipsychotics work. Decreasing D_2 can decrease psychosis but cause adverse effects elsewhere. Decreased D_2 in the nigrostriatal area can cause the movement side effects of EPS; decreased D_2 in the mesocortical area can worsen cognitive and negative symptoms of schizophrenia; decreased D_2 in the tuberoinfundibular area can increase the hormone prolactin leading to gynecomastia, galactorrhea, amenorrhea, and low libido (Stahl, 2008).

Clozapine. Clozapine (Clozaril) is an antipsychotic drug that is relatively free of the motor side effects of the phenothiazines and other second-generation antipsychotics. It is thought that clozapine preferentially blocks the dopamine 1 and 2 receptors in the mesolimbic system rather than those in the nigrostriatal area. This allows it to exert an antipsychotic action without leading to difficulties with EPS; however, it can cause a potentially fatal side effect in up to 0.8% of patients (McEvoy et al., 2006). Clozapine has the potential to suppress bone marrow and induce agranulocytosis. Any deficiency in white blood cells renders a person prone to serious infection; therefore, regular measurement of white blood cell count is required. Typically, the count is measured weekly for the first 6 months, every other week for the next 6 months, and every month thereafter.

Clozapine has the potential for inducing convulsions, a dose-related side effect, in 3.5% of patients. Caution should be used with other drugs that can increase the concentration of clozapine. There is also a potential for myocarditis that should be monitored, but the most common side effects of clozapine are drowsiness and sedation (39%), hypersalivation (31%) caused by its muscarinic M4 receptor activation, weight gain (31%), reflex tachycardia (25%) caused by M2 blockade, constipation (14%) caused by M1 blockade, and dizziness (19%) caused by α_1 blockade (Clozapine prescribing information, 2008).

Risperidone. Risperidone (Risperdal) has a low potential for inducing agranulocytosis or convulsions. However, high therapeutic dosages (more than 6 mg/day) may lead to motor difficulties. As a potent D_2 antagonist, it has the highest risk of EPS among the second-generation antipsychotics and may increase prolactin, which may lead to sexual dysfunction. Because risperidone blocks α_1 and H_1 receptors, it can cause orthostatic hypotension and sedation. Keep in mind that orthostatic hypotension can lead to falls, which are a serious problem among older adults. Weight gain, sedation, and sexual dysfunction are adverse effects that may affect adherence to the medication regimen and should be discussed with patients. Risperdal Consta is an injectable form of the drug that is administered every 2 weeks, providing an alternative to the depot form of first-generation antipsychotics. A rare but serious side effect is an increased risk of cerebrovascular accidents in older adults with dementia who are being treated for agitation.

Quetiapine. Quetiapine (Seroquel) has a broad receptor-binding profile. Its strong blockage of H_1 receptors accounts for the high sedation. The combination of H_1 and $5\text{-}HT_{2C}$ blockage leads to the weight gain associated with use of this drug and also to a moderate risk for metabolic syndrome. It causes moderate blockage of α_1 receptors and associated orthostasis. Quetiapine has a low risk for EPS or prolactin elevation from low D_2 binding due to rapid dissociation at D_2 receptors.

Other Second-Generation Antipsychotics

- Olanzapine is similar to clozapine in chemical structure. It is an antagonist of $5\text{-}HT_2$, D_2, H_1, α_1, and muscarinic receptors. Side effects include sedation, weight gain, hyperglycemia with new-onset type II diabetes, and higher risk for metabolic syndrome. Olanzapine is also available in a long-acting intramuscular agent under the trade name of Zyprexa Relprevv).
- Ziprasidone is a serotonin-norepinephrine reuptake inhibitor that also binds to multiple receptors: $5\text{-}HT_2$, D_2, α_1, and H_{1D}. The serotonin-norepinephrine reuptake inhibition and the binding to H_{1D} explain its potential antidepressant effects. The main side effects are dizziness and moderate sedation. Ziprasidone is contraindicated in patients with a known history of QT interval prolongation, recent acute myocardial infarction, or uncompensated heart failure.
- Aripiprazole is a unique second-generation antipsychotic known as a dopamine system stabilizer. It is a partial agonist at the D_2 receptor. In areas of the brain with excess dopamine, it lowers the dopamine level by acting as a receptor antagonist; however, in regions with low dopamine, it stimulates receptors to raise the dopamine level. Aripiprazole lacks H_1 and $5\text{-}HT_{2C}$ properties, which explains its lack of sedation and weight gain. Side effects include insomnia and akathisia.
- Paliperidone is the major active metabolite of risperidone. It has similar side effects such as EPS and prolactin elevation. Other than the D_2 and $5\text{-}HT_{2A}$ antagonistic properties as an antipsychotic, paliperidone is also an antagonist at α-1 receptors and H_1 receptors, which explains the side effects of orthostasis and sedation. The Osmotic Release Oral System (OROS) provides consistent 24-hour release of medication, leading to minimal peaks and troughs in plasma concentrations.
- Iloperidone (Fanapt), lurasidone (Latuda), and asenapine (Saphris) are the most recently approved second-generation antipsychotics in the United States.
- Iloperidone's therapeutic effects are also from the combination of D_2 and $5HT_{2A}$ blockade. Iloperidone possesses minimal binding affinity for histamine-1 receptors and has minimal affinity for cholinergic muscarinic receptors. The most common adverse effects are dizziness, dry mouth, somnolence, and dyspepsia. There was a significant increase in the mean QTc interval although no deaths or serious arrhythmias were noted in the clinical trials. Limitations to use of this medication include the risk of orthostatic hypotension and QT prolongation (Holmes, 2012)
- Lurasidone has high affinity for D_2 and $5\text{-}HT_{2A}$ receptors in addition to other serotonergic receptors such as $5\text{-}HT_{1A}$. It also has high affinity for noradrenaline receptors. It is recommended that lurasidone be administered with food to increase its bioavailability. Adverse effects include akathisia, nausea, sedation, and somnolence. Parkinsonism and agitation were also frequently reported in clinical trials (Holmes, 2012).
- Asenapine has similar pharmacological properties to the tetracyclic antidepressant mirtazapine. Asenapine has high affinity for serotonergic (such as $5HT_{2A}$ and $5HT_{2C}$), noradrenergic, and dopaminergic receptors (D_3 and D_4). There is minimal muscarinic receptor activity. Bioavailability of asenapine is reduced from 35% with sublingual administration to less than 2% with oral administration. Avoidance of food and water for 10 minutes following sublingual administration should be noted (Holmes, 2012). Adverse effects include akathisia, oral hypoesthesia (decreased oral sensitivity), and somnolence.

Third-Generation Antipsychotic

Aripiprazole (Abilify) is a unique antipsychotic known as a dopamine system stabilizer. It is a partial agonist at the D_2 receptor. In areas of the brain with excess dopamine, it lowers the dopamine level by acting as a receptor antagonist; however, in regions with low dopamine, it stimulates receptors to raise the dopamine level. Aripiprazole lacks H_1 and $5\text{-}HT_{2C}$ properties, which explains its lack of sedation and weight gain. Side effects include insomnia and akathisia.

Chapter 12 discusses the first-generation and second-generation antipsychotic drugs in detail, including the indications for use, adverse reactions, nursing implications, and patient and family teaching.

Drug Treatment for Attention Deficit Hyperactivity Disorder

Children and adults with attention deficit hyperactivity disorder (ADHD) show symptoms of short attention span, impulsivity, and overactivity. Paradoxically, psychostimulant drugs are the mainstay of treatment for this condition in children and increasingly in adults. Both methylphenidates (Ritalin and Daytrana, a transdermal system) and dextroamphetamines (Adderall and Vyvanse) are helpful in these conditions. They are sympathomimetic amines and have been shown to function as direct and indirect agonists at adrenergic receptor sites. Psychostimulants act directly at the postsynaptic receptor by mimicking the effects of norepinephrine or dopamine, blocking the reuptake of norepinephrine and dopamine into the presynaptic neuron, and increasing the release of these monoamines into the extraneuronal space. How this translates into clinical efficacy is far from understood, but it is thought that the monoamines may inhibit an overactive part of the limbic system.

Among many concerns with the use of psychostimulant drugs are side effects of agitation, exacerbation of psychotic thought processes, hypertension, and growth suppression, as well as their potential for abuse. The FDA has approved three non-stimulants for the treatment of ADHD: atomoxetine (Strattera), guanfacine (Intuniv), and clonidine (Kapvay). Atomoxetine is a norepinephrine reuptake inhibitor approved for use in children 6 years and older. Common side effects include decreased appetite and weight loss, fatigue, and dizziness. It is contraindicated for patients with severe cardiovascular disease due to its potential to increase blood pressure and heart rate.

Guanfacine and clonidine are centrally acting alpha$_2$ adrenergic agonists that have traditionally been used for hypertension. The FDA approved forms for ADHD are used in children ages 6 to 17. Both should be increased slowly and should not be discontinued abruptly. Guanfacine's most common side effects include sleepiness, trouble sleeping, low blood pressure, nausea, stomach pain, and dizziness. The drug's effectiveness with teenagers is questionable, and it probably works best in pre-teens. Clonidine extended-release tablets can be used alone or in addition to other ADHD drugs. Common side effects include fatigue, irritability, throat pain, insomnia, nightmares, emotional disorder, constipation, increased body temperature, dry mouth, and ear pain.

Drug Treatment for Alzheimer's Disease

The insidious and progressive loss of memory and other higher brain functions brought about by Alzheimer's disease is a great individual, family, and social tragedy. Because the disease seems to involve progressive structural degeneration of the brain, there are two major pharmacological directions in its treatment. The first is to attempt to prevent or slow the structural degeneration. Although actively pursued, this approach has been unsuccessful so far. The second is to attempt to maintain normal brain function for as long as possible.

Much of the memory loss in this disease has been attributed to insufficient acetylcholine, a neurotransmitter essential for learning, memory, and mood and behavior regulation. One class of drugs for Alzheimer's disease, **acetylcholinesterase inhibitors,** shows some efficacy in slowing the rate of memory loss and even improving memory. They work by inactivating the enzyme that breaks down acetylcholine, acetylcholinesterase, leading to less destruction of acetylcholine and, therefore, a higher concentration at the synapse. Four of the FDA-approved drugs for treatment of Alzheimer's disease are acetylcholinesterase inhibitors: tacrine (Cognex), donepezil (Aricept), galantamine (Razadyne, formerly named Reminyl), and rivastigmine (Exelon). Tacrine is no longer used extensively because of the risk of hepatic toxicity. These drugs are used for mild to moderate Alzheimer's and become less effective as the brain produces less acetylcholine.

Glutamate, an abundant excitatory neurotransmitter, plays an important role in memory function; however, too much glutamate is thought to be destructive to neurons. A fifth agent approved by the FDA for treatment of Alzheimer's disease is memantine, or Namenda and Namenda XR (an extended-release option), named for the receptor it blocks from glutamate, N-methyl-D-aspartate (NMDA). Normally, when glutamate binds to NMDA receptors, calcium flows freely and is essential to cell communication; however, pathological gray tangles of amyloid protein that build up in Alzheimer's brains, or amyloid plaques, are associated with excess glutamate. This excess glutamate results in excess calcium, which becomes toxic to surrounding brain cells. Memantine fills some of the NMDA receptor sites, reduces glutamate binding and calcium excess, and lessens damage. Memantine was shown to be effective in the treatment of moderate to severe Alzheimer's disease. Since memantine has a very different mechanism of action than the acetylcholinesterase inhibitors, they can be taken at the same time.

Refer to Chapter 23 for a more detailed discussion of these drugs as well as their nursing considerations and patient and family teaching.

Herbal Treatments

The growing interest in medicinal herbs is driven by a variety of factors. Many people believe that herbal treatments are safer because they are "natural" or that they may have fewer side effects than more costly traditional medications.

Herbal treatments have been researched in order to understand their mechanisms of action and have also been used in clinical trials to determine their safety and efficacy. This is especially true of St. John's wort. Many medicinal herbs have been found to be nontherapeutic and some even deadly if taken over long periods of time or in combination with other chemical substances and prescription drugs. The risk of bleeding may be increased in patients taking ginkgo biloba and warfarin, and kava may increase the risk of hepatotoxicity.

Among the major concerns of health care professionals are the potential long-term effects (e.g., nerve, kidney, and liver damage) of some herbal agents and the possibility of adverse chemical reactions when herbal agents are taken in conjunction with other substances, including conventional medications.

St. John's wort can have serious interactions with a number of conventional medications. Taking St. John's wort with other serotonergic agents (e.g., SSRIs, triptans) can cause serotonin syndrome. It may also reduce the effectiveness of other medications by increasing their rate of metabolism and reducing blood levels of these medications. St. John's wort is a cytochrome P450 (CYP450) 3A4 enzyme inducer. Patients taking CYP450 3A4 metabolized medications (e.g., oral contraceptives, most statin drugs, and some psychotropic medications) concurrently with St. John's wort may experience increased metabolism and subtherapeutic drug levels (Smith & Mischoulon, 2010).

Another key concern regarding the use of alternative herbs and nutrients is the quality of herbal supplements on the market. Many brands are of poor quality, have dosing inconsistencies, or are of questionable purity or stability. This is partly because herbal preparations are sold as dietary supplements rather than drugs; thus, they avoid regulation under the FDA's Federal Food, Drug, and Cosmetic Act. Health care professionals, and especially nurses, need to stay current using unbiased sources of product information in order to pass this information on to patients taking alternative agents. Independent evaluation of many brands with updates can be found at www.consumerlab.com. Recalls and warnings to stop use of certain brands are available at www.fda.gov/medwatch.

It is important that nurses explore the patient's use of herbal supplements in a nonjudgmental manner by asking, "What over-the-counter medications or herbs do you take to help your symptoms? Do they help? How much are you taking? How long have you been taking them?" Individuals taking medications or other supplements need to be aware of drug-substance interactions and product safety. Such discussion should be part of the initial and ongoing interviews with patients. Chapter 35 covers complementary and integrative therapies in more detail.

KEY POINTS TO REMEMBER

- All actions of the brain—sensory, motor, and intellectual—are carried out physiologically through the interactions of nerve cells. These interactions involve impulse conduction, neurotransmitter release, and receptor response. Alterations in these basic processes can lead to mental disturbances and physical manifestations.
- In particular, it seems that excess activity of dopamine is involved in the thought disturbances of schizophrenia, and deficiencies of norepinephrine, serotonin, or both underlie depression and anxiety. Insufficient activity of GABA also plays a role in anxiety.
- Pharmacological treatment of mental disturbances is directed at the suspected neurotransmitter-receptor problem. Thus, antipsychotic drugs decrease dopamine, antidepressant drugs increase synaptic levels of norepinephrine and/or serotonin, and antianxiety drugs increase the effectiveness of GABA or increase 5-HT and/or norepinephrine.
- Because the immediate target activity of a drug can result in many downstream alterations in neuronal activity, drugs with a variety of chemical actions may show efficacy in treating the same clinical condition. Newer drugs with novel mechanisms of action are thus being used in the treatment of schizophrenia, depression, and anxiety.
- Unfortunately, agents used to treat mental disease can cause various undesired effects. Prominent among these are sedation or excitement, motor disturbances, muscarinic blockage, α antagonism, sexual dysfunction, and weight gain. There is a continuing effort to develop new drugs that are effective, safe, and well-tolerated.

CRITICAL THINKING

1. Knowing that no matter where you practice nursing, many individuals under your care will be taking one psychotropic drug or another, how important is it for you to understand normal brain structure and function as they relate to mental disturbances and psychotropic drugs? Include the following in your answer:
   a. How nurses can use the knowledge about how normal brain function (control of peripheral nerves, skeletal muscles, the autonomic nervous system, hormones, and circadian rhythms) can be affected by either psychotropic drugs or psychiatric illness
   b. How brain imaging can help in understanding and treating people with mental disorders
   c. How your understanding of neurotransmitters may affect your ability to assess your patients' responses to specific medications
2. What specific information would you include in medication teaching based on your understanding of symptoms that may occur when the following neurotransmitters are altered?
   a. Dopamine D_2 (as with use of antipsychotic drugs)
   b. Blockage of muscarinic receptors (as with use of phenothiazines and other drugs)
   c. α_1 receptors (as with use of phenothiazines and other drugs)
   d. Histamine (as with use of phenothiazines and other drugs)
   e. MAO (as with use of an MAOI)
   f. GABA (as with use of benzodiazepines)
   g. Serotonin (as with the use of SSRIs and other drugs)
   h. Norepinephrine (as with the use of SNRIs)

CHAPTER REVIEW

1. A nurse administering a benzodiazepine should understand that the therapeutic effect of benzodiazepines results from potentiating the neurotransmitter:
   a. GABA
   b. dopamine
   c. serotonin
   d. acetylcholine
   e. a and c
2. Venlafaxine (Effexor) exerts its antidepressant effect by selectively blocking the reuptake of:
   a. GABA.
   b. dopamine
   c. serotonin
   d. norepinephrine
   e. c and d
3. The nurse administers each of the following drugs to various patients. The patient who should be most carefully assessed for fluid and electrolyte imbalance is the one receiving:
   a. lithium
   b. clozapine
   c. diazepam
   d. amitriptyline
4. Which drug group calls for nursing assessment for development of abnormal movement disorders among individuals who take therapeutic dosages?
   a. SSRIs
   b. Antipsychotics
   c. Benzodiazepines
   d. Tricyclic antidepressants
5. Blockage of dopamine transmission can lead to increased pituitary secretions of prolactin. In women, this hyperprolactinemia can result in:
   a. dry mouth
   b. amenorrhea
   c. increased production of testosterone
   d. blurred vision

Answers to Chapter Review
1. a; 2. e; 3. a; 4. b; 5. b.

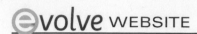

Visit the Evolve website for a posttest on the content in this chapter:
http://evolve.elsevier.com/Varcarolis

Post-Test interactive review

REFERENCES

American Psychiatric Association. (2008). *Practice guideline for the treatment of patients with bipolar disorder (2nd ed.).* Retrieved from http://psychiatryonline.org/content.aspx?bookid=28§ionid=1669577.

Bulechek, G. M., Butcher, H. K., Dochterman, J. M., & Wagner, C. (2013). *Nursing interventions classification (NIC)* (6th ed.). St. Louis, MO: Mosby.

Cruz, M. P. (2012). Vilazodone HCl (Viibryd): A serotonin partial agonist and reuptake inhibitor for the treatment of major depressive disorder. *Pharmacy & Therapeutics, 37,* 28–31.

Due, D. L., & Fitzgerald, L. S. (2006). A good night's rest-helping the patient with insomnia. *Pharmacy Times.* Retrieved from https://secure.pharmacytimes.com/lessons/200605-01.asp.

Herdman, T. H. (Ed.), (2012) *NANDA international nursing diagnoses: Definitions and classification, 2012-2014.* Oxford, UK: Wiley-Blackwell.

Holmes, J. C., & Zacher, J. L. (2012). Second-generation antipsychotics: a review of recently-approved agents and drugs in the pipeline. *Formulary, 47,* 106–121.

Karlsson, H. (2011). How psychotherapy changes the brain. *Psychiatric Times, 28*(8). Retrieved from http://www.psychiatrictimes.com/display/article/10168/1926705.

McEvoy, J. P., Lieberman, J. A., Stroup, T. S., Davis, S. M., Meltzer, H. Y., Rosenheck, R. A., et al. (2006). Effectiveness of clozapine versus olanzapine, quetiapine, and risperidone in patients with chronic schizophrenia who did not respond to prior atypical antipsychotic treatment. *American Journal of Psychiatry, 163,* 600–610.

Martinez, M., Marangell, L. B., & Martinez, J. M. (2011). Psychopharmacology. In R. E. Hales, S. C. Yudofsky, & G. O. Gabbard (Eds.), *Essentials of psychiatry* (pp. 455-524). Arlington, VA: American Psychiatric Publishing.

Moorhead, S., Johnson, M., Maas, M. L., & Swanson, E. (2013). *Nursing outcomes classification (NOC)* (5th ed.). St. Louis: Mosby.

Patel, D., & Goldman-Levine, J. D. (2011). Doxepin (Silenor) for insomnia. *American Family Physician, 84*(4), 453–454.

Smith, F. A., & Mischoulon, D. (2010). Drug-drug interactions in psychopharmacology. In T. A. Stern, G. L. Fricchione, N. H. Cassem, M. S. Jellinek, & J. F. Rosenbaum (Eds.), *Massachusetts General Hospital handbook of general hospital psychiatry* (6th ed., pp. 505-510). Philadelphia, PA: Elsevier.

Stahl, S.W. (2008). *Stahl's essential psychopharmacology* (3rd ed.). New York, NY: Cambridge University Press.

Stone, J. M., Howes, O. D., Egerton, A., et al. (2010). Altered relationship between hippocampal glutamate levels and striatal dopamine function in subjects at ultra high risk of psychosis. *Biological Psychiatry, 68,* 599–602.

United States Food and Drug Administration. (2012). *Prescribing information for Silenor.* Retrieved from http://www.accessdata.fda.gov/drugsatfda_docs/label/2010/022036lbl.pdf.

United States Food and Drug Administration. (2011). *Consumer health information.* Retrieved from http://www.fda.gov/downloads/ForConsumers/ConsumerUpdates/UCM279341.pdf?utm_campaign=Google2&utm_source=fdaSearch&utm_medium=website&utm_term=kapvay&utm_content=6.

United States Food and Drug Administration. (2010). *Oleptro medication guide.* Retrieved from http://www.fda.gov/downloads/Drugs/DrugSafety/UCM202202.pdf.

United States Food and Drug Administration. (2008). *Antidepressant use in children, adolescents, and adults.* Retrieved from http://www.fda.gov/cder/drug/antidepressants/default.htm.

CHAPTER

4

Settings for Psychiatric Care

Monica J. Halter, Christine Tebaldi, and Avni Cirpili

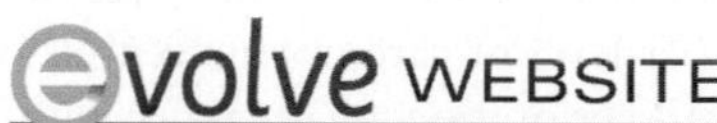

Visit the Evolve website for a pretest on the content in this chapter: http://evolve.elsevier.com/Varcarolis

Pre-Test interactive review

OBJECTIVES

1. Compare the process of obtaining care for physical problems with obtaining care for psychiatric problems.
2. Analyze the continuum of psychiatric care and the variety of care options available.
3. Describe the role of the primary care provider and the psychiatric specialist in treating psychiatric disorders.
4. Explain the purpose of patient-centered medical homes and implications for holistically treating individuals with psychiatric disorders.
5. Evaluate the role of community mental centers in the provision of community-based care.
6. Identify the conditions that must be met for reimbursement of psychiatric home care.
7. Discuss other community-based care providers including assertive community treatment (ACT) teams, partial hospitalization programs, and alternate delivery of care methods such as telepsychiatry.
8. Describe the nursing process as it pertains to outpatient settings.
9. List the standard admission criteria for inpatient hospitalization.
10. Discuss the purpose of identifying the rights of hospitalized psychiatric patients.
11. Explain how the multidisciplinary treatment team collaborates to plan and implement care for the hospitalized patient.
12. Discuss the process for preparing patients to return to the community for ongoing care and for promoting the continuation of treatment.

KEY TERMS AND CONCEPTS

admission criteria
assertive community treatment (ACT)
clinical pathway
codes
community mental health centers
continuum of psychiatric mental health care
decompensation
elopement
least restrictive environment
milieu
patient-centered medical (health) home
prevention
psychiatric case management
psychosocial rehabilitation
stabilization
stigma
triage

Obtaining traditional health care is pretty straightforward, and diagnoses tend to be based on objective measurements. For example, if you wake up with a sore throat, you know what to do and pretty much how things will progress. If you feel bad enough, you may go to see your primary care provider (PCP), be examined, and maybe get a throat culture to diagnose the problem. If the cause is bacterial, you will probably be prescribed an antibiotic. If you do not improve within a certain period of time, your PCP may order more tests or recommend that you visit an ear, nose, and throat specialist.

Compared to obtaining treatment for physical disorders, entry into the mental health care system for the treatment of psychiatric problems can be a mystery. Challenges in accessing and navigating this care system exist for several reasons. One reason is that the experience of others is unlikely to provide much of a benefit since having a psychiatric illness is often hidden. This is usually the result of embarrassment or concern of the stigma, or sense of responsibility, shame, and being flawed that is associated with these disorders. While you may know that when your grandmother had heart disease, she saw a cardiac specialist and had heart surgery, you probably will not know that she was also treated for depression by a psychiatrist after the surgery.

Seeking treatment for mental health problems is also complicated by the very nature of mental illness. At the most extreme, disorders with a psychotic component may disorganize thoughts and impede a person's ability to recognize the need for care or to follow logical paths in seeking care. Even major depression, a common psychiatric disorder, may interfere with motivation to seek care because the illness carries feelings of apathy, hopelessness, and anergia (lack of energy).

Mental health symptoms are also confused with other problems. For example, anxiety disorders often manifest in somatic (physical) symptoms such as a racing heart, sweaty palms, and dizziness, which could together be mistaken for cardiac problems. Ruling out physical causes is essential since diagnosing psychiatric illness is largely based on symptoms and not on objective measurements such as electrocardiograms (ECGs) and blood tests. Although necessary, the process of ruling out other illnesses often adds to treatment delays for mental illnesses.

The purpose of this chapter is to provide an overview of this system, to briefly examine the evolution of mental health care, and to explore different venues by which people receive treatment for mental health problems. Treatment options are roughly presented in order of acuteness, beginning with those in the least restrictive environment, or the setting that provides the necessary care allowing the greatest personal freedom. This chapter also explores funding sources for mental health care. Box 4-1 introduces the idea of influencing health care through advocacy initiatives.

BOX 4-1 POLICY AND POLITICS OF THE PROVISION OF PSYCHIATRIC CARE

Mental health advocates develop policies in order to create an ideal image of what we should be striving for in our health care delivery system. Organizations such as the World Health Organization (WHO) work hard at strategically planning policies that help direct the government's goals for health care. Improvements in mental health policy across the world are needed and impact how people with mental illness are treated. Policies can address various issues including availability and accessibility of care, discrimination, and basic human rights (WHO, 2012).

Grass-roots organizations, such as WHO, National Alliance on Mental Illness (NAMI), and American Nurses Association (ANA), along with groups specific to each state advocate for better mental healthcare. These organizations are able to share information with legislators about special interest issues. Nurses are encouraged to contact their legislators and work collaboratively on bills that may positively impact patient care and the profession of psychiatric mental health nursing. This is a special advocacy role for a nurse to engage in and provides a way to be involved in policymaking.

CONTINUUM OF PSYCHIATRIC MENTAL HEALTH CARE

What if you, your friend, or a family member needed psychiatric treatment or care? What would you do or recommend? Figure 4-1 presents a continuum of psychiatric mental health care that may help you to make a decision. Movement along the continuum is fluid and can go in either direction. For example, patients discharged from acute hospital care or a 24-hour supervised crisis stabilization unit (most acute level), may need intensive services to maintain their initial gains or to "step down" in care. Failure to follow up in outpatient treatment increases the likelihood of rehospitalization and other adverse outcomes. Patients may pass through the continuum of treatment in the reverse direction; that is, if symptoms do not improve, a lower-intensity service may refer the patient to a higher level of care in an attempt to prevent total decompensation (deterioration of mental health) and hospitalization.

The section that follows discusses care settings from least restrictive to most intensive. The notion of least restrictive interventions and settings is the foundational concept surrounding the care continuum. Ideally, the care setting will change to best address a patient's individual needs at any given moment, "meeting the patient where they are."

OUTPATIENT PSYCHIATRIC MENTAL HEALTH CARE

Primary Care Providers

Individuals with depression may notice that they don't really want to talk on the phone with friends, they've let their bedroom deteriorate to the point of being condemnable, nothing seems to be fun, their weight has crept up, and the ability to sleep is abysmal. These persons may wonder if they're seriously sick and may decide to see a primary care provider. In fact, psychiatric illness is often first detected during a primary care visit even though it is not usually the main reason the patient had scheduled the appointment.

In the example above, it is likely that these persons would make an appointment with complaints of fatigue or insomnia. Also, conditions such as cardiovascular disease, diabetes, menopause, and chronic pain are complicated by psychiatric conditions such as depression and anxiety and therefore warrant frequent psychiatric assessment. Ideally, primary care providers treat the patient as a whole and not just for specific conditions. Primary care providers recognize that psychiatric illness can be manifested by physical symptoms and also realize that psychiatric disorders can intensify preexisting conditions.

Registered nurses in primary care can maximize their effectiveness by using therapeutic communication, conducting thorough assessments, and providing essential teaching. Using therapeutic communication, such as listening, can help patients feel comfortable talking about their psychiatric symptoms so that they can be relayed to the primary care provider and therefore receive appropriate treatment. Assessing the patient's physical health concerns provides an opportunity to explore any mental health symptoms that the patient has not mentioned or maybe even recognized. Since many psychiatric disorders are discovered

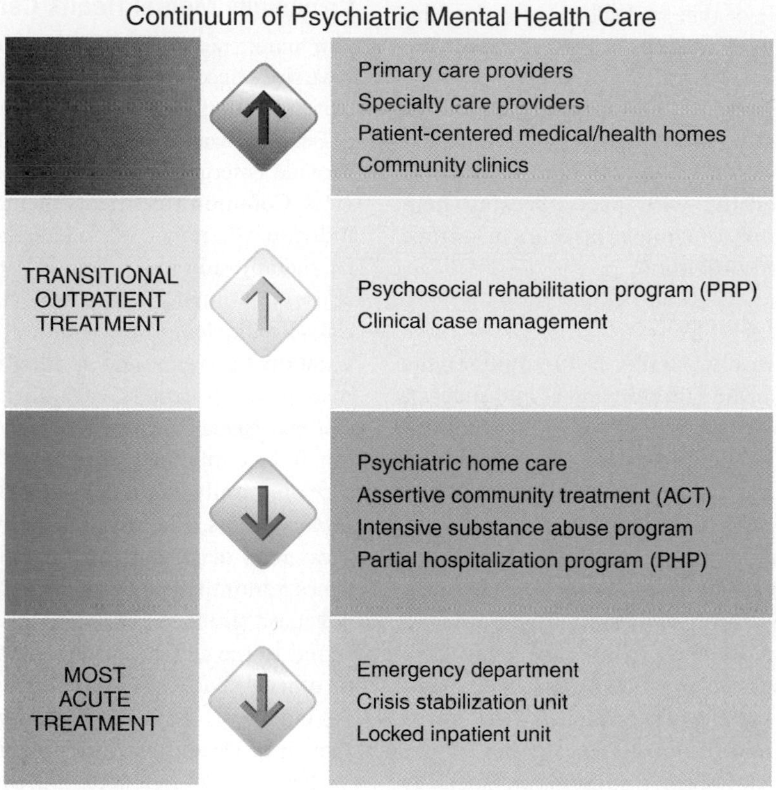

Continuum of Psychiatric Mental Health Care

	Primary care providers Specialty care providers Patient-centered medical/health homes Community clinics
TRANSITIONAL OUTPATIENT TREATMENT	Psychosocial rehabilitation program (PRP) Clinical case management
	Psychiatric home care Assertive community treatment (ACT) Intensive substance abuse program Partial hospitalization program (PHP)
MOST ACUTE TREATMENT	Emergency department Crisis stabilization unit Locked inpatient unit

FIG 4-1 The continuum of psychiatric mental health treatment.

in the primary care setting, it is an ideal time to screen and provide teaching about mental health and any psychiatric medications patients receive. This teaching can make the difference between success and failure for medication continuation.

Once the problem is identified, patients may be apprehensive about starting new medications and understanding them. Most importantly, if they know that many side effects are short-term, they may put up with them rather than discontinuing the medication prematurely. Proper education on why they are taking a medication, how it works, and the possible side effects (which ones are short-term and which ones are more serious) will likely make it easier for them to agree to continued treatment. It is also important to teach patients about their mental illness and its trajectory so that they can keep their provider informed of any changes in symptoms, whether they are getting better or worse.

The vignette in the next column demonstrates how a registered nurse working in a primary care setting can assist in the assessment and education of a patient with a psychiatric illness.

Specialty Psychiatric Care Providers

Although some primary care providers feel comfortable in treating common psychiatric illnesses such as uncomplicated depression, they may feel less comfortable when depression becomes suicidal or disorders are more severe. For more efficient, comprehensive psychiatric care, patients are directed to a specialized care provider. This is someone whose practice focuses solely on psychiatric care, such as an advanced practice psychiatric nurse (nurse practitioner or clinical nurse specialist), psychiatrist, psychologist, social worker, and a variety of licensed therapists.

VIGNETTE

Jayden Miller is a registered nurse at a primary care office where he works with a nurse practitioner. He greets his next patient, Mr. Newton, whom he has known for years and with whom he has established a solid rapport. He notices that even though Mr. Newton is pleasant, his affect is dull, and his voice is soft. He responds with vague, short answers, and has had poor eye contact, which is not usually how he acts. Mr. Newton reports that within the past year he has experienced increased fatigue, no enjoyment of anything, a chronic body ache, and has been craving carbohydrates uncontrollably.

After documenting his findings Jayden leans forward slightly on his stool and states in a caring tone, "Mr. Newton, I've known you for a while, and the change in your behavior has me concerned. Is there anything going on in your life that you'd like to talk about?" Mr. Newton hesitates but then tells Jayden that he was demoted at work last year and that he hasn't felt right since then.

The nurse practitioner assesses Mr. Newton and diagnoses him with major depressive disorder after ruling out possible medical conditions. He is prescribed fluoxetine (Prozac) 20 mg daily, educated about his diagnosis and new medication and provided with written material to take home. He is also given a list of referrals for therapy and support groups. After the visit, Jayden documents the education and Mr. Newton's response.

Specialized care providers can provide numerous services, such as prescribing medications, practicing individual psychotherapy ("talk" therapy), and leading group therapy. This type of provider is ideal for people looking for treatment specifically for their problem because these providers can have sub specialties they treat as well. An example of that would be a provider who specializes in working with war veterans with post traumatic stress disorder.

How does someone find one of these providers? One of the first steps is to inquire with a local care organization such as a primary care office, hospital, clinic, or therapy practice. Other ways include networking with peers, seeking help through support organizations, or contacting one's insurance company for a list of covered providers.

Patient-Centered Medical Homes

The Affordable Care Act (Health Affairs, 2010) outlines the concepts of patient-centered medical (health) homes and suggests the co-location of primary and specialty care in community-based mental health settings. The integration of primary care and behavioral health care is a common-sense approach that eliminates much of the stigma of seeking specialty care for psychiatric disorders.

Comprehensive and holistic care addresses mental and physical needs, supports acute and chronic illness interventions, and emphasizes prevention and wellness. This care requires a diverse team, including advanced practice nurses, physicians, physician assistants, nurses, social workers, pharmacists, nutritionists, care coordinators, and educators. Typically this team is in the same physical location; however, in some areas, especially rural areas, a virtual team linked electronically may serve the same purpose.

Patient-centered care in the health home refers to a whole-person orientation. It is an atmosphere of respect for the individual and family's unique culture, preferences, and values. It supports individual choices about how active a person is in organizing and managing his or her own health care. Central to patient-centered care is that patients and families are core members in developing a plan of care. The underlying values of the medical home include clear communication among patients and families, the home itself, and members of the health care system.

Outside services such as specialty care, home health care, hospitalization, and community services are coordinated through the patient-centered health homes. Coordination becomes especially important when changes are being made in care sites, such as when patients are discharged from the hospital.

Accessibility to service is central to this model. Imagine a system with shorter waiting time for urgent care, expanded clinical hours, and 24/7 telephone or electronic access to real people on the care team. The use of health information technology is also an essential aspect of this care (Meyers et al., 2010). Electronic health records will undoubtedly help these centers of care fully reach their potential.

Quality and quality improvement are key goals for patient-centered medical homes. This is accomplished through the use of evidence-based practice and clinical tools to guide decision making. Measuring patient experiences and patient satisfaction provides information by which improvements can be made. Publicly sharing the information gained from these quality improvement activities demonstrates a transparent commitment to quality.

Community Mental Health Centers

Community mental health centers were created in the 1960s and have since become the mainstay for those who have no access to private mental health care (Drake & Latimer, 2012). The range of services available at such centers varies, but generally they provide emergency services, adult services, and children's services. Common treatments include medication administration, individual therapy, psychoeducational and therapy groups, family therapy, and dual-diagnosis (mental health and substance abuse) treatment. A clinic may also be aligned with a psychosocial rehabilitation program that offers a structured day program, vocational services, and residential services. Some community mental health centers have an associated intensive psychiatric case management service to assist patients in finding housing or obtaining entitlements.

Community mental health centers also utilize multidisciplinary teams. The psychiatric mental health nurse may carry a caseload of 60 patients, each of whom is seen one to four times a month. The basic level nurse is often supervised by an advanced practice registered nurse (APRN). Patients are referred to the clinic for long-term follow-up by inpatient units or other providers of outpatient care at higher intensity levels. Patients may attend the clinic for years or be discharged when they improve and reach desired goals.

The following vignette illustrates part of a typical day for a nurse in a community mental health center.

VIGNETTE

Allen Morton is a registered nurse at a community mental health center. He is on the adult team and carries a caseload of patients diagnosed with chronic mental illness. An advanced practice registered nurse supervises him. His responsibilities include responding to crisis calls, seeing patients for regular assessment, administering medications, leading psychoeducation groups, and participating in staff meetings.

Today Allen's first patient is Mr. Enright, a 35-year-old man diagnosed with schizophrenia who has been in treatment at the clinic for 10 years. During their 30-minute counseling session, Allen assesses Mr. Enright for any exacerbation of psychotic symptoms (he has a history of grandiose delusions), eating and sleep habits, and social functioning in the psychosocial rehabilitation program that he attends 5 days a week, and today he presents as stable. Allen gives Mr. Enright his long-acting injectable (LAI) antipsychotic medication and schedules a return appointment for a month from now, reminding him of his psychiatrist appointment the following week.

Allen also leads a co-leads a medication group along with a social worker. This group consists of seven patients with chronic schizophrenia who have been attending biweekly group sessions for the past 5 years. Today, as Allen leads the group discussion, he asks the group to explain relapse prevention to a new member. He teaches significant elements, including adherence with the medication regimen and healthy habits. As group members give examples from their own experiences, he assesses each patient's mental status. At the end of the meeting, he gives members appointment cards for the next group session.

Psychiatric Home Care

Psychiatric home care was defined by Medicare regulations in 1979 as requiring four elements: (1) homebound status of the patient, (2) presence of a psychiatric diagnosis, (3) need for the skills of a psychiatric registered nurse, and (4) development of a plan of care under orders of a physician. Other payers besides Medicare also authorize home care services, but most follow Medicare's guidelines.

Homebound refers to the patient's inability to leave home independently to access community mental health care because of physical or mental conditions. Patients are referred to psychiatric home care following an acute inpatient episode—either psychiatric or somatic—or to prevent hospitalization. The psychiatric mental health nurse visits the patient one to three times per week for approximately 1 to 2 months. Although this is the ideal situation, some home care responsibilities are managed by caseworkers while the nurse's focus is more on the initial setup of treatment and medication adherence. By going to the patient's home, the nurse is better able to address the concerns of access to services and adherence with treatment. With the growing number of older adults being treated in the community for psychiatric and medical issues, the role of psychiatric home care is becoming even more important.

Family members or significant others are closely involved in most cases of psychiatric home care. Because many patients are older than 65, there are usually concurrent somatic illnesses to assess and monitor. The nurse acts as a case manager, coordinating all specialists (e.g., physical therapist, occupational therapist, and home health aide) involved in the patient's care, and is often supervised by an APRN team leader who is always available by telephone.

Boundaries become important in the home setting. Walking into a person's home creates a different set of dynamics than those commonly seen in a clinical setting. It may be important for the nurse to begin a visit informally by chatting about patient family events or accepting refreshments offered. Continuity of care in this type of situation can increase the level of comfort and has been shown to decrease levels of depression and anxiety (D'Errico & Lewis, 2010). There is great significance to the therapeutic use of self in such circumstances to establish a level of comfort for the patient and family; however, nurses must be aware of the boundaries between a professional relationship and a personal one. (See the vignette at the top of the next column.)

> **VIGNETTE**
> Emma Castillo is a registered nurse employed by a home care agency in a large rural county. She visits patients living in a radius of 50 miles from her home and has daily telephone contact with her supervisor. She stops by the office weekly to drop off paperwork and attends a team meeting once a month. The team includes her team leader, other field nurses, a team psychiatrist consultant, and a social worker. Emma chooses to make her visits from 8:00 AM until 3:30 PM and then completes her documentation at home.
>
> Emma spends an hour with Mr. Johnson, a 66-year-old man with a diagnosis of major depression after a stroke. His primary care physician referred him because of suicidal ideation. Emma has met with Mr. Johnson and his wife 3 times a week for the past 2 weeks. He denies suicidal ideation, plan, or intent and has been adherent to his antidepressant regimen. Today, she teaches the couple about stress-management techniques. Case-management responsibilities for Mr. Johnson include supervision of the home health aide, who helps him with hygiene, and coordination with the physical and occupational therapists who also treat him.

Assertive Community Treatment

Assertive community treatment (ACT) is an intensive type of case management developed in the 1970s in response to the oftentimes hard to engage, community-living needs of people with serious, persistent psychiatric symptoms and patterns of repeated hospitalization for services such as emergency room and inpatient care (Wright-Berryman, McGuire, & Salyers, 2011). Patients are referred to ACT teams by inpatient or outpatient providers because of a pattern of repeated hospitalizations with severe symptoms, along with an inability to participate in traditional treatment. ACT teams work intensively with patients in their homes or in agencies, hospitals, and clinics—whatever settings patients find themselves in. Creative problem solving and interventions are hallmarks of care provided by mobile teams. The ACT concept takes into account that people need support and resources after 5:00 PM; teams are on call 24 hours a day.

ACT teams are multidisciplinary and typically composed of psychiatric mental health registered nurses, social workers, psychologists, advanced practice registered nurses (APRNs), and psychiatrists. One of these professionals (often the registered nurse) serves as the case manager and may have a caseload of patients who require visits three to five times per week; the case manager is usually supervised by an APRN or psychiatrist. Length of treatment may extend to years, until the patient is ready to accept transfer to a more structured site for care.

The following vignette illustrates a typical day for a psychiatric mental health registered nurse on an ACT team.

> **VIGNETTE**
> Maria Rodriguez is a nurse who works on an ACT team at a large inner-city, university-based medical center. She had five years of inpatient experience before joining the ACT team, and she works with two social workers, two psychiatrists, and a mental health worker. She is supervised by an APRN.
>
> One of her two-hour home visits is to Ms. Abbott, a 53-year-old single woman with a diagnosis of schizoaffective disorder and hypertension. She lives alone in a senior citizen building and has no contact with family. The ACT team is now the payee for her Social Security check. Today, Maria will take Ms. Abbott to pay her bills and to her primary care provider. Ms. Abbott greets Maria warmly at the door, wearing excessive makeup and inappropriate summer clothing. With gentle encouragement, she agrees to wear warmer clothes. She gets irritable when Maria points out that she has not taken her morning medications. Observing the change in behavior and medication non adherence, Maria plans to return the following day to complete a follow-up assessment. By monitoring closely, she hopes to avoid a full decompensation that would require more intensive intervention.

Partial Hospitalization Programs

Partial hospitalization programs (PHPs) offer intensive, short-term treatment similar to inpatient care, except that the patient is able to return home each day. Typically, programs offer 5-6 hours per day utilizing individual and group psychotherapy treatment. The primary goals are symptom improvement, safety, education on clinical conditions, and medications and coping strategies. Referrals come from inpatient or outpatient providers. This level of care is designed to divert from an inpatient admission or a 'step-down'. The average length of stay is approximately 1 to 2 weeks, depending on the program, and the multidisciplinary team consists of at least a psychiatrist, registered nurse, and social worker.

Similar programs, called day treatment programs, are held at clinics or other community settings and focus less on therapy and more on social skill development, behavioral regulation, and community living. They serve all age groups and their aim is to reduce the number of hospitalizations by promoting self-awareness. Returning home each day allows the person to test out new skills and gradually reenter family and society.

Other Outpatient Venues for Psychiatric Care

Mobile mental health units have been developed in some service areas. In a growing number of communities, mental health programs are collaborating with other health or community services to provide integrated approaches to treatment. A prime example of this is the growth of dual-diagnosis programming at both mental health and substance abuse clinics.

Telephone crisis counseling, telephone outreach, and the Internet are being used to enhance access to mental health services. Although face-to-face interaction is still preferred, the new forms of treatment through technology, such as telepsychiatry, have shown immense patient satisfaction and no evidence of complications (Garcia-Lizana & Munoz-Mayorga, 2010). Access and overall health outcomes are expected to improve as models of care that include telehealth and other innovative practices advance.

PREVENTION IN COMMUNITY CARE

A distinct concept in the health care literature is that of treatment based on a public health model that takes a community approach to prevention. Primary, secondary, and tertiary prevention are levels at which interventions are directed. Primary prevention occurs before any problem is manifested and seeks to reduce the incidence, or rate of new cases. There is evidence (Brenner et al., 2010) that primary prevention may prevent or delay the onset of symptoms in genetically or otherwise vulnerable individuals. Although controversial, there is support for pharmacotherapy combined with cognitive-behavioral therapy for people at high risk for psychotic disorders such as schizophrenia. Coping strategies and psychosocial support for vulnerable young people are effective interventions in preventing mood and anxiety disorders.

Secondary prevention is also aimed at reducing the prevalence, or number of new and old cases at any point in time, of psychiatric disorders. Early identification of problems, screening, and prompt and effective treatment are hallmarks of this level. According to the Institute of Medicine (Katz & Ali, 2009), this level of prevention is the secondary defense against disease. While it does not stop the actual disorder from beginning, it may delay or avert progression to the symptomatic stage.

Tertiary prevention is the treatment of disease with a focus on preventing the progression to a severe course, disability, or even death. Tertiary prevention encompasses the term "rehabilitation," which aims to preserve or restore functional ability. In the case of treating major depression, the aim is to avoid loss of employment, reduce disruption of family processes, and prevent suicide.

OUTPATIENT AND COMMUNITY PSYCHIATRIC MENTAL HEALTH CARE

Psychiatric mental health nursing in the outpatient or community setting requires strong problem-solving and clinical skills, cultural competence, flexibility, solid knowledge of community resources, and comfort in functioning more autonomously than acute care nurses. Patients need assistance with problems related to individual psychiatric symptoms, family and support systems, and basic living needs, such as housing and financial support. Community treatment hinges on enhancing patient strengths in the daily environment, making individually tailored psychiatric care imperative. Treatment in the community permits patients and their support systems to learn new ways of coping with symptoms or situational difficulties. The result can be one of empowerment and self-management for patients.

Psychiatric mental health nurses may be the answer to transforming an illness-driven and dependency-oriented system into a system that emphasizes recovery and empowerment. Nurses are adept at understanding the system and coordinating care. They "can work between and within systems, connecting services and acting as an important safety net in the event of service gaps"(American Psychiatric Nurses Association [APNA] et al., 2007).

Over the past 30 years—with advances in psychopharmacological and psychosocial interventions—psychiatric care in the community has become more sophisticated, with a continuum of care that provides more settings and options for people with mental illness. The role of the outpatient or community psychiatric mental health registered nurse has grown to include service provision in a variety of these treatment settings, and nursing roles have developed outside traditional treatment sites.

For example, psychiatric needs are well known in the criminal justice system and the homeless population. Individuals suffering from a serious mental illness tend to cycle through the correctional systems and generally comprise more than 50% of the incarcerated population (Dumont et al., 2012). The nurse's role is not only to provide care to individuals as they leave the criminal justice system and re-enter the community, but also to educate police officers and justice staff in how to work with individuals entering the criminal system.

The percentage of homeless persons with serious mental illness has been estimated to be more than 26%, and it is speculated that the lack of mental health agencies has led to a greater number of homeless young adults (U.S. Department of Housing and Urban Development, 2011). The challenge to psychiatric mental health nurses is in making contact with these individuals who are outside the system but desperately in need of treatment.

Biopsychosocial Assessment

Assessment of the biopsychosocial needs and capacities of patients living in the community requires expansion of the general psychiatric mental health nursing assessment (refer to Chapter 7). To be able to plan and implement effective treatment, the nurse must also develop a comprehensive understanding of the patient's ability to cope with the demands of living in the community.

Key elements of this assessment are strongly related to the probability that the patient will experience successful outcomes. Problems in any of these areas require immediate attention because they can seriously impair the success of other treatment goals:

- Housing adequacy and stability: If a patient faces daily fears of homelessness, it is not possible to focus on other treatment issues.
- Income and source of income: A patient must have a basic income—whether from an entitlement, a relative, or other sources—to obtain necessary medication and meet daily needs for food and clothing.
- Family and support system: The presence of a family member, friend, or neighbor supports the patient's recovery and, with the patient's consent, gives the nurse a contact person.
- Substance abuse history and current use: Often hidden or minimized during hospitalization, substance abuse can be a destructive force, undermining medication effectiveness and interfering with community acceptance and procurement of housing.
- Physical well-being: Factors that increase health risks and decrease life span for individuals with mental illnesses include decreased physical activity, smoking, medication side effects, and lack of routine health exams.

Individual cultural characteristics are also very important to assess. For example, working with a patient who speaks a different language from the nurse requires the nurse to consider the implications of language and cultural background. The use of a translator or cultural consultant from the agency or from the family is essential when the nurse and patient speak different languages (refer to Chapter 5).

Treatment Goals and Interventions

Treatment goals and interventions are patient-centered and are therefore negotiated rather than imposed on the patient. To meet a broad range of needs, community psychiatric mental health nurses must approach interventions with flexibility and resourcefulness. The complexity of navigating the mental health and social service funding systems is often overwhelming to patients. Not unexpectedly, patient outcomes with regard to mental status and functional level have been found to be more positive and were achieved with greater cost effectiveness when the community psychiatric mental health nurse integrates case management into the professional role.

Differences in characteristics, treatment outcomes, and interventions between inpatient and community settings are outlined in Table 4-1. Note that all of these interventions fall within the practice domain of the basic level registered nurse.

TABLE 4-1 CHARACTERISTICS, TREATMENT OUTCOMES, AND INTERVENTIONS BY SETTING

OUTPATIENT/COMMUNITY MENTAL HEALTH SETTING	INPATIENT SETTING
Characteristics	
Intermittent supervision	24-hour supervision
Independent living environment with self-care, safety risks	Therapeutic milieu with hospital/staff supported healing environment
Treatment Outcomes	
Stable or improved level of functioning in community	Stabilization of symptoms and return to community
Interventions	
Establish long-term therapeutic relationship.	Develop short-term therapeutic relationship.
Develop comprehensive plan of care with patient and support system, with attention to sociocultural needs and maintenance of community living	Develop comprehensive plan of care, with attention to sociocultural needs of patient and focus on reintegration into the community
Encourage adherence with medication regimen.	Administer medication.
Teach and support adequate nutrition and self-care with referrals as needed.	Monitor nutrition and self-care with assistance as needed.
Assist patient in self-assessment, with referrals for health needs in community as needed.	Provide health assessment and intervention as needed.
Use creative strategies to refer patient to positive social activities.	Offer structured socialization activities.
Communicate regularly with family/support system to assess and improve level of functioning.	Plan for discharge with family/significant other with regard to housing and follow-up treatment.

Case Management

The role of the community psychiatric mental health nurse includes coordinating mental health, physical health, spiritual health, social service, educational service, and vocational realms of care for the mental health patient. The reality of community practice today is that few patients seeking treatment have uncomplicated symptoms of a single mental illness. The severity of illness has increased, and it is often accompanied by substance abuse, poverty, and stress. Repeated studies show that people with mental illnesses also have a higher risk for medical disorders than the general population (Robson & Gray, 2007).

The community psychiatric mental health nurse is in an excellent position to assist the team in bridging the gap between the psychiatric and physical needs of the patient. The nurse meets not only with the mental health treatment team but also with the patient's primary care team, serving as the liaison between the two. Integrating a nurse case manager to assist patients with primary care needs facilitates greater success with follow-up and adherence with appointments.

Promoting Continuation of Treatment

A significant number of patients treated in the community have problems continuing treatment and following through with prescribed treatments plans, particularly in taking medication. Formerly, these problems were called *noncompliance*, but this word is considered by many to be objectionable since it implies a medical "paternalism" (i.e., the patient is treated as a child who needs to be told what to do). Deegan and Drake (2006) contend that there are actually two experts involved in the care of people with mental illnesses. One is the health care professional—who has advanced skills and training in psychiatric disorders—and the other is the consumer of care, who has intimate knowledge of the disorder and its response to treatment. Shared decision making is the key to improving treatment adherence and success.

Patient-centered care is essential to shared decision making. A patient must be knowledgeable about the illness and treatment options. Research demonstrates that persons with mental illness want more than watered-down and simplistic information. (Imagine a pamphlet titled "Your Mental Illness and You.") To fully participate in the treatment plan, patients need current, evidence-based information about their illness and treatment options (Tanenbaum, 2008).

A successful life in the community is more likely when medications are taken as prescribed. Nurses are in a position to help the patient manage medication, recognize side effects, and be aware of interactions among drugs prescribed for physical illness and mental illness. Patient-family education and behavioral strategies, in the context of a therapeutic relationship with the clinician, promote adherence with the medication regimen.

Nursing Education

A baccalaureate degree is preferred in more autonomous community settings and will become increasingly in demand as the trend away from hospital-based acute care settings continues; however, educators believe that non-baccalaureate prepared nurses should be trained to meet the challenges of providing community care. Clinical experiences in community settings are valuable for all nursing students; they increase cultural sensitivity, teaching skills, and an appreciation for strong multidisciplinary teams.

Table 4-2 describes the educational preparation for a variety of outpatient and community roles.

Teamwork and Collaboration

The concept of using multidisciplinary treatment teams originated with the Community Mental Health Centers Act of 1963. Psychiatric nursing practice was identified as one of the core mental health disciplines, along with psychiatry, social work, and psychology. This recognition permitted the allocation of resources to educate psychiatric nurses and emphasized their unique contributions to the team.

In inter professional team meetings, the individual and discipline-specific expertise of each member is recognized. Generally, the composition of the team reflects the availability of fiscal and professional resources in the area. The community psychiatric team may include psychiatrists, nurses, social workers, psychologists, dual-diagnosis specialists, and mental health

TABLE 4-2 ROLES RELEVANT TO EDUCATIONAL PREPARATION IN OUTPATIENT AND COMMUNITY SETTINGS

ROLE	BASIC PRACTICE (DIPLOMA, AD, BS)	ADVANCED PRACTICE (MS, DNP, PHD)
Practice	Provide nursing care; assist with medication management as prescribed, under direct supervision	Nurse practitioner or clinical nurse specialist; manage consumer care and prescribe or recommend interventions independently
Consultation	Consult with staff about care planning and work with nurse practitioner or physician to promote health and mental health care; collaborate with staff from other agencies	Consultant to staff about plan of care, to consumer and family about options for care; collaborate with community agencies about service coordination and planning processes
Administration	Take leadership role within mental health treatment team	Administrative or contract consultant role within mental health agencies or mental health authority
Research and education	Participate in research at agency or mental health authority; serve as preceptor to undergraduate nursing students	Role as educator or researcher within agency or mental health authority

workers. Recognition of the ability of nurses to have an equal voice in team treatment planning with other professionals was novel at the time the team approach was implemented in the 1960s. This level of professional performance was later used as a model for other nursing specialties.

The nurse is able to integrate a strong nursing identity into the team perspective. At the basic or advanced practice level, the community psychiatric mental health nurse is in a critical position to link the biopsychosocial and spiritual components relevant to mental health care. The nurse also communicates in a manner that the patient, significant others, and other members of the team can understand. In particular, the management and administration of psychotropic medications have become significant tasks the community nurse is expected to perform.

Emergency Care and Crisis Stabilization

Patients and families seeking emergency care range from the worried well to those with acute symptoms. The primary goal in emergency services is to perform **triage** and **stabilization**. In reality, emergency department care often provides a bridge from the community to more intensive psychiatric services. Individuals may seek emergency care voluntarily; however, there are times when family, friends, treatment providers, schools, emergency medical personnel, or even law enforcement may suggest or require an individual to undergo emergency evaluation. When emergency evaluation and stabilization are needed, psychiatric clinicians, including psychiatric mental health nurses, will determine the correct interventions and level of care required. Refer to Chapter 6 for a more detailed discussion about involuntary treatment.

Emergency psychiatric care varies across the nation due to differences in state mental health system designs, access to care, and workforce. Despite these differences, emergency psychiatric care can be categorized into three major models:

1. **Comprehensive Emergency Service Model,** which is often affiliated with a full-service emergency department (ED) in a hospital or medical center setting. Typically, there is dedicated clinical space with specialty staffing. Psychiatric mental health nurses, psychiatric technicians/mental health specialists, social workers, mental health counselors, and psychiatrists generally make up the multidisciplinary workforce. The concepts of triage and stabilization are incorporated into the individualized care plan for each patient. Psychiatric mental health staffs manage the full scope of patient care, including medication reconciliation, physical care needs and safety checks.
2. **Hospital-Based Consultant Model** utilizes the concepts of the Comprehensive Model by incorporating triage and stabilization; however, there is generally not dedicated clinical space or comprehensive separate staffing. Psychiatric clinical staff members are assigned to a specific hospital and are on-site or on-call, serving as part of the medical ED/hospital staff. Psychiatric clinicians manage emergency psychiatric evaluations as requested. Clinicians complete a "level of care" assessment, attempt to stabilize patients, and arrange for discharge or transfer. The ED/hospital staff maintains responsibility for all immediate care needs.
3. **Mobile Crisis Team Model** is considered stabilization "in the field." While the teams vary in design, psychiatric mental health nurses, social workers, and counselors, in collaboration with a psychiatrist and/or an advanced practice nurse, often make up the care team. Clinicians are available to respond to where the crisis is and will conduct psychiatric evaluations in the community with a goal to assess and stabilize without a full ED visit. In some states, these teams complete evaluations in medical ED settings. Clinicians serve in a consultative function and facilitate patient access to necessary treatment.

Crisis Stabilization/Observation Units

Care models that prioritize rapid stabilization and short length of stay have become more prevalent in medical and psychiatric settings. Overnight short-term observation, often 1–3 days, are designed for individuals who have symptoms that are expected to remit in 72 hours or less or have a psychosocial stressor that can be addressed in that timeframe, maximizing their stability and allowing them to rapidly return to a community treatment setting.

At all levels of clinical care, contingencies are created for the management of behavioral crises. Planning ahead for the possibility of clinical destabilization can mitigate the effects of the crisis and maximize safety. The psychiatric mental health nurse is an integral part of the team working with patients, families, and systems to develop individualized crisis plans. Working with providers across the continuum of care, such as community-based treatment providers, pre-hospital care/Emergency Medical Service (EMS), and acute service providers can yield an effective crisis plan.

INPATIENT PSYCHIATRIC MENTAL HEALTH CARE

Inpatient psychiatric care has undergone significant changes over the past quarter century. During the 1980s, inpatient stays were at their peak as private and non-federal general hospital psychiatric units proliferated. However, by the mid-1990s, the number of patient days, psychiatric beds, and psychiatric facilities were dipping sharply. This decline was caused by improvements brought about by managed care, tougher limitations of covered days by insurance plans, and alternatives to inpatient care such as partial hospitalization programs and residential facilities. Lengths of stay decreased from weeks to days.

Hospitalization remains an option for the treatment of patients with mental disorders and emotional crises. In fact, 1.6 million patients were treated in hospitals in 2009 with a mental illness listed as their primary diagnosis (Centers for Disease Control and Prevention [CDC], 2012). The top five mental health diagnoses treated are mood disorders, substance-related disorders, delirium/dementia, anxiety disorders, and schizophrenia. Admission is commonly reserved for those people who are suicidal, homicidal, or extremely disabled and in need of short-term, acute care (Simon & Shuman, 2008).

Most inpatient treatment today takes place in general hospitals or private psychiatric hospitals. There are also state psychiatric hospitals that exist for longer-term care and for specialty populations, such as the most seriously mentally ill and forensic patients referred for evaluation or treatment by the court system. According to the National Association of Psychiatric Health Systems, in 2010 there were 2,257 inpatient psychiatric facilities within the United States (Dobson et al., 2010).

Ideally, treatment plans consist of individualized recovery-focused care. While there are a variety of inpatient models throughout the nation, one can expect similarities such as clinical management by an interprofessional treatment team in collaboration with patient and family. Rapid stabilization and reintegration to the community is a priority treatment goal from any inpatient setting. When intermediate or long-term treatment is required, treatment often occurs in a state hospital setting and stabilization goals may transition to more supportive treatment, health promotion, and generalized life skills education.

Entry to Acute Inpatient Care

Some patients are admitted directly to inpatient care based on a psychiatrist or primary care provider referral; however, the majority of patients receiving inpatient acute psychiatric care are admitted through an emergency department. Of the 12 million emergency department visits in the United States, nearly 13% are due to mental health and/or substance abuse conditions (as cited in Agency for Healthcare Research and Quality, 2010).

The average wait (commonly referred to as "boarding") in the emergency room for a patient in need of hospitalization can be lengthy and in some instances the delay can be days. Nurses that work on psychiatric units recognize the admission process can be stressful and consider any unique or increased support needs when developing the individualized care plan. A recommended wait time of less than six hours was made and even with the scrutiny that it has gotten and the push for more efficient care, few improvements have been made to our nation's hospitals (Horwitz, Green, & Bradley, 2010).

An emergency department physician and a psychiatric clinician (e.g., registered nurse, advanced practice registered nurse, social worker, or licensed counselor or psychiatrist) generally evaluate the patient to determine the correct level of care. The **admission criteria** to a hospital begin with the premise that the person is suffering from a mental illness, and there is evidence of one or more of the following:

1. Imminent danger of harming self
2. Imminent danger of harming others
3. Unable to care for basic needs and/or gross impairment of judgment, placing an individual at imminent risk based on inability to protect oneself

If symptoms meet the admission criteria, they are then given the option of being admitted on a voluntary basis, which means that they agree with the need for treatment and hospitalization. If patients do not wish to be hospitalized, but psychiatric mental health professionals feel that admission is necessary, they can be admitted against their wishes, commonly known as an *involuntary admission*. Involuntarily admitted patients still have rights and can petition the court for release. If the admission is contested, the treating psychiatrist—or in some states the advanced practice registered nurse—are required to present the case to the court, supporting hospitalization as necessary for the safety of the patient or others and explaining how the patient will benefit from treatment. The court then decides whether or not to continue hospitalization (refer to Chapter 6 for legal issues related to involuntary hospitalization).

The type of admission—voluntary vs. involuntary—is commonly referred to as legal status. Regardless of the legal status, a patient maintains his or her rights related to refusal of medication administration. Additionally, if the last resorts of medication restraint, mechanical restraint, or seclusion are used, the specific parameters of being imminently dangerous to self or others are outlined by regulatory agencies such as the Joint Commission or the Centers for Medicaid/Medicare.

VIGNETTE

Mr. Reese is a 22-year-old male who was brought to the emergency room by police after expressing thoughts of suicide. He is restless and irritable. When approached, he becomes very agitated and threatening to the nurses and physicians, stating that he wants to leave and does not understand why he needs to be here. He states that his mother and brother, who are only trying to have him admitted so they can take his money, tricked him. He is exhibiting poor judgment, insight, and impulse control. He stopped taking his antipsychotic medication 3 weeks ago because of side effects.

The psychiatric nurse in the ED approaches Mr. Reese in a non-threatening manner. She calmly asks him if he'd be more comfortable sitting while they speak with one another. Mr. Reese chooses to sit on the gurney and the nurse sits in a chair near the door. Mr. Reese already appears calmer after accepting a cold drink and nods as the nurse observes that he seems anxious. When asked if any medication ever helps him with feeling anxious, he responds that he has taken lorazepam (Ativan) before and it helps. The ED team writes an order for the medication and the psychiatric nurse provides Mr. Reese with education about the medication.

Rights of the Hospitalized Patient

Patients admitted to any psychiatric unit retain rights as citizens, which vary from state to state, and are entitled to certain privileges. Laws and regulatory standards require that patients' rights be explained in a timely fashion after an individual has been admitted to the hospital, and that the treatment team must always be aware of these rights. Any infringement by the team during the patient's hospitalization—such as a failure to protect patient safety—must be documented, and actions must be justifiable. All mental health facilities provide a written statement of patients' rights, often with copies of applicable state laws attached. Box 4-2 provides a sample list of patients' rights, and Chapter 6 offers a more detailed discussion of this issue.

BOX 4-2 TYPICAL ITEMS INCLUDED IN HOSPITAL STATEMENTS OF PATIENTS' RIGHTS

- Right to be treated with dignity
- Right to be involved in treatment planning and decisions
- Right to refuse treatment, including medications
- Right to request to leave the hospital, even against medical advice
- Right to be protected against harming oneself or others
- Right to a timely evaluation in the event of involuntary hospitalization
- Right to legal counsel
- Right to vote
- Right to communicate privately by telephone and in person
- Right to informed consent
- Right to confidentiality regarding one's disorder and treatment
- Right to choose or refuse visitors
- Right to be informed of research and to refuse to participate
- Right to the least restrictive means of treatment
- Right to send and receive mail and to be present during any inspection of packages received
- Right to keep personal belongings unless they are dangerous
- Right to lodge a complaint through a plainly publicized procedure
- Right to participate in religious worship

VIGNETTE

Ally Brennan is assigned as Mr. Reese's primary nurse, and Lisa Taylor is his evening shift nurse. Ally met with the treatment team to plan Mr. Reese's care during the hospitalization. The APRN's diagnosis was major depressive disorder with psychotic features. The priority issues the team identified, based on reports of the past 2 days and nursing assessments, were safety, paranoia, non-adherence with medications, and hypertension. Ally identified that the nursing diagnoses were risk for self-directed violence, disturbed thought processes, nonadherence, and deficient knowledge. Along with the treatment team, Ally identified the nursing education groups that Mr. Reese should participate in and recommended that suicide-precaution monitoring should be maintained due to Mr. Reese's level of risk and inability to maintain safety.

WORKING AS A TEAM IN INPATIENT CARE

Psychiatric mental health nurses are core members of a team of professionals and nonprofessionals who work together to provide care (Box 4-3). The team (including the patient) generally formulates a full treatment plan. The nurse's role in this process is often to lead the planning meeting. This nursing leadership reflects the holistic nature of nursing, as well as the fact that nursing is the discipline that is represented on the unit at all times. Nurses are in a unique position to contribute valuable information, such as continuous assessment findings, the patient's adjustment to the unit, and any health concerns, psycho educational needs, and deficits in self-care the patient may have. Additionally, nurses have an integral function to facilitate a patient's achievement of therapeutic goals by offering education and support in an individual or group format.

Ultimately, the treatment plan will be the guideline for the patient's care during the hospital stay. It is based on goals for the hospitalization and defines how achievement of the goals will be measured. Input from the patient and family (if available and desirable) is critical in formulating goals. Incorporating the patient's feedback in developing the treatment plan goals increases the likelihood of the success of the outcomes.

Members of each discipline are responsible for gathering data and participating in the planning of care. Newly admitted patients may find multiple professionals asking them similar questions to be extremely stressful or threatening. The urgency of the need for data should be weighed against the patient's ability to tolerate assessment. Often, assessments made by the intake worker and the nurse provide the basis for care. In most settings, the psychiatrist or advanced practice nurse evaluates the patient and provides orders within a limited time frame. Medical problems are usually referred to a primary care physician or specialist, who assesses the patient and consults with the unit physicians.

To provide standardization in treatment and improve outcomes, inpatient units use **clinical pathways**. They are document-based tools that provide suggestions and time frames for managing specific medical conditions (Kinsman et al., 2010). These tools provide an essential link between evidence-based knowledge and clinical practice. The treatment plan is revised if the patient's progress differs from the expected outcomes. Clinical pathways result in decreased costs, length of stay, and complications.

Therapeutic Milieu

Milieu is a word of French origin (mi "middle" + lieu "place") and refers to surroundings and physical environment. In a therapeutic context, it refers to the overall environment and interactions of the environment. Peplau (1989) referred to this as the therapeutic milieu. A well-managed milieu offers patients a sense of security and promotes healing. Structured aspects of the milieu include activities, unit rules, reality orientation practices, and unit environment.

In addition to the structured components of the milieu, Peplau described less tangible factors of the milieu, such as the interactions that occur among patients and staff, patients and patients, patients and visitors, and so forth. This is quite different from medical units where patients rarely interact with other patients. On psychiatric units, patients are in constant contact with their peers and staff. These interactions can help patients engage and increase the sense of social competence and worth

The therapeutic milieu can serve as a real-life training ground for practicing communication and coping skills to prepare for a return to the community. Even events that seemingly distract from the program of therapies can be

BOX 4-3 MEMBERS OF THE MULTIDISCIPLINARY TREATMENT TEAM

Psychiatric mental health registered nurses: Licensed registered nurses whose focus is on mental health and mental illness and who may or may not be certified in psychiatric mental health nursing. The registered nurse is typically the only 24-hours-a-day, 7-days-a-week, professional working in acute care. Among the responsibilities of the registered nurse are diagnosing and treating responses to psychiatric disorders, coordinating care, counseling, giving medication and evaluating responses, and providing education.

Psychiatric mental health advanced practice registered nurses: Licensed registered nurses who are prepared at the master's or doctoral level and hold specialty certification as either clinical nurse specialists or nurse practitioners. These nurses are qualified for clinical functions such as diagnosing psychiatric conditions, prescribing psychotropic medications and integrative therapy, and conducting psychotherapy; they are involved in case management, consulting, education, and research.

Psychiatrists: Depending on their specialty of preparation, psychiatrists may provide in-depth psychotherapy or medication therapy or head a team of mental health providers functioning as a private service based in the community. As physicians, psychiatrists may be employed by the hospital or may hold practice privileges in the facility. Because they have the legal power to prescribe and to write orders, psychiatrists often function as the leaders of the teams managing the care of patients individually assigned to them.

Psychologists: In keeping with their master's or doctoral degree preparation, psychologists conduct psychological testing, provide consultation for the team, and offer direct services such as specialized individual, family, or marital therapies.

Social workers: Basic level social workers help the patient prepare a support system that will promote mental health on discharge from the hospital. This includes contacts with day treatment centers, employers, sources of financial aid, and landlords. Licensed clinical social workers undergo training in individual, family, and group therapies, and often are primary care providers.

Counselors: Counselors prepared in disciplines such as psychology, rehabilitation counseling, and addiction counseling may augment the treatment plan by co-leading groups, providing basic supportive counseling, or assisting in psychoeducational and recreational activities.

Occupational, recreational, art, music, and dance therapists: Based on their specialist preparation, these therapists assist patients in gaining skills that help them cope more effectively, gain or retain employment, use leisure time to the benefit of their mental health, and express themselves in healthy ways.

Medical advanced practice nurses, medical doctors, and physician assistants: Medical professionals provide diagnoses and treatments on a consultation basis. Occasionally, a medical professional who is trained as an addiction specialist may play a more direct role on a unit that offers treatment for addictive disease.

Mental health workers (mental health specialists / psychiatric technicians): Mental health workers, including nursing assistants, function under the direction and supervision of registered nurses. They provide assistance to patients in meeting basic needs and also help the community to remain supportive, safe, and healthy.

Pharmacists: In view of the intricacies of prescribing, coordinating, and administering combinations of psychotropic and other medications, the consulting pharmacist can offer a valuable safeguard. Physicians and nurses collaborate with the pharmacist regarding new medications, which are proliferating at a steady rate.

turned into valuable learning opportunities for the members of the milieu. Psychiatric mental health nurses can support the milieu and intervene when necessary. They usually develop an uncanny ability to assess the mood of the unit (e.g., calm, anxious, disengaged, or tense) and predict environmental risk. Nurses observe the dynamics of interactions, reinforce adaptive social skills, and redirect patients during negative interactions. Reports from shift to shift provide information on the emotional climate and level of tension on the unit.

A number of measures are used to reduce barriers between patients and staff; these measures include a staff station in the center of the unit and accessible common areas. Many units also have incorporated the concepts of sensory integration into the environment. Some units have a specific room with sensory stimulation tools such as music, soothing fragrances, and weighted blankets, which help patients maximize their health and address symptoms they may be experiencing.

Managing Behavioral Crises

Behavioral crises can lead to patient violence toward self or others and usually, but not always, escalate through fairly predictable stages. Staff in most mental health facilities practice crisis prevention and management techniques. Many general and psychiatric hospitals have special teams made up of nurses, psychiatric technicians, and other professionals who respond to psychiatric emergencies called **codes**. Each member of the team takes part in the team effort to defuse a crisis in its early stages. If preventive measures fail and imminent risk of harm to self or others persists, each member of the team participates in a rapid, organized plan to safely manage the situation. The nurse is most often this team's leader, not only organizing the plan but also timing the intervention and managing the concurrent use of prn medications.

Seclusion, restraint, and medication over one's objection are actions of last resort, and the trend is to reduce or completely eliminate these practices whenever safely possible. The nurse can initiate such an intervention in the absence of a physician in most states but must secure a physician's order for restraint or seclusion within a specified time. The nurse also advocates for patients by ensuring that their legal rights are preserved, no matter how difficult their behavior may be for the staff to manage. Refer to Chapters 6 and 27 for further discussions and protocols for use of restraints and seclusion. The concept of "Trauma Informed Care" is a guiding principle for clinical interventions and unit philosophy and is addressed more comprehensively in Chapter 16.

Crises on the unit are upsetting and threatening to other patients as well. A designated staff member usually addresses their concerns and feelings. This person removes other patients from the area of crisis and helps them express their fears. Patients may be concerned for their own safety or the welfare of the patient involved in the crisis. They may fear that they too might experience such a loss of control.

Safety

A safe environment is an essential component of any inpatient setting. Protecting the patient is essential, but equally important is the safety of the staff and other patients. Safety needs are identified, and individualized interventions begin, on admission. Staff members check all personal property and clothing to prevent any potentially harmful items (e.g., medication, alcohol, or sharp objects) from being taken onto the unit. Some patients are at greater risk of suicide than others, and psychiatric mental health nurses are skillful in evaluating this risk through questions and observations.

The Joint Commission, an agency that accredits hospitals, developed National Patient Safety Goals (2012) specific to specialty areas within hospitals to promote patient safety. Table 4-3 lists safety goals specific to behavioral health care. Centers for Medicare and Medicaid Services (CMS) have also put more emphasis on patient safety and have identified several preventable hospital-acquired injuries for which they will not provide reimbursement. For example, they will not compensate health care organizations when a patient falls and fractures a hip; the rationale for not paying is that nearly all falls are preventable. It is likely that other health insurance providers will also begin to limit payment for preventable injuries under the regulatory concept of pay for performance.

Tracking patients' whereabouts and activities is done periodically or continuously, depending upon patients' risk for harming themselves or others. For actively suicidal patients, one-to-one observation is essential since even checking on a patient every 15 minutes may not prevent a suicide that takes only several minutes.

Visitors are another potential safety hazard. Although visitors can contribute to patients' healing through socialization, acceptance, and familiarity, visits may be overwhelming or distressing. Also, visitors may unwittingly or purposefully provide patients with unsafe items; unit staff should inspect bags and packages. Sometimes the unsafe items take the form of comfort foods from home or a favorite restaurant and should be monitored because they may be incompatible with diets or medications.

Intimate relationships between patients are discouraged or expressly prohibited. There are risks for sexually transmitted diseases, pregnancy, and emotional distress at a time when patients are vulnerable and may lack the capacity for consent.

Aggression and violence may also occur as a result of living in close quarters with reduced outlets to manage frustration. Psychiatric staff should have specialized training that promotes healthy, safe, and appropriate interactions. Most units are locked since some patients are hospitalized involuntarily, and **elopement** (escape) must be prevented in a way that avoids an atmosphere of imprisonment.

Unit Design to Promote Safety

The goal in designing psychiatric units is to provide a therapeutic and aesthetically pleasing environment while balancing the need for safety. Patients on inpatient psychiatric units are considered at risk for suicide. People who are considering suicide think about it for a long time and become extremely creative (Hunt & Sine, 2009). The Internet provides a disturbingly rich resource for methods; hangings from wardrobe doors have recently become popular due to advice obtained online.

TABLE 4-3 DIAGNOSES, WITH SAMPLE OUTCOMES AND INTERVENTIONS FOR PATIENTS DURING ADMISSION TO THE ACUTE CARE HOSPITAL

NURSING DIAGNOSES (NANDA INTERNATIONAL)	*NURSING OUTCOMES CLASSIFICATION (NOC)*	*NURSING INTERVENTIONS CLASSIFICATION (NIC)*
Risk for other-directed violence: At risk for behaviors in which an individual demonstrates that he or she can be physically, emotionally, and/or sexually harmful to others	*Aggression Self-Control:* Self-restraint of assaultive, combative, or destructive behaviors toward others	*Anger Control Assistance:* Facilitation of the expression of anger in an adaptive, nonviolent manner
Risk for self-directed violence: At risk for behaviors in which an individual demonstrates that he or she can be physically, emotionally, and/or sexually harmful to self	*Suicide Self-Restraint:* Personal actions to refrain from gestures and attempts at killing self	*Behavior Management: Self-Harm:* Assisting the patient to decrease or eliminate self-mutilating or self-abusive behaviors
Disturbed sensory perception (auditory): Change in the amount or patterning of incoming stimuli accompanied by a diminished, exaggerated, distorted, or impaired response to such stimuli	*Communication: Receptive:* Reception and interpretation of verbal and/or nonverbal messages	*Hallucination Management:* Promoting the safety, comfort, and reality orientation of a patient experiencing hallucinations

Data from North American Nursing Diagnosis Association. (2012). *NANDA nursing diagnoses: Definitions and classification 2012-14.* Philadelphia, PA: Author. Moorhead, S., Johnson, M., Maas, M., & Swanson, E. (Eds.). (2013). *Nursing outcomes classification (NOC)* (5th ed.). St. Louis, MO: Mosby. Bulechek, G. M., Butcher, H. K., Dochterman, J. M., & Wagner, C. (Eds.). (2013). *Nursing interventions classification (NIC)* (6th ed.). St. Louis, MO: Mosby.

In fact, the most frequent method of inpatient suicide is hanging, and about 75% of all hangings occur in the bathroom, bedroom, or closet. The bathroom is a choice location since most persons respect personal privacy there and it is locked (Knoll, 2012). Plumbing fixtures pose a serious risk, and almost any article of clothing can be tied to them. While we tend to think of hanging in the standard sense, patients frequently kneel or sit to complete this type of suicide.

Closets may be equipped with "break-bars" designed to hold a minimal amount of weight. Windows are locked and are made of safety glass, and safety mirrors are typically used. Showers may have non–weight-bearing showerheads. Beds are often platforms rather than mechanical hospital beds that can be dangerous because of their crushing potential or looping hazards. Standard hospital beds may be indicated, depending on patient physical health needs, but they are extremely dangerous and should be used with great caution.

Hunt and Sine (2009) recommend other important design elements on inpatient psychiatric units:

- Patient room doors should open out instead of in to prevent patients from barricading themselves in their rooms.
- Continuous hinges should be used on doors rather than three butt hinges to prevent hanging risk.
- Furniture should be anchored in place with the exception of a desk chair.
- Drapes should be mounted on a track that is firmly anchored to the ceiling rather than curtain rods.
- Mini blinds that are contained within window glass provide significantly more safety than those whose mountings are accessible.
- Bathroom towel bars should be eliminated in favor of breakable towel hooks.
- Steel boxes can be installed around plumbing.
- Mirrors should be polished stainless steel and not glass.

Inpatient Psychiatric Nursing Care

Being admitted to a hospital is anxiety-provoking for anyone, and anxiety can be severe for patients admitted to a psychiatric unit. Especially for the first-time patient, admission often summons preconceptions about psychiatric hospitals and the negative stigma associated with them. Patients may experience shame, and families may be reluctant to be forthcoming with pertinent information. Psychiatric mental health nurses can be most effective when they are sensitive to both the patient and family during the traumatizing effect of being hospitalized. In this initial encounter with the patient, psychiatric mental health nurses must try to provide reassurance and hope.

Assessment

The goal of the admission assessment is to gather information that will enable the treatment team to accurately develop a plan of care, ensure that safety needs are identified and addressed, identify the learning needs of the patient so that the appropriate information can be provided, and initiate a therapeutic relationship between the nurse and the patient. Chapter 7 presents a more detailed discussion of how to perform an admission assessment as well as a mental status examination. Table 4-4 illustrates common nursing diagnoses, sample nursing interventions, and sample nursing outcomes to guide the nurse in evidence-based practice during a patient's admission for acute psychiatric care.

Psychiatric nurses are in an excellent position to assess not only mental health but also physical health. A staggering number of individuals suffer from combinations of medical and psychiatric illness, and these conditions impact one another. For example, depressive symptoms may impair a patient's ability to cope with the added stress of a medical illness and negatively affect follow-up treatment recommendations. Conditions such as multiple sclerosis are often accompanied by depressive symptoms or even an actual diagnosis of major depressive disorder.

TABLE 4-4 NATIONAL PATIENT SAFETY GOALS IN BEHAVIORAL HEALTH CARE

GOAL	PROCESS	EXAMPLE
Identify patients correctly	Use at least two identifiers when providing care, treatment, or services.	Use the patient's name *and* date of birth for identification before drawing blood.
Use medicines safely	Maintain and communicate accurate medication information for the individual served.	Find out what medications the patient is taking and compare them to newly ordered medications.
Prevent infection	Use the hand cleaning guidelines from either the Centers for Disease Control (CDC) or the World Health Organization.	Wet hands first; apply an amount of product recommended by the manufacturer to hands, and rub hands together for at least 15 seconds, covering all surfaces of the hands and fingers. Rinse with water and dry thoroughly with a disposable towel. Use towel to turn off the faucet (CDC, 2002).
Identify patient safety risk	Determine which clients are most likely to try to commit suicide	Routinely administer a screening tool such as the Beck Scale for Suicidal Ideation, a 21-item tool that takes 5-10 minutes to complete.

From the Joint Commission (2012). Behavioral health care national safety goals. Retrieved from http://www.jointcommission.org/assets/1/6/2012_NPSG_BHC.pdf; Centers for Disease Control. (2002). Guideline for hand hygiene in health-care settings. Retrieved from http://www.cdc.gov/mmwr/preview/mmwrhtml/rr5116a1.htm; Pearson. (2012). Beck scale for suicidal ideation. Retrieved from http://www.pearsonassessments.com/HAIWEB/Cultures/en-us/Productdetail.htm?Pid=015-8018-443&Mode5summary.

Treatment Goals and Interventions

As in outpatient care, treatment goals and interventions are patient-centered and are developed collaboratively. Crisis stabilization, safety, and a focus on rapid discharge are the critical components of an acute inpatient stay. Inpatient care tends to be brief, and individuals are able to continue their recovery in their homes and communities, with community-based treatment and supports.

Interventions serve to support patients as they move toward stabilization. A general overview of inpatient interventions provided by psychiatric nurses is provided in the following paragraphs.

Therapeutic Groups

Psychiatric mental health nurses conduct specific, structured activities involving the therapeutic community, special groups, or families on most mental health units. Examples of these activities include morning goal-setting meetings and evening goal-review meetings. Daily community meetings may be held or scheduled at other times of the week. At these meetings, new patients are greeted, and departing patients are given farewells; ideas for unit activities are discussed; community problems or successes are considered; and other business of the therapeutic community is conducted.

Nurses also offer psychoeducational groups for patients and families on topics such as stress management, coping skills, grieving, medication management, and communication skills. Group therapy is a specialized therapy led by a mental health practitioner with advanced training. This therapy addresses communication and sharing, helps patients explore life problems and decrease their isolation and anxiety, and engages patients in the recovery process. Chapter 33 presents a more detailed discussion of therapeutic groups led by nurses.

Documentation

Documentation of patient progress is the responsibility of registered nurses and the entire mental health team. Although communication among team members and coordination of services are the primary goals when choosing a system for charting, practitioners in the inpatient setting must also consider professional standards, legal issues, requirements for reimbursement by insurers, and accreditation by regulatory agencies. Information must also be in a format that is retrievable for quality assurance monitoring, utilization management, peer review, and research. For nursing, the nursing process step of documentation is a guiding concern and is reflected in the different reporting formats commonly found in psychiatric hospitals. Chapter 7 gives an overview of documentation.

Medication Management

The safe administration of medications and the monitoring of their effects is a 24-hour responsibility for the nurse, who is expected to have detailed knowledge of psychoactive medications and the interactions and psychological side effects of other medications. The staff nurse is in a central position to monitor the patient's acceptance of the medication regimen, the presence or absence of side effects, and changes in the patient's behaviors. For example, a nurse may note that the patient is excessively sedated, communicate this observation, and receive an order for a decrease in the dosage of an antipsychotic medication.

Evaluating the need for medications that are prescribed on an as-needed (prn) basis is a skill that is developed by psychiatric mental health nurses. These evaluations are based on a combination of factors: the patient's wishes, the team's plan, attempts to use alternative methods of coping, and the nurse's judgments regarding timing and the patient's behavior. Documentation for administering each prn medication must include the rationale for its use.

Medication adherence is a common problem for persons taking psychotropic drugs, often because of side effects. Educating patients on how to recognize, report, and manage potential side effects can help empower patients and increase treatment success. This approach encourages the patient to seek out the nurse when it is time for medications to be administered and fosters responsibility and involvement in the treatment process.

Medical Emergencies

Mental health units, whether situated in a general hospital or independent facilities, must be able to stabilize the condition of a patient who experiences a medical crisis. Mental health or addictive disease units that manage detoxification (i.e., withdrawal from alcohol or other drugs) must anticipate several common medical crises associated with that process. Mental health units therefore store crash carts containing the emergency medications used to treat shock and cardiorespiratory arrest. Psychiatric nurses maintain their cardiopulmonary resuscitation skills and the ability to use basic emergency equipment. To be effective and practice at a high level of competency, nurses attend in-service sessions and workshops designed to teach and maintain skills.

Preparation for Discharge to the Community

Discharge planning begins on admission and is continuously modified as required by the patient's condition until the time of discharge. Typically, patients are discharged when serious symptoms are in control and there is a discharge plan in place. As members of the multidisciplinary team, nurses assist patients and their families to prepare for independent or assisted living in the community. Community-based programs provide patients with **psychosocial rehabilitation**, which moves the individual beyond stabilization toward recovery and a higher quality of life. This is especially important to the concept and practice of managed behavioral health care, which aims to reduce the length and frequency of hospital stays.

Nurses focus on precipitating factors that led to the crisis and hospital admission. Patients are assisted in learning coping skills and behaviors that will help them avert future crises. Psychoeducational groups, individual exploration of options and supports, and on-the-spot instruction (such as during medication administration) offer the patient numerous learning opportunities. Nurses encourage patients to use their everyday experiences on the unit to practice newly learned behavior.

The treatment plan or clinical pathway chosen for the patient should reflect this discharge planning emphasis as early as the day of admission. The patient is expected to begin to progress toward a resolution of acute symptoms, to assume personal responsibility, and to improve interpersonal functioning. Patients with prolonged mental illness benefit most from a seamless transition to community services. Collaboration with community mental health services and intensive case management programs facilitate this transition. Readiness for community re-entry should include preparation by members of the patient's support system for their role in enhancing the patient's mental health.

VIGNETTE

Lisa meets with Mr. Reese and his mother on the day of discharge to review the aftercare arrangements. Lisa reviews the goals that were established by the treatment team and Mr. Reese's own goal for hospitalization. She summarizes the accomplishments he made during the hospitalization, reinforces medication education, reviews each prescription, highlighting how the medication must be taken each day, and reminds Mr. Reese when and where the aftercare appointment is scheduled. Lisa answers Mr. Reese's and his mother's questions.

KEY POINTS TO REMEMBER

- The continuum of psychiatric treatment includes numerous community treatment alternatives with varying degrees of intensity of care.
- The community psychiatric mental health nurse needs access to resources to address ethical dilemmas encountered in clinical situations.
- Inpatient care has increasingly become more acute and short-term. Private insurers and a variety of governmental sources fund inpatient psychiatric care.
- Inpatient psychiatric mental health nursing requires strong skills in management, communication, and collaboration.
- The nurse plays a leadership role and also functions as a member of the multidisciplinary treatment team.
- The nurse advocates for the patient and ensures that the patient's rights are protected.
- Monitoring the environment and providing for safety are important components of good inpatient care. Psychiatric mental health nurses are skilled in protecting patients from suicidal impulses and aggressive behavior.
- Basic level nursing interventions include admission, providing a safe environment, psychiatric and physical assessments, milieu management, documentation, medication administration, and preparation for discharge to the community.
- Discharge planning begins on the day of admission and requires input from the treatment team and the community mental health provider.

CRITICAL THINKING

1. You are a nurse working at a local community mental health center. During an assessment of a 45-year-old single, male patient, he reports that he has not been sleeping and that his thoughts seem to be "all tangled up." Although he does not admit directly to being suicidal, he remarks, "I hope that this helps today because I don't know how much longer I can go on like this."
   He is disheveled and has been sleeping in homeless shelters. He has little contact with his family and becomes agitated when you suggest that it might be helpful to contact them. He reports a recent hospitalization at the local veterans' hospital and previous treatment at a dual-diagnosis facility, yet he denies substance abuse. When asked about his physical condition, he says that he has tested positive for hepatitis C and is "supposed to take" multiple medications that he cannot name.
   a. List your concerns about this patient in order of priority.
   b. Which of these concerns must be addressed before he leaves the clinic today?
   c. Do you feel there is an immediate need to consult with any other members of the multidisciplinary team today about this patient?
   d. Keeping in mind the concept of patient-centered care, how will you develop trust with the patient to increase his involvement with the treatment plan?
2. Imagine that you were asked for your opinion in regard to your patient's ability to make everyday decisions for himself. What sort of things would you consider as you weighed out safety versus autonomy and personal rights?
3. If nurses function as equal members of the multidisciplinary mental health team, what differentiates the nurse from the other members of the team?
4. How might the community be affected when patients with serious mental illness live in group homes? How would you feel about having a group home in your neighborhood?

CHAPTER REVIEW

1. Which of the following factors contribute to the movement of patients out of large state institutions and into community-based mental health treatment? *Select all that apply.*
   a. States desire to save money by moving the patients to the community, where the federal government would pick up more of the cost.
   b. The growing availability of generous mental health insurance coverage gave more patients the ability to seek private care in the community.
   c. A system of coordinated and accessible community care was developed by forward-thinking communities and offered more effective treatment.
   d. The Community Mental Health Centers Act of 1963 required states to develop and offer care in community-based treatment programs.
   e. Patient advocates exposed deficiencies of state hospitals and took legal actions, leading to the identification of a right to treatment in the least restrictive setting.

f. New psychotropic medications controlled symptoms more effectively, allowing many patients to live and receive care in less restrictive settings.

2. Levels of prevention strategies prominent in outpatient psychiatric care consist of primary prevention, secondary prevention, and ____________ prevention.

3. Anna, a patient at the community mental health center, tends to stop taking her medications at intervals, usually leading to decompensation. Which of the following interventions would most likely improve her adherence to her medications?
   a. Help Anna to understand her illness and share in decisions about her care.
   b. Advise Anna that if she stops her medications, her doctor will hospitalize her.
   c. Arrange for Anna to receive daily home care so that her use of medications is monitored.
   d. Discourage Anna from focusing on side effects and other excuses for stopping her pills.

4. A friend recognizes that his depression has returned and tells you he is suicidal and afraid he will harm himself. He wishes to be hospitalized but does not have health insurance. Which of the following responses best meets his immediate care needs and reflects the options for care a person in his position typically has?
   a. Provide emotional support and encourage him to contact his family to see if they can help him arrange and pay for inpatient care.
   b. Advise him that hospitals serve all persons regardless of their ability to pay, and immediately contact a Mobile Crisis team or accompany him to the nearest hospital emergency department.
   c. Help him apply for Medicaid coverage, arrange for him to be monitored by family and friends, and once Medicaid coverage is in place, take him to an emergency room for evaluation.
   d. Assist him in obtaining an outpatient counseling appointment at an area community mental health center, and call him frequently to assure he is safe until his appointment occurs.

5. Which of the following nursing actions is appropriate in maintaining a safe therapeutic inpatient milieu? *Select all that apply.*
   a. Interact frequently with both individuals and groups on the unit.
   b. Attempt to introduce patients with similar backgrounds to each other to form social bonds for after discharge.
   c. Initiate and support group interactions via therapeutic groups and activities.
   d. Provide and encourage opportunities to practice social and other life skills.
   e. Collaborate with housekeeping to provide a safe, pleasant environment.
   f. Assess patient belongings and the unit for any dangerous items that could be used by patients to hurt themselves or others.

6. The criteria for admission to an in patient psychiatric unit is that the patient:
   a. refuses to comply with the treatment team in regard to medication, counseling, living situation, or substance abuse abstinence.
   b. is in imminent danger of harming himself or others, or the patient cannot properly care for his basic needs and cannot protect himself from harm.
   c. refuses all psychotropic medication.
   d. is court-ordered by a judge specializing in mental health.

Answers to Chapter Review
1. a, c, d, e, f; 2. tertiary; 3. a; 4. d; 5. a, c, d, f; 6. b.

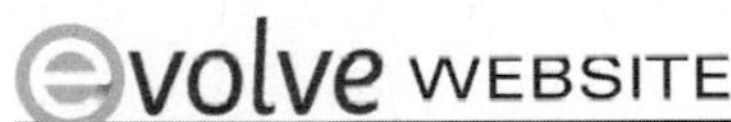

WEBSITE

Visit the Evolve website for a posttest on the content in this chapter: http://evolve.elsevier.com/Varcarolis

Post-Test interactive review

REFERENCES

Agency for Healthcare Research and Quality. (2010). *Statistical brief #92.* Retrieved from http://www.hcup-us.ahrq.gov/reports/statbriefs/sb92.pdf.

American Psychiatric Nurses Association, International Society of Psychiatric-Mental Health Nurses, & American Nurses Association. (2007). *Psychiatric-mental health nursing: Scope and standards of practice.* Silver Spring, MD: NurseBooks.org.

Brenner, R., Madhusoodanan, S., Puttichanda, S., & Chanrda, P. (2010). Primary prevention in psychiatry—Adult populations. *Annals of Clinical Psychiatry, 22*(4), 239–48.

Centers for Disease Control and Prevention. (2012). *Mental health.* Retrieved from http://www.cdc.gov/nchs/fastats/mental.htm.

Deegan P. E., & Drake R. E. (2006). Shared decision making and medication management in the recovery process. *Psychiatric Services, 57*, 1636–1639.

D'Errico, E. M., & Lewis, M. A. (2010). RN continuity in home health: Does it make a difference? *Home Health Care Management & Practice, 22*(6), 427–434.

Dobson, A., DaVanzo, J. E., Heath, S. H., Berger, G., El-Gamil, A. (2010). *The economic impact of inpatient psychiatric facilities: A national and state-level analysis.* Retrieved from http://www.naphs.org/news/documents/NAPHSFinalReport21910.2.pdf.

Drake, R., & Latimer, E. (2012). Lessons learned in developing community mental health care in North America. *World Psychiatry, 11*(1), 47–51. Retrieved from http://www.ncbi.nlm.nih.gov/pmc/articles/PMC3266763/?tool=pmcentrez.

Dumont, D., Brockmann, B., Dickman, S., Alexander, N., & Rich, J. (2012). Public health and the epidemic of incarceration. *Annual Review of Public Health, 33*, 325–339. doi:10.1146/annurev-publhealth-031811-124614.

Garcia-Lizana, F., & Munoz-Mayorga, I. (2010). What about telepsychiatry? A systematic review. *The Primary Care Companion to the Journal of Clinical Psychiatry, 12*(2). doi: 10.4088/PCC.09m00831whi.

Health Affairs. (2010). *Patient-centered medical homes.* Retrieved from http://www.healthaffairs.org/healthpolicybriefs/brief.php?brief_id=25.

Horwitz, L. I., Green, J., & Bradley, E. H. (2010). US emergency department performance on wait time and length of visit. *Annals of Emergency Medicine, 55*(2), 133–141.

Hunt, J. M., & Sine, D. M. (2009). Common mistakes in designing psychiatric facilities. *Academy Journal, 12*, 12–24. Retrieved from http://www.aia.org/groups/aia/documents/pdf/aiab090822.pdf.

The Joint Commission. (2012). *Behavioral health care: 2013 patient safety goals.* Retrieved from http://www.jointcommission.org/bhc_2013_npsg/.

Katz, D. L., & Ali, A. (2009). *Preventative medicine, integrative medicine, and the health of the public.* Presented at the IOM Summit on Integrative Medicine and the Health of the Public, Washington, DC. Retrieved from http://iom.edu/~/media/Files/Activity%20Files/Quality/IntegrativeMed/

Preventive%20Medicine%20Integrative%20Medicine%20and%20the%20Health%20of%20the%20Public.pdf.

Kinsman, R. T., El, J., Machotta, A., Gothe, H., Willis, J., Snow., P., & Kugler, J. (2010). Clinical pathways in hospitals. *Cochrane Database of Systematic Reviews, 3.* Retrieved from http://summaries.cochrane.org/CD006632/clinical-pathways-in-hospitals.

Knoll, J. L. (2012). Inpatient suicide: Identifying vulnerability in the hospital setting. *Psychiatric Times, 29*(5). Retrieved from http://www.psychiatrictimes.com/suicide/content/article/10168/2075044.

Meyers, D., Quinn, M., & Clancy, C. M. (2010). Health information technology: Turning the patient-centered medical home from concept to reality. *American Journal of Medical Quality, 26*(2), 154–6.

Peplau, H. E. (1989). Interpersonal constructs for nursing practice. In A. W. O'Toole & S. R. Welt (Eds.), *Interpersonal theory in nursing practice: Selected works of Hildegard E. Peplau* (pp. 42–55). New York, NY: Putnam.

Robson, D., & Gray, R. (2007). Serious mental illness and physical health problems: A discussion paper. *International Journal of Nursing Studies, 44*, 457–466.

Simon R. I., & Shuman, D. W. (2008). Psychiatry and the law. In R. E. Hales, S. C. Yudofsky, & G. O. Gabbard (Eds.), *Textbook of psychiatry* (pp. 1555–1959). Arlington, VA: American Psychiatric Publishing.

Tanenbaum, S. J. (2008). Consumer perspectives on information and other inputs to decision-making: implications for evidence-based practice. *Community Mental Health Journal, 44*(5), 331–335.

U.S. Department of Housing and Urban Development. (2011). *The 2010 Annual Homeless Assessment Report to Congress.* Washington, DC: Author.

World Health Organization. (2012). *Mental health policy, planning and service department.* Retrieved from http://www.who.int/mental_health/policy/services/en/index.html.

Wright-Berryman, J., McGuire, A., & Salyers, M. (2011). A review of consumer-provided services on assertive community treatment and intensive case management teams: Implications for future research and practice. *Journal of the American Psychiatric Association, 17*(1), 37–44.

CHAPTER

5

Cultural Implications for Psychiatric Mental Health Nursing

Rick Zoucha and Kimberly Gregg

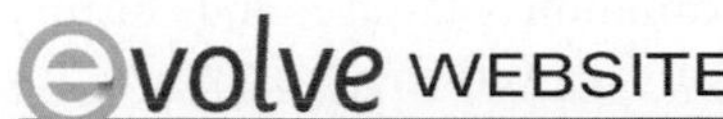

Visit the Evolve website for a pretest on the content in this chapter: http://evolve.elsevier.com/Varcarolis

Pre-Test interactive review

OBJECTIVES

1. Explain the importance of culturally relevant care in psychiatric mental health nursing practice.
2. Discuss potential problems in applying Western psychological theory to patients of other cultures.
3. Compare and contrast Western nursing beliefs, values, and practices with the beliefs, values, and practices of patients from diverse cultures.
4. Perform culturally sensitive assessments that include risk factors and barriers to quality mental health care that culturally diverse patients frequently encounter.
5. Develop culturally appropriate nursing care plans for patients of diverse cultures.

KEY TERMS AND CONCEPTS

acculturation
assimilation
cultural competence
culture
culture-bound syndromes
Eastern tradition
enculturation
ethnicity
ethnocentrism
indigenous culture
minority status
pharmacogenetics
race
refugee
somatization
stereotyping
Western tradition
worldview

Globally, how a society views mental health and mental illness has a tremendous impact on how care is allocated, whether individuals access mental health care, and how mental health care is funded. The United States has a relatively enlightened view regarding mental health care, yet we tend to consider it from the perspective of the dominant majority. According to Mental Health: Culture, Race, and Ethnicity—a 2001 report issued by the U.S. Surgeon General—cultural, racial, and ethnic minorities in America have not had the same access to quality mental health services as white Americans (U.S. Department of Health and Human Services [USDHHS], 2001). This report identifies culturally inappropriate services as one of the reasons minority groups in the United States do not receive and/or benefit from needed mental health services.

Psychiatric mental health nurses should practice culturally relevant nursing in order to meet the needs of culturally diverse patients. The goal of nursing is to promote health and well-being, and if we are to achieve this goal, mental health providers should strive to provide care that is as congruent as possible with patients' cultural beliefs, values, and practices—keeping in mind that certain cultural practices (e.g., sweat lodges, sun ceremonies, witchcraft) may be impractical, harmful, or even illegal. This kind of culturally competent care has been given other names: culturally appropriate care, culturally comfortable care, culturally sensitive care, and culturally congruent care. But whatever the name, *effective* care calls for adapting psychiatric mental health nursing assessments and interventions to each patient's cultural needs and preferences.

This chapter focuses on culture and how it affects the mental health and care of patients with mental illness. In this chapter you will learn about:

- Culture, race, ethnicity, minority status, and how they are related
- Demographic shifts, which make it essential that mental health nurses know how to provide culturally competent care
- The impact of cultural worldviews on mental health nursing
- Variations in cultural beliefs, values, and practices that affect mental health and care of patients with mental health problems
- Barriers to providing quality mental health services to culturally diverse patients
- Culturally diverse populations at increased risk of developing mental illness
- Techniques for providing culturally competent care to diverse populations

CULTURE, RACE, ETHNICITY, AND MINORITY STATUS

The 2001 Surgeon General's report discussed culture, race, and ethnicity in relation to minority groups (USDHHS, 2001). Although the definitions of these terms distinguish them from one another, they are related.

Minority status is connected more with economic and social standing in society than with cultural identity; however, many cultural, racial, and ethnic minority groups are also economically and socially disadvantaged groups.

Culture comprises the shared beliefs, values, and practices that guide a group's members in patterned ways of thinking and acting. Culture can also be viewed as a blueprint for guiding actions that impact care, health, and well-being (Leininger & McFarland, 2006). Culture is more than ethnicity and social norms; it includes religious, geographic, socioeconomic, occupational, ability- or disability-related, and sexual orientation–related beliefs and behaviors. Each group has cultural beliefs, values, and practices that guide its members in ways of thinking and acting. Cultural norms help members of the group make sense of the world around them and make decisions about appropriate ways to relate and behave. Because cultural norms prescribe what is "normal" and "abnormal," culture helps develop concepts of mental health and illness.

Ethnic groups have a common heritage and history (**ethnicity**). These groups share a **worldview**, a system for thinking about how the world works and how people should act, especially in relationship to one another. From this worldview, they develop beliefs, values, and practices that guide members of the group in how they should think and act in different situations.

Acknowledging the inadequacy of describing minority groups according to a single biological **race**, the U.S. Census Bureau used the 2000 census combined race-ethnicity categorization system for the 2010 census. Respondents are first asked whether they are of Hispanic, Latino, or Spanish origin; if not, they are asked to further identify their race. Federally defined racial groups were expanded from six categories in 2000 to fifteen in 2010 (U.S. Census Bureau, 2010). Respondents who do not identify with any of the predefined categories are encouraged to use blank spaces provided to classify their race (Figure 5-1).

The purpose of categorizing individuals according to racial-ethnic descriptions is to help the government understand the

Is Person 1 of Hispanic, Latino, or Spanish origin?
☐ No, not of Hispanic, Latino, or Spanish origin
☐ Yes, Mexican, Mexican Am., Chicano
☐ Yes, Puerto Rican
☐ Yes, Cuban
☐ Yes, another Hispanic, Latino, or Spanish origin — *Print origin, for example, Argentinean, Colombian, Dominican, Nicaraguan, Salvadoran, Spaniard, and so on.*

A

What is Person 1's race? *Mark* ☒ *one or more boxes.*
☐ White
☐ Black, African Am., or Negro
☐ American Indian or Alaska Native — *Print name of enrolled or principal tribe.*
☐ Asian Indian ☐ Japanese ☐ Native Hawaiian
☐ Chinese ☐ Korean ☐ Guamanian or Chamorro
☐ Filipino ☐ Vietnamese ☐ Samoan
☐ Other Asian — *Print race, for example, Hmong, Laotian, Thai, Pakistani, Cambodian, and so on.*
☐ Other Pacific Islander — *Print race, for example, Fijian, Tongan, and so on.*
☐ Some other race — *Print race.*

B

FIG 5-1 Race-ethnicity categorizations that were included in the 2010 U.S. Census. **A,** Respondents were first asked if they were of Hispanic, Latino, or Spanish origin. **B,** Respondents were asked to further identify their race.

needs of its citizens. The Surgeon General used data from the 2000 census classification system to identify disparities in mental health care along racial-ethnic lines. Recording these classifications also helps to determine when and how the health care needs of these populations are being met.

Despite the benefits, this convention of classifying groups of people can be confusing, confounding, and offensive. Consider the following:

- Each racial group contains multiple ethnic cultures. There are over 560 Native American and Alaskan tribes and over 40 countries in Asia and the Pacific Islands. The cultural norms of blacks or African Americans whose ancestors were brought to the United States centuries ago as slaves are very different from the norms of those who have recently immigrated from Africa or the Caribbean. Americans of European origin are a diverse group, some of whom have been in the United States for hundreds of years and some of whom are new immigrants.
- The Latino-Hispanic group is a cultural group based on a shared language, but all of its members are also members of a racial group or groups (white, black, and/or Native American) and may include Mexican Americans, Puerto Ricans, and Cuban Americans, just to name a few.
- Persons from the Middle East and the Arabian subcontinent are considered "white" in the classification system.
- Although children of multiracial, multicultural, and multiheritage marriages fall into more than one category, their unique identity is not distinguished and sometimes viewed as invisible.

Categorizing people according to a racial-ethnic system carries inherent problems. In psychiatric mental health nursing, we can assess patients further and make better decisions on their behalf if our focus is on *culture* rather than race.

DEMOGRAPHIC SHIFTS IN THE UNITED STATES

In 2043, the United States population is projected for the first time to become a majority-minority nation; that is, no one group will make up the majority (U.S. Census Bureau, 2012). Non-Hispanic whites will continue to remain the largest single group. A comparison of projected population composition in 2012 and 2060 is provided in Table 5-1.

TABLE 5-1 YEAR 2060 POPULATION PROJECTIONS (PERCENTAGE OF TOTAL POPULATION)*

	2012	2060
White, non-Hispanic	63	43
Black, non-Hispanic	13	15
Hispanic (of any race)	17	31
Asian	5	8
All other races	2	3

*Population percentages are rounded to the nearest 1%.
The Hispanic and Asian populations are growing at the fastest rates.
Data from U.S. Census Bureau. (2012). Population by race and Hispanic origin: 2012 and 2060. Retrieved from http://www.census.gov/newsroom/releases/img/racehispanic_graph.jpg.

These changing demographics mean that psychiatric nurses will likely be caring for culturally diverse patients. We need to know how to provide culturally relevant care and help reduce the problem of mental health disparities among culturally diverse populations.

WORLDVIEWS AND PSYCHIATRIC MENTAL HEALTH NURSING

Nursing theories, psychological theories, and the understanding of mental health and illness used by nurses in the United States have all grown out of a Western philosophical and scientific framework, which is in turn based on Western cultural ideals, beliefs, and values. Because psychiatric mental health nursing is grounded in Western culture, nurses should consider how their core assumptions about personality development, emotional expression, ego boundaries, and interpersonal relationships affect the nursing care of any patient.

A long history of Western science and European-American norms for mental health has shaped present-day American beliefs and values about people. Our understanding of how a person relates to the world and to other people is based on Greek, Roman, and Judeo-Christian thought. Other Western scientists and philosophers, such as Descartes (credited with the Western concept of body-mind dualism), have contributed to the Western scientific tradition. Nursing knowledge of psychology, development, and mental health and illness is based on this tradition.

However, a vast number of people throughout the world have very different philosophical histories and traditions from those of Western cultures (Table 5-2). The Eastern cultures of Asia are based on the philosophical thought of Chinese and Indian philosophers and the spiritual traditions of Confucianism, Buddhism, and Taoism. Diverse cultures found among Native Americans, African tribes, Australian and New Zealand aborigines, and tribal peoples on other continents frequently include rich cultural traditions based on deep personal connections to the natural world and the tribe.

In the **Western tradition**, one's identity is found in one's individuality, which inspires the valuing of autonomy, independence, and self-reliance. Mind and body are seen as two separate entities, so different practitioners treat disorders of the body and the mind. Disease is considered to have a specific, measurable, and observable cause, and treatment is aimed at eliminating the cause. Time is seen as linear, always moving forward, and waiting for no one. Success in life is obtained by preparing for the future.

Eastern tradition, however, sees the family as the basis for one's identity, so that family interdependence and group decision making are the norm. Body-mind-spirit are seen as a single entity; there is no sense of separation between

TABLE 5-2 WORLDVIEWS

World cultures have grown out of different worldviews and philosophical traditions. Worldview shapes how cultures perceive reality, the person, and the person in relation to the world and to others. Worldview also shapes perceptions about time, health and illness, and rights and obligations in society. The three worldviews compared here are broad categories and generalizations created to contrast some of the themes found in diverse world cultures. They do not necessarily fit any particular cultural group.

WESTERN (SCIENCE)	EASTERN (BALANCE)	INDIGENOUS (HARMONY)
Roman, Greek, Judeo-Christian; the Enlightenment; Descartes	Chinese and Indian philosophers: Buddha, Confucius, Lao-tse	Deep relationship with nature
The "real" has form and essence; reality tends to be stable.	The "real" is a force or energy; reality is always changing.	The "real" is multidimensional; reality transcends time and space.
Cartesian dualism: body and mind-spirit.	Mind-body-spirit unity.	Mind, body, and spirit are considered so united that there may not be words to indicate them as distinct entities.
Self is starting point for identity.	Family is starting point for identity.	Community is starting point for identity—a person is only an entity in relation to others. The self does not exist except in relation to others. There may be no concept of person or personal ownership.
Time is linear.	Time is circular, flexible.	Time is focused on the present.
Wisdom: preparation for the future.	Wisdom: acceptance of what is.	Wisdom: knowledge of nature.
Disease has a cause (pathogen, toxin, etc.) that creates the effect; disease can be observed and measured.	Disease is caused by a lack of balance in energy forces (e.g., yin-yang, hot-cold); imbalance between daily routine, diet, and constitutional type (Ayurveda).	Disease is caused by a lack of personal, interpersonal, environmental, or spiritual harmony; thoughts and words can shape reality; evil spirits exist.
Ethics of rights and obligations:	*Ethics of care:*	*Ethics of community:*
Based on the individual's right	Based on promoting positive relationships	Based on needs of the community
Value given to:	*Value given to:*	*Value given to:*
Right to decide Right to be informed Open communication Truthfulness	Sympathy, compassion, fidelity, discernment Action on behalf of those with whom one has a relationship Persons in need of health care considered to be vulnerable and to require protection from cruel truth	Contribution to community

a physical illness and a psychological one (Chan et al., 2006). Time is seen as circular and recurring, as in the belief in reincarnation. One is born into an unchangeable fate, with which one has a duty to comply. For the Chinese, disease is caused by fluctuations in opposing forces—the yin-yang energies.

The term **indigenous culture** refers to those people who have inhabited a country for thousands of years and includes such groups as New Zealand Maoris, Australian aborigines, American natives, and native Hawaiians. These groups place special significance on the place of humans in the natural world and frequently manifest a more dramatic difference from Western views (Cunningham & Stanley, 2003). Frequently, the basis of one's identity is the tribe. There may be no concept of person; instead, a person is an entity only in relation to others. The holism of body-mind-spirit may be so complete that there may be no adequate words in the language to describe them as separate entities. Disease is frequently seen as a lack of harmony of the individual with others or the environment.

Psychiatric mental health nursing theories and methods are themselves part of a cultural tradition and our nursing care is a culturally derived set of interventions designed to promote the verbalization of feelings, teach individually focused coping skills, and assist patients with behavioral and emotional self-control—all consistent with Western cultural ideals. When nurses understand that many of the concepts and methods found in psychiatric mental health nursing are based on different assumptions than those of our patients, the process of becoming *culturally competent* begins.

CULTURE AND MENTAL HEALTH

Diverse cultures have evolved from the three broad categories of worldview described in the previous section. Cultures developed norms consistent with their worldviews and

TABLE 5-3 SELECTED NONVERBAL COMMUNICATION PATTERNS

People perceive very strong messages from nonverbal communication patterns; however, the same nonverbal communication pattern can mean very different things to different cultures, as this table indicates. This table does not provide an exhaustive list of possible differences.

NONVERBAL COMMUNICATION PATTERN	PREDOMINANT PATTERNS IN THE UNITED STATES	PATTERNS SEEN IN OTHER CULTURES
Eye contact	Eye contact is associated with attentiveness, politeness, respect, honesty, and self-confidence.	Eye contact is avoided as a sign of rudeness, arrogance, challenge, or sexual interest.
Personal space	*Intimate space:* 0-1 ½ ft *Personal space:* 1½-3 ft In a personal conversation, if a person enters into the intimate space of the other, the person is perceived as aggressive, overbearing, and offensive. If a person stays more distant than expected, the person is perceived as aloof.	Personal space is significantly closer or more distant than in U.S. culture. *Closer*—Middle Eastern, Southern European, and Latin American cultures *Farther*—Asian cultures When closer is the norm, standing very close frequently indicates acceptance of the other.
Touch	Moderate touch indicates personal warmth and conveys caring.	Touch norms vary. *Low-touch cultures*—Touch may be considered an overt sexual gesture capable of "stealing the spirit" of another or taboo between women and men. *High-touch cultures*—People touch one another as frequently as possible (e.g., linking arms when walking or holding a hand or arm when talking).
Facial expressions and gestures	A nod means "yes." Smiling and nodding means "I agree." Thumbs up means "good job." Rolling one's eyes while another is talking is an insult.	Raising eyebrows or rolling the head from side to side means "yes." Smiling and nodding means "I respect you." Thumbs up is an obscene gesture. Pointing one's foot at another is an insult.

adapted to their own historical experiences and the influences of the "outside" world. Cultures are not static; they change and adjust, although usually very slowly. Each culture has different patterns of nonverbal communication (Table 5-3), etiquette norms (Box 5-1), beliefs and values that shape the culture (Table 5-4), and beliefs, values, and practices that influence how the culture understands health and illness (Table 5-5). For instance, in American culture, eye contact is a sign of respectful attention, but in many other cultures, it may be considered arrogant and intrusive. In Western culture, emotional expressiveness is valued, but in many other cultures, it may be a sign of immaturity. In American culture, independence and self-reliance are encouraged, and the family interdependence valued by other cultures may be seen as a symbiotic relationship or a pathological *enmeshment*.

The culture's worldview, beliefs, values, and practices are transmitted to its members in a process called **enculturation**. As children, we learn from our parents which behaviors, beliefs, values, and actions are "right" and which are "wrong." The individual is free to make choices, but the culture expects these choices to be made from its acceptable range of options.

Deviance from cultural expectations is considered to be a problem and frequently is defined by the cultural group as "illness." Mental health is often seen as the degree to which a

BOX 5-1 NORMS OF ETIQUETTE

People tend to feel offended when their rules for "polite" behavior are violated; however, the rules for polite behavior vary greatly from one culture to another. Unless we are aware of cultural differences in etiquette norms, we could infer rudeness on the part of a patient who is operating from a different set of cultural norms and believes his or her behavior is respectful.

Norms of etiquette that vary across cultures include:

- Whether "promptness" is expected and how important it is to be on time
- How formal one should be in addressing others
- Which people deserve recognition and honor and how respect is shown
- Whether shaking hands and other forms of social touch are appropriate
- Whether or not shoes can be worn in the home
- How much clothing should be worn to be "modest"
- What it means to accept or reject offers of food or drink and other gestures of hospitality
- What importance is given to "small talk" and how long it should continue before "getting down to business"
- Whether communication should be direct and forthright or circuitous and subtle
- What the tone of voice and pace of the conversation should be
- Which topics are considered taboo
- Whether or not the children in the home can be touched and admired

TABLE 5-4 CULTURAL BELIEF AND VALUE SYSTEMS

This table contrasts cultural beliefs and values that are predominant in the United States with those that are common in various other world cultures. Belief and value systems are best viewed as a continuum. The beliefs and values of cultures, and of the individuals within cultures, fall at various points along the continuum.

PREDOMINANT CULTURE PATTERNS AND CONCEPTS IN THE UNITED STATES	PATTERNS AND CONCEPTS IN VARIOUS OTHER CULTURES
Individualism	Familism
Independence, self-reliance	Interdependence of family
Autonomy, autonomous decision making	Interconnectedness Family decision making
Egalitarianis: Everyone has an equal voice and deserves equal opportunities.	Social hierarchy: Some deserve more honor or power than others because of their age, gender, occupation, or role in the family; family hierarchies can be patriarchal or matriarchal.
Youth	Age
Physical beauty	Wisdom
Competition	Cooperation
Achievement	Relationships
Materialistic orientation	Metaphysical orientation
Possessions	Spirituality, nature, relationships
Reason and logic	Meditation and intuition
Doing and activity	Being and receptivity
Mastery over nature	Harmony with nature
Latest technology	Natural, traditional ways
Master of one's fate: "I am the master of my destiny."	Fate is one's master: "Fate is responsible for my destiny."
Optimism	Fatalism
Internal locus of control: Life events and circumstances are the result of one's actions.	External locus of control: Life events and circumstances are beyond one's own control and rest in the hands of fate, chance, other people, or God.
Future orientation: "He who prepares for tomorrow will be successful."	Present orientation: "Live for today and let tomorrow take care of itself." Past orientation: Tradition
Punctuality ("clock time"): "Time waits for no one." "Time flies." "Time is money."	"People time": Time is flexible, indefinite; "Time starts when the group gathers." "Time walks. *El tiempo anda*."
Being on time is a sign of courtesy and responsibility.	Being on time can be a sign of compulsiveness and disregard for the people one was with before the appointment time.

person fulfills the expectations of the culture. The culture defines which differences are still within the range of normal (mentally healthy) and which are outside the range of normal (mentally ill).

The same thoughts and behaviors considered mentally healthy in one culture can be considered mentally ill in another. For example, many religious traditions view "speaking in tongues" as mentally healthy and a gift from God, whereas a different cultural group might consider this same behavior as psychosis and a sign of mental illness. Considering culture creates challenges for the psychiatric mental health nurse, and even if the nurse and patient agree the patient has a mental health problem, they may advocate very different ways of treating it.

All people are raised to view the world and everything in it through their own cultural lens, and nurses are no exception. We are products of our culture of professional socialization. Nurses may be tempted to think that the only "good care" is the care they have learned to believe in, value, and practice; however, this can lead to **ethnocentrism**, the universal tendency of humans to think their way of thinking and behaving is the only correct and natural way (Purnell, 2008). Most people are, to a certain degree, ethnocentric; but as nurses, we should examine our assumptions about other cultures to give the best and most culturally competent care possible. Imposing cultural norms on members of other cultural groups is known as cultural imposition (Leininger & McFarland, 2006).

BARRIERS TO QUALITY MENTAL HEALTH SERVICES

The first part of this chapter focused on the impact of culture on mental health and illness in a theoretical way. In the following sections, practice issues that nurses are likely to encounter when providing care to culturally diverse patients are presented, along with suggestions to overcome these barriers.

TABLE 5-5 CULTURAL BELIEFS AND VALUES ABOUT HEALTH AND ILLNESS

This table contrasts the views typically held by Western nurses and the views about health and illness their patients from diverse cultures may hold.

	WESTERN BIOMEDICAL PERSPECTIVE	PERSPECTIVE OF VARIOUS OTHER CULTURES
Health	Absence of disease Ability to function at a high level	Being in a state of balance Being in a state of harmony Ability to perform family roles
Disease causation	Measurable, observable cause that leads to measurable, observable effect Pathogens, mutant cells, toxins, poor diet	Frequently intangible, immeasurable cause Lack of balance (yin and yang) Lack of harmony with environment
Location of disorder	Body Mind	Whole entity: mind, body, and spirit are completely merged Disorder causing disease in the person may be in the family or environment
Decisions about care	Made by patient or holder of power of attorney Goals are autonomy and confidentiality Truth telling required so patient has information to make decisions	Made by the whole family or family head Goals are protection and support of patient Hope should be preserved; patient should be protected from painful truth
Sick role	Sick people should be as independent and self-reliant as possible Self-care is encouraged; one gets better by "getting up and getting going"	Sick people should be as passive as possible Family members should "take care of" and "do for" the sick person Passivity stimulates recovery
Best treatments	Physician-prescribed drugs and treatments Advanced medical technology	Regaining of lost balance or harmony by counteracting negative forces with positive ones and vice versa Treatment by folk healers and traditional remedies
Pain	Stoicism valued Pain described quantitatively Able to pinpoint location of pain In cultures in which negative feelings are not expressed freely, pain is kept as silent as possible: Northern European, Asian, Native American	Pain expressed vocally and dramatically Use of quantitative scales to measure pain is difficult Pain experienced globally In cultures in which emotional expression is encouraged, more dramatic pain expression is expected: Southern European, African, Middle Eastern
Ethics	Based on bioethical principles of autonomy, beneficence, justice, and confidentiality Informed consent requires truthfulness	Based on virtue or community needs Hope should be preserved, painful truth hidden Support and care should be provided Emphasis is on greatest good for the greatest number

Communication Barriers

Therapeutic communication is key to the care of patients with mental illness, yet often nurses and patients do not even speak the same language. The USDHHS Office of Minority Health (2007) states that health care organizations should offer and provide language assistance services, including an interpreter, at no cost to each patient with limited English proficiency at all points of contact and in a timely manner during all hours of operation and service. Patients with limited English proficiency are those who cannot speak English or do not speak English well enough to meet their communication needs.

When a professional interpreter is engaged, the interpreter should be matched to the patient as closely as possible in gender, age, social status, and religion. In addition to interpreting the language, the interpreter can alert the nurse to the meaning of nonverbal communication patterns and cultural norms that are relevant to the encounter. In this way, the interpreter acts as a cultural broker, interpreting not only the language but also the culture.

Interpreters should not be relatives or friends of the patient. The stigma of mental illness may prevent the openness needed during the encounter. Also, those close to the patient may not have the language skills necessary to meet the demands of interpretation, which is a very complex task. Languages frequently cannot be translated word for word; the literal translations of words in one language can carry many different connotations in the other language, and certain concepts are so culturally linked that an adequate translation is very difficult.

Even people who speak English well may have difficulty communicating emotional nuances in English; these may be more accessible to patients in their own languages. Idioms and figures of speech can be extremely confusing. For instance, the terms *feeling blue* or *feeling down* may have no meaning at all in the patient's literal understanding of English.

Nonverbal communication patterns may also be influenced by culture. Some Native American cultures use silence to a far greater degree than the dominant culture, and their silence can be mistaken for belligerence or sullenness, when in fact it is a common response to dealing with strangers and is even considered a sign of wisdom. The downcast eyes of an Asian woman may be viewed as a sign of evasiveness, when it is actually a sign of respect. Nonverbal communication patterns should be interpreted from within the patient's cultural perspective, not from the Western medical perspective (Munoz & Luckmann, 2005).

Stigma of Mental Illness

Mental illnesses are stigmatized disorders, and this stigma presents significant barriers to treatment. Many people in all sectors of society in the United States associate mental illness with moral weakness. Others express fear of, or bias against, those with mental health problems; however, in many cultural groups, the stigma of mental illness is more severe and prevalent than it generally is in the United States.

In cultural groups that emphasize the interdependence and harmony of the family, mental illness may be perceived as a failure of the family. In such groups, the pressures on both the individual with the mental illness and the family are increased. Both the individual and the whole family are perceived as ill, and the illness reflects badly on the character of all family members. Stigma and shame can lead to reluctance to seek help, so members of these cultural groups may enter the mental health care system at an advanced stage, when the family has exhausted its ability to cope with the problem.

Misdiagnosis

Another barrier to mental health care is misdiagnosis. Studies indicate that blacks and African Americans, Afro-Caribbean, and Latino-Hispanic Americans run a significant risk of being misdiagnosed with schizophrenia when the true diagnosis is bipolar disease or an affective disorder (Suite et al., 2007). Why does this happen? One reason for misdiagnosis is the use of culturally inappropriate psychometric instruments and other diagnostic tools. Most available tools have been validated using subjects of European origin. For instance, Kim (2002) states that although there are over 40 validated depression scales, they tend to be "linguistically irrelevant and culturally inappropriate" (p. 110) for some groups, and they fail to identify depression in Koreans. Kim argues that the current scales measure Western ways of expressing depression by focusing on the affective domain, whereas for Koreans more attention needs to be given to the somatic domain. To rectify this problem, Kim created and validated a depression scale for Korean Americans.

As this inadequacy of diagnostic tools suggests, psychological distress is manifested in different cultures in different ways. In cultures in which the body and mind are seen as one entity, or in cultures in which there is a high degree of stigma associated with mental health problems, individuals frequently somatize their feelings of psychological distress. In **somatization**, psychological distress is experienced as physical problems. Instead of perceiving the distress as emotional or affective, the psychological distress is perceived in the body. For example, a Cambodian woman may describe feelings of back pain, fatigue, and dizziness and say nothing about feelings of sadness or hopelessness (Henderson et al., 2008).

Somatization is just one example of how psychological distress is manifested. Just as we learn from our parents whether the appropriate way to deal with pain is either dramatic expressiveness or stoicism and denial, we learn different ways to manifest and express mental pain and pathology. Because of this, many cross-cultural mental health experts have been skeptical about using psychiatric diagnostic criteria that are based on studies with predominantly white American samples. Consideration for how ethnicity may affect a psychiatric diagnosis has been incorporated into the development of the American Psychiatric Association's diagnostic criteria for the fifth edition of the *Diagnostic and Statistical Manual of Mental Disorders (DSM-5)* (American Psychiatric Association, 2013a).

Furthermore, the *DSM-5* includes a standardized tool for taking into account cultural variations during the assessment phase of patient care. The "Cultural Formulation Interview" (American Psychiatric Association, 2013b) is a 14-question inventory that helps clinicians plan for care based on orientation, values, and assumptions that originate from particular cultures. It takes into consideration the meaning of the illness for the patient, the role of family and others as support, the patient's attempts to cope with previous illness, and expectations of current care.

Culture-bound syndromes are sets of signs and symptoms that are common in a limited number of cultures but virtually nonexistent in most other cultural groups (Henderson et al., 2008) (Box 5-2). In the most recent revision of the *Diagnostic and Statistical Manual*, experts have integrated issues related to culture and mental illness into the discussion of each disorder (American Psychiatric Association, 2013). This is a marked change from the previous edition of the manual, which segregated culture-bound syndromes into a separate section.

Culture-bound illnesses may seem exotic or irrational to nurses who have been trained within a Western medical framework. Symptoms may be shocking, and other-culture explanations regarding causation and treatment may be mystifying. These illnesses, however, are frequently well understood by the people within the cultural group; they know the name of the problem, its etiology, its course, and the way it should be treated. Frequently, when these illnesses are treated in culturally prescribed ways, the remedies are quite effective.

Many culture-bound syndromes have been identified. Some of these syndromes seem to be mental health problems that manifest in somatic ways. *Hwa-byung* and *neurasthenia* have many similarities to depression (Park et al., 2001), but because the somatic complaints are so prominent, and patients frequently deny feelings of sadness or depression, they may not fit the *DSM-IV* diagnostic criteria for depression.

Ataque de nervios and *ghost sickness* (see Box 5-2) belong to another group of culture-bound illnesses characterized by abnormal behaviors. These types of illness seem to be culturally acceptable ways for patients to express that they can no longer endure the stressors in their lives. People in the culture understand the patient is ill and provide support using culturally

BOX 5-2 EXAMPLES OF CULTURE-BOUND SYNDROMES

Because so many culture-bound syndromes have been identified, they cannot all be described in this chapter. However, the list here includes some of the syndromes the psychiatric mental health nurse might encounter.

Ataque de nervios: Latin American. Characterized by a sudden attack of trembling, palpitations, dyspnea, dizziness, and loss of consciousness. Thought to be caused by an evil spirit and related to intolerable stress. Treated by an espiritista (spiritual healer) and by the support of the family and community, who provide aid to the patient and consider the patient to be calling for help in a culturally acceptable way.

Ghost sickness: Navajo. Characterized by "being out of one's mind," dyspnea, weakness, and bad dreams. Thought to be caused by an evil spirit. Treated by overcoming the evil spirit with a stronger spiritual force the healer, a "singer," calls forth through a powerful healing ritual.

Hwa-byung: Korean. Characterized by epigastric pain, anorexia, palpitations, dyspnea, and muscle aches and pains. Thought to be caused by a lack of harmony in the body or in interpersonal relationships. Treated by reestablishing harmony. Some researchers feel that it is closely related to depression.

'Jin' possession: Somalian. Characterized by psychological distress and anxiety caused by the belief that one is possessed by a 'Jin' (a being that is able to see humans even though humans cannot see it, and that is capable of possessing a human's body when it is angry with the human). Intermittent, involuntary, abnormal body movements occur along with the psychological distress. Treated by exorcising the 'Jin' with the assistance of a religious leader, such as an Imam, who will ask the 'Jin' what the person has done to anger it so that the person can apologize and make amends. (Somali inpatient psychiatric nurse, personal communication, March 8, 2012).

Neurasthenia: Chinese. Characterized by somatic symptoms of depression (e.g., anorexia, weight loss, fatigue, weakness, trouble concentrating, insomnia), although feelings of sadness or depression are denied. Thought to be related to a lack of yin-yang balance.

Susto: Latin American. Characterized by a broad range of somatic and psychological symptoms. Thought to be related to a traumatic incident or fright that caused the patient's soul to leave the body. Treated by an espiritista (spiritual healer).

Wind illness: Chinese, Vietnamese. Characterized by a fear of cold, wind, or drafts. Derived from the belief that yin-yang and hot-cold elements must be in balance in the body or illness occurs. Treated by keeping very warm and avoiding foods, drinks, and herbs that are cold or considered to have a cold quality, as well as "cold" colors, emotions, and activities. Also treated by a variety of means designed to pull the "cold wind" out of the patient, such as by coining (vigorously rubbing a coin over the body) or cupping (applying a heated cup to the skin, creating a vacuum).

prescribed treatments, which actually relieve the stresses through remedies the patient finds helpful.

Another kind of culture-bound illness seems to be merely a cultural explanation of an illness Western medicine understands as having a biomedical cause. From a Western perspective, the patient may be experiencing depression, anxiety, or posttraumatic stress disorder, but the patient believes he is experiencing the illness as *susto,* or "soul loss," due to an extremely disturbing or frightening experience (Lim, 2006).

Culture-bound illnesses are frequently thought of as being found only in "other" (i.e., non-Western) cultures. However, some authors have pointed out that anorexia nervosa and bulimia seem to be bound to Western culture, apparently because other cultures do not value the thinness so prized by European and North American cultural groups (Marsella, 2003). It may be that all the psychiatric diagnoses used in the United States are culture-bound to Western patients since the criteria of these diagnoses were developed through studies of Western patients.

When we fail to consider culture in diagnosis and treatment, we are more likely to see culturally normal behavior as "abnormal" instead of merely different. In African American churches, it is common to talk about spiritual experiences in terms such as "I was talking to Jesus this morning." The speaker may have meant he was praying, but the clinician unfamiliar with the culture may misinterpret such a statement as delusional. If a Vietnamese father says he tried to take the "wind illness" out of his child by vigorously rubbing a coin down her back, the clinician may believe the father is a potential threat to the child.

When there is a cultural mismatch between the clinician and the patient, misdiagnosis and culturally inappropriate treatments frequently result in cultural imposition (Leininger & McFarland, 2006). One might be tempted to think that the only way to solve these problems is to ensure that patients have mental health providers who match the patient's culture; however, another way to solve the problem is to take the time to adapt the nursing care to meet the patient's cultural needs.

Genetic Variation in Pharmacodynamics

A third clinical practice issue that presents a barrier to quality mental health services for some groups is genetic variation in drug responses. There is a growing realization that many drugs vary in their action and effects along genetic and psychosocial lines (Lehne, 2010). What was found true in drug studies primarily performed with subjects of European origin may not be true in ethnically diverse populations. Genetic variations in drug metabolism have been documented for several classifications of drugs, including antidepressants and antipsychotics.

The relatively new field of **pharmacogenetics** focuses on how genes affect individual responses to medicines (National Institutes of Health [NIH], 2012). Genes carry recipes for making specific protein molecules. Medications interact with thousands of proteins, and the smallest difference in the quantities or composition of these molecules can make a big difference in how they work. By understanding how genes influence drug responses, we hope to one day prescribe drugs that are best suited for each person.

An important variation that impacts the ability to metabolize drugs relates to the more than 20 cytochrome P-450 (CYP) enzymes present in human beings (Henderson et al., 2008). Genetic variations in these enzymes may alter drug metabolism, and these variations tend to be propagated through racial and ethnic populations.

CYP enzymes metabolize most antidepressants and antipsychotics. Some genetic variations result in rapid metabolism, and if medications are metabolized too quickly, serum levels become too low, and therapeutic effects are minimized. Other variations may result in poor metabolism. If medications are metabolized too slowly, serum levels become too high, and the risk of intolerable side effects increases. One purpose of genetic testing of the future will be to enable clinicians to determine correct drugs and dosage using liver enzymes (NIH, 2012).

POPULATIONS AT RISK FOR MENTAL ILLNESS AND INADEQUATE CARE

Many people in the United States are subject to experiences that challenge their mental health in ways that members of the majority group do not have to face. Among these challenges are issues related to the experience of being an immigrant and the socioeconomic disadvantages of minority status.

Immigrants

Immigrants face many unknowns. Upon arriving in the United States, they may not speak English, yet they need to learn how to navigate new economic, political, legal, educational, transportation, and health care systems. Many who had status and skills in their homeland—jobs as teachers, administrators, or other professional positions—find that because of certification requirements or limited English skills, only menial jobs are open to them. After immigration, family roles may be upset, with wives finding jobs before their husbands. Immigrant families may find the struggle to live successfully in America arduous and wearisome. Long-honored cultural values and traditions, which once provided stability, are challenged by new cultural norms. During the period of adjustment, many immigrants find that the hope they felt on first immigrating turns into anxiety and depression.

Immigrants and their families embark on a process of **acculturation**—learning the beliefs, values, and practices of their new cultural setting—that sometimes takes several generations. Some immigrants adapt to the new culture quickly, absorbing the new worldview, beliefs, values, and practices rapidly until they are more natural than the ones they learned in their homeland (**assimilation**). Others attempt to maintain their traditional cultural ways. Some may become bicultural—able to move in and out of their traditional culture and their new culture, depending on where they are and with whom they associate. Some immigrants may suffer culture shock, finding the new norms disconcerting or offensive because they contrast so deeply with their traditional beliefs, values, and practices.

Many families find that the children assimilate the new culture at a rapid pace, whereas the elders maintain their traditional cultural beliefs, values, and practices. This sets the stage for intergenerational conflict. Children who are assimilating different values about family may challenge the traditional status of elders in a hierarchical family. Some children may feel lost between two cultures and unsure of where to place their cultural identity.

Refugees

A **refugee** is a special kind of immigrant. Whereas the immigrant generally values the new culture and wishes to enjoy a change in life circumstances, the refugee has left his or her own homeland to escape intolerable conditions and would have preferred to stay in the culture if that had been possible. Refugees do not perceive entry into the new culture as an active choice and may experience the stress of adjusting as imposed on them against their will. Many refugees from Southeast Asia, Central America, and Africa have been traumatized by war, genocide, torture, starvation, and other catastrophic events. Many have lost family members, a way of life, and a homeland to which they can never return. The degree of trauma and loss they have experienced may make them particularly vulnerable to a variety of psychiatric disorders, including major depressive disorder (MDD) and posttraumatic stress disorder (PTSD).

Cultural Minorities

Individuals who are considered "minorities" (non-whites) may be vulnerable to a variety of disadvantages, including poverty and limited opportunities for education and jobs. Cultural minority groups are frequent victims of bias, discrimination, and racism—subtle but pervasive forms of rejection that diminish self-esteem and self-efficacy and leave victims feeling excluded and marginalized.

In the United States, the incidence of various types of mental health disorders among cultural and racial minority groups is similar to that among whites *if* the poor and other vulnerable populations (e.g., homeless, institutionalized, children in foster care, victims of trauma) within the minority groups are excluded. If people in these vulnerable populations are included, however, the incidence of mental health problems among minorities increases. Therefore, the higher incidence of mental health problems is related to poverty not ethnicity (USDHHS, 2001).

People who live in poverty are two to three times more likely to develop mental illness than those who live above the poverty line. In 2011, 9.8% of non-Hispanic whites lived in poverty; 12.3% of Asian, 25.3% of Latino-Hispanic Americans, and 27.6% of blacks and African Americans lived below the poverty line (U.S. Census Bureau, 2012). Poverty is highly associated with other disadvantages, such as scarce educational and economic opportunities, which in turn are associated with substance abuse and violent crime. Persons who are poor are subject to a daily struggle for survival, and this takes its toll on mental health.

Persons from cultural minorities have reported that they perceived bias and experienced culturally uncomfortable care from health care providers, which made them less likely to seek medical services in the future. According to a report issued by the Institute of Medicine, *Unequal Treatment: Confronting Racial and Ethnic Disparities in Healthcare*, bias and discrimination taint the health care system, resulting in further stresses on the mental health of those in minority groups instead of delivering the help they need (Smedley et al., 2003).

CULTURALLY COMPETENT CARE

So far, this chapter has explained why the nursing needs of culturally diverse patient populations are so varied. Mental health and illness are biological, psychological, social, spiritual and *cultural* processes. Cultural competence is required of nurses if they are to assist patients in achieving mental health and well-being. How, exactly, are psychiatric mental health nurses to practice culturally competent care? The remainder of this chapter suggests techniques that answer this question.

The USDHHS Office of Minority Health (2007) defines culturally competent care as attitudes and behaviors that enable a nurse to work effectively *within* the patient's cultural context. Cultural and linguistic competence is a set of congruent behaviors, attitudes, and policies that come together in a system, agency, or among professionals and enable effective work in cross-cultural situations. **Cultural competence** means that nurses adjust *their* practices to meet their patients' cultural beliefs, practices, needs, and preferences. Having cultural sensitivity or awareness is an essential component of cultural competence. Culturally competent care goes beyond culturally sensitive care by adapting care to the patient's cultural needs and preferences (Narayan, 2006).

Campinha-Bacote (2008) recommends a blueprint for psychiatric mental health nurses in providing culturally effective care: the Process of Cultural Competence in the Delivery of Healthcare Services. In this model, nurses view themselves as *becoming* culturally competent rather than *being* culturally competent. This model suggests that nurses should constantly see themselves as learners throughout their careers—always open to, and learning from, the immense cultural diversity they will see among their patients. The model consists of five constructs that promote the process and journey of cultural competence:

1. Cultural awareness
2. Cultural knowledge
3. Cultural encounters
4. Cultural skill
5. Cultural desire

Cultural Awareness

Through cultural awareness, the nurse recognizes the enormous impact culture makes on what patients' health values and practices are, how and when patients decide they are ill and need care, and what treatments they will seek when illness occurs.

Cultural awareness should inspire nurses to first acknowledge themselves as cultural beings, so close to the norms of their own ethnic and professional cultures that these norms seem "right" (ethnocentrism) and not just "cultural." In accordance with the demands of cultural awareness, nurses should also examine all beliefs, values, and practices to ascertain which ones are cultural and which ones could be universally held (Campinha-Bacote, 2003). Through cultural awareness and cultural humility, nurses often discover that many norms are cultural, few are universal, and that they have an obligation to be open to and respectful of patients' cultural norms.

By practicing cultural awareness, nurses also examine their cultural assumptions and expectations about what constitutes mental health, a "healthy" self-concept, a "healthy" family, and the "right way" to behave in society. Assumptions and expectations about how people manifest psychological distress should also be examined. The culturally aware nurse questions whether the evidence-based guideline (derived from studies involving primarily subjects of European origin) should be modified to address the cultural aspects of a particular patient's life and illness (Campinha-Bacote, 2002).

A culturally aware nurse recognizes that three cultures are intersecting during any encounter with a patient: the culture of the patient, the culture of the nurse, and the culture of the setting (agency, clinic, hospital) (USDHHS, 2001). As a patient advocate, our job is to negotiate and support the patient's cultural needs and preferences.

Cultural Knowledge

Nurses can enhance their cultural knowledge in various ways. They can attend cultural events and programs, forge friendships with members of diverse cultural groups, and participate in in-service programs at which members of diverse groups talk about their cultural norms. Another way to obtain cultural knowledge is to study print or online resources designed for health care providers.

Cultural knowledge is proactive when it prevents nurses from assuming that they share a patient's underlying worldview and values; it highlights areas in which there may be cultural differences. Cultural knowledge can assist in understanding behaviors that might otherwise be misinterpreted. It helps nurses establish rapport, ask the right questions, avoid misunderstandings, and identify cultural variables that may need to be considered when planning nursing care (Narayan, 2002).

Available cultural guides and resources offer valuable information about various ethnic and religious cultures (Campinha-Bacote, 2002), including the following:

- Worldview, beliefs, and values that permeate the culture
- Nonverbal communication patterns, such as the meaning of eye contact, facial expressions, gestures, and touch
- Etiquette norms, such as the importance of punctuality, the pace of conversation, and the way respect and hospitality are shown
- Family roles and psychosocial norms, such as the way decisions are made and the degree of independence versus interdependence of family members
- Cultural views about mental health and illness, such as the degree of stigma and the nature of the "sick role"
- Patterns related to health and illness, including culture-bound syndromes, pharmacogenetic variations, and folk and herbal treatments frequently used within the culture

Cultural Encounters

Although obtaining cultural knowledge sets a foundation, cultural guides cannot tell us anything about a particular patient. According to Campinha-Bacote (2008), multiple cultural encounters with diverse patients deter nurses from stereotyping. Although generalizations can be made about cultures, stereotyping individuals within the group robs them of the individuality they possess and robs the culture of its diversity.

Stereotyping is the tendency to believe that every member of a group is like all other members. However, multiple cultural encounters enable us to experience the intra-ethnic diversity of cultural groups and to come to understand that although there are patterns that characterize a culture, individual members of the culture adhere to the culture's norms in diverse ways.

Each person is a unique blend of the many ethnic, spiritual, socioeconomic, geographic, educational, and occupational cultures to which he or she belongs. Each person brings a unique personality, life experiences, and creative thought to self-development and makes choices about which cultural norms to adopt or abandon. In the end, each person is a unique individual who never adheres to all (and may not adhere to any) of the norms of his or her culture of origin. The only way to know about the norms of a patient's culture is to ask the patient.

Cultural encounters help nurses develop confidence in cross-cultural interactions. Every nurse is likely to make cultural blunders and will need to recover from cultural mistakes. Cultural encounters help develop the skill of recognizing, avoiding, and reducing the cultural pain that can occur when nursing care causes the patient discomfort or offense by a failure to be sensitive to cultural norms (Kavanagh, 2008). Every nurse can learn to recognize signs of cultural pain, such as a patient's discomfort or alienation, and take measures to recover trust and rapport by asking what has caused the offense, apologizing for any lack of sensitivity, and expressing willingness to learn from the patient how care can be provided in a culturally sensitive way.

Cultural Skill

Cultural skill is the ability to perform a cultural assessment in a sensitive way (Campinha-Bacote, 2008). The first step is to ensure that meaningful communication can occur. If the patient is not proficient in English, a professional medical interpreter should be engaged.

Many cultural assessment tools are available (Andrews & Boyle, 2011; Purnell, 2008; Spector, 2004; Giger & Davidhizar, 2007; Narayan, 2003; Leininger, 2002). An appendix of the *DSM-IV-TR* (American Psychiatric Association, 2000), Outline for Cultural Formulation, recommends cultural assessment areas. A very useful mental health assessment tool is the classic set of questions proposed by Kleinman and colleagues (1978):

- What do you call this illness? *(diagnosis)*
- When did it start? Why then? *(onset)*
- What do you think caused it? *(etiology)*
- How does the illness work? What does it do to you? *(course)*
- How long will it last? Is it serious? *(prognosis)*
- How have you treated the illness? How do you think it should be treated? *(treatment)*

These questions allow the patient to feel heard and understood. They also help in eliciting culture-bound syndromes. They can be expanded to include questions such as:

- What are the chief problems this illness has caused you?
- What do you fear most about this illness? Do you think it is curable?
- Do you know others who have had this problem? What happened to them? Do you think this will happen to you?

Approaching these questions conversationally is generally more effective than using a direct, formal approach. One indirect technique is to ask the patient what another family member thinks is causing the problem. Instead of saying, "What do you call this illness?" and inquiring about how it started, the nurse can ask, "What does your family think is wrong? Why do they think it started? What do they think you should do about it?" After the patient describes what the family thinks, the nurse can simply ask in a nonjudgmental way if the patient agrees.

Another technique for promoting openness is to make a declaratory statement before asking the questions. For instance, before asking about cultural treatments the patient has tried, the nurse can first say, "Everyone has remedies they find help them when they are ill. Are there any special healers or treatments you have used or that you think might be helpful to you?"

There are some areas that deserve special attention during an assessment interview:

- Ethnicity, religious affiliation, and degree of acculturation to Western medical culture
- Spiritual practices that are important to preserving or regaining health
- Degree of proficiency in speaking and reading English
- Dietary patterns, including foods prescribed for sick people
- Attitudes about pain and experiences with pain in a Western medical setting
- Attitudes about and experience with Western medications
- Cultural remedies such as healers, herbs, and practices the patient may find helpful
- Whom the patient considers "family," who should receive health information, and how decisions are made in the family
- Cultural customs the patient feels are essential to preserve and is fearful will be violated in the mental health setting

The purpose of a culturally sensitive assessment is to develop a therapeutic plan that is mutually agreeable, culturally acceptable, and potentially productive of positive outcomes. While gathering assessment data, you should identify cultural patterns that may support or interfere with the patient's health and recovery process. Your professional knowledge can then be used to categorize the patient's cultural norms into three different groups:

1. Those that facilitate the patient's health and recovery, from the Western medical perspective
2. Those that are neither helpful nor harmful, from the Western medical perspective
3. Those that are harmful to the patient's health and well-being, from the Western medical perspective

Leininger and McFarland (2006) suggest a preservation/maintenance, accommodate/negotiate, repatterning/restructuring framework for care planning. Using this framework, effective nursing care preserves the aspects of the patient's culture that, from a Western perspective, promote health and well-being—such as a strong family support system and traditional values such as cooperation and emphasis on relationships.

Cultural values and practices that are neither helpful nor harmful are accommodated or may be negotiated. You may encourage the patient's use of neutral values and practices such as folk remedies and healers. By including these culture-specific interventions in the care as complementary interventions, nursing care builds on the patient's own coping and healing systems. For example, Native Americans with substance abuse problems may find tribal healing ceremonies helpful as a complement to the therapeutic program.

Finally, when cultural patterns are determined harmful, the nurse should make attempts to repattern/restructure them. For instance, if a patient is taking an herb that interferes with the prescription medication regimen, the nurse would do well to educate and negotiate with the patient until a mutually agreeable therapeutic program is developed.

Cultural Desire

The final construct in Campinha-Bacote's cultural competence model for psychiatric mental health nurses (2008) is cultural desire. Cultural desire indicates that the nurse is not acting out of a sense of duty but from a sincere and genuine concern for patients' welfare. This concern ideally leads to attempts to truly understand each patient's viewpoint. Nurses exhibit cultural desire through patience, consideration, and empathy. Giving the impression that you are willing to learn from the patient is the hallmark of cultural desire, as opposed to behaving as if you know what is best and are going to impose the "correct" treatment on the patient.

Cultural desire inspires openness and flexibility in applying nursing principles to meet the patient's cultural needs. Although it may be easier to establish a therapeutic relationship with someone who comes from a similar cultural background, cultural desire enables the nurse to achieve good outcomes with culturally diverse patients.

KEY POINTS TO REMEMBER

- Mental health and illness are biological, psychological, social, spiritual and cultural phenomena.
- As the diversity of the world and the United States increases, psychiatric mental health nurses will be caring for more and more people from diverse cultural groups.
- Nurses should learn to deliver culturally competent care, meaning culturally sensitive assessments and culturally congruent interventions.
- *Culture* is the shared beliefs, values, and practices of a group; it shapes the group's thinking and behavior in patterned ways. Cultural groups share these norms with new members of the group through *enculturation*.
- A group's culture influences its members' worldview, nonverbal communication patterns, etiquette norms, and ways of viewing the person, the family, and the "right" way to think and behave in society.
- The concept of mental health is formed within a culture, and deviance from cultural expectations can be defined as "illness" by other members of the group.
- Psychiatric mental health nursing is based on personality and developmental theories advanced by Europeans and Americans and grounded in Western cultural ideals and values.
- Nurses are as influenced by their own professional and ethnic cultures as patients are by theirs. Nurses should guard against ethnocentric tendencies when caring for patients, because cultural imposition does not promote patient health and well-being.
- Barriers to quality mental health care include communication barriers, ethnic variations in psychotropic drug metabolism, and misdiagnoses caused by culturally inappropriate diagnostic tools.
- Immigrants (especially refugees) and minority groups suffering from the effects of low socioeconomic status, including poverty and discrimination, are at particular risk for mental illness.
- Cultural competence consists of five constructs: cultural awareness, cultural knowledge, cultural encounters, cultural skill, and cultural desire.
- Through cultural awareness, nurses recognize that they, as well as patients, have cultural beliefs, values, and practices.
- Cultural knowledge is obtained by seeking cultural information from friends, participating in in-service programs, immersing oneself in the culture, or consulting print and online sources.
- Nurses experience intra-ethnic diversity through multiple cultural encounters, which prevents nurses from stereotyping their patients.
- Nurses demonstrate cultural skill by performing culturally sensitive assessment interviews and adapting care to meet patients' cultural needs and preferences.
- Care can be adapted by using the care planning preservation/maintenance, accommodate/negotiate, repatterning/restructure framework of Leininger & McFarland (2006) when creating the therapeutic plan.
- Cultural desire is a genuine interest in the patient's unique perspective; it enables nurses to provide considerate, flexible, and respectful care to patients of all cultures.

CRITICAL THINKING

1. Describe the cultural factors that have influenced the development of Western psychiatric mental health nursing practice. Contrast these Western influences with the cultural factors that influence patients who come from an Eastern or indigenous culture.
2. What do you think about the claim that mental illness, such as schizophrenia, is a cultural phenomenon and that individuals are judged to be mentally ill if they do not fit within the social definition of normal? What implications (good or bad) does a diagnosis of a mental illness have?
3. Analyze the effects cultural competence (or incompetence) can have on psychiatric mental health nurses and their patients.
4. How can barriers such as misdiagnosis and communication problems impede the promotion of competent psychiatric mental health care? What can the members of the health care team do to overcome such barriers?

CHAPTER REVIEW

1. In the *DSM-5*, a major change in how culture is viewed within each disorder is that:
   a. issues related to culture and mental illness are now integrated into the discussion of each disorder rather than separately discussing culture-bound syndromes.
   b. issues related to culture and mental illness are markedly absent in the discussion of each disorder.
   c. it is noted that it is impossible for health practitioners to be expected to be culturally aware with the increasing diversity of the United States.
   d. issues related to culture and mental illness are less important than previously thought in diagnostic criteria.
2. Julio is a 31-year-old patient who comes to your mental health outpatient clinic. Which of the following would alert you to the potential for somatization?
   a. Julio states, "I have been feeling sad for weeks."
   b. Julio shows you bottles of medication he has been prescribed for anxiety.
   c. Julio presents with concerns involving headaches, dizziness, and fatigue.
   d. Julio states, "I have been sleeping all the time."
3. You are caring for Maria, a patient who states that she has "ghost sickness." Which is the appropriate nursing response?
   a. "I have no idea what 'ghost sickness' is."
   b. "How does 'ghost sickness' make you feel?"
   c. "'Ghost sickness' is not listed in the manual of psychiatric disorders."
   d. "Let's talk about why you believe in evil spirits?"
4. Which nursing actions demonstrate cultural competence? *Select all that apply.*
   a. Planning mealtime around the patient's prayer schedule
   b. Advising a patient to visit with the hospital chaplain
   c. Researching foods that a lacto-ovo-vegetarian patient will eat
   d. Providing time for a patient's spiritual healer to visit
   e. Ordering standard meal trays to be delivered three times daily
5. The nurse is planning care for a patient of the Latin American culture. Which goal is appropriate?
   a. Patient will visit with spiritual healer once weekly.
   b. Patient will experience rebalance of yin-yang by discharge.
   c. Patient will identify sources that increase "cold wind" within 24 hours of admission.
   d. Patient will contact "singer" to provider healing ritual within 3 days of admission.

Answers to Chapter Review
1. a; 2. c; 3. b; 4. a, b, c, d; 5. a.

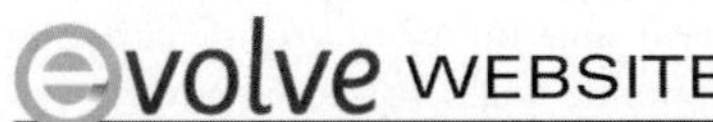
WEBSITE

Visit the Evolve website for a posttest on the content in this chapter: http://evolve.elsevier.com/Varcarolis

Post-Test interactive review

REFERENCES

American Psychiatric Association. (2013a). *Diagnostic and statistical manual of mental disorders* (5th ed). Washington, DC: Author.

American Psychiatric Association. (2013b). *DSM-5 cultural formulation interview.* Retrieved from http://www.dsm5.org/proposedrevision/Pages/Cult.aspx.

American Psychiatric Association. (2000). *Diagnostic and statistical manual of mental disorders* (4th ed., text rev.). Washington, DC: Author.

Andrews, M., & Boyle, J. (2011). *Transcultural concepts in nursing care* (6th ed.). Philadelphia, PA: Lippincott.

Bulechek, G. M., Butcher, H. K., Dochterman, J. M., & Wagner, C. (2013). *Nursing interventions classification (NIC)* (6th ed.). St. Louis, MO: Mosby.

Campinha-Bacote, J. (2002). Cultural competence in psychiatric nursing: Have you asked the right questions? *Journal of the American Psychiatric Nurses Association, 8*(6), 183–187.

Campinha-Bacote, J. (2003). *The process of cultural competence in the delivery of healthcare services* (4th ed.). Cincinnati, OH: Associates Press.

Campinha-Bacote, J. (2008). Cultural desire: 'Caught' or 'taught'? *Contemporary Nurse: Advances in Contemporary Transcultural Nursing, 28*(1-2), 141–148.

Chan, C. L. W., Ng, S. M., Ho, R. T. H., & Chow, Y. M. (2006). East meets West: Applying Eastern spirituality in clinical practice. *Journal of Clinical Nursing, 15,* 822–832.

Cunningham, C., & Stanley, F. (2003). Indigenous by definition, experience, and worldview. *British Medical Journal, 327*(7412), 403–404.

Giger, J. N., & Davidhizar, R. E. (2007).*Transcultural nursing: Assessment and intervention* (4th ed.). St. Louis: Mosby.

Henderson, D. C., Yeung, A., Fan, X., & Fricchione, G. L. (2008). Culture and psychiatry. In T. A. Stern, J. F. Rosenbaum, M. Fava, J. Biederman, & S. L. Rauch (Eds.), *Massachusetts General Hospital comprehensive clinical psychiatry* (pp. 907–916). St. Louis, MO: Mosby.

Herdman, T. H. (Ed.), (2012). *NANDA international nursing diagnoses: Definitions and classification, 2012-2014.* Oxford, UK: Wiley-Blackwell.

Kavanagh, H. K. (2008). Transcultural perspectives in mental health nursing. In M. M. Andrews, & J. S. Boyle (Eds.), *Transcultural concepts in nursing care* (pp. 226–260). Philadelphia, PA: Wolters.

Kim, M. (2002). Measuring depression in Korean Americans: development of the Kim Depression Scale for Korean Americans. *Journal of Transcultural Nursing, 13*(2), 109–117.

Kleinman, A., Eisenberg, L., & Good, B. (1978). Culture, illness and care: clinical lessons from anthropologic and cross-cultural research. *Annals of Internal Medicine, 88,* 251–258.

Leininger, M. (2002). Culture care assessments for congruent competency practices. In M. Leininger & M. McFarland (Eds.), *Transcultural nursing: Concepts, theories, research and practice* (pp. 117–144). New York, NY: McGraw-Hill.

Leininger, M., & McFarland, M. (2006). *Culture care diversity & universality: A worldwide nursing theory* (2nd ed.). Sudbury, MA: Jones & Bartlett.

Lehne, R. A. (2010). Individual variation in drug responses. In R .A. Lehne (Ed.), *Pharmacology for nursing care* (pp. 82–83). St. Louis, MO: Elsevier.

Lim, R. F. (2006). *Clinical manual of cultural psychiatry.* Arlington, VA: American Psychiatric Publishing.

Marsella, A .J. (2003). Cultural aspects of depressive experience and disorders. In W. J. Lonner, D. L. Dinnel, S. A. Hayes, & D. N. Sattler (Eds.), *Online readings in psychology and culture* (Unit 9, Chapter 4). Retrieved from http://www.wwu.edu/culture/Marsella.htm.

Moorhead, S., Johnson, M., Maas, M. L., & Swanson, E. (2013). *Nursing outcomes classification (NOC)* (5th ed.). St. Louis, MO: Mosby.

Munoz, C., & Luckmann, J. (2005). *Transcultural communication in nursing* (2nd ed.). Clifton Park, NJ: Delmar.

Narayan, M. C. (2002). Six steps to cultural competence: A clinician's guide. *Home Health Care Management and Practice, 14*, 378–386.

Narayan, M. C. (2003). Cultural assessment and care planning. *Home Healthcare Nurse, 21*, 611–618.

Narayan, M. C. (2006). Culturally relevant mental health nursing: A global perspective. In E. M. Varcarolis, V. B. Carson, & N. C. Shoemaker (Eds.), *Foundations of psychiatric mental health nursing* (pp. 99–113). Philadelphia, PA: Saunders.

National Institutes of Health. (2012). *Frequently asked questions about pharmacogenetics.* Retrieved from http://www.nigms.nih.gov/Research/FeaturedPrograms/PGRN/Background/pgrn_faq.htm.

Office of Minority Health. (2007). *National standards on culturally and linguistically appropriate services.* Washington, DC: U.S. Department of Health and Human Services, Office of Minority Health. Retrieved from http://www.omhrc.gov/templates/browse.aspx?lvl=2&lvlID=15.

Park, Y., Kim, H., Kang, H., & Kim, J. (2001). A survey of hwa-byung in middle-age Korean women. *Journal of Transcultural Nursing, 12*(2), 115–122.

Purnell, L. D. (2008). Transcultural diversity and health care. In L. D. Purnell, & B. J. Paulanka (Eds.), *Transcultural health care* (pp. 1–19). Philadelphia, PA: Davis.

Smedley, B., Stith A., & Nelson A. (2003). *Unequal treatment: Confronting racial and ethnic disparities in healthcare.* Washington, DC: National Academy Press.

Spector, R. E. (2004). *Cultural diversity in health and illness* (6th ed.). Upper Saddle River, NJ: Prentice-Hall.

Suite, D. H., LaBril, R., Primm, A., & Harrison-Ross, P. (2007). Beyond misdiagnosis, misunderstanding, and mistrust: Relevance of the historical perspective in the medical and mental health treatment of people of color. *Journal of the National Medical Association, 99*(8), 1–7.

United States Census Bureau. (2007). Minority population tops 100 million. *U.S. Census Bureau News.* Retrieved from http://www.census.gov/newsroom/releases/archives/population/cb07-70.html.

United States Census Bureau. (2012). *Income, poverty and health insurance coverage in the United States: 2011.* Retrieved from http://www.census.gov/newsroom/releases/archives/income_wealth/cb12-172.html#tablea.

United States Census Bureau. (2010). *Overview of race and Hispanic origin: 2010.* Retrieved from http://www.census.gov/prod/cen2010/briefs/c2010br-02.pdf.

Unites States Census Bureau. (2012). *U.S. Census Bureau projections show a slower growing, older, more diverse nation in a half century from now.* Retrieved from http://www.census.gov/newsroom/releases/archives/population/cb12-243.html.

United States Department of Health and Human Services. (2001). *Mental health: culture, race, and ethnicity: a supplement to Mental health: a report of the surgeon general.* Rockville, MD: U.S. Department of Health and Human Services, Substance Abuse and Mental Health Services Administration, Center for Mental Health Services.

CHAPTER

6

Legal and Ethical Guidelines for Safe Practice

Penny S. Brooke and Diane K. Kjervik

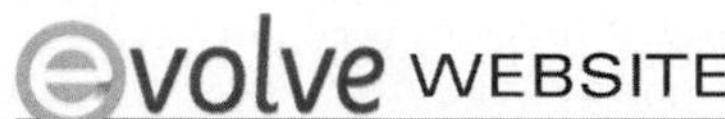

Visit the Evolve website for a pretest on the content in this chapter: http://evolve.elsevier.com/Varcarolis

Pre-Test interactive review

OBJECTIVES

1. Compare and contrast the terms *ethics* and *bioethics* and identify five principles of bioethics.
2. Discuss at least five patient rights, including the patient's right to treatment, right to refuse treatment, and right to informed consent.
3. Identify the steps nurses are advised to take if they suspect negligence or illegal activity on the part of a professional colleague or peer.
4. Apply legal considerations of patient privilege (a) after a patient has died, (b) if the patient tests positive for human immunodeficiency virus, or (c) if the patient's employer states a "need to know."
5. Provide explanations for situations in which health care professionals have a duty to break patient confidentiality.
6. Discuss a patient's civil rights and how they pertain to restraint and seclusion.
7. Develop awareness of the balance between the patient's rights and the rights of society with respect to the following legal concepts relevant in nursing and psychiatric mental health nursing: (a) duty to intervene, (b) documentation, and (c) confidentiality.
8. Identify legal terminology (e.g., torts, negligence, malpractice) applicable to psychiatric nursing and explain the significance of each term.

KEY TERMS AND CONCEPTS

assault
battery
bioethics
civil rights
competency
conditional release
confidentiality
duty to protect
duty to warn
ethical dilemma
ethics
false imprisonment
Health Insurance Portability and Accountability Act (HIPAA)
implied consent
informal admission
informed consent
intentional torts
involuntary admission
involuntary outpatient commitment
least restrictive alternative doctrine
long-term involuntary admission
malpractice
negligence
right to privacy
right to refuse treatment
right to treatment
temporary admission
tort
unconditional release
unintentional torts
voluntary admission
writ of habeas corpus

While a basic understanding of legal and ethical issues is important in every health care specialty area, the nature of the problems in psychiatric care elevates the significance of these issues. Patients in this population experience alterations in thought, mood, and behavior that may render them less able to make appropriate decisions regarding their care. On the other hand, individuals with mental illness may need their rights protected through the legal system. This chapter introduces current legal and ethical issues you may encounter in the practice of psychiatric mental health nursing.

ETHICAL CONCEPTS

Ethics is the study of philosophical beliefs about what is considered right or wrong in a society. The term **bioethics** is the study of specific ethical questions that arise in health care. The five basic principles of bioethics are:

1. **Beneficence**: The duty to act to benefit or promote the good of others (e.g., spending extra time to help calm an extremely anxious patient).
2. **Autonomy**: Respecting the rights of others to make their own decisions (e.g., acknowledging the patient's right to refuse medication promotes autonomy).
3. **Justice**: The duty to distribute resources or care equally, regardless of personal attributes (e.g., an ICU nurse devotes equal attention to someone who has attempted suicide as to someone who suffered a brain aneurysm).
4. **Fidelity** (nonmaleficence): Maintaining loyalty and commitment to the patient and doing no wrong to the patient (e.g., maintaining expertise in nursing skill through nursing education).
5. **Veracity**: One's duty to communicate truthfully (e.g., describing the purpose and side effects of psychotropic medications in a truthful and non-misleading way).

Laws tend to reflect the ethical values of society. It should be noted that, although nurses may feel obligated to follow ethical guidelines, these guidelines should not override laws. For example, you are aware of a specific rule created by your state's board of nursing that prohibits restraining patients. Even if you feel that you have an ethical obligation to protect the patient by using restraints, you would be wise to follow the law.

An **ethical dilemma** results when there is a conflict between two or more courses of action, each carrying favorable and unfavorable consequences. The response to these dilemmas is based partly on morals (beliefs of right or wrong) and values. Suppose you are caring for a pregnant woman with schizophrenia who wants to have the baby, but whose family insists she get an abortion. To promote fetal safety, her antipsychotic medication would need to be reduced, putting her at risk of exacerbating (making worse) the psychiatric illness; furthermore, there is a question as to whether she can safely care for the child. If you rely on the ethical principle of autonomy, you may conclude that she has the right to decide. Would other ethical principles be in conflict with autonomy in this case?

At times, your values may be in conflict with the value system of the institution. This situation further complicates the decision-making process and necessitates careful consideration of the patient's desires. For example, you may experience a conflict of values in a setting where older adult patients are routinely tranquilized to a degree you do not feel comfortable with. Whenever one's value system is challenged, increased stress results. Some nurses respond proactively by working to change the system or even advocate for legislation related to some particular issue.

MENTAL HEALTH LAWS

Federal and state legislatures have enacted laws to regulate the care and treatment of the mentally ill. Mental health laws—or statutes—vary from state to state; therefore, you are encouraged to review your state's code to better understand the legal climate in which you will be practicing. This can be accomplished by visiting the web page of your state mental health department or by doing an Internet search using the keywords "mental + health + statutes + (your state)."

Many of the state laws underwent substantial revision after the landmark Community Mental Health Centers Act of 1963 enacted under President John F. Kennedy (see Chapter 4) that promoted "de-institutionalization" of the mentally ill. The changes reflect a shift in emphasis from institutional care of the mentally ill to community-based care. There was an increasing awareness of the need to provide the mentally ill with humane care that respects their civil rights. Widespread, progressive use of psychotropic drugs in the treatment of mental illness enabled many patients to integrate more readily into the larger community.

Additionally, the legal system has begun to adopt a more therapeutic approach to persons with substance disorders and mental health disorders. There are now drug courts where the emphasis is more on rehabilitation than punishment (Armstrong, 2008; Schma, Kjervik, Petrucci, & Scott, 2005). Similarly, mental health courts handle criminal charges against the mentally ill by diverting them to community resources to prevent reoffending by, among other things, monitoring medication adherence.

Federal legislation providing parity for the mentally ill with other patients in terms of payments for services from health insurance plans also improves access to treatment. The Paul Wellstone and Pete Domenici Mental Health Parity and Addiction Equity Act, which went into effect in July 2010, and the Affordable Care Act, also enacted in 2010, provide for insurance funding for mental illness (Bazelton Center for Mental Health Law, 2012).

Civil Rights of Persons with Mental Illness

Persons with mental illness are guaranteed the same rights under federal and state laws as any other citizen. Most states specifically prohibit any person from depriving an individual receiving mental health services of his or her **civil rights**, including but not limited to the following:

- The right to vote
- The right to civil service ranking
- The right to receive, forfeit, or deny a driver's license

- The right to make purchases and enter contractual relationships (unless the patient has lost legal capacity by being adjudicated incompetent)
- The right to press charges against another person
- The right to humane care and treatment (medical, dental, and psychiatric needs must be met in accordance with the prevailing standards of these professions)
- The right to religious freedom and practice
- The right to social interaction
- The right to exercise and participate in recreational opportunities

Incarcerated persons with mental illness are afforded the same protections.

ADMISSION AND DISCHARGE PROCEDURES

Due Process in Involuntary Admission

The courts have recognized that involuntary admission (refer to Chapter 4) to a psychiatric inpatient setting is a "massive curtailment of liberty" (*Humphrey v. Cady*, 1972, p. 509), requiring due process protections in the civil commitment procedure. This right derives from the Fifth Amendment of the U.S. Constitution, which states that "no person shall . . . be deprived of life, liberty, or property without due process of law."

The Fourteenth Amendment explicitly prohibits *states* from depriving citizens of life, liberty, and property without due process of law. State civil commitment statutes, if challenged in the courts on constitutional grounds, must afford minimal due process protections to pass the court's scrutiny (*Zinernon v. Burch*, 1990). In most states, a patient can challenge commitments through a **writ of habeas corpus**, which means a "formal written order" to "free the person." The writ of habeas corpus is the procedural mechanism used to challenge unlawful detention by the government.

The writ of habeas corpus and the **least restrictive alternative doctrine** are two of the most important concepts applicable to civic commitment cases. The least restrictive alternative doctrine mandates that the least drastic means be taken to achieve a specific purpose. For example, if someone can be treated safely for depression on an outpatient basis, hospitalization would be too restrictive and unnecessarily disruptive.

Admission Procedures

Several types of admissions will be discussed in the following sections, all of which must be based on several fundamental guidelines:

- Neither voluntary nor involuntary admission determines a patient's ability to make informed decisions about his or her health care.
- A medical standard or justification for admission must exist.
- A well-defined psychiatric problem must be established, based on current illness classifications in the *Diagnostic and Statistical Manual of Mental Disorders, fifth edition (DSM-5)* (American Psychiatric Association [APA], 2013).
- The presenting illness should be of such a nature that it causes an immediate crisis situation or that other less-restrictive alternatives are inadequate or unavailable.
- There must be a reasonable expectation that the hospitalization and treatment will improve the presenting problems.

You are encouraged to become familiar with the laws in your state and provisions for admissions, discharges, patients' rights, and informed consent.

Informal Admission

Informal admission is one type of voluntary admission that is similar to any general hospital admission in which there is no formal or written application. The patient seeks an informal admission. Under this model, the normal doctor-patient relationship exists, and the patient is free to stay or leave, even against medical advice.

Voluntary Admission

Voluntary admission occurs when a patient applies in writing for admission to the facility. If the person is under 18, the parent, legal guardian, custodian, or next of kin may have authority to apply on the person's behalf. Voluntarily admitted patients have the right to request and obtain release; however, patients may be reevaluated and a decision may be made on the part of the care provider that an involuntary admission be initiated according to criteria established by state law.

Temporary Admission

Temporary admission is used (1) for people who are so confused or demented they cannot make decisions on their own or (2) for people who are so ill they need emergency admission. A physician initiates a temporary admission, and then a psychiatrist employed by the hospital must confirm the need for hospitalization. The primary purpose of this type of hospitalization is observation, diagnosis, and treatment of those who have mental illness or pose a danger to themselves or others. The length of time and procedures vary markedly from state to state; generally, patients can be held no more than 15 days under the temporary procedure.

Involuntary Admission

Involuntary admission is admission to a facility without the patient's consent. Generally, involuntary admission is necessary when a person is in need of psychiatric treatment, presents a danger to self or others, or is unable to meet his or her own basic needs. Involuntary admission requires that the patient retain freedom from unreasonable bodily restraints, the right to informed consent, and the right to refuse medications, including psychotropic or antipsychotic medications.

Involuntary admission procedures include that a specified number of physicians (usually two) certify that a person's mental health status justifies detention and treatment. Additionally, someone who is familiar with the individual and believes that he or she needs treatment usually makes a formal application for admission. This person might be a family member, legal guardian, custodian, treating psychiatrist, or someone who lives with the individual. Patients have the right of access to legal counsel and the right to take their case before a judge, who may order a release.

Patients can be kept involuntarily hospitalized for up to 60 days, with interim court appearances. After that time, a panel of professionals that includes psychiatrists, medical doctors, lawyers, and private citizens reviews their cases. A patient who believes that he is being held without just cause can file a petition for a writ of habeas corpus, which the hospital must immediately submit to the court. The court must then decide if the patient has been denied due process of law.

Forced treatment raises ethical dilemmas regarding autonomy versus paternalism, privacy rights, duty to protect, and right to treatment.

VIGNETTE

Elizabeth is a 50-year-old woman with a long history of admissions to psychiatric hospitals. During previous hospitalizations, she was diagnosed with paranoid schizophrenia. She has refused visits from her caseworker and quit taking medication, and her young-adult children have become increasingly concerned about her behavior. When they stop to visit, she is typically unkempt and smells bad, her apartment is filthy and filled with cats, there is no food in the refrigerator except for ketchup and an old container of yogurt, and they see that she is not paying her bills.

Elizabeth accuses her children of spying on her and of being in collusion with the government to get at her secrets of mind control and oil-rationing plans. She is making vague threats to the local officials, claiming that people who have caused the problems need to be "taken care of." Her daughter contacts her psychiatrist with this information, and a decision is made to begin emergency involuntary admission proceedings.

Long-Term Involuntary Admission. Long-term involuntary admission has as its primary purpose extended care and treatment of the mentally ill. Those who undergo extended involuntary hospitalization are admitted through medical certification, judicial review, or administrative action. Some states do not require a judicial hearing before involuntary long-term admission but often provide the patient with an opportunity for a judicial review after admission procedures. This type of involuntary hospitalization generally lasts 60 to 180 days, but it may also be for an indeterminate period.

Involuntary Outpatient Commitment. Involuntary outpatient commitment arose in the 1990s, when states began to pass legislation that permitted outpatient commitment as an alternative to forced inpatient treatment. More than 40 states now have this type of mandate. Involuntary outpatient commitment can be a preventive measure, allowing a court order before the onset of a psychiatric crisis that would result in an inpatient admission. The order for involuntary outpatient commitment is usually tied to receipt of goods and services provided by social welfare agencies, including disability benefits and housing. To access these goods and services, the patient is mandated to participate in treatment and may face inpatient admission if he or she fails to participate in treatment. Mental Health America (2012), an advocacy group, opposes the use of this type of involuntary treatment based on the belief that it is coercive and may be counterproductive by reducing personal responsibility and lowering self-esteem.

Discharge Procedures

Release from hospitalization depends on the patient's admission status. As previously discussed, voluntarily admitted patients have the right to request and receive release. Some states, however, do provide for conditional release of voluntary patients, which enables the treating physician or administrator to order continued treatment on an outpatient basis if the clinical needs of the patient warrant further care.

Conditional Release

Conditional release usually requires outpatient treatment for a specified period to determine the patient's adherence with medication protocols, ability to meet basic needs, and ability to reintegrate into the community. Generally, a voluntarily admitted patient who is conditionally released can only be involuntarily admitted through the usual methods described above; however, an involuntarily admitted patient who is conditionally released may be reinstitutionalized, although the commitment is still in effect without recommencement of formal admission procedures.

Unconditional Release

Unconditional release is the termination of a patient-institution relationship. This release may be court-ordered or administratively ordered by the institution's officials. Generally, the administrative officer of an institution has the discretion to discharge patients.

Release against Medical Advice (AMA)

In some cases, there is a disagreement between the mental health care providers and the patient as to whether continued hospitalization is necessary. In cases where treatment seems beneficial but there is no compelling reason (e.g., danger to self or others) to seek an involuntary continuance of stay, patients may be released against medical advice.

PATIENTS' RIGHTS UNDER THE LAW

Psychiatric facilities usually provide patients with a written list of basic rights derived from a variety of sources, especially legislation that came out of the 1960s. Since that time, rights have been modified to some degree, but most lists share commonalities described in the following sections.

Right to Treatment

With the enactment of the Hospitalization of the Mentally Ill Act in 1964, the federal statutory right to psychiatric treatment in public hospitals was created. The statute requires that medical and psychiatric care and treatment be provided to all persons admitted to a public hospital.

Although state courts and lower federal courts have decided that there may be a federal constitutional right to treatment, the U.S. Supreme Court has never clearly defined the right to treatment as a constitutional principle. Based on the decisions of a number of early court cases, treatment must meet the following criteria:

- The environment must be humane.
- Staff must be qualified and sufficient to provide adequate treatment.
- The plan of care must be individualized.

The initial cases presenting the psychiatric patient's right to treatment arose in the criminal justice system. An interesting case regarding the right to treatment is *O'Connor v. Donaldson* (1975). The court held that a "state cannot constitutionally confine a non-dangerous individual who is capable of surviving safely in freedom by himself or with the help of willing and responsible family members or friends" (*O'Connor v. Donaldson*, 1975, p. 576). Such court cases provide an interesting history of the evolution and shortcomings of our mental health delivery system and its intersection with the law.

Right to Refuse Treatment

Just as patients have the right to receive treatment, they also have the right to refuse it. Patients may withhold consent or withdraw consent at any time. Retraction of consent previously given must be honored whether it is a verbal or written retraction; however, the patient's **right to refuse treatment** with psychotropic drugs has been debated in the courts, based partly on the issue of patients' competency to give or withhold consent to treatment and their status under the civil commitment statutes. Early cases—initiated by state hospital patients—considered medical, legal, and ethical considerations such as basic treatment problems, the doctrine of informed consent, and the bioethical principle of autonomy. Tables 6-1 and 6-2 summarize the evolution of two landmark sets of cases regarding the patient's right to refuse treatment.

Does commitment mean that a person will be forced to take medication?

No, people who have been committed retain their right to refuse treatment.

TABLE 6-1 RIGHT TO REFUSE TREATMENT: EVOLUTION FROM MASSACHUSETTS CASE LAW TO PRESENT LAW

CASE	COURT	DECISION
Rogers v. Okin, 478 F. Supp. 1342 (D. Mass. 1979)	Federal district court	Ruled that involuntarily hospitalized patients with mental illness are competent and have the right to make treatment decisions. Forcible administration of medication is justified in an emergency if needed to prevent violence and if other alternatives have been ruled out. A guardian may make treatment decisions for an incompetent patient.
Rogers v. Okin, 634 F.2nd 650 (1st Cir. 1980)	Federal court of appeals	Affirmed that involuntarily hospitalized patients with mental illness are competent and have the right to make treatment decisions. The staff has substantial discretion in an emergency. Forcible medication is also justified to prevent the patient's deterioration. A patient's rights must be protected by judicial determination of competency or incompetency.
Mills v. Rogers, 457 U.S. 291 (1982)	U.S. Supreme Court	Set aside the judgment of the court of appeals, with instructions to consider the effect of an intervening state court case.
Rogers v. Commissioner of the Department of Mental Health, 458 N.E.2d 308 (Mass. 1983)	Massachusetts Supreme Judicial Court answering questions certified by federal court of appeals	Ruled that involuntarily hospitalized patients are competent and have the right to make treatment decisions unless they are judicially determined to be incompetent.

TABLE 6-2 RIGHT TO REFUSE TREATMENT: EVOLUTION FROM NEW JERSEY CASE LAW TO PRESENT LAW

CASE	COURT	DECISION
Rennie v. Klein, 476 F. Supp. 1292 (D. N.J. 1979)	Federal district court	Ruled that involuntarily hospitalized patients with mental illness have a qualified constitutional right to refuse treatment with antipsychotic drugs. Voluntarily hospitalized patients have an absolute right to refuse treatment with antipsychotic drugs under New Jersey law.
Rennie v. Klein, 653 F.2d 836 (3d Cir. 1981)	Federal court of appeals	Ruled that involuntarily hospitalized patients with mental illness have a constitutional right to refuse antipsychotic drug treatment. The state may override a patient's right when the patient poses a danger to self or others. Due process protections must be complied with before forcible medication of patients in nonemergency situations.
Rennie v. Klein, 454 U.S. 1078 (1982)	U.S. Supreme Court	Set aside the judgment of the court of appeals, with instructions to consider the case in light of the U.S. Supreme Court decision in *Youngberg v. Romeo*.
Rennie v. Klein, 720 F.2d 266 (3d Cir. 1983)	Federal court of appeals	Ruled that involuntarily hospitalized patients with mental illness have the right to refuse treatment with antipsychotic medications. Decisions to forcibly medicate must be based on "accepted professional judgment" and must comply with due process requirements of the New Jersey regulations.

Under what circumstances can someone be medicated against his or her will?

In an emergency to prevent a person from causing serious and imminent harm to self or others, a person may be medicated without a court hearing.

Following a court hearing, a person can be medicated if he or she meets all of the following criteria: (1) the person has a serious mental illness; (2) the person's ability to function is deteriorating or he or she is suffering or exhibiting threatening behavior; (3) the benefits of treatment outweigh the harm; (4) the person lacks the capacity to make a reasoned decision about the treatment; and (5) less restrictive services have been found inappropriate.

For persons who are hospitalized, this bill amends the conditions under which involuntary medication or other treatment can be authorized to include "current" deterioration "as compared to the recipient's ability to function prior to the current onset of symptoms of the mental illness or disability for which treatment is presently sought."

Medication can be considered a chemical restraint. Is forcing medication an infringement on a person's liberty similar to an involuntary admission? Cases involving the right to refuse psychotropic drug treatment are still evolving, and without clear direction from the Supreme Court, there will continue to be different case outcomes in different jurisdictions. The numerous cases involving the right to refuse medication have illustrated the complex and difficult task of translating social policy concerns into a clearly articulated legal standard.

Right to Informed Consent

The principle of informed consent is based on a person's right to self-determination, as enunciated in the landmark case of *Canterbury v. Spence* (1972):

> *The root premise is the concept, fundamental in American jurisprudence, that every human being of adult years and sound mind has a right to determine what shall be done with his own body. . . . True consent to what happens to one's self is the informed exercise of choice, and that entails an opportunity to evaluate knowledgeably the options available and the risks attendant on each. (p. 780)*

Proper orders for specific therapies and treatments are required and must be documented in the patient's medical record. Consent for surgery, electroconvulsive treatment, or the use of experimental drugs or procedures must be obtained. In some state institutions, consent is required for each medication addition or change. Patients have the right to refuse participation in experimental treatments or research and the right to voice grievances and recommend changes in policies or services offered by the facility, without fear of punishment or reprisal.

For consent to be effective legally, it must be informed. Generally, the physician or other health professional must obtain the informed consent of the patient before a treatment or procedure is performed. Patients must be informed of the following:

- The nature of their problem or condition
- The nature and purpose of a proposed treatment
- The risks and benefits of that treatment
- The alternative treatment options
- The probability that the proposed treatment will be successful
- The risks of not consenting to treatment

It is important that psychiatric mental health nurses know that the presence of psychotic thinking does not mean that the patient is incompetent or incapable of understanding.

Competency is the capacity to understand the consequences of one's decisions. Patients are considered legally competent until they have been declared incompetent through a formal legal proceeding. If found incompetent, the patient may be appointed a legal guardian or representative who is legally responsible for giving or refusing consent for the patient, while always considering the patient's wishes.

Guardians are typically selected from among family members. The order of selection is usually (1) spouse, (2) adult children or grandchildren, (3) parents, (4) adult siblings, and (5) adult nieces and nephews. In the event a family member is either unavailable or unwilling to serve as guardian, the court may also appoint a court-trained and approved social worker, representing the county, state, or member of the community.

Many procedures nurses perform have an element of implied consent attached. For example, if you approach the patient with a medication in hand, and the patient indicates a willingness to receive the medication, implied consent has occurred. It should be noted that many institutions—particularly state psychiatric hospitals—have a requirement to obtain informed consent for every medication given. A general rule for you to follow is that the more intrusive or risky the procedure, the higher the likelihood that informed consent must be obtained. The fact that you may not have a legal duty to be the person to inform the patient of the associated risks and benefits of a particular medical procedure does not excuse you from clarifying the procedure to the patient and ensuring his or her expressed or implied consent.

Rights Regarding Involuntary Admission and Advance Psychiatric Directives

Patients concerned that they may be subject to involuntary admission can prepare an advance psychiatric directive document that will express their treatment choices. Health care providers should follow the advance directive for mental health decision making when the patient is not competent to make informed decisions. This document can clarify the patient's choice of a surrogate decision maker and instructions about hospital choices, medications, treatment options, provider preferences, and emergency interventions. Identification of persons who are to be notified of the patient's hospitalization and who may have visitation rights is especially helpful, given the privacy demands of the Health Insurance Portability and Accountability Act (HIPAA).

Rights Regarding Restraint and Seclusion

The history of restraint and seclusion is marked by abuse, overuse, and even a tendency to use restraint as punishment. This was especially true prior to the 1950s when there were no effective chemical treatments. Legislation has dramatically reduced this problem by mandating strict guidelines.

The American Psychiatric Nurses Association (APNA) identifies psychiatric nurses as leaders in promoting a culture of minimal use of seclusion and restraint (APNA, 2007). As previously mentioned, the use of the least restrictive means of restraint for the shortest duration is always the general rule. According to the Centers for Medicare and Medicaid (CMS, 2008), in emergencies less restrictive measures do not necessarily have to have been tried, but in the staff's professional judgment they should have been considered ineffective.

Physical causes of agitation, confusion, and combative behavior include drug interaction, drug side effects, temperature elevation, hypoglycemia, hypoxia, and electrolyte imbalances. Addressing these problems can reduce or eliminate the need for restraint or seclusion. Verbal interventions or asking the patient for cooperation, reducing stimulation, active listening, diversionary approaches, and offering PRN medications are considered prior to using seclusion and restraint.

While we tend to think of classical restraining devices, a restraint can actually be any mechanical or physical device, equipment, or material that prevents or reduces movement of the patient's legs, arms, body, or head. Even side rails could be considered a restraint if they are used to prevent the patient from exiting the bed.

Restricting a patient's movement by holding him or her is considered to be a restraint. So-called *therapeutic holds* have resulted in the deaths of many patients. A 16-year-old boy in a residential treatment center for disturbed youth in New York recently died after being placed in a therapeutic hold by several staff members (Bernstein, 2012). According to witnesses the boy had complained he could not breathe and then became unresponsive.

A restraint may also be chemical in nature. Chemical restraints are defined as medications or doses of medication that are not being used for the patient's condition. Chemical interventions are usually considered less restrictive than physical or mechanical interventions, but they can have a greater impact on the patient's ability to relate to the environment because psychotropic medication alters the ability to think and produces other side effects. When used judiciously, however, psychopharmacology is extremely effective and helpful as an alternative to physical methods of restraint. An example of an improper use of chemical restraint is to medicate a patient with sundown syndrome with a high dose of a sedative to knock him out and get him to stay in bed.

Seclusion is confining a patient alone in an area or a room and preventing the patient from leaving. It is used only when a patient is demonstrating violent or self-destructive behavior that jeopardizes the safety of others or the patient. Even if the door is not locked, making threats if the patient tries to leave the room is still considered seclusion; however, a person who is physically restrained in an open room is not considered to be in seclusion.

Seclusion should be distinguished from **timeout**. This is an intervention in which a patient chooses to spend time alone in a specific area for a certain amount of time. The patient can leave the timeout area at any point.

Orders and Documentation

In an emergency, a nurse may place a patient in seclusion or restraint but must obtain a written or verbal order as soon as possible thereafter. Orders for restraint or seclusion are never written as a PRN or as a standing order. These orders to manage self-destructive or violent behavior may be renewed for a total of 24 hours with limits depending upon the patient's age (CMS, 2008). Adults 18 years or older are limited to 4 hours; children and adolescents 9 to 17 years old are limited to 2 hours; and children under 9 years old have a 1-hour limit. After 24 hours, a physician or other licensed person responsible for the patient's care must personally assess the patient. Restraint or seclusion must be discontinued as soon as safer and quieter behavior begins. Once a patient is removed from restraints or seclusion, a new order is required to reinstitute the intervention.

The nurse should carefully document restraint or seclusion in the treatment plan or plan of care, including noting *the* behavior leading to restraint or seclusion, and the time the patient is placed in and released from restraint. The patient in restraint must be assessed at regular and frequent intervals (e.g., every 15 to 30 minutes) for physical needs (e.g., food, hydration, and toileting), safety, and comfort; these observations must also be documented every 15 to 30 minutes. While in restraints, the patient must be protected from all sources of harm.

Agencies continue to revise their policies and procedures regarding restraint and seclusion, further limiting their use after recent changes in laws. Many practitioners accustomed to using restraint and seclusion have grave concerns about reducing or abolishing these practices. They believe that out-of-control patients pose a danger to themselves and others and that there are times when these physical measures are warranted; however, most agencies, which have reduced the use of restraints and seclusion, have found no negative impact, and alternative methods of therapy and cooperation with the patient have proved successful.

Nurses should also be aware that the use of seclusion or restraints is sometimes contraindicated (Box 6-1).

Rights Regarding Confidentiality

Confidentiality of care and treatment remains an important right for all patients, particularly psychiatric patients. Any

BOX 6-1 CONTRAINDICATIONS TO SECLUSION AND RESTRAINT

- Extremely unstable medical and psychiatric conditions*
- Delirium or dementia leading to inability to tolerate decreased stimulation*
- Severe suicidal tendencies*
- Severe drug reactions or overdoses or need for close monitoring of drug dosages*
- Desire for punishment of patient or convenience of staff*

*Unless close supervision and direct observation are provided.
From Simon, R. I. (2001). *Concise guide to psychiatry and law for clinicians* (3rd ed., p. 117). Washington, DC: American Psychiatric Press.

discussion or consultation involving a patient should be conducted discreetly and only with individuals who have a need and a right to know this privileged information. The legal privilege of confidentiality can be waived only by the patient.

VIGNETTE

Sharing information may be tempting. Imagine that your mom's best friend who is also a longtime family friend was admitted to the psychiatric unit while you were a nursing student there.

You hear in report that she is going through a horrendous divorce and also learn that she has breast cancer. Though you are uncomfortable and uncertain, you approach her, give her a hug, and ask how she's doing. She seems relieved to have a familiar person around and openly shares what is happening. When you suggest that she call your mom so that she can visit, her eyes widen, she shakes her head adamantly, and says, "I don't want anyone to know I'm here; I'm so ashamed." As a friend, you believe that your mom would be hurt if she didn't know and would also provide strong social support. As a future nurse, you know that you cannot say a word to your mom, and you do not.

The American Nurses Association's (ANA's) *Code of Ethics for Nurses* (2001) asserts that it is a duty of the nurse to protect confidential patient information (Box 6-2). Failure to provide this protection may harm the nurse-patient relationship, as well as the patient's well being; however, the code clarifies that this duty is not absolute. In some situations, disclosure may be necessary to protect the patient, other persons, or the public health.

Health Insurance Portability and Accountability Act (HIPAA)

The psychiatric patient's right to receive treatment and to have medical records kept confidential is legally protected by the Health Insurance Portability and Accountability Act (HIPAA), enacted in 1996. The fundamental principle underlying the ANA code on confidentiality is a person's constitutional right to privacy. Generally, your legal duty to maintain confidentiality is to protect the patient's right to privacy.

The HIPAA Privacy Rule took effect on April 14, 2003. According to this rule, you may not, without the patient's consent, disclose information obtained from the patient or the medical record to anyone except those persons for whom it is necessary for implementation of the patient's treatment plan. HIPAA also gives special protection to notes taken during psychotherapy that are kept separate from the patient's health information. Discussions about a patient in public places such as elevators and the cafeteria—even if the patient's name is not mentioned—can lead to disclosures of confidential information and liability for you and the facility.

For example, giving information to a patient's employer about his or her condition without the patient's consent is a breach of confidentiality that subjects you to liability for the tort of invasion of privacy as well as a HIPAA violation. On the other hand, discussion of a patient's history with other staff members to determine a consistent treatment approach is not a breach of confidentiality.

BOX 6-2 CODE OF ETHICS FOR NURSES

The House of Delegates of the American Nurses Association approved these nine provisions of the *Code of Ethics for Nurses* at its June 30, 2001, meeting in Washington, DC. In July of 2001, the Congress of Nursing Practice and Economics voted to accept the new language of the interpretive statements, resulting in a fully approved revised *Code of Ethics for Nurses with Interpretive Statements.*

The nurse, in all professional relationships, practices with compassion and respect for the inherent dignity, worth, and uniqueness of every individual, unrestricted by considerations of social or economic status, personal attributes or the nature of health problems.

The nurse's primary commitment is to the patient, whether an individual, family, group, or community.

The nurse promotes, advocates for, and strives to protect the health, safety, and rights of the patient.

The nurse is responsible and accountable for individual nursing practice and determines the appropriate delegation of tasks consistent with the nurse's obligation to provide optimum patient care.

The nurse owes the same duties to self as to others, including the responsibility to preserve integrity and safety, to maintain competence, and to continue personal and professional growth.

The nurse participates in establishing, maintaining, and improving health care environments and conditions of employment conducive to the provision of quality health care and consistent with the values of the profession through individual and collective action.

The nurse participates in the advancement of the profession through contributions to practice, education, administration, and knowledge development.

The nurse collaborates with other health professionals and the public in promoting community, national, and international efforts to meet health needs.

The profession of nursing, as represented by associations and their members, is responsible for articulating nursing values, for maintaining the integrity of the profession and its practice, and for shaping social policy.

From American Nurses Association. (2001). *Code of ethics for nurses with interpretive statements.* Washington, DC: American Nurses Publishing.

Generally, a patient–health professional relationship must exist before information is privileged, and the information must concern the care and treatment of the patient. The health professional may refuse to disclose information to protect the patient's privacy; however, the right to privacy is the patient's right, and health professionals cannot invoke confidentiality for their own defense or benefit.

Confidentiality after Death

A person's reputation can be damaged even after death; therefore, it is important that you do not divulge information after a person's death that you could not legally share before the death. In the courtroom setting the Dead Man's Statute protects confidential information about individuals when they are not alive to speak for themselves. About half the states have such a law; the laws vary from state to state.

Confidentiality of Professional Communications

A legal privilege exists as a result of specific laws and exists to protect the confidentiality of certain professional communications (e.g., nurse-patient [in some states], physician-patient, attorney-patient). The theory behind providing a privilege is to ensure that patients will speak frankly and be willing to disclose personal information about themselves when they know that their confidential conversations will not be repeated or distributed.

In some states the legal privilege of confidentiality has not been extended to nurses. There, you must answer a court's inquiries regarding the patient's disclosures, even if this information implicates the patient in a crime. In these states, the confidentiality of communications cannot be guaranteed.

Notwithstanding issues of confidentiality if a duty to report exists, you may be required to divulge private information shared with you by the patient.

Confidentiality and Human Immunodeficiency Virus Status

Some states have enacted mandatory or permissive statutes that direct health care providers to warn a spouse if a partner tests positive for human immunodeficiency virus (HIV). Nurses must understand the laws in their jurisdiction of practice regarding privileged communications and duty to warn of infectious disease exposure, including that of HIV status.

Exceptions to the Rule

Duty to Warn and Protect Third Parties. The California Supreme Court, in its 1974 landmark decision *Tarasoff v. Regents of University of California*, ruled that a psychotherapist has a **duty to warn** a patient's potential victim of potential harm. A university student who was in counseling at the University of California was despondent over being rejected by Tatiana Tarasoff, whom he had once kissed. The psychologist notified police verbally and in writing that the young man might pose a danger to Tarasoff. The police questioned the student, found him to be rational, and secured his promise to stay away from his love interest. The student killed Tarasoff two months later.

This case created much controversy and confusion in the psychiatric and medical communities over issues concerning (1) breach of patient confidentiality and its impact on the therapeutic relationship in psychiatric care and (2) the ability of the psychotherapist to predict when a patient is truly dangerous.

The *Tarasoff* case acknowledged that generally there is no common-law duty to aid third persons who may become victims of crime. The court found an exception when special relationships exist, and the court found the patient-therapist relationship sufficient to create a duty of the therapist to aid Ms. Tarasoff, the victim. The duty to protect the intended victim from danger arises when the therapist determines or, pursuant to professional standards, should have determined that the patient presents a serious danger to another.

The California Supreme Court held a second hearing in 1976 in the case of *Tarasoff v. Regents of the University of California* (now known as *Tarasoff II*), and it broadened the earlier duty to warn. When a therapist determines that a patient presents a serious danger of violence to another, the therapist has the **duty to protect** that other person. In fulfilling this duty the therapist may be required to call and warn the intended victim, the victim's family, or the police or to take whatever steps are reasonably necessary under the circumstances.

Most states currently have similar laws regarding the duty to protect third parties of potential life threats. The duty to protect usually includes the following:

- Assessing and predicting the patient's danger of violence toward another
- Identifying the specific persons being threatened
- Taking appropriate action to protect the identified victims

Implications for psychiatric mental health nursing. Even though the psychiatric community objected, this trend toward finding a therapist's duty to warn third persons of potential harm continues to gain wider acceptance. It is important for students and nurses to understand its implications for nursing practice. Although none of these cases have dealt with nurses, it is fair to assume that in jurisdictions that have adopted the *Tarasoff* doctrine, the duty to warn third persons may apply to advanced practice psychiatric mental health nurses in private practice who engage in individual therapy. If, however, a staff nurse—who is a member of a team of psychiatrists, psychologists, psychiatric social workers, and other psychiatric nurses—does not report to other members of the team a patient's threats of harm against specified victims or classes of victims, this failure is likely to be considered substandard nursing care.

Failure to communicate and record relevant information from police, relatives, or the patient's old records might also be deemed negligent. Breach of patient-nurse confidentiality should not pose ethical or legal dilemmas for nurses in these situations because a team approach to the delivery of psychiatric care presumes communication of pertinent information to other staff members to develop a treatment plan in the patient's best interest.

Statutes for Reporting Child and Elder Abuse. All 50 states and the District of Columbia have child abuse reporting statutes. Although these statutes differ from state to state, they generally include a definition of child abuse, a list of persons required or encouraged to report abuse, and the governmental agency designated to receive and investigate the reports. Most statutes include civil penalties for failure to report. Many states specifically require nurses to report cases of suspected abuse. Refer to Box 6-3 for a possible example of how to report abuse.

BOX 6-3 HOW DOES A NURSE GO ABOUT REPORTING CHILD ABUSE?

Institutions usually have policies for reporting abuse. Often the responsibility goes to social workers, who have expertise in these matters and know how to navigate the system. However, if you are caring for a child covered in old and new bruises or who has a broken bone and decaying teeth, and if you suspect abuse, it is your legal and ethical responsibility to make a report to your state's child welfare agency. You should also let the child's parents/guardians know that you are filing the report. Whether the physician or your peers agree with you or not, if you report suspected child abuse in good faith, you will be protected from criminal or civil liability. More importantly, you may save one child from further suffering.

There is a conflict between federal and state laws with respect to child abuse reporting when the health care professional discovers child abuse or neglect during the suspected abuser's alcohol or drug treatment. Federal laws and regulations governing confidentiality of patient records, which apply to almost all drug abuse and alcohol treatment providers, prohibit any disclosure without a court order. In this case, federal law supersedes state reporting laws although compliance with the state law may be maintained under the following circumstances:

- If a court order is obtained
- If a report can be made without identifying the abuser as a patient in an alcohol or drug treatment program
- If the report is made anonymously (some states, to protect the rights of the accused, do not allow anonymous reporting)

States may require health professionals to report other kinds of abuse. A growing number of states have enacted **elder abuse reporting statutes**, which require registered nurses and others to report cases of abuse of adults 65 and older. Agencies that receive federal funding (e.g., Medicare or Medicaid) must follow strict guidelines for reporting and preventing elder abuse.

These laws also apply to dependent or disabled adults—adults between the ages of 18 and 64 whose physical or mental limitations restrict their ability to carry out normal activities or to protect themselves—when the registered nurse has actual knowledge that the person has been the victim of physical abuse. Under most state laws, a person who is required to report suspected abuse, neglect, or exploitation of a disabled adult and willfully fails to do so is guilty of a misdemeanor crime. Most state statutes protect one who makes a report in good faith by providing immunity from civil liability.

You may also report knowledge of or reasonable suspicion of mental abuse or suffering. Both dependent adults and elders are protected by the law from purposeful physical or fiduciary neglect or abandonment. **Because state laws vary, students are encouraged to become familiar with the requirements of their states.**

TABLE 6-3 **COMMON LIABILITY ISSUES**

ISSUE	EXAMPLES
Patient safety	Failure to notice or take action on suicide risks Failure to use restraints properly or monitor the patient Miscommunication Medication errors Violation of boundaries (e.g., sexual misconduct) Misdiagnosis
Intentional torts May carry criminal penalties Punitive damages may be awarded Not covered by malpractice insurance	Voluntary acts intended to bring a physical or mental consequence Purposeful acts Recklessness Not obtaining patient consent *Note:* Self-defense or protection of others may serve as a defense to charges of an intentional tort.
Negligence/ malpractice	Carelessness Foreseeability of harm
Assault and battery	Person apprehensive (assault) of harmful/offensive touching (battery) Threat to use force (words alone are not enough) with opportunity and ability Treatment without patient's consent
False imprisonment	Intent to confine to a specific area Indefensible use of seclusion or restraints Detention of voluntarily admitted patient, with no agency or legal policies to support detaining
Defamation of character Slander (spoken) Libel (written)	Sharing private information with people who are not directly involved with care Confidential documents shared with people who are not directly involved with care
Supervisory liability (vicarious liability)	Inappropriate delegation of duties Lack of supervision of those supervising

Failure to Protect Patients

Another common legal issue in psychiatric mental health nursing concerns the failure to protect the safety of patients (Table 6-3). For example, if a suicidal patient is left alone with the means of self-harm, the nurse who has a duty to protect the patient will be held responsible for any resultant injuries. Leaving a suicidal patient alone in a room on the sixth floor with an open window is an example of unreasonable judgment on the part of a nurse.

Miscommunications and medication errors are common in all areas of nursing, including psychiatric care; since most psychiatric patients are ambulatory, carefully checking identification prior to medicating is essential.

Another common area of liability in psychiatry arises from the abuse of the therapist-patient relationship. Issues of sexual misconduct during the therapeutic relationship have been a source of concern in the psychiatric community. This is particularly significant given the connection that exists between care providers and patients and the power differential between them. Misdiagnosis is also frequently charged in legal suits.

Precautions to prevent harm also must be taken whenever a patient is restrained since there is a risk of strangulation from the restraints or even from other patients, given the restrained patient's vulnerable state. Many psychiatric nurses attest to hearing of incidents of rape while patients are restrained. Even without restraints, patients should be protected from other patients. One patient sued a hospital when she was beaten unconscious by another patient who entered her room looking for a fight. Her lawsuit alleged that there was inadequate staffing to monitor and supervise the patients under the hospital's care.

Potential threats from the patient's family or friends present another source of concern for patient safety. Patients may come from families where domestic violence is common. The nurse may witness controlling behavior by these family members that is based in fear, anxiety, and possibly guilt (Boudreaux, 2010). The nurse should protect the patient and himself or herself by remaining calm, listening carefully, and assuring family members of the importance of their contributions to the patient's welfare. Where domestic violence is reported to the nurse or witnessed by the nurse, objective documentation of the information or event is also necessary and may need to be reported to authorities (Lentz, 2010).

Tort Law

An injured party (the plaintiff) may seek money damages from the responsible party (the defendant) in the form of a **tort**. The injury can be to person, property, or reputation. Because tort law applies generally to nursing practice, this section may contain a review of material previously covered elsewhere in your nursing curriculum.

Intentional Torts

Nurses in psychiatric settings may encounter provocative, threatening, or violent behavior that may require the use of restraint or seclusion; however, use of such interventions must be carefully determined and used only in the most extreme situations. As discussed earlier in this chapter, restraint and seclusion historically were used with little regard to patients' rights, and overuse and abuses were common. Stories of patients restrained and left to lie in their own excrement or locked in seclusion for days have resulted in strict laws. Accordingly, the nurse in the psychiatric setting should understand **intentional torts**, which are willful or intentional acts that violate another person's rights or property. Some examples of intentional torts include **assault**, **battery**, and **false imprisonment** (see Table 6-3).

Other types of intentional torts may hurt a person's sense of self or financial status. They are **invasion of privacy** and **defamation of character**. Invasion of privacy in health care has to do with breaking a person's confidences or taking photographs without explicit permission. Defamation of character includes slander (verbal), such as talking about patients on the elevator with others around, and libel (printed), where written information about the patient is shared with people outside the professional setting.

Unintentional Torts

Unintentional torts are unintended acts against another person that produce injury or harm. **Negligence** is the failure to use ordinary care in any professional or personal situation when you have a duty to do so. For example, you have a duty to drive safely. If you do not and cause an accident, you may be charged with negligence. When health care professionals fail to act in accordance with professional standards, or when they fail to foresee consequences that other similar professionals with similar skills and education would be expected to foresee, they can be liable for their professional negligence, or **malpractice**. Malpractice is an act or omission to act that breaches the duty of due care and results in or is responsible for a person's injuries. The five elements required to prove negligence are (1) duty, (2) breach of duty, (3) cause in fact, (4) proximate cause, and (5) damages. Foreseeability or likelihood of harm is also evaluated.

Duty. When nurses represent themselves as being capable of caring for psychiatric patients and accept employment, a **duty** of care has been assumed. As a nurse, you have the duty to understand the theory and medications used in the specialty care of psychiatric patients. The staff nurse assigned to a psychiatric unit must be knowledgeable enough to assume a reasonable duty of care for the patients. Persons who represent themselves as possessing superior knowledge and skill, such as advanced practice psychiatric nurses, are held to a higher standard of care in the practice of their profession.

Breach of Duty. If you do not meet the standard of care that other nurses would be expected to supply under similar circumstances, you have breached the duty of care. A **breach of duty** occurs if the nursing conduct falls below the standard of care and exposes the patient to an unreasonable risk of harm. This breach of duty includes doing something that results in harm (an act of *commission*) or failing to do something that results in harm (an act of *omission*).

Cause in Fact, Proximate Cause, and Damages. **Cause in fact** may be evaluated by asking the question, "If it were not for what this nurse did (or failed to do), would this injury have occurred?" **Proximate cause**, or legal cause, may be evaluated by determining whether there were any intervening actions or persons that were, in fact, the causes of harm to the patient.

Damages include actual damages (e.g., loss of earnings, medical expenses, and property damage), as well as pain and suffering. They also include incidental or consequential damages. For example, giving a patient the wrong medication may have actual damage of a complicated hospital stay, but it also may result in permanent disability, requiring such things as special education needs and special accommodations in the home. Furthermore, incidental damages may deprive others of the benefits of the injured person, such as losing a normal relationship with a husband or father.

Foreseeability of harm evaluates the likelihood of the outcome under the circumstances. If the average, reasonable nurse could foresee that injury would result from the action or inaction, then the injury was foreseeable.

Box 6-4 gives a description of a case of false imprisonment, negligence, and malpractice.

STANDARDS FOR NURSING CARE

State boards of nursing, professional associations, policies and procedures from various institutions, and even historical customs influence how nurses practice. They contribute standards by which nurses are measured and are important in determining legal responsibility and liability. Nursing boards are state governmental agencies that regulate nursing practice and whose primary goal is to protect the health of the public by overseeing the safe practice of nursing. They have the authority to license nurses who meet a minimum competency score on board examinations and also the power to revoke licenses. Each state has its own Nurse Practice Act that identifies the qualifications for registered nurses, identifies the titles that registered nurses will use, defines what nurses are legally allowed to do (Scope of Practice), and describes the actions that are followed if nurses do not follow the nursing law (National Council of State Boards of Nursing, 2012).

BOX 6-4 FALSE IMPRISONMENT, NEGLIGENCE, AND MALPRACTICE: *PLUMADORE V. STATE OF NEW YORK* (1980)

Delilah Plumadore was admitted to Saranac Lake General Hospital for a gallbladder condition. During her medical workup, she confessed that marital problems had resulted in suicide attempts several years before her admission. After a series of consultations and tests, the attending surgeon scheduled gallbladder surgery for later that day. After the surgeon's visit, a consulting psychiatrist who examined Mrs. Plumadore told her to dress and pack her belongings because she was going to be admitted to a state hospital at Ogdensburg.

Subsequently, two uniformed state troopers handcuffed Mrs. Plumadore and strapped her into the back seat of a patrol car and transported her to the state hospital. On arrival, the admitting psychiatrist realized that the referring psychiatrist lacked the authority to order this involuntary admission. He therefore requested that Mrs. Plumadore sign a voluntary admission form, which she refused to do. Despite Mrs. Plumadore's protests regarding her admission to the state hospital, the psychiatrist assigned her to a ward without physical or psychiatric examination. She did not even have the opportunity to contact her family or her medical doctor and remained in the hospital for the weekend.

The court awarded $40,000 to Mrs. Plumadore for malpractice and false imprisonment on the part of health care professionals and negligence on the part of the troopers. This settlement was greatly influenced by the fact that she had an acute medical illness that was left untreated for days due to being locked in a psychiatric ward.

As a profession, nursing also self-regulates through professional associations. A professional association's primary focus is to elevate the practice of its members by setting standards of excellence. Two of the main nursing associations that influence psychiatric nursing are the American Nurses Association (ANA) and the American Psychiatric Nurses Association (APNA), each with individual state chapters. The ANA fosters high standards of nursing practice, promotes the rights of nurses, projects a positive view of nursing, and represents nurses in legislative issues. The ANA's *Scope and Standard of Practice and Professional Performance* (2010) provides parameters for nursing practice through 15 standards and outlines the role of nurses regardless of level, setting, or specialty area.

APNA is a professional association that is organized to advance the science and education of psychiatric-mental health nursing. More specific guidelines for psychiatric nursing practice are provided in *Psychiatric-Mental Health Nursing: Scope and Standards of Practice* (2007). This publication is a joint effort of the ANA, APNA, and the International Society of Psychiatric Mental Health Nurses. A summary of this publication is provided on the inside back cover of this book.

Hospital policies and procedures define institutional criteria for care, and these criteria may be introduced in legal proceedings to prove that a nurse met or failed to meet them. The weakness of this method is that the hospital's policy may be substandard. For example, an institution may determine that patients can be kept in seclusion for up to 6 hours, based on the original physician's order, but state licensing laws for institutions might set a limit of 4 hours. **Substandard institutional policies may put nurses at risk of liability, so professional standards of nursing care should be followed.** As advocates for patients and the profession, nurses should address questionable policies and bring about positive change.

Custom can also be used as evidence of a standard of care. In the absence of a written policy on the use of restraint, testimony might be offered regarding the customary use of restraint in emergency situations in which the combative, violent, or confused patient poses a threat of harm to self or others. Using custom to establish a standard of care may have the same weakness as in using hospital policies and procedures; custom may not comply with the laws, recommendations of the accrediting body, or other recognized standards of care. Custom must be carefully and regularly evaluated to ensure that substandard routines have not developed. Substandard customs do not protect you when a psychiatric patient charges that a right has been violated or that harm has been caused by the staff's common practices.

Nurses are held to a basic standard of care. This standard is based on what other nurses who possess the same degree of skill or knowledge in the same or similar circumstances would do. Psychiatric patients, whether they are in a large, small, rural, or urban facility, have the right to receive the level of care recognized by bodies governing nursing.

GUIDELINES FOR ENSURING ADHERENCE TO STANDARDS OF CARE

Negligence, Irresponsibility, or Impairment

In your professional life, you may suspect negligence on the part of a peer. In most states, you have a legal duty to intervene and to report such risks of harm to the patient. It is also important to document the evidence clearly and accurately before making serious accusations against a peer. If you question a fellow nurse's or physician's orders or actions, it is usually wise to communicate these concerns directly to the person involved. If this fails, you have an obligation to communicate your concerns to a supervisor, who should then intervene to ensure that the patient's rights and well-being are protected. If the supervisor does not rectify a dangerous situation, and if there is no time to resolve the issue through the normal process, the nurse has no choice but to act to protect the patient's life. If you do not intervene and the patient is injured, you may be liable for any resulting injuries because of your failure to act with professional nursing judgment. If the problem is not life-threatening, you have a duty to report your concerns to the appropriate authority, such as the state board of nursing.

The problem of reporting impaired colleagues causes deep concerns, especially if you have not observed direct harm to a patient. Nurses may adopt a code of silence regarding substance abuse among health professionals because of concerns for professional reputations and personal privacy; however, several states now require you to report impaired or incompetent colleagues to professional licensing boards. In the absence of such a legal mandate, the questions of whether to report and to whom to report become ethical ones. The American Nurses Association (2001) identifies "acting on questionable practice" as being part of a nurse's professional responsibility. As a patient advocate, the nurse should be alert and take proper actions in cases of impaired colleagues.

The issues are less complex when a professional colleague's conduct (including that of a student nurse) is criminally unlawful. Specific examples include the diversion of drugs from the hospital and sexual misconduct with patients. You must immediately report any such criminal behavior.

VIGNETTE

Amanda is a new nurse on the crisis management unit. She completed the hospital and unit orientations two weeks ago and has begun to care for patients independently. As she prepares to give the 5:00 PM medications, Amanda notices that Greg Thorn, a 55-year-old man admitted after a suicide attempt, has been ordered the antidepressant sertraline (Zoloft). Amanda remembers that Mr. Thorn had been taking phenelzine (Nardil) prior to his admission and seems to recall something dangerous about mixing these two medications. She looks the antidepressants up in her drug guide and realizes that Nardil is a monoamine oxidase inhibitor (MAOI) and that adding this second antidepressant within two weeks of discontinuing the Nardil could result in severe side effects and a potentially lethal response.

After clarifying with Mr. Thorn that he had been on Nardil and discussing the issue with another nurse, Amanda puts the medication on hold and contacts Mr. Thorn's psychiatrist, Dr. Cruz, by phone. Amanda begins by saying, "I see that Mr. Thorn has been ordered Zoloft. His nursing admission assessment says that he had been taking Nardil up until a few days ago. However, I don't see it listed on the assessment that was done by the medical resident."

First Possible Outcome

Dr. Cruz responds, "Really? Wow, thanks for calling that to my attention. When I make rounds in the morning, I'll decide what to do with his medications. For now, I definitely agree that we hold the Zoloft." Amanda clarifies what Dr. Cruz has said, writes the order, and documents what happened in the nurses notes.

Second Possible Outcome

Dr. Cruz responds, "It sounds like you have must have gotten a medical degree. If it wasn't on my resident's assessment, then he wasn't taking it. A nurse must have made a mistake—again. I wrote an order for Nardil. Give it to him." She hangs up on Amanda, who then documents the exchange, determines that the safest and most appropriate response is to continue to hold the medication, and contacts her nursing supervisor. The supervisor supports her decision and follows up with the chief of psychiatry.

When the nurse is given an assignment to care for a patient, the nurse must provide the care or ensure that the patient is safely reassigned to another nurse. Abandonment, a legal concept, occurs if a nurse does not deliver a patient safely to another health professional before discontinuing treatment. Abandonment issues arise when a nurse does not provide accurate, timely, and thorough reporting or when follow-through of patient care, on which the patient is relying, has not occurred.

The same principles apply for the psychiatric mental health nurse working in a community setting. For example, if a suicidal patient refuses to come to the hospital for treatment, you must take the necessary steps to ensure the patient's safety. These actions may include enlisting the assistance of the law in involuntarily admitting the patient on a temporary basis.

DOCUMENTATION OF CARE

The purposes of the medical record are to provide accurate and complete information about the care and treatment of patients and to give health care personnel a means of communicating with one another, allowing continuity of care. A record's usefulness is determined by how accurately and completely it portrays the patient's behavioral status at the time it was written. The patient has the right to see the medical record, but it belongs to the institution. The patient must follow appropriate protocol to view his or her records.

For example, if a psychiatric patient describes intent to harm himself or another person and his or her nurse fails to document the information—including the need to protect the patient or the identified victim—the information will be lost when the nurse leaves work. If the patient's plan is carried out, the harm caused could be linked directly to the nurse's failure to communicate the patient's intent. Even though documentation takes time away from patient care, its importance in communicating and preserving the nurse's assessment and memory cannot be overemphasized.

Medical Records and Quality Improvement

The medical record has many other uses aside from providing information on the course of the patient's care and treatment by health care professionals. According to the Institute of Medicine (2011), quality improvement is a key goal for the future of nursing and health care. A retrospective medical record review provides valuable information to the facility on the quality of care provided and on ways to improve that care. A facility may conduct reviews for risk management purposes to determine areas of potential liability for the facility and to evaluate methods used to reduce the facility's exposure to liability. For example, risk managers often review documentation of the use of restraints and seclusion for psychiatric patients. Accordingly, the medical record may be used to evaluate care for quality assurance or peer review. Utilization review analysts evaluate the medical record to determine appropriate use of hospital and staff resources consistent with reimbursement schedules. Insurance companies and other reimbursement agencies rely on the medical record in determining what payments they will make on the patient's behalf.

Medical Records as Evidence

From a legal perspective, the medical record is a recording of data and opinions made in the normal course of the patient's hospital care. Courts deem it good evidence because it is presumed to be true, honest, and untainted by memory lapses. Accordingly, the medical record finds its way into a variety of legal cases for a variety of reasons. Some examples of its use include determining (1) the extent of the patient's damages and pain and suffering in personal injury cases, such as when a psychiatric patient attempts suicide while under the protective care of a hospital, (2) the nature and extent of injuries in child abuse or elder abuse cases, (3) the nature and extent of physical or mental disability in disability cases, and (4) the nature and extent of injury and rehabilitative potential in workers' compensation cases.

Medical records may also be used in police investigations, civil conservatorship proceedings, competency hearings, and involuntary admission procedures. In states that mandate mental health legal services or a patients' rights advocacy program, audits may be performed to determine the facility's compliance with state laws or violation of patients' rights. Finally, medical records may be used in professional and hospital negligence cases.

During the initial, or discovery, phase of litigation, the medical record is a pivotal source of information for attorneys in determining whether a cause of action exists in a professional negligence or hospital negligence case. Evidence of the nursing care will be found in the nurses' documentation.

Guidelines for Electronic Documentation

Informatics provides the health care system with essential technology to manage knowledge, communicate, reduce error, and facilitate decision making (Quality and Safety Education for Nurses, 2012), yet electronic record keeping creates challenges for protecting the confidentiality of the records of psychiatric patients. Institutions must protect against intrusions into the privacy of patient record systems. Sensitive information regarding treatment for mental illness can adversely impact patients who are seeking employment, insurance, and credit.

Federal laws address concerns for the privacy of patients' records and provide guidelines for agencies that use electronic documentation. Only staff members who have a legitimate need to know about the patient are authorized to access a patient's electronic medical record. Guidelines for compliance include the recommendation that staff be assigned a unique password for entering patients' records in order to identify staff members who have gained access to confidential patient information. There are penalties, including termination of employment, if a staff member enters a record without authorization.

It is reasonable to assume that your password should remain private; never allow someone else to access a record using your password. If a classmate forgets her password and asks for yours, you should only offer to help her retrieve her own from the appropriate source. You are responsible for all entries into records using your password. The various systems allow specific time frames within which the nurse must make corrections if a documentation error is made.

Documentation methods that improve communication between care providers should be encouraged. Courts assume that nurses and physicians read each other's notes on patient progress. They also assume that if care is not documented, it did not occur. Your notes may serve as a valuable memory refresher if the patient sues years after the care is rendered. In providing complete and timely information on the care and treatment of patients, the medical record enhances communication among health professionals. Internal institutional audits of the record can improve the quality of care rendered.

FORENSIC NURSING

The new and evolving specialty of forensic nursing includes the application of nursing principles in a court of law to assist in reaching a decision on a contested issue. The nurse acts as an advocate, educating the court about the science of nursing. The witness applies nursing knowledge to the facts in the lawsuit and may provide opinions using appropriate nursing standards. Examples of psychiatric mental health forensic nursing may include testimony related to patient competency, fitness to stand trial, involuntary admission, or responsibility for a crime. Forensic nurses may also focus on victims and perpetrators of crime and violence, the collection of evidence, and the provision of health care in prison settings. Refer to Chapter 32 for a complete discussion of forensic nursing.

VIOLENCE IN THE PSYCHIATRIC SETTING

Nurses must protect themselves in both institutional and community settings. Employers are not typically held responsible for employee injuries due to violent patient behavior. It is therefore important for nurses to participate in setting policies that create and maintain a safe working environment. Good judgment while on the job means avoiding a potentially violent situation.

Nurses, as citizens, have the same rights as patients not to be threatened or harmed. Appropriate security support should be readily available. When you work in community settings, you must avoid placing yourself unnecessarily in dangerous environments, especially when alone at night. You should use common sense and enlist the help of local law enforcement officers when needed. A violent patient is not being abandoned if placed safely in the hands of the authorities.

In 2009, registered nurses reported 2050 violent acts with about four days of lost work per incident (United States Bureau of Labor Statistics, 2011). Although emergency room nurses are more likely to be assaulted, psychiatric nurses also have fairly high rates. Recent legislation has addressed the topic of workplace violence by imposing enhanced criminal charges and penalties for striking a nurse and other health care workers. Usually, a prosecutor will not bring charges against disoriented, delirious, psychotic, or otherwise mentally impaired patients; however, violent patients, friends of patients, and family members who are aware of their actions can be charged with serious crimes. Figure 6-1 identifies states with workplace violence legislation (American Nurses Association, 2012).

The psychiatric mental health nurse must also be aware of the potential for violence in the community when a patient is discharged following a short-term stay. The duty of the nurse to

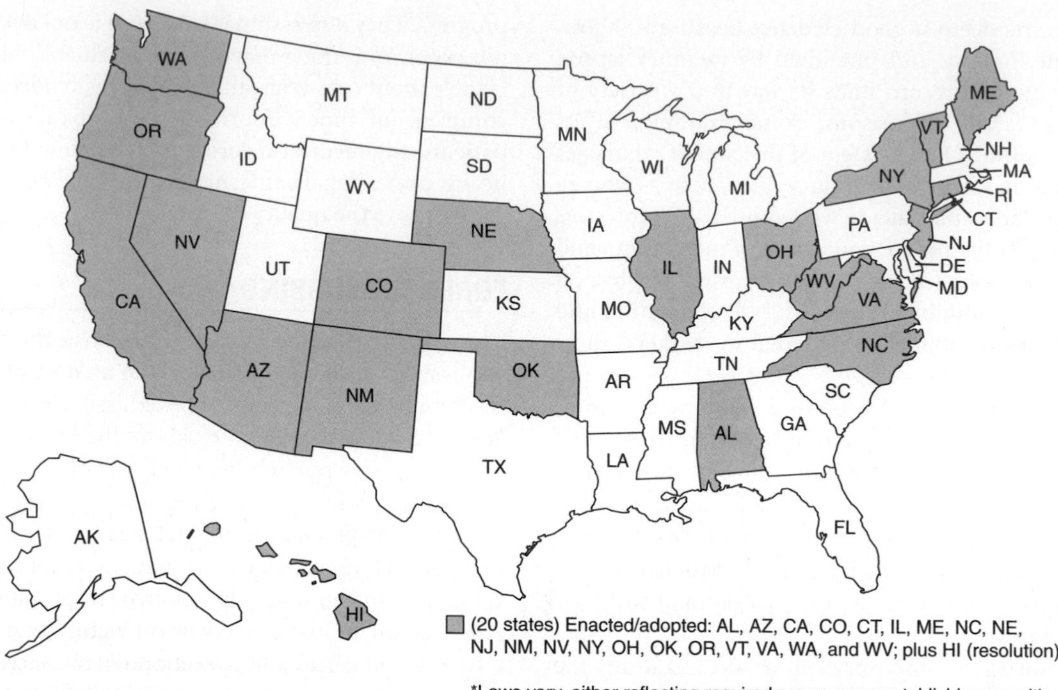

FIG 6-1 The American Nurses Association's Nationwide State Legislative Agenda, which identifies states with workplace violence legislation. (Reprinted with permission from the American Nurses Association.)

protect the patient and warn others who may be threatened by the violent patient is discussed earlier in this chapter. The nurse's assessment of the patient's potential for violence must be documented and acted on if there is legitimate concern regarding discharge of a patient who is discussing or exhibiting potentially violent behavior. The psychiatric mental health nurse must communicate his or her observations to the medical staff when discharge decisions are being considered.

KEY POINTS TO REMEMBER

- The states have the power to enact laws for public health and safety and for the care of those unable to care for themselves
- Psychiatric mental health nurses frequently encounter problems requiring ethical choices.
- The nurse's privilege to practice carries with it the responsibility to practice safely, competently, and in a manner consistent with state and federal laws.
- Knowledge of the law, the ANA's *Code of Ethics for Nurses*, and the Standards of Practice and Professional Performance from the *Psychiatric-Mental Health Nursing: Scope and Standards of Practice* (ANA et al., 2007) are essential for providing safe, effective psychiatric mental health nursing care and will serve as a framework for ethical decision making.

CRITICAL THINKING

1. Joe and Beth are registered nurses who have worked together on the psychiatric unit for two years. Beth confided to Joe that her marital situation has become particularly difficult over the last six months. He expressed concern and shared his observation that she seems to be distracted and less happy lately. As Joe prepares the medication for the evening shift, he notices that two of his patients' medications are missing; both are bedtime Ativan (lorazepam). When he phones the pharmacy to send up the missing medications, the pharmacist responds, "You people need to watch your carts more carefully because this has become a pattern." Shortly after, another patient complains to Joe that he did not receive his 5 P.M. Xanax (alprazolam). On the medication administration record Beth has recorded that she has given the drugs. Joe suspects that Beth may be diverting the drugs.

   Should Joe confront Beth with his suspicions?

   If Beth admits that she has been diverting the drugs, should Joe's next step be to report Beth to the supervisor or to the board of nursing?

   When Joe talks to the nursing supervisor, should he identify Beth or should he state his suspicions in general terms?

   How does the nature of the drugs affect your responses? That is, if the drugs were to treat a "physical" condition such as hypertension, would you be more concerned?

   What does the Nurse Practice Act in your state mandate regarding reporting the illegal use of drugs by a nurse?
2. Linda has been employed in a psychiatric setting for five years. One day she arrives at work and is informed that the staffing office has

requested that a nurse from the psychiatric unit assist the intensive care unit (ICU) staff in caring for an agitated car accident victim with a history of schizophrenia. Linda goes to the ICU and joins a nurse named Corey in providing care for the patient. Eventually, the patient is stabilized and goes to sleep, and Corey leaves the unit for a break. Since Linda is unfamiliar with the telemetry equipment, she fails to recognize that the patient is having an arrhythmia, and the patient experiences a cardiopulmonary arrest. Although he is successfully resuscitated after six minutes, he suffers permanent brain damage.

Can Linda legally practice in this situation? (That is, does her RN license permit her to practice in the intensive care unit?)

Does the ability to practice legally in an area differ from the ability to practice competently in that area?

Did Linda have any legal or ethical grounds to refuse the assignment to the intensive care unit?

What are the risks in accepting an assignment in an area of specialty in which you are professionally unprepared to practice?

What are the risks in refusing an assignment in an area of specialty in which you are professionally unprepared to practice?

Would there have been any way for Linda to minimize the risk of retaliation by the employer had she refused the assignment?

What action could Linda have taken to protect the patient and herself when Corey left the unit for a break?

If Linda is negligent, is the hospital liable for any harm to the patient caused by her?

3. A 40-year-old man is admitted to the emergency department for a severe nosebleed and has both of his nostrils packed. Because of a history of alcoholism and the possibility for developing delirium tremens (withdrawal), the patient is transferred to the psychiatric unit. His physician orders a private room, restraints, continuous monitoring, and 15-minute checks of vital signs and other indicators. At the next 15-minute check, the nurse discovers that the patient does not have a pulse or respiration. The patient had apparently inhaled the nasal packing and suffocated.

   Does it sound as if the nurse was responsible for the patient's death?

   Was the order for the restraint appropriate for this type of patient?

   What factors did you consider in making your determination?

4. Assume that there are no mandatory reporting laws for impaired or incompetent colleagues in the following clinical situation. A 15-year-old boy is admitted to a psychiatric facility voluntarily at the request of his parents because of violent, explosive behavior. This behavior began after his father's recent remarriage following his parents' divorce. In group therapy, he has become incredibly angry in response to a discussion about weekend passes for Mother's Day. "Everyone has abandoned me; no one cares," he screamed. Several weeks later, on the day before his discharge, he convinces his nurse to keep his plan to kill his mother confidential. Consider the ANA *Code of Ethics for Nurses* on patient confidentiality, the principles of psychiatric nursing, the statutes on privileged communications, and the duty to warn third parties in answering the following questions:

   Did the nurse use appropriate judgment in promising confidentiality?

   Does the nurse have a legal duty to warn the patient's mother of her son's threat?

   Is the duty owed to the patient's father and stepmother?

   Would a change in the admission status from voluntary to involuntary protect the patient's mother without violating the patient's confidentiality?

   What nursing action, if any, should the nurse take after the disclosure by the patient?

CHAPTER REVIEW

1. A nurse makes a post on a social media page about his peer taking care of a patient with a crime-related gunshot wound during his shift in the emergency department. He does not use the name of the patient. It can be concluded that:
   a. the nurse has not violated confidentiality laws because he did not use the patient's name.
   b. the nurse cannot be held liable for violating confidentiality laws because he was not the primary nurse for the patient.
   c. the nurse has violated confidentiality laws and can be held liable.
   d. the nurse cannot be held liable because postings on a social media site are excluded from confidentiality laws.
2. Brian, a patient with schizophrenia, has been ordered an antipsychotic medication. The medication will likely benefit him, but there are side effects; in a small percentage of patients, it may cause a dangerous side effect. After medication teaching, Brian is unable to identify side effects and responds, "I won't have any side effects because I am iron and cannot be killed." Which response would be most appropriate under these circumstances?
   a. Administer the medication because Brian has made a decision to take the medication, and care should be patient-centered.
   b. Petition the court to appoint a guardian as a substitute for Brian, as he is unable to comprehend the proposed treatment.
   c. Administer the medication because Brian's need for treatment is the clear priority.
   d. Withhold the medication until Brian is able to identify the benefits and risks of both consenting and refusing consent to the medications.
3. A family who is worried that an adult female might hurt herself asks for her to be admitted to the hospital. An assessment indicates moderate depression with no risk factors for suicide other than a depressed mood. The patient denies any intent or thoughts about self-harm. The family agrees that the patient has not done or said anything to suggest that she might be a danger to herself. Which of the following responses is consistent with the concept of "least restrictive alternative" doctrine?
   a. Admit the patient as a temporary inpatient admission.
   b. Persuade the patient to agree to a voluntary inpatient admission.
   c. Admit the patient involuntarily to an inpatient mental health treatment unit.
   d. Arrange for an outpatient counseling appointment the next day.
4. David has an overnight pass, and he plans to spend this time with his sister and her family. As you meet with the patient and his sister just prior to the pass, the sister mentions that she has missed her brother and needs him to babysit. You notice that the patient becomes visibly agitated when she says this. How do you balance safety and the patient's right to confidentiality?
   a. Cancel the pass without explanation to the sister, and reschedule it for a time when babysitting would not be required of the patient.
   b. Suggest that the sister make other arrangements for child care, but withhold the information the patient shared regarding his concerns about harming children.
   c. Speak with the patient about the safety risk involved in babysitting, seeking his permission to share this information and advising against the pass if he declines to share the information.
   d. Meet with the patient's sister, sharing with her the patient's previous disclosure about his anger toward children and the resultant risk that his babysitting would present.

5. Gina is admitted for treatment of depression with suicidal ideation triggered by marital discord. Her spouse visits one night and informs Gina that he has decided to file for divorce. The staff are aware of the visit and the husband's intentions regarding divorce but take no further action, feeling that the q15-minute suicide checks Gina is already on are sufficient. Thirty minutes after the visit ends, staff make rounds and discover Gina has hanged herself in her bathroom, using hospital pajamas she had tied together into a rope. Which of the following statements best describes this situation? *Select all that apply.*
   - **a.** The nurses have created liability for themselves and their employer by failing in their duty to protect Gina.
   - **b.** The nurses have breached their duty to reassess Gina for increased suicide risk after her husband's visit.
   - **c.** Given Gina's history, the nurses should have expected an increased risk of suicide after the husband's announcement.
   - **d.** The nurses correctly reasoned that suicides cannot always be prevented and did their best to keep Gina safe through checks every 15 minutes.
   - **e.** The nurses are subject to a tort of professional negligence for failing to prevent the suicide by increasing the suicide precautions in response to Gina's increased risk.
   - **f.** Had the nurses restricted Gina's movements or increased their checks on her, they would have been liable for false imprisonment and invasion of privacy, respectively.

Answers to Chapter Review
1. c; 2. b; 3. d; 4. d; 5. a, b, c, e.

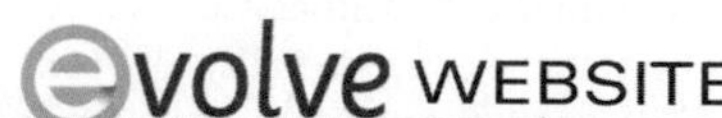

Visit the Evolve website for a posttest on the content in this chapter: http://evolve.elsevier.com/Varcarolis

Post-Test interactive review

REFERENCES

American Nurses Association. (2001). *Code of ethics for nurses with interpretive statements.* Washington, DC: American Nurses Publishing.

American Nurses Association, American Psychiatric-Mental Health Nurses Association, & International Society of Psychiatric-Mental Health Nurses. (2007). *Psychiatric mental health nursing: Scope and standards of practice.* Silver Spring, MD: American Nurses Association.

American Psychiatric Association. (2013). *Diagnostic and statistical manual of mental disorders (DSM-5)* (5th ed.). Washington, DC: Author.

Armstrong, E. (2008). The drug court as postmodern justice. *Critical Criminology, 16,* 271–284. doi:10.1007/s10612-008-9061-9.

Bazelton Center for Mental Health Law. (2012). *Where we stand: Mental health parity.* Retrieved from http://www.bazelton.org/Where-We-Stand?Access-to-Services/Mental-Health-Parity.aspx.

Berstein, N. (2012, April 20). Restrained youth's death in Yonkers is investigated. *New York Times.* Retrieved from http://www.nytimes.com/2012/04/21/nyregion/death-of-youth-at-leake-watts-center-in-yonkers-is-investigated.html?_r=0.

Boudreaux, A. (2010). Keeping cool with difficult family members. *Nursing 2010, 40*(12), 48–51.

Canterbury v. Spence, 464 F.2d 722 (D.C. Cir. 1972), quoting Schloendorf v. Society of N.Y. Hosp., 211 N.Y. 125 105 N.E.2d 92, 93 (1914).

Centers for Medicare and Medicaid Services. (2008). *Hospitals—Restraint/seclusion interpretive guidelines and updated state operations manual.* Retrieved from http://www.cms.gov/Medicare/Provider-Enrollment-and-Certification/SurveyCertificationGenInfo/downloads/SCLetter08-18.pdf.

Health Insurance Portability and Accountability Act, U.S.C.45C.F.R § 164.501 (2003).

Humphrey v. Cady, 405 U.S. 504 (1972).

Illinois v. Russell, 630, N.E.2d 794 Ill. Sup. Ct. (1994).

Institute of Medicine. (2011). *The future of nursing: Focus on education.* Retrieved from http://www.iom.edu/Reports/2010/The-Future-of-Nursing-Leading-Change-Advancing-Health/Report-Brief-Education.aspx

Lentz, L. (2010). 10 tips for documenting domestic violence. *Nursing 2010, 40*(9), 53–55.

Mental Health America. (2012). *Position statement 22: Involuntary outpatient commitment.* Retrieved from http://www.nmha.org/go/position-statements/p-36.

National Council of State Boards of Nursing. (2012). *Boards of nursing.* https://www.ncsbn.org/boards.htm.

O'Connor v. Donaldson, 422 U.S. 563 (1975).

Plumadore v. State of New York, 427 N.Y.S.2d 90 (1980).

Quality and Safety Education for Nurses. (2012). *Competency knowledge, skills, and attitudes.* Retrieved from http://www.qsen.org/ksas_prelicensure.php#informatics.

Sadock, B. J., & Sadock, V.A. (2008). *Concise textbook of clinical psychiatry* (3rd ed.) Philadelphia, PA: Lippincott, Williams & Wilkins.

Schma, W., Kjervik, D., Petrucci, C., & Scott, C. (2005). Therapeutic jurisprudence: using the law to improve the public's health. *Journal of Law, Medicine & Ethics, 33*(4), 59–63.

Tarasoff v. Regents of University of California, 529 P.2d 553, 118 Cal Rptr 129 (1974).

Tarasoff v. Regents of University of California, 551 P.2d 334, 131 Cal Rptr 14 (1976).

United States Bureau of Labor Statistics. (2011). *Illnesses, injuries, and fatalities.* Retrieved from http://www.bls.gov/iif/.

Zinernon v. Burch, 494 U.S. 113, 108 L.Ed.2d 100, 110 S. Ct. 975 (1990).

CHAPTER

7

The Nursing Process and Standards of Care for Psychiatric Mental Health Nursing

Elizabeth M. Varcarolis

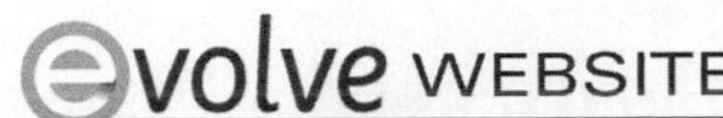

Visit the Evolve website for a pretest on the content in this chapter: http://evolve.elsevier.com/Varcarolis

Pre-Test interactive review

OBJECTIVES

1. Compare the different approaches you would consider when performing an assessment with a child, an adolescent, and an older adult.
2. Differentiate between the use of an interpreter and a translator when performing an assessment with a non–English speaking patient.
3. Conduct a mental status examination (MSE).
4. Perform a psychosocial assessment, including brief cultural and spiritual components.
5. Explain three principles a nurse follows in planning actions to reach agreed-upon outcome criteria.
6. Construct a plan of care for a patient with a mental or emotional health problem.
7. Identify three advanced practice psychiatric mental health nursing interventions.
8. Demonstrate basic nursing interventions and evaluation of care following the ANA's Standards of Practice.
9. Compare and contrast *Nursing Interventions Classification (NIC)*, *Nursing Outcomes Classification (NOC)*, and evidence-based practice (EBP).

KEY TERMS AND CONCEPTS

evidence-based practice (EBP)
health teaching
mental status examination (MSE)
milieu therapy
Nursing Interventions Classification (NIC)
Nursing Outcomes Classification (NOC)
outcome criteria
psychosocial assessment
self-care activities

The nursing process is a six-step problem-solving approach intended to facilitate and identify appropriate, safe, culturally competent, developmentally relevant, and quality care for individuals, families, groups, or communities. Psychiatric mental health nursing practice bases nursing judgments and behaviors on this accepted theoretical framework (Figure 7-1). Theoretical paradigms such as developmental theory, psychodynamic theory, systems theory, holistic theory, cognitive theory, and biological theory are some examples. Whenever possible, interventions are also supported by scientific theories when we apply evidence-based research to our nursing plans and actions of care (refer to Chapter 1).

The nursing process is also the foundation of the Standards of Practice as presented in *Psychiatric-Mental Health Nursing: Scope and Standards of Practice* (ANA et al., 2007), which in turn provide the basis for the:

- Criteria for certification
- Legal definition of nursing, as reflected in many states' nurse practice acts
- National Council of State Boards of Nursing Licensure Examination (NCLEX-RN®)

Safety and quality care for patients has become the new standard for nursing education. As of the late 1990s, the Institute of Medicine (IOM; based on their *Quality Chasm* reports) and

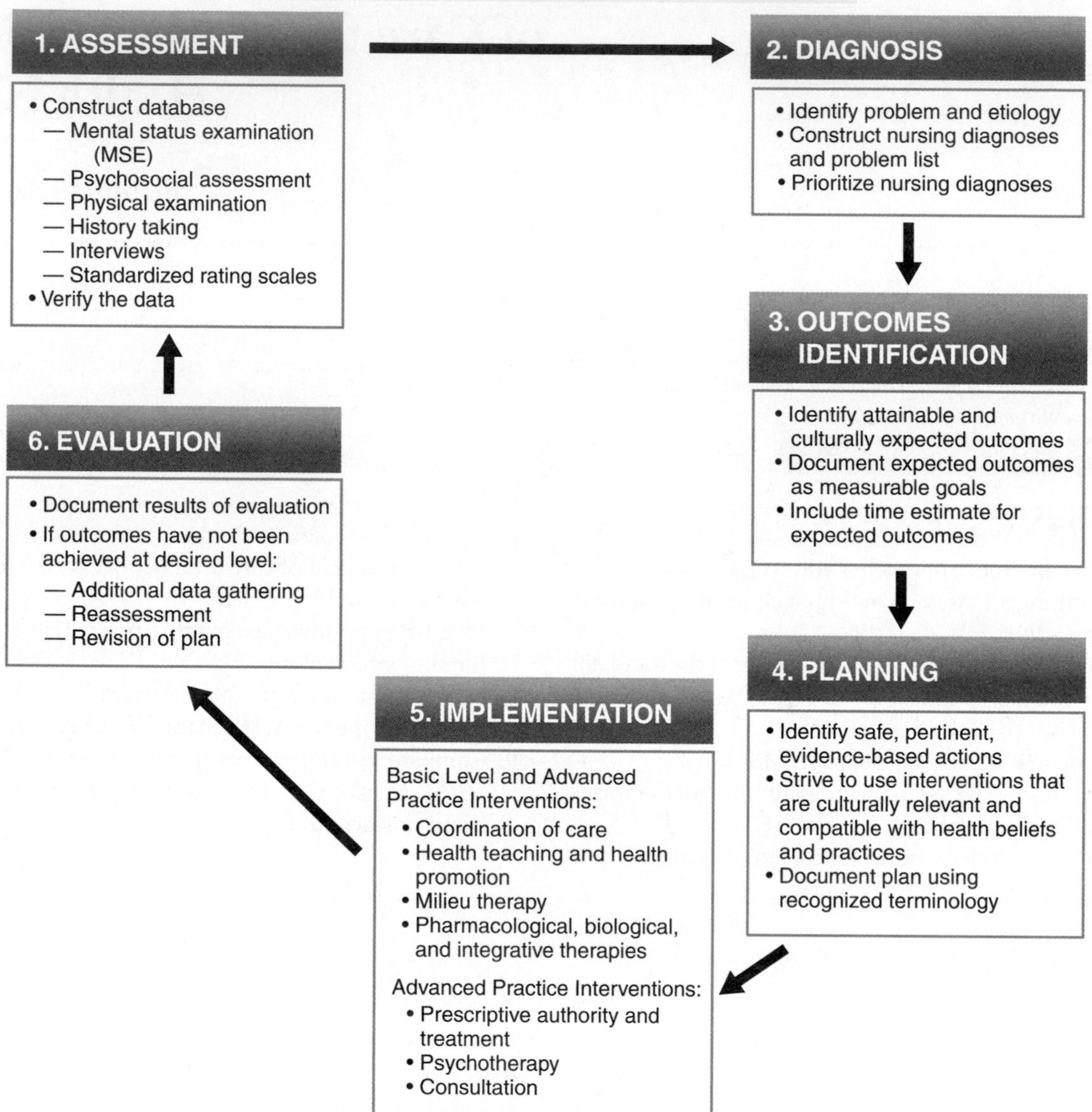

NURSING ASSESSMENT
The assessment interview requires culturally effective communication skills and encompasses a large database (e.g., significant support system; family; cultural and community system; spiritual and philosophical values, strengths, and health beliefs and practices; as well as many other factors).
1. ASSESSMENT
• Construct database
— Mental status examination (MSE)
— Psychosocial assessment
— Physical examination
— History taking
— Interviews
— Standardized rating scales
• Verify the data
2. DIAGNOSIS
• Identify problem and etiology
• Construct nursing diagnoses and problem list
• Prioritize nursing diagnoses
3. OUTCOMES IDENTIFICATION
• Identify attainable and culturally expected outcomes
• Document expected outcomes as measurable goals
• Include time estimate for expected outcomes
4. PLANNING
• Identify safe, pertinent, evidence-based actions
• Strive to use interventions that are culturally relevant and compatible with health beliefs and practices
• Document plan using recognized terminology
5. IMPLEMENTATION
Basic Level and Advanced Practice Interventions:
• Coordination of care
• Health teaching and health promotion
• Milieu therapy
• Pharmacological, biological, and integrative therapies
Advanced Practice Interventions:
• Prescriptive authority and treatment
• Psychotherapy
• Consultation
6. EVALUATION
• Document results of evaluation
• If outcomes have not been achieved at desired level:
— Additional data gathering
— Reassessment
— Revision of plan

FIG 7-1 The nursing process in psychiatric mental health nursing.

other organizations found a need to improve the quality and safety outcomes of health care delivery. As nursing practice focused more on quality and safety issues, it became evident that graduating nursing students were missing critical competencies for safety and quality of care.

The context and approach of nursing education is changing, and new models of education are needed (Valiga & Champagne, 2011). The competencies mandated by the IOM require changes throughout health professionals' education to better prepare students with the responsibilities and realities in the health care setting. There is now a strong national focus on improving patient safety and quality that is known as *Quality and Safety Education in Nursing (QSEN)* (Sullivan, 2010). The primary goal of QSEN is to prepare future nurses with the knowledge, skills, and attitudes (KSAs) required to enhance quality, care, and safety in the health care settings in which they are employed (Cronenwett et al., 2007). QSEN bases their work on six competencies (Box 7-1). These competencies are integrated into this chapter and throughout the textbook.

QSEN has underscored the need to increase knowledge about patient safety practices and the value of redesigning student learning experiences to improve the integration of this content (Sherwood & Hicks, 2011). Clinical simulations using sophisticated mannequins, combined with instructors who can

BOX 7-1 QUALITY AND SAFETY EDUCATION FOR NURSES (QSEN) COMPETENCIES

Patient-centered care: Recognize the patient or designee as the source of control and full partner in providing compassionate and coordinated care based on respect for the patient's preferences, values, and needs.

Quality improvement: Use data to monitor the outcomes of care processes and use improvement methods to design and test changes to continuously improve the quality and safety of health care systems.

Safety: Minimize risk of harm to patients and provide optimal health care through both system effectiveness and individual performance.

Informatics: Use information and technology to communicate, manage knowledge, mitigate error, and support decision making.

Teamwork and collaboration: Function effectively within nursing and interprofessional teams, fostering open communication, mutual respect, and shared decision making to achieve quality patient care.

Evidence-based practice (EBP): Integrate best current evidence with clinical expertise and patient/family preferences and values for delivery of optimal health care.

Cronenwett, L., Sherwood, G., Barnsteiner, J., Disch, J., Johnson, J., Mitchell, P., Sullivan, D., & Warren, J. (2007). Quality and safety education for nurses. *Nursing Outlook, 55*(3), 122–131.

provide realistic case scenarios and provide debriefing through videotaped patient care sessions are useful in safely identifying and reinforcing quality care concepts. Self-directed computer-based simulation programs are also popular and effective. These programs portray virtual clinical settings and may use avatars to offer students a chance to implement their knowledge, skills, and attitudes without the potential for patient harm (Durham & Sherwood, 2008).

Suggestions for the use of QSEN competencies in the discussion of Standards of Practice can be found in "Competency Knowledge, Skills, Attitudes (KSAs) (Pre-Licensure)" at the website www.qsen.org/competencies/pre-licensure-ksas/.

The following sections describe the Standards of Practice, which "describe a competent level of psychiatric-mental health nursing care as demonstrated by the critical thinking model known as the nursing process (ANA et al., 2007)." The Standards of Practice and Professional Performance are listed on the inside back cover of this book.

STANDARD 1: ASSESSMENT

A view of the individual as a complex blend of many parts is consistent with nurses' holistic approach to care. Nurses who care for people with physical illnesses ideally maintain a holistic view that involves an awareness of psychological, social, cultural, and spiritual issues. Likewise, nurses who work in the psychiatric mental health field need to assess or have access to past and present medical history, a recent physical examination, and any physical complaints, as well as document any observable physical conditions or behaviors (e.g., unsteady gait, abnormal breathing patterns, wincing as if in pain, doubling over to relieve discomfort).

The assessment process begins with the initial patient encounter and continues throughout the care of the patient. To develop a basis for the plan of care and in preparation for discharge, every patient should have a thorough, formal nursing assessment on entering treatment. Subsequent to the formal assessment, data is collected continually and systematically as the patient's condition changes and—hopefully—improves. Perhaps the patient came into treatment actively suicidal, and the initial focus of care was on protection from injury; through regular assessment, it may be determined that although suicidal ideation has diminished, negative self-evaluation is still certainly a problem.

Assessments are conducted by a variety of professionals, including nurses, psychiatrists, social workers, dietitians, and other therapists. Virtually all facilities have standardized nursing assessment forms to aid in organization and consistency among reviewers. These forms may be paper or electronic versions, according to the resources and preferences of the institution. The time required for the nursing interview—a standard aspect of the formal nursing assessment—varies, depending on the assessment form and the patient's response pattern (e.g., a patient who is lengthy or rambling, is prone to tangential thought, has memory disturbances, or gives markedly slowed responses). Refer to Chapter 9 for sound guidelines for setting up and conducting a clinical interview.

In emergency situations, immediate intervention is often based on a minimal amount of data. In all situations, however, the patient, who must also receive a copy of the Health Insurance Portability and Accountability Act (HIPAA) guidelines, gives legal consent. Essentially, the purpose of the HIPAA privacy rule is to ensure that an individual's health information is properly protected, while at the same time allowing health care providers to obtain personal health information for the purpose of providing and promoting high-quality health care (USDHHS, 2003). HIPAA was first enacted in 1996, but compliance was not mandated until April 14, 2003. Chapter 7 has a more detailed discussion of HIPAA. Visit www.hhs.gov/ocr/privacy/hipaa/understanding/index.html for a full overview.

In patient-centered care, the nurse's *primary source* for data collection is the patient; however, there may be times when it is necessary to supplement or rely completely on another for the assessment information. These *secondary sources* can be invaluable when caring for a patient experiencing psychosis, muteness, agitation, or catatonia. Such secondary sources include members of the family, friends, neighbors, police, health care workers, and medical records.

The best atmosphere in which to conduct an assessment is one of minimal anxiety; therefore, if an individual becomes upset, defensive, or embarrassed regarding any topic, the topic should be abandoned. The nurse can acknowledge that the subject makes the patient uncomfortable and suggest within the medical record that the topic be discussed when the patient feels more comfortable. It is important that nurses not probe, pry, or push for information that is difficult for the patient to discuss; however, it should be recognized that increased anxiety about any subject is data in itself. The nurse can note this in the assessment without obtaining any further information.

Age Considerations

Assessment of Children

An effective interviewer working with children should have familiarity with basic cognitive and social/emotional developmental theory and have some exposure to applied child development (Sommers-Flanagan & Sommers-Flanagan, 2009).

The role of the caretaker is central in the interview; however, when assessing children, it is important to gather data from a variety of sources. Although the child is the best source in determining inner feelings and emotions, the caregivers (parents or guardians) often can best describe the behavior, performance, and conduct of the child. Caregivers also are helpful in interpreting the child's words and responses, but a separate interview is advisable when an older child is reluctant to share information, especially in cases of suspected abuse (Arnold & Boggs, 2011).

Developmental levels should be considered in the evaluation of children. One of the hallmarks of psychiatric disorders in children is the tendency to regress (i.e., return to a previous level of development). Although it is developmentally appropriate for toddlers to suck their thumbs, such a gesture is unusual in an older child.

One study found that children felt more comfortable if their health care provider was the same gender (Bernzweig et al., 1997). Another study indicated that although 60% of parents preferred that a man care for their children, 79% of the children, regardless of gender, requested that a female physician care for them (Waseem & Ryan, 2005). Age-appropriate communication strategies are perhaps the most important factor in establishing successful communication (Arnold & Boggs, 2011).

Assessment of children should be accomplished by a combination of interview and observation. Watching children at play provides important clues to their functioning. From a psychodynamic view, play is a safe area for the child to act out thoughts and emotions and can serve as a safe way in which children can release pent-up emotions—for example, having a child act out their story with the use of anatomically correct dolls or tell a story of their family using a family of dolls. Asking the child to tell a story, draw a picture, or engage in specific therapeutic games can be a useful assessment tool when determining critical concerns and painful issues a child may have difficulty expressing. Usually, a clinician with special training in child and adolescent psychiatry works with young children.

Assessment of Adolescents

Adolescents are especially concerned with confidentiality and may fear that anything they say to the nurse will be repeated to their parents. Lack of confidentiality can become a barrier of care with this population. Adolescents need to know that their records are private; they should receive an explanation as to how information will be shared among the treatment team. Questions related to such topics as substance abuse and sexual abuse demand confidentiality (Arnold & Boggs, 2011); however, threats of suicide, homicide, sexual abuse, or behaviors that put the patient or others at risk for harm must be shared with other professionals, as well as with the parents. Because identifying risk factors is one of the key objectives when assessing adolescents, it is helpful to use a brief, structured interview technique such as the HEADSSS interview (Box 7-2).

> **BOX 7-2 THE HEADSSS PSYCHOSOCIAL INTERVIEW TECHNIQUE**
>
> **H** Home environment (e.g., relations with parents and siblings)
> **E** Education and employment (e.g., school performance)
> **A** Activities (e.g., sports participation, after-school activities, peer relations)
> **D** Drug, alcohol, or tobacco use
> **S** Sexuality (e.g., whether the patient is sexually active, practices safe sex, or uses contraception)
> **S** Suicide risk or symptoms of depression or other mental disorder
> **S** "Savagery" (e.g., violence or abuse in home environment or in neighborhood)

Assessment of Older Adults

As we get older, our five senses (taste, touch, sight, hearing, and smell) and brain function begin to diminish, but the extent to which this affects each person varies. Your patient may be a spry and alert 80-year-old or a frail and confused 60-year-old; therefore, it is important not to stereotype older adults and expect them to be physically and/or mentally deficient. For example, the tendency may be to jump to the conclusion that someone who is hard of hearing is cognitively impaired. By the same token, many older adults often need special attention. The nurse needs to be aware of any physical limitations—any sensory condition (difficulty seeing or hearing), motor condition (difficulty walking or maintaining balance), or medical condition (back pain, cardiac or pulmonary deficits)—that could cause increased anxiety, stress, or physical discomfort for the patient during assessment of mental and emotional needs.

It is wise to identify any physical deficits at the onset of the assessment and make accommodations for them. If the patient is hard of hearing, speak a little more slowly in clear, louder tones (but not too loud), and seat the patient close to you without invading his or her personal space. Often, a voice that is lower in pitch is easier for older adults to hear, although a higher-pitched voice may convey anxiety to some. Refer to Chapter 30 for more on assessing and communicating with the older adult.

Language Barriers

It is becoming more and more apparent that psychiatric mental health nurses can best serve their patients if they have a thorough understanding of the complex cultural and social factors that influence health and illness. Awareness of individual cultural beliefs and health care practices can help nurses minimize stereotyped assumptions that can lead to ineffective care and interfere with the ability to evaluate care. There are many opportunities for misunderstandings when assessing a patient from a different cultural or social background from your own, particularly if the interview is conducted in English and the patient speaks a different language or a different form of English (Fontes, 2008).

Often health care professionals require a translator to understand the patient's history and health care needs. There is a difference between an *interpreter* and a *translator*. An interpreter is more likely to unconsciously try to make sense of (interpret) what the patient is saying and therefore inserts his or her own understanding of the situation into the database. A professional translator, on the other hand, tries to avoid interpreting. DeAngelis (2010) strongly advises against the use of untrained interpreters such as family members, friends, and neighbors. These individuals might censor or omit certain content (e.g. profanity, psychotic thoughts, and sexual topics) due to fear or a desire to protect the patient. They can also make subjective interpretations based on their own feelings, share confidential details with outsiders, or leave out traumatic topics because they hit too close to home for them.

For patients who do not speak English or have language difficulties, federal law mandates the use of a trained translator (Arnold & Boggs, 2011). In fact, Poole and Higgo state that the "use of a trained translator is essential wherever the patient's first language is not spoken English (even where the person has some English)" (2006, p. 135). A professionally trained translator is proficient in both English and the patient's spoken language, maintains confidentiality, and follows specific guidelines. Unfortunately, professional translators are not always readily available in many health care facilities.

Psychiatric Mental Health Nursing Assessment

The purpose of the psychiatric mental health nursing assessment is to:

- Establish rapport
- Obtain an understanding of the current problem or chief complaint
- Review physical status and obtain baseline vital signs
- Assess for risk factors affecting the safety of the patient or others
- Perform a mental status examination
- Assess psychosocial status
- Identify mutual goals for treatment
- Formulate a plan of care

Gathering Data

Review of Systems. The mind-body connection is significant in the understanding and treatment of psychiatric disorders. A primary care provider also gives many patients who are admitted for treatment of psychiatric conditions a thorough physical examination. Likewise, most nursing assessments include a baseline set of vital statistics, a historical and current review of body systems, and a documentation of allergic responses.

Poole and Higgo (2006) point out that several medical conditions and physical illnesses may mimic psychiatric illnesses (Box 7-3); therefore, physical causes of symptoms must be ruled

BOX 7-3 SOME MEDICAL CONDITIONS THAT MAY MIMIC PSYCHIATRIC ILLNESS

Depression

Neurological disorders:
- Cerebrovascular accident (stroke)
- Alzheimer's disease
- Brain tumor
- Huntington's disease
- Epilepsy (seizure disorder)
- Multiple sclerosis
- Parkinson's disease

Infections:
- Mononucleosis
- Encephalitis
- Hepatitis
- Tertiary syphilis
- Human immunodeficiency virus (HIV) infection

Endocrine disorders:
- Hypothyroidism and hyperthyroidism
- Cushing's syndrome
- Addison's disease
- Parathyroid disease

Gastrointestinal disorders:
- Liver cirrhosis
- Pancreatitis

Cardiovascular disorders:
- Hypoxia
- Congestive heart failure

Respiratory disorders:
- Sleep apnea

Nutritional disorders:
- Thiamine deficiency
- Protein deficiency
- B_{12} deficiency
- B_6 deficiency
- Folate deficiency

Collagen vascular diseases:
- Lupus erythematosus
- Rheumatoid arthritis

Cancer

Anxiety

Neurological disorders:
- Alzheimer's disease
- Brain tumor
- Stroke
- Huntington's disease

Infections:
- Encephalitis
- Meningitis
- Neurosyphilis
- Septicemia

Endocrine disorders:
- Hypothyroidism and hyperthyroidism
- Hypoparathyroidism
- Hypoglycemia
- Pheochromocytoma
- Carcinoid

Metabolic disorders:
- Low calcium
- Low potassium
- Acute intermittent porphyria
- Liver failure

Continued

BOX 7-3 SOME MEDICAL CONDITIONS THAT MAY MIMIC PSYCHIATRIC ILLNESS—cont'd

Cardiovascular disorders:
- Angina
- Congestive heart failure
- Pulmonary embolus

Respiratory disorders:
- Pneumothorax
- Acute asthma
- Emphysema

Drug effects:
- Stimulants
- Sedatives (withdrawal)

Lead, mercury poisoning

Psychosis

Medical conditions:
- Temporal lobe epilepsy
- Migraine headaches
- Temporal arteritis
- Occipital tumors
- Narcolepsy
- Encephalitis
- Hypothyroidism
- Addison's disease
- HIV infection

Drug effects:
- Hallucinogens (e.g., LSD)
- Phencyclidine
- Alcohol withdrawal
- Stimulants
- Cocaine
- Corticosteroids

out. Conversely, psychiatric disorders can result in physical or somatic symptoms such as stomachaches, headaches, lethargy, insomnia, intense fatigue, and even pain. When depression is secondary to a known medical condition, it often goes unrecognized and thus untreated. All patients who come into the health care system need to have both a medical and mental health evaluation to ensure a correct diagnosis and appropriate care.

Some people with certain physical conditions may be more prone to psychiatric disorders such as depression. It is believed, for example, that the disease process of multiple sclerosis or other autoimmune diseases may actually bring about depression. Other medical diseases typically associated with depression are coronary artery disease, diabetes, and stroke. A recent study demonstrated that women with both depression and diabetes have a significantly higher risk for mortality and cardiovascular disease than do women with either depression or diabetes alone (Brauser & Barclay, 2011). Individuals need to be evaluated for any medical origins of their depression or anxiety.

When evidence suggests the presence of mental confusion or organic mental disease, a mental status examination should be performed.

Laboratory Data. Hypothyroidism may have the clinical appearance of depression, and hyperthyroidism may appear to be a manic phase of bipolar disorder; a simple blood test can usually differentiate between depression and thyroid problems. Abnormal liver enzyme levels can explain irritability, depression, and lethargy. People who have chronic renal disease often suffer from the same symptoms when their blood urea nitrogen and electrolyte levels are abnormal. Results of a toxicology screen for the presence of either prescription or illegal drugs also may provide useful information.

Mental Status Examination. Fundamental to the psychiatric mental health nursing assessment is a **mental status examination (MSE)**. In fact, an MSE is part of the assessment in all areas of medicine. The MSE in psychiatry is analogous to the physical examination in general medicine, and the purpose is to evaluate an individual's current cognitive processes. For acutely disturbed patients, it is not unusual for the mental health clinician to administer MSEs every day. Sommers-Flanagan and Sommers-Flanagan (2009) advise anyone seeking employment in the medical–mental health field to be competent in communicating with other professionals via MSE reports. Box 7-4 is an example of a basic MSE.

The MSE, by and large, aids in collecting and organizing objective data. The nurse observes the patient's physical behavior, nonverbal communication, appearance, speech patterns, mood and affect, thought content, perceptions, cognitive ability, and insight and judgment.

Psychosocial Assessment. A **psychosocial assessment** provides additional information from which to develop a plan of care. It includes the following information about the patient:

- Central or chief complaint (in the patient's own words)
- History of violent, suicidal, or self-mutilating behaviors
- Alcohol and/or substance abuse
- Family psychiatric history
- Personal psychiatric treatment, including medications and complementary therapies
- Stressors and coping methods
- Quality of activities of daily living
- Personal background
- Social background, including support system
- Weaknesses, strengths, and goals for treatment
- Racial, ethnic, and cultural beliefs and practices
- Spiritual beliefs or religious practices

The patient's psychosocial history is most often the **subjective** part of the assessment. The focus of the history is the *patient's perceptions and recollections* of current lifestyle and life in general (family, friends, education, work experience, coping styles, and spiritual and cultural beliefs).

A psychosocial assessment elicits information about the systems in which a person operates. To conduct such an assessment, the nurse should have fundamental knowledge of growth and development, basic cultural and religious practices, pathophysiology, psychopathology, and pharmacology. Box 7-5 provides a basic psychosocial assessment tool.

BOX 7-4 MENTAL STATUS EXAMINATION

Appearance
- Grooming and dress
- Level of hygiene
- Pupil dilation or constriction
- Facial expression
- Height, weight, nutritional status
- Presence of body piercing or tattoos, scars, etc.
- Relationship between appearance and age

Behavior
- Excessive or reduced body movements
- Peculiar body movements (e.g., scanning of the environment, odd or repetitive gestures, level of consciousness, balance, and gait)
- Abnormal movements (e.g., tardive dyskinesia, tremors)
- Level of eye contact (keep cultural differences in mind)

Speech
- Rate: slow, rapid, normal
- Volume: loud, soft, normal
- Disturbances (e.g., articulation problems, slurring, stuttering, mumbling)
- Cluttering (e.g., rapid, disorganized, tongue-tied speech)

Mood
- Affect: flat, bland, animated, angry, withdrawn, appropriate to context
- Mood: sad, labile, euphoric

Disorders of the Form of Thought
- Thought process (e.g., disorganized, coherent, flight of ideas, neologisms, thought blocking, circumstantiality)
- Thought content (e.g., delusions, obsessions)

Perceptual Disturbances
- Hallucinations (e.g., auditory, visual)
- Illusions

Cognition
- Orientation: time, place, person
- Level of consciousness (e.g., alert, confused, clouded, stuporous, unconscious, comatose)
- Memory: remote, recent, immediate
- Fund of knowledge
- Attention: performance on serial sevens, digit span tests
- Abstraction: performance on tests involving similarities, proverbs
- Insight
- Judgment

Ideas of Harming Self or Others
- Suicidal or homicidal thoughts
- Presence of a plan
- Means to carry out the plan
- Opportunity to carry out the plan

BOX 7-5 PSYCHOSOCIAL ASSESSMENT

Previous hospitalizations

Educational background

Occupational background
- Employed? Where? What length of time?
- Special skills

Social patterns
- Describe family.
- Describe friends.
- With whom does the patient live?
- To whom does the patient go in time of crisis?
- Describe a typical day.

Sexual patterns
- Sexually active? Practices safe sex? Practices birth control?
- Sexual orientation
- Sexual difficulties

Interests and abilities
- What does the patient do in his or her spare time?
- What sport, hobby, or leisure activity is the patient good at?
- What gives the patient pleasure?

Substance use and abuse
- What medications does the patient take? How often? How much?
- What herbal or over-the-counter drugs does the patient take (caffeine, cough medicines, St. John's wort)? How often? How much?
- What psychotropic drugs does the patient take? How often? How much?
- How many drinks of alcohol does the patient take per day? Per week?
- What recreational drugs does the patient use (club drugs, marijuana, psychedelics, steroids)? How often? How much?
- Does the patient overuse prescription drugs (benzodiazepines, pain medications)?
- Does the patient identify the use of drugs as a problem?

Coping abilities
- What does the patient do when he or she gets upset?
- To whom can the patient talk?
- What usually helps to relieve stress?
- What did the patient try this time?

Spiritual assessment
- What importance does religion or spirituality have in the patient's life?
- Do the patient's religious or spiritual beliefs relate to the way the patient takes care of himself or herself or the illness? How?
- Does the patient's faith help the patient in stressful situations?
- Whom does the patient see when he or she is medically ill? Mentally upset?
- Are there special health care practices within the patient's culture that address his or her particular mental problem?

Spiritual/Religious Assessment. The importance of spirituality and religious beliefs is an often overlooked element of patient care although numerous empirical studies have suggested that being part of a spiritual community is helpful to people coping with illness and recovering from surgery (Kling, 2011). Spirituality and religious beliefs have the potential to exert an influence on how people understand meaning and purpose in their lives and how they use critical judgment to solve problems (e.g., crises of illness).

The terms *spirituality* and *religion* are different in their meanings, although not mutually exclusive. **Spirituality** is more of an internal phenomenon and is often understood as addressing universal human questions and needs. Spirituality can be expressed as having three dimensions: (1) *cognitive* (beliefs, values, ideals, purpose, truth, wisdom), (2) *experiential* (love, compassion, connection, forgiveness, altruism), and (3) *behavioral* (daily behavior, moral obligations, life choices, and medical choices) (Anandarajab, 2008). Spirituality is the part of us that seeks to understand life and may or may not be connected with the community or religious rituals. The term spirituality is more about the believer's faith being more personal, less dogmatic, and more inclusive, considering the belief that there are many spiritual paths and no one "real path." It has been found that spirituality has the potential to increase healthy behaviors, social support, and a sense of meaning, which are linked to decreased overall mental and physical illness.

In contrast, **religion** is an external system that includes beliefs, patterns of worship, and symbols. An individual connects personal, spiritual beliefs with a larger organized group or institution. Belonging to a religious community can provide support during difficult times. For many individuals, prayer is a source of hope, comfort, and support in healing. Although religion is often concerned with spirituality, religious groups are social entities and are often characterized by other non spiritual goals as well (cultural, economic, political, social,)

O'Rioran (2010), in an interview with Dr. Donald Lloyd-Jones (Northwestern University Fienberg School of Medicine, Chicago), quoted him as saying:

"In general, from the perspective of overall health, health care utilization, and outcomes, the suggestion has been from some of the studies that greater religiosity, in terms of participation or spirituality, is typically associated with better health outcomes."

Delgado (2007) notes that nurses and other health care providers may be uncomfortable with assessing for, or discussing spiritual issues with, patients, even though their proximity with patients and intimate patient needs gives them a unique opportunity to develop spiritual care theory and practices.

The following questions may be included in a spiritual or religious assessment:

- Who or what supplies you with strength and hope?
- Do you have a religious affiliation?
- Do you practice any spiritual activities (yoga, tai chi, meditation)?
- Do you participate in any religious activities?
- What role does religion or spiritual practice play in your life?
- Does your faith help you in stressful situations?
- Do you pray or meditate?
- Has your illness affected your religious/spiritual practices?
- Would you like to have someone from your church/synagogue/temple or from our facility visit?

Cultural and Social Assessment. Because of the cultural diversity in most societies, there is a need for nursing assessments, diagnoses, and subsequent care to be planned around the unique cultural health care beliefs, values, and practices of each individual patient. Chapter 5 has a detailed discussion of the cultural implications for psychiatric mental health nursing and how to conduct a cultural and social assessment.

Some questions we can ask to help with a cultural and social assessment are:

- What is your primary language? Would you like a translator?
- How would you describe your cultural background?
- Whom are you close to?
- Whom do you seek in times of crisis?
- Whom do you live with?
- Whom do you seek when you are medically ill? Mentally upset or concerned?
- What do you do to get better when you have physical problems?
- What are the attitudes toward mental illness in your culture?
- How is your current problem viewed by your culture? Is it seen as a problem that can be fixed? A disease? A taboo? A fault or curse?
- Are there special foods that you eat?
- Are there special health care practices within your culture that address your particular mental or emotional health problem?
- Are there any special cultural beliefs about your illness that might help me give you better care?

After the cultural and social assessment, it is useful to summarize pertinent data with the patient. This summary provides patients with reassurance that they have been heard and gives them the opportunity to clarify any misinformation. The patient should be told what will happen next. For example, if the initial assessment takes place in the hospital, you should tell the patient who else he or she will be seeing. If a psychiatric mental health nurse in a mental health clinic conducted the initial assessment, the patient should be told when and how often he or she would meet with the nurse to work on the patient's problems. If you believe a referral is necessary, this should be discussed with the patient.

Validating the Assessment

To gain an even clearer understanding of your patient, it is helpful to look to outside sources. Ideally, patients would have electronic medical records where all health care information would be available. We have not reached that degree of sophistication, but informatics have made gathering this information easier. Emergency department records can be a valuable resource in understanding an individual's presenting behavior and problems. Police reports may be available in cases in which hostility and legal altercations occurred. Old medical records, most now accessible by computer, are a great help in validating information you already have or in adding new information to your database. If the patient was admitted to a psychiatric unit in the past, information about the patient's previous level of functioning and behavior gives you a baseline for making clinical judgments. Occasionally, consent forms may have to be signed by the patient or an appropriate relative to obtain access to records.

Using Rating Scales

A number of standardized rating scales are useful for psychiatric evaluation and monitoring. A clinician often administers rating scales, but many are self-administered. Table 7-1 lists some of the common ones in use. Many of the clinical chapters in this book include a rating scale.

TABLE 7-1 STANDARDIZED RATING SCALES*

USE	SCALE
Depression	Beck Inventory Brief Patient Health Questionnaire (Brief PHQ) Geriatric Depression Scale (GDS) Hamilton Depression Scale Zung Self-Report Inventory Patient Health Questionnaire-9 (PHQ-9)
Anxiety	Brief Patient Health Questionnaire (Brief PHQ) Generalized Anxiety Disorder–7 (GAD-7) Modified Spielberger State Anxiety Scale Hamilton Anxiety Scale
Substance use disorders	Addiction Severity Index (ASI) Recovery Attitude and Treatment Evaluator (RAATE) Brief Drug Abuse Screen Test (B-DAST)
Obsessive-compulsive behavior	Yale Brown Obsessive Compulsive Scale (Y-BOCS)
Mania	Mania Rating Scale
Schizophrenia	Scale for Assessment of Negative Symptoms (SANS) Brief Psychiatric Rating Scale (BPRS)
Abnormal movements	Abnormal Involuntary Movement Scale (AIMS) Simpson Neurological Rating Scale
General psychiatric assessment	Brief Psychiatric Rating Scale (BPRS) Global Assessment of Functioning Scale (GAF)
Cognitive function	Mini-Mental State Examination (MMSE) St. Louis University Mental Status Examination (SLUMS) Cognitive Capacity Screening Examination (CCSE) Alzheimer's Disease Rating Scale (ADRS) Memory and Behavior Problem Checklist Functional Assessment Screening Tool (FAST) Global Deterioration Scale (GDS)
Family assessment	McMaster Family Assessment Device
Eating disorders	Eating Disorders Inventory (EDI) Body Attitude Test Diagnostic Survey for Eating Disorders

* These rating scales highlight important areas in psychiatric assessment. Because many of the answers are subjective, experienced clinicians use these tools as a guide when planning care and also draw on their knowledge of their patients.

STANDARD 2: DIAGNOSIS

A nursing diagnosis is a clinical judgment about a patient's response, needs, actual and potential psychiatric disorders, mental health problems, and potential comorbid physical illnesses. An accurate and clear, standardized nursing diagnosis is the basis for selecting therapeutic outcomes and interventions. NANDA International, Inc. (NANDA-I) provides evidence-based diagnoses for nursing care (Herdman, 2012). See the last page of this text (opposite the inside back cover) for a list of NANDA-I 2012-2014 approved nursing diagnoses.

Diagnostic Statements

Nursing diagnostic statements are made up of the following structural components:

1. Problem/potential problem
2. Related factors
3. Defining characteristics

The **problem**, or unmet need, describes the state of the patient at present. Problems that are within the nurse's domain to treat are termed *nursing diagnoses*. The nursing diagnostic label states what should change. For example: *Hopelessness*. For health promotion diagnoses, what is diagnosed is readiness for enhancing specific health behaviors that can occur at any point on the health-illness continuum. For example: *Readiness for enhanced decision-making*.

Related factors are linked to the diagnostic label with the words *related to*. The related factors usually indicate what needs to be addressed to effect change through nursing interventions. In the case of *hopelessness related to long-term stress* the nurse would work with the patient to reduce or prevent the negative impacts of stress. However, in the case of *hopelessness related to abandonment,* there may be nothing the nurse can do to change the abandonment; in that case, the focus would be on symptom management by addressing the defining characteristics.

Defining characteristics include signs (objective and measurable) and symptoms (subjective and reported by the patient). They may be linked to the diagnosis and with the words *as evidenced by*. The previous example would then become: *Hopelessness related to abandonment as evidenced by stating, "Nothing will change," lack of involvement with family and friends, and lack of motivation to care for self or environment.*

Types of Nursing Diagnoses

Actual diagnoses are problems that currently exist. This category of nursing diagnosis is accompanied by defining characteristics that are clustered into patterns that constitute etiology, or "related to." (Formula: Problem + Related Factors + Defining Characteristics)

Health promotion diagnoses refer to the desire or motivation to improve health standing. Defining characteristics support this type of diagnosis; related factors are not used in this problem statement since they would always be the same, that is, motivated to improve health standing. Health promotion diagnoses always begin with the phrase "readiness for enhanced . . . " An example of this type of diagnosis is *readiness for enhanced coping as evidenced by seeking social support and knowledge of new strategies.* (Formula: Problem + Defining Characteristics)

Risk diagnoses pertain to vulnerability that carries a high probability of developing problematic experiences or responses. Common problems in this category include preventable occurrences such as falls, self-injury, pressure ulcers, and infection; these problems are directly linked with quality improvement and patient safety (QSEN).

This category of diagnosis always begins with the phrase "risk for," followed by the problem. Since the problem has not yet happened, there is controversy over whether we can cite causation in the form of related factors; others believe that since the problem has not yet happened we cannot have evidence or defining characteristics.

Herdman (personal communication, 2012) supports problem statements that omit related factors and include defining characteristics (risk factors) such as, *risk for self-mutilation as evidenced by impulsivity, inadequate coping, isolation, and unstable self-esteem* (Formula: Problem + Defining Characteristics/Risk Factors).

Syndromes refer to a group of two or more nursing diagnoses that typically happen together, that can be addressed with similar interventions. Defining characteristics support these diagnoses; related factors are used if necessary to clarify the definition. An example of this type of syndrome diagnosis is post trauma syndrome, which includes fear, anxiety, pain, and grief. (Formula: Problem +/- Related Factors + Defining Characteristics)

STANDARD 3: OUTCOMES IDENTIFICATION

Outcome criteria are the hoped-for outcomes that reflect the maximal level of patient health that can realistically be achieved through nursing interventions. Whereas nursing diagnoses identify nursing problems, outcomes reflect the desired change. The expected outcomes provide direction for continuity of care (ANA et al., 2007). Outcomes should take into account the patient's culture, values, and ethical beliefs. Specifically, outcomes are stated in attainable and measurable terms and include a time estimate for attainment (ANA et al., 2007). Therefore, outcome criteria are patient-centered, geared to each individual, and documented as obtainable goals.

Moorhead and colleagues (2013) have compiled a standardized list of nursing outcomes in *Nursing Outcomes Classification (NOC)* (refer to Chapter 1). *NOC* includes standardized outcomes that provide a mechanism for communicating the effect of nursing interventions on the well-being of patients, families, and communities. Each outcome has an associated group of indicators used to determine patient status in relation to the outcome. Table 7-2 provides suggested *NOC* indicators for the outcome of *Suicide Self-Restraint,* along with the Likert scale that quantifies the achievement on each indicator from 1 (never demonstrated) to 5 (consistently demonstrated).

TABLE 7-2 *NOC* INDICATORS FOR SUICIDE SELF-RESTRAINT

Definition: Personal actions to refrain from gestures and attempts at killing self
Outcome target rating: Maintain at _________ Increase to _________

SUICIDE SELF-RESTRAINT OVERALL RATING	NEVER DEMONSTRATED 1	RARELY DEMONSTRATED 2	SOMETIMES DEMONSTRATED 3	OFTEN DEMONSTRATED 4	CONSISTENTLY DEMONSTRATED 5	
Expresses feelings	1	2	3	4	5	NA
Expresses sense of hope	1	2	3	4	5	NA
Maintains connectedness in relationships	1	2	3	4	5	NA
Obtains assistance as needed	1	2	3	4	5	NA
Verbalizes suicidal ideas	1	2	3	4	5	NA
Controls impulses	1	2	3	4	5	NA
Refrains from gathering means for suicide	1	2	3	4	5	NA
Refrains from giving away possessions	1	2	3	4	5	NA
Refrains from inflicting serious injury	1	2	3	4	5	NA
Refrains from using unprescribed mood-altering substances	1	2	3	4	5	NA
Discloses plan for suicide if present	1	2	3	4	5	NA
Upholds suicide contract	1	2	3	4	5	NA

TABLE 7-2 *NOC* INDICATORS FOR SUICIDE SELF-RESTRAINT—cont'd

SUICIDE SELF-RESTRAINT OVERALL RATING	NEVER DEMONSTRATED 1	RARELY DEMONSTRATED 2	SOMETIMES DEMONSTRATED 3	OFTEN DEMONSTRATED 4	CONSISTENTLY DEMONSTRATED 5	
Maintains self-control without supervision	1	2	3	4	5	NA
Refrains from attempting suicide	1	2	3	4	5	NA
Obtains treatment for depression	1	2	3	4	5	NA
Obtains treatment for substance abuse	1	2	3	4	5	NA
Reports adequate pain control for chronic pain	1	2	3	4	5	NA
Uses suicide prevention resources	1	2	3	4	5	NA
Uses social support group	1	2	3	4	5	NA
Uses available mental health care services	1	2	3	4	5	NA
Plans for future	1	2	3	4	5	NA

Modified from Moorhead, S., Johnson, M., Maas, M., & Swanson, E. (2013). *Nursing outcomes classification (NOC)* (5th ed.). St. Louis, MO: Mosby.

NOC is a useful resource for specific patient care outcomes, especially with objective measurement scales. Students are encouraged to use these resources whenever possible. In terms of planning care, short- and long-term outcomes, often stated as goals, are suggested for assessing the effectiveness of nursing interventions and for teaching and learning purposes. The use of goals guides nurses in building incremental steps toward meeting the desired outcome. All outcomes (goals) are written in positive terms, following the criteria set out by the Standards of Practice. The clinical chapters in this book will include these short- and long-term outcomes. Table 7-3 shows how specific outcome criteria might be stated for a suicidal individual with a nursing diagnosis of *Risk for suicide related to depression and suicide attempt.*

STANDARD 4: PLANNING

Inpatient and community-based facilities increasingly are using standardized care plans or clinical pathways for patients with specific diagnoses. Standardizing pathways or plans of care allows for inclusion of evidence-based practice and newly tested interventions as they become available. They are more time efficient, although less focused on the specific individual patient needs. Other health care facilities continue to devise individual plans of care. Whatever the care planning procedures in a specific institution, the nurse considers the following specific principles when planning care:

- **Safe:** Interventions must be safe for the patient as well as for other patients, staff, and family.

TABLE 7-3 EXAMPLES OF LONG- AND SHORT-TERM GOALS FOR A SUICIDAL PATIENT

LONG-TERM GOALS OR OUTCOMES	SHORT-TERM GOALS OR OUTCOMES
Patient will remain free from injury throughout the hospital stay.	Patient will state he or she understands the rationale and procedure of the unit's protocol for suicide precautions shortly after admission. Patient will sign a "no-suicide" contract for the next 24 hours, renewable at the end of every 24-hour period (if approved for use by the mental health facility). Patient will seek out staff when feeling overwhelmed or self-destructive during hospitalization.
By discharge, patient will state he or she no longer wishes to die and has at least two persons to contact if suicidal thoughts arise.	Patient will meet with social worker to find supportive resources in the community before discharge and work on trigger issues (e.g., housing, job). By discharge, patient will state the purpose of medication, time and dose, adverse effects, and whom to call for questions or concerns. Patient will have the written name and telephone numbers of at least two people to turn to if feeling overwhelmed or self-destructive. Patient will have a follow-up appointment to meet with a mental health professional by discharge.

- **Compatible and appropriate:** Interventions must be compatible with other therapies and with the patient's personal goals and cultural values as well as with institutional rules.
- **Realistic and individualized:** Interventions should be (1) within the patient's capabilities, given the patient's age, physical strength, condition, and willingness to change; (2) based on the number of staff available; (3) reflective of the actual available community resources; and (4) within the student's or nurse's capabilities.
- **Evidence-based:** Interventions should be based on scientific evidence and principles when available.

Using evidence-based interventions and treatments as they become available is the gold standard in health care (refer to Chapter 1). There are many definitions for evidence-based practice, but David Sackett's (an original founder of evidence-based medicine) definition remains among the most useful in today's practice. His definition clearly considers patient values and clinical experience together with the best research evidence (Sackett, 2000). **Evidence-based practice (EBP)** for nurses is a combination of clinical skill and the use of clinically relevant research in the delivery of effective patient-centered care. The combined use of the best available research, patient preferences, and sound clinical judgment and skills makes for an optimal patient-centered nurse-patient relationship (Sackett et al., 2000). Box 7-6 lists several online resources for evidence-based practice. Keep in mind that whatever interventions are planned, they must be acceptable and appropriate to the individual patient.

The ***Nursing Interventions Classification (NIC)*** (Bulechek et al., 2013) is a research-based, standardized listing of interventions reflective of current clinical practices the nurse can use to plan care (refer to Chapter 1). This evidence-based approach to care is consistent with QSEN standards. Nurses in all settings can use *NIC* to support quality patient care and incorporate evidence-based nursing actions. Although many safe and appropriate interventions may not be included in *NIC*, it is a useful guide for standardized care. Individualizing interventions to meet a patient's special needs should always be part of the planning.

BOX 7-6 USEFUL EVIDENCE-BASED PRACTICE WEBSITES

- Academic Center for Evidence-Based Practice (ACE): www.acestar.uthscsa.edu
- Center for Research & Evidence Based Practice: www.son.rochester.edu/son/research/centers/research-evidenced-based-practice
- Centre for Evidence-Based Mental Health (CEBMH): www.cebmh.com
- The Cochrane Collaboration: www.cochrane.org
- The Joanna Briggs Institute: www.joannabriggs.edu.au
- The Sarah Cole Hirsh Institute for Best Nursing Practice Based on Evidence: http://fpb.case.edu/Centers/Hirsh/
- Evidence-Based Practice: An Interprofessional Tutorial: http://www.biomed.lib.umn.edu/learn/ebp/

STANDARD 5: IMPLEMENTATION

Psychiatric-Mental Health Nursing: Scope and Standards of Practice (ANA et al., 2007) identifies seven areas for intervention. Recent graduates and practitioners new to the psychiatric setting will participate in many of these activities with the guidance and support of more experienced health care professionals. The following four interventions are performed by both the psychiatric mental health registered nurse (RN-PMH) and the psychiatric mental health advanced practice registered nurse (APRN-PMH). (Refer to Chapter 1 for further discussion of these nursing roles.)

The basic implementation skills are accomplished through the nurse-patient relationship and therapeutic interventions. The nurse implements the plan using evidence-based practice whenever possible, uses community resources, and collaborates with nursing colleagues.

Basic Level Interventions

Standard 5A: Coordination of Care

The psychiatric mental health nurse coordinates the implementation of the plan and provides documentation.

Standard 5B: Health Teaching and Health Promotion

Psychiatric mental health nurses use a variety of health teaching methods adaptive to the patient's needs (e.g., age, culture, ability to learn, readiness, etc.), integrating current knowledge and research and seeking opportunities for feedback and effectiveness of care. **Health teaching** includes identifying the health education needs of the patient and teaching basic principles of physical and mental health, such as giving information about coping, interpersonal relationships, social skills, mental disorders, the treatments for such illnesses and their effects on daily living, relapse prevention, problem-solving skills, stress management, crisis intervention, and self-care activities. The last of these, **self-care activities**, assists the patient in assuming personal responsibility for activities of daily living (ADL) and focuses on improving the patient's mental and physical well-being.

Standard 5C: Milieu Therapy

Milieu therapy is an extremely important consideration in helping patients feel comfortable and safe. Milieu management includes orienting patients to their rights and responsibilities, selecting specific activities that meet patients' physical and mental health needs, and ensuring that patients are maintained in the least restrictive environment safety permits. It also includes informing patients in a culturally competent manner about the need for limits and the conditions necessary to remove them (refer to Chapter 6). The milieu is the environment in which teamwork and collaboration occur to provide the most comprehensive care possible.

Standard 5D: Pharmacological, Biological, and Integrative Therapies

Nurses need to know the intended action, therapeutic dosage, adverse reactions, and safe blood levels of medications being administered and must monitor them when appropriate (e.g., blood levels for lithium). The nurse is expected to discuss and provide medication teaching tools to the patient and family regarding drug action, adverse side effects, dietary restrictions, and drug interactions and to provide time for questions. The nurse's assessment of the patient's response to psychobiological interventions is communicated to other members of the multidisciplinary mental health team. Interventions are also aimed at alleviating untoward effects of medication.

Advanced Practice Interventions

The following three interventions can be carried out by the APRN-PMH only.

Standard 5E: Prescriptive Authority and Treatment

The APRN-PMH is educated and clinically prepared to prescribe psychopharmacological agents for patients with mental health or psychiatric disorders in accordance with state and federal laws and regulations. Such prescriptions take into account individual variables such as culture, ethnicity, gender, religious beliefs, age, and physical health.

Standard 5F: Psychotherapy

The APRN-PMH is educationally and clinically prepared to conduct individual, couples, group, and family psychotherapy, using evidence-based psychotherapeutic frameworks and nurse-patient therapeutic relationships (ANA, 2007). Refer to Chapter 2 for an overview of various psychotherapies, Chapter 33 for a discussion of therapeutic groups, Chapter 34 for a discussion of family interventions, and Chapter 35 for a discussion of integrative therapies.

Standard 5G: Consultation

The APRN-PMH works with other clinicians to provide consultation, influence the identified plan, enhance the ability of other clinicians, provide services for patients, and effect change.

STANDARD 6: EVALUATION

Unfortunately, evaluation of patient outcomes is often the most neglected part of the nursing process. Evaluation of the individual's response to treatment should be systematic, ongoing, and criteria-based. Supporting data are included to clarify the evaluation. Ongoing assessment of data allows for revisions of nursing diagnoses, changes to more realistic outcomes, or identification of more appropriate interventions when outcomes are not met.

DOCUMENTATION

Documentation could be considered the seventh step in the nursing process. Keep in mind that medical records are legal documents and may be used in a court of law. Besides the evaluation of stated outcomes, the medical record should include changes in patient condition, informed consents (for medications and treatments), reaction to medication, documentation of symptoms (verbatim when appropriate), concerns of the patient, and any untoward incidents in the health care setting. Documentation of patient progress is the responsibility of the entire mental health team.

Although communication among team members and coordination of services are the primary goals when choosing a system for documentation, practitioners in all settings must also consider professional standards, legal issues, requirements for reimbursement by insurers, and accreditation by regulatory agencies.

Information also must be in a format that is retrievable for quality improvement monitoring, utilization management, peer review, and research. Documentation—using the nursing process as a guide—is reflected in two of the formats commonly used in health care settings and described in Table 7-4. Informatics in general and electronic medical records specifically are increasingly used in both inpatient and outpatient settings. Nurses need to be trained to use these technologies in the medical setting, and we should be prepared to provide further training for nurses in the use of terminology, progress notes relating to needs assessment, nursing interventions, and nursing diagnoses (Hayrinen, 2010). Whatever format is used, documentation must be focused, organized, pertinent, and conform to certain legal and other generally accepted principles (Box 7-7)

TABLE 7-4 NARRATIVE VERSUS PROBLEM-ORIENTED CHARTING

	NARRATIVE CHARTING	PROBLEM-ORIENTED CHARTING: SOAPIE
Characteristics	A descriptive statement of patient status written in chronological order throughout a shift. Used to support assessment findings from a flow sheet. In charting by exception, narrative notes are used to indicate significant symptoms, behaviors, or events that are exceptions to norms identified on an assessment flow sheet.	Developed in the 1960s for physicians to reduce inefficient documentation. Intended to be accompanied by a problem list. Originally SOAP, with IE added later. The emphasis is on problem identification, process, and outcome. S:Subjective data (patient statement) O: Objective data (nurse observations) A: Assessment (nurse interprets *S* and *O* and describes either a problem or a nursing diagnosis) P: Plan (proposed intervention) I: Interventions (nurse's response to problem) E: Evaluation (patient outcome)

Continued

TABLE 7-4 NARRATIVE VERSUS PROBLEM-ORIENTED CHARTING—cont'd

	NARRATIVE CHARTING	PROBLEM-ORIENTED CHARTING: SOAPIE
Example	(Date/time/discipline) Patient was agitated in the morning and pacing in the hallway. Blinked eyes, muttered to self, and looked off to the side. Stated heard voices. Verbally hostile to another patient. Offered 2 mg haloperidol (Haldol) prn and sat with staff in quiet area for 20 minutes. Patient returned to community lounge and was able to sit and watch television.	(Date/time/discipline) S: "I'm so stupid. Get away, get away." "I hear the devil telling me bad things." O: Patient paced the hall, mumbling to self and looking off to the side. Shouted derogatory comments when approached by another patient. Watched walls and ceiling closely. A: Patient was having auditory hallucinations and increased agitation. P: Offered patient haloperidol prn. Redirected patient to less stimulating environment. I: Patient received 2 mg haloperidol PO prn. Sat with patient in quiet room for 20 minutes. E: Patient calmer. Returned to community lounge, sat and watched television.
Advantages	Uses a common form of expression (narrative writing) Can address any event or behavior Explains flow-sheet findings Provides multidisciplinary ease of use	Structured Provides consistent organization of data Facilitates retrieval of data for quality assurance and utilization management Contains all elements of the nursing process Minimizes inclusion of unnecessary data Provides multidisciplinary ease of use
Disadvantages	Unstructured May result in different organization of information from note to note Makes it difficult to retrieve quality assurance and utilization management data Frequently leads to omission of elements of the nursing process Commonly results in inclusion of unnecessary and subjective information	Requires time and effort to structure the information Limits entries to problems May result in loss of data about progress Not chronological Carries negative connotation

BOX 7-7 LEGAL CONSIDERATIONS FOR DOCUMENTATION OF CARE

Do

- Chart in a timely manner all pertinent and factual information.
- Be familiar with the nursing documentation policy in your facility and make your charting conform to this standard. The policy generally states the method, frequency, and pertinent assessments, interventions, and outcomes to be recorded. If your agency's policies and procedures do not encourage or allow for quality documentation, bring the need for change to the administration's attention.
- Chart legibly in ink.
- Chart facts fully, descriptively, and accurately.
- Chart what you see, hear, feel, and smell.
- Chart pertinent observations: psychosocial observations, physical symptoms pertinent to the medical diagnosis, and behaviors pertinent to the nursing diagnosis.
- Chart follow-up care provided when a problem has been identified in earlier documentation. For example, if a patient has fallen and injured a leg, describe how the wound is healing.
- Chart fully the facts surrounding unusual occurrences and incidents.
- Chart *all* nursing interventions, treatments, and outcomes (including teaching efforts and patient responses) and safety and patient-protection interventions.
- Chart the patient's expressed subjective feelings.
- Chart each time you notify a physician and record the reason for notification, the information that was communicated, the accurate time, the physician's instructions or orders, and the follow-up activity.
- Chart physicians' visits and treatments.
- Chart discharge medications and instructions given for use, as well as all discharge teaching performed, and note which family members were included in the process.

Don't

- Do *not* chart opinions that are not supported by facts.
- Do *not* defame patients by calling them names or making derogatory statements about them (e.g., "an unlikable patient who is demanding unnecessary attention").
- Do *not* chart before an event occurs.
- Do *not* chart generalizations, suppositions, or pat phrases (e.g., "patient in good spirits").
- Do *not* obliterate, erase, alter, or destroy a record. If an error is made, draw one line through the error, write "mistaken entry," the date, and initial. Follow your agency's guidelines closely.
- Do *not* leave blank spaces for chronological notes. If you must chart out of sequence, chart "late entry." Identify the time and date of the entry and the time and date of the occurrence.
- If an incident report is filed, *do not note in the chart that one was filed.* This form is generally a privileged communication between the hospital and the hospital's attorney. Describing it in the chart may destroy the privileged nature of the communication.

KEY POINTS TO REMEMBER

- The nursing process is a six-step problem-solving approach to patient care.
- The Institute of Medicine (IOM) and Quality and Safety Education for Nurses (QSEN) faculty have established mandates to prepare future nurses with the knowledge, skills, and attitudes (KSAs) necessary for achieving quality and safety as they engage in the six competencies of nursing: patient-centered care, teamwork and collaboration, evidence based practice (EBP), quality improvement (QI), safety, and informatics.
- The *primary source* of assessment is the patient. *Secondary sources* of information include family members, neighbors, friends, police, and other members of the health team.
- A professional translator often is needed to prevent serious misunderstandings during assessment, treatment, and evaluation with non–English-speaking patients.
- The assessment interview includes gathering objective data (mental or emotional status) and subjective data (psychosocial assessment).
- Medical examination, history, and systems review round out a complete assessment.
- Assessment tools and standardized rating scales may be used to evaluate and monitor a patient's progress.
- Determination of the nursing diagnosis (NANDA-I) defines the practice of nursing, improves communication between staff members, and assists in accountability of care.
- Nursing diagnoses always include a problem. Depending upon the type of diagnosis (e.g., actual or risk), related factors and defining characteristics are included in the diagnostic statement.
- Outcomes are variable, measurable, and stated in terms that reflect a patient's actual state. *NOC* provides standardized outcomes. Planning involves determining desired outcomes.
- Behavioral goals support outcomes. Goals are short, specific, and measurable; indicate the desired patient behavior(s); and include a set time for achievement.
- Planning nursing actions (using *NIC* or other sources) to achieve outcomes includes the use of specific principles. The plan should be (1) safe, (2) compatible with and appropriate for implementation with other therapies, (3) realistic and individualized, and (4) evidence-based whenever possible. *NIC* provides nurses with 542 standardized nursing interventions applicable for use in all settings.
- Psychiatric mental health nursing practice includes four basic-level interventions: coordination of care, health teaching and health promotion, milieu therapy, and pharmacological, biological, and integrative therapies.
- A nurse who is educated at the master's level or higher carries out advanced practice interventions. Nurses certified for advanced practice psychiatric mental health nursing can prescribe certain medications, practice psychotherapy, and perform consulting work.
- The evaluation of care is a continual process of determining to what extent the outcome criteria have been achieved. The plan of care may be revised based on the evaluation.
- Documentation of patient progress through evaluation of the outcome criteria is crucial. The medical record is a legal document and should accurately reflect the patient's condition, medications, treatment, tests, responses, and any untoward incidents.

CRITICAL THINKING

Pedro Gonzales, a 37-year-old Hispanic man, arrives by ambulance from a supermarket where he had fallen. On his arrival to the emergency department (ED), his breath smells "fruity." He appears confused and anxious, saying that "they put the evil eye on me, they want me to die, they are drying out my body . . . it's draining me dry . . . they are yelling, they are yelling . . . no, no, I'm not bad . . . oh, God, don't let them get me!" When his mother arrives in the ED, she tells the staff, through the use of a translator, that Pedro is a severe diabetic, has a diagnosis of paranoid schizophrenia, and this happens when he doesn't take his medications. In a group or in collaboration with a classmate, respond to the following:

1. A number of nursing diagnoses are possible in this scenario. Given the above information, formulate at least two nursing diagnoses (problems), and include "related to" and "as evidenced by" as appropriate.
2. For each of your nursing diagnoses, write out one long-term outcome (the problem, what should change, etc.). Include a time frame, desired change, and three criteria that will help you evaluate whether the outcome has been met, not met, or partially met.
3. What specific needs might you take into account when planning nursing care for Mr. Gonzales?
4. Using the SOAPIE format (see Table 7-4), formulate an initial nurse's note for Mr. Gonzales.

CHAPTER REVIEW

1. You are assessing a 6-year-old patient. When assessing a child's perception of a difficult issue, which methods of assessment are appropriate? *Select all that apply.*
   a. Engage the child in a specific therapeutic game.
   b. Ask the child to draw a picture.
   c. Provide the child with an anatomically correct doll to act out a story.
   d. Allow the child to tell a story.
2. Which are the purposes of a thorough mental health nursing assessment? *Select all that apply.*
   a. Establish a rapport between the nurse and patient.
   b. Assess for risk factors affecting the safety of the patient or others.
   c. Allow the nurse the chance to provide counseling to the patient.
   d. Identify the nurse's goals for treatment.
   e. Formulate a plan of care.
3. You are performing a spiritual assessment on a patient. Which patient statement would indicate that there is an experiential concern in the patient's spiritual life?
   a. "I really believe that my spouse loves me."
   b. "My sister will never forgive me for what I did."
   c. "I try to find time every day to pray, even though it's not easy."
   d. "I am happy with my life choices, even if my mother is not."

4. A patient states he has "given up on life." His wife left him, he was fired from his job, and he is four payments behind on his mortgage, meaning he will soon lose his house. Which nursing diagnosis is appropriate?
   a. Anxiety related to multiple losses
   b. Defensive coping related to multiple losses
   c. Ineffective denial related to multiple losses
   d. Hopelessness related to multiple losses
5. A 43-year-old female patient is brought to the emergency department with complaints of bizarre speech, visual hallucinations, and changes in behavior. She has no psychiatric history. Before ordering a psychiatric consultation, the emergency room physician orders a battery of blood tests as well as an MRI of the brain. The rationale for this is:
   a. To avoid a lawsuit.
   b. Medical conditions and physical illnesses may mimic psychiatric illnesses; therefore, physical causes of symptoms must be ruled out
   c. Emergency room physicians are required to order a certain number of tests for the emergency room visit to be reimbursed.
   d. To comply with hospital standards of care.

Answers to Chapter Review
1. a, b, c, d; 2. a, b, d, e; 3. b; 4. d; 5. b.

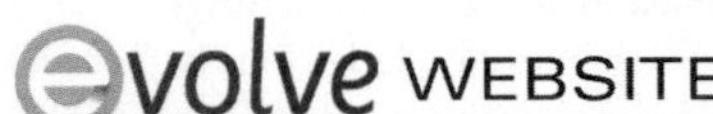
WEBSITE

Visit the Evolve website for a posttest on the content in this chapter: http://evolve.elsevier.com/Varcarolis

Post-Test interactive review

REFERENCES

American Nurses Association, American Psychiatric Nurses Association, & International Society of Psychiatric-Mental Health Nurses. (2007). *Psychiatric-mental health nursing: Scope and standards of practice.* Washington, DC: Nursesbooks.org.

Anandarajab, G. (2008). The 3 H and BMSEST models for spirituality in multicultural whole-person medicine. *Annals of Family Medicine, 6*(5), 448–458.

Arnold, E. C. & Boggs, K. U. (2011). *Interpersonal relationships: Professional communication skills for nurses* (5th ed.). St. Louis, MO: Saunders.

Bernzweig, J., Takayama, J. I., Phibbs, C., Lewis, C., & Pantell, R. H. (1997). Gender differences in physician-patient communication. *Archives of Pediatric and Adolescent Medicine, 151*(6), 586–591.

Brauser, D., & Barclay, X. (2011). Deadly combination of depression and diabetes doubles mortality risk. *Medscape Nurses Education.* Retrieved from http://www.medscape.org/viewarticle/735714.

Bulechek, G. M., Butcher, H. K., Dochterman, J. M., & Wagner, C. (2013). *Nursing interventions classification (NIC)* (6th ed.). St. Louis, MO: Mosby.

Cronenwett, L., Sherwood, G., Barnsteiner, J., Disch, J., Johnson, J., Mitchell, P., Sullivan, D., & Warren, J. (2007). Quality and safety education for nurses. *Nursing Outlook, 55*(3), 122–131.

DeAngelis, T. (2010). Found in translation. *Monitor on Psychology, 41*(2), 52.

Delgado, C. (2007). Meeting clients' spiritual needs. *Nursing Clinics of North America, 42*(2), 279–293.

Durham, C. F., & Sherwood, G. D. (2008). Education to bridge the quality gap: A case to study approach. *Urologic Nursing, 28*(6), 431–438.

Hayrinen, K. (2010). Evaluation of electronic nursing documentation—Nursing process model and standardized terminologies as key to visible and transparent nursing. *International Journal of Medical Informatics, 79*(8), 554–564.

Herdman, T. H. (Ed.), (2012). *NANDA international nursing diagnoses: Definitions and classification, 2012-2014.* Oxford, UK: Wiley-Blackwell.

Kling, J. (2011). *Spirituality an important component of patient care. Medscape Nurses News.* Retrieved from http://www.medscape.com/viewarticle/738237.

Lenburg, C. E. (2011). The influence of contemporary trends and issues in nursing education. In B. Cherry & S. R. Jacob (Eds.), *Contemporary nursing: Issues, trends, & management* (pp. 41–70). St Louis, MO: Elsevier.

Mian, A. I., Al-Mateen, C. S., & Cerda, G. (2010). Training child and adolescent psychiatrist to be culturally competent. *Child and Adolescent Psychiatric Clinics of North America, 19*(4), 7–31.

Fontes, L. A. (2008). *Interviewing across cultures.* New York, NY: Guilford Press.

Moorhead, S., Johnson, M., Maas, M. L., & Swanson, E. (2013). *Nursing outcomes classification (NOC)* (5th ed.). St Louis, MO: Mosby.

Poole, R., & Higgo, R. (2006). *Psychiatric interviewing and assessment.* Liverpool, UK: Cambridge University Press.

Sackett, D. L., Straus, S. E.. Richardson, W. S., Rosenberg, W., & Haynes, R.B. (2000). *Evidence-based medicine: how to practice and teach EBMB.* London, UK: Churchill Livingstone.

Sommers-Flanagan, J., & Sommers-Flanagan, R. (2009). *Clinical interviewing* (4th ed.). Hoboken, NJ: Wiley.

U.S. Department of Health and Human Services. (2003). *Summary of the HIPAA Privacy Act.* Washington, DC: Author.

Waseem, M. & Ryan, M. (2005). "Doctor" or "doctora": Do patients care? *Pediatric Emergency Care, 21*, 515–517.

CHAPTER

8

Therapeutic Relationships

Elizabeth M. Varcarolis

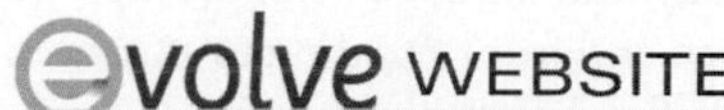

Visit the Evolve website for a pretest on the content in this chapter: http://evolve.elsevier.com/Varcarolis

Pre-Test interactive review

OBJECTIVES

1. Explain the three phases of the nurse-patient relationship.
2. Compare and contrast a social relationship and a therapeutic relationship regarding purpose, focus, communications style, and goals.
3. Identify at least four patient behaviors a nurse may encounter in the clinical setting.
4. Explore qualities that foster a therapeutic nurse-patient relationship and qualities that contribute to a nontherapeutic nursing interactive process.
5. Define and discuss the roles of empathy, genuineness, and positive regard on the part of the nurse in a nurse-patient relationship.
6. Identify two attitudes and four actions that may reflect the nurse's positive regard for a patient.
7. Analyze what is meant by boundaries and the influence of transference and countertransference on boundary blurring.
8. Understand the use of attending behaviors (e.g., eye contact, body language, vocal qualities, and verbal tracking).
9. Discuss the influences of disparate values and cultural beliefs on the therapeutic relationship.

KEY TERMS AND CONCEPTS

clinical supervision
contract
countertransference
empathy
genuineness
orientation phase
patient-centered care
rapport
social relationship
termination phase
therapeutic encounter
therapeutic relationship
therapeutic use of self
transference
values
working phase

Psychiatric mental health nursing is in many ways based on principles of *science*. A background in anatomy, physiology, and chemistry is the basis for providing safe and effective biological treatments. Knowledge of pharmacology—a medication's mechanism of action, indications for use, and adverse effects, based on evidence-based studies and trials—is vital to nursing practice. However, it is the caring relationship and the development of the interpersonal skills needed to enhance and maintain such a relationship that make up the *art* of psychiatric nursing. Human beings are social creatures. A therapeutic relationship creates a space where caring and healing can occur.

CONCEPTS OF THE NURSE-PATIENT RELATIONSHIP

The health care community has increasingly grown to accept the concept of **patient-centered care** as the gold standard. The core concepts of patient- and family-centered care consist of (1) dignity and respect, (2) information sharing, (3) patient and family participation, and (4) collaboration in policy and program development (Institute for Patient- and Family-Centered Care, 2010). These tenets are familiar to members of the nursing profession as the nurse-patient relationship.

The nurse-patient relationship is the basis of all psychiatric mental health nursing treatment approaches, regardless of the specific goals. The very first connections between nurse and patient are to establish an understanding that the nurse is safe, confidential, reliable, and consistent, and that the relationship will be conducted within appropriate and clear boundaries.

It is true that many psychiatric disorders, such as schizophrenia, bipolar disorder, and major depression, have strong biochemical and genetic components; however, many accompanying emotional problems such as poor self-image, low self-esteem, and difficulties with adherence to a treatment regimen can be significantly improved through a therapeutic nurse-patient relationship. All too often, patients entering treatment have taxed or exhausted their familial and social resources and find themselves isolated and in need of emotional support.

The nurse-patient relationship is a creative process and unique to each nurse. Each of us has distinct gifts that we can learn to use creatively to form positive bonds with others, historically referred to as the **therapeutic use of self**. Travelbee (1971) defined therapeutic use of self as "the ability to use one's personality consciously and in full awareness in an attempt to establish relatedness and to structure nursing interventions" (p. 19). The efficacy of this therapeutic use of self has been scientifically substantiated as an evidence-based intervention. Randomized clinical trials have repeatedly found that development of a positive alliance (therapeutic relationship) is one of the best predictors of positive outcomes in therapy (Gordon et al., 2010; Kopta et al., 1999). On the other hand, nonadherence with treatment and poor outcomes in therapy are related to a patient feeling unheard, disrespected, or otherwise unconnected with the clinician/health care worker (Gordon et al., 2010).

A successful therapeutic alliance is greatly influenced by the personal characteristics of the clinician and the patient, not necessarily the particular process employed. Furthermore, evidence suggests that psychotherapy (talk therapy) within a therapeutic partnership actually changes brain chemistry in much the same way as medication (Hollon & Ponniah, 2010; Serfaty et al., 2009). Thus the best treatment for most psychiatric problems (less so with psychotic disorders) is a combination of medication and psychotherapy. Cognitive-behavioral therapy, in particular, has met with great success in the treatment of depression, phobias, obsessive-compulsive disorders, and others.

Establishing a therapeutic relationship with a patient takes time. Skills in this area gradually improve with guidance from those with more skill and experience.

Goals and Functions

The nurse-patient relationship is often loosely defined, but a therapeutic nurse-patient relationship has specific goals and functions, including the following:

- Facilitating communication of distressing thoughts and feelings
- Assisting patients with problem solving to help facilitate activities of daily living
- Helping patients examine self-defeating behaviors and test alternatives
- Promoting self-care and independence

Social Versus Therapeutic

A relationship is an interpersonal process that involves two or more people. Throughout life, we meet people in a variety of settings and share a variety of experiences. With some individuals, we develop long-term relationships; with others, the relationship lasts only a short time. Naturally, the kinds of relationships we enter vary from person to person and from situation to situation. Generally, relationships can be defined as *intimate, social,* or *therapeutic.* Intimate relationships occur between people who have an emotional commitment to each other. Within intimate relationships, mutual needs are met, and intimate desires and fantasies are shared. For our purposes in this chapter, we will limit our exploration to the aspects of social and therapeutic relationships.

Social Relationships

A **social relationship** can be defined as a relationship that is primarily initiated for the purpose of friendship, socialization, enjoyment, or accomplishment of a task. Mutual needs are met during social interaction (e.g., participants share ideas, feelings, and experiences). Communication skills may include giving advice and (sometimes) meeting basic dependency needs, such as lending money and helping with jobs. Often, the content of the communication remains superficial. During social interactions, roles may shift. Within a social relationship, there is little emphasis on the evaluation of the interaction, as in the following example:

Patient: "Oh, I just hate to be alone. It's getting me down, and sometimes it hurts so much."

Nurse: "I know just how you feel. I don't like it either. What I do is get a friend and go to a movie or something. Do you have someone to hang out with?" *(In this response the nurse is minimizing the patient's feelings and giving advice prematurely.)*

Patient: "No, not really, but often I don't even feel like going out. I just sit at home feeling scared and lonely."

Nurse: "Most of us feel like that at one time or another. Maybe if you took a class or joined a group you could meet more people. I know of some great groups you could join. It's not good to be stuck in the house by yourself all of the time." *(Again, the nurse is not "hearing" the patient's distress and is minimizing her pain and isolation. The nurse goes on to give the patient unwanted and unhelpful advice, thus closing off the patient's feelings and experience.)*

Therapeutic Relationships

In a **therapeutic relationship**, the nurse maximizes his or her communication skills, understanding of human behaviors, and personal strengths to enhance the patient's growth. Patients more easily engage in the relationship when the clinician's interactions address their concerns, respect the patient as a partner in decision making, and use language that is straightforward (Gordon et al., 2010). These interactions are evidence that the focus of the relationship is on the patient's ideas, experiences, and feelings. Inherent in a therapeutic relationship is the nurse's focus on significant personal issues introduced by the patient during the clinical interview. The nurse and the patient identify areas that need exploration and periodically evaluate the degree of change in the patient.

Although the nurse may assume a variety of roles (e.g., teacher, counselor, socializing agent, liaison), the relationship is consistently focused on the patient's problem and needs. Nurses' needs must be met outside the relationship. When nurses begin to want the patient to "like them," "do as they suggest," "be nice to them," or "give them recognition," the needs of the patient cannot be adequately met, and the interaction could be detrimental (nontherapeutic) to the patient.

Working under clinical supervision is an excellent way to keep the focus and boundaries clear. Communication skills and knowledge of the stages and phenomena in a therapeutic relationship are crucial tools in the formation and maintenance of that relationship. Within the context of a therapeutic relationship, the following occur:

- The needs of the patient are identified and explored.
- Clear boundaries are established.
- Alternate problem-solving approaches are taken.
- New coping skills may be developed.
- Behavioral change is encouraged.

Just like staff nurses, nursing students may struggle with the boundaries between social and therapeutic relationships because there is a fine line between the two. In fact, students often feel more comfortable "being a friend" because it is a more familiar role, especially with patients close to their own age. When this occurs, the nurse or student needs to make it clear (to themselves and the patient) that the relationship is a therapeutic one. This does *not* mean that the nurse is not friendly toward the patient, and it does *not* mean that talking about everyday topics (e.g., television, weather, and children's pictures) is forbidden. It *does* mean, however, that the nurse must follow the prior stated guidelines regarding a therapeutic relationship; essentially, the focus is on the patient, and the relationship is not designed to meet the nurse's needs. The patient's problems and concerns are explored, both patient and nurse discuss potential solutions, and the patient, as in the following example, implements solutions:

Patient: "Oh, I just hate to be alone. It's getting me down, and sometimes it hurts so much."

Nurse: "Loneliness can be painful. What is going on now that you are feeling so alone?"

Patient: "Well, my mom died 2 years ago, and last month, my—oh, I am so scared." *(Patient takes a deep breath, looks down, and looks as if she might cry.)*

Nurse: *(Sits in silence while the patient recovers.)* "Go on."

Patient: "My boyfriend left for Afghanistan. I haven't heard from him, and they say he's missing. He was my best friend, and we were going to get married, and if he dies, I don't want to live."

Nurse: "That must be scary not knowing what is going on with your boyfriend. Have you thought of harming yourself?"

Patient: "Well, if he dies, I will. I can't live without him."

Nurse: "Have you ever felt like this before?"

Patient: "Yes, when my mom died. I was depressed for about a year until I met my boyfriend."

Nurse: "It sounds as if you're going through a very painful and scary time. Perhaps you and I can talk some more and come up with some ways for you to feel less anxious, scared, and overwhelmed. Would you be willing to work on this together?"

The ability of the nurse to engage in interpersonal interactions in a goal-directed manner to assist patients with their emotional or physical health needs is the foundation of the therapeutic nurse-patient relationship. Necessary behaviors of health care workers, including nurses, include the following:

- **Accountability**: Nurses assume responsibility for their conduct and the consequences of their actions.
- **Focus on patient needs**: The interest of the patient rather than the nurse, other health care workers, or the institution is given first consideration. The nurse's role is that of patient advocate.
- **Clinical competence**: The criteria on which the nurse bases his or her conduct are principles of knowledge and those that are appropriate to the specific situation. This involves awareness and incorporation of the latest knowledge made available from research (evidence-based practice).
- **Delaying judgment**: Ideally, nurses refrain from judging patients and avoid transferring their own values and beliefs on others.
- **Supervision**: Supervision by a more experienced clinician or team is essential to developing one's competence in establishing therapeutic nurse-patient relationships.

Nurses interact with patients in a variety of settings: emergency departments, medical-surgical units, obstetric and pediatric units, clinics, community settings, schools, and patients' homes. Nurses who are sensitive to patients' needs and have effective assessment and communication skills can significantly help patients confront current problems and anticipate future choices.

Sometimes the type of relationship that occurs may be informal and not extensive, such as when the nurse and patient meet for only a few sessions. Even though it is brief, the relationship may be substantial, useful, and important for the patient. This limited relationship is often referred to as a therapeutic encounter. When the nurse shows genuine concern for another's circumstances (has positive regard and empathy), even a short encounter can have a powerful effect.

At other times, the encounters may be longer and more formal, such as in inpatient settings, mental health units, crisis centers, and mental health facilities. This longer time span allows the therapeutic nurse-patient relationship to be more fully developed.

Relationship Boundaries and Roles

Establishing Boundaries

According to Fox (2008), boundaries can be thought of in terms of the following:

- **Physical boundaries**: General environment, office space, treatment room, conference room, corner of the day room, and other such places
- **The contract**: Set time, confidentiality, agreement between nurse and patient as to roles, money, if involved with a licensed therapist
- **Personal space**: Physical space, emotional space, space set by roles, and so forth

Blurring of Boundaries

A well-defined therapeutic nurse-patient relationship allows the establishment of clear boundaries that provide a safe space in which the patient can explore feelings and treatment issues. Theoretically, the nurse's role in the therapeutic relationship can be stated rather simply as follows: The patient's needs are separated from the nurse's needs, and the patient's role is different from that of the nurse; therefore, the boundaries of the relationship are well defined. Boundaries are constantly at risk of blurring, and a shift in the nurse-patient relationship may lead to nontherapeutic dynamics. Two common circumstances in which boundaries are blurred are (1) when the relationship is allowed to slip into a social context and (2) when the nurse's needs (for attention, affection, and emotional support) are met at the expense of the patient's needs.

Boundaries are primarily necessary to protect the patient. The most egregious boundary violations are those of a sexual nature (Wheeler, 2008). This type of violation results in high levels of malpractice actions and the loss of professional licensure on the part of the nurse. Other boundary issues are not as obvious. Table 8-1 illustrates some examples of patient and nurse behaviors that reflect blurred boundaries.

Blurring of Roles

Blurring of roles in the nurse-patient relationship is often a result of unrecognized transference or countertransference.

Transference. Transference is a phenomenon originally identified by Sigmund Freud when he used psychoanalysis to treat patients. Transference occurs when the patient unconsciously and inappropriately displaces (transfers) onto the nurse feelings and behaviors related to significant figures in the patient's past. The patient may even say, "You remind me of my (mother, sister, father, brother, etc.)."

Patient: "Oh, you are so high and mighty. Did anyone ever tell you that you are a cold, unfeeling machine, just like others I know?"

Nurse: "Tell me about one person who is cold and unfeeling toward you." *(In this example, the patient is experiencing the nurse in the same way she experienced significant other[s] during her formative years. In this case, the patient's mother was very aloof, leaving the patient with feelings of isolation, worthlessness, and anger.)*

Although transference occurs in all relationships, it seems to be intensified in relationships of authority. This may occur because parental figures were the original figures of authority. Physicians, nurses, and social workers all are potential objects of transference. This transference may be positive or negative. If a patient is motivated to work with you, completes assignments between sessions, and shares feelings openly, it is likely the patient is experiencing positive transference (Wheeler, 2008).

Positive transference does not need to be addressed with the patient, whereas negative transference that threatens the nurse-patient relationship may need to be explored. Common forms of transference include the desire for affection or respect and the gratification of dependency needs. Other transferential feelings are hostility, jealousy, competitiveness, and love.

Sometimes patients experience positive or negative thoughts, feelings, and reactions that are realistic and appropriate and *not* a result of transference onto the health care worker. For example, if a nurse makes promises to the patient that are not kept, such as not showing up for a meeting, the patient may feel resentment and mistrust toward the nurse.

Countertransference. Countertransference occurs when the nurse unconsciously and inappropriately displaces onto the patient feelings and behaviors related to significant figures in the nurse's past. Frequently the patient's transference evokes countertransference in the nurse. For example, it is normal to feel angry when attacked persistently, annoyed when frustrated unreasonably, or flattered when idealized. A nurse might feel extremely important when depended on exclusively by a patient. If the nurse does not recognize his or her own omnipotent feelings as countertransference, encouragement of independent growth in the patient might be minimized at best.

Recognizing countertransference maximizes our ability to *empower* our patients. When we fail to recognize countertransference, the therapeutic relationship stalls, and essentially we *disempower* our patients by experiencing them not as individuals but rather as extensions of ourselves. Example:

Patient: "Yeah, well I decided not to go to that dumb group. 'Hi, I'm so-and-so, and I'm an alcoholic.' Who cares?" *(Patient sits slumped in a chair chewing gum, nonchalantly looking around.)*

Nurse: *(In an impassioned tone)* "You always sabotage your chances. You need AA to get in control of your life. Last week you were going to go, and now you've disappointed everyone." *(Here the nurse is reminded of her mother, who was an alcoholic. The nurse had tried everything to get her mother into treatment and took it as a personal failure and deep disappointment that her mother never sought recovery.*

TABLE 8-1 PATIENT AND NURSE BEHAVIORS THAT REFLECT BLURRED BOUNDARIES

WHEN THE NURSE IS OVERLY INVOLVED	WHEN THE NURSE IS NOT INVOLVED
More frequent requests by the patient for assistance, which causes increased dependency on the nurse	Patient's increased verbal or physical expression of isolation (depression)
Inability of the patient to perform tasks of which he or she is known to be capable prior to the nurse's help, which causes regression	Lack of mutually agreed-upon goals
Unwillingness on the part of the patient to maintain performance or progress in the nurse's absence	Lack of progress toward goals
Expressions of anger by other staff who do not agree with the nurse's interventions or perceptions of the patient	Nurse's avoidance of spending time with the patient
Nurse's keeping of secrets about the nurse-patient relationship	Failure of the nurse to follow through on agreed-upon interventions

Data from Pilette, P. C., Berck, C. B., & Achber, L. C. (1995). Therapeutic management of helping boundaries. *Journal of Psychosocial Nursing and Mental Health Services, 33*(1), 40–47.

After the nurse sorts out her thoughts and feelings and realizes the frustration and feelings of disappointment and failure belonged with her mother and not the patient, the nurse starts out the next session with the following approach.)

Nurse: "Look, I was thinking about last week, and I realize the decision to go to AA or find other help is solely up to you. It's true that I would like you to live a fuller and more satisfying life, but it's your decision. I'm wondering, however, what happened to change your mind about going to AA."

If the nurse feels either a strongly positive or a strongly negative reaction to a patient, the feeling most often signals countertransference. One common sign of countertransference is overidentification with the patient. In this situation, the nurse may have difficulty recognizing or objectively seeing patient problems that are similar to the nurse's own. For example, a nurse who is struggling with an alcoholic family member may feel disinterested, cold, or disgusted toward an alcoholic patient. Other indicators of countertransference are when the nurse gets involved in power struggles, competition, or arguments with the patient. Table 8-2 lists some common countertransference reactions.

Identifying and working through various transference and countertransference issues is crucial if we are to achieve professional and clinical growth and allow for positive change in the patient. Supervision by peers or by the therapeutic team can help work through transference and countertransference, as well as numerous other issues. Besides helping with boundaries, supervision supplies practical and emotional support, education, and guidance regarding ethical issues. Regularly scheduled supervision sessions provide the nurse with the opportunity to increase self-awareness, clinical skills, and growth as well as allow for continued growth of the patient. No matter how hard clinicians may try to examine their interactions objectively, professional support and help from an experienced supervisor are essential to good practice (Fox, 2008).

Self-Check on Boundaries

It is useful for all of us to take time out to be reflective and aware of our thoughts and actions with patients as well as with colleagues, friends, and family. Figure 8-1 is a helpful boundary

TABLE 8-2 COMMON COUNTERTRANSFERENCE REACTIONS

As a nurse, you will sometimes experience countertransference feelings. Once you are aware of them, use them for self-analysis to understand those feelings that may inhibit productive nurse-patient communication.

REACTION TO PATIENT	BEHAVIORS CHARACTERISTIC OF THE REACTION	SELF-ANALYSIS	SOLUTION
Boredom (indifference)	Showing inattention. Frequently asking the patient to repeat statements. Making inappropriate responses.	Is the content of what the patient presents uninteresting? Or is it the style of communication? Does the patient exhibit an offensive style of communication? Have you anything else on your mind that may be distracting you from the patient's needs? Is the patient discussing an issue that makes you anxious?	Redirect the patient if he or she provides more information than you need or goes "off track." Clarify information with the patient. Confront ineffective modes of communication.
Rescue	Reaching for unattainable goals. Resisting peer feedback and supervisory recommendations. Giving advice.	What behavior stimulates your perceived need to rescue the patient? Has anyone evoked such feelings in you in the past? What are your fears or fantasies about failing to meet the patient's needs? Why do you want to rescue this patient?	Avoid secret alliances. Develop realistic goals. Do not alter meeting schedule. Let the patient guide interaction. Facilitate patient problem solving.
Overinvolvement	Coming to work early, leaving late. Ignoring peer suggestions, resisting assistance. Buying the patient clothes or other gifts. Accepting the patient's gifts. Behaving judgmentally at family interventions. Keeping secrets. Calling the patient when off duty.	What particular patient characteristics are attractive? Does the patient remind you of someone? Who? Does your current behavior differ from your treatment of similar patients in the past? What are you getting out of this situation? What needs of yours are being met?	Establish firm treatment boundaries, goals, and nursing expectations. Avoid self-disclosure. Avoid calling the patient when off duty.
Overidentification	Having special agenda, keeping secrets. Increasing self-disclosure. Feeling omnipotent. Experiencing physical attraction.	With which of the patient's physical, emotional, cognitive, or situational characteristics do you identify? Recall similar circumstances in your own life. How did you deal with the issues now being created by the patient?	Allow the patient to direct issues. Encourage a problem-solving approach from the patient's perspective. Avoid self-disclosure.

Continued

TABLE 8-2 **COMMON COUNTERTRANSFERENCE REACTIONS—cont'd**

REACTION TO PATIENT	BEHAVIORS CHARACTERISTIC OF THE REACTION	SELF-ANALYSIS	SOLUTION
Misuse of honesty	Withholding information. Lying.	Why are you protecting the patient? What are your fears about the patient's learning the truth?	Be clear in your responses and aware of your hesitation; do not hedge. If you can provide information, tell the patient and give your rationale. Avoid keeping secrets. Reinforce the patient with regard to the multidisciplinary nature of treatment.
Anger	Withdrawing. Speaking loudly. Using profanity. Asking to be taken off the case.	What patient behaviors are offensive to you? What dynamic from your past may this patient be re-creating?	Determine the origin of the anger (nurse, patient, or both). Explore the roots of patient anger. Avoid contact with the patient if the anger is not understood.
Helplessness or hopelessness	Feeling sadness.	Which patient behaviors evoke these feelings in you? Has anyone evoked similar feelings in the past? Who? What past expectations were placed on you (verbally and nonverbally) by this patient?	Maintain therapeutic involvement. Explore and focus on the patient's experience rather than on your own.

Data from Aromando, L. (1995). *Mental health and psychiatric nursing* (2nd ed.). Springhouse, PA: Springhouse.

NURSING BOUNDARY INDEX SELF-CHECK

Please rate yourself according to the frequency with which the following statements reflect your behavior, thoughts, or feelings within the past 2 years while providing patient care.*

1. Have you ever received any feedback about your behavior being overly intrusive with patients and their families?	Never ____	Rarely ____	Sometimes ____	Often ____
2. Do you ever have difficulty setting limits with patients?	Never ____	Rarely ____	Sometimes ____	Often ____
3. Do you ever arrive early or stay late to be with your patient for a longer period?	Never ____	Rarely ____	Sometimes ____	Often ____
4. Do you ever find yourself relating to patients or peers as you might to a family member?	Never ____	Rarely ____	Sometimes ____	Often ____
5. Have you ever acted on sexual feelings you have for a patient?	Never ____	Rarely ____	Sometimes ____	Often ____
6. Do you feel that you are the only one who understands the patient?	Never ____	Rarely ____	Sometimes ____	Often ____
7. Have you ever received feedback that you get "too involved" with patients or families?	Never ____	Rarely ____	Sometimes ____	Often ____
8. Do you derive conscious satisfaction from patients' praise, appreciation, or affection?	Never ____	Rarely ____	Sometimes ____	Often ____
9. Do you ever feel that other staff members are too critical of "your" patient?	Never ____	Rarely ____	Sometimes ____	Often ____
10. Do you ever feel that other staff members are jealous of your relationship with your patient?	Never ____	Rarely ____	Sometimes ____	Often ____
11. Have you ever tried to "match-make" a patient with one of your friends?	Never ____	Rarely ____	Sometimes ____	Often ____
12. Do you find it difficult to handle patients' unreasonable requests for assistance, verbal abuse, or sexual language?	Never ____	Rarely ____	Sometimes ____	Often ____

*Any item that is responded to with "Sometimes" or "Often" should alert the nurse to a possible area of vulnerability. If the item is responded to with "Rarely," the nurse should determine whether it is an isolated event or a possible pattern of behavior.

FIG 8-1 Nursing Boundary Index Self-Check. (From Pilette, P., Berck, C., & Achber, L. [1995]. Therapeutic management. *Journal of Psychosocial Nursing, 33*[1], 45.)

self-test you can use throughout your career, no matter what area of nursing you choose.

VALUES, BELIEFS, AND SELF-AWARENESS

Values are abstract standards and represent an ideal, either positive or negative. It is crucial that we have an understanding of our own values and attitudes so we may become aware of the beliefs or attitudes we hold that may interfere with establishing positive relationships with those under our care.

When working with patients, it is important for nurses to understand that our values and beliefs are not necessarily right and certainly are not right for everyone. It is helpful to realize that our values and beliefs (1) reflect our own culture/subculture, (2) are derived from a range of choices, and (3) are those we have *chosen* for ourselves from a variety of influences and role models. These chosen values (religious, cultural, societal) guide us in making decisions and taking actions that we hope will make our lives meaningful, rewarding, and fulfilled.

Interviewing others whose values, beliefs, cultures, or lifestyles are radically different from our own can be a challenge (Fontes, 2008). Several topics that cause controversy in society in general—including religion, gender roles, abortion, war, politics, money, drugs, alcohol, sex, and corporal punishment—also can cause conflict between nurses and patients (Fontes, 2008). Although we emphasize that the patient and nurse should identify outcomes together, what happens when the nurse's values, beliefs, and interpretive system are very different from those of a patient? Consider the following examples of possible conflicts:

- The patient wants an abortion, which is against the nurse's values.
- The nurse believes the patient who was raped should get an abortion, but the patient refuses.
- The patient engages in unsafe sex with multiple partners, which is against the nurse's values.
- The nurse cannot understand a patient who refuses medications on religious grounds.
- The patient puts material gain and objects far ahead of loyalty to friends and family, in direct contrast with the nurse's values.
- The nurse is deeply religious, whereas the patient is a nonbeliever who shuns organized religion.
- The patient's lifestyle includes taking illicit drugs, which is against the nurse's values.

How can nurses develop working relationships and help patients solve problems when patients' values, goals, and interpretive systems are so different from their own? Self-awareness requires that we understand what we value and those beliefs that guide our behavior. It is critical that, as nurses, we not only understand and accept our own values and beliefs but also are sensitive to and accepting of the unique and different values and beliefs of others. This is another area in which supervision by an experienced colleague can prove invaluable.

PEPLAU'S MODEL OF THE NURSE-PATIENT RELATIONSHIP

Hildegard Peplau introduced the concept of the nurse-patient relationship in 1952 in her groundbreaking book *Interpersonal Relations in Nursing*. This model of the nurse-patient relationship is well accepted in the United States and Canada and is an important tool for all nursing practice. A **professional nurse-patient relationship** consists of a nurse who has skills and expertise and a patient who wants to alleviate suffering, find solutions to problems, explore different avenues to increased quality of life, and/or find an advocate (Fox, 2008).

Peplau (1952) proposed that the nurse-patient relationship "facilitates forward movement" for both the nurse and the patient (p. 12). This interactive nurse-patient process is designed to facilitate the patient's boundary management, independent problem solving, and decision making that promotes autonomy.

Peplau (1952, 1999) described the nurse-patient relationship as evolving through three distinct interlocking and overlapping phases. An additional preorientation phase, during which the nurse prepares for the orientation phase, has been identified. The four phases are as follows:

1. Preorientation phase
2. Orientation phase
3. Working phase
4. Termination phase

Most likely, you will not have time to develop all phases of the nurse-patient relationship in your brief psychiatric mental health nursing rotation; however, it is important to be aware of these phases in order to recognize and use them later. It is also important to remember that *any* contact that is caring, respectful, and demonstrative of concern for the situation of another person can have an enormous positive impact.

Preorientation Phase

Even before the first meeting, the nurse may have many thoughts and feelings related to the first clinical session. Beginning health care professionals usually have many concerns and experience anxiety on their first clinical day. These universal concerns include being afraid of persons with psychiatric problems, of saying "the wrong thing," and of not knowing what to do in response to certain patient behaviors. Table 8-3 identifies common patient behaviors (e.g., crying, asking the nurse to keep a secret, threatening to commit suicide, giving a gift, wanting physical contact with the nurse) and gives examples of possible reactions by the nurse and suggested responses.

Talking with the instructor and participating in the supervised peer group discussion will promote confidence, feedback, and suggestions. Refer to Chapter 9 for a detailed discussion of communication strategies used in clinical practice.

Most experienced psychiatric mental health nursing faculty and staff monitor the unit atmosphere and have a sixth sense for behaviors that indicate escalating tension. They are trained in crisis interventions, and formal security is often available onsite to give the staff support. Your instructor will set the ground rules for safety during the first clinical day. For example, don't

TABLE 8-3 COMMON PATIENT BEHAVIORS, POSSIBLE NURSE REACTIONS, AND SUGGESTED NURSE RESPONSES

POSSIBLE REACTIONS	USEFUL RESPONSES
IF THE PATIENT THREATENS SUICIDE	
The nurse may feel overwhelmed or responsible for "talking the patient out of it." The nurse may pick up some of the patient's feelings of hopelessness.	The nurse assesses whether the patient has a plan and the lethality of the plan. The nurse tells the patient that this is serious, that the nurse does not want harm to come to the patient, and that this information needs to be shared with other staff: "This is very serious, Mr. Lamb. I don't want any harm to come to you. I'll have to share this with the other staff." The nurse can then discuss with the patient the feelings and circumstances that led up to this decision. (Refer to Chapter 25 for strategies in suicide intervention.).
IF THE PATIENT ASKS THE NURSE TO KEEP A SECRET.	
The nurse may feel conflict because the nurse wants the patient to share important information but is unsure about making such a promise.	The nurse *cannot* make such a promise. The information may be important to the health or safety of the patient or others: "I cannot make that promise. It might be important for me to share it with other staff." The patient then decides whether to share the information.
IF THE PATIENT ASKS THE NURSE A PERSONAL QUESTION.	
The nurse may think that it is rude not to answer the patient's question. A new nurse may feel relieved to put off having to start the interview. The nurse may feel put on the spot and want to leave the situation. New nurses are often manipulated by a patient into changing roles. This keeps the focus off the patient and prevents the building of a relationship.	The nurse may or may not answer the patient's query. If the nurse decides to answer a natural question, he or she answers in a word or two, then refocuses back on the patient:. **Patient:** Are you married? **Nurse:** Yes. Do you have a spouse? **Patient:** Do you have any children? **Nurse:** This time is for you. Tell me about yourself. **Patient:** You can just tell me if you have any children. **Nurse:** This is your time to focus on your concerns. Tell me something about your family.
IF THE PATIENT MAKES SEXUAL ADVANCES	
The nurse feels uncomfortable but may feel conflicted about "rejecting" the patient or making him or her feel "unattractive" or "not good enough."	The nurse needs to set clear limits on expected behavior: "I'm not comfortable having you touch (kiss) me. This time is for you to focus on your problems and concerns." Frequently restating the nurse's role throughout the relationship can help maintain boundaries. If the patient doesn't stop, the nurse might say: "If you can't stop this behavior, I'll have to leave. I'll be back at [time] to spend time with you then." Leaving gives the patient time to gain control. The nurse returns at the stated time.
IF THE PATIENT CRIES	
The nurse may feel uncomfortable and experience increased anxiety or feel somehow responsible for making the person cry.	The nurse should stay with the patient and reinforce that it is all right to cry. Often it is at that time that feelings are closest to the surface and can be best identified: "You seem ready to cry." "You are still upset about your brother's death." "What are you thinking right now?" The nurse offers tissues when appropriate.
IF THE PATIENT LEAVES BEFORE THE SESSION IS OVER	
The nurse may feel rejected, thinking it was something that he or she did. The nurse may experience increased anxiety or feel abandoned by the patient.	Some patients are not able to relate for long periods without experiencing an increase in anxiety. On the other hand, the patient may be testing the nurse: "I'll wait for you here for 15 minutes, until our time is up." During this time, the nurse does not engage in conversation with any other patient or even with the staff. When the time is up, the nurse approaches the patient, says the time is up, and restates the day and time the nurse will see the patient again.

TABLE 8-3 COMMON PATIENT BEHAVIORS, POSSIBLE NURSE REACTIONS, AND SUGGESTED NURSE RESPONSES—cont'd

POSSIBLE REACTIONS	USEFUL RESPONSES
IF THE PATIENT DOES NOT WANT TO TALK	
The nurse new to this situation may feel rejected or ineffectual.	At first, the nurse might say something to this effect: "It's all right. I would like to spend time with you. We don't have to talk." The nurse might spend short, frequent periods (e.g., 5 minutes) with the patient throughout the day: "Our 5 minutes is up. I'll be back at 10 am and stay with you 5 more minutes." This gives the patient the opportunity to understand that the nurse means what he or she says and is back on time consistently. It also gives the patient time between visits to assess how he or she feels, what he or she thinks about the nurse, and perhaps to feel less threatened.
IF THE PATIENT GIVES THE NURSE A PRESENT	
The nurse may feel uncomfortable when offered a gift. The meaning needs to be examined. Is the gift (1) a way of getting better care, (2) a way to maintain self-esteem, (3) a way of making the nurse feel guilty, (4) a sincere expression of thanks, or (5) a cultural expectation?	Possible guidelines: If the gift is expensive, the only policy is to graciously refuse. If it is inexpensive, then (1) if it is given at the end of hospitalization when a relationship has developed, graciously accept; (2) if it is given at the beginning of the relationship, graciously refuse and explore the meaning behind the present:"Thank you, but it is our job to care for our patients. Are you concerned that some aspect of your care will be overlooked?" If the gift is money, it is always graciously refused.
IF ANOTHER PATIENT INTERRUPTS DURING TIME WITH YOUR CURRENT PATIENT	
The nurse may feel a conflict. The nurse does not want to appear rude. Sometimes the nurse tries to engage both patients in conversation.	The time the nurse had contracted with a selected patient is that patient's time. By keeping his or her part of the contract, the nurse demonstrates that the nurse means what he or she says and views the sessions as important: "I am with Mr. Rob for the next 20 minutes. At 10 AM, after our time is up, I can talk to you for 5 minutes."

go into a patient's room alone, know whether there are any patients not to engage, stay where others are around in an open area, and know the signs and symptoms of escalating anxiety.

There are actions a nurse can take if a patient's anger begins to escalate, many of which are presented in Table 8-4. Chapter 27 offers a more detailed discussion of maintaining personal safety, recognizing potential agitation, and intervening with angry or aggressive patients. You should always trust your own instincts. If you feel uncomfortable for any reason, excuse yourself for a moment, and discuss your feelings with your instructor or a staff member. In addition to getting reassurance and support, students can often provide valuable information about the patient's condition by sharing these perceptions.

Orientation Phase

The orientation phase can last for a few meetings or extend over a longer period. It is the first time the nurse and the patient meet and is the phase in which the nurse conducts the initial interview (refer to Chapter 9). When strangers meet, they interact according to their own backgrounds, standards, values, and experiences. The fact that each person has a unique frame of reference underlies the need for self-awareness on the part of the nurse. The initial interview includes the following aspects:

- An atmosphere is established in which rapport can grow.
- The nurse's role is clarified, and the responsibilities of both the patient and the nurse (parameters) are defined.
- The contract containing the time, place, date, and duration of the meetings is discussed.
- Confidentiality is discussed and assumed.
- The terms of termination are introduced (these are also discussed throughout the orientation phase and beyond).
- The nurse becomes aware of transference and countertransference issues.
- Patient problems are articulated, and mutually agreed-upon goals are established.

Establishing Rapport

A major emphasis during the first few encounters with the patient is on providing an atmosphere in which trust and understanding, or rapport, can grow. As in any relationship, rapport can be nurtured by demonstrating genuineness and empathy, developing positive regard, showing consistency, and offering assistance in problem solving and providing support.

TABLE 8-4 GUIDELINES FOR MAINTAINING SAFETY WHEN A PATIENT'S ANGER ESCALATES

NURSING INTERVENTION	RATIONALE
Pay attention to angry and aggressive behavior. Respond as early as possible.	Minimization of angry behaviors and ineffective limit setting are the most frequent factors contributing to the escalation of violence.
Assess for and provide for personal safety. Pay attention to the environment: Leave door open or use hallway. Choose a quiet place that is visible to staff. Have a quick exit available. The more angry the patient, the more space he/she will need to feel comfortable. Never turn your back on an angry patient. Leave immediately if there are signs behavior is escalating out of control or if you are uncomfortable. State, "I am leaving now, I will be back in 10 minutes," and seek out your clinical instructor or other staff member right away.	Exercising basic caution is essential to protecting yourself. Although the risk for violence may be minimal, it is easier to prevent a problem than to get out of a bad situation. These precautions are similar to using universal precautions (gloves, masks, gowns, etc.) on medical floors.
Appear calm and in control.	The perception that someone is in control can be comforting and calming to an individual whose anxiety is beginning to escalate.
Speak softly in a nonprovocative, nonjudgmental manner	When tone of voice is low and calm and the words are spoken slowly, anxiety levels in others may decrease.
Demonstrate genuineness and concern.	Even the most psychotic individual with schizophrenia may respond to nonprovocative interpersonal contact and expressions of concern and caring.
If patient is willing, both nurse and patient should sit at a 45-degree angle. Do not tower over or stare at the patient.	Sitting at a 45-degree angle puts you both on the same level but allows for frequent breaks in eye contact. Avoid towering over or staring at a patient, which can be interpreted as threatening or controlling by paranoid individuals.
When patient begins to talk, listen. Use clarification.	Allows patient to feel heard and understood, helps build rapport, and energy can be channeled productively.

Parameters of the Relationship

The patient needs to know about the nurse (who the nurse is and the nurse's background) and the purpose of the meetings. For example, a student might furnish the following information:

> **Student**: "Hello, Mrs. Chang, I am Jacob Thompson from the community college. I am in my psychiatric rotation and will be coming here for the next six Thursdays. I would like to spend time with you each Thursday if you are still here. I'm here to be a support person for you as you work on your treatment goals."

Formal or Informal Contract

A contract emphasizes the patient's participation and responsibility because it shows that the nurse does something *with* the patient rather than *for* the patient. The **contract**, either stated or written, contains the place, time, date, and duration of the meetings. During the orientation phase, the patient may begin to express thoughts and feelings, identify problems, and discuss realistic goals. Mutual agreement on those goals is also part of the contract.

> **Student**: "Mrs. Chang, we will meet at 10 AM each Thursday in the consultation room at the clinic for 45 minutes from September 15 to October 27. We can use that time for further discussion of your feelings of loneliness and anger and explore some things you could do to make the situation better for yourself."

Confidentiality

The patient has a right to know (1) who else will be given the information shared with the nurse and (2) that the information may be shared with specific people, such as a clinical supervisor, the physician, the staff, or other students in conference. The patient also needs to know that the information will not be shared with relatives, friends, or others outside the treatment team, except in extreme situations. Extreme situations include (1) child or elder abuse, (2) threats of self-harm or harm to others, or (3) intention not to follow through with the treatment plan.

If information must be shared with others, this is usually done by the physician, according to legal guidelines (refer to Chapter 6). The nurse must be aware of the patient's right to confidentiality and must not violate that right. Safeguarding the privacy and confidentiality of patients is not only an ethical obligation but a legal responsibility as well (Erickson & Miller, 2005).

> **Student**: "Mrs. Chang, I will be sharing some of what we discuss with my nursing instructor, and at times I may discuss certain concerns with my peers in conference or with the staff. However, I will *not* be sharing this information with your husband or any other members of your family or anyone outside the hospital without your permission."

Terms of Termination

Termination is that last phase in Peplau's model, but planning for termination actually begins in the orientation phase. It also may be mentioned when appropriate during the working phase if the nature of the relationship is time limited (e.g., six or nine sessions). The date of the termination phase should be clear from the beginning. In some situations, the nurse-patient contract may be renegotiated when the termination date has been reached. In other situations, when the therapeutic nurse-patient relationship is an open-ended one, the termination date is not known.

Student: "Mrs. Chang, as I mentioned earlier, our last meeting will be on October 27. We will have three more meetings after today."

Working Phase

The development of a strong working relationship can allow the patient to experience increased levels of anxiety and demonstrate dysfunctional behaviors in a safe setting while trying out new and more adaptive coping behaviors. Specific tasks of the **working phase** of the nurse-patient relationship are to:

- Maintain the relationship.
- Share information.
- Gather further data.
- Promote the patient's problem-solving skills, self-esteem, and use of language.
- Facilitate behavioral change.
- Evaluate progress.
- Support the practice and expression of alternative adaptive behaviors.

During the working phase, the nurse and patient together identify and explore areas that are causing problems in the patient's life. Often, the patient's present ways of handling situations stem from earlier means of coping devised to survive in a chaotic and dysfunctional family environment. Although certain coping methods may have worked for the patient at an earlier age, they now interfere with the patient's interpersonal relationships and prevent attainment of current goals. The patient's dysfunctional behaviors and basic assumptions about the world are often defensive, and the patient is usually unable to change the dysfunctional behavior at will. Therefore, most of the problem behaviors or thoughts continue because of unconscious motivations and needs that are beyond the patient's awareness.

The nurse can work with the patient to identify unconscious motivations and assumptions that keep the patient from finding satisfaction and reaching potential. Describing, and often reexperiencing, old conflicts generally awakens high levels of anxiety. Patients may use various defenses against anxiety and displace their feelings onto the nurse; therefore, during the working phase, intense emotions such as anxiety, anger, self-hate, hopelessness, and helplessness may surface. Defense mechanisms, such as acting out on anger inappropriately, withdrawing, intellectualizing, manipulating, and denying are to be expected.

During the working phase, the patient may unconsciously transfer strong feelings that belong to significant others from the past into the present and onto the nurse (transference). The emotional responses and behaviors in the patient may also awaken strong countertransference feelings in the nurse. The nurse's awareness of personal feelings and reactions to the patient are vital for effective interaction with the patient.

Termination Phase

The **termination phase** is the final, integral phase of the nurse-patient relationship. Termination is discussed during the first interview and again during the working stage at appropriate times. Termination may occur when the patient is discharged or when the student's clinical rotation ends. Basically, the tasks of termination include the following:

- Summarizing the goals and objectives achieved in the relationship
- Discussing ways for the patient to incorporate into daily life any new coping strategies learned
- Reviewing situations that occurred during the nurse-patient relationship
- Exchanging memories, which can help validate the experience for both nurse and patient and facilitate closure of that relationship

Termination can stimulate strong feelings in both nurse and patient. Termination of the relationship signifies a loss for both although the intensity and meaning of termination may be different for each. If a patient has unresolved feelings of abandonment, loneliness, being unwanted, or rejection, these feelings may be reawakened during the termination process. This process can be an opportunity for the patient to express these feelings, perhaps for the first time.

Important reasons for the student or nurse to address the termination phase include the following:

- Feelings are aroused in both the patient and the nurse with regard to the experience they have had; when these feelings are recognized and shared, patients learn that it is acceptable to feel sadness and loss when someone they care about leaves.
- Termination can be a learning experience; patients can learn that they are important to at least one person, and nurses learn continually from each clinical experience and patient encounter.
- By sharing the termination experience with the patient, the nurse demonstrates caring for the patient.
- This may be the first successful termination experience for the patient.

If a nurse has been working with a patient for a while, it is important for the nurse to recognize that separation may be difficult for the patient. A general question—such as "How do you feel about being discharged?"—may provide the opening necessary for the patient to describe feelings associated with the termination of the relationship. Both new practitioners and students in the psychiatric setting need to give serious thought to their last clinical experience with a patient and work with their supervisors or instructors to facilitate communication during this time.

A common response of beginning practitioners and students is feeling guilty about terminating the relationship. These feelings may, in rare cases, be manifested by the student's giving the patient his or her telephone number, making plans to get together for coffee after the patient is discharged, continuing to see the patient afterward, or exchanging letters. Maintaining contact after discharge is not acceptable and is in opposition to the goals of a therapeutic relationship. Often this is in response to the student's need to (1) feel less guilty for "using the patient for learning needs," (2) maintain a feeling of being "important" to the patient, or (3) sustain the illusion that the student is the only one who "understands" the patient, among other student-centered rationales.

Indeed, part of the termination process may be to explore—after discussion with the patient's case manager—the patient's plans for the future: where the patient can go for help, which agencies to contact, and which people may best help the patient find appropriate and helpful resources.

WHAT HINDERS AND WHAT HELPS THE NURSE-PATIENT RELATIONSHIP

Not all nurse-patient relationships follow the classic phases outlined by Peplau. Some start in the orientation phase and move to a mutually frustrating phase and finally to mutual withdrawal (Figure 8-2).

Forchuk and associates (2000) conducted a qualitative study of the nurse-patient relationship. They examined the phases of both therapeutic and nontherapeutic relationships. From this study, they identified certain behaviors that were beneficial to the progression of the nurse-patient relationship as well as those that hampered the development of this relationship. The study emphasized the importance of consistent, regular, and private interactions with patients as essential to the development of a therapeutic relationship. Nurses in this study stressed the importance of consistency, pacing, and listening. Specifically, the study found evidence that the following factors enhanced the nurse-patient relationship, allowing it to progress in a mutually satisfying manner:

- **Consistency** includes ensuring that a nurse is always assigned to the same patient and that the patient has a regular routine for activities. Interactions are facilitated when they are frequent and regular in duration, format, and location. Consistency also refers to the nurse's being honest and consistent (congruent) in what is said to the patient.
- **Pacing** includes letting the patient set the pace and letting the pace be adjusted to fit the patient's moods. A slow approach helps reduce pressure, and at times it is necessary to step back and realize that developing a strong relationship may take a long time.
- **Listening** includes letting the patient talk when needed. The nurse becomes a sounding board for the patient's concerns and issues. **Listening is perhaps the most important skill for nurses to master.** Truly listening to another person (i.e., attending to what is behind the words) is a learned skill.
- **Initial impressions**, especially positive initial attitudes and preconceptions, are significant considerations in how the relationship will progress. Preconceived negative impressions and feelings toward the patient usually bode poorly for the positive growth of the relationship. In contrast, the nurse's feeling that the patient is "interesting" or a "challenge" and a positive attitude about the relationship are usually favorable signs for the developing therapeutic relationship.
- **Promoting patient comfort** and **balancing control** usually reflect caring behaviors. *Control* refers to keeping a balance in the relationship: not too strict and not too lenient.
- **Patient factors** that seem to enhance the relationship include **trust** on the part of the patient and the patient's **active participation** in the nurse-patient relationship.

In relationships that did not progress to therapeutic levels, there seemed to be two major factors that hampered the development of positive relationships: inconsistency and unavailability (e.g., lack of contact, infrequent meetings, meetings in the hallway) on the part of the nurse, patient, or both. When nurse and patient are reluctant to spend time together and when meeting times become sporadic or superficial, the term *mutual avoidance* is used. This is clearly a lose-lose situation.

The nurse's personal feelings and lack of self-awareness are major elements that contribute to the lack of progression of positive relationships. Negative preconceived ideas and feelings (e.g., discomfort, dislike, fear, and avoidance) about the patient seem to be a constant in relationships that end in frustration and mutual withdrawal. Sometimes these feelings are known, and sometimes the nurse is only vaguely aware of them.

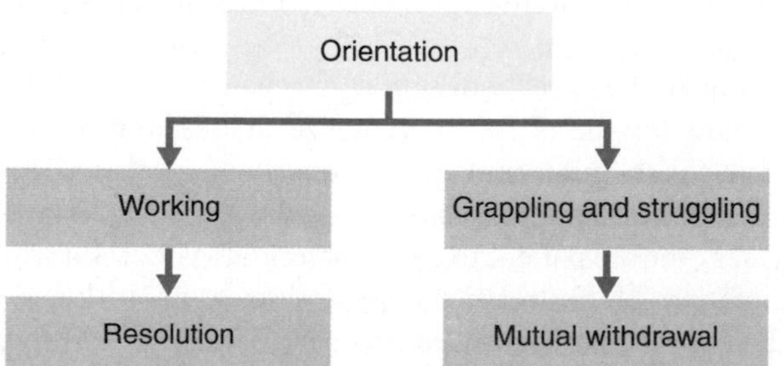

FIG 8-2 Phases of therapeutic and nontherapeutic relationships. (From Forchuk, C., Westwell, J., Martin, M., Bamber-Azzapardi, W., Kosterewa-Tolman, D., & Hux, M. [2000]. The developing nurse-client relationship: Nurses' perspectives. *Journal of the American Psychiatric Nurses Association, 6*[1], 3–10.)

FACTORS THAT ENCOURAGE AND PROMOTE PATIENTS' GROWTH

Rogers and Truax (1967) identified three personal characteristics of the nurse that help promote change and growth in patients—factors still valued today as vital components for establishing a therapeutic relationship: (1) genuineness, (2) empathy, and (3) positive regard. These are some of the intangibles that are at the heart of the art of nursing and patient-centered care.

Genuineness

Genuineness, or self-awareness of one's feelings as they arise within the relationship and the ability to communicate them when appropriate, is a key ingredient in building trust. When a person is genuine, one gets the sense that what is displayed on the outside of the person is congruent with the internal processes. Nurses convey genuineness by listening to and communicating clearly with patients. Being genuine in a therapeutic relationship implies the ability to use therapeutic communication tools in an appropriately spontaneous manner, rather than rigidly or in a parrot like fashion.

Empathy

Empathy is a complex multidimensional concept in which the helping person attempts to understand the world from the patient's perspective. It does not mean that the nurse condones or approves of the patient's actions but rather is nonjudgmental or uncritical of the patient's choices (Arkowitz et al., 2008). Essentially it means "temporarily living in the other's life, moving about in it delicately without making judgments" (Rogers, 1980, p. 142). Ward and colleagues (2012) define empathy as a cognitive rather than emotional skill "that includes the ability to understand a patient's experience and communicate in a manner that conveys recognition of patient concerns and perspectives."

Ward and colleagues (2012) state that empathy has been found to be consistent with improved patient outcomes and increased patient satisfaction with care. In a study of 214 undergraduate nursing students who had previously earned a degree in another discipline, the cohort group of nurses over a year's time demonstrated more a lack of empathy rather than an increase in empathy. These findings seem to be consistent with those of medical students as they progress through years of school.

Can empathy be taught? With increased use of simulation-based education, learners can "practice necessary skills in an environment that allows for error and professional growth without risking patient safety" (Galloway, 2009). Chaffin (2010) demonstrated that simulated exercises may help students increase their range and depth of understanding another's experience. Chaffin's study proposes a demonstration with the use of simulation to help develop empathy in nursing students during the psychiatric rotation. Students were asked to listen with headphones to a CD that simulated the voices heard by a person with schizophrenia while the students' lab partners were performing a mental status exam on them. The study's findings were that students experience:

- Annoyance
- Distraction
- Frustration
- Sometimes anger
- Fatigue
- Desire for simple quiet
- Overwhelming desire to stop the CD

The result of this experiment over a four-semester period created a paradigm shift among those students who participated in the lab. The clinical experience after the lab found students were:

- Choosing more patients in 1:1 interactions
- More willing to wait for patients to answer
- Desired a therapeutic relationship with patient
- More understanding
- More focused
- More caring

Can the use of clinical simulation provide more depth in understanding and a more lasting impression of patient experience? Future surveys and studies will attempt to bear this out. For all the pros and cons of clinical simulation in nursing education, it seems by many to be a profound adjunct to interactive teaching and a more engaging way for many students to learn.

Empathy Versus Sympathy

There is much confusion regarding empathy versus sympathy. A simple way to distinguish them is that in empathy, we *understand* the feelings of others, and in sympathy, we *feel* the feelings of others. When a helping person is feeling sympathy for another, objectivity is lost, and the ability to assist the patient in solving a personal problem ceases; furthermore, sympathy is associated with feelings of pity and commiseration. Although these are considered nurturing human traits, they may not be particularly useful in a therapeutic relationship. When people express sympathy, they express agreement with another, which in some situations may discourage further exploration of a person's thoughts and feelings.

The following examples are given to clarify the distinction between empathy and sympathy. A friend tells you that her mother was just diagnosed with inoperable cancer. Your friend then begins to cry and pounds the table with her fist.

> **Sympathetic response**: "I feel so sorry for you. I know exactly how you feel. My mother was hospitalized last year, and it was awful. I was so depressed. I still get upset just thinking about it." *(You go on to tell your friend about the incident.)*

Sometimes when nurses try to be sympathetic, they are apt to project their own feelings onto the patient's, which thus limits the patient's range of responses. A more useful response might be as follows:

> **Empathetic response**: "How upsetting this must be for you. Something similar happened to my mother last year, and I had so many mixed emotions. What thoughts and feelings are you having?" *(You continue to stay with your friend and listen to his or her thoughts and feelings.)*

Empathy is not a technique but rather an attitude that conveys respect, acceptance, and validation of the patient's strengths. In the practice of psychotherapy or counseling, empathy is one of the most important factors in building a trusting and therapeutic relationship (Wheeler, 2008).

Positive Regard

Positive regard implies respect. It is the ability to view another person as being worthy of caring about and as someone who has strengths and achievement potential. Positive regard is usually communicated indirectly by attitudes and actions rather than directly by words.

Attitudes

One attitude that might convey positive regard, or respect, is willingness to work with the patient. That is, the nurse takes the patient and the relationship seriously. The experience is viewed not as "a job," "part of a course," or "time spent talking" but as an opportunity to work with patients to help them develop personal resources and actualize more of their potential in living.

Actions

Some actions that manifest an attitude of respect are attending, suspending value judgments, and helping patients develop their own resources.

Attending. Attending behavior is the foundation of interviewing. To succeed, nurses must pay attention to their patients in culturally and individually appropriate ways. *Attending* is a special kind of listening that refers to an intensity of presence, or being with the patient. At times, simply being with another person during a painful time can make a difference.

Posture, eye contact, and body language are nonverbal behaviors that reflect the degree of attending and are highly culturally influenced. Refer to Chapter 9 for a more detailed discussion of the cultural implications of the clinical interview.

Suspending Value Judgments. Although we will always have personal opinions, nurses are more effective when they guard against using their own value systems to judge patients' thoughts, feelings, or behaviors. For example, if a patient is taking drugs or is involved in risky sexual behavior, the nurse may recognize that these behaviors are hindering the patient from living a more satisfying life, posing a potential health threat, or preventing the patient from developing satisfying relationships; however, labeling these activities as bad or good is not useful. Rather, the nurse should focus on exploring the behavior and work toward identifying the thoughts and feelings that influence this behavior. Judgment on the part of the nurse will most likely interfere with further exploration.

The first steps in eliminating judgmental thinking and behaviors are to (1) recognize their presence, (2) identify how or where you learned these responses to the patient's behavior, and (3) construct alternative ways to view the patient's thinking and behavior. Denying judgmental thinking will only compound the problem.

Patient: "I guess you could consider me an addictive personality. I love to gamble when I have money and spend most of my time in the casino. It seems like I'm hooking up with a different woman every time I'm there, and it always ends in sex. This has been going on for at least 3 years."

A judgmental response would be:

Nurse A: "So your compulsive gambling and promiscuous sexual behaviors really haven't brought you much happiness, have they? You're running away from your problems and could end up with AIDS and broke."

A more helpful response would be:

Nurse B: "So your sexual and gambling activities are part of the picture also. You sound as if these activities are not making you happy."

In this example, Nurse B focuses on the patient's behaviors and the possible meaning they might have to the patient. Nurse B does not introduce personal value statements or prejudices regarding promiscuous behavior, as does Nurse A. Empathy and positive regard are essential qualities in a successful nurse-patient relationship.

Helping Patients Develop Resources. The nurse becomes aware of patients' strengths and encourages patients to work at their optimal level of functioning. It can be seen as one form of collaboration with the patient. The nurse does not act for patients unless absolutely necessary and then only as a step toward helping them act on their own. It is important that patients remain as independent as possible to develop new resources for problem solving. The following are examples of helping the patient to develop independence:

Patient: "This medication makes my mouth so dry. Could you get me something to drink?"

Nurse: "There is juice in the refrigerator. I'll wait here for you until you get back" *or* "I'll walk with you while you get some juice from the refrigerator."

Patient: "Could you ask the doctor to let me have a pass for the weekend?"

Nurse: "Your doctor will be on the unit this afternoon. I'll let her know that you want to speak with her."

Consistently encouraging patients to use their own resources helps minimize the patients' feelings of helplessness and dependency and validates their potential for change.

KEY POINTS TO REMEMBER

- The nurse-patient relationship is well defined, and the roles of the nurse and the patient must be clearly stated.
- It is important that the nurse be aware of the differences between a therapeutic relationship and a social or intimate relationship. In a therapeutic nurse-patient relationship, the focus is on the patient's needs, thoughts, feelings, and goals. The nurse is expected to meet personal needs outside this relationship in other professional, social, or intimate arenas.
- Although the boundaries and roles of the nurse-patient relationship generally are clearly defined, they can become blurred; this blurring can be insidious and may occur on an unconscious level. Usually, transference and countertransference phenomena are operating when boundaries are blurred.
- It is important to have a grasp of common countertransference feelings and behaviors and of the nursing actions to counteract these phenomena.
- Supervision aids in promoting both the professional growth of the nurse and the nurse-patient relationship, allowing the patient's goals to be worked on and met.
- The phases of the nurse-patient relationship include orientation, working, and termination.
- Genuineness, empathy, and positive regard are personal strengths of the helping person; they foster growth and change in others.

CRITICAL THINKING

1. On your first clinical day, you are assigned to work with an older adult, Mrs. Schneider, who is depressed. Your first impression is, "Oh, my, she looks like my nasty Aunt Elaine. She even dresses like her." You approach her with a vague feeling of uneasiness and say, "Hello, Mrs. Schneider. My name is Alisha. I am a nursing student, and I will be working with you today." She tells you that "a student" could never understand what she is going through. She then says, "If you really want to help me, you would help me get me a good job after I leave here."
   - **a.** Identify transference and countertransference issues in this situation. What is your most important course of action?
   - **b.** What other information will you give Mrs. Schneider during this first clinical encounter? Be specific.
   - **c.** What are some useful responses you could give Mrs. Schneider regarding her concern about whether you could understand what she was going through?
   - **d.** Analyze Mrs. Schneider's request that you help her find a job. Keeping in mind the aim of Peplau's interactive nurse-patient process, describe some useful ways you could respond to this request.
2. You are interviewing Tom Stone, a 17-year-old who was admitted to a psychiatric unit after a suicide attempt. How would you best respond to each of the following patient requests and behaviors?
   - **a.** "I would feel so much better if you would sit closer to me and hold my hand."
   - **b.** "I will tell you if I still feel like killing myself, but you have to promise not to tell anyone else. If you do, I just can't trust you, ever."
   - **c.** "I don't want to talk to you. I have absolutely nothing to say."
   - **d.** "I will be going home tomorrow, and you have been so helpful and good to me. I want you to have my watch to remember me by."
   - **e.** Tom breaks down and starts sobbing.

CHAPTER REVIEW

1. Which of the following actions best represents the basis or foundation of all other psychiatric nursing care?
   - **a.** The nurse assesses the patient at regular intervals.
   - **b.** The nurse administers psychotropic medications.
   - **c.** The nurse spends time sitting with a withdrawn patient.
   - **d.** The nurse participates in team meetings with other professionals.
2. A male patient frequently inquires about the female student nurse's boyfriend, social activities, and school experiences. Which of the following initial responses by the student best addresses the issue raised by this behavior?
   - **a.** The student requests assignment to a patient of the same gender as the student.
   - **b.** She limits sharing personal information and stresses the patient-centered focus of the conversation.
   - **c.** She tells him that she will not talk about her personal life.
   - **d.** She explains that if he persists in focusing on her, she cannot work with him.
3. Amanda was raised by a rejecting and abusive father and had a difficult childhood. As an inpatient, she frequently comments on how hard her nurse, Jane, works and on how other staff members do not seem to care as much about their patients as Jane does. Jane finds herself agreeing with Amanda. Jane appreciates her insightfulness, and realizes that the other staff members do not appreciate how hard she works and take her for granted. Jane enjoys the time she spends with Amanda and seeks out opportunities to interact with her. What phenomenon is occurring here, and which response by Jane would most benefit her and the patient?
   - **a.** Amanda is experiencing transference; Jane should help Amanda to understand that she is emphasizing in Jane those qualities that were missing in her father.
   - **b.** Jane is idealizing Amanda, seeing in her strengths and abilities that Amanda does not possess; Jane should temporarily distance herself somewhat from Amanda.
   - **c.** Amanda is overidentifying with Jane, seeing similarities that do not in reality exist; Jane should label and explore this phenomenon in her interactions with Amanda.
   - **d.** Jane is experiencing countertransference in response to Amanda's meeting Jane's needs for greater appreciation; Jane should seek clinical supervision to explore these dynamics.
4. A student nurse exhibits the following behaviors or actions while interacting with her patient. Which of these are appropriate as part of a therapeutic relationship?
   - **a.** Sitting attentively in silence with a withdrawn patient until the patient chooses to speak.
   - **b.** Offering the patient advice on how he could cope more effectively with stress.
   - **c.** Controlling the pace of the relationship by selecting topics for each interaction.
   - **d.** Limiting the discussion of termination issues so as not to sadden the patient unduly.
5. Emily is a 28-year-old nurse on the psychiatric unit. She has been working with Jenna, a 27-year-old who was admitted with depression. Emily and Jenna find they have much in common, including each having a 2-year-old daughter and each having graduated from the same high school. Emily and Jenna discuss getting together for lunch with their daughters after Jenna is discharged. This situation reflects:
   - **a.** Successful termination
   - **b.** Promoting interdependence
   - **c.** Boundary blurring
   - **d.** A strong therapeutic relationship

Answers to Chapter Review

1. a; 2. b; 3. a; 4. a; 5. c.

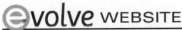
WEBSITE

Visit the Evolve website for a posttest on the content in this chapter: http://evolve.elsevier.com/Varcarolis

Post-Test interactive review

REFERENCES

Arkowitz, H., Westra, H. A., Miller, W. R., & Rollnick, R. (2008). *Motivational interviewing in the treatment of psychosocial problems*. New York, NY: Guilford Press.

Butler Center for Research. (2006). *Therapeutic alliance: Improving treatment outcome. Research update*. Hazelden Foundation. Retrieved from www.hazelden.org/web/public/bcrup1006.pdf.

Chaffin, A.J. (2010). *Use of a psychiatric nursing skills lab simulation to develop empathy in nursing students*. Retrieved from http://www.cinhc.org/wordpress/wp-content/uploads/2009/09/23-Use-of-a-Psychiatric-Nursing-Chaffin.pdf.

Erickson, J. I., & Miller, S. (2005). Caring for patients while respecting their privacy: Renewing our commitment. *Online Journal of Issues in Nursing, 10*(2). Retrieved from http://www.nursingworld.org/MainMenuCategories/ANAMarketplace/ANAPeriodicals/OJIN/TableofContents/Volume102005/No2May05/tpc27_116017.aspx.

Fontes, L. A. (2008). *Interviewing clients across cultures*. New York, NY: Guilford Press.

Forchuk, C., Westwell, J., Martin, M., Bamber-Azzapardi, W., Kosterewa-Tolman, D., & Hux, M. (2000). The developing nurse-client relationship: Nurse's perspectives. *Journal of the American Psychiatric Nurses Association, 6*(1), 3–10.

Fox, S. (2008). *Relating to clients*. Philadelphia, PA: Kingsley.

Galloway, S. (2009). *Simulation techniques to bridge the gap between novice and competent health care professionals*. Retrieved from http://nursingworld.org/MainMenuCategories/ANAMarketplace/ANAPeriodicals/OJIN/TableofContents/Vol142009/No2May09/Simulation-Techniques.html.

Gordon, C., Phillips, M., & Bereson, E. V. (2010). The doctor-patient relationship. In T. A. Stern, G. L. Fricchione, N. H. Cassen, M. S. Jellinek, & J. F. Rosenbaum (Eds.), *Massachusetts General Hospital handbook of general hospital psychiatry* (6th ed., pp. 15–24). Philadelphia, PA: Saunders.

Hollon, S. D., & Ponniah, K. (2010). A review of empirically supported psychological therapies for mood disorders in adults. *Depression and Anxiety, 27*(10), 891–932.

Institute for Patient- and Family-Centered Care. (2010). *Frequently asked questions*. Retrieved from http://www.ipfcc.org/faq.html.

Kopta, S. M., Saunders, S. M., Lueger, R. L., & Howard, K. I. (1999). Individual psychotherapy outcome and process research: Challenge leading to great turmoil or positive transition? *Annual Review of Psychology, 50*, 441–469.

Korn, M. L. (2001). *Cultural aspects of the psychotherapeutic process*. Retrieved from http://doctor.medscape.com/viewarticle/418608.

Peplau, H. E. (1952). *Interpersonal relations in nursing: A conceptual frame of reference for psychodynamic nursing*. New York, NY: Putnam.

Peplau, H. E. (1999). *Interpersonal relations in nursing: A conceptual frame of reference for psychodynamic nursing*. New York, NY: Springer.

Rogers, C. R. (1980). *A way of being*. Boston, MA: Houghton Mifflin.

Rogers, C. R., & Truax, C. B. (1967). The therapeutic conditions antecedent to change: A theoretical view. In C. R. Rogers (Ed.), *The therapeutic relationship and its impact*. Madison, WI: University of Wisconsin Press.

Serfaty, M. A., Haworth, D., Blanchard, M., Buszewicz, M., Murad, S., & King, M. (2009). Clinical effectiveness of individual cognitive behavioral therapy for depressed older people in primary care: A randomized controlled trial. *Archives of General Psychiatry, 66*(12), 1332–1340.

Travelbee, J. (1971). *Interpersonal aspects of nursing* (2nd ed.). Philadelphia, PA: F. A. Davis.

Ward, J., Cody, J., Schaal, M., & Hojat, M. (2012). The empathy enigma: An empirical study of decline in empathy among undergraduate nursing students. *Journal of Professional Nursing, 28*, 34–40.

Wheeler, K. (2008). *Psychotherapy for the advanced practice psychiatric nurse*. St. Louis, MO: Mosby.

CHAPTER

9

Communication and the Clinical Interview

Elizabeth M. Varcarolis

evolve WEBSITE

Visit the Evolve website for a pretest on the content in this chapter: http://evolve.elsevier.com/Varcarolis

Pre-Test interactive review

OBJECTIVES

1. Describe the communication process.
2. Identify three personal and two environmental factors that can impede communication.
3. Discuss the differences between verbal and nonverbal communication.
4. Identify two attending behaviors the nurse might focus on to increase communication skills.
5. Compare and contrast the range of verbal and nonverbal communication of different cultural groups in the areas of (a) communication style, (b) eye contact, and (c) touch. Give examples.
6. Relate problems that can arise when nurses are insensitive to cultural aspects of patients' communication styles.
7. Demonstrate the use of four techniques that can *enhance* communication, highlighting what makes them *effective*.
8. Demonstrate the use of four techniques that can *obstruct* communication, highlighting what makes them *ineffective*.
9. Identify and give rationales for suggested (a) setting, (b) seating, and (c) methods for beginning the nurse-patient interaction.
10. Explain to a classmate the importance of clinical supervision.

KEY TERMS AND CONCEPTS

- active listening
- closed-ended questions
- cultural filters
- double messages
- double-bind messages
- feedback
- nontherapeutic communication techniques
- nonverbal behaviors
- nonverbal communication
- open-ended questions
- patient-centered
- therapeutic communication techniques
- verbal communication

Humans have a built-in need to relate to others, and our advanced ability to communicate with others gives substance and meaning to our lives. Our need to express ourselves to others is powerful; it is the foundation on which we form happy and productive relationships in our adult lives. By the same token, stress and negative feelings within a relationship are often the result of ineffective communication. All our actions, words, and facial expressions convey meaning to others. It has been said that we cannot *not* communicate. Even silence can convey acceptance, anger, or thoughtfulness.

In the provision of nursing care, communication takes on a new emphasis. Just as social relationships are different from therapeutic relationships, *basic communication* is different from professional, patient-centered, goal-directed, and scientifically based *therapeutic communication.*

The ability to form patient-centered therapeutic relationships/partnerships is fundamental and essential to effective nursing care. Patient-centered refers to the patient as a full partner in his care whose values, preferences, and needs are respected (Quality and Safety Education, 2012). Therapeutic communication is crucial to the formation of patient-centered therapeutic relationships. Determining levels of pain in the postoperative patient, listening as parents express feelings of fear concerning their child's diagnosis, or understanding, without words, the needs of the intubated patient in the intensive care unit are essential skills in providing quality nursing care.

Ideally, therapeutic communication is a professional skill you learn and practice early in your nursing curriculum. But in psychiatric mental health nursing, communication skills take on a different and new emphasis. Psychiatric disorders cause not only physical symptoms (e.g., fatigue, loss of appetite, insomnia) but also emotional symptoms (e.g., sadness, anger, hopelessness, euphoria) that affect a patient's ability to relate to others.

It is often during the psychiatric rotation that students discover the utility of therapeutic communication and begin to rely on techniques they once considered artificial. For example, restating may seem like a funny thing to do. Using it in a practice session between students ("I felt sad when my dog ran away." "You felt sad when your dog ran away?") can derail communication and end the seriousness with laughter. Yet in the clinical setting, restating can become a powerful and profound tool:

Patient: "At the moment they told me my daughter would never be able to walk like her twin sister, I felt like I couldn't go on."

Student: *(after a short silence)* "You felt like you couldn't go on."

The technique, and the empathy it conveys, is appreciated in such a situation. Developing therapeutic communication skills takes time, and with continued practice, you will develop your own style and rhythm. Eventually, these techniques will become a part of the way you instinctively communicate with others in the clinical setting.

Novice psychiatric practitioners are often concerned that they may say the wrong thing, especially when learning to apply therapeutic techniques. Will you say the wrong thing? Yes, you probably will, but that is how we all learn to find more useful and effective ways of helping individuals reach their goals. The challenge is to recover from your mistakes and use them for learning and growth (Sommers-Flanagan & Sommers-Flanagan, 2013).

One of the most common concerns students have is that they will say the one thing that will "push the patient over the edge" or maybe cause the patient to give up all hope. This is highly unlikely. Consider that symptoms of psychiatric disorders, such as irritability, agitation, negativity, disinterest in communication, or hypertalkativeness, often frustrate and alienate friends and family. It is likely that the interactions the patient had been having were not always pleasant and supportive. Patients often see a well-meaning person who conveys genuine acceptance, respect, and concern for their well-being as a gift. Even if mistakes in communication are made or when the "wrong thing" is said, there is little chance that the comments will do actual harm.

THE COMMUNICATION PROCESS

Communication is an interactive process between two or more persons who send and receive messages to one another. The following is a simplified model of communication (Berlo, 1960):

1. One person has a need to communicate with another (stimulus) for information, comfort, or advice.
2. The person sending the message (sender) initiates interpersonal contact.
3. The message is the information sent or expressed to another. The clearest messages are those that are well-organized and expressed in a manner familiar to the receiver.
4. The message can be sent through a variety of media, including auditory (hearing), visual (seeing), tactile (touch), olfactory (smell), or any combination of these.
5. The person receiving the message (receiver) then interprets the message and responds to the sender by providing **feedback**.

Validating the accuracy of the sender's message is extremely important. The nature of the feedback often indicates whether the receiver has correctly interpreted the meaning of the message sent. An accuracy check may be obtained by simply asking the sender, "Is this what you mean?" or "I notice you turn away when we talk about your going back to college. Is there a conflict there?"

Figure 9-1 shows this simple model of communication, along with some of the many factors that affect it.

Effective communication in therapeutic relationships depends on nurses' (1) knowing what they are trying to convey (the purpose of the message), (2) communicating what is really meant to the patient, and (3) comprehending the meaning of what the patient is intentionally or unintentionally conveying (Arnold & Boggs, 2011). Peplau (1952) identified two main principles that can guide the communication process during the nurse-patient interview, which is discussed in detail later in this chapter: (1) clarity, which ensures that the meaning of the message is accurately understood by both parties "as the result of joint and sustained effort of all parties concerned," and (2) continuity, which promotes connections among ideas "and the feelings, events, or themes conveyed in those ideas" (p. 290).

FACTORS THAT AFFECT COMMUNICATION

Personal Factors

Personal factors that can impede accurate transmission or interpretation of messages include emotional factors (e.g., mood, responses to stress, personal bias), social factors (e.g., previous experience, cultural differences, language differences), and cognitive factors (e.g., problem-solving ability, knowledge level, language use).

Environmental Factors

Environmental factors that may affect communication include physical factors (e.g., background noise, lack of privacy, uncomfortable accommodations) and societal determinants (e.g., the presence of others; expectations of others; sociopolitical, historical, and economic factors).

Relationship Factors

Relationship factors refer to the status of individuals in terms of social standing, power, relationship type, age, etc. Communication is influenced by this status. Consider how you would describe your day in the clinical setting to your instructor, compared to how you would describe it to your friend. The fact that your instructor has more education than you and is in an

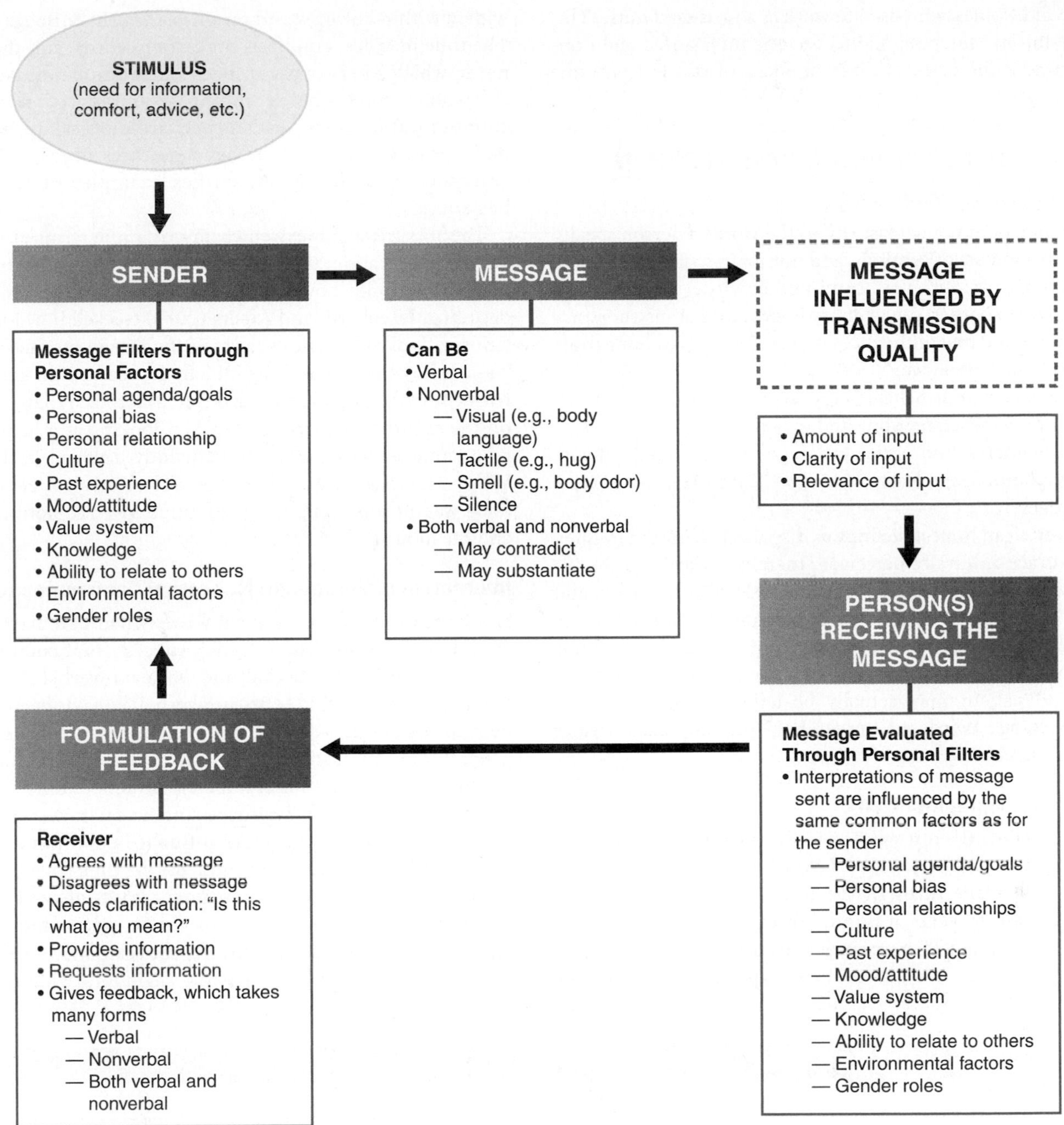

FIG 9-1 Operational Definition of Communication. (Data from Ellis, R., & McClintock, A. [1990]. *If you take my meaning*. London: Arnold.)

evaluative role would likely influence how much you share and your choice of words.

Now think about the relationship between you and your patient. Your patient may be older or younger than you are, more or less educated, richer or poorer, successful at work or unemployed. These factors play into the dynamics of the communication, whether at a conscious or an unconscious level, and recognizing their influence is important. It may be difficult for you to work with a woman your mother's age, or you may feel impatient with a patient who is unemployed and an alcoholic.

It is sometimes difficult for students to grasp or remember that patients, regardless of their relationship factors, are in a position of vulnerability. The presence of a hospital identification band is a formal indication of a need for care, and as a caregiver, you are viewed in a role of authority. Part of the art of therapeutic communication is in finding a balance between your role as a professional and your role as a human being who has been socialized into complex patterns of interactions based, at least in part, on status.

Students sometimes fall back into time-tested and comfortable roles. One of the most common responses nursing students have is in treating the patient as a buddy. Imagine a male nursing student walking onto the unit, seeing his assigned patient, and saying, "Hey, how's it going today?" while giving the patient a high-five. Or consider the female nursing student assigned to the

60-year-old woman who used to work as a registered nurse. This relationship has the potential to become unbalanced and nontherapeutic if the patient shifts the focus of concern onto the student.

VERBAL AND NONVERBAL COMMUNICATION

Verbal Communication

Verbal communication consists of all the words a person speaks. We live in a society of symbols, and our main social symbols are words. Talking is our most common activity. It is our public link with one another, the primary instrument of instruction, a need, an art, and one of the most personal aspects of our private lives. When we speak, we:

- Communicate our beliefs and values
- Communicate perceptions and meanings
- Convey interest and understanding *or* insult and judgment
- Convey messages clearly *or* convey conflicting or implied messages
- Convey clear, honest feelings *or* disguised, distorted feelings

Words are culturally perceived; therefore, clarifying the intent of certain words is very important. Even if the nurse and patient have a similar cultural background, the mental image that each has for a given word may not be exactly the same. Although they believe they are talking about the same thing, the nurse and patient may actually be talking about two quite different things. Words are the symbols for emotions as well as mental images.

Nonverbal Communication

It is often said, "It's not what you say but how you say it." In other words, it is the nonverbal behaviors that may be sending the "real" message through the tone or pitch of the voice. It is important to keep in mind, however, that culture influences the pitch and the tone a person uses. For example, the tone and pitch of a voice used to express anger can vary widely within cultures and families (Arnold & Boggs, 2011). The tone of voice, emphasis on certain words, and the manner in which a person paces speech are examples of nonverbal communication. Other common examples of nonverbal communication (often called *cues*) are physical appearance, body posture, eye contact, hand gestures, sighs, fidgeting, and yawning. Table 9-1 identifies examples of nonverbal behaviors.

Facial expression is extremely important in terms of nonverbal communication; the eyes and the mouth seem to hold the biggest clues into how people are feeling through emotional decoding. Eisenbarth and Alpers (2011) tracked how long participants looked at various parts of the face in response to different emotions. Participants initially focused on the eyes more frequently when looking at a sad face, and they initially focused on the mouth more frequently when looking at a happy face. Like sadness, anger was more frequently decoded in the eyes. When presented with either a fearful or neutral expression, there was an equal amount of attention given to both the eyes and the mouth.

Interaction of Verbal and Nonverbal Communication

Shawn Shea (1998), a nationally renowned psychiatrist and communication workshop leader, suggests that communication is roughly 10% verbal and 90% nonverbal. The high percentage he attributes to nonverbal behaviors may best describe our understanding of feelings and attitudes and not general communication. After all, it would be difficult to watch a foreign film and completely understand its meaning based solely on body language and vocal tones; however, nonverbal behaviors and cues influence communication to a surprising degree. Communication thus involves two radically different but interdependent kinds of symbols.

Spoken words represent our public selves and can be straightforward or used to distort, conceal, deny, or disguise true feelings. Nonverbal behaviors include a wide range of

TABLE 9-1 NONVERBAL BEHAVIORS

BEHAVIOR	POSSIBLE NONVERBAL CUES	EXAMPLE
Body behaviors	Posture, body movements, gestures, gait	The patient is slumped in a chair, puts her face in her hands, and occasionally taps her right foot.
Facial expressions	Frowns, smiles, grimaces, raised eyebrows, pursed lips, licking of lips, tongue movements	The patient grimaces when speaking to the nurse; when alone, he smiles and giggles to himself.
Eye expression and gaze behavior	Lowering brows, intimidating gaze	The patient's eyes harden with suspicion
Voice-related behaviors	Tone, pitch, level, intensity, inflection, stuttering, pauses, silences, fluency	The patient talks in a loud sing-song voice.
Observable autonomic physiological responses	Increase in respirations, diaphoresis, pupil dilation, blushing, paleness	When the patient mentions discharge, she becomes pale, her respirations increase, and her face becomes diaphoretic.
Personal appearance	Grooming, dress, hygiene	The patient is dressed in a wrinkled shirt, his pants are stained, his socks are dirty, and he is unshaven.
Physical characteristics	Height, weight, physique, complexion	The patient is grossly overweight, and his muscles appear flabby.

human activities, from body movements to facial expressions to physical reactions to messages from others. How a person listens and uses silence and sense of touch may also convey important information about the private self that is not available from conversation alone, especially in consideration of cultural norms.

Some elements of nonverbal communication, such as facial expressions, seem to be inborn and are similar across cultures (Matsumoto, 2006; Matsumoto & Sung Hwang 2011). Some cultural groups (e.g., Japanese, Russians) may control their facial expressions in public while others (e.g., Americans) tend to be open with facial expressions. Gender also plays a role in facial expressions; men are more likely to hide surprise and fear while women control disgust, contempt, and anger.

Other types of nonverbal behaviors, such as how close people stand to each other when speaking, depend on cultural conventions. Some nonverbal communication is formalized and has specific meanings (e.g., the military salute, the Japanese bow).

Messages are not always simple; they can appear to be one thing when in fact they are another. Often persons have greater conscious awareness of their verbal messages than their nonverbal behaviors. The verbal message is sometimes referred to as the *content* of the message (what is said), and the nonverbal behavior is called the *process* of the message (nonverbal cues a person gives to substantiate or contradict the verbal message).

When the content is congruent with the process, the communication is more clearly understood and is considered healthy. For example, if a student says, "It's important that I get good grades in this class," that is *content.* If the student has bought the books, takes good notes, and has a study buddy, that is *process.* Therefore, the content and process are congruent and straightforward, and there is a "healthy" message. If, however, the verbal message is not reinforced or is in fact contradicted by the nonverbal behavior, the message is confusing. For example, if the student does not have the books, skips several classes, and does not study, that is *process.* Here the student is sending two different messages.

Messages are sent to create meaning but also can be used defensively to hide what is actually going on, create confusion, and attack relatedness (Ellis et al., 2003). Conflicting messages are known as **double messages** or *mixed messages.* One way a nurse can respond to verbal and nonverbal incongruity is to reflect and validate the patient's feelings. For example, the nurse could say, "You say you are upset you did not pass this semester, but I notice you look relaxed. What do you see as some of the pros and cons of not passing the course this semester?"

Bateson and colleagues (1956) coined the term **double-bind messages**. They are characterized by two or more mutually contradictory messages given by a person in power. Opting for either choice will result in displeasure of the person in power. Such messages may be a mix of content (what is said) and process (what is conveyed nonverbally) that has both nurturing and hurtful aspects. The following vignette gives an example.

VIGNETTE

A 21-year-old female who lives at home with her chronically ill mother wants to go out for an evening with her friends. She is told by her frail but not helpless mother: "Oh, go ahead, have fun. I'll just sit here by myself, and I can always call 911 if I don't feel well. You go ahead and have fun." The mother says this while looking sad, eyes downcast, slumped in her chair, and letting her cane drop to the floor.

The recipient of this double-bind message is caught inside contradictory statements, so she cannot decide what is right. If she goes, the implication is that she is being selfish by leaving her sick mother alone, but if she stays, the mother could say, "I told you to go have fun." If she does go, the chances are she will not have much fun, so the daughter is trapped in a no-win situation.

With experience, nurses become increasingly aware of patients' verbal and nonverbal communication. Nurses can compare patients' dialogue with their nonverbal behaviors to gain important clues about the real message. What individuals do may either express and reinforce or contradict what they say. So, as in the saying "actions speak louder than words," *actions* often reveal the true meaning of a person's intent, whether the intent is conscious or unconscious.

COMMUNICATION SKILLS FOR NURSES

Therapeutic Communication Techniques

Peplau emphasized the art of communication to highlight the importance of nursing interventions in facilitating achievement of quality patient care and quality of life (Haber, 2000). The nurse must establish and maintain a therapeutic relationship in which the patient will feel safe and hopeful that positive change is possible.

Once a therapeutic relationship is established, specific needs and problems can be identified, and the nurse can work with the patient on increasing problem-solving skills, learning new coping behaviors, and experiencing more appropriate and satisfying ways of relating to others. To do this, the nurse must have a sound knowledge of communication skills; therefore, nurses must become more aware of their own interpersonal methods, eliminating obstructive, nontherapeutic communication techniques and developing additional responses that maximize nurse-patient interactions and increase the use of helpful **therapeutic communication techniques**. Useful tools for nurses when communicating with their patients are (1) silence, (2) active listening, (3) clarifying techniques, and (4) questions.

Using Silence

Students and practicing nurses alike may find that when the flow of words stops, they become uncomfortable. They may rush to fill the void with "questions or chatter," thus cutting off potentially important thoughts and feelings the patient might be taking time to think about before articulating. Silence is not the absence of communication but a specific channel for transmitting and receiving messages; therefore, the practitioner needs to understand that silence is a significant means of influencing and being influenced by others.

Talking is a highly individualized practice. Some people find the telephone a nuisance whereas others believe they cannot live without their cell phones on their persons at all times. In the initial interview, patients may be reluctant to speak because of the newness of the situation, the fact that the nurse is a stranger, or feelings of distrust, self-consciousness, embarrassment, or shyness. The nurse must recognize and respect individual differences in styles and tempos of responding. People who are quiet, those who have a language barrier or speech impediment, older adults, and those who lack confidence in their ability to express themselves may communicate a need for support and encouragement through their silence.

Although there is no universal rule concerning how much silence is too much, silence has been said to be worthwhile only as long as it is serving some function and not frightening the patient. Knowing when to speak during the interview largely depends on the nurse's perception about what is being conveyed through the silence. Icy silence may be an expression of anger and hostility; being ignored or given "the silent treatment" is recognized as an insult and is a particularly hurtful form of communication.

Silence may provide meaningful moments of reflection for both participants and gives an opportunity to contemplate thoughtfully what has been said and felt, weigh alternatives, formulate new ideas, and gain a new perspective on the matter under discussion. If the nurse waits to speak and allows the patient to break the silence, the patient may share thoughts and feelings that would otherwise have been withheld. Nurses who feel compelled to fill every void with words often do so because of their own anxiety, self-consciousness, and embarrassment. When this occurs, the nurse's need for comfort has taken priority over the needs of the patient.

It is crucial to recognize that some psychiatric disorders, such as major depression and schizophrenia, and medications may cause an overall slowing of thought processes. This slowing may be so severe that it may seem like an eternity before the patient responds. Patience and gentle prompting (e.g., "You were saying that you would like to get a pass this weekend to visit your niece") can help patients gather their thoughts.

Conversely, silence is not always therapeutic. Prolonged and frequent silences by the nurse may hinder an interview that requires verbal articulation. Although a less-talkative nurse may be comfortable with silence, this mode of communication may make the patient feel like a fountain of information to be drained dry. Moreover, without feedback, patients have no way of knowing whether what they said was understood. Additionally, children and adolescents in particular tend to feel uncomfortable with silence.

Active Listening

People want more than just a physical presence in human communication. Most people want the other person to be there for them psychologically, socially, and emotionally. Active listening in the nurse-patient relationship includes the following aspects:

- Observing the patient's nonverbal behaviors
- Understanding and reflecting on the patient's verbal message
- Understanding the patient in the context of the social setting of the patient's life
- Detecting "false notes" (e.g., inconsistencies or things the patient says that need more clarification)
- Providing feedback about himself or herself of which the patient might not be aware

Sommers-Flanagan and Sommers-Flanagan (2013) advise students, as well as experienced clinicians, to learn to quiet themselves: "They need to rein in any natural urges to help, personal needs, and anxieties" (p. 5). Relaxation techniques may help some before an interview with the patient (e.g., closing one's eyes and breathing slowly for a few minutes or using mindfulness training/meditation). This usually results in more concentration on the patient and less distraction by personal worries or personal thoughts of what to say next.

Effective interviewers learn to become active listeners when the patient is talking as well as when the patient becomes silent. During active listening, nurses carefully note verbal and nonverbal patient responses and monitor their own nonverbal responses. Using silence effectively and learning to listen actively—to both the patient and your own thoughts and reactions—are key ingredients in effective communication. Both skills take time to develop but can be learned; you will become more proficient with guidance and practice.

Active listening helps strengthen the patient's ability to solve problems. By giving the patient undivided attention, the nurse communicates that the patient is not alone. This kind of intervention enhances self-esteem and encourages the patient to direct energy toward finding ways to deal with problems. Serving as a sounding board, the nurse listens as the patient tests thoughts by voicing them aloud. This form of interpersonal interaction often enables the patient to clarify thinking, link ideas, and tentatively decide what should be done and how best to do it.

Clarifying Techniques

Understanding depends on clear communication, which is aided by verifying the nurse's interpretation of the patient's messages. The nurse can request feedback on the accuracy of the message received from verbal and nonverbal cues. The use of clarifying techniques helps both participants identify major differences in their frame of reference, giving them the opportunity to correct misperceptions before they cause any serious misunderstandings. The patient who is asked to elaborate on or clarify vague or ambiguous messages needs to know that the purpose is to promote mutual understanding.

Paraphrasing. Paraphrasing is accomplished by restating in different (often fewer) words the basic content of a patient's message. Using simple, precise, and culturally relevant terms, the nurse may readily confirm interpretation of the patient's previous message before the interview proceeds. By prefacing statements with a phrase such as "I'm not sure I understand" or "In other words, you seem to be saying . . . ," the nurse helps the patient form a clearer perception of what may be a bewildering mass of details. After paraphrasing, the nurse must validate the accuracy of the restatement and its helpfulness to the discussion. The patient may confirm or deny the perceptions through nonverbal cues or by direct response to a question such as "Was I correct in saying . . . ?" As a result, the patient is made aware that the interviewer is actively involved in the search for understanding.

Restating. In restating, the nurse mirrors the patient's overt and covert messages, so the technique may be used to echo feeling as well as content. Restating differs from paraphrasing in that it involves repeating the same key words the patient has just spoken. If a patient remarks, "My life is empty . . . it has no meaning," additional information may be gained by restating, "Your life has no meaning?" The purpose of this technique is to explore more thoroughly subjects that may be significant; however, patients may interpret frequent and indiscriminate use of restating as inattention or disinterest.

It is easy to overuse this tool so that its application becomes mechanical. Parroting or mimicking what another has said may be perceived as poking fun at the person; therefore, the use of this nondirective approach can become a definite barrier to communication. To avoid overuse of restating, the nurse can combine restatements with direct questions that encourage descriptions: "What does your life lack?" "What kind of meaning is missing?" "Describe a day in your life that appears empty to you."

Reflecting. Reflection is a means of assisting patients to better understand their own thoughts and feelings. Reflecting may take the form of a question or a simple statement that conveys the nurse's observations of the patient when sensitive issues are being discussed. The nurse might then describe briefly to the patient the apparent meaning of the emotional tone of the patient's verbal and nonverbal behavior. For example, to reflect a patient's feelings about his or her life, a good beginning might be, "You sound as if you have had many disappointments."

When you share observations with a patient, it demonstrates acceptance and that the patient has your full attention. When you reflect, you make the patient aware of inner feelings and encourage the patient to own them. For example, you may say to a patient, "You look sad." Perceiving your concern may allow the patient to spontaneously share feelings. The use of a question in response to the patient's question is another reflective technique (Arnold & Boggs, 2007). For example:

Patient: "Nurse, do you think I really need to be hospitalized?"
Nurse: "What do you think, Kelly?"
Patient: "I don't know; that's why I'm asking you."
Nurse: "I'll be willing to share my impression with you at the end of this first session. However, you've probably thought about hospitalization and have some feelings about it. I wonder what they are."

Exploring. A technique that enables the nurse to examine important ideas, experiences, or relationships more fully is exploring. For example, if a patient tells you he does not get along well with his wife, you will want to further explore this area. Possible openers include the following:

"*Tell me more* about your relationship with your wife."
"*Describe* your relationship with your wife."
"*Give me an example* of how you and your wife don't get along."

Asking for an example can greatly clarify a vague or generic statement made by a patient.

Patient: "No one likes me."
Nurse: "Give me an example of one person who doesn't like you."
or
Patient: "Everything I do is wrong."
Nurse: "Give me an example of one thing you do that you think is wrong."

Table 9-2 lists more examples of therapeutic communication techniques.

Questions

Open-Ended Questions. Open-ended questions encourage patients to share information about experiences, perceptions, or responses to a situation. For example:

- "What do you perceive as your biggest problem right now?"
- "What is an example of some of the stresses you are under right now?"
- "How would you describe your relationship with your wife?"

Since open-ended questions are not intrusive and do not put the patient on the defensive, they help the clinician elicit information, especially in the beginning of an interview or when a patient is guarded or resistant to answering questions. They are particularly useful when establishing rapport with a person.

Closed-Ended Questions. Nurses are usually urged to ask open-ended questions to elicit more than a "yes" or "no" response; however, closed-ended questions, when used sparingly, can give you specific and needed information. Closed-ended questions are most useful during an initial assessment or intake interview or to ascertain results, as in "Are the medications helping you?" "When did you start hearing voices?" "Did you seek therapy after your first suicide attempt?" Care needs to be exercised with this technique. Frequent use of closed-ended questions during time spent with patients can close an interview down rapidly; this is especially true with guarded or resistant patients.

Projective Questions. Projective questions usually start with a "*what if*" to help people articulate, explore, and identify thoughts and feelings. They are surprisingly strong in their ability to think about problems differently and to identify priorities. Projective questions can also help people imagine thoughts, feelings, and behaviors they might have in certain situations (Sommers-Flanagan & Sommers-Flanagan, 2013):

- If you had three wishes, what would you wish for?
- What if you could go back and change how you acted in (X situation/significant life event); what would you do differently now?
- What would you do if you were given $1 million, no strings attached?

Presupposition Questions. Presupposition questions, also known as the miracle questions, are useful tools. Suppose you woke up in the morning and a miracle happened and this problem had gone away. What would be different? How would it change your life? These two questions can reveal a lot about a person that can be used in identifying goals that the patient may be motivated to pursue, and they often get to the crux of what might be the most important issues in a person's thinking/life.

TABLE 9-2 THERAPEUTIC COMMUNICATION TECHNIQUES

THERAPEUTIC TECHNIQUE	DESCRIPTION	EXAMPLE
Silence	Gives the person time to collect thoughts or think through a point.	Encouraging a person to talk by waiting for the answers.
Accepting	Indicates that the person has been understood. An accepting statement does not necessarily indicate agreement but is nonjudgmental.	"Yes." "Uh-huh." "I follow what you say."
Giving recognition	Indicates awareness of change and personal efforts. Does not imply good or bad, right or wrong.	"Good morning, Mr. James." "You've combed your hair today." "I see you've eaten your whole lunch."
Offering self	Offers presence, interest, and a desire to understand. Is not offered to get the person to talk or behave in a specific way.	"I would like to spend time with you." "I'll stay here and sit with you awhile."
Offering general leads	Allows the other person to take direction in the discussion. Indicates that the nurse is interested in what comes next.	"Go on." "And then?" "Tell me about it."
Giving broad openings	Clarifies that the lead is to be taken by the patient. However, the nurse discourages pleasantries and small talk.	"Where would you like to begin?" "What are you thinking about?" "What would you like to discuss?"
Placing the events in time or sequence	Puts events and actions in better perspective. Notes cause-and-effect relationships and identifies patterns of interpersonal difficulties.	"What happened before?" "When did this happen?"
Making observations	Calls attention to the person's behavior (e.g., trembling, nail biting, restless mannerisms). Encourages patient to notice the behavior and describe thoughts and feelings for mutual understanding. Helpful with mute and withdrawn people.	"You appear tense." "I notice you're biting your lips." "You appear nervous whenever John enters the room."
Encouraging description of perception	Increases the nurse's understanding of the patient's perceptions. Talking about feelings and difficulties can lessen the need to act them out inappropriately.	"What do these voices seem to be saying?" "What is happening now?" "Tell me when you feel anxious."
Encouraging comparison	Brings out recurring themes in experiences or interpersonal relationships. Helps the person clarify similarities and differences.	"Has this ever happened before?" "Is this how you felt when . . .?" "Was it something like . . .?"
Restating	Repeats the main idea expressed. Gives the patient an idea of what has been communicated. If the message has been misunderstood, the patient can clarify it.	*Patient:* "I can't sleep. I stay awake all night." *Nurse:* "You have difficulty sleeping?" or *Patient:* "I don't know . . . he always has some excuse for not coming over or keeping our appointments." *Nurse:* "You think he no longer wants to see you?"
Reflecting	Directs questions, feelings, and ideas back to the patient. Encourages the patient to accept his or her own ideas and feelings. Acknowledges the patient's right to have opinions and make decisions and encourages the patient to think of self as a capable person.	*Patient:* "What should I do about my husband's affair?" *Nurse:* "What do you think you should do?" *or* *Patient:* "My brother spends all of my money and then has the nerve to ask for more." *Nurse:* "You feel angry when this happens?"
Focusing	Concentrates attention on a single point. It is especially useful when the patient jumps from topic to topic. If a person is experiencing a severe or panic level of anxiety, the nurse should not persist until the anxiety lessens.	"This point you are making about leaving school seems worth looking at more closely." "You've mentioned many things. Let's go back to your thinking of 'ending it all.'"
Exploring	Examines certain ideas, experiences, or relationships more fully. If the patient chooses not to elaborate by answering no, the nurse does not probe or pry. In such a case, the nurse respects the patient's wishes.	"Tell me more about that." "Would you describe it more fully?" "Could you talk about how it was that you learned your mom was dying of cancer?"

TABLE 9-2 THERAPEUTIC COMMUNICATION TECHNIQUES—cont'd

THERAPEUTIC TECHNIQUE	DESCRIPTION	EXAMPLE
Giving information	Makes facts the person needs available. Supplies knowledge from which decisions can be made or conclusions drawn. For example, the patient needs to know the role of the nurse, the purpose of the nurse-patient relationship, and the time, place, and duration of the meetings.	"My purpose for being here is . . ." "This medication is for . . ." "The test will determine . . ."
Seeking clarification	Helps patients clarify their own thoughts and maximize mutual understanding between nurse and patient.	"I am not sure I follow you." "What would you say is the main point of what you just said?" "Give an example of a time you thought everyone hated you."
Presenting reality	Indicates what is real. The nurse does not argue or try to convince the patient, just describes personal perceptions or facts in the situation.	"That was Dr. Todd, not a man from the Mafia." "That was the sound of a car backfiring." "Your mother is not here; I am a nurse."
Voicing doubt	Undermines the patient's beliefs by not reinforcing the exaggerated or false perceptions.	"Isn't that unusual?" "Really?" "That's hard to believe."
Seeking consensual validation	Clarifies that both the nurse and patient share mutual understanding of communications. Helps the patient become clearer about what he or she is thinking.	"Tell me whether my understanding agrees with yours."
Verbalizing the implied	Puts into concrete terms what the patient implies, making the patient's communication more explicit.	*Patient:* "I can't talk to you or anyone else. It's a waste of time." *Nurse:* "Do you feel that no one understands?"
Encouraging evaluation	Aids the patient in considering other persons and events from the perspective of the patient's own set of values.	"How do you feel about . . .?" "What did it mean to you when he said he couldn't stay?"
Attempting to translate into feelings	Responds to the feelings expressed, not just the content. Often termed *decoding*.	*Patient:* "I am dead inside." *Nurse:* "Are you saying that you feel lifeless? Does life seem meaningless to you?"
Suggesting collaboration	Emphasizes working with the patient, not doing things for the patient. Encourages the view that change is possible through collaboration.	"Perhaps you and I can discover what produces your anxiety." "Perhaps by working together, we can come up with some ideas that might improve your communications with your spouse."
Summarizing	Brings together important points of discussion to enhance understanding. Also allows the opportunity to clarify communications so that both nurse and patient leave the interview with the same ideas in mind.	"Have I got this straight?" "You said that . . ." "During the past hour, you and I have discussed . . ."
Encouraging formulation of a plan of action	Allows the patient to identify alternative actions for interpersonal situations the patient finds disturbing (e.g., when anger or anxiety is provoked).	"What could you do to let anger out harmlessly?" "The next time this comes up, what might you do to handle it?" "What are some other ways you can approach your boss?"

Adapted from Hays, J. S., & Larson, K. (1963). *Interacting with patients.* New York, NY: Macmillan. Copyright © 1963 by Macmillan Publishing Company.

Nontherapeutic Communication Techniques

Although people may use "nontherapeutic" or ineffective communication techniques in their daily lives, they can cause problems for nurses because they tend to impede or shut down nurse-patient interaction. Table 9-3 describes **nontherapeutic communication techniques** and suggests more helpful responses.

Excessive Questioning

Excessive questioning—asking multiple questions (particularly closed-ended) consecutively or rapidly—casts the nurse in the role of interrogator who demands information without respect for the patient's willingness or readiness to respond. This approach conveys a lack of respect for and sensitivity to the patient's

TABLE 9-3 NONTHERAPEUTIC COMMUNICATION TECHNIQUES

NONTHERAPEUTIC TECHNIQUE	DESCRIPTION	EXAMPLE	MORE HELPFUL RESPONSE
Giving premature advice	Assumes the nurse knows best and the patient can't think for self. Inhibits problem solving and fosters dependency.	"Get out of this situation immediately."	**Encouraging problem solving**: "What are the pros and cons of your situation?" "What were some of the actions you thought you might take?" "What are some of the ways you have thought of to meet your goals?"
Minimizing feelings	Indicates that the nurse is unable to understand or empathize with the patient. Here the patient's feelings or experiences are being belittled, which can cause the patient to feel small or insignificant.	*Patient:* "I wish I were dead." *Nurse:* "Everyone gets down in the dumps." "I know what you mean." "You should feel happy you're getting better." "Things get worse before they get better."	**Empathizing and exploring**: "You must be feeling very upset. Are you thinking of hurting yourself?"
Falsely reassuring	Underrates a person's feelings and belittles a person's concerns. May cause the patient to stop sharing feelings if the patient thinks he or she will be ridiculed or not taken seriously.	"I wouldn't worry about that." "Everything will be all right." "You will do just fine, you'll see."	**Clarifying the patient's message:** "What specifically are you worried about?" "What do you think could go wrong?" "What are you concerned might happen?"
Making value judgments	Prevents problem solving. Can make the patient feel guilty, angry, misunderstood, not supported, or anxious to leave.	"How come you still smoke when your wife has lung cancer?"	**Making observations:** "I notice you are still smoking even though your wife has lung cancer. Is this a problem?"
Asking "why" questions	Implies criticism; often has the effect of making the patient feel defensive.	"Why did you stop taking your medication?"	**Asking open-ended questions; giving a broad opening:** "Tell me some of the reasons that led up to your not taking your medications."
Asking excessive questions	Results in the patient's not knowing which question to answer and possibly being confused about what is being asked.	*Nurse:* "How's your appetite? Are you losing weight? Are you eating enough?" *Patient:* "No."	**Clarifying:** "Tell me about your eating habits since you've been depressed."
Giving approval, agreeing	Implies the patient is doing the *right* thing—and that not doing it is wrong. May lead the patient to focus on pleasing the nurse or clinician; denies the patient the opportunity to change his or her mind or decision.	"I'm proud of you for applying for that job." "I agree with your decision."	**Making observations:** "I noticed that you applied for that job." "What factors will lead up to your changing your mind?" **Asking open-ended questions; giving a broad opening**: "What led to that decision?"
Disapproving, disagreeing	Can make a person defensive.	"You really should have shown up for the medication group." "I disagree with that."	**Exploring**: "What was going through your mind when you decided not to come to your medication group?" "That's one point of view. How did you arrive at that conclusion?"
Changing the subject	May invalidate the patient's feelings and needs. Can leave the patient feeling alienated and isolated and increase feelings of hopelessness.	*Patient:* "I'd like to die." *Nurse:* "Did you go to Alcoholics Anonymous like we discussed?"	**Validating and exploring:** *Patient:* "I'd like to die." *Nurse:* "This sounds serious. Have you thought of harming yourself?"

Adapted from Hays, J. S., & Larson, K. (1963). *Interacting with patients.* New York, NY: Macmillan.

needs. Excessive questioning controls the range and nature of the responses, can easily result in a therapeutic stall, or may completely shut down an interview. It is a controlling tactic and may reflect the interviewer's lack of security in letting the patient tell his or her own story. It is better to ask more open-ended questions and follow the patient's lead. For example:

Excessive questioning: "Why did you leave your wife? Did you feel angry with her? What did she do to you? Are you going back to her?"
More therapeutic approach: "Tell me about the situation between you and your wife."

Giving Approval or Disapproval

"You look great in that dress." "I'm proud of the way you controlled your temper at lunch." "That's a great quilt you made." What could be bad about giving someone a pat on the back once in a while? Nothing, if it is done without conveying a positive or negative judgment. We often give our friends and family approval when they do something well, but giving praise and approval becomes much more complex in a nurse-patient relationship.

A patient may be feeling overwhelmed, experiencing low self-esteem, feeling unsure of where his or her life is going, and desperate for recognition, approval, and attention. Yet when people are feeling vulnerable, a value comment might be misinterpreted. For example:

Giving approval: "You did a great job in group telling John just what you thought about how rudely he treated you."

This message implies that the nurse was pleased by the manner in which the patient talked to John. The patient then sees such a response as a way to please the nurse by doing the right thing. To continue to please the nurse (and get approval), the patient may continue the behavior. The behavior might be useful for the patient, but when a behavior is being done to please another person, it is not coming from the individual's own volition or conviction. Also, when the other person the patient needs to please is not around, the motivation for the new behavior might not be there either. Thus, the new response really is not a change in behavior as much as a ploy to win approval and acceptance from another.

Giving approval also cuts off further communication.

More therapeutic approach: "I noticed that you spoke up to John in group yesterday about his rude behavior. How did it feel to be more assertive?"

This opens the way for finding out if the patient was scared, was comfortable, wants to work more on assertiveness, etc. It also suggests that this was a self-choice the patient made. The patient is given recognition for the change in behavior, and the topic is also opened for further discussion.

Giving disapproval implies that the nurse has the right to judge the patient's thoughts or feelings. Again, an observation should be made instead.

Giving disapproval: "You really should not cheat, even if you think everyone else is doing it."
More therapeutic approach: "Can you give me two examples of how cheating could negatively affect your goal of graduating?"

Giving Advice

Although we ask for and give advice all the time in daily life, giving advice to a patient is rarely helpful. Often when we ask for advice, our real motive is to discover whether we are thinking along the same lines as someone else. When a nurse gives advice to a patient, the nurse is interfering with the patient's ability to make personal decisions. When a nurse offers the patient solutions, the patient eventually begins to think the nurse does not view him or her as capable of making effective decisions. People often feel inadequate when they are given no choices over decisions in their lives. Giving advice to patients also can foster dependency ("I'll have to ask the nurse what to do about . . .") and undermine the patient's sense of competence and adequacy.

However, people do need information to make informed decisions. Often you can help a patient define a problem and identify what information might be needed to come to an informed decision. A useful approach would be to ask, "What do you see as some possible actions you can take?" It is much more constructive to encourage problem solving by the patient. At times you might suggest several alternatives a patient might consider (e.g., "Have you ever thought of telling your friend about the incident?"). The patient is then free to give you a yes or no answer and make a decision from among the suggestions.

Asking "Why" Questions

Why demands an explanation and implies wrong doing. "Why did you come late?" "Why didn't you go to the funeral?" "Why didn't you study for the exam?" Such questions often imply criticism. We may ask our friends or family such questions, and in the context of a solid relationship, the *why* may be understood more as "What happened?" With people we do not know—especially those who may be anxious or overwhelmed—a *why* question from a person in authority (e.g., nurse, physician, and teacher) can be experienced as intrusive and judgmental, which serves only to make the person defensive.

It is much more useful to ask what is happening rather than why it is happening. Questions that focus on who, what, where, and when often elicit important information that can facilitate problem solving and further the communication process. See Table 9-3 for additional ineffective communication techniques as well as statements that would better facilitate interaction and patient comfort.

Cultural Considerations

The United States Census Bureau (2012) announced that for the first time in history, 50.4% of children under the age of 1 were minorities. Health care professionals need to be familiar with the cultural meaning of certain verbal and nonverbal communications. Cultural awareness in initial face-to-face encounters with a patient can lead to the formation of positive therapeutic alliances with members of a diverse society or lead to frustration and misunderstanding by both the nurse and the patient. Always assess the patient's ability to speak and understand English well and provide an interpreter when needed.

Unrecognized differences in cultural identities can result in assessment and interventions that are not optimally respectful of the patient and can be inadvertently biased or prejudiced. Health care workers need to have not only knowledge of various patients' cultures but also awareness of their own cultural identities. Especially important are nurses' attitudes and beliefs toward those from cultures other than their own because these will affect their relationships with patients (Kavanaugh, 2011). Four areas that may prove problematic for the nurse interpreting specific verbal and nonverbal messages of the patient include the following:

1. Communication style
2. Use of eye contact
3. Perception of touch
4. Cultural filters

Communication Style

People may communicate in an intense and highly emotional manner. Some may consider it normal to use dramatic body language when describing emotional problems, and others may perceive such behavior as being out of control or reflective of some degree of pathology. For example, within the Hispanic community, intensely emotional styles of communication often are culturally appropriate and expected (Kavanaugh, 2011). French and Italian Americans typically show animated facial expressions and expressive hand gestures during communication, which can be misinterpreted by others.

In other cultures, a calm facade may mask severe distress. For example, in many Asian cultures, expression of positive or negative emotions is a private affair, and open expression of them is considered to be in bad taste and possibly a weakness. A quiet smile by an Asian American may express joy, an apology, stoicism in the face of difficulty, or even anger (USDHHS, 2001). In general, Asian individuals exercise emotional restraint, and interpersonal conflicts are not directly addressed or even allowed (Arnold & Boggs, 2011). German and British Americans also tend to value highly the concept of self-control and may show little facial emotion in the presence of great distress or emotional turmoil.

Eye Contact

Fontes (2008) warns that the presence or absence of eye contact should not be used to assess attentiveness, judge truthfulness, or make assumptions on the degree of engagement one has with a patient. Cultural norms dictate a person's comfort or lack of comfort with direct eye contact. Some cultures consider direct eye contact disrespectful and improper. For example, Hispanic individuals have traditionally been taught to avoid eye contact with authority figures such as nurses, physicians, and other health care professionals. Avoidance of direct eye contact is seen as a sign of respect to those in authority, but it could be misinterpreted as disinterest or even as a lack of respect.

In Japan, direct eye contact is considered to show lack of respect and to be a personal affront; preference is for shifting or downcast eyes or focus on the speaker's neck. With many Chinese, gazing around and looking to one side when listening to another is considered polite; however, when speaking to an older adult, direct eye contact is used (Kavanaugh, 2011). Filipino Americans may try to avoid eye contact; however, once it is established, it is important to return and maintain eye contact. In some Middle Eastern cultures, for a woman to make direct eye contact with a man may imply a sexual interest or even promiscuity.

Many Native Americans also believe it is disrespectful or even a sign of aggression to engage in direct eye contact, especially if the speaker is younger. Direct eye contact by members of the dominant culture in the health care system can and does cause discomfort for some patients and is considered a sign of disrespect, while listening is considered a sign of respect and essential to learning about the other individual (Kalbfleisch, 2009; Kavanaugh, 2011).

On the other hand, among German Americans, direct and sustained eye contact indicates that the person listens or trusts, is somewhat aggressive, or, in some situations, is sexually interested. Russians also find direct, sustained eye contact the norm for social interactions (Giger, 2012). In Haiti, it is customary to hold eye contact with everyone but the poor (Kavanaugh, 2011; USDHHS, 2001). French, British, and many African Americans maintain eye contact during conversation; avoidance of eye contact by another person may be interpreted as being disinterested, not telling the truth, or avoiding the sharing of important information. In Greece, staring in public is acceptable (Kavanaugh, 2011).

Touch

The therapeutic use of touch is a basic aspect of the nurse-patient relationship and is generally considered a gesture of warmth and friendship; however, the degree to which a patient is comfortable with the use of touch is often culturally determined. People from some cultures, Hispanic for example, are accustomed to frequent physical contact. Holding a patient's hand in response to a distressing situation or giving the patient a reassuring pat on the shoulder may be experienced as supportive and thus help facilitate openness (Kavanaugh, 2011). People from Italian and French backgrounds may also be accustomed to frequent touching during conversation, and in the Russian culture, touch is an important part of nonverbal communication, used freely with intimate and close friends (Giger, 2012).

However, personal touch within the context of an interview may be perceived as an invasion of privacy or experienced as patronizing, intrusive, aggressive, or sexually inviting in other cultures. Among German, Swedish, and British Americans, touch practices are infrequent although a handshake may be common at the beginning and end of an interaction. Chinese Americans may not like to be touched by strangers.

Even among people from similar cultures, the use of touch has different interpretations and rules regarding gender and class. Students are urged to find out if their facility has a "no touch" policy, particularly with adolescents and children who have experienced inappropriate touch and may not know how to interpret therapeutic touch from the health care worker.

Cultural Filters

It is important to recognize that it is impossible to listen to people in an unbiased way. In the process of socialization, we develop **cultural filters** through which we listen to the world around us (Egan, 2009). Cultural filters are a form of cultural bias or cultural prejudice that determines what we pay attention to and what we ignore. Egan stated that we need these cultural filters to provide structure for our lives and help us interpret and interact with the world. These cultural filters, however, also unavoidably introduce various forms of bias into our communication, because they are bound to influence our personal, professional, familial, and sociological values and interpretations.

We all need a frame of reference to help us function in our world, but the trick is to understand that other peoples use many other frames of reference to help them function in their worlds. Acknowledging that everyone views the world differently and understanding that these various views impact each person's beliefs and behaviors can go a long way toward minimizing our personal distortions in listening. Building acceptance and understanding of cultural diversity is a skill that can be learned. Chapter 5 has a more in-depth discussion of cultural considerations in nursing.

TELEHEALTH THROUGH INFORMATION COMMUNICATION TECHNOLOGIES

E-health/e-medicine, telehealth technology has found widespread uses within the United States and is still evolving, but it has only recently been adopted for behavioral health and mental health care (Ryan, 2011). Telehealth is used as a live interactive mechanism, as a way to track clinical data and to provide access to people who otherwise might not receive good medical or psychosocial help. It is a valuable tool for consumers as well as practitioners to access current psychiatric and medical breakthroughs, diagnoses, and treatment options (Arnold & Boggs, 2011). As information communication technologies (ICTs) advance, it is possible that electronic house calls, Internet support groups, and virtual health examination may well be the wave of the future, eliminating office visits altogether (Arnold & Boggs, 2011; Kinsella, 2003).

Castelli (2010) states that, besides providing better health care for those in rural areas or for those who cannot travel, telehealth helps relieve the impending nursing shortage. Nursing schools are having a difficult time meeting the nursing shortage because of a decrease in financial resources and retiring faculty (Castelli, 2010). The use of telehealth/telehome care technologies allows nurses to monitor patients' vital signs, including lung sounds, and to identify changes in patients' physiological states. Clinicians can conduct remote physical assessment and consults, which are especially helpful in facilities that have limited nursing resources, including schools, prisons, health clinics, or rural hospitals (Castelli, 2010).

Essentially, "Telehealth is the use of electronic information and telecommunication technologies to support long-distance clinical health care, patient and professional health-related education, public health and health administration. Technologies include videoconferencing, the Internet, store-and-forward imaging, streaming media, and terrestrial and wireless communications" (USDHHS-HRSA, 2011). Ryan (2011) states that one in four adults could be diagnosed with a mental health issue. It could be anxiety, stress, marital issues, depression, or substance abuse. Most of these mental health issues are not addressed because of the fear of stigma, the scarcity of health care providers in remote areas, or problems with transportation (e.g., because of anxiety, physical limitations, or lack of transportation). The consequences of not seeking help can be significant. For example, consequences can range from problems at work to domestic violence, increased depression, and suicide—consequences that can result in a host of other ramifications (Joch, 2008).

The U.S. Department of Defense is particularly interested in implementing and expanding the use of these technologies because, according to Weckerlein (2011), up to 25% of service members screened positive for mental health concerns. These technologies can be used for telepsychiatric appointments ranging from treating posttraumatic stress disorder and depression to providing wellness and resiliency interventions, especially in rural areas (Weckerlein, 2011).

Because the practices of psychiatry, psychology, counseling, and nursing are based on human interaction, there still remains a need for "human to human sensitivity, acknowledgment, and respect for the patient care experience" (Malloch, 2010, p. 1).

Evaluation of Communication Skills

After you have had some introductory clinical experience, you may find the facilitative skills checklist in Figure 9-2 useful for evaluating your progress in developing interviewing skills. Note that some of the items might not be relevant for some of your patients (e.g., numbers 11 through 13 may not be possible when a patient is experiencing psychosis [disordered thought, delusions, and/or hallucinations]). Self-evaluation of clinical skills is a way to focus on therapeutic improvement. Role-playing can help prepare you for clinical experience and practice effective and professional communication skills.

THE CLINICAL INTERVIEW

Ideally, the content and direction of the clinical interview are decided and led by the patient. The nurse employs communication skills and active listening to better understand the patient's situation.

Preparing for the Interview

Pace

Helping a person with an emotional or medical problem is rarely a straightforward task, and the goal of assisting a patient to regain psychological or physiological stability can be difficult to achieve. Extremely important to any kind of counseling is permitting the patient to set the pace of the interview, no matter how slow or halting the progress may be (Arnold & Boggs, 2011).

FACILITATIVE SKILLS CHECKLIST

Instructions: Periodically during your clinical experience, use this checklist to identify areas where growth is needed and progress has been made. Think of your clinical client experiences. Indicate the extent of your agreement with each of the following statements by marking the scale: *SA,* strongly agree; *A,* agree; *NS,* not sure; *D,* disagree; *SD,* strongly disagree.

1. I maintain good eye contact.	SA	A	NS	D	SD
2. Most of my verbal comments follow the lead of the other person.	SA	A	NS	D	SD
3. I encourage others to talk about feelings.	SA	A	NS	D	SD
4. I am able to ask open-ended questions.	SA	A	NS	D	SD
5. I can restate and clarify a person's ideas.	SA	A	NS	D	SD
6. I can summarize in a few words the basic ideas of a long statement made by a person.	SA	A	NS	D	SD
7. I can make statements that reflect the person's feelings.	SA	A	NS	D	SD
8. I can share my feelings relevant to the discussion when appropriate to do so.	SA	A	NS	D	SD
9. I am able to give feedback.	SA	A	NS	D	SD
10. At least 75% or more of my responses help enhance and facilitate communication.	SA	A	NS	D	SD
11. I can assist the person to list some alternatives available.	SA	A	NS	D	SD
12. I can assist the person to identify some goals that are specific and observable.	SA	A	NS	D	SD
13. I can assist the person to specify at least one next step that might be taken toward the goal.	SA	A	NS	D	SD

FIG 9-2 Facilitative Skills Checklist. (Adapted from Myrick, D., & Erney, T. [2000]. *Caring and sharing* [2nd ed., p. 168]. Copyright © 2000 by Educational Media Corporation, Minneapolis, Minnesota.)

Setting

Effective communication can take place almost anywhere. However, the quality of the interaction—whether in a clinic, a clinical unit, an office, or the patient's home—depends on the degree to which the nurse and patient feel safe; establishing a setting that enhances feelings of security is important to the therapeutic relationship. A health care setting, a conference room, or a quiet part of the unit that has relative privacy but is within view of others is ideal, but when the interview takes place in the patient's home, it offers the nurse a valuable opportunity to assess the patient in the context of everyday life.

Seating

In all settings, chairs should be arranged so that conversation can take place in normal tones of voice and so that eye contact can be comfortably maintained or avoided. A nonthreatening physical environment for both nurse and patient would involve:

- Assuming the same height, either both sitting or both standing
- Avoiding a face-to-face stance when possible; a 90- to 120-degree angle or side-by-side position may be less intense, and patient and nurse can look away from each other without discomfort
- Providing safety and psychological comfort in terms of exiting the room. The patient should not be positioned between the nurse and the door, nor should the nurse be positioned in such a way that the patient feels trapped in the room.
- Avoiding a desk barrier between the nurse and the patient

Introductions

In the orientation phase, students tell the patient who they are, what the purpose of the meeting is, and how long and at what time they will be meeting with the patient. The issue of confidentiality is brought up during the initial interview. Remember that all health care professionals must respect the private, personal, and confidential nature of the patient's communication, except in the specific situations outlined earlier (e.g., harm to self or others, child abuse, elder abuse). What is discussed with staff and your clinical group in conference should not be discussed outside with others, no matter who they are (e.g., patient's relatives, news media, friends, etc.). The patient needs to know that whatever is discussed will stay confidential unless permission is given for it to be disclosed. Refer to Chapter 8 to review the nurse's responsibilities in the orientation phase.

Ask the patient how he or she would like to be addressed. This question conveys respect and gives the patient direct control over an important ego issue. (Some patients like to be called by their last names; others prefer being on a first-name basis with the nurse) (Arnold & Boggs, 2011).

Initiating the Interview

Once introductions have been made, you can turn the interview over to the patient by using one of a number of open-ended questions or statements:

- "Where should we start?"
- "Tell me a little about what has been going on with you."
- "What are some of the stresses you have been coping with recently?"
- "Tell me a little about what has been happening in the past couple of weeks."

- "Perhaps you can begin by letting me know what some of your concerns have been recently."
- "Tell me about your difficulties."

Communication can be facilitated by appropriately offering leads (e.g., "Go on"), making statements of acceptance (e.g., "Uh-huh"), or otherwise conveying interest.

Tactics to Avoid

Certain behaviors (Moscato, 1988) are counterproductive and should be avoided. For example:

DO NOT:	TRY TO:
Argue with, minimize, or challenge the patient.	Keep focus on facts and the patient's perceptions.
Give false reassurance.	Make observations of the patient's behavior: "Change is always possible."
Interpret to the patient or speculate on the dynamics.	Listen attentively, use silence, and try to clarify the patient's problem.
Question or probe patients about sensitive areas they do not wish to discuss.	Pay attention to nonverbal communication. Strive to keep the patient's anxiety to a minimum.
Try to sell the patient on accepting treatment.	Encourage the patient to look at pros and cons.
Join in attacks patients launch on their mates, parents, friends, or associates.	Focus on facts and the patient's perceptions. Be aware of nonverbal communication.
Participate in criticism of another nurse or any other staff member.	Focus on facts and the patient's perceptions. Check out serious accusations with the other nurse or staff member. Have the patient meet with the nurse or staff member in question in the presence of a senior staff member/clinician and clarify perceptions.

Helpful Guidelines

Classic guidelines for conducting the initial interview have been supplied by Meier and Davis (2001). In the interview:

- Speak briefly.
- When you do not know what to say, say nothing.
- When in doubt, focus on feelings.
- Avoid advice.
- Avoid relying on questions.
- Pay attention to nonverbal cues.
- Keep the focus on the patient.

Attending Behaviors: The Foundation of Interviewing

Engaging in attending behaviors and actively listening are two key principles of counseling on which almost everyone can agree (Sommers-Flanagan & Sommers-Flanagan, 2013). Positive attending behaviors serve to open up communication and encourage free expression whereas negative attending behaviors are more likely to inhibit expression. All behaviors must be evaluated in terms of cultural patterns and past experiences of both the interviewer and the interviewee. There are no universals; however, there are guidelines students can follow.

Eye Contact

As previously discussed, cultural and individual variations influence a patient's comfort with eye contact. For some patients and interviewers, sustained eye contact is normal and comfortable. For others, it may be more comfortable and natural to make brief eye contact but look away or down much of the time. A general rule of communication and eye contact is that it is appropriate for nurses to maintain more eye contact when the patient speaks and less constant eye contact when the nurse speaks.

Body Language

Body language involves two elements: kinesics and proxemics. *Kinesics* is associated with physical characteristics, such as body movements and postures. Facial expressions, eye contact or lack thereof, the way someone holds the head, legs, and shoulders, and so on convey a multitude of messages. A person who slumps in a chair, rolls the eyes, and sits with arms crossed in front of the chest can be perceived as resistant and unreceptive to what another wants to communicate. On the other hand, a person who leans in slightly toward the speaker, maintains a relaxed and attentive posture, makes appropriate eye contact, makes hand gestures that are unobtrusive and smooth while minimizing the number of other movements, and who matches facial expressions to personal feelings or to the patient's feelings can be perceived as open to and respectful of the communication.

Proxemics refers to the study of **personal space** and the significance of the physical distance between individuals. Proxemics takes into account that these distances may be different for different cultural groups. **Intimate distance** in the United States is 0 to 18 inches and is reserved for those we trust most and with whom we feel most safe. **Personal distance** (18 to 40 inches) is for personal communications such as those with friends or colleagues. **Social distance** (4 to 12 feet) applies to strangers or acquaintances, often in public places or formal social gatherings. **Public distance** (12 feet or more) relates to public space (e.g., public speaking). In public space, one may hail another, and the parties may move about while communicating.

Vocal Quality

Vocal quality, or paralinguistics, encompasses voice loudness, pitch, rate, and fluency. Sommers-Flanagan and Sommers-Flanagan (2013) report that vocal qualities can improve rapport, demonstrate empathy and interest, and add emphasis to words or concepts. Paralinguistics provides a perfect example of "It's not *what* you say, but *how* you say it." Speaking in soft and gentle tones is apt to encourage a person to share thoughts and feelings whereas speaking in a rapid, high-pitched tone may convey anxiety and create it in the patient. Consider, for example, how tonal quality can affect communication in a simple sentence like "I will see you tonight."

1. "*I* will see you tonight." (I will be the one who sees you tonight.)
2. "I *will* see you tonight." (No matter what happens, or whether you like it or not, I will see you tonight.)
3. "I will see *you* tonight." (Even though others are present, it is you I want to see.)
4. "I will see you *tonight*." (It is definite; tonight is the night we will meet.)

Clinical Supervision

Communication and interviewing techniques are acquired skills. You will learn to increase these abilities through practice and clinical supervision. In clinical supervision, the focus is on the nurse's behavior in the nurse-patient relationship; nurse and supervisor have opportunities to examine and analyze the nurse's feelings and reactions to the patient and the way they affect the relationship.

Farkas-Cameron (1995) observed that clinical supervision could be a therapeutic process for the nurse. During the process, feelings and concerns are ventilated as they relate to the developing nurse-patient relationship. The opportunity to examine interactions, obtain insights, and devise alternative strategies for dealing with various clinical issues enhances clinical growth and minimizes frustration and burnout. Clinical supervision is a necessary professional activity that fosters professional growth and helps minimize the development of nontherapeutic nurse-patient relationships.

Process Recordings

The best way to increase communication and interviewing skills is to review your clinical interactions exactly as they occur. This process offers the opportunity to identify themes and patterns in both your own and your patients' communications. As students, clinical review helps you learn to deal with the variety of situations that arise in the clinical interview.

Process recordings are written records of a segment of the nurse-patient session that reflect as closely as possible the verbal and nonverbal behaviors of both patient and nurse. Process recordings have some disadvantages because they rely on memory and are subject to distortions; however, they can be a useful tool for identifying communication patterns. Sometimes an observing clinician takes notes during the interview, but this practice also has disadvantages in that it may be distracting for both interviewer and patient. Some patients (especially those with a paranoid disorder) may resent or misunderstand the student's intent.

Although the use of process recordings is decreasing in many schools of nursing, they remain a useful tool for students and new clinicians to reflect on the interview, examine the process, and consider more appropriate responses, thereby improving communication skills.

Table 9-4 gives an example of a process recording.

TABLE 9-4 EXAMPLE OF A PROCESS RECORDING

NURSE	PATIENT	COMMUNICATION TECHNIQUE	STUDENT'S THOUGHTS AND FEELINGS
"Good morning, Mr. Long."		**Therapeutic.** Giving recognition. Acknowledging a patient by name can enhance self-esteem and communicates that the patient is viewed as an individual by the nurse.	I was feeling nervous. He had attempted suicide, and I didn't know if I could help him. Initially I was feeling somewhat overwhelmed.
	"Who are you, and where the devil am I?" Gazes around with a confused look on his face—quickly sits on the edge of the bed.		
"I am Ms. Rodriguez. I am a student nurse from the college, and you are at Mount Sinai Hospital. I would like to spend some time with you today."		**Therapeutic.** Giving information. Informing the patient of facts needed to make decisions or come to realistic conclusions. **Therapeutic.** Offering self. Making oneself available to the patient.	
	"What am I doing here? How did I get here?" (*Spoken in a loud, demanding voice.*)		I felt a bit intimidated when he raised his voice.

TABLE 9-4 EXAMPLE OF A PROCESS RECORDING—cont'd

NURSE	PATIENT	COMMUNICATION TECHNIQUE	STUDENT'S THOUGHTS AND FEELINGS
"You were brought in by your wife last night after swallowing a bottle of aspirin. You had to have your stomach pumped."		**Therapeutic.** Giving information. Giving needed facts so that the patient can orient himself and better evaluate his situation.	
	"Oh . . . yeah." Silence for 2 minutes. Shoulders slumped, Mr. Long stares at the floor and drops his head and eyes.		I was uncomfortable with the silence, but since I didn't have anything useful to say, I stayed with him in silence for the 2 minutes.
"You seem upset, Mr. Long. What are you thinking about?"		**Therapeutic.** Making observations. He looks sad. **Therapeutic.** Giving broad openings in an attempt to get at his feelings.	I began to feel sorry for him; he looked so sad and helpless.
	"Yeah, I just remembered. . . . I wanted to kill myself." *(Said in a low tone almost to himself.)*		
"Oh, Mr. Long, you have so much to live for. You have such a loving family."		**Nontherapeutic.** Defending. **Nontherapeutic.** Introducing an unrelated topic.	I felt overwhelmed. I didn't know what to say—his talking about killing himself made me nervous. I could have said, "You must be very upset" *(verbalizing the implied)* or "Tell me more about this" *(exploring).*
	"What do you know about my life? You want to know about my family? . . . My wife is leaving me, that's what." *(Faces the nurse with an angry expression on his face and speaks in loud tones.)*		Again, I felt intimidated by his anger, but now I linked it with his wife's leaving him, so I didn't take it as personally as I did the first time.
"I didn't know. You must be terribly upset by her leaving."		**Therapeutic.** Reflective. Observing the angry tone and content of the patient's message and reflecting back the patient's feelings.	I really felt for him, and now I thought that encouraging him to talk more about this could be useful for him.

KEY POINTS TO REMEMBER

- Knowledge of communication and interviewing techniques is the foundation for developing any nurse-patient relationship. Goal-directed professional communication is referred to as *therapeutic communication.*
- Communication is a complex process. Berlo's communication model has five parts: stimulus, sender, message, medium, and receiver. Feedback is a vital component of the communication process for validating the accuracy of the sender's message.
- A number of factors can minimize, enhance, or otherwise influence the communication process: culture, language, knowledge level, noise, lack of privacy, presence of others, and expectations.
- There are verbal and nonverbal elements in communication; the nonverbal elements often play the larger role in conveying a person's message. Verbal communication consists of all words a person speaks. Nonverbal communication consists of the behaviors displayed by an individual, in addition to the actual content of speech.
- Communication has two levels: the content level (verbal speech) and the process level (nonverbal behavior). When content is congruent with process, the communication is said to be *healthy*. When the verbal message is not reinforced by the communicator's actions, the message is ambiguous; we call this a *double (or mixed) message.*
- Cultural background (as well as individual differences) has a great deal to do with what nonverbal behavior means to different individuals. The degree of eye contact and the use of touch are two nonverbal behaviors that can be misunderstood by individuals of different cultures.
- There are a number of therapeutic communication techniques nurses can use to enhance their nursing practices.

- There are also a number of nontherapeutic communication techniques that nurses can learn to avoid to enhance their effectiveness with people.
- Most nurses are most effective when they use nonthreatening and open-ended communication techniques.
- Effective communication is a skill that develops over time and is integral to the establishment and maintenance of a therapeutic relationship.
- The clinical interview is a key component of psychiatric mental health nursing, and the nurse must establish a safe setting and plan for appropriate seating, introductions, and initiation of the interview.
- Attending behaviors (e.g., eye contact, body language, and vocal qualities) are key elements in effective communication.
- A meaningful therapeutic relationship is facilitated when values and cultural influences are considered. It is the nurse's responsibility to seek to understand the patient's perceptions.

CRITICAL THINKING

1. Keep a written log of a conversation you have with a patient. In your log, identify the therapeutic and nontherapeutic techniques you noticed yourself using. Rewrite the nontherapeutic communications and replace them with statements that would better facilitate discussion of thoughts and feelings. Share your log and discuss the changes you are working on with one classmate.
2. Role-play with a classmate at least five nonverbal communications and have your partner identify the message he or she was receiving.
3. With the other students in your class watching, plan and role-play a nurse-patient conversation that lasts about three minutes. Use both therapeutic and nontherapeutic techniques. When you are finished, have your other classmates try to identify the techniques that you used.
4. Demonstrate how the nurse would use touch and eye contact when working with patients from three different cultural groups.

CHAPTER REVIEW

1. You have been working closely with a patient for the past month. Today he tells you he is looking forward to meeting with his new psychiatrist but frowns and avoids eye contact while reporting this to you. Which of the following responses would most likely be therapeutic?
   - **a.** "A new psychiatrist is a chance to start fresh; I'm sure it will go well for you."
   - **b.** "You say you look forward to the meeting, but you appear anxious or unhappy."
   - **c.** "I notice that you frowned and avoided eye contact just now; don't you feel well?"
   - **d.** "I get the impression you don't really want to see your psychiatrist—can you tell me why?"
2. Which student behavior is consistent with therapeutic communication?
   - **a.** Offering your opinion when asked in order to convey support.
   - **b.** Summarizing the essence of the patient's comments in your own words.
   - **c.** Interrupting periods of silence before they become awkward for the patient.
   - **d.** Telling the patient he did well when you approve of his statements or actions.
3. Which statement about nonverbal behavior is accurate?
   - **a.** A calm expression means that the patient is experiencing low levels of anxiety.
   - **b.** Patients respond more consistently to therapeutic touch than to verbal interventions.
   - **c.** The meaning of nonverbal behaviors varies with cultural and individual differences.
   - **d.** Eye contact is a reliable measure of the patient's degree of attentiveness and engagement.
4. A nurse stops in to interview a patient on a medical unit and finds the patient lying supine in her bed with the head elevated at 10 degrees. Which initial response(s) would most enhance the chances of achieving a therapeutic interaction? *Select all that apply.*
   - **a.** Apologize for the differential in height and proceed while standing to avoid delay.
   - **b.** If permitted, raise the head of the bed and, with the patient's permission, sit on the bed.
   - **c.** If permitted, raise the head of the bed to approximate the nurse's height while standing.
   - **d.** Sit in whatever chair is available in the room to convey informality and increase comfort.
   - **e.** Locate a chair or stool that would place the nurse at approximately the level of the patient.
   - **f.** Remain standing and proceed so as not to create distraction by altering the arrangements.
5. James is a 42-year-old patient with schizophrenia. He approaches you as you arrive for day shift and anxiously reports, "Last night demons came to my room and tried to rape me." Which response would be most therapeutic?
   - **a.** "There are no such things as demons; what you saw were hallucinations."
   - **b.** "It is not possible for anyone to enter your room at night; you are safe here."
   - **c.** "You seem very upset; please tell me more about what you experienced last night."
   - **d.** "That must have been very frightening, but we'll check on you at night and you'll be safe."

Answers to Chapter Review

1. b; 2. b; 3. c; 4. e; 5. c.

evolve WEBSITE

Visit the Evolve website for a posttest on the content in this chapter: http://evolve.elsevier.com/Varcarolis

Post-Test interactive review

REFERENCES

Arnold, E. C., & Boggs, K. U. (2011). *Interpersonal relationships: Professional communication skills for nurses* (5th ed.). St. Louis, MO: Saunders.

Bateson, G., Jackson, D., & Haley, J. (1956). Toward a theory of schizophrenia. *Behavioral Sciences, 1*(4), 251–264.

Berlo, D. K. (1960). *The process of communication*. San Francisco, CA: Reinhart Press.

Egan, G. (2009). *The skilled helper: A systematic approach to effective helping* (9th ed.). Pacific Grove, CA: Brooks/Cole.

Eisenbarth, H., & Halpers, G. W. (2011). Happy mouth and sad eyes: Scanning emotional facial expressions. *Emotion, 11*(4), 860–865.

Ellis, R. B., Gates, B., & Kenworthy, N. (2003). *Interpersonal communication in nursing* (2nd ed.). London: Churchill Livingstone.

Farkas-Cameron, M. M. (1995). Clinical supervision in psychiatric nursing. *Journal of Psychosocial Nursing and Mental Health Services, 33*(2), 40–47.

Fontes, L. A. (2008). *Interviewing clients across cultures: A practitioner's guide*. New York, NY: Guilford.

Giger, J. N. (2012). *Transcultural nursing: Assessment and intervention* (6th ed.). St. Louis, MO: Mosby.

Haber, J. (2000). Hildegard E. Peplau: The psychiatric nursing legacy of a legend. *Journal of the American Psychiatric Nursing Association, 6*, 510–562.

Kavanaugh, K. H. (2011). Transcultural perspectives in mental health nursing. In M. M. Andrews, & J. S. Boyle (Eds.), *Transcultural concepts in nursing care* (pp. 226-261). Philadelphia, PA: Lippincott Williams & Wilkins.

Malloch, K. (2010). Innovation leadership: New perspectives for new work. *Nursing Clinics of North America, 45*(1), 1–9.

Matsumoto, D. (2006). Culture and nonverbal behavior. In V. L. Manusov, & M. L. Patterson, (Eds.), *The Sage handbook of nonverbal communication* (pp. 219–235). Newbury Park, CA: Sage.

Meier, S. T., & Davis, S. R. (2001). *The elements of counseling* (4th ed.). Pacific Grove, CA: Brooks/Cole.

Moscato, B. (1988). Psychiatric nursing. In H. S. Wilson, & C. S. Kneisel (Eds.), *The one-to-one relationship*. Menlo Park, CA: Addison-Wesley.

Peplau, H. E. (1952). *Interpersonal relations in nursing: A conceptual frame of reference for psychodynamic nursing*. New York, NY: Putnam.

Quality and Safety Education for Nurses. (2012). *Patient centered care*. Retrieved from http://www.qsen.org/definition.php?id=1.

Shea, S. C. (1998). *Psychiatric interviewing: The art of understanding* (2nd ed.). Philadelphia, PA: Saunders.

Sommers-Flanagan, J. & Sommers-Flanagan, R. (2013). *Clinical interviewing* (5th ed.). Hoboken, NJ: Wiley.

United States Census Bureau. (2012). *Most children younger than age 1 are minorities, Census Bureau reports*. Retrieved from http://www.census.gov/newsroom/releases/archives/population/cb12-90.html.

CHAPTER

10

Understanding and Managing Responses to Stress

Margaret Jordan Halter and Elizabeth M. Varcarolis

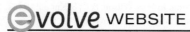

Visit the Evolve website for a pretest on the content in this chapter: http://evolve.elsevier.com/Varcarolis

Pre-Test interactive review

OBJECTIVES

1. Recognize the short- and long-term physiological consequences of stress.
2. Compare and contrast Cannon's (fight-or-flight), Selye's (general adaptation syndrome), and psychoneuroimmunological models of stress.
3. Describe how responses to stress are mediated through perception, personality, social support, culture, and spirituality.
4. Assess stress level using the Recent Life Changes Questionnaire.
5. Identify and describe holistic approaches to stress management.
6. Teach a classmate or patient a behavioral technique to help lower stress and anxiety.
7. Explain how cognitive techniques can help increase a person's tolerance for stressful events.

KEY TERMS AND CONCEPTS

biofeedback
cognitive reframing
coping styles
distress
eustress
fight-or-flight response
general adaptation syndrome (GAS)
guided imagery
humor
journaling
meditation
mindfulness
physical stressors
progressive muscle relaxation (PMR)
psychological stressors
psychoneuroimmunology
relaxation response
stressors

Before turning our attention to the clinical disorders presented in the chapters that follow, we will explore the subject of stress. Stress is natural, and humans have evolved with a capacity to respond to internal and external situations. A classic definition of stress is that it is a negative emotional experience that results in predictable biochemical, physiological, cognitive, and behavioral changes directed at adjusting to the effects of the stress or altering the stress itself (Baum, 1990).

Stress and our responses to it are central to psychiatric disorders and the provision of mental health care. The interplay among stress, the development of psychiatric disorders, and the exacerbation (worsening) of psychiatric symptoms has been widely researched. The old adage "what doesn't kill you will make you stronger" does not hold true with the development of mental illness; early exposure to stressful events actually sensitizes people to stress in later life. In other words, we know that people who are exposed to high levels of stress as children—especially during stress-sensitive developmental periods—have a greater incidence of all mental illnesses as adults (Taylor, 2010). We do not know, however, if severe stress causes a vulnerability to mental illness or if vulnerability to mental illness influences the likelihood of adverse stress responses.

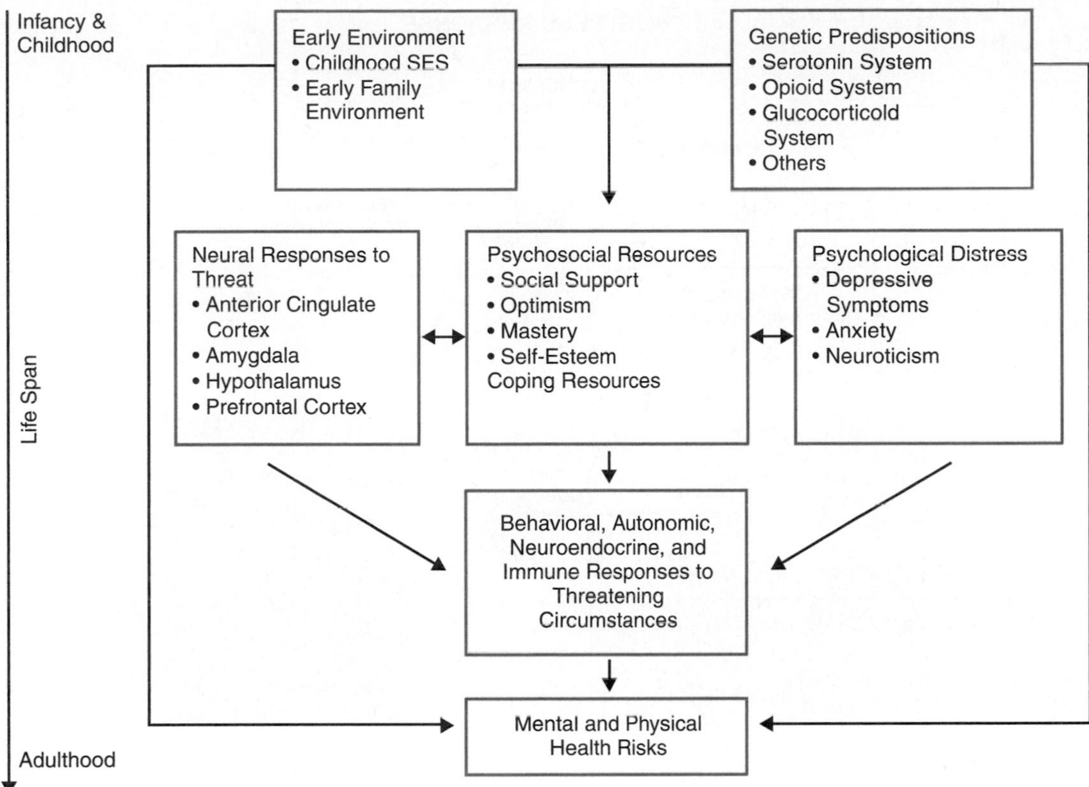

FIG 10-1 Early life stress and adult mental health outcomes. *SES,* Socioeconomic status. (From Taylor. S. [2010]. *Mechanisms linking early life stress to adult health outcomes.* Proceedings of the National Academy of Sciences of the United States of America. doi: 10.1073/pnas.1003890107.)

It is most important to recognize that severe stress is unhealthy and can weaken biological resistance to psychiatric pathology in any individual; however, stress is especially harmful for those who have a genetic predisposition to these disorders.

Figure 10-1 illustrates stress and health across the life span. It first takes into account nurture (environment) and nature (inborn qualities), responses to stressors (biological, social, and psychological), resultant physiological responses to stressors, and, finally, mental and physical health risks.

While an understanding of the connection between stress and mental illness is essential in the psychiatric setting, it is also important when developing a plan of care for any patient, in any setting, with any diagnosis. Imagine having an appendectomy and being served with an eviction notice on the same day. How well could you cope with either situation, let alone both simultaneously? The nurse's role is to intervene to reduce stress by promoting a healing environment, facilitating successful coping, and developing future coping strategies. In this chapter, we will explore how we are equipped to respond to stress, what can go wrong with the stress response, and how to care for our patients and even ourselves during times of stress.

RESPONSES TO AND EFFECTS OF STRESS

Early Stress Response Theories

The earliest research into the stress response (Figure 10-2) began as a result of observations that stressors brought about physical disorders or made existing conditions worse. **Stressors** are psychological or physical stimuli that are incompatible with current functioning and require adaptation. Walter Cannon (1871–1945) methodically investigated the sympathetic nervous system as a pathway of the response to stress, known more commonly as *fight* (aggression) *or flight* (withdrawal). The well-known **fight-or-flight response** is the body's way of preparing for a situation an individual perceives as a threat to survival. This response results in increased blood pressure, heart rate, and cardiac output.

While groundbreaking, Cannon's theory has been criticized for being simplistic, since not all animals or people respond by fighting or fleeing. In the face of danger, some animals become still (think of a deer) to avoid being noticed or to observe the environment in a state of heightened awareness. Also, Cannon's theory was developed primarily based on responses of animals and men. New research indicates that women may have unique physiological responses to stress. Physically, women have a lower hypothalamic-pituitary-adrenal axis and lower autonomic responses to stress at all ages, especially during pregnancy, and researchers hypothesize that estrogen exposure may regulate stress responses (Kajantie & Phillips, 2006). Men and women also have different neural responses to stress. While men experience altered prefrontal blood flow and increased salivary cortisol in response to stress, women experience increased limbic (emotional) activity and less significantly altered salivary cortisol (Wang et al., 2007).

Hans Selye (1907–1982) was another pioneer in stress research who introduced the concept of stress into both the scientific and popular literature. He expanded Cannon's theory

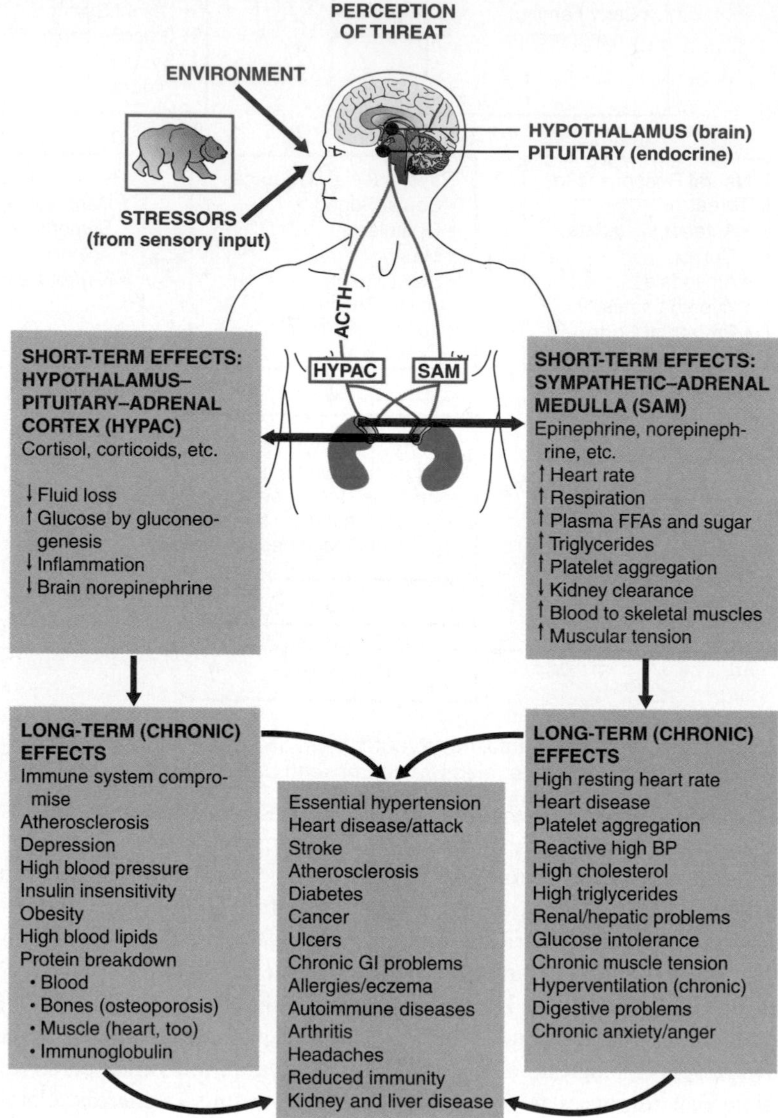

FIG 10-2 The stress response. *ACTH*, Adrenocorticotropic hormone; *BP*, blood pressure; *FFAs*, free fatty acids; *GI*, gastrointestinal. (From Brigham, D. D. [1994]. *Imagery for getting well: Clinical applications of behavioral medicine*. New York, NY: W. W. Norton.)

of stress in 1956 in his formulation of the **general adaptation syndrome (GAS)**. The GAS occurs in three stages:

1. The *alarm* (or *acute stress*) stage is the initial, brief, and adaptive response (fight or flight) to the stressor. During the alarm stage, there are three principle responses.
   - Sympathetic. The brain's cortex and hypothalamus signal the adrenal glands to release the catecholamine adrenalin. This increases sympathetic system activity (e.g., increased heart rate, respirations, and blood pressure) to enhance strength and speed. Pupils dilate for a broad view of the environment, and blood is shunted away from the digestive tract (resulting in dry mouth) and kidneys to more essential organs.
   - Corticosteroids. The hypothalamus also sends messages to the adrenal cortex. The adrenal cortex produces corticosteroids to help increase muscle endurance and stamina whereas other nonessential functions (e.g., digestion) are decreased. Unfortunately, the corticosteroids also inhibit functions such as reproduction, growth, and immunity.
   - Endorphins. Endorphins are released to reduce sensitivity to pain and injury. These polypeptides interact with opioid receptors in the brain to limit the perception of pain.

   The alarm stage is extremely intense, and no organism can sustain this level of reactivity and excitement for long. If the organism survives, the resistance stage follows.
2. The *resistance* stage could also be called the *adaptation stage* because it is during this time sustained and optimal resistance to the stressor occurs. Usually, stressors are successfully overcome; however, when they are not, the organism may experience the final exhaustion stage.

3. The *exhaustion* stage occurs when attempts to resist the stressor prove futile. At this point, resources are depleted, and the stress may become chronic, producing a wide array of psychological and physiological responses and even death.

One of the most important concepts of this theory is that regardless of the threat, the body responds the same physiologically. It is a matter of individual perception. The threat may be real or only perceived. It does not matter if the threat is physical, psychological, or social; the physiological response is the same.

Additionally, the body cannot differentiate between the energy generated by positive and negative stimuli. Lazarus and colleagues (1980) described these reactions as *distress* and *eustress:*

- **Distress** is a negative, draining energy that results in anxiety, depression, confusion, helplessness, hopelessness, and fatigue. Distress may be caused by such stressors as a death in the family, financial overload, or school/work demands.
- **Eustress** ('*eu*' Greek for well, *good* + *stress*) is a positive, beneficial energy that motivates and results in feelings of happiness, hopefulness, and purposeful movement. Eustress is the result of a positive perception toward a stressor. Examples of eustress are a much-needed vacation, playing a favorite sport, the birth of a baby, or the challenge of a new job. Since the same physiological responses are in play with stress and eustress, eustress can still tax the system, and down-time is important.

Selye's GAS remains a popular theory, but it has been expanded and reinterpreted since the 1950s. Some researchers question the notion of "nonspecific responses" and believe that different types of stressors bring about different patterns of responses, and that it is the *degree* of stress that is important (Koolhaas et al., 2011). Stress seems to be characterized by a reduced recovery. The magnitude of the stress response is determined by unpredictability or uncontrollability of the neuroendocrine reaction.

Furthermore, the GAS is most accurate in the description of how males respond when threatened. Females do not typically respond to stress by fighting or fleeing but rather by tending and befriending, a survival strategy that emphasizes the protection of the young and a reliance on the social network for support. , Women are more vulnerable to stress-related disorders. This may be due to females being more sensitive to even low levels of corticotropin-releasing factor (CRF), a peptide hormone released from the hypothalamus in response to stress. Additionally, females seem to be less able to adapt to high levels of CRF as compared to men (Bangasser et al., 2010).

Increased understanding of the exhaustion stage of the GAS has revealed that illness results from not only the depletion of reserves but also the stress mediators themselves. For example, people experiencing chronic distress have wounds that heal more slowly. Table 10-1 describes some reactions to acute and prolonged (chronic) stress.

TABLE 10-1 SOME REACTIONS TO ACUTE AND PROLONGED (CHRONIC) STRESS

ACUTE STRESS CAN CAUSE	PROLONGED (CHRONIC) STRESS CAN CAUSE
Uneasiness and concern	Anxiety and panic attacks
Sadness	Depression or melancholia
Loss of appetite	Anorexia or overeating
Suppression of the immune system	Lowered resistance to infections, leading to increase in opportunistic viral and bacterial infections
Increased metabolism and use of body fats	Insulin-resistant diabetes
Hypertension	
Infertility	Amenorrhea or loss of sex drive
Impotence, anovulation	
Increased energy mobilization and use	Increased fatigue and irritability
Decreased memory and learning	
Increased cardiovascular tone	Increased risk for cardiac events (e.g., heart attack, angina, and sudden heart-related death)
Increased risk of blood clots and stroke	
Increased cardiopulmonary tone	Increased respiratory problems

Neurotransmitter Stress Responses

Serotonin is a brain catecholamine that plays an important role in mood, sleep, sexuality, appetite, and metabolism. It is one of the main neurotransmitters implicated in depression, and many medications used to treat depression do so by increasing the availability of serotonin. During times of stress, serotonin synthesis becomes more active. This stress-activated turnover of serotonin is at least partially mediated by the corticosteroids, and researchers believe this activation may dysregulate (impair) serotonin receptor sites and the brain's ability to use serotonin. The influence of stressful life events on the development of depression is well documented, but researchers still do not understand fully the relationship. This neurotransmitter stress response research sheds some new light on the process.

Immune Stress Responses

Cannon and Selye focused on the physical and mental responses of the nervous and endocrine systems to acute and chronic stress. Later work revealed that there was also an interaction between the nervous system and the immune system that occurs during the alarm phase of the GAS. In one study, rats were given a mixture of saccharine along with a drug that reduces the immune system (Ader & Cohen, 1975). Afterward, when given *only* the saccharine, the rats continued to have decreased immune responses, which indicated that stress itself negatively impacts the body's ability to produce a protective structure.

Psychoneuroimmunology focuses on the interaction between psychological process and nervous and immune functions. Researchers continue to find evidence that stress, through the hypothalamic-pituitary-adrenal and sympathetic-adrenal medullary axes, can induce changes in the immune system. This model helps explain what many researchers and clinicians have believed and witnessed for centuries: There are links among stress (biopsychosocial), the immune system, and disease—a clear mind-body connection that may alter health outcomes. Stress may result in malfunctions in the immune system that are implicated in autoimmune disorders, immunodeficiency, and hypersensitivities.

Stress influences the immune system in several complex ways. Stress can enhance the immune system and prepare the body to respond to injury by fighting infections and healing wounds. Immune cells normally release cytokines, which are proteins and glycoproteins used for communication between cells, when a pathogen is detected; they serve to activate and recruit other immune cells. During times of stress, these cytokines are released, and immunity is profoundly activated, but the activation is limited since the cytokines stimulate further release of corticosteroids, which inhibits the immune system.

The immune response and the resulting cytokine activity in the brain raise questions regarding their connection with psychological and cognitive states such as depression. Researchers have found concentrations of cytokines that cause systemic inflammation, especially tumor necrosis factor (TNF)-α and interleukin-6, to be significantly higher in depressed subjects compared with control subjects (Dowlati et al., 2010). Cancer patients are often treated with cytokine molecules known as *interleukins*; unfortunately, but understandably, these chemotherapy drugs tend to cause or increase depression (National Cancer Institute, 2011).

Research in this field is promising. Investigators are examining how psychosocial factors, such as optimism and social support, moderate the stress response. They are mapping the biological and cellular mechanisms by which stress affects the immune system and are testing new theories.

MEDIATORS OF THE STRESS RESPONSE

Stressors

Many dissimilar situations (e.g., emotional arousal, fatigue, fear, loss, humiliation, loss of blood, extreme happiness, unexpected success) are capable of producing stress and triggering the stress response (Selye, 1993). No individual factor can be singled out as the cause of the stress response; however, stressors can be divided into two categories: physical and psychological. **Physical stressors** include environmental conditions (e.g., trauma and excessive cold or heat) as well as physical conditions (e.g., infection, hemorrhage, hunger, and pain). **Psychological stressors** include such things as divorce, loss of a job, unmanageable debt, the death of a loved one, retirement, and fear of a terrorist attack as well as changes we might consider positive, such as marriage, the arrival of a new baby, or unexpected success.

Perception

Have you ever noticed that something that upsets your friend doesn't bother you at all? Or that your professor's habit of going over the allotted class time drives you up a wall, yet (to your annoyance) your best friend in class doesn't seem to notice? Researchers have looked at the degree to which various life events upset a specific individual and have, not surprisingly, found that the *perception* of a stressor determines the person's emotional and psychological reactions to it (Rahe, 1995).

Responses to stress and anxiety are affected by factors such as age, gender, culture, life experience, and lifestyle, all of which may work to either lessen or increase the degree of emotional or physical influence and the sequelae (consequence or result) of stress. For example, a man in his 40s who has a new baby, has just purchased a home, and is laid off with 6 months' severance pay may feel the stress of the job loss more intensely than a man in his 60s who is financially secure and is asked to take an early retirement.

Individual Temperament

As mentioned earlier, part of the response to stressors is based on our own individual perceptions, which are colored by a variety of factors, including genetic structure and vulnerability, childhood experiences, coping strategies, and personal outlook on life and the world. All these factors combine to form a unique personality with specific strengths and vulnerabilities.

Social Support

The benefit of social support cannot be emphasized enough, whether it is for you or for your patients. Humans once lived in close communities with extended family sharing the same living quarters; essentially, neighbors were the therapists of the past. Suburban life may result in isolated living spaces where neighbors may interact sporadically; in fact, you may not even know your neighbors. People in crowded cities often live in isolation, where eye contact and communication may be considered an invasion of privacy.

Strong social support from significant others can enhance mental and physical health and act as a significant buffer against distress. A shared identity—whether with a family, social network, religious group, or colleagues—helps people overcome stressors more adaptively (Haslam & Reicher, 2006; Ysseldyk et al, 2010). Numerous studies have found a strong correlation between lower mortality rates and intact support systems; people, and even animals, without social companionship risk early death and have higher rates of illness (Taylor, 2010).

Support Groups

The proliferation of self-help groups attests to the need for social supports, and the explosive growth of a great variety of support groups reflects their effectiveness for many people. Many of the support groups currently available are for people going through similar stressful life events: Alcoholics Anonymous (a prototype for 12-step programs), Gamblers Anonymous, Reach for Recovery (for cancer patients), and Parents Without Partners, to note but a few. The proliferation of online support groups provides cost-effective, anonymous, and easily accessible self-help for people with every disorder imaginable (McCormack, 2010). A Google search for online + support + groups yielded nearly 60 million hits; there has to be a group out there for everyone although quality and fit are always factors to be considered.

Culture

Each culture not only emphasizes certain problems of living more than others but also interprets emotional problems differently from other cultures. Although Western European and North American cultures tend to subscribe to a psychophysiological view of stress and somatic distress, this is not the dominant view in other cultures. The overwhelming majority of Asians, Africans, and Central Americans tend to express distress in somatic terms and actually experience it physically.

Spirituality and Religious Beliefs

Many spiritual and religious beliefs help persons cope with stress, and these deserve closer scientific investigation. Studies have demonstrated that spiritual practices can enhance the immune system and sense of well-being (Koenig et al., 2012). Some scholars propose that spiritual well-being helps people deal with health issues, primarily because spiritual beliefs help people cope with issues of living. Thus, people with spiritual beliefs have established coping mechanisms they employ in normal life and can use when faced with illness. People who include spiritual solutions to physical or mental distress often gain a sense of comfort and support that can aid in healing and lowering stress. Even prayer, in and of itself, can elicit the relaxation response (discussed later in this chapter) that is known to reduce stress physically and emotionally and to reduce stress on the immune system.

Figure 10-3 operationally defines the process of stress and the positive or negative results of attempts to relieve stress, and Box 10-1 identifies several stress busters that can be incorporated into our lives with little effort.

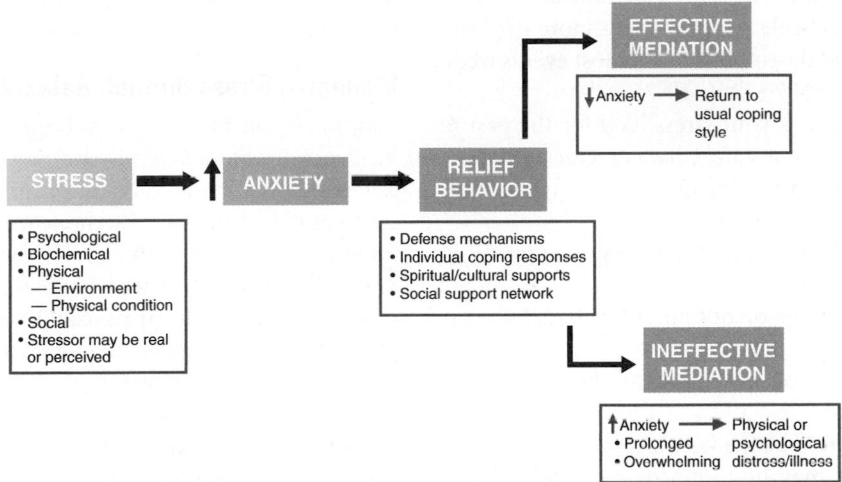

FIG 10-3 Stress and anxiety operationally defined.

BOX 10-1 EFFECTIVE STRESS BUSTERS

Sleep
- Chronically stressed people are often fatigued, so going to sleep 30 to 60 minutes early each night for a few weeks is suggested.
- If fatigue persists, try going to bed another 30 minutes earlier.
- Sleeping later in the morning is not helpful and can disrupt body rhythms.

Exercise (Aerobic)
- Exercise can dissipate chronic and acute stress.
- It may decrease levels of anxiety, depression, and sensitivity to stress.
- It can decrease muscle tension and increase endorphin levels.
- A recommended level of exercise is at least 30 minutes, three or more times a week.
- It is best to exercise at least 3 hours before bedtime.

Reduction or Cessation of Caffeine Intake
- Lowering or stopping caffeine intake can lead to more energy, fewer muscle aches, and greater relaxation.
- Slowly wean off coffee, tea, colas, and chocolate drinks.

Music (Classical or Soft Melodies of Choice)
- Listening to music increases the sense of relaxation.
- Increased healing effects may result.
- Therapeutically, music can decrease agitation and confusion in older adults.
- Quality of life in hospice settings is enhanced.

Pets
- Pets can bring joy and reduce stress.
- They can be an important social support.
- Pets can alleviate medical problems aggravated by stress.

Massage
- Massage can slow the heart rate and relax the body.
- Alertness may actually increase.

NURSING MANAGEMENT OF STRESS RESPONSES

Measuring Stress

In 1967, Holmes and Rahe published the Social Readjustment Rating Scale. This life-change scale measures the level of positive or negative stressful life events over a 1-year period. The level, or life-change unit, of each event is assigned a score based on the degree of severity and/or disruption. This questionnaire has been rescaled twice, first in 1978 and again in 1997 when it was adapted as the Recent Life Changes Questionnaire.

Since the scale was developed in 1967, life seems to have become more demanding and stressful. For example, travel is perceived as much more stressful now compared to 30 years ago. In 2007, online interviews were conducted to collect data from 1306 participants and then compared to data collected in the original study by Holmes and Rahe (First30Days, 2008). Although some life-change events were viewed as more stressful in 1967 (such as divorce and death of spouse), most events were viewed as more stressful in 2007 (Table 10-2).

Take a few minutes to assess your stress level for the past 6 to 12 months using the Recent Life Changes Questionnaire (Table 10-3). When you administer the questionnaire, take into account the following:

- Not all events are perceived to have the same degree of intensity or disruptiveness.
- Culture may dictate whether or not an event is stressful or how stressful it is.
- Different people may have different thresholds beyond which disruptions occur.
- The questionnaire equates change with stress.

Other stress scales that may be useful to nursing students have been developed. You might like to try the Perceived Stress Scale, the most widely used scale to measure perceived stress (Figure 10-4). Although there are no absolute scores, this scale measures how relatively uncontrollable, unpredictable, and overloaded you find your life. You might try this scale alone or suggest that it be used in a clinical post-conference for comparison and discussion.

TABLE 10-2 PERCEPTION OF LIFE STRESSORS IN 1967 AND 2007

LIFE CHANGE EVENT	1967	2007
Death of spouse	100	80
Death of family member	63	70
Divorce/separation	73/65	66
Job lay off or firing	47	62
Birth of child/pregnancy	40	60
Death of friend	50	50
Marriage	50	50
Retirement	45	49
Marital reconciliation	45	48
Change job field	36	47
Child leaves home	29	43

Data from First30Days. (2008). *Making changes today considered more difficult to handle than 30 years ago.* Retrieved from http://www.first30days.com/pages/press_changereport.html.

Assessing Coping Styles

People cope with life stressors in a variety of ways, and a number of factors can act as effective mediators to decrease stress in our lives. Rahe (1995) identified four discrete personal attributes (**coping styles**) people can develop to help manage stress:

1. Health-sustaining habits (e.g., medical compliance, proper diet, relaxation, pacing one's energy)
2. Life satisfactions (e.g., work, family, hobbies, humor, spiritual solace, arts, nature)
3. Social supports
4. Effective and healthy responses to stress

Examining these four coping categories can help nurses identify areas to target for improving their patients' responses to stress.

Managing Stress through Relaxation Techniques

Poor management of stress has been correlated with an increased incidence of a number of physical and emotional conditions, such as heart disease, poor diabetes control, chronic pain, and significant emotional distress. Psychoneuroimmunology provides the foundation for several integrative therapies, also referred to as *mind-body therapies*. There is now considerable evidence that many mind-body therapies can be used as effective adjuncts to conventional medical treatment for a number of common clinical conditions. Chapter 35 offers a more detailed discussion of holistic, mind-body, and integrative therapies.

Nurses should be aware of the conditions that can benefit from stress- and anxiety-reduction techniques. Problems that are known to benefit from stress reduction are anxiety, depression, headache, and pain (National Center for Complementary and Alternative Medicine, 2011). Stress- and anxiety-reduction techniques may also have benefits for some other disorders, including high blood pressure, asthma, nausea, fibromyalgia, irritable bowel syndrome, heart disease and heart symptoms, and insomnia. Although the results are not clear, there is some evidence to indicate that stress-reduction techniques may aid in smoking cessation and may improve temporomandibular disorder, ringing in the ears, overactive bladder, nightmares, and hot flashes associated with menopause. Current research is investigating the usefulness of stress-reduction techniques for back pain.

Because no single stress-management technique feels right for everyone, employing a mixture of techniques brings the best results. All are useful in a variety of situations for specific individuals, and all are evidence-based (Varvogli & Darviri, 2011). Essentially, there are stress-reducing techniques for every personality type, situation, and level of stress. Give them a try. Practicing relaxation techniques will help you to help your patients reduce their stress levels and also help you manage your own physical responses to stressors. These techniques result in reduced heart and breathing rates, decreased blood pressure, improved oxygenation to major muscles, and reduced muscle tension. They also help manage subjective anxiety and improve appraisals of reality.

TABLE 10-3 RECENT LIFE CHANGES QUESTIONNAIRE

LIFE-CHANGING EVENT	LIFE CHANGE UNIT*
HEALTH	
An injury or illness that:	
Kept you in bed a week or more or sent you to the hospital	74
Was less serious than above	44
Major dental work	26
Major change in eating habits	27
Major change in sleeping habits	26
Major change in your usual type and/or amount of recreation	28
WORK	
Change to a new type of work	51
Change in your work hours or conditions	35
Change in your responsibilities at work:	
More responsibilities	29
Fewer responsibilities	21
Promotion	31
Demotion	42
Transfer	32
Troubles at work:	
With your boss	29
With co-workers	35
With persons under your supervision	35
Other work troubles	28
Major business adjustment	60
Retirement	52
Loss of job:	
Laid off from work	68
Fired from work	79
Correspondence course to help you in your work	18
HOME AND FAMILY	
Major change in living conditions	42
Change in residence:	
Move within the same town or city	25
Move to a different town, city, or state	47
Change in family get-togethers	25
Major change in health or behavior of family member	55
Marriage	50
Pregnancy	67
Miscarriage or abortion	65
Gain of a new family member:	
Birth of a child	66
Adoption of a child	65
A relative moving in with you	59
Spouse beginning or ending work	46
Child leaving home:	
To attend college	41
Due to marriage	41
For other reasons	45
Change in arguments with spouse	50
In-law problems	38
Change in the marital status of your parents:	
Divorce	59
Remarriage	50
Separation from spouse:	
Due to work	53
Due to marital problems	76
Divorce	96
Birth of grandchild	43
Death of spouse	119
Death of other family member:	
Child	123
Brother or sister	102
Parent	100
PERSONAL AND SOCIAL	
Change in personal habits	26
Beginning or ending of school or college	38
Change of school or college	35
Change in political beliefs	24
Change in religious beliefs	29
Change in social activities	27
Vacation	24
New close personal relationship	37
Engagement to marry	45
Girlfriend or boyfriend problems	39
Sexual differences	44
"Falling out" of a close personal relationship	47
An accident	48
Minor violation of the law	20
Being held in jail	75
Death of a close friend	70
Major decision regarding your immediate future	51
Major personal achievement	36
FINANCIAL	
Major change in finances:	
Increase in income	38
Decrease in income	60
Investment and/or credit difficulties	56
Loss or damage of personal property	43
Moderate purchase	20
Major purchase	37
Foreclosure on a mortgage or loan	58

*One-year totals ≧ 500 life change units are considered indications of high recent life stress.

From Miller, M. A., & Rahe, R. H. (1997). Life changes scaling for the 1990s. *Journal of Psychosomatic Research, 43*(3), 279–292.

Instructions: The questions in this scale ask you about your feelings and thoughts during the last month. In each case, please indicate with a check how often you felt or thought a certain way.

1. In the last month, how often have you been upset because of something that happened unexpectedly?
   ___0 never ___1 almost never ___2 sometimes ___3 fairly often ___4 very often
2. In the last month, how often have you felt that you were unable to control the important things in your life?
   ___0 never ___1 almost never ___2 sometimes ___3 fairly often ___4 very often
3. In the last month, how often have you felt nervous and "stressed"?
   ___0 never ___1 almost never ___2 sometimes ___3 fairly often ___4 very often
4. In the last month, how often have you felt confident about your ability to handle your personal problems?
   ___0 never ___1 almost never ___2 sometimes ___3 fairly often ___4 very often
5. In the last month, how often have you felt that things were going your way?
   ___0 never ___1 almost never ___2 sometimes ___3 fairly often ___4 very often
6. In the last month, how often have you found that you could not cope with all the things that you had to do?
   ___0 never ___1 almost never ___2 sometimes ___3 fairly often ___4 very often
7. In the last month, how often have you been able to control irritations in your life?
   ___0 never ___1 almost never ___2 sometimes ___3 fairly often ___4 very often
8. In the last month, how often have you felt that you were on top of things?
   ___0 never ___1 almost never ___2 sometimes ___3 fairly often ___4 very often
9. In the last month, how often have you been angered because of things that were outside of your control?
   ___0 never ___1 almost never ___2 sometimes ___3 fairly often ___4 very often
10. In the last month, how often have you felt difficulties were piling up so high that you could not overcome them?
   ___0 never ___1 almost never ___2 sometimes ___3 fairly often ___4 very often

Perceived stress scale scoring
Items 4, 5, 7, and 8 are the positively stated items. PSS-10 scores are obtained by reversing the scores on the positive items, e.g., 0=4, 1=3, 2=2, etc. and then adding all 10 items.

FIG 10-4 Perceived Stress Scale–10 Item (PSS-10). (Modified from the John D. and Catherine T. MacArthur Research Network on Socioeconomic Status and Health. Retrieved from www.macses.ucsf.edu/Research/Psychosocial/notebook/PSS10.html.)

Deep Breathing Exercises

According to the National Health Interview Survey (2007), the most common relaxation technique used in the United States is **deep breathing exercises.** Nearly 13% of respondents used this technique as a mainstay or a quick fix to calm down. This technique is simple and easy to remember, even when anxiety begins to escalate.

One breathing exercise that has proved helpful for many people coping with anxiety and anxiety disorders has two parts (Box 10-2). The first part focuses on abdominal breathing while the second part helps patients interrupt trains of thought, thereby quieting mental noise. With increasing skill, breathing becomes a tool for dampening the cognitive processes likely to induce stress and anxiety reactions.

Progressive Muscle Relaxation

In 1938, Edmund Jacobson, a Harvard-educated physician, developed a rather simple procedure that elicits a relaxation response, which he coined progressive muscle relaxation (PMR). This technique can be done without any external gauges or feedback and can be practiced almost anywhere by anyone. The premise behind PMR is that since anxiety results in tense muscles, one way to decrease anxiety is to nearly eliminate muscle contraction. This is accomplished by deliberately tensing groups of muscles (beginning with feet and ending with face, or vice versa) as tightly as possible for about 8 seconds and then releasing the tension you have created.

BOX 10-2 DEEP BREATHING EXERCISE

- Find a comfortable position.
- Relax your shoulders and chest; let your body relax.
- Shift to relaxed, abdominal breathing. Take a deep breath through your nose, expanding the abdomen. Hold it for 3 seconds and then exhale slowly through the mouth; exhale completely, telling yourself to relax.
- With every breath, turn attention to the muscular sensations that accompany the expansion of the belly.
- As you concentrate on your breathing, you will start to feel focused.
- Repeat this exercise for 2 to 5 minutes.

Considerable research supports the use of PMR as helpful for a number of medical conditions, such as "tension headaches" and psychiatric disorders, especially those with anxiety components (Conrad & Roth, 2006).

There are many free PMR scripts, audios, and videos on the Internet, and some of them can be quite lengthy. An abbreviated example of a PMR script that focuses on key muscle tension areas is listed in Box 10-3. Many people prefer to hear their own voice reciting the script, so you may want to make a tape of yourself.

Relaxation Response

Herbert Benson (1975, 1996) expanded on Jacobson's work by incorporating a state of mind that is conducive to relaxation. His techniques are influenced by Eastern practices and are achieved by adopting a calm and passive attitude and focusing on a pleasant mental image in a calm and peaceful environment. The stress response is counteracted by the relaxation response and allows the patient to switch from the sympathetic mode of the autonomic nervous system (fight-or-flight response) to a state of relaxation (the parasympathetic mode). Follow the steps in Box 10-4 to practice the relaxation response. Benson and Henry's (2000) techniques have been combined successfully with meditation and visual imagery to treat numerous disorders, such as high blood pressure, chronic pain, irregular heartbeats, premenstrual syndrome, insomnia, anxiety, depression, infertility, and migraine headaches.

Meditation

Meditation follows the basic guidelines described for the relaxation response. It is a discipline for training the mind to develop greater calm and then using that calm to bring penetrative insight into one's experience. Meditation can be used to help people reach their deep inner resources for healing, calm their minds, and help them operate more efficiently in the world. It can help people develop strategies to cope with stress, make sensible adaptive choices under pressure, and feel more engaged in life.

Meditation elicits a relaxation response by creating a hypometabolic state of quieting the sympathetic nervous system. Some people meditate using a visual object or a sound to help them focus. Others may find it useful to concentrate on their breathing while meditating. There are many meditation techniques, some with a spiritual base, such as Siddha meditation or prayer. Meditation is easy to practice anywhere. Some students find that meditating the morning of a test helps them focus and lessens anxiety. Keep in mind that meditation, like most other skills, must be practiced to produce the relaxation responses.

Mindfulness, a centuries-old form of meditation that dates back to Buddhist tradition, has received increased attention among health care professionals. Farb and colleagues (2007) describe mindfulness from a neuroscience perspective and identify two different networks for experiencing the world. One is a default network that includes the medial prefrontal cortex and memory regions such as the hippocampus. In this state we operate on a sort of mental autopilot or "mind wandering." You are thinking about what to make for dinner, how your hair looks, and continually compiling the narrative of your life and people you know. Research indicates that we may engage in mind wandering nearly half of our waking hours (Killingsworth & Gilbert, 2010).

The other network is the direct experience network that is the focus of mindfulness. Several areas of the brain are activated in this state. The insular cortex is active and makes us aware of bodily sensation and a sense of self. The anterior cingulate cortex is active and is central to attention and focuses us on what is happening around us. In this state you are in tune with your

BOX 10-3 SHORT PROGRESSIVE MUSCLE RELAXATION

Tense and relax each area listed below. When you tense the area, do not cause any pain. Tighten only until you feel tension. If you feel any discomfort, stop or ease up.

- The first key area is your neck and shoulders: Raise your shoulders up toward your ears . . . tighten the muscles there . . . hold . . . feel the tension there . . . and now release. Let your shoulders drop to a lower, more comfortable position.
- The next key area is your hands: Tighten your hands into fists. Very, very tight . . . as if you are squeezing a rubber ball very tightly in each hand . . . hold . . . feel the tension in your hands and forearms . . . and now release. Shake your hands gently, shaking out the tension. Feel how much more relaxed your hands are now.
- Now, your forehead: Raise your eyebrows, feeling the tight muscles in your forehead. Hold that tension. Now tightly lower your eyebrows and scrunch your eyes closed, feeling the tension in your forehead and eyes. Hold it tightly. And now, relax . . . let your forehead be relaxed and smooth, your eyelids gently resting.
- Your jaw is the next key area: Tightly close your mouth, clamping your jaw shut, very tightly. Your lips will also be tight and tense across the front of your teeth. Feel the tension in your jaws. Hold . . . and now relax. Release all of the tension. Let your mouth and jaw be loose and relaxed.
- There is only one more key area to relax, and that is your breathing: Breathe in deeply, and hold that breath. Feel the tension as you hold the air in. Hold . . . and now relax. Let the air be released through your mouth. Breathe out all the air.
- Once more, breathe in . . . and now hold the breath. Hold . . . and relax. Release the air, feeling your entire body relax. Breathe in . . . and out . . . in . . . and out . . .
- Continue to breathe regular breaths.
- You have relaxed all of the key areas where tension can build up. Remember to relax these areas a few times each day, using this quick progressive muscle relaxation script, to prevent stress symptoms.

From Inner Health Studio. (2011). *Quick progressive muscle relaxation script: Key areas.* Retrieved from http://www.innerhealthstudio.com/quick-progressive-muscle-relaxation.html.

BOX 10-4 THE BENSON-HENRY PROTOCOL

Phase I

- Choose a focus word (e.g., *love, peace, one),* phrase, image, or short prayer. You may choose to focus only on your breathing.
- Sit in a comfortable position in a calm place.
- Close your eyes.
- Progressively relax all your muscles, beginning at your feet and moving up to your face.
- Breathe through your nose. Be aware of your breathing. As you breathe out, say your word or phrase or picture your image. For example, breathe in . . . out (phrase), in . . . out (phrase), and so forth. Or simply focus on your breathing. Breathe easily and naturally.
- You may notice other thoughts but do not judge or react to them. Gently ignore them and go back to your word or phrase.
- Continue for 12 to 15 minutes once or twice a day for at least 8 weeks.
- When you finish, sit quietly for several minutes, at first with your eyes closed and then with your eyes open. Do not stand up for a few minutes.

Phase II

For 8 to 10 minutes focus on imagery of a peaceful scene where you are free from whatever health problem or negative condition you are experiencing. The focusing will promote healing expectations, beliefs, and memories.

From Benson, H., & Proctor, W. (2000). *Relaxation revolution.* New York, NY: Scribner.

environment, live in the moment, and take a break from planning, strategizing, and setting goals.

Being mindful includes being in the moment by paying attention to what is going on around you—what you are seeing, feeling, hearing. Imagine how much you miss during an ordinary walk to class if you spend it staring straight ahead as your mind wanders from one concern to the next. You miss the pattern of sunlight filtered through the leaves, the warmth of the sunshine on your skin, and the sounds of birds calling out to one another. By focusing on the here and now, rather than past and future, you are practicing mindfulness.

Mindfulness has been formalized as the Mindfulness Based Stress Reduction Program and is extremely popular. It is discussed in the bestselling book *Wherever You Go, There You Are* (2005) by Jon Kabat-Zinn. The goal of this program is to make mindfulness a continuous process. With practice, people can gradually learn to let go of internal dialogue and reactiveness. Practicing mindfulness can be done at any time, and proponents suggest that it become a way of life. One mindfulness technique can be found in Box 10-5.

Guided Imagery

Native Americans and other traditions, including Hindu, Judeo-Christian, and traditional Chinese medicine, have used **guided imagery** (Academy for Guided Imagery, 2010). Consider that long before we can speak, our experience is based on mental images—envisioning images that are both calming and health enhancing. If a person has dysfunctional images, he or she can be helped to generate more effective and functional coping images to replace the depression- or anxiety-producing ones. For example, athletes have discovered that the use of images of positive coping and success can lead to improvement in performance (Aetna InteliHealth, 2008). See Box 10-6 for a sample script for guided imagery.

BOX 10-5 A MINDFULNESS TECHNIQUE

Creating space to come down from the worried mind and back into the present moment has been shown to be enormously helpful to people. When we are present, we have a firmer grasp of all our options and resources that often make us feel better. Next time you find your mind racing with stress, try the acronym S.T.O.P.

S – Stop what you are doing; put things down for a minute.

T – Take a breath. Breathe normally and naturally and follow your breath coming in and out of your nose. You can even say to yourself "in" as you're breathing in and "out" as you're breathing out if that helps with concentration.

O – Observe your thoughts, feelings, and emotions. You can reflect about what is on your mind and also notice that thoughts are not facts, and they are not permanent. If the thought arises that you are inadequate, just notice the thought, let it be, and continue on. Notice any emotions that are there and just name them. Just naming your emotions can have a calming effect. Then notice your body. Are you standing or sitting? How is your posture? Any aches and pains?

P – Proceed with something that is important to you in the moment, whether that is talking with a friend, appreciating your children, or walking while paying attention to the world.

From Goldstein, E. (2012). *The now effect.* New York, NY: Atria Books.

BOX 10-6 SCRIPT FOR GUIDED IMAGERY

- Imagine releasing all the tension in your body . . . letting it go.
- Now, with every breath you take, feel your body drifting down deeper and deeper into relaxation . . . floating down . . . deeper and deeper.
- Imagine a peaceful scene. You are sitting beside a clear, blue mountain stream. You are barefoot, and you feel the sun-warmed rock under your feet. You hear the sound of the stream tumbling over the rocks. The sound is hypnotic, and you relax more and more. You see the tall pine trees on the opposite shore bending in the gentle breeze. Breathe the clean, scented air, with each breath moving you deeper and deeper into relaxation. The sun warms your face.
- You are very comfortable. There is nothing to disturb you. You experience a feeling of well-being.
- You can return to this peaceful scene by taking time to relax. The positive feelings can grow stronger and stronger each time you choose to relax.
- You can return to your activities now, feeling relaxed and refreshed.

Imagery techniques are a useful tool in the management of medical conditions and are an effective means of relieving pain for some people. Inducing muscle relaxation and focusing the mind away from the pain reduce pain. For some, imagery techniques are healing exercises in that they not only relieve the pain but also, in some cases, diminish the source of the pain. Cancer patients use guided imagery to help reduce high levels of cortisol, epinephrine, and catecholamines—which prevent the immune system from functioning effectively—and to produce β-endorphins—which increase pain thresholds and enhance lymphocyte proliferation.

Often, audio recordings are made specifically for patients and their particular situations; however, many generic guided-imagery CDs and MP3s are available to patients and health care workers online.

Biofeedback

Through the use of sensitive instrumentation, biofeedback provides immediate and exact information regarding muscle activity, brain waves, skin temperature, heart rate, blood pressure, and other bodily functions. Indicators of the particular internal physiological process are detected and amplified by a sensitive recording device. An individual can achieve greater voluntary control over phenomena once considered to be exclusively involuntary if he or she knows instantaneously, through an auditory or visual signal, whether a somatic activity is increasing or decreasing.

Using biofeedback requires special training, and the technique is thought to be most effective for people with low-to-moderate hypnotic ability. For people with higher hypnotic ability, meditation, PMR, and other cognitive-behavioral therapy techniques produce the most rapid reduction in clinical symptoms.

With increasing recognition of the role of stress in a variety of medical illnesses, including diseases affected by immune dysfunction, biofeedback has emerged as an effective strategy for stress management. The necessity of using the complex instrumentation required to detect minute levels of muscle tension or certain patterns of electroencephalographic activity is uncertain, but it has been confirmed that teaching people to relax deeply and to apply these skills in response to real-life stressors can be helpful in lowering stress levels.

Physical Exercise

Physical exercise can lead to protection from the harmful effects of stress on both physical and mental states. Regular physical activity was associated with lower incidence of all psychiatric disorders except bipolar disorder and of comorbid conditions in subjects aged 14 to 24 in a study by Strohle and colleagues (2007). Older adults who engage in regular physical activity have some protection from anxiety and depressive disorder (Pasco et al., 2011). Researchers have been particularly interested in the influence exercise has over depression. Blumenthal and colleagues (2007) found that patients who had either 4 months of treatment with a selective serotonin reuptake inhibitor antidepressant or with aerobic exercise had similar relief of depression. Yoga, an ancient form of exercise, has been found to be helpful for depression when used in conjunction with medication (Shapiro et al., 2007). Other popular forms of exercise that can decrease stress and improve well-being are walking, tai chi, dancing, cycling, aerobics, and water exercise.

Cognitive Reframing

The goal of cognitive reframing (also known as *cognitive restructuring*) is to change the individual's perceptions of stress by reassessing a situation and replacing irrational beliefs ("I can't pass this course") with more positive self-statements ("If I choose to study for this course, I will increase my chances of success). A positive correlation has been found between cognitive reframing and improved affect and higher self-esteem (Billingsley, Collins, & Miller, 2007). We can learn from most situations by asking ourselves the following:

- "What positive things came out of this situation or experience?"
- "What did I learn in this situation?"
- "What would I do in a different way?"

The desired result is to reframe a disturbing event or experience as less disturbing and to give the patient a sense of control over the situation. When the perception of the disturbing event is changed, there is less stimulation to the sympathetic nervous system, which in turn reduces the secretion of cortisol and catecholamines that destroy the balance of the immune system.

Cognitive distortions often include overgeneralizations ("He always . . . " or "I'll never . . . ") and "should" statements ("I should have done better" or "He shouldn't have said that"). Table 10-4 shows some examples of cognitive reframing of anxiety-producing thoughts. Often, cognitive reframing is used along with progressive muscle relaxation, mindfulness, and guided imagery to reduce stress.

Journaling

Writing in **a journal** (journaling) is an extremely useful and surprisingly simple method of identifying stressors. It is a technique that can ease worry and obsession, help identify hopes and fears, increase energy levels and confidence, and facilitate the grieving process. Keeping an informal diary of daily events and activities can reveal surprising information on sources of daily stress. Simply noting which activities put a strain on energy and time, which trigger anger or anxiety, and which precipitate a negative physical experience (e.g., headache, backache, fatigue) can be an important first step in stress reduction. Writing down thoughts and feelings is helpful not only in dealing with stress and stressful events but also in healing both physically and emotionally.

Humor

The use of humor as a cognitive approach is a good example of how a stressful situation can be "turned upside down." The intensity attached to a stressful thought or situation can be dissipated when it is made to appear absurd or comical. Essentially, the bee loses its sting.

TABLE 10-4 COGNITIVE REFRAMING OF IRRATIONAL THOUGHTS

IRRATIONAL THOUGHT	POSITIVE STATEMENTS
"I'll never be happy until I am loved by someone I really care about."	"If I do not get love from one person, I can still get it from others and find happiness that way." "If someone I deeply care for rejects me, that will seem unfortunate, but I will hardly die." "If the only person I truly care for does not return my love, I can devote more time and energy to winning someone else's love and probably find someone better for me." "If no one I care for ever cares for me, I can still find enjoyment in friendships, in work, in books, and in other things."
"He should treat me better after all I do for him."	"I would like him to do certain things to show that he cares. If he chooses to continue to do things that hurt me after he understands what those things are, I am free to make choices about leaving or staying in this hurtful relationship."

Adapted from Ellis, A., & Harper, R. A. (1975). *A new guide to rational living.* North Hollywood, CA: Wilshire.

KEY POINTS TO REMEMBER

- Stress is a universal experience and an important concept when caring for any patient in any setting.
- The body responds similarly whether stressors are real or perceived and whether the stressor is negative or positive.
- Physiologically, the body reacts to anxiety and fear by arousal of the sympathetic nervous system. Specific symptoms include rapid heart rate, increased blood pressure, diaphoresis, peripheral vasoconstriction, restlessness, repetitive questioning, feelings of frustration, and difficulty concentrating.
- Cannon introduced the fight-or-flight model of stress, and Selye introduced the widely known general adaptation syndrome (GAS).
- The psychoneuroimmunology model describes the immune system's response to stress and effect on neural pathways in the brain.
- Prolonged stress can lead to chronic psychological and physiological responses when not mitigated at an early stage.
- There are basically two categories of stressors: physical (e.g., heat, hunger, cold, noise, trauma) and psychological (e.g., death of a loved one, loss of job, schoolwork, humiliation).
- Age, gender, culture, life experience, and lifestyle all are important in identifying the degree of stress a person is experiencing.
- Lowering the effects of chronic stress can alter the course of many physical conditions; decrease the need for some medications; diminish or eliminate the urge for unhealthy and destructive behaviors such as smoking, insomnia, and drug addiction; and increase a person's cognitive functioning.
- An extremely important factor to assess is a person's support system. Studies have shown that high-quality social and intimate supports can go a long way toward minimizing the long-term effects of stress.
- Cultural differences exist in the extent to which people perceive an event as stressful and in the behaviors they consider appropriate to deal with a stressful event.
- Spiritual practices have been found to lead to an enhanced immune system and a sense of well-being.
- A variety of relaxation techniques are available to reduce the stress response and elicit the relaxation response, which results in improved physical and psychological functioning.

CRITICAL THINKING

1. Assess your level of stress using the Recent Life Changes Questionnaire found in Table 10-3, and evaluate your potential for illness in the coming year. Identify stress-reduction techniques you think would be useful to learn.
2. Teach a classmate the deep-breathing exercise identified in this chapter (see Box 10-2).
3. Assess a classmate's coping styles and have the same classmate assess yours. Discuss the relevance of your findings.
4. Using Figure 10-2, explain to a classmate the short-term effects of stress on the sympathetic–adrenal medulla system, and identify three long-term effects if the stress is not relieved. How would you use this information to provide patient teaching? If your classmate were the patient, how would his or her response indicate that effective learning had taken place?
5. Using Figure 10-2, have a classmate explain to you the short-term effects of stress on the hypothalamus–pituitary–adrenal cortex and the eventual long-term effects if the stress becomes chronic. Summarize to your classmate your understanding of what was presented. Using your knowledge of the short-term effects of stress on the hypothalamus–pituitary–adrenal cortex and the long-term effects of stress, develop and present a patient education model related to stress for your clinical group.
6. In postconference discuss a patient you have cared for who had one of the stress-related effects identified in Figure 10-2. See if you can identify some stressors in the patient's life and possible ways to lower chronic stress levels.

CHAPTER REVIEW

1. You are caring for a patient who is experiencing a crisis. Which symptoms would indicate that the patient is in the stage of alarm?
   a. Constricted pupils
   b. Dry mouth
   c. Decrease in heart rate
   d. Sudden drop in blood pressure
2. If it is determined that a patient will benefit from guided imagery, what teaching should you provide?
   a. Focus on a visual object or sound.
   b. Become acutely aware of your breathing pattern.
   c. Envision an image of a place that is peaceful.
   d. Develop deep abdominal breathing.
3. Neal, age 30, will be undergoing biofeedback. Which statement by Neal indicates a need for further teaching?
   a. "This will measure my muscle activity, heart rate, and blood pressure."
   b. "It will help me recognize how my body responds to stress."
   c. "I will feel a small shock of electricity if I tell a lie."
   d. "The instruments will know if my skin temperature changes."
4. Your 39- year-old patient, Samantha, who was admitted with anxiety, asks you what the stress-relieving technique of mindfulness is. The best response is:
   a. Mindfulness is focusing on an object and repeating a word or phrase while deep breathing
   b. Mindfulness is progressively tensing, then relaxing, body muscles
   c. Mindfulness is focusing on the here and now, not the past or future, and paying attention to what is going on around you
   d. Mindfulness is a memory system to assist you in short-term memory recall
5. Which of the following are believed to help individuals mediate, or lessen, the effects of stress? *Select all that apply.*
   a. Spirituality and/or religious beliefs
   b. Wealth
   c. Higher education level
   d. Social support
   e. Culture

Answers to Chapter Review
1. b; 2. c; 3. b; 4. c; 5. a, d, e.

evolve WEBSITE

Visit the Evolve website for a posttest on the content in this chapter: http://evolve.elsevier.com/Varcarolis

Post-Test interactive review

REFERENCES

Academy for Guided Imagery. (2010). *History of the Academy for Guided Imagery.* Retrieved from http://www.academyforguidedimagery.com/abouttheacademy/page13/page13.html.

Ader, R., & Cohen, N. (1975). Behaviorally conditioned immunosuppression. *Psychosomatic Medicine, 37*, 333–340.

Aetna InteliHealth. (2008). *Guided imagery*. Retrieved from http://www.intelihealth.com/IH/ihtIH/WSIHW000/8513/34968/358820.html?d5dmtContent.

Bangasser, A., Curtis, A., Reyes, B. A. S., Bethea, T. T., Parastatidis I., Ischiropoulos H., Van Bockstaele, E. J., & Valentino, R. J. (2010). Sex differences in corticotropin-releasing factor receptor signaling and trafficking: Potential role in female vulnerability to stress-related psychopathology. *Molecular Psychiatry, 15*, 896–904. doi:10.1038/mp.2010.66.

Baum, A. (1990). Stress, intrusive imagery, and chronic distress. *Health Psychology, 9*, 653–675.

Benson, H. (1975). *The relaxation response* (2nd ed.). New York, NY: William Morrow & Company.

Benson, H., & Stark, M. (1996). *Timeless healing*. New York, NY: Scribner.

Billingsley, S. K., Collins, A. M., & Miller, M. (2007). Healthy student, healthy nurse: A stress management workshop. *Nurse Educator, 32*(2), 49–51.

Blumenthal, J. A., Babyak, M. A., Doraiswamy, P. M., Watkins, L., Hoffman, B. M., Barbour, K.A., . . . Sherwood, A. (2007). Exercise and pharmacotherapy in the treatment of major depressive disorder. *Psychosomatic Medicine, 69*, 587–596.

Conrad, A., & Roth, W. T. (2006). Muscle relaxation therapy for anxiety disorders: It works but how? *Journal of Anxiety Disorders, 21*(3), 243–264.

First30Days. (2008). *First30days' the change report: Making changes today considered more difficult to handle than 30 years ago.* Retrieved from http://www.first30days.com/pages/press_changereport.html.

Dowlati, Y., Herrmann, N., Swardfager, W., Liu, H., Sham, L., Reim, E. K., & Lanctot, K. L. (2010). A meta-analysis of cytokines in major depression. *Biological Psychiatry, 67*(5), 446–457.

Farb, N. A., Segal, Z. V., Mayberg, H., Bean, J., McKeon, D., Fatima, Z., & Anderson, K. (2007). Attending to the present: Mindfulness meditation reveals distinct neural modes of self-reference. *Social Cognitive and Affective Neuroscience, 2*(4), 313–322. doi: 10.1093/scan/nsm030.

Haslam, S. A., & Reicher, S. (2006). Stressing the group: Social identity and the unfolding dynamics of responses to stress. *Journal of Applied Psychology, 91*, 1037–1052.

Holmes, T. H., & Rahe, R. H. (1967). The social readjustment rating scale. *Journal of Psychosomatic Research, 11*, 213.

Kabat-Zinn, J. (2005). *Wherever you go, there you are* (10th ed.). New York, NY: Hyperion.

Kajantie, E., & Phillips, D.I. (2006). The effects of sex and hormonal status on the physiological response to acute psychosocial stress. *Psychoneuroendocrinology, 31*, 151–178.

Killingsworth, M. A., & Gilbert, D. T. (2010). A wandering mind is an unhappy mind. *Science, 330*(6006), 932. doi: 10.1126/science.1192439.

Koenig, H. G., King, D. E. & Carson, V. B. (2012). *Handbook of religion and health* (2nd ed). New York, NY: Oxford University Press.

Koolhaus, J. M., Bartolomucci, A., Buwalda, B., de Boer, S. F., Flugge, G., Korte, S. M., . . . Fuchs, E. (2011). Stress revisited: A critical evaluation of the stress concept. *Neuroscience & Biobehavioral Reviews, 35*(5), 1291–1301.

Lazarus, R. S., & DeLongis, A. (1983). Psychological stress and coping in aging. *American Psychologist, 38*, 245.

McCormack, A. (2010). Individuals with eating disorders and the use of online support groups as a form of social support. *Computers Informatics Nursing, 28*(1), 12–19. doi: 10.1097/NCN.0b013e3181c04b06.

National Cancer Institute. (2011). *Depression.* Retrieved from http://www.cancer.gov/cancertopics/pdq/supportivecare/depression/HealthProfessional/page2#Reference2.3.

National Center for Complementary and Alternative Medicine. (2011). *Relaxation techniques for health: An introduction.* Retrieved from http://nccam.nih.gov/health/stress/relaxation.htm.

Pasco, J. A., Williams, L. J., Jacka, F. N., Henry, M. J., Coulson, C. E., Brennan, S. L., . . . Berk, M. (2011). Habitual physical activity and the risk for depressive and anxiety disorders among older men and women. *International Psychogeriatrics, 23*(2), 292–298.

Rahe, R. H. (1995). Stress and psychiatry. In H.I. Kaplan, & B.J. Sadock, (Vol. Eds.), *Comprehensive textbook of psychiatry/VI: Vol. 2* (pp. 1545–1559). Baltimore, MD: Williams & Wilkins.

Sadock, V. A., & Sadock, B. J. (2008). *Kaplan and Sadock's concise textbook of clinical psychiatry* (3rd ed.). Philadelphia, PA: Lippincott, Williams & Wilkins.

Selye, H. (1974). *Stress without distress.* Philadelphia, PA: Lippincott.

Selye, H. (1993). History of the stress concept. In L. Goldberger & S. Breznitz (Eds.), *Handbook of stress: Theoretical and clinical aspects* (pp. 7–17). New York, NY: Free Press.

Shapiro, D., Cook, I. A., Davydov, D. M., Ottaviani, C., Leuchter, A. F., & Abrams, M. (2007). Yoga as a complementary treatment of depression: Effects of traits and moods on treatment outcome. Evidenced Based *Complementary and Alternative Medicine.* Retrieved from http://ecam.oxfordjournals.org/cgi/content/abstract/nel114v1.

Strohle, A., Hofler, M., Pfister, H., Muller, A., Hoyer, J., Wittchen, H., & Lieb, R. (2007). Physical activity and prevalence and incidence of mental disorders in adolescents and young adults. *Psychological Medicine, 37,* 1657–1666.

Taylor, S. (2010). Mechanisms linking early life stress to adult health outcomes. *Proceedings of the National Academy of Sciences of the United States of America, 107*(19), 8507-8512. doi: 10.1073/pnas.1003890107.

Wang, J., Korczykowski, M., Rao, H., Fan, Y., Pluta, J., Gur, R. C., Detre, J. (2007). Gender difference in neural response to psychological stress. *Social Cognitive and Affective Neuroscience Advance Access, 2*(3), 227–239.

Ysseldyk, R., Matheson, K., & Anisman, H. (2010). Religiosity as identity: Toward an understanding of religion from a social identity perspective. *Personality and Social Psychology Review, 14*(1), 60–71. doi: 10.1177/1088868309349693.

CHAPTER

11

Childhood and Neurodevelopmental Disorders

Cindy Parsons and Elizabeth Hite Erwin

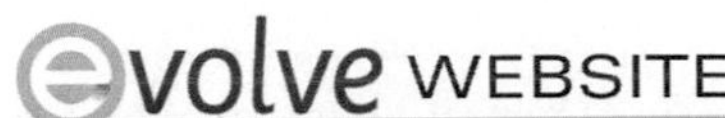

Visit the Evolve website for a pretest on the content in this chapter: http://evolve.elsevier.com/Varcarolis

Pre-Test interactive review

OBJECTIVES

1. Identify the significance of psychiatric disorders in children and adolescents.
2. Explore factors and influences contributing to neurodevelopmental disorders.
3. Identify characteristics of mental health and factors that promote resilience in children and adolescents.
4. Describe the specialty area of psychiatric mental health nursing.
5. Discuss the holistic assessment of a child or adolescent.
6. Compare and contrast at least six treatment modalities for children and adolescents with neurodevelopmental disorders.
7. Describe clinical features and behaviors of at least three child and adolescent psychiatric disorders.
8. Formulate one nursing diagnosis, stating patient outcomes and interventions for patients with intellectual development disorder, autism spectrum disorder, and attention deficit hyperactivity disorder.

KEY TERMS AND CONCEPTS

attention deficit hyperactivity disorder
autism spectrum disorders
bibliotherapy
communication disorders
early intervention programs
intellectual development disorder
motor disorders
play therapy
principle of least restrictive intervention
resilience
specific learning disorders
temperament
therapeutic games

We tend to think of mental illness as a phenomenon of adulthood, but in one large study more than 75% of young adults with a psychiatric disorder were first diagnosed between 11 and 18 years of age (Copeland et al., 2009). It is estimated that 20% of children and adolescents in the United States suffer from a major mental illness that causes significant impairment at home, at school, with peers, and in the community (Merekangas et al., 2010).

Because of their timing, these disorders can disrupt the normal pattern of childhood development and may carry devastating consequences in terms of academic, social, and psychological functioning. These disorders not only affect the child but also can cause significant stress for families and disrupt family functioning. Stigma and misconceptions can cause patients and families to attempt to conceal the conditions or even limit help seeking and professional care. Fortunately, this often silent public health epidemic is being addressed by increasingly sophisticated screening and treatment methods that show promise in reducing the impact of mental illness in children and on into adolescence and adulthood.

Younger children are more difficult to diagnose than older children because of limited language skills and cognitive and emotional development. Additionally, children undergo more rapid psychological, neurological, and physiological changes over a briefer period than adults. The rapidity and complexity of this development must be considered during assessment for psychiatric disorders. Clinicians and parents often wait to see whether symptoms are the result of a developmental lag or trauma response that will eventually correct itself; therefore, intervention may be delayed. Considering all the developmental changes, associated vulnerabilities, and resiliencies that occur during adolescence, it is clear that this is an optimal time to target intervention.

Unfortunately, lack of services and premature termination of treatment are two main problems, especially for vulnerable populations (poor children with single mothers, minority children, and those with serious presenting problems at intake) (Children's Defense Fund, 2011). The suffering experienced by children and adolescents with mental disorders is significant, and the cost to society is high.

The U.S. government's recognition of childhood and adolescent mental health problems and efforts toward identifying effective treatments were first identified in *Mental Health: A Report of the Surgeon General* (U.S. Department of Health and Human Services [USDHHS], 1999). More than two decades later, there continue to be barriers to assessment and treatment including: (1) lack of consensus and clarity about conditions for screening children; (2) lack of coordination among multiple systems; (3) lack of community-based resources and long waiting lists for services; (4) lack of mental health providers; and (5) cost and inadequate reimbursement (Children's Defense Fund, 2011).

The passage of the Mental Health Parity Act of 2011 has created opportunities to improve funding, access to care, and research to understand the reasons for underutilization and early termination of services. The Substance Abuse and Mental Health Services Administration (SAMHSA) has created an ambitious 3-year plan to improve the use of resources in the prevention, early detection, treatment, and recovery services for individuals with mental or substance abuse disorders (SAMHSA, 2011).

In this chapter, we will begin with an overview of overall discussion of the risk factors of psychiatric disorders in children, overall assessments, general interventions, and an overview of the specialty of child-adolescent psychiatric nursing. Several neurodevelopmental disorders – communication disorder, learning disorder, and motor disorder—are described briefly. Other disorders in this group—intellectual developmental disorder, autism spectrum disorders, attention deficit hyperactivity disorder—will be discussed in greater depth.

ETIOLOGY

Experts believe that the course of mental illness may be less severe if early detection and effective intervention are implemented. A genetic vulnerability coupled with the parent's inability to model effective coping strategies can lead to learned helplessness, creating anxiety or apathy and an inability to master the environment.

Biological Factors

Genetic

Hereditary factors are implicated in numerous childhood-onset psychiatric disorders. Because not all genetically vulnerable

EVIDENCE-BASED PRACTICE

Substance Abuse as a Family Problem

Caldwell, R., Silver, N.C., & Strada, M. (2010). Substance abuse, familial factors, and mental health: Exploring racial and ethnic differences among African American, Caucasian and Hispanic juvenile offenders. *The American Journal of Family Therapy, 38,* 310-321.

Purpose of Study

This study examined a high-risk population (juvenile offenders) to determine if there is a relationship between family composition, exposure to substance abuse, and mental health issues of self-esteem and depression as a function of race.

Method

The study consisted of 438 participants, ranging in age from 11-18, who were incarcerated in juvenile facilities in the western part of the U.S. The racial mix was 34% African American, 28% Caucasian, and 38% Hispanic. The study used a demographic questionnaire to determine a key variable— family composition, which was defined as intact, reconstituted, single-parent household, or other (living with grandparents or siblings etc.). Questionnaires were used as well to determine participant's family history of substance abuse; individual substance abuse was measured using a 32-question, Likert scale Substance Abuse Index. Mental symptoms were measured with the Major Depression Sub-Scale Psychopathology Scale Short Form (APS-SF) (Reynolds 2000) and the Rosenberg Self Esteem Scale (Rosenberg, 1965).

Key Findings

Family composition was correlated with race, depression, self-esteem, and substance use. Those coming from intact families had higher self-esteem than those from single-parent or reconstituted families. The study findings showed negative correlations between depression and self-esteem for African Americans and Hispanics, with Caucasians having a stronger negative correlation between depression and self-esteem.

African Americans reported lower cocaine use than Caucasians and Hispanics while Caucasians had more severe methamphetamine use. Caucasians also indicated greater severity of narcotic/barbiturate use than African Americans and Hispanics. Females indicated greater use of cigarettes than males, and Caucasians used cigarettes most. This study did not find differences in substance abuse as a function of family composition among the three racial and ethnic groups.

Implications for Nursing Practice

The study findings demonstrate a significant difference in mental health as a function of family composition. These findings highlight the critical importance of identifying family composition, race, and cultural values when assessing, diagnosing, and treating adolescents who exhibit symptoms congruent with mental health or substance abuse disorders.

children develop mental disorders, it is assumed that factors such as resilience, intelligence, and a supportive environment aid in avoiding the development of mental disorders.

Neurobiological

Dramatic changes occur in the brain during childhood and adolescence, including a declining number of synapses (they peak at age 5), myelination of brain fibers, changes in the relative volume and activity level in different brain regions, and interactions of hormones (Blakemore et al., 2010). Myelination increases the speed of information processing, improves the conduction speed of nerve impulses, and enables faster reactions to occur. The teen years are also marked by changes in the frontal and prefrontal cortex regions, leading to improvements in executive functions, organization and planning skills, and inhibiting responses (Evans & Seligman, 2005). These changes, including cerebellum maturation and hormonal changes, reflect the emotional and behavioral fluctuations characteristic of adolescence. Early adolescence is typically characterized by low emotional regulation and intolerance for frustration; emotional and behavioral control usually increases over the course of adolescence.

Psychological Factors

Temperament

Temperament is the style of behavior a child habitually uses to cope with the demands and expectations of the environment. This style is present in infancy, modifies with maturation, and develops in the context of the social environment (Gemelli, 2008). All people have temperaments, and the fit between the child and parent's temperament is critical to the child's development. The caregiver's role in shaping that relationship is of primary importance, and the nurse can intervene to teach parents ways to modify their behaviors to improve the interaction. If there is incongruence between parent and child temperament and the caregiver is unable to respond positively to the child, there is a risk of insecure attachment, developmental problems, and future mental disorders.

By the time children enter grade school, temperament and behavioral traits can be powerful predictors of substance use and abuse in later life. These traits include shyness, aggressiveness, and rebelliousness. External risk factors for substance abuse include peer or parental substance use and involvement in legal problems such as truancy or vandalism. Researchers have also identified childhood protective factors that shield some children from drug use, including self-control, parental monitoring, academic achievement, anti–drug-use policies, and strong neighborhood attachment (National Institute on Drug Abuse, 2008).

Resilience

Many children with risk factors for the development of mental illness develop normally. The phenomenon of **resilience** has been used to describe the relationship between a child's inborn strengths and that child's success in handling stressful environmental factors. Studies have shown that resilience is influenced by internal and external factors such as self-concept, future expectations, social competence, problem-solving skills, family, and school and community interactions. The *resilient child* has the following characteristics (Bellin & Kovacs, 2006):

1. Adaptability to changes in the environment
2. Ability to form nurturing relationships with other adults when the parent is not available
3. Ability to distance self from emotional chaos
4. Good social intelligence
5. Good problem-solving skills
6. Ability to perceive a long-term future

Environmental Factors

To a far greater degree than adults, children are dependent on others. During childhood, the main context is the family. Parents model behavior and provide the child with a view of the world. If parents are abusive, rejecting, or overly controlling, the child may suffer detrimental effects at the developmental point(s) at which the trauma occurs. Familial risk factors correlate with child psychiatric disorders; these risk factors include severe marital discord, low socioeconomic status, large families and overcrowding, parental criminality, maternal psychiatric disorders, and foster-care placement.

Witnessing violence is traumatizing and a well-documented risk factor for many mental health problems, including depression, anxiety, PTSD, aggressive and delinquent behavior, drug use, academic failure, and low self-esteem (Farrell et al., 2007). Children who have experienced abuse are at risk for identifying with their aggressor and may act out, bully others, become abusers, or develop dysfunctional interpersonal relationships in adulthood.

Neglect is the most prevalent form of child abuse in the United States. According to the National Child Abuse and Neglect Data System, there were 1.7 million reports of child abuse and neglect in 2010. Of the substantiated cases, 15% were physical abuse, 9% sexual abuse, and 75% neglect. Although neglect has a much higher incidence rate than physical or sexual abuse, research into its effect on children's mental health has been studied less.

Girls are more frequently the victims of sexual abuse. Boys are also sexually abused, but the numbers are likely underreported due to shame and stigma. Sexual abuse varies from fondling to forcing a child to observe lewd acts to sexual intercourse. All instances of sexual abuse are devastating to a child who lacks the mental capacity or emotional maturation to consent to this type of a relationship. Nurses are required to report suspected abuse of a minor child to the local child protective services.

Bullying is also a risk factor for such problems as depression and suicide disorder. Children may bully and act violently toward one another, and gang involvement is a growing problem among adolescents. It is estimated there are 21,500 gangs and 73,100 members across the United States (U.S. Department of Justice, 2010). The targeted age group for gang initiation seems to be 11-13, a time of particular developmental vulnerability. Decision-making capacities are not fully formed at this stage, and they may look up to older peers for status and belonging.

HEALTH POLICY

Cyberbullying Legislation: Why Education is Preferable to Regulation

Cyberbullying is a phenomenon of increasing concern for those working with teens. Compared to previous fears about online predation, which have been greatly overblown, concerns about cyberbullying are more well-founded. There is sufficient evidence to support that the incidence is increasing. The effects of this form of bullying are as damaging as that done face to face and can have severe emotional consequences.

In the wake of a handful of high-profile cyberbullying incidents that resulted in teen suicides, some state lawmakers introduced legislation to address the issue. More recently, two very different federal approaches have been proposed. One approach is focused on the creation of a new federal felony to punish cyberbullying, which would include fines and jail time for violators. The other legislative approach is education-based and would create an Internet safety education grant program to address the issue in schools and communities.

Criminalizing what is mostly child-on-child behavior will not likely solve the age-old problem of kids mistreating one another, a problem that has traditionally been dealt with through counseling and rehabilitation at the local level. Moreover, criminalization could raise thorny free speech and due process issues related to legal definitions of harassing or intimidating speech. To the extent criminal sanctions are pursued as a solution, it may be preferable to defer to state experimentation with varying models at this time. In contrast, education and awareness-based approaches have a chance of effectively reducing truly harmful behavior, especially over the long haul. These approaches have the added benefit of avoiding court challenges or other legal entanglements. At this time it is clear that regulation is, at best, premature and that education is the better approach. If federal criminal law has a role to play, it is in punishing clear cases of harassment of minors by adults.

Szoka, B. M., & Thierer, A. D. (2009). Cyberbullying legislation: Why education is preferable to regulation. *Progress on Point, 16*(12). Retrieved from http://www.pff.org/interstitial/index.php?url=issues-pubs/pops/2009/pop16.12-cyberbullying-education-better-than-regulation.pdf.

CONSIDERING CULTURE

The Experience of Attention Deficit Hyperactivity Disorder in African-American Youth

It has long been recognized that cultural factors influence an individual's perception of health or illness, need for health care, and self-efficacy in symptom management, yet this is an area that has not been well researched. This qualitative study sought to explore how African American teenagers describe and narrate their lived experience with attention deficit hyperactivity disorder (ADHD) as well as how their culture influenced their encounters with health care providers. Previous studies have suggested that ADHD in African American youth is undiagnosed and untreated. Youth with ADHD are at higher risk for impulsive risk-taking behavior, dropping out of high school, and involvement with the juvenile justice system; historically, African American youth already are at higher risk for the latter. In regard to their encounters with health care providers, lack of effective communication (including the cultural and societal context) can adversely affect care.

Narrative expression serves an important function in the context of African American cultural traditions. Oral narratives traditionally served as a means to preserve and transmit historical events, guide and shape individual behavior to conform to societal expectations, and nurture spirituality. Common characteristics of the oral tradition can be seen to affirm the dignity of the African people, bring good to the community, and reflect on the constant resistance to a system of oppression and past enslavement. Linguistics and music have been intertwined to serve as a means of social entertainment and expression; thus, contemporary hip-hop and rap have served the role of oral narrative.

This study was conducted as part of an ongoing mixed-method longitudinal project studying youth identified as high risk for ADHD during school screenings performed between the school years of kindergarten and fifth grade. Children with developmental disabilities or autism were excluded, and only one child per household was included in the sample. Study subjects were interviewed over the course of three months, and after the initial interview the subjects initiated contact and provided their narrative stories.

Study findings reveal that the teen's narratives, while acknowledging that they behaved in problematic ways, rarely identified this as specific ADHD symptoms. Both males and females discussed particular behaviors such as "forgetfulness" (inattention); emotional reactivity, such as bad attitude and short temper (impulsiveness); and fidgeting or talking and disrupting peers during class (hyperactivity), which are consistent with ADHD diagnostic criteria. The narratives do provide insight into the teen's awareness of problematic behavior, yet their experience perceived the difficulty to exist with unrealistic adult expectations or lack of flexibility. Further exploration identified that family or caregivers did not identify the symptoms that interfere with social or academic functioning as sufficiently problematic to warrant medical care. The authors propose that African American teenagers can be useful informants of their symptoms; however, providers must become educated about their linguistics and culture so as to accurately translate this and provide congruent care. Providers need to take the time to discover culturally relevant meanings and experiences through studying narratives, which will lead to improved communication. Providers must modify communication and care to be culturally relevant, leading to recognition of behavioral symptoms and the meaning to the individual.

Koro-Ljunberg, M., Bussing, R., Williamson, P., Wilder J., & Mills, T. (2008). *Journal of Child and Family Studies, 17*, 467-485.

Cultural

Differences in cultural expectations, presence of stressors, and lack of support by the dominant culture may have profound effects on children and increase the risk of mental, emotional, and academic problems. Working with children and adolescents from diverse backgrounds requires an increased awareness of one's own biases as well as the patient's needs. The social and cultural context of the patient, including factors such as age, ethnicity, gender, sexual orientation, worldview, religiosity, and socioeconomic status should be considered when assessing and planning care.

CHILD AND ADOLESCENT PSYCHIATRIC MENTAL HEALTH NURSING

In 2007, the American Nurses Association (ANA), together with the American Psychiatric Nurses Association (APNA) and International Society of Psychiatric-Mental Health Nurses (ISPN), defined the basic-level functions in the combined child and adult *Psychiatric-Mental Health Nursing: Scope and Standards of Practice*. Child psychiatric mental health nurses utilize evidence-based psychiatric practices to provide care that is responsive to the patient and family's specific problems, strengths, personality, sociocultural context, and preferences. Another important publication for this specialty area is the *New Practice Parameters for Child/Adolescent Psychiatric Inpatient Treatment* (ISPN, 2007).

Assessing Development and Functioning

A child or adolescent with mental illness is one whose progressive personality development and functioning are hindered or arrested due to biological, psychosocial, and spiritual factors, resulting in functional impairments. In comparison, a child or adolescent who does not have a mental illness matures with only minor regressions, coping with the stressors and developmental tasks of life. Learning and adapting to the environment and bonding with others in a mutually satisfying way are signs of mental health (Box 11-1). The degree of mental health and illness can be viewed on a continuum, with one's level on the continuum changing over time.

Assessment Data

The type of data collected to assess mental health depends on the setting, the severity of the presenting problem, and the availability of resources. Box 11-2 identifies essential assessment data, including history of the present illness; medical, developmental, and family history; mental status; and neurological developmental characteristics. Agency policies determine which data are collected, but a nurse should be prepared to make an independent judgment about what to assess and how to assess it. In all cases, a physical examination is part of a complete assessment for serious mental problems.

BOX 11-1 CHARACTERISTICS OF A MENTALLY HEALTHY CHILD OR ADOLESCENT

- Trusts others and sees his or her world as being safe and supportive
- Correctly interprets reality and makes accurate perceptions of the environment and one's ability to influence it through actions (e.g., self-determination)
- Behaves in a way that is developmentally appropriate and does not violate social norms
- Has a positive, realistic self-concept and developing identity
- Adapts to and copes with anxiety and stress using age-appropriate behavior
- Can learn and master developmental tasks and new situations
- Expresses self in spontaneous and creative ways
- Develops and maintains satisfying relationships

Data Collection

Methods of collecting data include interviewing, screening, testing (neurological, psychological, intelligence), observing, and interacting with the child or adolescent. Histories are taken from multiple sources, including parents, teachers, other caregivers, and the child or adolescent when possible. Parents and teachers can complete structured questionnaires and behavior checklists. A genogram can document family composition, history, and relationships (refer to Chapter 34). Numerous assessment tools and rating scales are available, and with training, nurses can use them to effectively monitor symptoms and behavioral change.

The observation-interaction part of a mental health assessment begins with a semistructured interview in which the nurse asks the young person about the home environment, parents, and siblings and the school environment, teachers, and peers. In this format, the child is free to describe current problems and give information about his or her developmental history. Play activities, such as **therapeutic games**, drawings, and puppets are used for younger children who cannot respond to a direct approach. The initial interview is key to observing interactions among the child, caregiver, and siblings (if available) and building trust and rapport.

Mental Status Examination

Assessment of mental status of children is similar to that of adults, adapted to be appropriate for the child's cognitive capabilities and verbal skills. It provides information about the mental state at the time of the examination and identifies problems with thinking, feeling, and behaving. Broad categories to assess include safety, general appearance, socialization, activity level, speech, coordination and motor function, affect, manner of relating, intellectual function, thought processes and content, and characteristics of play.

Developmental Assessment

The developmental assessment provides information about the child or adolescent's maturational level. These data are then reviewed in relation to the child's chronological age to identify developmental strengths or deficits. The Denver II Developmental Screening Test is a popular assessment tool. For adolescents, tools may be tailored to specific areas of assessment, such as neuropsychological, physical, hormonal, and biochemical. The Youth Risk Behavior Survey for children and adolescents is conducted annually by the Centers for Disease Control and provides data as to the prevalence of risky behaviors in the population, helping the nurse to be aware of trends or increased risk.

Abnormal findings in the developmental and mental status assessments may be related to stress and adjustment problems or to more serious disorders. Nurses need to evaluate behaviors indicative of stress, as well as those of more serious psychopathology, and identify the need for further evaluation or referral. Stress-related behaviors or minor regressions may be handled by working with parents; however, the development and consistent use of maladaptive coping behaviors increases the risk of developing mental disorders. Serious psychopathology requires evaluation by an advanced practice nurse, in collaboration with clinicians from other specialty disciplines.

BOX 11-2 **TYPES OF ASSESSMENT DATA**

History of Present Illness
- Chief complaint
- Development and duration of problems
- Help sought and results
- Effect of problem on child's life at home and school
- Effect of problem on family and siblings' lives

Developmental History
- Pregnancy, birth, neonatal data
- Developmental milestones
- Description of eating, sleeping, and elimination habits and routines
- Attachment behaviors
- Types of play
- Social skills and friendships
- Sexual activity

Developmental Assessment
- Psychomotor skills
- Language skills
- Cognitive skills
- Interpersonal and social skills
- Academic achievement
- Behavior (response to stress, to changes in environment)
- Problem-solving and coping skills (impulse control, delay of gratification)
- Energy level and motivation

Neurological Assessment
- Cerebral functions
- Cerebellar functions
- Sensory functions
- Reflexes

NOTE: Functions can be observed during developmental assessment and while playing games involving a specific ability (e.g., "Simon says, 'Touch your nose.'")

Medical History
- Review of body systems
- Traumas, hospitalizations, operations, and child's response
- Illnesses or injuries affecting central nervous system
- Medications (past and current)
- Allergies

Family History
- Illnesses in related family members (e.g., seizures, mental disorders, mental retardation, hyperactivity, drug and alcohol abuse, diabetes, cancer)
- Background of family members (occupation, education, social activities, religion)
- Family relationships (separation, divorce, deaths, contact with extended family, support system)

Mental Status Assessment
- General appearance
- Activity level
- Coordination and motor function
- Affect
- Speech
- Manner of relating
- Intellectual functions
- Thought processes and content
- Characteristics of play

General Interventions for Children and Adolescents

The interventions described in this section can be used in a variety of settings: inpatient, residential, outpatient, day treatment, outreach programs in schools, and home visits. Many of the modalities can encompass activities of daily living, learning activities, multiple forms of play and recreational activities, and interactions with adults and peers.

Family Therapy

The family is critical to improving the function of a young person with a psychiatric illness; family counseling is often a key component of treatment. In family therapy, specific goals are defined for each member, identifying ways to improve and work to achieve the goals for the family or subunits within the family (e.g., parental, sibling). Homework assignments are often used for family members to practice newly learned skills outside the therapeutic environment. In addition, multiple-family therapy may prove useful for (1) learning how other families solve problems and build on strengths, (2) developing insight and improved judgment about their own family, (3) learning and sharing new information, and (4) developing lasting and satisfying relationships with other families.

Group Therapy

Group therapy for younger children uses play to introduce ideas and work through issues. For grade-school children, it combines play, learning skills, and talking about the activity. The child learns social skills by taking turns and sharing with peers. For adolescents, group therapy involves learning skills and talking, focusing largely on peer relationships and working through specific problems. Adolescent group therapy might use a popular media event or personality as the basis for a group discussion. Groups have been used effectively to deal with specific issues in a child's life (e.g., bereavement, physical abuse, substance use, dating, or chronic illnesses such as juvenile diabetes).

Behavioral Therapy

Behavior modification involves rewarding desired behavior to reduce maladaptive behaviors. Behavioral therapy and milieu management follow principles based on respecting individual rights and are classified according to the level of restrictiveness and intrusiveness. To ensure that the civil and legal rights of individuals are maintained, techniques are selected according to the **principle of least restrictive intervention**. This principle requires that more-restrictive interventions should be used *only* after less restrictive interventions have been attempted to manage the behavior and have been unsuccessful. Nurses use clinical knowledge, skills, and judgment to develop a plan for managing behaviors that present imminent danger to self or others. Restrictive techniques (such as the use of seclusion or physical restraints) are implemented to manage behavior and maintain safety only when very severe or dangerous behaviors are exhibited.

Most child and adolescent treatment settings use a behavior modification program to motivate and reward age-appropriate behaviors. One popular method is the point and level system, in which points are awarded for desired behaviors and increasing levels of privileges can be earned. The value for specific behaviors and privileges for each level are spelled out, and daily points earned are recorded. Children who work on individual behavioral goals (e.g., seeking help in problem solving) can earn additional points. Points are used to obtain a specific reward, which can be part of the system or be negotiated on an individual or group basis. These point systems can easily be applied to the home setting and used by parents and teachers to continue to assist the child in learning new skills.

Cognitive-Behavioral Therapy

Cognitive-behavioral therapy (CBT) is an evidence-based treatment approach. Simply put, it is based on the premise that negative and self-defeating thoughts lead to psychiatric pathology and that learning to replace these thoughts with more realistic and accurate appraisals results in improved functioning. Researchers and clinicians have discovered that CBT is also successful in treating children with anxiety or depressive disorders (Abernethy & Schlozman, 2008).

Disruptive Behavior Management

Controversy continues over the use of a locked seclusion room and physical restraint in managing dangerous behavior, and evidence suggests both are psychologically harmful and can be physically harmful. Deaths have resulted, primarily by asphyxiation due to physical holds during restraints; however, a child's behavior may be so destructive or dangerous that physical restraint or seclusion is required for the safety of all. All members of the treatment team who use therapeutic holding, locked seclusion, or physical restraint of children and adolescents must receive training to decrease the risk of injury to the young person and themselves. In general, seclusion is viewed as less restrictive than restraint, where all movement is constrained.

Guidelines and standards of practice for the use of seclusion or restraint have been created by the Centers for Medicare and Medicaid Services (CMS), State Mental Health Acts, and professional nursing organizations such as the International Society for Psychiatric Mental Health Nursing (ISPN) and the American Psychiatric Nursing Association (APNA). These interventions require prompt, firm, nonretaliatory protective restraint that is gentle and safe and reduces the risk of injury to self or others. Children are released as soon as they are no longer dangerous, usually after a few minutes, and adhering to best practices most facilities strive to avoid the use of all intensive interventions that restrict movement.

The decision to restrain or seclude a child is often made by the registered nurse who is working with the patient. A physician, nurse practitioner, or other advanced level practitioner must authorize this action, according to facility policy and state regulation. All patients in seclusion or restraints must be monitored constantly. Vital signs and range of motion in extremities must be monitored every 15 minutes. Hydration, elimination, comfort, and other psychological and physical needs should be monitored. The patient's family should be informed of any incident of seclusion or restraint, and family members should be encouraged to discuss the event with their child and reinforce the treatment plan to reduce the likelihood of future incidents (Masters, 2009).

Once the child is calm, the staff should discuss what happened with the patient. This helps to strengthen the nurse-patient relationship, which may have been disrupted. Debriefings provide an opportunity for staff members to discuss the event and if it could have been prevented, evaluate their emotional responses, review the plan of care, and enhance their clinical skills.

Time-out. Asking or directing a child or adolescent to take a time-out from an activity is another method for intervening to halt disruptive behaviors, allow for self-reflection, or encourage self-control. It has been found to be a less restrictive alternative to seclusion and restraint (Bowers et al., 2012). Taking a time-out may require going to a designated room or sitting on the periphery of an activity until self-control is regained and the episode is reviewed with a staff member. Time-out is used as an integral part of the treatment plan, and the child and family's input are considered in including this modality. The child's individual behavioral goals are considered in setting limits on behavior and using time-out periods. If they are overused or used as an automatic response to a behavioral infraction, time-outs lose their effectiveness.

Quiet Room. A unit may have an unlocked quiet room for a child who needs an area with decreased stimulation for regaining and maintaining self-control. The types of quiet rooms have evolved and incorporate principles of trauma-informed care. These can include the feelings room, which is carpeted and supplied with soft objects that can be punched and thrown, and the sensory room, which contains items for relaxation and meditation, such as music and yoga mats. The child is encouraged to express freely and work through feelings of anger or sadness in privacy and with staff support. The vignette on the next page shows how, through the use of time-out and a sensory room, a child begins to develop improved coping skills and decrease self-injurious behavior.

Play Therapy

Play is often described as the work of childhood through which the child learns to master impulses and adapt to the environment. Play is a medium of communication that can be used to assess developmental and emotional status, determine diagnosis, and institute therapeutic interventions. Melanie Klein (1955) and Anna Freud (1965) were the first to use play as a therapeutic tool in their psychoanalysis of children in the 1920s and 1930s. Axline

> **VIGNETTE**
> Levi, a school-aged child, was admitted to the hospital from his foster home placement. He has been in foster care since his mother died from a drug overdose; his father is currently incarcerated for armed robbery and drug-related offenses. Levi has a history of self-injurious behavior that includes biting and pinching himself and hitting his head against the wall when he is frustrated. The nurse and activity therapist have worked to teach Levi to request time in the sensory room when he begins to feel upset or anxious. He has been able to identify certain triggers and to request time in the sensory room, decreasing his episodes of self-injury over the last week.

(1969) identified the guiding principles of play therapy, which are still used by mental health professionals:

- Accept children as they are and follow their lead.
- Establish a warm, friendly relationship that fosters the expression of feelings completely.
- Recognize the child's feelings and reflect them back to promote insight.
- Accept the child's ability to solve personal problems.
- Set limits only to provide reality and security.

Play therapy occurs in playrooms that are equipped with a range of developmentally appropriate toys for both genders, including art supplies, clay or play dough, dolls and dollhouses, hand puppets, toys, building blocks, and trucks and cars. Through the use of an appropriate medium, a child can express thoughts or emotions that he or she may not be able to express verbally. The dolls, puppets, and dollhouse provide the child with opportunities to act out conflicts and situations involving the family, work through feelings, and develop more adaptive ways of coping. The following vignette shows how, through the use of play therapy, a child begins to cope with a significant life event.

> **VIGNETTE**
> Hannah, a 5-year-old with autism spectrum disorder, began having separation anxiety, excessive crying, and nightmares after she started school. Her enrollment in school was her first experience in a formal, structured classroom. The parents were referred to a play therapist. During play therapy the therapist used dolls and playhouses to help Hannah communicate her fears and anxieties. After five sessions she is able to place dolls in the model classroom and move them from room to room without becoming anxious or tearful.

Bibliotherapy

Bibliotherapy involves using literature to help the child express feelings in a supportive environment, gain insight into feelings and behavior, and learn new ways to cope with difficult situations. When children listen to or read a story, they unconsciously identify with the characters and experience a catharsis of feelings. The stories and books should be selected to reflect the situations or feelings the child is experiencing. It should be selected with consideration of the child's cognitive and developmental level and emotional readiness for the particular topic. A children's librarian has access to a large collection of stories and knows which books are written specifically to help children deal with particular subjects; however, the nurse should read the book first to be sure the content is age-appropriate and fits with the treatment plan. Whenever possible, the nurse consults with the family to make sure the books do not violate the family's belief systems. A choice of several books is offered, and a book is never forced on the child.

Therapeutic Drawing

The therapeutic use of art and drawing provides a non verbal means of expressing difficult or confusing emotions. Drawing and painting may illustrate the thoughts, feelings, and tensions children cannot express verbally, are unaware of, or are denying. Children who have experienced trauma will often show the traumatic event in their drawing when asked to draw whatever they wish. For some, however, this modality may be too threatening or not engaging. Children and adolescents can be encouraged to draw themes, such as people, families, themselves, or more abstract themes such as feelings. To use this modality, the nurse needs to be familiar with the drawing capabilities expected of children at particular developmental levels, and additional training is recommended.

Journaling

Another effective technique when working with younger persons, particularly teenagers, is using a journal. Journaling is a tangible way of recording and viewing emotions and may be a way to begin a dialogue with others. The use of a daily journal is also effective in setting goals and evaluating progress.

Music Therapy

The healing power of music has been recognized for centuries. Music has been used adjunctively to treat diverse physical and psychological disorders in various cultures throughout the world. The Bonny Guided Imagery Method (GIM) integrates Freudian and Jungian principles with imagery techniques (Bonny & Wyatt, 2009). It uses 18 different music programs to help patients access their unconscious, reduce defenses, and facilitate insight and to develop new coping skills to manage psychiatric symptoms. During a session the therapist guides the patient in exploring images and feelings inspired by the music selection chosen by the therapist. Bonny GIM has been used successfully in patients with post traumatic stress disorder, cancer, rheumatoid arthritis, and depression.

Psychopharmacology

The treatment of mental illness in children requires a multimodal approach, which may include the use of medication. Medicating children typically works best when combined with another treatment such as cognitive-behavioral therapy (Sadock & Sadock, 2008). Medications that target specific symptoms can make a real difference in a family's ability to cope and in quality of life, and they can enhance the child or adolescent's potential for growth. Medications will be discussed along with specific disorders in the following pages.

Teamwork and Safety

Children and adolescents with neurodevelopmental disorders may require intensive teamwork to promote safety on inpatient units, long-term residential care, or intensive outpatient care. Nurses collaborate with other health care providers in structuring and maintaining the therapeutic environment to provide physical safety and psychological security and improve coping. The multidisciplinary team shares and articulates a philosophy regarding how to provide physical and psychological security, promote personal growth, and work with problematic behaviors.

NEURODEVELOPMENTAL DISORDERS: CLINICAL PICTURE

According to the American Psychiatric Association (2013), the following disorders are considered under the umbrella of neurodevelopmental disorders and will be discussed now:

- Communication disorder
- Learning disorder
- Motor disorders
- Intellectual developmental disorder
- Autism spectrum disorder
- Attention deficit hyperactivity disorder

COMMUNICATION DISORDER

Communication disorders are a deficit in language skills acquisition that creates impairments in academic achievement, socialization, or self-care. Broadly, we consider speech and language as being two subcategories for evaluation communication. *Speech disorders* have to do with problems in making sounds. Children may have trouble making certain sounds such as "no" for "snow" or "wabbit" for rabbit; they may distort, add, or omit sounds. Another aspect of speech that may be disturbed is fluency, which is manifested as a stutter comprised of hesitations and repetition. While all children may have mild and transient symptoms of speech problems, speech disorders significantly impact a child's ability to communicate.

Language disorders result in difficulty understanding or in using words in context and appropriately. Difficulty understanding may be evident by inability to follow directions. Expressive language disorder is impairment in the ability to develop skills to communicate verbally or through sign language. The child demonstrates difficulty learning words or an inability to speak in complete, coherent sentences. Some children have a mixture of both problems and can neither understand others nor communicate properly themselves. These disorders range from mild to severe (National Institutes of Health, 2012).

While some children have no problem with language and no problem speaking, they may have problems relating with other people (Tomblin et al., 2004). In *social communication disorder* children have problems using verbal and nonverbal means for interacting socially with others. Impairments are also evident in written communication where the child is trying to relate to others. Autism spectrum disorders need to be ruled out in order to receive this diagnosis.

About 6% of children have some sort of communication disorder. Language disorders may be present from birth or may happen later. Causes include hearing loss, neurological disorders, intellectual disabilities, drug abuse, brain injury, physical problems such as cleft palate or lip, and vocal abuse or misuse. Frequently, the cause is unknown.

The Disabilities Education Act provides for early intervention services in every state for toddlers up to age 3 (National Dissemination Center for Children with Disabilities, 2011). Service providers will meet with the family to develop a treatment plan. Special education and services are also available for individuals ages 3 to 21. Typically, the first step in the plan is a hearing test.

SPECIFIC LEARNING DISORDER

Children with **specific learning disorders** are identified during the school years. A learning disorder is diagnosed when a child demonstrates persistent difficulty in the acquisition of reading (dyslexia), mathematics (dyscalculia), and/or written expression (dysgraphia), and their performance is well below the expected performance of their peers. Diagnosis of a learning disorder is made through the evaluation of multiple assessments, including formal psychological evaluations, and is not better explained in the context of another mental illness (American Academy of Pediatrics, 2012).

The lifetime prevalence of learning disorders is nearly 10% (Altarac & Saroha, 2007). They affect children with special health needs at more than 25% compared with about 5% in average developing children. Some factors associated with this problem are lower family education, poverty, and male gender. Learning disabilities account for the largest percentage of children receiving special education services. Long-term outcomes for children with learning disorders include low self-esteem, poor social skills, higher rates of school dropout, difficulties with attaining and maintaining employment, and poorer social adjustment (Pierangolo, & Giuliano, 2006).

Screening for learning disorders is essential for early interventions that may be beneficial. Most students with this type of disability are eligible for assistance at a school that is supported by Disabilities Education Improvement Act. This assistance involves careful monitoring of progress, special education intervention, and the establishment of an Individual Education Program.

MOTOR DISORDER

A key feature of childhood growth and development is the acquisition of gross and fine motor skills and coordination. The ability to practice, exposure to new tasks, experience, and environment are factors that play a role in motor development. Impairments in skill development, or coordination below what would be expected for the child's developmental age and severe enough to interfere with academic achievement or activities of daily living, are features of developmental coordination disorder. Serious impairments in skills development or coordination are usually apparent to all involved with the child; however, those with less severe impairments may exhibit reluctance to engage in certain tasks or activities because of embarrassment or feelings of incompetence. Two **motor disorders** will be discussed in this chapter—stereotypic movement disorder and Tourette's disorder.

Stereotypic movement disorder is manifested through repetitive, purposeless movements (e.g., hand waving, rocking, head banging, nail biting, and teeth grinding) for a period of four weeks or greater (American Academy of Pediatrics, 2012). The diagnosis of either disorder is determined by the severity of impairment in daily living and is not a symptom in the context of another disorder. Evaluation and diagnosis of motor skills occur in the context of a child's chronological and developmental age, his or her style, and strengths and weaknesses.

This disorder is more common in boys than in girls. Other disorders such as Tourette's syndrome or other tic disorders, autism spectrum disorder, or stimulant abuse are ruled out prior to receiving a stereotypic movement disorder diagnosis.

Interventions for this disorder focus on safety and prevention of injury. Helmets may be required for children who have the potential for head injury. Behavioral therapy includes habit-reversal techniques such as folding the arms when the urge to wave hands begins. Naltrexone, an opioid antagonist, may block euphoric responses from these behaviors, thereby reducing their occurrence.

Tourette's disorder is characterized by motor and verbal tics appearing between ages 2 and 7 that cause marked distress and significant impairment in social and occupational functioning (American Academy of Pediatrics, 2012). Motor tics usually involve the head but can involve the torso or limbs, and they change in location, frequency, and severity over time. Other motor tics are tongue protrusion, touching, squatting, hopping, skipping, retracing steps, and twirling when walking. Vocal tics include spontaneous production of words and sounds. Despite the Hollywood characterization of Tourette's disorder as a kid with a foul mouth, coprolalia (uttering of obscenities) occurs in fewer than 10% of cases. A child or adolescent with tics may have low self-esteem as a result of feeling ashamed, self-conscious, and rejected by peers and may severely limit behavior in public situations for fear of displaying tics.

The disorder is usually permanent, but periods of remission may occur, and symptoms often diminish during adolescence and sometimes disappear by early adulthood. A familial pattern exists in about 90% of cases. Tourette's disorder often coexists with depression, obsessive-compulsive disorder, and attention deficit hyperactivity disorder (ADHD) (Flaherty, 2008). Central nervous system stimulants increase severity of tics, so medications must be carefully monitored in children with coexisting ADHD.

The only drugs with FDA approval for treating the tics associated with Tourette's disorder are conventional antipsychotics haloperidol (Haldol) and pimozide (Orap). Aripiprazole (Abilify), an atypical antipsychotic, is being used investigationally for both tics and explosive outbursts (Packer, 2011). Clonidine hydrochloride (Catapres), an alpha 2-adrenergic agonist used to treat hypertension, is prescribed for tics. While less effective and far slower acting than the antipsychotics, it has fewer side effects. The antianxiety drug clonazepam (Klonopin) is used as a supplement to other medications; it may work by reducing anxiety and resultant tics. Botulinum Toxin Type A (Botox) injections are used to calm the muscle(s) associated with tics.

Behavioral techniques have been found to reduce tic expression (Packer, 2011). They are referred to as habit reversal, and the most promising form is called Comprehensive Behavior Intervention for Tics. It works by making the patient aware of the urge to tic building up and then using a muscular response that is in competition to or incompatible with the tic.

A sort of pacemaker for the brain, deep brain stimulation (DBS) is used when more conservative treatments fail. A fine wire is threaded into affected areas of the brain and connected to a small device implanted under the collarbone that delivers electrical impulses. Users of DBS can turn the device on to control tics or shut it off when they go to sleep.

INTELLECTUAL DEVELOPMENT DISORDER

Intellectual development disorders (IDD), previously called mental retardation, are disorders that are characterized by deficits in three areas. The first, intellectual functioning, is characterized by deficits in reasoning, problem solving, planning, judgment, abstract thinking, and academic ability as compared to same-age peers. The second, social functioning, is impaired in terms of communication and language, interpreting and acting on social cues, and regulating emotions. Finally, practical aspects of daily life are impacted by a deficit in managing age-appropriate activities of daily living, functioning at school or work, and performing self-care. Impairments must be evidenced during childhood development, range from mild to severe, and include the consideration of the person's level of dependence on others for ongoing care and support (Carulla et. al, 2011).

The incidence of IDD has been estimated at about 1% to 2% of the population. The etiology of IDDs may be primarily biological, psychosocial, or a combination of both. The factors that have been correlated with IDD are heredity, problems with pregnancy or perinatal development, environmental influences, or a direct result of a medical condition. Hereditary factors can include chromosomal disorders such as Fragile X, Down or Klinefelter's syndrome, inborn errors of metabolism such as phenylketonuria, or genetic abnormalities. These are implicated in about 5% of cases. Approximately 10% are due to problems during pregnancy or birth and include malnutrition, chronic maternal substance abuse, maternal infection, and complications of pregnancy such as toxemia, placenta previa, or trauma to the head during birth. In addition, up to 20% of cases are attributed to environmental or social factors such as impoverished social environments that don't foster the development of social or linguistic skills or a lack of a nurturing relationship. IDDs can also be associated with other mental disorders such as autism spectrum disorders.

APPLICATION OF THE NURSING PROCESS

ASSESSMENT

ASSESSMENT GUIDELINES

Intellectual Development Disorders

1. Assess for delays in cognitive and physical development or lack of ability to perform tasks or achieve milestones in relation to peers. Gather information from family, caregivers, or others actively involved in the child's life.
2. Assess for delays in cognitive, social, or personal functioning, focusing on strengths and abilities.

ASSESSMENT GUIDELINES—cont'd

Intellectual Development Disorders

3. Assess for areas of independent functioning and the need for support/assistance to meet requirements of daily living (examples are hygiene, dressing, or feeding).
4. Assess for physical and emotional signs of potential neglect or abuse. Be aware that children with behavioral and developmental problems are at risk for abuse.
5. Be knowledgeable about community resources or programs that can provide family and caregivers with the needed resources and support to meet the child's need for intellectual and social development and the family's need for education and emotional support.

DIAGNOSIS

The child with IDD has impairments in conceptual, social, and practical functioning, ranging from mild to severe. The severity of impairment is evidenced in the ability to communicate effectively, meet one's self-care and safety needs, and socialize in an age-appropriate manner. Due to the increased need for supervision and assistance with daily living and the chronic nature of the disorder, families or caregivers may experience significant stress and be at risk for impaired family functioning. Table 11-1 lists potential nursing diagnoses.

TABLE 11-1 NURSING DIAGNOSES IN NEURODEVELOPMENTAL DISORDERS

SIGNS AND SYMPTOMS	NURSING DIAGNOSIS
Lack of responsiveness or interest in others, empathy, or sharing	*Impaired social interaction* *Risk for impaired attachment*
Lack of cooperation or imaginative play with peers	*Activity intolerance* *Situational low self-esteem*
Language delay or absence, stereotyped or repetitive use of language	*Impaired verbal communication*
Inability to feed, bathe, dress, or toilet self at age-appropriate level	*Delayed growth and development*
Head banging, face slapping, hand biting	*Risk for trauma*
Frequent disregard for bodily needs	*Self-care deficit* *Risk for situational low self-esteem*
Failure to follow age-appropriate social norms	*Ineffective coping*
Depression	*Stress overload* *Spiritual distress*
Refusal to attend school	*Ineffective coping* *Readiness for enhanced parenting*
Inability to concentrate, withdrawal, difficulty in functioning, feeling down, change in vegetative symptoms	*Risk for suicide*

Herdman, T.H. (Ed.). *Nursing diagnoses—Definitions and classification 2012-2014.*

OUTCOMES IDENTIFICATION

Nursing Outcomes Classification (NOC) (Moorhead et al., 2013) identifies a number of outcomes appropriate for the child with IDD:

- Using spoken language to make or respond to requests
- Engaging in simple social interactions and accepting assistance or feedback regarding behavior without frustration.
- Tolerating social interaction for short periods of time without becoming disruptive or frustrated.
- Refraining from acting impulsively toward self or others when frustrated.

Additionally, the family may be in denial over the diagnosis. A family outcome would be for the family to acknowledge the existence of impairment and its potential to alter family routines.

IMPLEMENTATION

Psychosocial Interventions

Nurses may provide services to children with IDDs in a variety of settings. Children with IDDs may be cared for in the community through services determined and coordinated by early intervention programs or public school programs as they reach school age. Federal legislation, the Individuals with Disabilities in Education Act (IDEA), requires that public schools provide services to assist children with emotional or developmental disorders to participate in school (U.S. Department of Education). IDEA provides a definition of children with disabilities or impairments who require special services or assistance, and it requires state public schools to provide these services either through an Individualized Education Plan (IEP) or Section 504 of the Rehabilitation Act. Individuals may also require short-term hospitalization related to socially impaired behaviors such as aggression, self-harm, or severe self-care deficits.

Treatment plans should be individualized and realistic, using intervention designed to assist the child to achieve his or her potential. Although the care plan is developed for the child, family members or caregivers should be included in the process as they will be involved in the ongoing care of the child. Supportive education should be ongoing regarding the scope and nature of the illness; conceptual, social, and practical deficits; and realistic assessment of the child's potential. Long-term planning should include consideration of continuing care needs as the child ages and matures into adulthood.

EVALUATION

In evaluating the family and child with IDD, it is important for nurses to use a strength-based perspective. In the assessment, we identify both the areas of need and capabilities, focusing on how to maximize the family resources and link to services where need exists. Areas to evaluate at the individual level will be multifaceted as the needs for direct care and services vary greatly among individual clients. Specific areas to evaluate include linkage with all the necessary service providers. Are the child and family receiving timely and efficient services? Is the care patient-and family-centered, allowing for the family to take a lead role in directing the plan of care? For the child with an IDD, personal and environmental safety is of utmost importance and should be an ongoing component of the evaluation process. Cognitive capacity, progress, and potential will influence resource allocation and short-term goals as well as long-term treatment planning. In addition, evaluation of the individual's capabilities to manage activities of daily living and social relationships will be factors that require continuous evaluation and treatment plan modifications. Persons with IDD require lifelong services that range in intensity dependent on the severity of symptomatology.

Families may require a great deal of education and ongoing reinforcement to achieve realistic expectations for the child. Due to the chronic nature of IDDs, comparative measures of family and individual development will guide treatment. While the individual may be the direct recipient of care, the family system may have been disrupted. Families, for the most part, possess the ability to adapt to and solve their own problems, given access to the appropriate resources. If interventions are unsuccessful, rather than labeling the family or individual resistant or noncompliant, the nurse must carefully inquire as to the decision-making process and appreciate the reasons for modifying or choosing not to use a particular intervention. Families and individuals with IDDs require lifelong support, so our evaluations will focus on both short- and long-term goals. Gauging the progress toward normalization will help the nurse to plan for greater assumption of direct care and coordination of services by the family. As treatment progresses, it is important for all members of the multidisciplinary team and the family to include long-term planning, with a goal of transitioning the child to a level of supervised or assisted care as he or she ages into adulthood.

AUTISM SPECTRUM DISORDERS

Autism spectrum disorders (ASDs) are complex neurobiological and developmental disabilities that typically appears during a child's first three years of life. Autism affects the normal development of the brain in social interaction and communication skills. It ranges in severity from mild to moderate to severe. Symptoms associated with autism spectrum disorders include significant deficits in social relatedness, including communication, nonverbal behavior, and age-appropriate interaction. There are deficits in developing and maintaining relationships. Other behaviors include stereotypical repetitive speech, use of objects, overadherence to routines or rituals, fixations with particular objects, hyper- or hypo-reactivity to sensory input, and extreme resistance to change. The symptoms will first occur in childhood and cause impairments in everyday functioning.

About 5% of individuals with autism spectrum disorder have a single gene direct inheritance form of the disorder; they are Fragile X, tuberous sclerosis, and Rett Syndrome (Insel, 2012). There is a genetic component to autism. The concordance rate for identical twins is 70% to 90% (Smoller et al., 2008). Autism is four times more common in boys than girls (Sadock & Sadock, 2008). It has no racial, ethnic, or social boundaries and is not influenced by family income, educational levels, or lifestyles.

Without intensive intervention, individuals with severe autism may not be able to live and work independently, and only about one third achieve partial independence with restricted interests and activities. Early intervention for children with autism can greatly enhance their potential for a full, productive life. Unfortunately, many families with an autistic child may not recognize the deficits in social and communicative skills and seek help early. Problems with left hemispheric functions (e.g. language, logic, and reasoning) are evident, yet music and visual-spatial activities may, in rare cases, be enhanced such as in savant syndrome (Ursano et al., 2008). Often, symptoms are first noticed when the infant fails to be interested in others or to be socially responsive through eye contact and facial expressions. Some children show improvement during development, but puberty can be a turning point toward either improvement or deterioration.

APPLICATION OF THE NURSING PROCESS

ASSESSMENT

ASSESSMENT GUIDELINES

Autism Spectrum Disorders

1. Assess for developmental delays, uneven development, or loss of acquired abilities. Use baby books and diaries, photographs, videotapes, or anecdotal reports from nonfamily caregivers.
2. Assess the parent-child relationship for evidence of bonding, anxiety, tension, and fit of temperaments.
3. Assess for physical and emotional signs of possible abuse. Be aware that children with behavioral and developmental problems are at risk for abuse.
4. Be knowledgeable about community programs providing support services for parents and children, including parent education, counseling, and after-school programs.

DIAGNOSIS

The child with ASD has severe impairments in social interactions and communication skills, often accompanied by stereotypical behavior, interests, and activities. The stress on the family can be severe, owing to the chronic nature of the disease. The severity of the impairment is evident in the degree of responsiveness to or interest in others, the presence of associated behavioral problems (e.g., head banging), and the ability to bond with peers. Table 11-1 lists potential diagnoses.

OUTCOMES IDENTIFICATION

NOC (Moorhead et al., 2013) identifies a number of outcomes appropriate for the child with ASD.

IMPLEMENTATION

Psychosocial Interventions

Children with ASD are referred to **early intervention programs** once communication and behavioral symptoms are identified, typically in the second or third year of life. Through case management and coordination of care, they may be treated in therapeutic nursery schools, day treatment programs, and special education classes in public or specialized private schools. Their education and treatment with therapeutic modalities are mandated under the Children with Disabilities Act.

Treatment plans include behavior management with a reward system, teaching parents to provide structure, rewards, consistency in rules, and expectations at home in order to shape and modify behavior and foster the development of socially appropriate skills. Children with ASD may receive physical, occupational, and speech therapy as part of the plan of care.

As with all patient care, especially with the management of chronic health conditions, it is important that the nurse recognize and capitalize on the individual's and family's strengths. Also, the family's goals and priorities should influence the plan of care. It is the job of the multidisciplinary team to assist the family in making realistic goals.

Psychobiological Interventions

Pharmacological

Pharmacological agents target specific symptoms and may be used to improve relatedness and decrease anxiety, compulsive behaviors, or agitation. The unconventional agents such as risperidone, olanzapine, quietiapine, and aripiprazole have been shown to reduce harmful behaviors. The SSRIs are the most popular psychotropic agent used in this population, improving mood and reducing anxiety thereby allowing the patient a higher degree of tolerance for new situations.

EVALUATION

ASDs yield deficits in communication and social skills in the individual with the level of severity varying from person to person; therefore, evaluation will be individualized. The broad measures will include the individual's communication and social skills with family, peers, and other care providers, especially those within the academic setting. Due to the variations in severity, using a strength-based perspective assists the multidisciplinary team in planning goals that are realistic for both the individual and family. For children with milder forms of ASD, it is reasonable to expect greater participation and input from the child; however, with those with more severe impairments, there will be greater reliance on the family. Family members must have clear and realistic expectations of the long-term needs of their child and be linked with the appropriate health care and community resources to assist with long-term planning.

Evaluation measurements should include access to the timely, efficient, and effective provision of all needed support services and the family's awareness of how to advocate for appropriate service provision. Has the early intervention program been accessed? How are the child and family coordinating appointments? For the school-aged child, is the IEP or 504 plan reflective of realistic educational goals? The nurse should monitor both the individual and the family for the effects of stress related to treatment by multiple providers and the subsequent disruptions or intrusions that can occur. Increased stress may interfere with the family's ability to utilize resources, or family members may find the coordination and integration of services to be overwhelming. In managing chronic conditions the role of the health care team needs to be viewed as supportive rather than authoritative and responsible for all aspects of care. The ultimate goal is to create an informed, activated patient and family with adequate support for decision making and self-management.

ATTENTION DEFICIT HYPERACTIVITY DISORDER

Individuals with **attention deficit hyperactivity disorder** (ADHD) show an inappropriate degree of inattention, impulsiveness, and hyperactivity. Some children can have attention deficit disorder without hyperactivity (ADD). In order to diagnose a child with ADHD symptoms must be present in at least two settings (e.g., at home and school) and occur before age twelve. In adults, fewer symptoms are necessary to gain a diagnosis. The disorder is most often detected when the child has difficulty adjusting to elementary school. Attention problems and hyperactivity contribute to low frustration tolerance, temper outbursts, labile moods, poor school performance, peer rejection, and low self-esteem.

It is estimated that nearly 8% of children between the ages of 5 and 11 have ADHD and about 12% of adolescents aged 12 and 17 have ADHD (CDC, 2010). Boys have more than twice the rate as girls. Children in poor health are more than twice as likely to have ADHD (8% versus 21%). The median age of onset is 7 years old. While symptoms of the disorder emerge in childhood or adolescence, they may go undiagnosed until functional impairments become noticeable in adulthood.

Children with ADHD are often diagnosed with comorbid disorders such as oppositional defiant disorder or conduct disorder. The behaviors and symptoms associated with ADHD can include hyperactivity, difficulty taking turns or maintaining social relationships, high levels of impulsivity, poor social boundaries, intrusive behaviors, or frequently interrupting others. Those with inattentive type of ADHD may exhibit high degrees of distractibility and disorganization; they may be unable to complete challenging or tedious tasks, become easily bored, lose things frequently, or require frequent prompts to complete tasks.

APPLICATION OF THE NURSING PROCESS

ASSESSMENT

ASSESSMENT GUIDELINES

Attention Deficit Hyperactivity Disorder

1. Observe for level of physical activity, attention span, talkativeness, frustration tolerance, impulse control, and the ability to follow directions and complete tasks without need for frequent redirection. Assess for developmental variance in these behaviors.
2. Assess social skills, friendship history, problem-solving skills, and school performance. Academic failure and poor peer relationships lead to low self-esteem, depression, and further acting out.
3. Assess for associated comorbidities, such as anxiety and depression.

DIAGNOSIS

Children and adolescents with ADHD can be overactive and may display disruptive behaviors that are impulsive, angry, aggressive, and often dangerous. They may have difficulty with maintaining attention in situations that require sustained attention and have difficulty following simple rules required for board games or team activities. In addition, their behaviors negatively impact their ability to develop fulfilling peer and family relationships. They are often in conflict with others, are noncompliant, do not follow age-appropriate social norms, and may use inappropriate ways to meet their needs. Refer to Table 11-1 for potential nursing diagnoses.

OUTCOMES IDENTIFICATION

NOC identifies a number of outcomes appropriate for the child with ADHD. *NOC* outcomes target hyperactivity, impulse self-control, the development of self-identity and self-esteem, positive coping skills, and family functioning.

IMPLEMENTATION

Psychosocial Interventions

Interventions for patients with ADHD focus on correcting the faulty personality (ego and superego) development, which includes firmly entrenched patterns, such as blaming others and denial of responsibility for their actions. Children and adolescents with these disorders also must generate more mature and adaptive coping mechanisms and pro-social goals, a process that is gradual and cannot be accomplished during short-term treatment.

Treatment may include hospitalization for those who present an imminent danger to self or others but is predominantly on an outpatient basis, using individual, group, and family therapy, with an emphasis on parenting issues. Children whose behavior requires longer-term intensive treatment may be referred to residential treatment or group home placement.

To control the aggressive behaviors found with these disorders, a wide variety of pharmacological agents have been tried, including antipsychotics, lithium, anticonvulsants, and antidepressants. Psychostimulants must be used judiciously as they appear to have a dose-dependent effect; low doses stimulate aggressive behaviors while moderate to high doses suppress aggression. This appears to be most effective in those patients with ADHD and associated aggressive behavior. Mood stabilizers such as lithium and anticonvulsants reduce aggressive behavior and are recommended for impulsivity, explosive temper, and mood lability. Adrenolytic medications such as clonidine are also useful in reducing agitation and rage and in increasing frustration tolerance. Antipsychotic medications have reduced violent behavior, hyperactivity, and social unresponsiveness. Due to the risk of tardive dyskinesia associated with long-term use, antipsychotic medications are recommended for use only in severely aggressive conduct disorder (Perepletchikova & Kazdin, 2005). Cognitive-behavioral therapy is used to change the pattern of misconduct by fostering the development of internal controls and working with the family to improve coping and support. Development of problem solving, conflict resolution, empathy, and social skills is an important component of the treatment program.

Families are actively engaged in therapy and given support in using parenting skills to provide nurturance and set consistent limits. They are taught techniques for modifying behavior, monitoring medication for effects, collaborating with teachers to foster academic success, and setting up a home environment that is consistent, structured, and nurturing and that promotes achievement of normal developmental milestones. If families are abusive, drug dependent, or highly disorganized, the child may require out-of-home placement.

Techniques for managing disruptive behaviors are listed in Box 11-3.

Psychobiological Interventions

Psychopharmacology

Paradoxically, the mainstay of treatment for ADHD is the use of psychostimulant drugs. Responses to these drugs can be dramatic and can quickly increase attention and task-directed behavior while reducing impulsivity, restlessness, and distractibility (Lehne, 2010). Methylphenidate (Ritalin) and amphetamine salts (Adderall) are the most widely used psychostimulants because of their relative safety and simplicity of use. As with any controlled substance, however, there is a risk of abuse and misuse, such as the sale of the medication on the street or the use by people for whom the medication was not intended.

Insomnia is a common side effect while taking the stimulant ADHD medications (Lehne, 2010). Treating with the minimum effective dose is essential, as is administering the medication no later than 4:00 in the afternoon. The extended-release formulations of these medications have improved dosing and scheduling, allowing for a morning administration with sustained release of the medication over the course of the day and with a decreased incidence of insomnia. Other common side effects include appetite suppression, headache, abdominal pain, and lethargy. A nonstimulant selective norepinephrine reuptake inhibitor, atomoxetine (Strattera), is approved for childhood and adult ADHD (primarily inattentive).

Therapeutic responses develop slowly, and it may take up to 6 weeks for full improvement (Lehne, 2010). Strattera should be used with extreme caution in those patients with comorbid depression or anxiety as its use has been associated with an increased incidence of suicidal ideation. The most common side effects are gastrointestinal disturbances, reduced appetite, weight loss, urinary retention, dizziness, fatigue, and insomnia. It may also cause liver injury in some patients and a small increase in blood pressure and heart rate. Ongoing monitoring of vital signs and regular screening of liver function are key aspects of assessment. Rarely, serious allergic reactions occur. Patients and their families should be clearly educated on the risks and benefits of treatment prior to starting this medication.

BOX 11-3 TECHNIQUES FOR MANAGING DISRUPTIVE BEHAVIORS

Behavioral contract: A verbal or written agreement between the patient and nurse or other parties (e.g., family, treatment team, teacher) about behaviors, expectations, and needs. The contract is periodically evaluated and reviewed and typically coupled with rewards and other contingencies, positive and negative.

Counseling: Verbal interactions, role playing, and modeling to teach, coach, or maintain adaptive behavior and provide positive reinforcement. Best used with motivated youth and those with well-developed communication and self-reflective skills.

Modeling: A method of learning behaviors or skills by observation and imitation that can be used in a wide variety of situations. It is enhanced when the modeler is perceived to be similar (e.g., age, interests) and attending to the task is required.

Role playing: A counseling technique in which the nurse, the patient, or a group of youngsters acts out a specified script or role to enhance their understanding of that role, learn and practice new behaviors or skills, and practice specific situations. It requires well-developed expressive and receptive language skills.

Planned ignoring: When behaviors are determined by staff to be attention seeking and not dangerous, they may be ignored. Additional interventions may be used in conjunction (e.g., positive reinforcement for on-task actions).

Use of signals or gestures: Use a word, a gesture, or eye contact to remind the child to use self-control. To help promote behavioral change, this may be used in conjunction with a behavioral contract and a reward system. An example is placing your finger to your lips and making eye contact with a child who is talking during a quiet drawing activity.

Physical distance and touch control: Moving closer to the child for a calming effect, perhaps putting an arm around the child (with permission). Evaluate the effect of this, because some children may find this more agitating and may need more space and less physical closeness. It also may involve putting the nurse or a staff member between certain children who have a history of conflict.

Redirection: A technique used following an undesirable or inappropriate behavior to engage or re-engage an individual in an appropriate activity. It may involve the use of verbal directives (e.g., setting firm limits), gestures, or physical prompts.

Additional affection: Involves giving a child planned emotional support for a specific problem or engaging in an enjoyable activity. It can be used to redirect a child away from an undesirable activity as well. This shows acceptance of the child while ignoring the behavior and can increase rapport in the nurse-patient relationship.

Use of humor: Use well-timed, appropriate kidding about some external, nonpersonal (to the child) event as a diversion to help the child save face and relieve feelings of guilt or fear.

Clarification as intervention: Breaking down a problem situation that a child experiences can help the child understand the situation, the roles of others, and his or her own motivation for the behavior. This can be done verbally and using worksheets, depending on the age and functional level of the child.

Restructuring: Changing an activity in a way that will decrease the stimulation or frustration (e.g., shorten a story or change to a physical activity). This requires flexibility and planning and an alternative if the activity is not going well.

Limit setting: Involves giving direction, stating an expectation, or telling a child what to do or where to go. This should be done firmly, calmly, without judgment or anger, preferably in advance of any problem behavior occurring, and should be used consistently by all staff in a treatment setting. An example would be, "I would like for you to stop turning the light on and off."

Simple restitution: Refers to a procedure in which an individual is required or expected to correct the adverse environmental or relational effects of his or her misbehavior by restoring the environment to its prior state, making a plan to correct his or her actions with the nurse, and implementing the plan (e.g., apologizing to the persons harmed, fixing the chairs that are upturned).

Physical restraint: Use therapeutic holding to control and protect the child from impulses to act out and hurt self or others.

The dosing schedule of these medications is important. Drug preparations vary in their onset of action and duration of action. This may result in dosing once a day (in the morning) or up to three times a day. Once-a-day dosing provides convenience and limits missed doses and potential stigma of taking medications at school, so long-acting medications should be used when possible. See Table 11-2 for a summary of the FDA-approved medications used to treat ADHD.

EVALUATION

For the family and child with ADHD, evaluation will focus on the symptom patterns and severity. For those with ADHD, inattentive type, the focus of evaluation will be academic performance, activities of daily living, social relationships, and personal perception. For those with ADHD, hyperactive-impulsive type or combined type, the focus will be on both academic and behavioral responses.

Evaluation of the response to pharmacotherapy is important; stimulant medications are quite effective in symptom management yet can yield very troublesome side effects. Monitoring and managing the timing and administration of medication is dependent on ongoing evaluation of efficacy or side effect. Medication adjustments once the child has stabilized on a pharmacotherapy regimen may occur; however, these tend to be infrequent and are often associated with the child's physical growth and development. As the child responds positively to a pharmacotherapy regimen, the individual and family members become familiar with intended effects and quickly identify when a need for medication evaluation is required.

For all children with neurobiological disorders, safety is a major emphasis; for those with ADHD of any subtype, maintenance of personal safety requires ongoing evaluation. Children with ADHD can have difficulties in assessing the environment or realistically assessing risks of danger. They

TABLE 11-2 **DRUG TREATMENT OF PATIENTS WITH ADHD**

CLASSIFICATION	TRADE NAME	INDICATIONS	DURATION	SCHEDULE
Methylphenidate	Ritalin	Ages 6-12	3-5 hours	2 or 3 times a day
Immediate release	Methylin	Ages 6 and older	3-5 hours	
Extended or sustained release	Ritalin SR	Ages 6-12	6-8 hours	1 or 2 times a day
	Metadate ER	Ages 6-15	6-8 hours	1 or 2 times a day
	Metadate CD	Ages 6-15	6-8 hours	Once a day
	Ritalin LA	Ages 6-12	7-9 hours	Once a day
	Concerta	Ages 6-65	Up to 14	Once a day
Transdermal patch	Daytrana	Ages 6-12	10-12 hours (up to 3 hours after removal)	Once a day
Dexmethylphenidate SR	Focalin	Ages 6 and older	4-5 hours	2 times a day
Extended release	Focalin XR	Ages 6 and older	6-8 hours	Once a day
Dextroamphetamine	Dexedrine	Ages 3-16	4-6 hours	2 or 3 times a day
Short acting				
Intermediate acting	Dexedrine Spansules	Ages 6-16	6-10 hours	1 or 2 times a day
Lisdexamfetamine dimesylate	Vyvanse	Ages 6-12	10-12 hours	Once a day
Amphetamine mixture	Adderall	Ages 6 and older	4-6 hours	2 times a day
Intermediate acting				
Extended release	Adderall–XR	Ages 6 and older	10-12 hours	1 or 2 times a day
Atomoxetine	Strattera	Ages 6-65	24 hours	Once a day
Extended release				

Data from Lehne, R. A. (2010). *Pharmacology for nursing care* (7th ed.). Philadelphia, PA: Saunders; Huffman, J. C., & Stern, T. A. (2008). Side effects of psychotropic medications. In T. S. Stern, J. F. Rosenbaum, M. Fava, J. Biederman, & S. L. Rauch (Eds.), *Massachusetts General Hospital comprehensive clinical psychiatry* (pp. 705-720). St. Louis, MO: Mosby.

may increase the risk of harm to self or others due to aggressive or disruptive behaviors. The nurse should take into consideration the developmental level of the child and evaluate for appropriateness of action and impulse control.

At the family system level the nurse will assess the level of understanding of symptoms and symptom management by family members. Unrealistic expectations can result in frustration for both the individual and family and yield unfulfilling or negative interpersonal relationships. What is the family's perception of the problem? What type of services do they need to support their attempts in implementing effective behavioral plans? Has the family system stabilized, and are family developmental tasks the focus of family member's energies, or is the child's illness continuing to tax family resources?

Finally, long-term planning and goal setting should be a core evaluation measure; ADHD is chronic and unremitting in nature, and symptoms frequently persist into adulthood. Are the patient and family setting realistic expectations as the child prepares to transition to postsecondary education or a vocation? Has the patient assumed primary responsibility for treatment planning and symptom management? Supporting the patient and family in the decision-making process and linking them with any additional resources needed can assist in a smooth transition. Satisfaction with treatment and their interaction with the multidisciplinary team can foster a positive ongoing relationship leading to improved outcomes.

QUALITY IMPROVEMENT

As we learn about the assessment and management of children with neurodevelopmental and mental health disorders, we must include ongoing assessment of the efficacy, safety, and outcomes of care. Quality assessment and measurement is an important aspect of continuous quality improvement and includes the establishment of indicators of care and outcomes measures that are monitored regularly and evaluated to validate evidence-based practice or to provide information that guides program revisions.

Currently, there is a lack of reliable quality measures designed for child and adolescent mental health; however, the Center for Quality Assessment and Improvement in Mental Health (2007) identifies the following measures for child and adolescent mental health:.

- Access to child specialty care for treatment of depression
- Family involvement in the treatment of ADHD
- Stimulant medication treatment for ADHD
- Antipsychotic treatment for childhood psychoses
- Completion of treatment for substance use disorders
- Referral to post-detoxification treatment services

These measures are based primarily on expert opinion or consensus; therefore, more data collection and analysis are required to develop valid and reliable measures. Psychiatric mental health nurses can play a key role in assisting with this through the use of tools and involvement in quality assessment and measurement activities in the wide variety of work settings where child and adolescent mental health services are delivered.

KEY POINTS

- One in five children and adolescents in the United States suffers from a major mental illness that causes significant impairments at home, at school, with peers, and in the community.
- An estimated two thirds of all young persons with mental health problems are not receiving proper treatment.
- Factors known to affect the development of mental and emotional problems in children and adolescents include genetic influences, biochemical (prenatal and postnatal) factors, temperament, psychosocial developmental factors, social and environmental factors, and cultural influences.
- The characteristics of a resilient child include an adaptable temperament, the ability to form nurturing relationships with surrogate parental figures, the ability to distance the self from emotional chaos in parents and family, good social intelligence, the ability to perceive a future, and problem-solving skills.
- Seclusion and restraint should be used as last resorts after less restrictive interventions have failed and only in the case of dangerous behavior toward self or others. Seclusion and restraint require continuous monitoring by trained staff and must not be punitive. Parents/guardians should be notified if such measures are used.
- Communication disorders are a deficit in language skills acquisition that creates impairments in academic achievement, socialization, or getting self-care.
- Learning disorders may be in the areas of reading, mathematics, or written expression with performance in those areas below the level expected for the age and cognitive level. Interventions are designated in an Individualized Education Plan (IEP) and provided through special education in public schools.
- Motor disorders are manifested by impairments in gross and fine motor skill acquisition. They can range from mild to profound in severity. Stereotypic movement disorders are characterized by purposeless, repetitive movements that interfere with daily living activities. Tourette's disorder is characterized by motor and vocal tics that interfere with the child's social and academic functioning.
- Autism spectrum disorders typically occur within the first three years of life, yielding deficits in social interaction and communication skills. Children with ASDs are referred to early intervention programs and continue to receive school-based services as they enter the public education system.
- Attention deficit hyperactivity disorders are evidenced by symptoms of inattentiveness and/or hyperactivity and impulsivity that are developmentally inappropriate and cause the child problems in a number of settings, such as home, school, and community. ADHD is treated primarily with stimulant medications and behavioral therapies.
- Treatment of childhood and adolescent disorders requires a multimodal approach in almost all instances, and family involvement is seen as critical to improvement in outcomes.
- Nurses can be important advocates for children with severe emotional and behavioral disorders.
- Cognitive-behavioral therapies, social skills groups, family therapy, parent training in behavioral techniques, and individual therapy focused on self-esteem issues have been found useful.
- Skills training may focus on a variety of areas, depending on the child's or adolescent's presenting symptoms, and requires an individualized assessment to determine each child's need.

CRITICAL THINKING EXERCISES

1. Chris, a 5-year-old boy, has been diagnosed with autism spectrum disorder (ASD).
   a. Describe the specific behavioral data you would find on assessment in terms of (1) communication, (2) social interactions, (3) behaviors and activities.
   b. Name at least three realistic outcomes for a child with ASD.
   c. Which interventions do you think are the most important for a child with ASD? Identify at least six.
   d. What kinds of support should the family receive?
2. Joe is an 8-year-old boy in the third grade who has been diagnosed with attention deficit hyperactivity disorder (ADHD).
   a. What clinical behaviors might he be exhibiting at home and in the classroom? Give behavioral examples of his (1) inattention, (2) hyperactivity, and (3) impulsivity.
   b. Identify at least six intervention strategies one might use for him, including a discussion of the use of medication management. Identify at least two different medications that could be used, and identify their intended effect, potential side effects, and key patient teaching information.
   c. Describe the concept of time-out and how it could be used therapeutically with Joe.
3. Samantha is a 6-year-old girl who has been diagnosed with intellectual development disorder and has been biting and hitting herself in the face when frustrated.
   a. Explain to one of your classmates the assessment data that would be relevant in terms of (1) school performance, (2) socialization with peers, (3) activities of daily living, and (4) coping with frustration.
   b. What are the normal developmental milestones for a 6-year-old child?
   c. What are three ways you could support Samantha's parents? Where could you refer this family within your own community?
   d. What is the overall prognosis for children with this disorder?

CHAPTER REVIEW

1. The nurse is developing a care plan for a teenage patient with attention deficit hyperactivity disorder who is at high risk for self-harm due to poor judgment, high risk-taking behaviors, and impulsivity. Which of the following is the priority nursing intervention?
   a. Schedule a regular nurse-patient session daily, and encourage her to explore stressors that may worsen her depressed mood.
   b. Develop a "no self-harm" contract with the patient, and encourage her to engage in all unit activities
   c. Assign a staff member one-to-one close observation until the treatment team determines she is no longer a risk for self-harm.
   d. The patient is to wear hospital-issue clothing (pajamas) and sit/sleep within view of staff until the physician determines she is no longer a risk for self-harm.

2. The nurse is preparing to assess a child who primarily speaks Spanish but is fluent in English. Which is the appropriate method for gathering information?
   a. Begin the assessment in English.
   b. Utilize a Spanish dictionary to ask questions of the child.
   c. Ask the child if he understands English.
   d. Obtain an interpreter who is fluent in Spanish
3. The nurse educator is teaching a new nurse about seclusion and restraint. Order the following interventions from least (1) to most (4) restrictive:
   a. Allowing the patient to sit in the sensory room
   b. Placing the patient in physical restraints
   c. Placing the patient in a locked seclusion room
   d. Offering a PRN medication by mouth
4. A 7-year-old male without any other diagnosed problem engages in jaw clenching and rocking back and forth. Which condition should the nurse anticipate?
   a. Attention deficit hyperactivity disorder
   b. Tourette's disorder
   c. Stereotypic movement disorder
   d. Autism spectrum disorder
5. The nurse is caring for a patient with attention deficit hyperactivity disorder. The child has been prescribed methylphenidate (Ritalin). Which of the following symptoms are side effects the nurse will monitor for? *(Select all that apply.)*
   a. Hypotension
   b. Decreased appetite
   c. Sedation
   d, Insomnia
   e. Headache
   f. Seizure

Answers to Chapter Review
1. c; 2. a; 3. a = 1, b = 4, c = 3, d = 2; 4. d; 5. b, d, e.

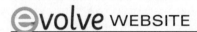

Visit the Evolve website for a posttest on the content in this chapter: http://evolve.elsevier.com/Varcarolis

Post-Test interactive review

REFERENCES

Abernethy, R. S., & Schlozman, S. C. (2008). An overview of the psychotherapies. In T. S. Stern, J. F. Rosenbaum, M. Fava, J. Biederman, & S. L. Rauch (Eds.), *Massachusetts General Hospital comprehensive clinical psychiatry* (pp. 129–140). St. Louis, MO: Mosby.

Ackley, B. J., & Ladwig, G. B. (2008). *Nursing diagnosis handbook: An evidence-based guide to planning care.* St. Louis, MO: Mosby.

Altarac, M., & Saroha, E. (2007). Lifetime prevalence of learning disability among U.S. children. *Pediatrics, 11*,9(suppl 1):2, 77–83.

American Academy of Pediatrics. (2013). *Diagnosing a learning disability.* Retrieved from http://www.healthychildren.org/English/health-issues/conditions/learning-disabilities/Pages/Diagnosing-a-Learning-Disability.aspx.

American Academy of Pediatrics. (2012). *Learning, motor skills, and communication disorders.* Retrieved from http://www.healthychildren.org/English/health-issues/conditions/adhd/Pages/Learning-Motor-Skills-and-Communication-Disorders.aspx.

American Academy of Pediatrics. (2012). *Tics, Tourette's syndrome and OCD.* Retrieved from http://www.healthychildren.org/English/health-issues/conditions/emotional-problems/Pages/Tics-Tourette-Syndrome-and-OCD.aspx.

American Nurses Association [ANA], American Psychiatric-Mental Health Nurses Association [APNA], & International Society of Psychiatric-Mental Health Nurses [ISPN] (2007). *Psychiatric mental health nursing: Scope and standards of practice.* Silver Spring, MD: American Nurses Association.

American Psychiatric Association. (2013). *DSM-5 table of contents.* Retrieved from http://www.psychiatry.org/dsm5.

Axline, V. (1969). *Play therapy.* New York, NY: Ballantine Books.

Beebe, L., & Wyatt, T. (2009). Using the Bonny Method to evoke emotion and access the unconscious. *Journal of Psychosocial Nursing, 47*(1), 29–33.

Bellin, M., & Kovacs, P. (2006). Fostering resilience in siblings of youth with a chronic health condition: A review of the literature. *Health and Social Work, 31*(3), 209–216.

Blakemore, S. J., Burnett, S., & Dahl, R. E. (2010). The role of puberty in the developing adolescent brain. *Human Brain Mapping, 31*(6), 926–933. doi: 10.1002/hbm.21052

Bowers, L., Ross, J., Nijman, H., Muir-Cochrane, E., Noorthoorn, E., & Stewart, D. The scope for replacing seclusion with time out in acute inpatient psychiatry in England. *Journal of Advanced Nursing, 68*(4), 826–35. doi: 10.1111/j.1365-2648.2011.0578x.

Bulechek, G. M., Butcher, H. K., Dochterman, J. M., & Wagner, C. (2013). *Nursing interventions classification (NIC)* (6th ed). St. Louis, MO: Mosby.

Caldwell, R., Silver, N. C., & Strada, M. (2010). Substance abuse, familial factors and mental health: Exploring racial and ethnic differences among African American, Caucasian and Hispanic juvenile offenders. *The American Journal of Family Therapy, 38*, 310–321.

Carulla, L. S., Reed, G. M., Vaez-Azizi, L. M., Cooper, S., Leal, R. M., Bertelli, M., . . . Saxena, S. (2011). Intellectual development disorders: Towards a new name, definition and framework for "mental retardation/intellectual disability" in ICD-11. *World Psychiatry, 10*(3), 175–180.

Centers for Disease Control and Prevention. (2012). *Prevalence of autism spectrum disorders.* Retrieved from http://www.cdc.gov/mmwr/preview/mmwrhtml/ss6103a1.htm?s_cid=ss6103a1_w.

Centers for Disease Control and Prevention. (2012). *Attention-deficit/hyperactivity disorder (ADHD).* Retrieved from http://www.cdc.gov/ncbddd/adhd/data.html.

Centers for Disease Control and Prevention. (2010). *Summary health statistics for U.S. children: National Health Interview Survey, 2009.* Retrieved from http://www.cdc.gov/nchs/data/series/sr_10/sr10_247.pdf.

Centers for Disease Control and Prevention. (2009). *Key findings: Trends in the prevalence of developmental disabilities in U.S. children, 1997-2008.* Retrieved from http://www.cdc.gov\ncbdd\featuresbirthdefects-dd-keyfindings.htm.

Center for Quality Assessment and Improvement in Mental Health (2007). *Quality Measure Inventory.* Retrieved from http://www.cqaimh.org/index.html.

Children's Defense Fund (2011). *The state of America's children 2011.* Washington, DC: Author.

Evans, D., & Seligman., M. E. P. (2005). Introduction. In D. Evans, E. Foa, R. Gur, H. Hendin, C. O'Brien, M. Seligman, & B. T. Walsh (Eds.), *Treating and preventing adolescent mental health disorders.* New York: Oxford University Press.

Farrell, A., Erwin, E., Allison, K., Meyer, A., Sullivan, T., Camou, S., . . . Espisito, E. (2007). Problematic situations in the lives of urban African American middle school students: A qualitative study. *Journal of Research on Adolescence, 17*(2), 413–454.

Flaherty, A. W. (2008). Movement disorders. In T. A. Stern, J. F. Rosenbaum, M. Fava, J. Biederman, & S. L. Rauch (Eds.), *Massachusetts General Hospital comprehensive clinical psychiatry* (pp. 1091–1105). St. Louis, MO: Mosby.

Freud, A. (1965). *Normality and pathology in childhood: Assessments of development.* New York, NY: International Universities Press.

Gemelli, R. J. (2008). Normal child and adolescent development. In R. E. Hales, S. C. Yudofsky, & G. O. Gabbard (Eds.), *Textbook of psychiatry* (pp. 245–300). Washington, DC: American Psychiatric Publishing.

Herdman, T. H. (Ed.), (2012). *NANDA international nursing diagnoses: Definitions and classification, 2012-2014.* Oxford, UK: Wiley-Blackwell.

International Society of Psychiatric Nurses. (2007). *Practice parameters: Child and adolescent inpatient psychiatric treatment.* Retrieved from http://www.ispn-psych.org/docs/PracticeParameters.pdf.

Klein, M. (1955). The psychoanalytic play technique. *American Journal of Orthopsychiatry, 25,* 223–237.

Koro-Ljunberg, M., Bussing, R., Williamson, P., Wilder, J., & Mills, T. (2008). African American teenagers' stories of attention deficit hyperactivity disorder, *Journal of Child and Family Studies, 17,* 467–485.

Lehne, R. A. (2010). *Pharmacology for nursing care* (7th ed.). Philadelphia, PA: Saunders.

Masters, K. (2009). Risk management: Part 1: Seclusion and restraint. *Audio Digest Psychiatry, 38*(6), Retrieved from http://www.cme-ce-summaries.com/psychiatry/ps3806.html.

Merikangas, K. R., He, J., Burstein, M., Swanson, S.A., Avenevoli, S., Cui, L., Benjet, C., Georgiades, K., & Swendsen, J. (2010). Lifetime prevalence of mental disorders in U. S. adolescents: Results from the National Comorbidity Study-Adolescent Supplements (NCS-A). *Journal of the Academy of Child and Adolescent Psychiatry, 49*(10), 980–989.

Moorhead, S., Johnson, M., Maas, M.L., & Swanson, E. (2013). *Nursing outcomes classification (NOC)* (5th ed.). St Louis, MO: Mosby.

National Child Abuse and Neglect Data System. (2010). *Child abuse and neglect statistics.* Retrieved from http://www.childwelfare.gov/systemwide/statistics/can.cfm.

National Dissemination Center for Children with Disabilities. (2011). *Speech and language impairments.* Retrieved from http://nichcy.org/disability/specific/speechlanguage.

National Institute of Health. (2012). *Speech and communication disorders.* Retrieved from http://www.nlm.nih.gov/medlineplus/speechandcommunicationdisorders.html.

National Institute on Drug Abuse. (2008). *Preventing drug abuse among children and adolescents.* Retrieved from http://www.nida.nih.gov/Prevention/risk.html.

Packer, L. E. (2011). *Treatment of Tourette's syndrome.* Retrieved from http://www.tourettesyndrome.net/disorders/tourette%E2%80%99s-syndrome/treatment-of-tourettes-syndrome/.

Perepletchikova, F., & Kazdin, A. Oppositional defiant disorder and conduct disorder. In K. Cheng & K. Myers (Eds.), *Child and adolescent psychiatry: The essentials.* Philadelphia, PA: Lippincott, Williams & Wilkins.

Pierangolo, R., & Giuliano, G. (2006). *Learning disabilities: A practical approach to foundations, assessment, diagnosis and teaching.* Boston, MA: Pearson, Allyn and Bacon.

Sadock, B. J., & Sadock, A. (2008). *Kaplan & Sadock's concise textbook of clinical psychiatry* (3rd ed.). Philadelphia, PA: Lippincott, Williams & Wilkins.

Smoller, J. W., Sheidley, B. R., & Tsuang, M. T. (2008). *Psychiatric genetics: Applications in clinical practice.* Arlington, VA: American Psychiatric Publishing.

Substance Abuse and Mental Health Services Administration. (2011). *Leading change: A plan for SAMHSA's roles and actions 2011-2014.* Retrieved from http://www.samhsa.gov/product/SMA11-4629.

Szoka, B. M., & Thierer, A. D. (2009). *Cyberbullying legislation: Why education is preferable to regulation* [SSRN Working Paper Series]. Retrieved from http://papers.ssrn.com/sol3/papers.cfm?abstract_id=1422577.

Tomblin, J. B., Zhang, X., Weiss, A., Catts, H., & Ellis Weismer, S. (2004). Dimensions of individual differences in communication skills among primary grade children. In M. L. Rice & S. F. Warren (Eds.), *Developmental language disorders: From phenotypes to etiologies* (pp. 53–76). Mahwah, NJ: Lawrence Erlbaum.

U.S. Department of Education, Office of Special Education Programs. (2007). *U.S. Department of Education and Rehabilitative Services history: 25 years of progress in educating children with disabilities through IDEA.* Retrieved from www.ed.gov/policy/speced/leg/idea/history.pdf.

U.S. Department of Health & Human Services. (1999). *Mental health: A report of the surgeon general.* Rockville, MD: U.S. Department of Health & Human Services, Center for Mental Health Services, National Institutes of Health. Retrieved from http://www.surgeongeneral.gov/library/mentalhealth/ toc.html#chapter3.

U.S. Department of Justice. (2010). *Highlights of the 2008 national youth gang survey.* Retrieved from http://www.ncjrs.gov/pdffiles1/ojjdp/229249.pdf.

Ursano, A. M., Kartheiser, P. H., & Barnhill, L. J. (2008). Disorders usually first diagnosed in infancy, childhood, or adolescence. In R. E. Hales, S. C. Yudofsky, & G. O. Gabbard (Eds.), *Textbook of psychiatry* (pp. 861–920). Washington, DC: American Psychiatric Publishing.

CHAPTER

12

Schizophrenia and Schizophrenia Spectrum Disorders

Edward A. Herzog

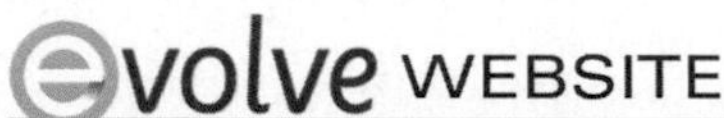

Visit the Evolve website for a pretest on the content in this chapter: http://evolve.elsevier.com/Varcarolis

Pre-Test interactive review

OBJECTIVES

1. Identify the schizophrenia spectrum disorders.
2. Describe the symptoms, progression, nursing care, and treatment needs for the prepsychotic through maintenance phases of schizophrenia.
3. Discuss at least three of the neurobiological-anatomical-genetic findings that indicate that schizophrenia is a brain disorder.
4. Differentiate among the positive and negative symptoms of schizophrenia in terms of treatment and effect on quality of life.
5. Discuss how to deal with common reactions the nurse may experience while working with a patient with schizophrenia.
6. Develop teaching plans for patients taking first-generation (e.g., haloperidol [Haldol]) and second-generation (e.g., risperidone [Risperdal]) antipsychotic drugs.
7. Compare and contrast the first-generation and second-generation antipsychotics.
8. Create a nursing care plan incorporating evidence-based interventions for symptoms of psychosis, including hallucinations, delusions, paranoia, cognitive disorganization, anosognosia, and impaired self-care.
9. Role-play intervening with a patient who is hallucinating, delusional, and exhibiting disorganized thinking.

KEY TERMS AND CONCEPTS

acute dystonia
affect
affective symptoms
akathisia
ambivalence
anosognosia
associative looseness
clang association
cognitive symptoms
command hallucinations
concrete thinking
delusions
depersonalization
derealization
echolalia
echopraxia
executive functioning
extrapyramidal side effects (EPSs)
first-generation antipsychotics
hallucinations
ideas of reference
illusions
metabolic syndrome
negative symptoms
neologisms
neuroleptic malignant syndrome (NMS)
paranoia
positive symptoms
pseudoparkinsonism
reality testing
recovery model
second-generation antipsychotics
stereotyped behaviors
tardive dyskinesia (TD or TDK)
third-generation antipsychotics
word salad

Schizophrenia spectrum and other psychotic disorders disturb the fundamental ability to determine what is or is not real. In this chapter we will be reviewing concepts important to these disorders. The spectrum disorders are described in Box 12-1; they are listed, in general, from least to most severe. While clinicians contend that the boundaries are so unclear that separate diagnostic labels are not necessarily warranted, for the most current edition of the *Diagnostic and Statistical Manual* (American Psychiatric Association, 2013), the distinctions remain.

The most severe disorder in this category is schizophrenia and it is the major focus of this chapter. Understanding the concepts important to this specific diagnosis will help in understanding the others. Schizophrenia is a potentially devastating brain disorder that affects a person's thinking, language, emotions, social behavior, and ability to perceive reality accurately. It affects over 3.5 million persons in the United States and is among the most disruptive and disabling of mental disorders.

CLINICAL PICTURE

Children who later go on to be diagnosed with schizophrenia often have unusual characteristics years before psychotic symptoms become apparent (Minzenberger et al., 2011). They tend to do less well in school than their siblings, are less socially engaged, less positive, and exhibit unusual motor development. Actual childhood schizophrenia is extremely rare, carries a worse prognosis than the adult-onset version, and is diagnosed before the age of 12.

Adolescents who are later diagnosed with schizophrenia often experience prodromal symptoms (i.e., early symptoms that indicate that a problem may be developing) for a few months or a few years (Minzenberger et al., 2011). Adolescents may experience social withdrawal, irritability, and depression and become antagonistic. Conduct problems and academic decline often bring them to the attention of school and community clinicians. Suspiciousness and

BOX 12-1 PSYCHOTIC DISORDERS OTHER THAN SCHIZOPHRENIA

Schizotypal Personality Disorder

The patient demonstrates a personality alteration characterized by altered interpersonal boundaries, eccentric behavior, eccentric use of language, restricted or socially inappropriate expression of emotion, increased mistrust and sensitivity regarding the intent or responses of others, and difficulty setting goals, determining their own beliefs, and other alterations in identity. Although such persons may appear eccentric or odd, they do not exhibit the frank psychotic features seen in psychotic disorders, such as hallucinations and delusions. Refer to Chapter 24 for further discussion of this disorder.

Delusional Disorder

A person with delusional disorder experiences nonbizarre delusions (e.g., situations that could occur in real life, such as being followed, being loved by another, or having a disease). Apart from the delusion, functioning is not significantly impaired and there are no other symptoms of psychosis. A related disorder, Capgras Syndrome, involves a delusion about a significant other (e.g., family member or pet) being replaced by an imposter; this disorder may be due to psychiatric or organic brain disease (Christodoulou et al., 2009).

Brief Psychotic Disorder

This disorder involves an acute onset of psychosis (delusions, hallucinations, disorganized speech) or grossly disorganized or catatonic behavior in response to extreme stress. It lasts less than 1 month, and a full recovery usually occurs.

Substance-Induced Psychotic Disorder

Psychosis induced by drugs of abuse, alcohol, medications, or toxins.

Psychosis or Catatonia Associated with Another Medical Condition

Psychosis or catatonia caused by a medical condition (e.g., delirium, neurological or metabolic conditions, hepatic or renal diseases, and many others). Medical conditions and substance abuse must always be ruled out before a diagnosis of schizophrenia or other psychotic disorder can be made.

Schizophreniform Disorder

Schizophreniform disorder is the diagnosis used in situations in which a person has many of the features of schizophrenia but has had these for a period of less than six months. It may or may not develop into schizophrenia.

Schizoaffective Disorder

When an episode of major depression, mania, or mixed depression and mania occurs in the presence of symptoms of schizophrenia, it is called schizoaffective disorder.

Psychotic or Catatonic Disorder Not Otherwise Specified

Disorders that involve psychotic features such as impaired reality testing or bizarre behavior but do not meet the criteria for diagnosis as specific psychotic disorders are diagnosed as Psychosis Not Otherwise Specified (NOS). Similarly, persons exhibiting gross changes in the rate of motor behavior but who do not meet the criteria for Catatonic Disorder are categorized as Catatonic Disorder NOS.

low-level distortions in thought seem be especially linked to subsequent schizophrenia.

All people diagnosed with schizophrenia have at least one psychotic symptom, such as hallucinations, delusions, and/or disorganized speech. In children the symptoms are severe enough to interrupt normal childhood activities, such as schooling, or to disrupt important age-appropriate milestones. Adults have extreme difficulty or are unable to function in their family, social, or occupational lives. Basic needs such as hygiene and nutrition are often neglected. During a six-month period individuals may have times when they are not experiencing psychotic symptoms, but in those times they tend to be apathetic or depressed.

VIGNETTE

Sam, a 25-year-old man soon to be discharged from the hospital, constantly tells his family he wants his own apartment. When Sam is told that an apartment has been found for him, he asks, "But who will take care of me?" Sam is acting out his **ambivalence** between his desire to be independent and his desire to be taken care of.

EPIDEMIOLOGY

The prevalence of childhood-onset schizophrenia is about 1 in 10,000 children. In adults, the lifetime prevalence of schizophrenia is 1% worldwide with no differences related to race, social status, or culture. It is diagnosed more frequently in males (1.4:1) and among persons growing up in urban areas (Tandon et al., 2008). Schizophrenia usually presents during the late teens and early twenties. Childhood schizophrenia, although rare, does exist, occurring in 1 out of 40,000 children. Early-onset schizophrenia (18 to 25 years) occurs more often in males and is associated with poor functioning before onset, more structural brain abnormality, and increased levels of apathy. Individuals with a later onset (25 to 35 years) are more likely to be female, to have less structural brain abnormality, and to have better outcomes.

COMORBIDITY

Substance abuse disorders occur in nearly 50% of persons with schizophrenia and are associated with treatment nonadherence, relapse, incarceration, homelessness, violence, suicide, and a poorer prognosis (Gottlieb et al., 2012). These disorders may represent a maladaptive way of coping with schizophrenia. **Nicotine dependence** rates in schizophrenia range from 70% to 90% and contribute to an increased incidence of cardiovascular and respiratory disorders (D'Souza & Markou, 2012).

Anxiety, depression, and suicide co-occur frequently in schizophrenia. Anxiety may be a response to symptoms (e.g., hallucinations) or circumstances (e.g., isolation, overstimulation) and may worsen schizophrenia symptoms and prognosis. Approximately 10% of persons with schizophrenia commit suicide, a rate 8.5 times that of the general population; both depression and suicide attempts can occur at any point in the illness (Kasckow, Felmet, & Zisook, 2011).

Physical health illnesses are more common among people with schizophrenia than in the general population. The risk of premature death is 1.6 to 2.8 times greater than that in the general population; on average, patients with schizophrenia die 28 years prematurely due to disorders such as hypertension (22%), obesity (24%), cardiovascular disease (21%), diabetes (12%), chronic obstructive pulmonary disease (COPD) (10%), and trauma (6%) (Miller et al., 2007).

Persons with psychotic disorders may be at greater risk due to apathy (a symptom of schizophrenia), poor health habits, medications (see the discussion of metabolic syndrome later in this chapter), poverty, limited access to health care, and failure to recognize signs of illness. Owing to poverty, stigma, or stereotyping (e.g., emergency department personnel assuming that because a patient has a psychotic disorder, his chest pain is imaginary), they may not receive adequate health care.

Polydipsia can lead to fatal water intoxication (indicated by hyponatremia, confusion, worsening psychotic symptoms, and ultimately coma). Polydipsia occurs in upwards of 20% of persons with schizophrenia and a seemingly insatiable thirst that results causes hyponatremia in 2-5%; contributing factors include antipsychotic medication (causes dry mouth), compulsive behavior, and neuroendocrine abnormalities (Goldman, 2009).

ETIOLOGY

Schizophrenia is a complicated disorder. In fact, what we call "schizophrenia" actually may be a group of disorders with common but varying features and multiple, overlapping etiologies. What is known is that brain chemistry, structure, and activity are different in a person with schizophrenia.

The scientific consensus is that schizophrenia occurs when multiple inherited gene abnormalities combine with nongenetic factors (e.g., viral infections, birth injuries, environmental stressors, prenatal malnutrition), altering the structures of the brain, affecting the brain's neurotransmitter systems, and/or injuring the brain directly (Tandon et al., 2008). This is called the *diathesis-stress model of schizophrenia* (Walker & Tessner, 2008).

Biological Factors

Genetic

Schizophrenia and schizophrenia-like symptoms, such as eccentric thinking, occur at an increased rate in relatives of individuals with schizophrenia. According to Giegling and colleagues (2010):

- Compared to the usual 1% risk in the population, having a first-degree relative with schizophrenia increases the risk to nearly 10%.
- Concordance rates in twins (how often one twin will have the disorder when the other one has it) is about 50% for identical twins and about 15% for fraternal twins.
- The degree to which genetics plays a role in causing schizophrenia is estimated at 65-80%

Evidence suggests that multiple genes on different chromosomes interact with each other in complex ways to create vulnerability for schizophrenia. Genes potentially linked to schizophrenia continue to be identified, suggesting a high degree of complexity (Tandon et al., 2008).

Neurobiological

Dopamine Theory. The first antipsychotic drugs are known as *conventional* (or *first-generation*) *antipsychotics* (e.g., haloperidol and chlorpromazine). These drugs block the activity of dopamine-2 (D_2) receptors in the brain, limiting the activity of dopamine and reducing some of the symptoms of schizophrenia. Cocaine, methylphenidate (Ritalin), and levodopa increase the activity of dopamine in the brain and, in biologically susceptible persons, may bring on schizophrenia. Amphetamines can be used to induce a model of schizophrenia in persons without schizophrenia and can precipitate the disorder; in fact, almost any drug of abuse, including marijuana, can lead to schizophrenia in biologically vulnerable persons (Callaghan et al., 2012). Because the dopamine-blocking agents do not alleviate all the symptoms of schizophrenia, it seems likely that other neurotransmitters or other factors may be involved.

Other Neurochemical Hypotheses. *Second-generation (unconventional) antipsychotics* block serotonin (5-hydroxytryptamine 2A, or 5-HT2A) as well as dopamine, which suggests that serotonin may play a role in schizophrenia as well. If we can better understand how second-generation agents modulate the expression and targeting of serotonin and its receptors, we may better understand schizophrenia.

Researchers have long been aware that phencyclidine piperidine (PCP) induces a state closely resembling schizophrenia. This observation led to interest in the *N*-methyl-D-aspartate (NMDA) receptor complex and the possible role of **glutamate** in the pathophysiology of schizophrenia. Glutamate is a crucial neurotransmitter during periods of neuromaturation; abnormal maturation of the central nervous system (CNS) is considered to be a central factor contributing to information-processing deficits in schizophrenia (Kegeles et al., 2012). Acetylcholine (Ach), active in the muscarinic system, is another implicated neurotransmitter and is emerging as an important target for future treatment (Jones, Byun, & Bubser, 2012).

Brain Structure Abnormalities

Disruptions in communication pathways in the brain are thought to be severe in schizophrenia. It is possible that structural abnormalities cause such disruption. Using brain imaging techniques—computed tomography (CT), magnetic resonance imaging (MRI), and positron emission tomography (PET)—researchers (Hulshoff et al., 2012; Wang et al., 2011; van Haren et al., 2011) have provided substantial evidence that some people with schizophrenia have structural brain abnormalities, including the following:

- Enlargement of the lateral cerebral ventricles, third ventricle dilation, and/or ventricular asymmetry
- Reduced cortical, frontal lobe, hippocampal and/or cerebellar volumes
- Increased size of the sulci (fissures) on the surface of the brain
- Reduced cortical thickness
- Reduced connectivity in various brain regions

PET scans also show a lowered rate of blood flow and glucose metabolism in the frontal lobes, which govern planning, abstract thinking, social adjustment, and decision making, all of which are affected in schizophrenia. Figure 3-5 in Chapter 3 shows a PET scan demonstrating reduced brain activity in the frontal lobe of a patient with schizophrenia. Such structural changes may worsen as the disorder continues. Postmortem studies on individuals with schizophrenia reveal a reduced volume of gray matter in the brain, especially in the temporal and frontal lobes; those with the most tissue loss had the worst symptoms (e.g., hallucinations, delusions, bizarre thoughts, and depression).

Psychological and Environmental Factors

A number of biological, chemical, and environmental stressors, particularly those occurring prenatally and during other vulnerable periods of neurological development, are believed to combine with genetic vulnerabilities to produce schizophrenia.

Prenatal Stressors

A history of pregnancy or birth complications is associated with an increased risk for schizophrenia. Prenatal risk factors include poor nutrition (e.g., folate deficiency) and hypoxia. Infectious agents such as human herpes virus 2 and human endogenous retrovirus 2 are also implicated (Arias et al., 2011). Psychological trauma to the mother during pregnancy (e.g., the death of a relative) can also contribute to the development of schizophrenia (Khashan et al., 2008). Other risk factors include a father older than 35 at the child's conception and being born during late winter or early spring (Tandon et al., 2008).

Psychological Stressors

Stress increases cortisol levels, impeding hypothalamic development and causing other changes that may precipitate the illness in vulnerable individuals. Schizophrenia often manifests at times of developmental and family stress, such as beginning college or moving away from one's family. Social, psychological, and physical stressors may play a significant role in both the severity and course of the disorder and the person's quality of life. Other factors increasing the risk of schizophrenia include childhood sexual abuse, exposure to social adversity (e.g., living in chronic poverty or high-crime environments), migration to or growing up in a foreign culture, and exposure to psychological trauma or social defeat (Tandon et al., 2008).

Environmental Stressors

Environmental factors such as toxins, including the solvent tetrachloroethylene (used in dry cleaning and to line water pipes and sometimes found in drinking water) are also believed to contribute to the development of schizophrenia in vulnerable persons (Aschengrau et al., 2012).

Course of the Disorder

The onset of symptoms or forewarning (prodromal) symptoms may appear a month to more than a year before the first psychotic break or full-blown manifestations of the illness; such symptoms represent a clear deterioration from previous functioning. The course thereafter typically includes recurrent exacerbations separated by periods of reduced or dormant symptoms. Occasionally a person will have a single episode of schizophrenia without recurrences or will have several episodes and none thereafter. For most patients, however, schizophrenia is a chronic or recurring disorder that, like diabetes or heart disease, is managed but rarely cured.

Frequently, prior to the illness, a person with schizophrenia was socially awkward, lonely, perhaps depressed, and expressed himself or herself in vague, odd, or eccentric ways. In this prodromal phase, anxiety, phobias, obsessions, dissociation, and compulsions may be noted. As anxiety mounts, indications of a thought disorder become evident: Concentration, memory, and completion of school- or job-related work deteriorate. Intrusive thoughts, "mind wandering," and the need to devote more time to maintaining one's thoughts are reported.

The person may feel that something "strange" or "wrong" is happening. Routine stimuli such as traffic noise or voices in a café can become overwhelming. Events are misinterpreted, and mystical or symbolic meanings may be given to ordinary events. For example, the patient may think that certain colors have special powers or that a song on the radio is a message from God intended just for him. Discerning others' emotions from facial expression or tone of voice becomes more difficult, and others' actions or words may be mistaken for signs of hostility or evidence of harmful intent (Gold et al., 2012).

Prognostic Considerations

For the majority of patients, most symptoms can be at least somewhat controlled through medications and psychosocial interventions. With support and effective treatments, many people with schizophrenia experience a good quality of life and success within their families, occupations, and other roles. Associates may not even realize the person has schizophrenia.

In most cases, however, schizophrenia does not respond fully to available treatments, leaving residual symptoms and causing varying degrees of dysfunction or disability. Some persons require repeated or lengthy inpatient care or institutionalization. An abrupt onset of symptoms is usually a favorable prognostic sign, and those with good premorbid social and occupational functioning have a greater chance for a good remission or a complete recovery. Factors associated with a less positive prognosis include a slow, insidious onset (e.g., over 2 to 3 years); younger age at onset; longer duration between first symptoms and first treatment; longer periods of untreated illness; and more negative symptoms.

Phases of Schizophrenia

Schizophrenia usually progresses through predictable phases, although the presenting symptoms during a given phase and the length of the phase can vary widely; these phases are (Chung et al., 2008):

- **Phase I—Acute:** Onset or exacerbation of florid, disruptive symptoms (e.g., hallucinations, delusions, apathy, withdrawal) with resultant loss of functional abilities; increased care or hospitalization may be required.
- **Phase II—Stabilization:** Symptoms are diminishing, and there is movement toward one's previous level of functioning (baseline); partial hospitalization or care in a residential crisis center or a supervised group home may be needed.
- **Phase III—Maintenance:** The patient is at or nearing baseline (or premorbid) functioning; symptoms are absent or diminished; level of functioning allows the patient to live in the community. Ideally, recovery with reduced or no residual symptoms has occurred.

Some clinicians also designate an earlier Prodromal (or Prepsychotic) Phase in which subtle symptoms or deficits associated with schizophrenia are present; such symptoms may or may not herald the later onset of schizophrenia.

APPLICATION OF THE NURSING PROCESS

ASSESSMENT

Nursing assessment of patients who may have a psychotic disorder focuses largely on symptoms, coping, functioning, and safety. Assessment involves interviewing the patient and observing behavior and other outward manifestations of the disorder; information from others who know the patient is also important as patients may conceal or minimize symptoms when under scrutiny. Assessment also should include a mental status examination, along with review of spiritual, cultural, biological, psychological, social, and environmental elements that might be affecting the presentation (or that could be potential resources for recovery). Sound therapeutic communication skills, an understanding of the disorder and the ways patients may be experiencing their world, and establishing trust in a therapeutic nurse-patient relationship all strengthen the assessment.

Prepsychotic Phase

Early detection and treatment of symptoms is believed to lessen the risk of developing the disorder (or reduce the severity of the disorder if it does develop). A delay in diagnosis and treatment allows the psychotic process to become more entrenched; it can also result in maladaptive coping (e.g., drinking) and relational, work, housing, and school problems.

Therefore, early assessment plays a key role in improving the prognosis for persons with schizophrenia (Chung et al., 2008). This form of primary prevention involves monitoring those at high risk (e.g., children of parents with schizophrenia) for symptoms such as abnormal social development and cognitive dysfunction. Intervening to reduce stressors (i.e., reduce or avoid exposure to triggers), enhancing social and coping skills (i.e., build resiliency), and administering prophylactic antipsychotic medication may also be of benefit.

Research suggests that with each relapse of psychosis, there is an increase in residual dysfunction and deterioration (Crespo-Facorro et al., 2010). Recognition of the early warning signs of relapse—such as reduced sleep and concentration—followed by close monitoring and intensification of treatment is essential. For this reason, adherence to antipsychotics can be more important than the risk of side effects because most side effects are reversible whereas the consequences of relapse may not be.

General Assessment

Not all people with schizophrenia (or even people with the same subtype of the disorder) have the same symptoms, and some of the symptoms of schizophrenia are also found in other disorders. Figure 12-1 describes the four main symptom groups of schizophrenia:

1. **Positive symptoms:** The presence of something that is not normally present (e.g., hallucinations, delusions, bizarre behavior, paranoia, abnormal movements, gross errors in thinking)

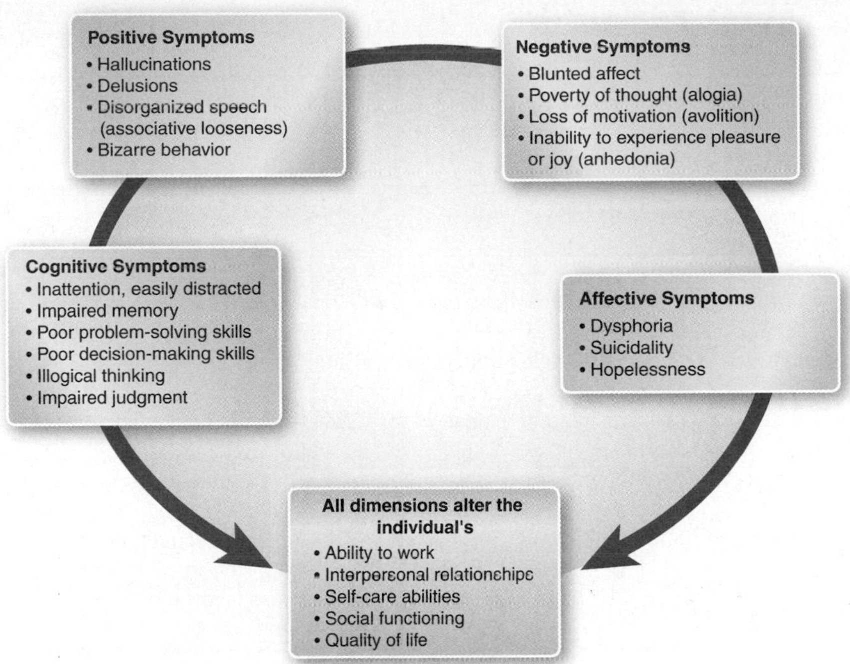

Positive Symptoms
• Hallucinations
• Delusions
• Disorganized speech (associative looseness)
• Bizarre behavior
Negative Symptoms
• Blunted affect
• Poverty of thought (alogia)
• Loss of motivation (avolition)
• Inability to experience pleasure or joy (anhedonia)
Cognitive Symptoms
• Inattention, easily distracted
• Impaired memory
• Poor problem-solving skills
• Poor decision-making skills
• Illogical thinking
• Impaired judgment
Affective Symptoms
• Dysphoria
• Suicidality
• Hopelessness
All dimensions alter the individual's
• Ability to work
• Interpersonal relationships
• Self-care abilities
• Social functioning
• Quality of life

FIG 12-1 Four main symptom groups of schizophrenia.

2. Negative symptoms: The absence of something that should be present (e.g., interest in hygiene, motivation, ability to experience pleasure)
3. Cognitive symptoms: Often subtle changes in memory, attention, or thinking (e.g. impaired executive functioning [the ability to set priorities or make decisions])
4. Affective symptoms: Symptoms involving emotions and their expression

The positive symptoms usually appear early in the illness, and their dramatic nature captures our attention and often precipitates hospitalization. They are also the symptoms most laypersons connect with insanity, making schizophrenia the disorder most associated with being "crazy." Positive psychotic symptoms, however, are perhaps less important prognostically and usually respond to antipsychotic medication. The negative symptoms tend to be more persistent and crippling because they reduce motivation and limit social and vocational success.

Positive Symptoms

Positive symptoms are associated with an acute onset. These symptoms tend to respond well to medication, and individuals commonly function normally during remission. The positive symptoms presented here are categorized as alterations in thought, speech, perception, and behavior.

Alterations in Thought. We all experience thoughts that are irrational or exaggerated, yet we can usually catch and correct the error by using intact reality testing. This is an often automatic and unconscious process by which we sort out what is and is not real. People with impaired reality testing, however, make, maintain, and build upon errors in thinking, which contribute to delusions.

Delusions are false fixed beliefs that cannot be corrected by reasoning. About 75% of people with schizophrenia experience delusions at some time. Student nurses sometimes try unsuccessfully to reason a patient out of delusions by offering evidence of reality. This is counterproductive as an even stronger defense is developed for the position. Also, this may irritate the patient and slow the development of a therapeutic relationship.

The most common delusions are persecutory, grandiose, or those involving religious or hypochondriacal ideas. Table 12-1 provides definitions and examples of types of delusions. A delusion may be a response to anxiety or reflect areas of concern; for example, someone with poor self-esteem may believe he is Beethoven or an emissary of God, leading him to feel more powerful or important. Looking for and addressing such underlying themes or needs can be a key nursing intervention.

Just because someone has delusions does not mean that every story that sounds improbable is untrue. One patient repeatedly told the staff that the Mafia was out to kill him. The staff later learned that he had been selling drugs and had not paid his contacts and that gang members *were* trying to hurt or even kill him.

Concrete thinking refers to an impaired ability to think abstractly. For example, a nurse might ask what brought the patient to the hospital, and the patient might answer, concretely, "a cab" (rather than explaining that he had attempted suicide). Concreteness is often assessed through the patient's interpretation of proverbs; a concrete interpretation of "The grass is always greener on the other side of the fence" would be "That side gets more sun, so it's greener there." Concreteness reduces one's ability to understand and address abstract concepts such as love or the passage of time.

Alterations in Speech. Associations are the mental threads that tie one thought logically to another. In associative looseness, these threads are interrupted or disjointed; thinking becomes haphazard, illogical, and difficult to follow. Here's an

TABLE 12-1 SUMMARY OF DELUSIONS*

DELUSION	DEFINITION	EXAMPLE
Control	Believing that another person, group of people, or external force controls thoughts, feelings, impulses, or behavior	Brian covered his apartment walls with aluminum foil to block governmental efforts to control his thoughts.
Ideas of Reference	Giving personal significance to unrelated or trivial events; perceiving events as relating to you when they are not	Barbara believes that the birds sing when she walks down the street just for her.
Persecution	Believing that one is being singled out for harm by others; this belief often takes the form of a plot by people in power	Peter believed that the Secret Service was planning to kill him by poisoning his food; therefore, he would eat only prepackaged food.
Grandeur	Believing that one is a very powerful or important person	Sam believed he was a famous playwright and tennis pro.
Somatic Delusions	Believing that the body is changing in unusual ways (e.g., rotting inside)	David said his heart had stopped and was rotting away.
Erotomanic	Believing that another person desires you romantically	Although he barely knew her, Patti insisted that Eric would marry her if only his current wife would stop interfering.
Jealousy	Believing that one's mate is unfaithful	Sally wrongly accused her spouse of going out with other women. Her proof was that he twice came home from work late (even though his boss explained that everyone had worked late).

*A false belief held and maintained as true regardless of evidence to the contrary. This does not include sharing unusual beliefs maintained by one's culture or subculture.

example: "I need to get a Band-Aid for my paper cut. My friend was talking about AIDs. Friends talk about French fries and how can you trust the French? They won't let you take pictures of the menu at McDonald's."

Clang association is choosing words based on their sound rather than their meaning, often rhyming or having a similar beginning sound ("On the track . . . have a Big Mac"; "Click, clack, clutch, close"). Clanging may also be seen in neurological disorders.

Word salad (schizophasia) is a jumble of words that is meaningless to the listener—and perhaps to the speaker as well—because of an extreme level of disorganization. ("Throat hoarse strength of policy dreadfully essential Brazilian highlighters on a boat reigning supreme!")

Neologisms are made-up words (or idiosyncratic uses of existing words) that have meaning for the patient but a different or nonexistent meaning to others. ("I was going to tell him the *mannerologies* of his hospitality won't do.") This eccentric use of words represents disorganized thinking and interferes with communication.

Echolalia is the pathological repeating of another's words and is often seen in catatonia.

> **Nurse:** Mary, come get your medication.
> **Mary:** Come get your medication.

Other disorders of thought or speech include:

- **Religiosity:** An excessive preoccupation with religious themes.
- **Magical thinking:** Believing that one's thoughts or actions can affect others; this is common in children (e.g., wearing pajamas inside out to make it snow).
- **Paranoia:** An irrational fear of others, ranging from mild (wariness, guardedness) to profound (believing that another person intends to kill you). Note that persons who fear others may sometimes act defensively, harming the other person before that person harms the patient; this creates a risk to others.
- **Circumstantiality:** Including unnecessary and often tedious details in one's conversation (e.g., describing your breakfast when asked how your day is going).
- **Tangentiality:** Leaving the main topic to talk about less important information; going off on tangents in a way that takes the conversation off-topic.
- **Cognitive retardation:** A generalized slowing in the pace of thinking, represented by delays in responding to questions or difficulty finishing one's thoughts.
- **Alogia**, or **poverty of speech:** A reduction in spontaneity or volume of speech, represented by a lack of spontaneous comments and overly brief responses.
- **Rapid or pressured speech**
- **Flight of ideas:** Moving rapidly from one thought to the next, making it difficult for others to follow the conversation.
- **Thought blocking:** A reduction in the amount of thinking; an abrupt stoppage of thought that derails conversation.
- **Thought insertion:** Feeling that one's thoughts are not one's own or that they were inserted into one's mind.
- **Thought deletion:** A belief that one's thoughts have been taken or are missing.
- **Illogical, disorganized or bizarre thinking**
- **Inability to maintain attention:** Represented by easy distractibility, off-topic comments in group, or unfinished tasks.

Alterations in Perception. Alterations in perception involve errors in how one perceives reality. Hallucinations are the most common form of altered perception; other alterations in perception include the following:

- **Depersonalization:** A feeling that one is somehow different or unreal or has lost his identity. People may feel that body parts do not belong to them or may sense that their body has drastically changed (e.g., a patient may see her fingers as being smaller or more distant, or not her own).

- Derealization: A false perception that the environment has changed (e.g., everything seems bigger or smaller, or familiar surroundings seem somehow strange and unfamiliar).

Hallucinations involve perceiving a sensory experience for which no external stimulus exists (e.g., hearing a voice when no one is speaking). Hallucinations differ from illusions in that illusions are *misperceptions or misinterpretations of a real experience*. For example, a man sees a coat on a shadowy coat rack and believes it is a bear; he sees something real, but misinterprets what it is.

Causes of hallucinations include psychiatric disorders, drug abuse, medications, organic disorders, hyperthermia, toxicity (e.g., digitalis), and other conditions. Types of hallucination include the following:

- **Auditory**: Hearing voices or sounds
- **Visual**: Seeing persons or things
- **Olfactory**: Smelling odors
- **Gustatory**: Experiencing tastes
- **Tactile**: Feeling bodily sensations

Auditory hallucinations are experienced by 60% of people with schizophrenia at some time during their lives (Riddle, Mason & Wykes, 2011). They may be vague sounds or indistinct or clear "voices." Voices typically seem to come from outside the person's head, and auditory processing areas of the brain are activated during auditory hallucinations just as they are when a genuine external sound is heard. This abnormal activation may cause hallucinations, but another leading theory is that "voices" are a misperception of one's internally generated conversation.

John Nash, the world-renowned mathematician with schizophrenia portrayed in the film *A Beautiful Mind* (2001), describes the voices he heard:

> I thought of the voices as . . . something a little different from aliens. I thought of them more like angels . . . It's really my subconscious talking; it was really that . . . I know that now.

Voices may be of person's familiar or unknown, single or multiple. They may be perceived as supportive and pleasant or derogatory and frightening. Voices commenting on the person's behavior or conversing with the person are most common. A person who hears voices struggles to understand the experience, sometimes developing related delusions to explain the voices (e.g., believing the voices are from God, the devil, or deceased relatives). Persons with chronic hallucinations may attempt to cope by drowning them out with loud music or by competing with them by talking loudly, and such auditory competition may in fact reduce hallucinations and serve as a recommended intervention (Na, 2009).

Command hallucinations direct the person to take an action. All hallucinations must be assessed and monitored carefully, because the voices may command the person to hurt self or others; for example, telling a patient to "jump out the window" or "hit that nurse." Command hallucinations are often terrifying and may herald a psychiatric emergency. It is essential to assess *what* the patient hears, his ability to *recognize the hallucination as "not real,"* and his ability to resist any commands. Patients may falsely deny hallucinations, requiring observation for behavioral indications of hallucinations; these include tracking movements (e.g., turning or tilting the head as if to listen to someone), suddenly stopping current activity as if interrupted, talking to oneself, and moving the lips silently.

Visual hallucinations occur less frequently in schizophrenia and are more likely to occur in organic disorders such as acute alcohol withdrawal or dementia. Olfactory, tactile, or gustatory hallucinations are unusual; when present, other causes should be investigated.

Alterations in Behavior. Alterations in behavior include bizarre and agitated behaviors involving stilted, rigid demeanor or eccentric dress, grooming, and rituals. Other behavioral changes seen in schizophrenia include the following:

- **Catatonia**: A pronounced increase or decrease in the rate and amount of movement; the most common form is stuporous behavior in which the person moves little or not at all.
- **Motor retardation**: A pronounced slowing of movement.
- **Motor agitation**: Excited behavior such as running or pacing rapidly, often in response to internal or external stimuli; it can pose a risk to the patient (e.g., exhaustion, collapse, and even death) or others (being knocked down).
- Stereotyped behaviors: Repeated motor behaviors that do not serve a logical purpose.
- **Waxy flexibility**: The extended maintenance of posture, usually seen in catatonia. For example, the nurse raises the patient's arm, and the patient continues to hold this position in a statue like manner.
- Echopraxia: The mimicking of movements of another. It is also seen in catatonia.
- **Negativism**: Akin to resistance but may not be intentional. The patient does the opposite of what he or she is told to do (*active negativism*) or fails to do what is requested (*passive negativism*).
- **Impaired impulse control**: A reduced ability to resist one's impulses. Examples include interrupting in group or throwing unwanted food on the floor.
- **Gesturing or posturing**: Assuming unusual and illogical expressions (often grimaces) or positions.
- **Boundary impairment**: An impaired ability to sense where one's body or influence ends and another's begins. For example, a patient might stand too close to others or might drink another's beverage, believing that, because it is near him, it is his.

Negative Symptoms

Negative symptoms develop slowly and are those that most interfere with a person's adjustment and ability to cope. Negative symptoms impede one's ability to do the following:

- Initiate and maintain conversations and relationships
- Obtain and maintain employment
- Make decisions and follow through on plans
- Maintain adequate hygiene and grooming

Negative symptoms contribute to poor social functioning and social withdrawal. During the acute phase, they are difficult to assess because positive symptoms (such as delusions and hallucinations) dominate. See Table 12-2 for these and other negative symptoms.

Affect is the outward expression of a person's internal emotional state. In schizophrenia, affect may not always coincide

TABLE 12-2 NEGATIVE SYMPTOMS OF SCHIZOPHRENIA

NEGATIVE SYMPTOM	DESCRIPTION
Affective blunting	A reduction in the expression, range, and intensity of affect (In *flat affect,* no facial expression is present.)
Anergia	Lack of energy; passivity, lack of persistence at work or school
Anhedonia	Inability to experience pleasure in activities that usually produce it
Avolition	Reduced motivation and spontaneous activity; inability to initiate tasks such as social contacts, grooming, and other activities of daily living (ADLs)
Poverty of content of speech	While adequate in amount, speech conveys little information because of vagueness or superficiality
Poverty of speech	Reduced spontaneity and amount of speech; rarely initiates speech and responds in brief or one-word answers
Thought blocking	A sudden interruption in the thought process, usually due to internal stimuli. *Example:* A patient abruptly stops talking in the middle of a sentence and remains silent. Nurse: What just happened now? Patient: I forgot what I was saying. Something took my thoughts away.

with inner emotions. Affect in schizophrenia can usually be categorized in one of four ways:

- **Flat:** Immobile or blank facial expression
- **Blunted:** Reduced or minimal emotional response
- **Inappropriate:** Incongruent with the actual emotional state or situation (e.g., a man laughs when a peer threatens him)
- **Bizarre:** Odd, illogical, grossly inappropriate, or unfounded; includes grimacing and giggling

Cognitive Symptoms

Cognitive symptoms represent the third symptom group and are evident in most persons with schizophrenia. They involve difficulty with attention, memory, information processing, cognitive flexibility, and executive functions (e.g., decision making, judgment, planning, and problem solving). These impairments can lead to poor judgment and leave the patient less able to cope, learn, manage his health, or hold a job.

Affective Symptoms

Affective symptoms, the fourth group, are common and increase patients' suffering. Mood may be depressed, elated, unstable, erratic, or hostile. Assessment for depression is crucial because depression may:

- Herald an impending relapse
- Increase substance abuse
- Increase suicide risk
- Further impair functioning

Self-Assessment

Working with individuals with schizophrenia produces strong emotional reactions (called *countertransference*) in most health care workers. Some of these reactions are positive, and many persons find work with this population challenging and extremely rewarding. Some may decide to make this their career. For others, the patient's bizarre, irrational, disorganized, or fearful presentation brings on uncomfortable and frightening emotions. The chronicity, repeated exacerbations, and slow response to treatment many patients experience can lead to feelings of helplessness and powerlessness in staff.

Without support and a willingness to explore these feelings with more experienced staff, the nurse may adopt nontherapeutic responses: denial, withdrawal, patient avoidance, and anger. These behaviors reduce the patient's progress and undermine the nurse's self-esteem. Comments such as "These patients are hopeless" and "All you can do is babysit in this rotation" are indications of unrecognized, unresolved countertransference that, if left uncorrected, interfere with both treatment and work satisfaction. Examining whether one's expectations of patients are realistic and seeking new ways of helping patients can help staff overcome feelings of helplessness and reduce countertransference.

Fear, stigma, or shame about their mental illness can cause patients to conceal some aspects of their experience. Negativism and alogia (reduced verbalization) can also reduce responsiveness. Many persons with schizophrenia experience **anosognosia**, an inability to realize they are ill (which is caused by the illness itself). The resulting lack of insight can make assessment (and treatment) challenging, requiring additional nursing skill.

ASSESSMENT GUIDELINES

Schizophrenia and Other Psychotic Disorders

1. Determine if the patient has had a medical workup. Assess for indications of medical problems that might mimic psychosis (e.g., digitalis or anticholinergic toxicity, brain trauma, drug intoxication, delirium, fever).
2. Assess for drug or alcohol abuse or dependency.
3. Determine risk to self or others.
4. Assess for command hallucinations (e.g., voices telling the person to harm self or another). If present, ask the patient:
   - Do you recognize the voices?
   - Do you believe the voices are real?
   - Do you plan to follow the command? (A "yes" to any of these questions suggests an increased risk that the patient will act on the commands.)
5. Assess the patient for delusions. If present, are they firmly held? Is the patient able to reality test (determine what is real)? Also ask:
   - Does the patient believe that he or loved ones are being threatened or in danger?

ASSESSMENT GUIDELINES—cont'd

Schizophrenia and Other Psychotic Disorders

- Does the patient feel the need to act against a person or organization to protect or avenge himself or others? (A positive response to either of these questions suggests an increased risk of danger to others.)

6. Assess for suicide risk (refer to Chapter 25).
7. Assess for ability to ensure personal safety:
   - Adequate food and fluid intake?
   - Hygiene and self-care?
   - Ability to move about safely? (e.g., falls, walking into traffic)
   - Impulse control and judgment intact?
   - Safe dress for weather conditions?
9. Assess prescribed medications, whether and how they are taken, and what factors (e.g., costs, mistrust of staff, side effects) are affecting adherence.
10. Complete a mental status examination, noting which symptoms are present, how they affect functioning, and how the patient is managing them.
11. Assess the patient's insight, knowledge of the illness, relationships and support systems, other coping resources, and strengths.
12. Assess the family's knowledge of and response to the patient's illness and its symptoms. Are family members overprotective? Hostile? Anxious? Are they familiar with family support groups and respite resources?

CONSIDERING CULTURE

The Stigma of Schizophrenia

Mrs. Chou, a young Chinese-American woman, learned that her mother died from pneumonia. Mrs. Chou commented that her mother would not have become ill if she had been a better daughter, and that evil would now come to their family as a result.

After the funeral Mrs. Chou became increasingly lethargic, staring into space and mumbling to herself. When Mr. Chou asked whom she was talking to, she answered, "My mother." Mr. Chou knew something was wrong with his wife but was reluctant to seek help. In his culture there is strong stigma against mental illness, and it is often perceived as a punishment.

When Mrs. Chou quit eating and taking care of herself and their child, Mr. Chou took her to an herbalist. The herbalist convinced Mr. Chou to take her to a hospital. During her admission, the unkempt and pale Mrs. Chou sat motionless and mute.

Mr. Chou apologized for burdening others with her care and asked that her treatment be kept secret. Mr. Nolan helped Mr. Chou recognize that Mrs. Chou had a physical illness that affected her thinking and behavior, that treatment would help her, and that this was acceptable in the American culture.

Mr. Chou's calmed as he realized others would help care for his wife. As Mrs. Chou improved, she and Mr. Chou came to attribute the illness to fate and stress, reducing their guilt. They met with a Chinese-American healer who helped them integrate their beliefs with the beliefs and resources of their adopted culture, further reducing their distress.

Tung, W-C. (2011). Cultural barriers to mental health services among Asian Americans. *Home Health Care Management and Practice, 23*(4), 303-305.

DIAGNOSIS

People with schizophrenia have multiple disturbing and disabling symptoms that require a multifaceted approach to care and treatment of both the patient and the family. Table 12-3 lists potential nursing diagnoses for a person with schizophrenia.

OUTCOMES IDENTIFICATION

Desired outcomes vary with the phase of the illness. *Nursing Outcomes Classification (NOC)* (Moorhead et al., 2013) is a useful guide. Outcomes should focus on illness management, coping, and maximizing one's quality of life. Outcomes should be consistent with the **recovery model** (refer to Chapter 31), which stresses hope, living a full and productive life, and eventual recovery rather than focusing on controlling symptoms and adapting to disability.

Phase I: Acute

For the acute phase, the overall goal is **patient safety and stabilization.** If the patient is at risk for violence to self or others, initial outcome criteria address safety issues (e.g., *patient refrains from self injury*). Another outcome is *patient consistently labels hallucinations as "not real—a symptom of an illness."*

Phase II: Stabilization

Outcome criteria during phase II focus on helping the patient understand the illness and treatment, become stabilized on medications, and control or cope with symptoms. The outcomes target the negative symptoms and may address the ability to succeed in social, vocational, or self-care activities.

Phase III: Maintenance

Outcome criteria for phase III focus on maintaining achievement, adhering to treatment, preventing relapse, and achieving independence and a satisfactory quality of life.

PLANNING

The planning of appropriate interventions is guided by the phase of the illness and the strengths and needs of the patient. Cultural considerations, available resources, and patient preferences influence planning.

Phase I: Acute

Hospitalization is indicated if the patient is considered a danger to self or others (e.g., refuses to eat or drink or is too disorganized or otherwise impaired to function safely in the community without supervision). Planning focuses on the best strategies to ensure patient safety and control symptoms.

In discharge planning, the patient and multidisciplinary treatment team identify needs for follow-up and support. The nurse considers not only external factors, such as the patient's living arrangements, economic resources, social supports, and family relationships, but also internal factors such as resilience and range of coping skills. Because relapse can be devastating

TABLE 12-3 POTENTIAL NURSING DIAGNOSES FOR SCHIZOPHRENIA

SYMPTOM	NURSING DIAGNOSES
Positive Symptoms	
Hears voices that others do not *(auditory hallucinations)*	*Disturbed sensory perception: auditory/visual*
Hears voices telling him or her to hurt self or others *(command hallucinations)*	*Risk for self-directed/other-directed violence*
Delusions	
Shows loose association of ideas *(associative looseness)*	*Impaired verbal communication*
Conversation is derailed by unnecessary and tedious details *(circumstantiality)*	
Negative Symptoms	
Uncommunicative, withdrawn	*Social isolation*
Expresses feelings of rejection or aloneness (lies in bed all day, positions back to door)	*Impaired social interaction* *Risk for loneliness*
Talks about self as "bad" or "no good"	*Chronic low self-esteem*
Feels guilty because of "bad thoughts"; extremely sensitive to real or perceived slights	*Risk for self-directed violence*
Shows lack of energy *(anergia)*	*Ineffective coping*
Shows lack of motivation *(avolition)*, unable to initiate tasks (social contact, grooming, and other aspects of daily living)	*Self-care deficit (bathing/hygiene, dressing/grooming)* *Constipation*
Other	
Families and significant others become confused or overwhelmed, lack knowledge about disorder or treatment, feel powerless in coping with patient	*Compromised family coping* *Caregiver role strain* *Deficient knowledge*
Stops taking medication (because of anosognosia, side effects, drugs costs, mistrust of staff), stops going to therapy, is not supported in treatment by significant others	*Nonadherence*

Herdman, T.H. (Ed.). *Nursing diagnoses—Definitions and classification 2012-2014.*

(resulting in loss of employment, housing, and relationships) and worsen the long-term prognosis, vigorous efforts are made to *connect the patient and family with* (not simply refer them to) community resources that provide therapeutic programming and social, financial, and other needed support.

Phase II: Stabilization and Phase III: Maintenance

Planning during the stabilization and maintenance phases focuses on providing patient and family education and skills training (psychosocial education). **Relapse prevention skills (see** Box 12-2) **are vital.** Planning identifies interpersonal, coping, health care, and vocational needs and addresses how and where these needs can best be met within the community.

IMPLEMENTATION

Interventions are geared toward the phase of the disorder. For example, during the acute phase, the clinical focus is on crisis intervention, medication for symptom stabilization, and safety. Interventions are often hospital-based; however, to reduce costs and provide treatment in the least restrictive setting, many patients in the acute stage increasingly are being treated in the community.

BOX 12-2 CAN SCHIZOPHRENIA BE PREVENTED?

Factors such as smoking tobacco or marijuana, drug abuse, or prenatal malnutrition or infection increase the risk of developing schizophrenia. Primary prevention to reduce the development of schizophrenia could focus on such factors, but not all risk factors can be avoided. If genetics leaves one vulnerable to schizophrenia, what can be done? Apart from avoiding triggers, such as environmental stressors, and interventions to promote resiliency and coping in children and families, research suggests at least two additional options: prophylactic treatment with antipsychotic medications and supplemental essential fatty acids.

Early assessment of prodromal symptoms (such as eccentric or magical thinking, cognitive disorganization, or quasi-hallucinations) is accomplished via tools such as the Structured Interview for Psychosis-Risk Syndrome (McGlashan & Woods, 2011). Research suggests that antipsychotic medications could be used preventively during the prodromal phase to reduce the development or severity of schizophrenia. The downside: Only one third of those deemed "at risk" of schizophrenia actually develop the disorder, so some would be unnecessarily experiencing the not-insignificant side effect risks of antipsychotics (Barnes, 2011; Brown & McGrath, 2011).

More promising: omega -3 and omega-6 polyunsaturated fatty acids (found in fish oils and oily fish, e.g. tuna, salmon, sardines). These fats are abnormally low in the brains of people with schizophrenia. They reduce inflammation and free radicals in the brain and contribute to ACH and serotonin stability. Although it is not clear that these fatty acids reduce symptomatology in schizophrenia (as has been reported), preliminary evidence suggests that they reduce the conversion from "at risk" to actually having schizophrenia (Atker et al., 2011).

EVIDENCE-BASED PRACTICE

Transcranial Magnetic Stimulation in Pharmacologically Unresponsive Patients with Schizophrenia

Oh, S-Y, & Kim, Y-K. (2011). Adjunctive treatment of bimodal repetitive transcranial magnetic stimulation in pharmacologically non-responsive patients with schizophrenia: A preliminary study. *Progress in Neuro-Psychopharmacology & Biological Psychiatry, 35*(2011), 1938-1943.

Problem

Antipsychotics are of limited value to a significant number of persons with schizophrenia; 5% to 10% do not respond at all, and 20% to 45% respond only partially.

Purpose of Study

This study sought to determine whether repeated application of magnetic energy to the brain through the cranium (transcranial magnetic stimulation, or TMS) would produce significant improvement in a population of patients who responded inadequately to antipsychotic medication. TMS can increase or decrease neural excitability in targeted areas of the brain depending on the frequency of the magnetic impulses.

Methods

A sample of 10 patients who had not responded adequately to antipsychotics was given a series of 15 transcranial magnetic stimulation sessions over a 3-week period. Symptom levels were assessed before and after this intervention. TMS in this study was modified based on earlier research findings to provide stimulation to two sections of the brain in series (bimodal TMS) during each session, an approach not previously studied.

Key Findings

The bimodal TMS treatments produced measured improvement in symptoms significantly exceeding that achieved by medications alone.

Implications for Nursing Practice

Alternative or adjunctive treatments to help those who respond poorly to psychopharmacology are sorely needed to reduce suffering and promote recovery. This new approach to treatment holds promise for helping those not adequately helped by antipsychotics.

Phase I: Acute

Settings

A number of factors that affect the choice of treatment setting include the following:

- Level of care/restrictiveness needed to prevent harm to self or others
- Needs for external structure and support (e.g., others guiding the patient's activities)
- Ability to cooperate with treatment
- Need for a treatment available only in particular settings
- Need for treatment of a concurrent medical condition
- Availability of third-party information and treatment history required so that staff can reliably assess the patient's needs

Interventions

Acute phase interventions include the following:

- Psychiatric, medical, and neurological evaluation
- Psychopharmacology
- Support, psychoeducation, and guidance
- Supervision and structure in a therapeutic environment (milieu)
- Monitor fluid intake

The length of hospitalization or other intensive treatment programs during the acute phase is often short (days), ending when acute symptoms have been stabilized; however, this does not necessarily take into account the extended time needed for recovery from serious mental illness, making continued care in the community all the more important after discharge (Moller & Zauszniewski, 2011). Community-based services provide such care during the stabilization and maintenance phases.

Phase II: Stabilization and Phase III: Maintenance

Effective long-term care of persons with schizophrenia relies on a three-pronged approach: medication administration/adherence, relationships with trusted care providers, and community-based therapeutic services. **Family psychoeducation, a key role of the nurse, is essential**. All care is geared to the patient's strengths, culture, personal preferences, and needs.

Community-based programs may include group and individual psychotherapy, supervised activities, and training (e.g. social or coping skills). Staff must be aware of such community resources and provide this information to discharged patients and their families, ideally by directly connecting them with these resources. Patients and family members should be given telephone numbers and addresses of local support groups such as the National Alliance on Mental Illness (NAMI) (www.nami.org).

Other community resources include community mental health centers (usually providing medication services, day treatment, access to 24-hour emergency services, psychotherapy, psychoeducation, and case management), home health services, supported employment programs (wherein patients receive services from job training to on-site coaches who help them learn to succeed in the work environment, often via the Bureau of Vocational Rehabilitation [BVR]), peer-led services (e.g., drop-in centers, sometimes called "clubhouses," that offer social contact, constructive activities, and sometimes employment opportunities), family educational/skills groups (e.g., NAMI's "Family-to-Family" program), and respite care for caregivers.

Teamwork and Safety

Effective care provides (1) protection from undue stress and (2) structure—a planned routine and external limits that create a sense of security. This therapeutic structure promotes a faster recovery than would occur in an unstructured setting such as one's residence. Hospital alternatives (e.g., crisis centers) also provide a structured milieu in a less restrictive setting. A therapeutic milieu is consciously designed to provide a physical and social environment that maximizes safety, opportunities for learning and practicing skills such as conflict resolution, stress reduction, and symptom management techniques, and therapeutic activities (e.g., games that promote socialization).

Activities and Groups

Participation in activities and groups appropriate to the patient's level of functioning may decrease withdrawal, enhance motivation, modify unacceptable behaviors, facilitate support and feedback from staff and peers, and increase social competence. Drawing, reading poetry, journaling, and listening to music focus conversations and promote the recognition and expression of feelings. Self-esteem is enhanced via task completion and participation in activities for which there is a high likelihood of success. Recreational activities such as picnics and outings to stores or restaurants are not simply diversions; they teach constructive leisure skills, increase social comfort, build social concern and interactional skills, and improve boundaries. Outpatient group therapy can provide necessary structure after discharge.

Working with an Aggressive Patient

A small percentage of patients with schizophrenia, especially during the acute phase, may exhibit a risk for physical violence, typically in response to hallucinations (especially command hallucinations), delusions, paranoia, and impaired judgment or impulse control. When the potential for violence exists, measures to protect the patient and others become the priority. Interventions include increasing supervision, reducing stimulation (e.g., noise, patient involvement in unit activities), addressing paranoia and other contributing symptoms, providing constructive diversion and outlets for physical energy, teaching and practicing coping skills, using cognitive-behavioral approaches to correct unrealistic expectations or selectively extinguish aggression, de-escalating tension verbally, and, when necessary, using seclusion or chemical (medication) or physical restraints.

Refer to Chapter 27 for a more information on caring for the aggressive patient. Another significant safety concern for persons experiencing psychosis is the risk of suicide. Schizophrenia is typically a chronic disorder that significantly alters a person's quality of life. This can contribute to depression and despair, which in combination with limited coping skills and reduced access to support persons can result in suicide. Suicide and self-injury can also result from delusional thinking or hallucinatory experience; for example, a person may hear voices directing him to amputate his genitalia due to the delusion that he has sexually assaulted others. Please refer to Chapter 25 for more information on assessing and reducing suicide risk.

Counseling and Communication Techniques

Therapeutic communication techniques for patients with schizophrenia aim to lower the patient's anxiety, build trust, encourage clear communication, increase self-awareness, encourage interaction, enhance self-esteem, and enhance skills such as reality testing and assertiveness. It is important to remember that patients with schizophrenia may have memory impairment and require repetition. Persons who think concretely also benefit from concrete examples during education (e.g., counting out the number of sugar cubes in a bottle of cola to show its sugar content). Shorter (<30 minutes) but more frequent interactions may be less stimulating and better tolerated than fewer, longer interactions.

Hallucinations

When a patient is hallucinating, the nurse focuses on understanding the patient's experiences and responses. Suicidal or homicidal themes or commands necessitate appropriate safety measures. For example, "voices" that tell a patient that a peer plans to harm him may lead him to act aggressively against that person; one-to-one supervision of the patient, or transfer of the potential victim to another unit, is often essential.

Hallucinations are real to the person who is experiencing them and may be distracting during nurse-patient interactions. Call the patient by name, speak simply and loudly enough to be understood amidst the hallucinations, present in a nonthreatening and supportive manner, maintain eye contact, and redirect the patient's focus to your conversation as needed. Box 12-3 lists other techniques for communicating with patients experiencing hallucinations.

BOX 12-3 HELPING PATIENTS WHO ARE EXPERIENCING HALLUCINATIONS

- Ask the patient directly about the hallucinations. Example: "What are you hearing?"
- Watch the patient for cues that he or she is hallucinating, such as eyes tracking an unheard speaker, muttering, talking to self, appearing distracted, or watching a vacant area of the room.
- Avoid referring to hallucinations as if they are real.
- Do not negate the patient's experience, but offer your own perceptions and convey empathy. Example: "I don't hear the angry voices, but that must be very frightening for you."
- Focus on reality-based, "here-and-now" activities such as conversations or simple projects. Tell the patient, "The voice you hear is part of your illness; it cannot hurt you. Try to listen to me and the others you can see around you."
- Be alert to signs of anxiety in the patient, which may indicate that hallucinations are increasing.
- Encourage the use of competing auditory stimuli such as listening to music through headphones
- Address any underlying emotion, need, or theme that seems to be indicated by the hallucination, such as fear with menacing voices or guilt with accusing voices.

Data from Farhall, J., Greenwood, K. M., & Jackson, H. J. (2007). Coping with hallucinated voices in schizophrenia: A review of self-initiated strategies and therapeutic interventions. *Clinical Psychology Review, 27*, 476–493.

Delusions

Delusions may be the patient's attempts to understand confusing and distorted experiences. Impaired reality testing prevents self-correction when one misperceives his circumstances. When the nurse attempts to see the world through the patient's eyes, it becomes easier to understand the patient's delusion. For example:

> **Patient:** You people are all alike . . . all in on the FBI plot to destroy me.
> **Nurse:** I don't want to hurt you, Tom. Thinking that people are out to destroy you must be very frightening.

In this example, the nurse acknowledges the patient's experience, conveys empathy about the patient's fearfulness, avoids questioning the content of the delusion (FBI and plot to destroy), and labels the patient's feelings so they can be explored (as tolerated). Note that talking about the feelings and underlying themes is helpful, but extended focus on delusional material is not.

Until reality testing improves it is *never* useful to debate or attempt to dissuade the patient from the delusion. This can intensify the irrational beliefs and cause the patient to view you as rejecting or a threat; however, it *is* helpful to clarify misinterpretations of the environment and gently suggest, as tolerated, a more reality-based perspective. For example:

> **Patient:** I see the doctor is here; he wants to kill me.
> **Nurse:** It is true the doctor wants to see you, but he wants to talk to you about your treatment. Would you feel more comfortable talking with him in the day room than his office?

Focusing on specific reality-based activities and events occurring in the present helps to minimize the focus on delusions. The more time spent engaged in activities or with people, the more opportunities there are to receive feedback about and become comfortable with reality.

Work with the patient to find out which coping strategies help and how the patient can make the best use of them. Box 12-4 lists techniques for communicating with patients experiencing delusions, and Box 12-5 presents patient and family education for coping with hallucinations and delusions.

Associative Looseness

Associative looseness often mirrors the patient's idiosyncratic and disorganized thinking. An increase in looseness of associations often follows increased anxiety or overwhelming internal and external stimuli. The nurse may respond to the patient's disorganization with confusion and frustration. These guidelines are useful when a patient's speech is confused and disorganized:

- Do *not* pretend (or allow the patient to think) that you understand the patient when you don't; supportively state that you do not understand.
- Place the difficulty in understanding on yourself, *not* on the patient. Example: "I'm having trouble following what you are saying," *not* "You're not making any sense."
- Tell the patient what you *do* understand, and reinforce clear communication and accurate expression of needs, feelings, and thoughts.
- Look for recurring topics and *themes* in the patient's communications, and *tie these to events and timelines.* Example: "You've mentioned trouble with your brother several times, usually after your family has visited. Tell me about your brother and your visits with him."
- Summarize or paraphrase the patient's communications to role-model clearer communication and to give the patient a chance to correct anything you may have misunderstood.
- Reduce stimuli in the vicinity, and speak concisely, clearly, and concretely in sentences rather than paragraphs.

Health Teaching and Health Promotion

Education is essential and includes teaching the patient and family about the illness: causes, medications and side effects, coping strategies, what to expect, and relapse prevention. This knowledge and skill helps the patient and family to appreciate the impact of stress and the importance of treatment to a good outcome. It encourages involvement in (and support of) therapeutic activities and identifies resources for ongoing help in dealing with the illness.

BOX 12-4 GUIDELINES FOR COMMUNICATION WITH PATIENTS EXPERIENCING DELUSIONS

- To build trust, be open, honest, genuine, and reliable.
- Respond to suspicion in a matter-of-fact, empathic, supportive, and calm manner.
- Ask the patient to describe his beliefs. Example: "Tell me more about someone trying to hurt you."
- Avoid debating the delusional content, but interject doubt where appropriate. Example: "It seems as if it would be hard for a girl that small to hurt you."
- Validate if part of the delusion is real. Example: "Yes, there was a man at the nurse's station, but I did not hear him talk about you."
- Focus on the feelings or theme that underlie or flow from the delusions. Example: "You seem to wish you could be more powerful" or "It must feel frightening to believe others want to hurt you."
- Once trust has been established, acknowledge that, while the belief seems very real to the patient, illnesses can sometimes make things seem true even though they aren't. Introducing this obliquely can make it less confrontational: "I wonder if that might be what is happening here, because what seems true to you does not seem true to others."
- Once the patient has begun to question the delusion and/or understand the concept of delusions, label subsequent delusions to help the patient recognize them as well.
- Do not dwell excessively on the delusion. Instead, refocus onto reality-based topics. If the patient obsesses about delusions, set limits on the amount of time you will talk about them, and explain your reason.
- Observe for events that trigger delusions. If possible, help the patient find ways to avoid such triggers or reduce associated anxiety.
- Promote improved reality testing by guiding the patient to question his beliefs: "I wonder if there might be any other explanation why others might be avoiding you? Instead of hating you, might they simply be busy?"

Data from Farhall, J., Greenwood, K. M., & Jackson, H. J. (2007). Coping with hallucinated voices in schizophrenia: A review of self-initiated strategies and therapeutic interventions. *Clinical Psychology Review, 27*, 476–493.

BOX 12-5 PATIENT AND FAMILY TEACHING: COPING WITH AUDITORY HALLUCINATIONS OR DELUSIONS

Use Competing Auditory Stimuli
- Listen to music
- Read aloud
- Count backwards from 100
- Talk with others

Promote Reality Testing
- Look at others; do they seem to be hearing/seeing what you are?
- Ask others if they are experiencing what you are.
- If not, you can safely ignore the voices/images.

Engage in Activity
- Walk
- Clean the house
- Take a relaxing bath
- Play music or an instrument, or sing
- Go to the mall (or any place you enjoy being, where others will be present)

Talk to Yourself
- Tell the voices or thoughts to go away
- Tell yourself that the voices and thoughts are a symptom and aren't real
- Tell yourself that no matter what you hear, voices can be safely ignored

Make Contact With Others
- Talk to a trusted friend or relative
- Call a help line or going to a drop-in center
- Visit a favorite place or a comfortable public place

Do Something Physical
- Take extra medication when ordered (call your prescriber)
- Go for a walk or do other exercise
- Use breathing exercises and other relaxation methods

Data from Ruddle, A., Mason, O., & Wykes T. (2011). A review of hearing voices groups: Evidence and mechanisms of change. *Clinical Psychology Review, 31*, 757-766; Na, H.J. (2009). Effects of listening to music on auditory hallucinations and psychiatric symptoms in people with schizophrenia. *Journal of Korean Academy of Nursing, 39*(1) 62-71.

Including family members in any strategies aimed at reducing psychotic symptoms reduces family anxiety and distress and enables the family to reinforce the patient's and staff's efforts. The patient who returns to a warm, concerned, and supportive environment is less likely to experience relapse. When significant others are critical, controlling or intrusive, relapse increases and outcomes are poorer.

Lack of understanding of the disease and its symptoms can lead others to misinterpret the patient's apathy and lack of drive as laziness, resulting in frustration or anger in family members or others and leading to provocative and possibly dangerous conflicts. Public education about schizophrenia can thus reduce tensions in families as well as communities. The most effective education is provided when the family is most receptive and occurs over time (rather than all at once). Box 12-6 offers guidelines for patient and family teaching about schizophrenia.

Psychobiological Interventions

Drugs used to treat psychotic disorders, **antipsychotics**, first became available in the late 1950s. Previously available medications provided only sedation, not treatment of the disorder itself. Until the 1960s, patients who had even one episode of schizophrenia usually spent months or years in state or private hospitals. Psychotic episodes resulted in great emotional and financial burdens to patients, families, and society. Antipsychotic drugs at last provided symptom control and allowed patients to live and be treated in the community.

Three groups of antipsychotic drugs exist: **first-generation antipsychotics** (traditional dopamine antagonists [D_2 dopamine receptor antagonists]), also known as *conventional antipsychotics* or *neuroleptics*; **second-generation antipsychotics** (serotonin-dopamine antagonists [5-HT_{2A} receptor antagonists]), and newer **third-generation antipsychotics** such as aripiprazole (Abilify). Other drugs such as anticonvulsants are used to augment antipsychotics for the approximately 30% of patients who do not respond fully, and agents that target the glutamate system such as glycine, D-cycloserine, and D-serine—an amino acid that enhances NMDA activity—have been shown to increase the effectiveness of selected antipsychotics (de Bartolomeis et al., 2012).

All antipsychotics are effective for exacerbations and relapse prevention of schizophrenia (Lehne, 2010). The first-generation antipsychotics affect primarily the positive symptoms of schizophrenia (e.g., hallucinations, delusions, disordered thinking, etc.). The second- and third-generation antipsychotics can improve negative symptoms (e.g., asociality, blunted affect, lack of motivation) as well.

All antipsychotic agents usually take effect 2 to 6 weeks after the regimen is started, and all may require significant dosage adjustment in order to obtain an optimal balance between effectiveness and side effects. In cases where patients fail to respond satisfactorily to an antipsychotic drug after an adequate trial and dosage, an adjunctive medication may be used to improve the response, or another antipsychotic can be tried. Note that each medication change can be very trying for the patient due to the long time required to achieve optimal response.

All antipsychotics may increase mortality in elderly patients with dementia. No antipsychotics are addictive, though there may be a rebound effect characterized by a temporary increase in psychotic symptoms. All antipsychotics are unlikely to be lethal in overdose situations. A lesser-known risk of all antipsychotic meds, due to dopamine blockade, is impaired swallowing; this places patients at risk of choking and may require meal monitoring and diet adjustments (Allen et al., 2012). Finally,

BOX 12-6 PATIENT AND FAMILY TEACHING: SCHIZOPHRENIA

Further information can be found in the Substance Abuse and Mental Health Services Administration (SAMHSA) pamphlet *Developing A Recovery And Wellness Lifestyle: A Self-Help Guide*, available at http://mentalhealth.samhsa.gov/publications/allpubs/SMA-3718 or via the Wellness Recovery Action Plan (WRAP) website (M. A. Copeland and staff): www.mentalhealthrecovery.com

1. Learn all you can about the illness.
   - Attend educational and support groups.
   - Join the National Alliance on Mental Illness (NAMI).
   - Read books about mental illness such as *Surviving Schizophrenia: A Manual for Families, Patients, and Providers* by E. Fuller Torrey.
   - Access trusted websites such as the National Institute of Mental Health (www.nimh.nih.gov).
2. Develop a relapse prevention plan.
   - Know the early warning signs of relapse (e.g., avoiding others, trouble sleeping, troubling thoughts).
   - Make a list of whom to call, what to do, and where to go if signs of relapse appear. Keep it with you.
   - Relapse is part of the illness, not a sign of failure.
3. Participate in family, group, and individual therapy.
4. Learn new ways to act and coping skills to help handle family, work, and social stress. Get information from your nurse, case manager, doctor, NAMI, community mental health groups, or a hospital. Everyone needs a place to talk about fears and losses and to learn new ways of coping.
5. Have a plan, on paper, of what to do to cope with stressful times.
6. Adhere to treatment. People who adhere to treatment that works for them are more likely to get better and stay better.
   - Engaging in struggles over adherence does not help, but tying adherence to the patient's own goals does. ("Staying in treatment will help you keep your job and avoid trouble with the police.")
   - Share concerns about troubling side effects or concerns (e.g., sexual problems, weight gain, "feeling funny") with your nurse, case manager, doctor, or social worker; most side effects can be helped.
   - Keeping side effects a secret or stopping medication can prevent you from having the life you want.
7. Avoid alcohol and/or drugs; they can act on the brain and cause a relapse.
8. Keep in touch with supportive people.
9. Keep healthy and stay in balance.
   - Taking care of one's diet, health, and hygiene helps prevent medical illnesses.
   - Maintain a regular sleep pattern.
   - Keep active (hobbies, friends, groups, sports, job, special interests).
   - Nurture yourself, and practice stress-reduction activities daily.

Data from *Beyond symptom control: Moving towards positive patient outcomes.* Paper presented at the American Psychiatric Association 55th Institute on Psychiatric Services, October 29 to November 2, 2003, Boston, MA. Retrieved from www.medscape.com/viewprogram/2835_pnt. Further information can be found in the Substance Abuse and Mental Health Services Administration (SAMHSA) pamphlet *Developing a recovery and wellness lifestyle: A self-help guide,* available at http://mentalhealth.samhsa.gov/publications/allpubs/SMA-3718, or via the Wellness Recovery Action Plan (WRAP) website (M. A. Copeland and staff) at www.mentalhealthrecovery.com.

persons with impaired cognition are at increased fall risk, a problem worsened by sedating medications (Allen et al., 2012).

Some antipsychotics are available in long-acting injectable formulations that require special administration techniques; by requiring interaction with medications less frequently, adherence can be improved and conflict with others about taking medications can be reduced. Liquid or fast-dissolving forms can make it difficult for a person to "cheek" his medicine (hide it in his cheek and spit it out later), also increasing adherence.

First-Generation Antipsychotics

First-generation antipsychotics are used less in schizophrenia because of their minimal impact on negative symptoms and their wide range of side effects; however, they are effective against positive symptoms and are much less expensive than second-generation antipsychotics; for patients who can tolerate the side effects, this class of drugs remains an appropriate choice, especially when cost or metabolic syndrome (described later in this chapter) is a concern.

First-generation antipsychotics are dopamine D_2 antagonists in both the limbic and motor centers. This blockage of D_2 dopamine receptors in the motor areas causes **extrapyramidal side effects (EPSs)**. Three of the more common EPSs are **acute dystonia** (acute sustained contraction of muscles, usually of the head and neck), **akathisia** (psychomotor restlessness evident as pacing or fidgeting, sometimes pronounced and very distressing to patients), and **pseudoparkinsonism** (a medication-induced, temporary constellation of symptoms associated with Parkinson's disease: tremor, reduced accessory movements, impaired gait, and stiffening of muscles).

Lowering dosages can usually minimize EPSs, and adding antiparkinsonian drugs, especially centrally acting anticholinergic drugs such as trihexyphenidyl (Artane) and benztropine mesylate (Cogentin). Diphenhydramine hydrochloride (Benadryl) and amantadine hydrochloride (Symmetrel) are also useful. Lorazepam, a benzodiazepine, may be helpful in reducing akathisia, as can relaxation exercises. Table 12-4 identifies drugs most commonly used to treat EPSs. Most patients develop tolerance to EPSs after a few months.

The first-generation antipsychotics are divided into low-potency and high-potency drugs on the basis of their anticholinergic (ACh) side effects, EPSs, and sedative profiles. Table 12-5 provides more detailed information, but in general the following applies:

Low potency = high sedation + high ACh + low EPSs
High potency = low sedation + low ACh + high EPSs

Other adverse reactions include anticholinergic effects (including anticholinergic toxicity, which can be fatal, and can be mistaken for a worsening of the patient's psychosis),

TABLE 12-4 SIDE EFFECTS OF CONVENTIONAL ANTIPSYCHOTICS AND RELATED NURSING INTERVENTIONS

SIDE EFFECT	ONSET	NURSING INTERVENTIONS
Anticholinergic Symptoms		
Dry mouth		Provide frequent sips of water, ice chips, and sugarless candy or gum. If severe, provide Xero-Lube or other saliva substitute.
Urinary retention and hesitancy		Check voiding; check for distended bladder. Try running water and warm towel on abdomen, and consider catheterization if no result.
Constipation		Ensure adequate fluid and fiber intake. May use stool softener, laxative, or dietary laxatives (e.g., prune juice).
Blurred vision		Usually abates in 1 to 2 weeks. May require use of reading or magnifying glasses. If intolerable, consider consult regarding medication change.
Photosensitivity		Encourage patient to wear sunglasses, sunscreen, sun-blocking clothing. Limit exposure to sunlight.
Dry eyes		Use artificial tears. Avoid wind exposure.
Sexual dysfunction		Consult prescriber—patient may need alternative medication. Artificial lubricants for vaginal dryness.
Anticholinergic toxicity: dry mucous membranes; reduced or absent peristalsis; mydriasis; nonreactive pupils; hot, dry, red skin; hyperpyrexia without diaphoresis; tachycardia; agitation; unstable vital signs; worsening of psychotic symptoms; delirium; urinary retention; seizure; repetitive motor movements		***Potentially life-threatening medical emergency*** Consult prescriber immediately. Hold all medications. Implement emergency cooling measures as ordered (cooling blanket, alcohol, or ice bath). Implement urinary catheterization prn. Administer benzodiazepines or other prn sedation as ordered. Physostigmine may be ordered.
Extrapyramidal Side Effects (EPSs)		
Pseudoparkinsonism: masklike facies, stiff and stooped posture, shuffling gait, drooling, tremor, "pill-rolling" phenomenon	5 hours-30 days	Administer prn antiparkinsonian agent (e.g., trihexyphenidyl or benztropine) If intolerable, consult prescriber regarding medication change. Provide towel or handkerchief to wipe excess saliva. Teach how to reduce fall risk (holding onto rails, arise gradually).
Acute dystonic reactions: acute contractions of tongue, face, neck, and back (usually tongue and jaw first) Opisthotonos: tetanic heightening of entire body, head and belly up Oculogyric crisis: eyes locked upward Laryngeal dystonia: could threaten airway (rare)	1-5 days	Administer antiparkinsonian agent as above (IM for faster response). Also consider diphenhydramine hydrochloride (Benadryl) 25-50 mg IM/IV. Relief usually occurs in 5-15 minutes. Prevent further dystonias with antiparkinsonian agent (see Table 12-9). Experience can be frightening, and patient may fear choking. Stay with the patient; accompany to quiet area to provide comfort and support. Assist patient to understand the event and avert distortion or mistrust of medications. Monitor airway.
Akathisia: motor inner-driven restlessness (e.g., tapping foot incessantly, rocking forward and backward in chair, shifting weight from side to side)	2 hours-60 days	Consult prescriber regarding possible medication change. Give antiparkinsonian agent. Tolerance to akathisia does not develop, but akathisia usually subsides when antipsychotic is discontinued. Propranolol (Inderal), lorazepam (Ativan), or diazepam (Valium) may be used. In severe cases, may cause great distress and contribute to suicidality.

TABLE 12-4 SIDE EFFECTS OF CONVENTIONAL ANTIPSYCHOTICS AND RELATED NURSING INTERVENTIONS—cont'd

SIDE EFFECT	ONSET	NURSING INTERVENTIONS
Tardive dyskinesia (TD): *Face:* protruding and rolling tongue, blowing, smacking, licking, spastic facial distortion, smacking movements *Limbs:* Choreic: rapid, purposeless, and irregular movements Athetoid: slow, complex, and serpentine movements *Trunk:* neck and shoulder movements, dramatic hip jerks and rocking, twisting pelvic thrusts Possibly 20% of patients taking these drugs for >2 years may develop TD.	Months to years	No known treatment. Discontinuing the drug rarely relieves symptoms. Nurses and doctors should screen for TD at least every 3 months. Onset may merit reconsideration of meds. Changes in appearance may contribute to stigmatizing response by others. Provide support. Teach patient actions to conceal involuntary movements (e.g., holding one hand with the other, as purposeful muscle contraction overrides involuntary tardive movements).
α_2 Block: Cardiovascular Effects		
Hypotension and postural hypotension		Check blood pressure before giving agent. Hold dose and consult prescriber if systolic pressure is < 80 mm Hg when standing. Advise patient to arise slowly to prevent dizziness and to hold onto railings/furniture while arising to reduce falls. Effect usually subsides when drug is stabilized in 1 to 2 weeks. Assure adequate hydration. Elastic bandages may prevent pooling. If condition is dangerous, consult prescriber regarding medication change, volume expanders, or pressure agents.
Tachycardia		Always evaluate patients with existing cardiac problems before antipsychotic drugs are administered. Abnormal Q-T interval can be a contraindication for certain antipsychotics.
Rare and Toxic Effects		
Agranulocytosis: symptoms include sore throat, fever, malaise, mouth sores, increased infections, and reduced white blood cell and neutrophil counts. It is rare but a possibility the nurse should be aware of; any flulike symptoms should be carefully evaluated	Usually during the first 12 weeks of therapy. Occurs suddenly.	***Potentially dangerous blood dyscrasia*** Clozaril blood work usually done every week for 6 months, then less frequently. Physician may order blood work to determine presence of leukopenia or agranulocytosis. If test results are positive, the drug is discontinued, and reverse isolation may be initiated. Mortality is high if the drug is continued and treatment is not initiated. Teach patient to observe for signs of infection.
Cholestatic jaundice: rare, reversible, and usually benign if caught in time; early symptoms are fever, malaise, nausea, and abdominal pain; jaundice appears 1 week later.		Consult prescriber regarding possible medication change. Bed rest and high-protein, high-carbohydrate diet if ordered. Liver function tests should be performed every 6 months.

Continued

TABLE 12-4 SIDE EFFECTS OF CONVENTIONAL ANTIPSYCHOTICS AND RELATED NURSING INTERVENTIONS—cont'd

SIDE EFFECT	ONSET	NURSING INTERVENTIONS
Neuroleptic malignant syndrome (NMS): rare, potentially fatal *Severe extrapyramidal:* severe muscle rigidity, oculogyric crisis, dysphasia, flexor-extensor posturing, cogwheeling, decreased responsiveness. *Hyperpyrexia is a cardinal feature:* temperature over 103 ° F or 39 ° C Autonomic dysfunction: hypertension, tachycardia, diaphoresis, incontinence Delirium, stupor, coma	Can occur in the first week of drug therapy, but often occurs later. Rapidly progresses over 2 to 3 days after initial manifestation Risk Factors: Concomitant use of other psychotropics Older age Female gender (3:2) Presence of a mood disorder (40%) Rapid dose titration	***Acute, life-threatening medical emergency*** Stop neuroleptic. Transfer STAT to a critical care unit Bromocriptine (Parlodel) can relieve muscle rigidity and reduce fever. Dantrolene (Dantrium) may reduce muscle spasms. Cool body to reduce fever (cooling blankets, alcohol, cool water, or ice bath as ordered). Maintain hydration with oral and IV fluids; correct electrolyte imbalance. Arrhythmias should be treated. Small doses of heparin may decrease possibility of pulmonary emboli. Early detection increases patient's chance of survival.

Data from Lehne, R.A. (2010). *Pharmacology for nursing care* (7th ed.). St. Louis: Saunders; Howland, R.H. (2012). Drugs to treat bipolar disorder. *Journal of Psychosocial Nursing, 50*(6), 9-10; Kemmerer, D. A. (2007). Anticholinergic syndrome. *Journal of Emergency Nursing, 33*(1), 76–78.

TABLE 12-5 ANTIPSYCHOTIC DRUGS: CLASSIFICATION, ROUTE, AND SIDE-EFFECT PROFILE

CLASSIFICATION GENERIC (BRAND)	ROUTE	EPSs	SEDATION	OH	ACH	WEIGHT GAIN	DIABETES
First-Generation Antipsychotics (Treat Positive Symptoms)							
Low Potency							
Chlorpromazine (Thorazine)	PO, IM, IV, R	Moderate	High	High	Moderate	Moderate	Moderate
Thioridazine (Mellaril)	PO	Low	High	High	High	Moderate	Moderate
Medium Potency							
Loxapine (Loxitane)	PO	Moderate	Moderate	Low	Low	Low	Low
Molindone (Moban)	PO	Moderate	Moderate	Low	Low	Low	Low
Perphenazine (Trilafon)	PO	Moderate	Moderate	Low	Low	—	—
High Potency							
Trifluoperazine (generic only)	PO, IM	High	Low	Low	Low	—	—
Thiothixene (Navane)	PO	High	Low	Moderate	Low	—	Moderate
Fluphenazine (Prolixin)	PO, IM	High	Low	Low	Low	—	—
Haloperidol (Haldol)	PO, IM	High	Low	Low	Low	—	Moderate
Pimozide (Orap)	PO	High	Moderate	Low	Moderate	—	—
Second-Generation Antipsychotics (Treat Positive and Negative Symptoms)							
Asenapine (Saphris)	SL	*	*	*	*	*	*
Clozapine (Clozaril)	PO	Very low	High	Moderate	High	High	High
Iloperidone (Fanapt)	PO	*	*	*	*	*	*
Lurasidone (Latuda)	PO	*	*	*	*	*	*
Olanzapine (Zyprexa)	PO, IM	Very low	High	Moderate	High	High	High
Paliperidone (Invega)	PO	Very low	*	*	*	*	Moderate
Quetiapine (Seroquel)	PO	Very low	Moderate	Moderate	None	Moderate	Moderate
Risperidone (Risperdal)	PO, IM	Very low	Low	Low	None	Moderate	Moderate
Ziprasidone (Geodon)	PO, IM	Very low	Moderate	Moderate	None	Low	Low
Third-Generation Antipsychotic							
Aripiprazole (Abilify)	PO	Very low	Low		None	Low	Low

*Data unavailable.

ACh, Anticholinergic side effects; *EPSs,* extrapyramidal side effects; *OH,* orthostatic hypotension.

Data from Martinez, M., Marangell, L. B., & Martinez, J. M. (2008). Psychopharmacology. In R. E. Hales, S. C. Yudofsky, & G. O. Gabbard (Eds.), *Textbook of psychiatry.* Arlington, VA: American Psychiatric Publishing; Lehne, R. A. (2010). *Pharmacology for nursing care* (7th ed.). St. Louis, MO: Saunders.

orthostasis, photosensitivity, and lowered seizure threshold. Unfortunately, antiparkinsonian drugs can cause significant anticholinergic side effects and worsen the anticholinergic side effects of first-generation antipsychotics and other anticholinergic medications. These side effects include urinary retention, dilated pupils, constipation, reduced visual accommodation (blurred vision), dry mucous membranes, reduced peristalsis, and cognitive impairment.

Tardive dyskinesia (TD or TDK) is a persistent EPS that usually appears in 10% or more of patients after prolonged treatment and persists even after the medication has been discontinued. TDK consists of involuntary choreoathetoid (writhing, worm like) movements especially of the tongue and face; a slow, worm like movement of the tongue (fasciculations), lip-smacking movements, and in-and-out tongue protrusion are typical. TDK involving the tongue and mouth can interfere with chewing, swallowing, and speaking. As TDK progresses, similar movements can be seen in the fingers, toes, neck, trunk, or pelvis; in advanced cases, a flapping motion occurs. More common in women, TDK varies from mild to severe and can be disfiguring or incapacitating; its appearance can contribute to the stigmatization of mentally ill persons.

No reliable treatment exists for tardive dyskinesia. The National Institute of Mental Health (NIMH) developed the Abnormal Involuntary Movement Scale (AIMS), a brief test for the tracking of tardive dyskinesia and other involuntary movements (Figure 12-2). It examines facial, oral, extremity, and trunk movement. Regular administration of the AIMS exam is a key nursing role.

Other troubling side effects of first-generation anti psychotics include weight gain, sexual dysfunction, endocrine disturbances (e.g., galactorrhea, amenorrhea, gynecomastia), drooling, and tardive dyskinesia, discussed in the following section. Weight gain can be more than 100 pounds; therefore, changing the antipsychotic may be necessary. Impotence, anorgasmia, and other sexual dysfunctions may also necessitate a medication change.

Table 12-4 identifies common side effects of the first-generation antipsychotic medications, their usual times of onset, and related nursing and medical interventions.

Second-Generation Antipsychotics

Second-generation antipsychotics include risperidone (Risperdal), olanzapine (Zyprexa), quetiapine (Seroquel), and ziprasidone (Geodon). They first emerged in the early 1990s with clozapine (Clozaril). Unfortunately, clozapine produces agranulocytosis in 0.8% to 1% of those who take it and also increases the risk for seizures. Clozapine produced dramatic improvement in some patients whose disorder had been resistant to the earlier antipsychotics. Due to the risk for agranulocytosis, however, patients taking clozapine must have weekly white blood cell counts for the first 6 months, then frequent monitoring thereafter, to obtain the medication. As a result, after the development of additional second-generation antipsychotics, clozapine use is declining.

Second-generation antipsychotics are often chosen as first-line antipsychotics because they treat both the positive and negative symptoms of schizophrenia; furthermore, they produce minimal extrapyramidal side effects (EPSs) or tardive dyskinesia. Reduced side effects translate into improved medication adherence.

Unlike Clozaril, other second-generation antipsychotics rarely cause agranulocytosis; however, with the exception of ziprasidone and aripiprazole, they have a tendency to cause significant weight gain. Metabolic syndrome—which includes weight gain, dyslipidemia, and altered glucose metabolism thought to be due to increased insulin resistance—is a significant concern in most second-generation antipsychotics and increases the risk of diabetes, hypertension, and atherosclerotic heart disease. Table 12-5 lists the classification, route, and side-effect profile of the anti-psychotic drugs.

Third-Generation Antipsychotics

Third-generation antipsychotics have different mechanisms of action than first-generation antipsychotics and second-generation antipsychotics. Aripiprazole [Abilify] is the first and only agent in this class. Sometimes described as a dopamine system stabilizer, it has a better safety profile than second-generation antipsychotics but may be less effective than some. It improves positive and negative symptoms and cognitive function while appearing to produce little risk of EPSs or TDK. Unlike second-generation antipsychotics, aripiprazole is unlikely to cause significant metabolic effects, hypotension, or prolactin release; it also has little anticholinergic effect and does not seem to cause dysrhythmias. Cariprazine is an investigational antipsychotic drug that acts as a D_2 and D_3 receptor antagonist, with high selectivity toward the D_3 receptor; preliminary research suggests efficacy and a side effect profile similar to the second-generation antipsychotics (Potkin et al., 2009).

Potentially Dangerous Responses to Antipsychotics

Nurses need to know about some rare—but serious and potentially fatal—effects of antipsychotic drugs, including anticholinergic toxicity, neuroleptic malignant syndrome, agranulocytosis, and liver impairment. In addition, some second-generation antipsychotics possess unique and dangerous side effects: Asenapine maleate (Saphris) can cause a dangerous anaphylactic reaction, and risperidone (Risperdal) may cause a prolonged Q-T interval, increasing the risk of potentially fatal dysrhythmias in at-risk individuals.

Anticholinergic toxicity is a potentially life-threatening medical emergency caused by antipsychotics or other medications with anticholinergic effects, including many antiparkinsonian drugs. Usually seen in older adults or those on multiple anticholinergic drugs, symptoms include hyperthermia, hot/dry/red skin, reduced bowel sounds, paralytic ileus, agitation, delirium, fluctuating vital signs, tachycardia, marked mydriasis, confusion, mental status changes, worsening of psychotic symptoms, and coma.

Neuroleptic malignant syndrome (NMS) occurs in about 0.2% to 1% of patients who have taken first-generation antipsychotics but can occur with second-generation antipsychotics as well. Caused by excessive dopamine receptor blockage, NMS is a life-threatening medical emergency that is fatal in about 10% of cases. It usually occurs early in therapy but has been reported in patients after

ABNORMAL INVOLUNTARY MOVEMENT SCALE (AIMS)

Public Health Service
Alcohol, Drug Abuse, and Mental Health Administration
National Institute of Mental Health

Name: ______________________
Date: ______________________
Prescribing Practitioner: ______________

Code: 0 = None
1 = Minimal, may be extreme normal
2 = Mild
3 = Moderate
4 = Severe

Instructions: Complete Examination Procedure before making ratings.

Movement ratings: Rate highest severity observed. Rate movements that occur upon activation one *less* than those observed spontaneously. Circle movement as well as code number that applies.		Rater Date	Rater Date	Rater Date	Rater Date
Facial and Oral Movements	**1. Muscles of facial expression** (e.g., movements of forehead, eyebrows, periorbital area, cheeks, including frowning, blinking, smiling, grimacing)	0 1 2 3 4	0 1 2 3 4	0 1 2 3 4	0 1 2 3 4
	2. Lips and perioral area (e.g., puckering, pouting, smacking)	0 1 2 3 4	0 1 2 3 4	0 1 2 3 4	0 1 2 3 4
	3. Jaw (e.g., biting, clenching, chewing, mouth opening, lateral movement)	0 1 2 3 4	0 1 2 3 4	0 1 2 3 4	0 1 2 3 4
	4. Tongue: Rate only increases in movement both in and out of mouth — *not* inability to sustain movement. Darting in and out of mouth.	0 1 2 3 4	0 1 2 3 4	0 1 2 3 4	0 1 2 3 4
Extremity Movements	**5. Upper (arms, wrists, hands, fingers):** Include choreic movements (i.e., rapid, objectively purposeless, irregular, spontaneous) and athetoid movements (i.e., slow, irregular, complex, serpentine). *Do not include tremor* (i.e., repetitive, regular, rhythmic).	0 1 2 3 4	0 1 2 3 4	0 1 2 3 4	0 1 2 3 4
	6. Lower (legs, knees, ankles, toes) (e.g., lateral knee movement, foot tapping, heel dropping, foot squirming, inversion and eversion of foot)	0 1 2 3 4	0 1 2 3 4	0 1 2 3 4	0 1 2 3 4
Trunk Movements	**7. Neck, shoulder, hips** (e.g., rocking, twisting, squirming, pelvic gyrations)	0 1 2 3 4	0 1 2 3 4	0 1 2 3 4	0 1 2 3 4
Global Judgments	**8. Severity of abnormal movements overall**	0 1 2 3 4	0 1 2 3 4	0 1 2 3 4	0 1 2 3 4
	9. Incapacitation due to abnormal movements	0 1 2 3 4	0 1 2 3 4	0 1 2 3 4	0 1 2 3 4
	10. Patient's awareness of abnormal movements: Rate only patient's report. No awareness 0 Aware, no distress 1 Aware, mild distress 2 Aware, moderate distress 3 Aware, severe distress 4	0 1 2 3 4	0 1 2 3 4	0 1 2 3 4	0 1 2 3 4
Dental Status	**11. Current problems with teeth and/or dentures**	No Yes	No Yes	No Yes	No Yes
	12. Are dentures usually worn?	No Yes	No Yes	No Yes	No Yes
	13. Edentia	No Yes	No Yes	No Yes	No Yes
	14. Do movements disappear in sleep?	No Yes	No Yes	No Yes	No Yes

FIG 12-2 Abnormal Involuntary Movement Scale (AIMS).

AIMS Examination Procedure
Either before or after completing the Examination Procedure, observe the patient unobtrusively, at rest (e.g., in waiting room).

The chair to be used in this examination should be a hard, firm one without arms.

1. Ask patient to remove shoes and socks.
2. Ask patient whether there is anything in his or her mouth (e.g., gum, candy) and, if there is, to remove it.
3. Ask patient about the *current* condition of his or her teeth. Ask patient if he or she wears dentures. Do teeth or dentures bother the patient *now?*
4. Ask patient whether he or she notices any movements in mouth, face, hands, or feet. If yes, ask to describe and to what extent they *currently* bother patient or interfere with his or her activities.
5. Have patient sit in chair with hands on knees, legs slightly apart, and feet flat on floor. Look at entire body movements while in this position.
6. Ask patient to sit with hands hanging unsupported: if male, between legs; if female and wearing a dress, hanging over knees. Observe hands and other body areas.
7. Ask patient to open mouth. Observe tongue at rest within mouth. Do this twice.
8. Ask patient to protrude tongue. Observe abnormalities of tongue movement. Do this twice.
9. Ask patient to tap thumb, with each finger, as rapidly as possible for 10 to 15 seconds, separately with right hand, then with left hand. Observe each facial and leg movement.
10. Flex and extend patient's left and right arms (one at a time). Note any rigidity.
11. Ask patient to stand up. Observe in profile. Observe all body areas again, hips included.
12. Ask patient to extend both arms outstretched in front with palms down. Observe trunk, legs, and mouth.
13. Have patient walk a few paces, turn, and walk back to chair. Observe hands and gait. Do this twice.

FIG 12-2, cont'd

20 years of treatment. NMS is characterized by reduced consciousness, increased muscle tone (muscular rigidity), and autonomic dysfunction—including marked hyperpyrexia, labile hypertension, tachycardia, tachypnea, diaphoresis, and drooling. Treatment consists of early detection, discontinuation of the antipsychotic, management of fluid balance, rapid temperature reduction (cooling blankets, ice water or alcohol baths), and monitoring for complications such as deep vein thrombosis and rhabdomyolysis. Mild cases of neuroleptic malignant syndrome are treated with bromocriptine (Parlodel). More severe cases are treated with intravenous dantrolene (Dantrium).

Agranulocytosis, most often seen with clozapine (Clozaril) but possible with most antipsychotics, is a serious blood dyscrasia that can be fatal. Monitoring for total WBC counts below 3000/mm3 or neutropenia (ANC below 1500/mm3), and for signs of infection (e.g., sore throats) or increased susceptibility to infection, is essential. **Liver impairment** may also occur, making monitoring of liver function values essential. Nurses need to be aware of the prodromal signs and symptoms of these side effects and teach them to their patients and patients' families (see Table 12-4).

Adjuncts to Antipsychotic Drug Therapy

Disorders co-occurring with schizophrenia should be actively treated. Depression, which is common in schizophrenia, should typically be treated with **antidepressants** (refer to Chapter 14 for a discussion of depression and antidepressants).

Mood stabilizing agents may enhance the effectiveness of antipsychotics. Valproate is used during acute exacerbations of psychosis to hasten response to antipsychotics (Freudenriech et al., 2008). Lamotrigine may be given along with clozapine to improve therapeutic effects. Mood stabilizers and/or antidepressants are especially important for persons with schizoaffective disorder.

Augmentation with **benzodiazepines** (e.g., lorazepam [Ativan]) can reduce anxiety and agitation and contribute to improvement in positive and negative symptoms.

Case Study and Nursing Care Plan 12-1 discusses a patient with schizophrenia.

Advanced Practice Interventions

Services that may, in most locations, be provided by advanced practice registered nurses (APRNs) include individual and group psychotherapy (e.g. cognitive-behavioral therapy [CBT]), psychoeducation (e.g., social skills training), medication prescription and monitoring, basic health assessment, cognitive remediation, and family therapy. Family therapy is one of the most important interventions the APRN can implement for the patient with schizophrenia.

Family Therapy

Family therapy is usually delivered by APRNs or other independently licensed personnel. Families of persons with schizophrenia often endure considerable hardship while coping with the acute and residual symptoms of the illness, particularly if they are direct caregivers. The patient and family may become isolated from other relatives, communities, and support systems. In fact, until the 1970s (and sometimes even today) families were often blamed for causing schizophrenia in the affected family member. NAMI and the National Alliance for Research in Schizophrenia and Depression (NARSD) are actively involved in countering this image and in making families full partners in the treatment process.

12-1 CASE STUDY AND NURSING CARE PLAN

Schizophrenia

Tom, 42, is a patient in a Veterans Administration hospital. He has been in and out of hospitals for 13 years. Tom is a former Marine who first "heard voices" at the age of 19 while he was serving in the Gulf War. He subsequently received a medical discharge. He has been separated from his wife and four children for 3 years.

This hospitalization was precipitated by auditory hallucinations and paranoia worsened by drug abuse. "I thought people were following me. I hear voices, usually a woman's voice, and she's nasty. People say that it happens because I don't take my medications. The medications make me tired, and I can't have sex." Tom also uses marijuana, which he knows increases his paranoia. "It makes me feel good, and not much else does." Tom left high school in the 11th grade. He says he has no close friends. He spent 5 years in prison for manslaughter and was abusing alcohol and drugs when the crime occurred.

Sarah is Tom's nurse. Tom is dressed in pajamas; his hygiene is good, and he is well nourished. He does not sleep much because "the voices get worse at night." Sarah notes in Tom's chart that he has had two episodes of suicidal ideation, during which the voices were telling him to jump off a building. During the first interview, Tom rarely makes eye contact and speaks in a low monotone. At times, he glances about the room as if distracted, mumbles to himself, and appears upset.

Nurse: *Tom, my name is Sarah. I will be your nurse while you're in the hospital. If it is okay with you, we will meet every day for 20 minutes. We can talk about anything that concerns you.*

Tom: *Well . . . don't believe what they say about me. I want to start . . . . Are you married?*

Nurse: *This time is for you to talk about your concerns.*

Tom: *(scans the room, then lowers his eyes) I think someone is trying to kill me . . . .*

Nurse: *You seem to be focusing on something other than our conversation.*

Tom: *Voices tell me things . . . I can't say . . . .*

Nurse: *That must be disturbing. Tell me what is happening, and I will try to help you.*

After acknowledging his distress, Sarah keeps the 1:1 with Tom short and focused on the here and now and what is happening on the unit. As Tom attends more to the conversation, his thoughts become more connected; he concentrates more, and appears less distracted.

Self-Assessment

On the day of admission Tom shoved a male patient against a wall. He said that he thought that the other patient was the one who wanted to kill him.

This action frightens Sarah. She is worried that Tom may hurt her, especially when he's hallucinating and highly delusional. An experienced nurse suggests that Sarah meet with Tom in an open area of the unit until he demonstrates more control and less suspicion of others and that Sarah focus on building trust and rapport with Tom. After 5 days Tom is calmer, and the sessions are moved to an interview room. By understanding her own fear and consulting a colleague, Sarah was able to manage the situation effectively.

Assessment

Objective Data

Speaks in low monotone
Poor eye contact
Clean, bathed, clothes match
Impaired reality testing
Thoughts scattered when anxious

Subjective Data

No close friends
"I hear voices"
"Someone is trying to kill me."
"I don't take my medications. They make me tired, and I can't have sex."
"The voices get worse at night, and I can't sleep."
"(Drugs) make me feel good . . . not much else does."
Voices have told him to "jump off rooftops."

Chart Data

Separated from wife and children
History of drug abuse (cocaine, marijuana)
First hospitalized at age 19, has not worked since that time
Has had suicidal impulses twice, both associated with command hallucinations
Imprisoned for 5 years for manslaughter, assaulted a peer in the hospital

Diagnosis

1. *Acute confusion* related to neurological dysfunction, as evidenced by persecutory hallucinations and paranoia:
   - Voices have told him to "jump off rooftops."
   - "Someone is trying to kill me, I think."
   - Abuses cocaine and marijuana (although these increase paranoia) because "They make me feel good."
2. *Nonadherence to medication regimen* related to side effects of therapy, as evidenced by verbalization of nonadherence and persistence of symptoms:
   - Failure to take prescribed medications because "They make me tired, and I can't have sex."
   - History of recurrent relapses

Outcomes Identification

- Tom consistently refrains from acting upon his "voices" and suspicions.
- Tom consistently refrains from substance abuse.

Planning

- Sarah plans intervention that will (1) help Tom deal with his disturbing thoughts and (2) minimize drug abuse and adverse effects of medication to increase adherence and decrease the potential for relapse and violence.

Implementation

- **Nursing diagnosis:** Acute confusion R/T schizophrenia AEB patient stating, "Voices are scaring me."
- **Outcome:** Tom consistently refrains from acting upon his "voices" and suspicions when they occur.

12-1 CASE STUDY AND NURSING CARE PLAN—cont'd

Schizophrenia

SHORT-TERM GOAL	INTERVENTION	RATIONALE	EVALUATION
1. By the end of the first week, Tom will recognize the presence of hallucinations and identify one or more contributing factors, as evidenced by telling his nurse when they occur and what preceded them.	1a. Meet with Tom each day for 30 minutes to establish trust and rapport. 1b. Explore those times when voices are most threatening and disturbing, noting the circumstances that precede them. 1c. Provide noncompetitive activities that focus on the here and now.	1a. Short, consistent meetings help decrease anxiety and establish trust. 1b. Identifies events that increase anxiety and trigger "voices"; by learning to manage triggers, hallucinations can be reduced. 1c. Increased time spent in reality-based activities decreases focus on hallucinations.	**GOAL MET** By the end of the first week, Tom tells the nurse when he is experiencing hallucinations.
2. By the end of the first week, Tom will recognize hallucinations as "not real" and ascribe them to his illness.	2a. Explore content of hallucinations with Tom. 2b. Educate Tom about the nature of hallucinations and ways to determine if "voices" are real.	2a. Identifies suicidal or aggressive themes or command hallucinations. 2b. Improves Tom's reality testing and helps him begin to attribute his experiences to schizophrenia.	**GOAL MET** Tom identifies that the voices tell him he is a loser and he needs to be careful "because someone is after me." He identifies that the voices are worse at nighttime. He notes that others do not seem to hear what he hears and also states that smoking marijuana and taking cocaine produce very threatening voices.
3. By discharge, Tom will consistently report a decrease in hallucinations.	3. Explore with Tom possible actions that can minimize anxiety and/or reduce hallucinations, such as whistling or reading aloud.	3. Offers alternatives while anxiety level is relatively low.	**GOAL MET** Tom states that he is hearing voices less, and they are less threatening to him. Tom identifies that if he whistles or sings, he stays calm and can control the voices.

- **Nursing diagnosis:** Nonadherence
- **Outcome:** Tom consistently adheres to medication regimen.

SHORT-TERM GOAL	INTERVENTION	RATIONALE	EVALUATION
1. By the end of week 1, Tom will discuss his concerns about medication and its side effects with staff.	1a. Evaluate medication response and side-effect issues. 1b. Evaluate medication change to olanzapine (Zyprexa). 1c. Educate Tom regarding side effects—how long they last and what actions can be taken.	1a. Identify drugs and dosages that have increased therapeutic value and decreased side effects. 1b. Olanzapine causes no known sexual difficulties. 1c. Reduces patient distress and resulting resistance caused by side effects, increasing patient's sense of control.	**GOAL MET** Tom identifies the reasons for stopping his medication. He agrees to try olanzapine because he trusts staff's assurances that the side effects will be reduced. Tom states that he sleeps better at night but is still tired during the day.
2. By the end of week 2, Tom will develop peer support in the community.	2. Connect Tom with the local National Alliance of Mentally Ill (NAMI) support group.	2. Provides peer support and a chance to hear from others (further along in recovery) how medications can be helpful and side effects can be managed. NAMI group can also offer suggestions for dealing with his loneliness and other problems.	**GOAL MET** Week 1: Tom attends meeting. Week 2: He speaks in the group about "not feeling good." Several group members say they understand and try to help him figure out why he is not feeling good. Peers say how taking medication has helped them feel better.

Evaluation

By discharge, Tom expresses hope that the medicines will help him feel better and avoid problems like jail. He has a better understanding of his medications and what to do for side effects. He knows that marijuana and cocaine increase his symptoms and explains that when he gets lonely, he now has ideas of things other than drugs he can do to "feel good." Tom continues with the support group and outpatient counseling, stating that it's because Ms. Lally really cared about him; this made him want to get better and led him to trust what staff told him. He reports sleeping much better and says that he has more energy during the day.

Family education and therapy improve the quality of life for the patient and reduce the relapse rate for many. The following example shows how a family came to distinguish between "Martha's problem" and "the problem caused by schizophrenia."

"It was a good idea, us all meeting in our own home to discuss my sister's illness. We were all able to say how it felt, and for the first time I realized that I knew very little about what she was suffering or how much—the word *schizophrenia* meant nothing to me before. I used to think she was just being lazy until she told me what it was really like" (Gamble & Brennan, 2000, p. 192).

Programs that provide support, education, coping skills training, and social network development are extremely effective. This **psychoeducational** approach brings educational and behavioral approaches into family treatment and recognizes families as secondary victims of a biological illness (hence the name secondary consumers for families). In family therapy sessions, fears, faulty communication patterns, and distortions are identified, problem-solving skills are taught, healthier alternatives to conflict are explored, and guilt and anxiety can be lessened.

EVALUATION

Evaluating progress requires an understanding of the recovery process for schizophrenia. Staff should remember that improvement is a process that is highly individualized; progress in some may occur erratically or slowly, and gains may be small and difficult to discern. Setting small, step-wise goals makes it easier to identify progress that may occur in small increments.

Patients' progress should be reevaluated regularly and treatment adjusted when needed. Active staff involvement and interest in the patient's progress communicates concern and caring, helps the patient to maximize progress, promotes treatment adherence, and reduces staff feelings of helplessness and burnout. Involving the patient as a true member of the team, in a partnership with staff, is consistent with the Recovery Model and will increase patient motivation, trust, and cooperation, in turn speeding recovery and improving outcomes. Staff must stay abreast of developing treatments and assure that care is evidence-based.

QUALITY IMPROVEMENT

Patient care and outcomes can be improved by examining outcomes data (Quality and Safety Education for Nurses, 2012). The American Psychiatric Association and similar organizations have promulgated standards of practice for schizophrenia. Such standards typically include the use of evidence-based performance measures regarding assessment, treatment, and evaluating care, including the following:

- The use of effective, affordable medications titrated to effective dosages, including second-generation antipsychotics for persons with prominent negative symptoms
- Assessment for risk of suicide
- Assessment for substance abuse
- Weight monitoring
- Monitoring for extrapyramidal effects (EPSs) and addressing them through adjunctive medications and symptom treatment
- Screening for involuntary movement and metabolic syndrome
- Screening for hyperlipidemia when an unconventional antipsychotic is prescribed
- Involving the patient in active case management services to assure coordination of care and prevent "falling through the cracks"
- Involving the patient in cognitive remediation treatment (a series of interventions, often designed as computer games, that enhance and remediate cognitive skills such as attentiveness and memory)
- Promoting involvement in self-help and support groups, such as the National Alliance on Mental Illness (NAMI.org), and in other activities and resources consistent with the Recovery Model

Assessment forms, recommended standards of care, and similar materials are available through online sites such as the American Psychiatric Association (www.psych.org/practice/clinical-practice-guidelines) and the Agency for Healthcare Research and Quality (www.ahrq.gov/clinic/schzrec.htm). Figure 12-2 is an example of an assessment form used to track abnormal, involuntary movements caused by antipsychotic medications.

KEY POINTS TO REMEMBER

- Schizophrenia spectrum disorders are biological disorders of the brain; they are a group of disorders with overlapping symptoms and treatments, and are categorized from least severe to most severe (schizophrenia).
- Schizophrenia varies in terms of which symptoms dominate, their severity, the impairment in affect and cognition, and the impact on social and other areas of functioning.
- Symptoms vary considerably among patients and fluctuate over time.
- Psychotic symptoms are often more pronounced and obvious than symptoms of other disorders, making schizophrenia more apparent to others and increasing stigmatization.
- Neurochemical, genetic, and neuroanatomical findings help explain the symptoms of schizophrenia; however, no one theory accounts fully for the complexities of schizophrenia.
- *Positive symptoms* of schizophrenia (e.g., hallucinations, delusions, associative looseness) are easier to recognize and respond best to antipsychotic drug therapy.
- *Negative symptoms* of schizophrenia (e.g., social withdrawal and dysfunction, lack of motivation, reduced affect) respond less well to antipsychotic therapy and can be more debilitating. Psychosocial interventions such as support groups improve negative symptoms.
- Cognitive impairment varies; it warrants careful assessment and active intervention to increase the patient's ability to function and maximize the ultimate quality of life.
- Comorbid depression must be identified and treated to reduce the potential for suicide, substance abuse, nonadherence, and relapse.
- Some applicable nursing diagnoses include *Disturbed sensory perception, Acute confusion, Impaired communication, Ineffective coping, Risk for self-directed or other-directed violence, and Impaired family coping.*
- Outcomes are chosen based on the phase of schizophrenia and the patient's individual symptoms, needs, strengths, and level of functioning. Short-term and intermediate indicators are also developed to better track the incremental progress typical of schizophrenia.
- Interventions for people with schizophrenia include trust-building and therapeutic communication: support; assistance with self-care, nutrition and sleep; promoting independence and stress management; promoting socialization; psycho-education about the illness and its treatment; milieu management; on-going risk assessment.
- Therapeutic interventions for schizophrenia include cognitive-behavioral interventions, cognitive enhancement/remediation (evidence-based, highly structured, classes that educate patients about cognitive skills and provide computer-based and interpersonal practice of cognitive skills).
- Improving and promoting reality testing are essential in care for people with schizophrenia.
- Antipsychotic medications are essential in patients with schizophrenia. Nurses must understand the properties, desired and undesired effects, and dosages of first-, second-, and third-generation antipsychotics and other medications used.
- Schizophrenia can produce countertransference responses in staff; clinical supervision and self-assessment help the nurse remain objective and therapeutic.

CRITICAL THINKING

1. Jamie, age 24, is hospitalized after an abrupt onset of psychosis and is diagnosed with schizophrenia. Jamie is recently divorced and works as a legal secretary. Her work had become erratic, and her suspiciousness was upsetting colleagues. Jamie is being discharged in two days to her mother's care until she is able to resume her job. Jamie's mother is overwhelmed and asks how she is going to cope: "I can hardly talk to Jamie without upsetting her. She is still mad at me because I called 911 and had her admitted. She says there is nothing wrong with her, and I'm worried she'll stop her medication once she is home. What am I going to do?"
   a. Explain Jamie's behavior and symptoms to a classmate as you would to Jamie's mother.
   b. How would you respond to the mother's immediate concerns?
   c. What priority concerns should the nurse address before discharge?
   d. Identify interventions that are consistent with the Recovery Model.
   e. What community resources can help support this family? Describe how each could be helpful.
   f. What do you think of the prognosis for Jamie? Support your position with data regarding Jamie's diagnosis and the treatment you have planned.

CHAPTER REVIEW

1. Mark, a 32-year-old patient with schizophrenia, is found in a closet with an empty 2-liter bottle of cola taken from the staff refrigerator. The bottle had been full. The patient has also been drinking more from the hallway water cooler and taking drinks from his peers' dinner trays. Recently, staff has noticed an increase in auditory hallucinations and the onset of confusion. Which response is most appropriate?
   a. Place Mark on every-15-minute checks to identify any further deterioration.
   b. Restrict his access to fluids, and evaluate for water intoxication via daily weights.
   c. Attempt to distract the patient from excess fluid intake and other bizarre behavior.
   d. Request an increase in antipsychotic medication, owing to the worsening of his psychosis.
2. Jordan is a 21-year-old who was recently diagnosed with schizophrenia. He has had to drop out of college as the positive symptoms of his disease have made it impossible for him to pursue his dream of being an architect. He presents to the emergency department with flat affect, depressed mood, and having auditory hallucinations telling him he is "no good to anyone anymore." Which of the following statement is true regarding depression and schizophrenia?
   a. Anxiety and substance abuse are comorbid with schizophrenia, but not depression or dysphoria.
   b. It is important to assess for depression in patients with schizophrenia, but suicide rarely occurs in this population of clients.
   c. Assessing for depression and suicidal ideation in patients with schizophrenia is important since almost half of people with schizophrenia will attempt suicide.
   d. The medications that will be given to control the positive symptoms of schizophrenia, such as auditory hallucinations, will alleviate any depressive symptoms a patient may have.
3. Tony, a 45-year-old patient with schizophrenia, sometimes moves his lips silently or murmurs to himself when he does not realize others are watching. Sometimes when talking to others, he suddenly stops, appears distracted for a moment, and then resumes. Based on these observations, Tony most likely is experiencing:
   a. Illusions
   b. Delusional thinking
   c. Auditory hallucinations
   d. Impaired reality testing
4. Julia, a 28-year-old diagnosed with schizophrenia, is encouraged to attend groups but stays in her room instead. Staff and peers encourage her participation, but without success. Her hygiene is poor despite encouragement to shower and brush her teeth. She does not seem concerned that others wish she would behave differently. Which is the most likely explanation for Julia's failure to respond to others' efforts to help her behave in a more adaptive fashion? *Select all that apply.*
   a. She is displaying avolition.
   b. She is displaying anergia.
   c. She is displaying negativism.
   d. She is exhibiting paranoid delusions.
   e. She is being resistant or oppositional.
   f. She is apathetic due to her schizophrenia.
5. Kyle, a 23-year-old patient with schizophrenia, has been admitted to the psychiatric unit for one week. He has begun to take the first-generation antipsychotic haloperidol (Haldol). One day you find him sitting very stiffly and not moving. He is diaphoretic, and when you ask if he is okay he seems unable to turn towards you or to respond verbally. You obtain vital signs, which are as follows: BP 170/100, P 110, T 103. What are the priority nursing interventions? *Select all that apply.*
   a. Begin to wipe him with a washcloth wet with cold water or alcohol.
   b. Hold his medication, and contact his provider stat.
   c. Administer a medication such as benztropine IM to correct his dystonic reaction.
   d. Reassure him that although there is no treatment for his tardive dyskinesia, it will pass.
   e. Explain that he has anticholinergic toxicity, hold his meds, and give IM physostigmine.
   f. Hold his medication tonight, and consult his provider after completing medication rounds.

Answers to Chapter Review

1. b; 2. c; 3. c; 4. a, b, f; 5. a, b.

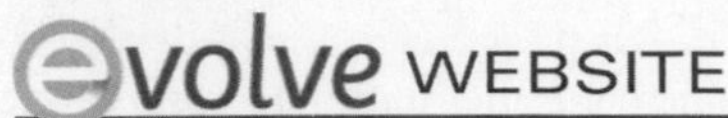

Visit the Evolve website for a posttest on the content in this chapter: http://evolve.elsevier.com/Varcarolis

Post-Test interactive review

REFERENCES

Allen, D. E., de Nesnera, A., & Robinson, D. A. (2012). Psychiatric patients are at increased risk of falling and choking. *Journal of the American Psychiatric Nurses Association, 18*(2) 91–95.

American Psychiatric Association. (2013). *DSM-5 table of contents.* Retrieved from http://www.psychiatry.org/dsm5.

Barnes, T. R. E., & the Schizophrenia Consensus Group of the British Association for Psychopharmacology. (2011). Evidence-based guidelines for the pharmacological treatment of schizophrenia. *Journal of Psychopharmacology, 25*(5), 567–620.

de Bartolomeis, A., Sarappa, C., Magara, S., & Iasevoli F. (2011). Targeting glutamate system for novel antipsychotic approaches: Relevance for residual psychotic symptoms and treatment resistant schizophrenia. *European Journal of Pharmacology, 682,* 1–11.

Brown, A., & McGrath, J. (2011). The prevention of schizophrenia. *Schizophrenia Bulletin, 37*(2), 257–261.

Bulechek, G. M., Butcher, H. K., Dochterman, J. M., & Wagner, C. (2013). *Nursing interventions classification (NIC)* (6th ed). St. Louis, MO: Mosby.

Callaghan, R. C., Cunningham, J. K., Allebeck, P., Arenovich, T., Sajeev, G., Remington, G., . . . Kish, S. J. (2012). Methamphetamine use and schizophrenia: A population-based cohort study in California. *American Journal of Psychiatry, 169*(4), 389–396.

Christodoulou, G. N., Margariti, M., Kontaxakis, V. P., & Christodoulou, N. G. (2009). The delusional misidentification syndromes: Strange, fascinating, and instructive. *Current Psychiatry Reports, 11,* 185–189.

Chung, Y. S., Kang, D., Shin, N. Y., Yu, S. Y., & Kwon, J. S. (2008). Deficit of theory of mind in individuals at ultra-high risk for schizophrenia. *Schizophrenia Research, 99,* 111–118.

Crespo-Facorro, B., Perez-Iglesias, R., Mata, I., Caseiro, O., Martinez-Garcia, O., Pardo, G., . . . Vazquez-Barquero, J. L. (2011). Relapse prevention and remission attainment in first episode non-affective psychosis: A randomised, controlled 1-year follow-up comparison of haloperidol, risperidone and olanzapine. *Journal of Psychiatric Research, 45,* 763–769.

D'Souza, M. S., & Markou, A. (2012). Schizophrenia and tobacco smoking comorbidity: nAChR agonists in the treatment of schizophrenia-associated cognitive deficits. *Neuropharmacology, 62,* 1564–1573.

Gamble, C., & Brennan, G. (2000). Working with families and informed careers. In C. Gamble & G. Brennan (Eds.), *Working with serious mental illness: A manual for clinical practice.* London, UK: Baillière Tindall.

Giegling, I., Genius, J., Benninghoff, J., & Rujesci, D. (2010). Genetic findings in schizophrenia patients related to alterations in intracellular Ca-homeostasis. *Progress in Neuro-Psychopharmacology and Biological Psychiatry, 34,* 1375–1380.

Gold, R., Butler, P., Revheim, N., Leitman, D., Hansen, J.A., Gur, R., . . . Javitt, D.C. (2012). Auditory emotion recognition impairments in schizophrenia: Relationship to acoustic features and cognition. *American Journal of Psychiatry, 169*(4), 424–432.

Goldman, M. B. (2009). The mechanism of life-threatening water imbalance in schizophrenia and its relationship to underlying illness. *Brain Research Reviews, 61,* 210–220.

Gottlieb, J. D., Mueser, K. T., & Glynn, S. M. (2012). Family therapy for schizophrenia: Co-occurring psychotic and substance use disorders. *Journal of Clinical Psychology: In Session, 68*(5), 490–501.

Herdman, T. H. (Ed.) (2012). *NANDA International nursing diagnoses: Definitions and classification, 2012-2014.* Oxford, UK: Wiley-Blackwell.

Hulshoff, H. E., van Baal, G. C. M., Schnack, H. G., Brans, R. G. H., van der Schot, A. C., Brouwer, R. M., . . . Kahn, R. S. (2012). Overlapping and segregating structural brain abnormalities in twins with schizophrenia or bipolar disorder. *Archives of General Psychiatry, 69*(4), 349–359.

Jones, C., Byun, N., & Bubser, M. (2011). Muscarinic and nicotinic acetylcholine receptor agonists and allosteric modulators for the treatment of schizophrenia. *Neuropsychopharmacology Reviews, 37,* 16–42.

Kasckow, J., Felmet, K., & Zisook, S. (2011). Managing suicide risk in a patient with schizophrenia. *CNS Drugs, 25*(2), 129–143.

Kegeles, L. S., Mao, X., Stanford, A. D., Girgis, R., Ojeil, N., Xu, X., . . . Shungu, D. C. (2012). Elevated prefrontal cortex y-aminobutyric acid and glutamate levels in schizophrenia measured in vivo with proton magnetic resonance spectroscopy. *Archives of General Psychiatry online.* Retrieved from http://archpsyc.ama-assn.org/cgi/content/abstract/archgenpsychiatry.2011.1519v1?maxtoshow=&hits=10&RESULTFORMAT=&fulltext=elevated+prefrontal+cortext&searchid=1&FIRSTINDEX=0&resourcetype=HWCIT.

Khashan, A. S., Abel, K. M., McNamee, R., Pedersen, M. G., Webb, R. T., Baker, P. N., . . . Mortensen, P. B. (2008). Higher risk of offspring schizophrenia following antenatal maternal exposure to severe adverse life events. *Archives of General Psychiatry, 65*(2), 146–152.

Lehne, R. (2010). *Pharmacology for nursing care* (7th ed.). St. Louis, MO: Saunders.

McGlashan, T., & Woods, S. (2011). Early antecedents and detection of schizophrenia. *Psychiatric Times, 28*(3). Retrieved from http://www.psychiatrictimes.com/schizophrenia/content/article/10168/1822847.

Miller, B. J., Paschall, C. B., & Svendsen, D. P. (2007). *Mortality and medical co-morbidity in patients with serious mental illness.* Poster presentation at the 8th Annual All-Ohio Institute on Community Psychiatry, March 16, 2007.

Minzenberger, M. J., Yoon, J. H., & Carter, C. S. (2011). Schizophrenia. In R. E. Hales, S. C. Yudofsky, & G. O. Gabbard (Eds.), *Essentials of psychiatry*. Washington, DC: American Psychiatric Publishing.

Moller, M., & Zauszniewski, J. (2011). Psychophenomenology of the postpsychotic adjustment process. *Archives of Psychiatric Nursing, 25*(4) 253–268.

Moorhead, S., Johnson, M., Maas, M. L., & Swanson, E. (2013). *Nursing outcomes classification (NOC)* (5th ed.). St Louis, MO: Mosby.

Nash, J. (2008). *John Nash quotes.* Retrieved from http://thinkexist.com/quotes/john_nash/.

Potkin, S., Keator, D., Mukherjee, J., Preda, A., Highum, D., Gage, A., . . . Laszlovsky, I. (2009). Dopamine D3 and D2 receptor occupancy of Cariprazine in schizophrenic patients. *European Neuropsychopharmacology, 19*(supplement 3), S316.

Tandon, R., Keshavan, M. S., & Nasrallah, H. A. (2008). Schizophrenia, "just the facts": What we know in 2008. Part 2: Epidemiology and etiology. *Schizophrenia Research, 102*(1–3), 1–18.

van Haren, N. E. M., Schnack, H. G., Cahn, W., van den Heuvel, M. P., Lepage, C., Collins, L., . . . Kahn, R. S. (2011). Changes in cortical thickness during the course of schizophrenia. *Archives of General Psychiatry, 68*(9), 871–880.

Walker, E., & Tessner, K. (2008). Schizophrenia. *Perspectives on Psychological Science, 3*(1), 30–37.

Wang, Q., Deng, W., Huang, C., Li, M., Ma, X., Wang, W., . . . Li, T. (2010). Abnormalities in connectivity of white-matter tracts in patients with familial and non-familial schizophrenia. *Psychological Medicine, 41,* 1691–1700.

CHAPTER

13

Bipolar and Related Disorders

Margaret Jordan Halter

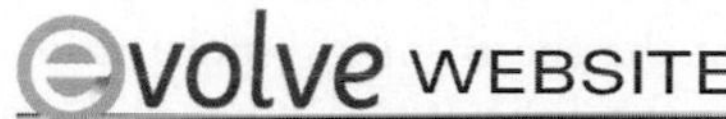

Visit the Evolve website for a pretest on the content in this chapter: http://evolve.elsevier.com/Varcarolis

Pre-Test interactive review

OBJECTIVES

1. Assess a patient with mania for (a) mood, (b) behavior, and (c) thought processes, and be alert to possible dysfunction.
2. Formulate three nursing diagnoses appropriate for a patient with mania, and include supporting data.
3. Explain the rationales behind five methods of communication that may be used with a patient experiencing mania.
4. Teach a classmate at least four expected side effects of lithium therapy.
5. Distinguish between signs of early and severe lithium toxicity.
6. Write a medication care plan specifying five areas of patient teaching regarding lithium carbonate.
7. Compare and contrast basic clinical conditions that may respond better to anticonvulsant therapy with those that may respond better to lithium therapy.
8. Evaluate specific indications for the use of seclusion for a patient experiencing mania.
9. Defend the use of electroconvulsive therapy for a patient in specific situations.
10. Review at least three of the items presented in the patient and family teaching plan (see Box 13-2) for a patient with bipolar disorder.
11. Distinguish the focus of treatment for a person in the acute manic phase from the focus of treatment for a person in the continuation or maintenance phase.

KEY TERMS AND CONCEPTS

acute phase
anticonvulsant drugs
bipolar I disorder
bipolar II disorder
clang association
continuation phase
cyclothymic disorder
dysphoric mania
electroconvulsive therapy (ECT)
euphoric mania
flight of ideas
grandiosity
hypomania
lithium carbonate
maintenance phase
mania
mood stabilizers
rapid cycling
seclusion protocol

Once commonly known as *manic-depression*, bipolar disorder is a chronic, recurrent illness that must be carefully managed throughout a person's life. Bipolar disorder frequently goes unrecognized, and people suffer for years before receiving a proper diagnosis and treatment. Up to 21% of patients with major depression in primary care may actually have an undiagnosed bipolar disorder; lack of specific treatment for the bipolar disorder is associated with worse outcomes (Smith et al., 2011).

Bipolar disorders are part of a larger umbrella of disorders, mood disorders, which refer to disturbances in how people feel.

Most of us spend our time in moderate moods, neither very high nor very low, but most persons with mood disorders will only experience a depressed mood. A minority of people will experience the opposite of a depressed mood—a manic episode, which is a shocking thing to witness. Persons with **mania** are the happiest, most excited, and most optimistic people you could meet. They feel euphoric and energized; they don't sleep or eat, and they talk constantly. Since they feel so important and powerful, they take horrific chances and do foolish things. As the disorder intensifies, psychosis ensues, and persons with mania begin to hear voices, sometimes the voice of God.

Bipolar disorder is marked by shifts in mood, energy, and ability to function. The course of the illness is variable, and symptoms range from severe mania—an exaggerated euphoria or irritability—to severe depression. Periods of normal functioning may alternate with periods of illness (highs, lows, or a combination of both); however, many individuals continue to experience chronic interpersonal or occupational difficulties even during remission. The mortality rate for bipolar disorder is severe; 25% to 60% of individuals with bipolar disorder will make a suicide attempt at least once in their lifetime, and nearly 20% of all deaths among this population are from suicide (Tondo, 2006).

CLINICAL PICTURE

The three types of bipolar disorder currently identified are listed from most to least severe (American Psychiatric Association, 2013):

Bipolar I disorder: Bipolar I is a mood disorder that is characterized by at least one week-long manic episode that results in excessive activity and energy (Angst et al., 2012). Manic episodes may alternate with depression or a mixed state of agitation and depression. Though people with bipolar I disorder may have periods of time when they may be symptom-free, it is such a severe disorder that the person experiencing it tends to have difficulty in maintaining social connections and employment. Psychosis (hallucinations, delusions, and dramatically disturbed thoughts) may occur during manic episodes. Additionally, the presence of three of the following behaviors constitutes mania:

- Extreme drive and energy
- Inflated sense of self-importance
- Drastically reduced sleep requirements
- Excessive talking combined with pressured speech
- Personal feeling of racing thoughts
- Distraction by environmental events
- Unusually obsessed with and overfocused on goals
- Purposeless arousal and movement
- Dangerous activities such as indiscriminate spending, reckless sexual encounters, or risky investments

Mania can be euphoric or dysphoric. **Euphoric mania** feels wonderful in the beginning, but it turns scary and dark as it progresses toward loss of control and confusion. **Dysphoric mania** is also referred to as a mixed state or agitated depression, with depressive symptoms along with mania. A person with dysphoric mania may be irritable, angry, suicidal, or hypersexual and may experience panic attacks, pressured speech, agitation, severe insomnia or grandiosity as well as persecutory delusions and confusion.

Bipolar II disorder: In bipolar II disorder, low-level mania alternates with profound depression. We call this low-level symptomatology **hypomania**. The hypomania of bipolar II disorder tends to be euphoric and often increases functioning. Like mania, hypomania is accompanied by excessive activity and energy for at least four days and involves at least three of the behaviors listed under mania. Unlike mania, psychosis is never present in hypomania although it may be present in the depressive side of the disorder (Mazzarini et al., 2010). The disorder is not usually severe enough to cause serious impairment in occupational or social functioning, and hospitalization is rare; however, the depressive symptoms tend to put those who suffer from it at particular risk for suicide.

Cyclothymic disorder: Symptoms of hypomania alternate with symptoms of mild to moderate depression for at least two years in adults and one year in children. Neither set of symptoms constitutes an actual diagnosis of either disorder, yet the symptoms are disturbing enough to cause social and occupational impairment. As part of the spectrum of bipolar disorders, cyclothymic disorder may be difficult to distinguish from bipolar II disorder (Baldessarini et al., 2011). Individuals with cyclothymic disorder tend to have irritable hypomanic episodes. In children, cyclothymic disorder is marked by irritability and sleep disturbance (VanMeter et al., 2011).

Some persons experience **rapid cycling** and may have at least four mood episodes in a 12-month period. The cycling can also occur within the course of a month or even a 24-hour period. Rapid cycling is associated with more severe symptoms, such as poorer global functioning, high recurrence risk, and resistance to conventional somatic treatments. It is estimated to be present in 12% to 24% of patients who go to specialized clinics for mood disorders (Bauer, 2008).

EPIDEMIOLOGY

Among children and teens bipolar disorder has a rate of about 1% (American Academy of Child and Adolescent Psychiatry, 2010). The lifetime risk, or the percentage of the population that will have a bipolar disorder by age 75, is 5.1% (Kessler, 2005).

The median age of onset for bipolar I is 18 years; for bipolar II, the median age of onset is 20 years (Merikangas, 2007). Bipolar I tends to begin with a depressive episode—in women 75% of the time and in men 67% of the time (Sadock & Sadock, 2008). The episodes tend to increase in number and severity during the course of the illness.

Women who experience a severe postpartum psychosis within two weeks of giving birth have a four times greater chance of subsequent conversion to bipolar disorder (Munk-Olsen et al., 2011). Researchers believe that giving birth may act as a trigger for the first symptoms of bipolar disorder, although few are diagnosed with this disorder during that episode. Hormone changes and sleep deprivation may be causative.

Bipolar I disorder seems to be somewhat more common among males, but bipolar II disorder (characterized by the milder form of mania—hypomania—and increased depression), rapid cycling, mixed states, and depressive episodes are more common among females (Ketter, 2010). Women with bipolar disorders are more likely to abuse alcohol, commit suicide, and develop thyroid disease; men with bipolar disorder are more likely to have legal problems and commit acts of violence.

Among children, researchers are actively studying the difference between attention deficit/hyperactivity disorder (ADHD) and bipolar disorder. Symptoms present in both ADHD and bipolar disorder include impulsivity, inattention, and hyperactivity. It may be that ADHD is overdiagnosed and bipolar disorder is underdiagnosed. This difference in diagnosis may be due to our uncertainty of how bipolar disorder looks or manifests itself in childhood since it does not tend to be diagnosed until adolescence or early adulthood.

Among adults, bipolar II disorder is believed to be underdiagnosed and is often mistaken for major depression or personality disorders, when it actually may be the most common form of bipolar disorder (Vieta & Suppes, 2008). Clinicians may downplay bipolar II and consider it to simply be the milder version of bipolar disorders; however, it is a source of significant morbidity and mortality, particularly due to the occurrence of severe depression. Anyone with major depression should be assessed for symptoms of hypomania since these symptoms are frequently associated with a progression to bipolar disorder (Fiedorowicz et al., 2011).

Cyclothymic disorder usually begins in adolescence or early adulthood. There is a 15% to 50% risk that an individual with this disorder will subsequently develop bipolar I or bipolar II disorder.

COMORBIDITY

One large-scale study with 9,282 participants revealed that more than half of people with bipolar disorder have another psychiatric disorder (Merikangas, 2007). Within a lifetime, the most commonly co-occurring disorders for all bipolar disorders were panic attacks (62%), alcohol abuse (39%), social phobia (38%), oppositional defiant disorder (37%), specific phobia (35%), and seasonal affective disorder (35%). Substance use disorders were much higher in bipolar I than in bipolar II disorders. Substance abuse and bipolar disorder should be treated at the same time whenever possible.

The incidence of borderline personality disorder occurring along with bipolar disorder is high. Patients who have borderline personality disorder have a 19.4% higher rate of bipolar disorder than do people with other personality disorders (Gunderson, 2006). An important consideration is that this combination may result in higher levels of impulsiveness and aggressiveness and may be a risk factor for suicidality (Carpiniello et al., 2011).

With advances in a global scientific database, trends are emerging that were previously unknown. One such trend is the relationship between psychiatric illnesses and physically based illnesses. In a study of nearly 37,000 people, several physical disorders were found to be associated with bipolar I (McIntyre, 2006). The rates of the following disorders were significantly higher: chronic fatigue syndrome, asthma, migraine, chemical sensitivity, hypertension, bronchitis, and gastric ulcers. The presence of these diseases further complicates the lives of persons with bipolar I by impairing their ability to work, increasing their dependence on others, and increasing their need for health care.

ETIOLOGY

Bipolar disorders are thought to be distinctly different from one another; for example, bipolar I disorder, bipolar II disorder, and cyclothymic disorder have different characteristics. Other variants of bipolar disease, including a number of other diseases whose end result is bipolar symptomatology, are currently being evaluated (Baum, 2008).

When the disorder starts in childhood or during the teen years, it is called early-onset bipolar disorder and is more severe than the forms that first appear in older teens and adults (Birmaher et al., 2006). Young persons with bipolar disorder have more frequent mood switches, have more mixed episodes, are sick more often, and are at a greater risk of suicide attempts.

Episodes of depression in bipolar disorders are different from unipolar depression (i.e., depression without episodes of mania—refer to Chapter 14). Depressive episodes in bipolar disorder affect younger people, produce more episodes of illness, and require more frequent hospitalization. They are also characterized by higher rates of divorce and marital conflict.

Theories of the development of bipolar disorders focus on biological, psychological, and environmental factors. Most likely, multiple independent variables contribute to the occurrence of bipolar disorder. For this reason, a biopsychosocial approach will likely be the most successful approach to treatment.

Biological Factors

Genetic

The bipolar disorders have a strong heritability (i.e., the influence of genetic factors is much greater than the influence of external factors). Bipolar disorders are 80% to greater than 90% heritable whereas Parkinson's disease, for example, is only 13% to 30% heritable (Burmeister, McInnis, & Zollner, 2008). The rate of bipolar disorders may be as much as 5 to 10 times higher for people who have a relative with bipolar disorder than the rates found in the general population.

It is likely that bipolar disorder is a polygenic disease, which means that a number of genes contribute to its expression. In a landmark study at the National Institute of Mental Health (NIMH), researchers found a connection between bipolar disorder and a genome that encodes an enzyme called *diacylglycerol kinase eta* (DGKH). Lithium is the first-line therapy for bipolar disorder, and DGKH is a crucial part of a lithium-sensitive pathway (Baum, 2008). Other research has focused on abnormal circadian genes that may result in a superfast biological clock, which manifests itself in extreme insomnia (McClung, 2007). Genetically, rapid cyclers tend to look a bit different. The circadian clock gene *CRY2* is associated with rapid cycling in bipolar disorder (Sjöholm et al., 2010).

The scientific community has been increasingly drawn to the concept of bipolar disorders and schizophrenia having similar genetic origins and pathology (Ivleva, 2010). Both disorders exhibit irregularities on chromosomes 13 and 15. It may be that the genotype has more to do with the specific expression of psychoses (altered thought, delusions, and hallucinations) than is reflected in traditional classification systems. Current psychiatric diagnostic systems will undoubtedly be modified as advances are made in molecular genetics, which will revolutionize our understanding and treatment of many psychotic disorders.

Neurobiological

Neurotransmitters (norepinephrine, dopamine, and serotonin) have been studied since the 1960s as causal factors in mania and depression. One simple explanation is that too few of these chemical messengers will result in depression, and an oversupply will cause mania; however, proportions of neurotransmitters in relation to one another may be more important. Receptor site insensitivity could also be at the root of the problem; even if there is enough of a certain neurotransmitter, it is not going where it needs to go.

Additional research has found that the interrelationships in the neurotransmitter system are complex, and more elaborate theories have been developed since the amine hypotheses were originally proposed. Mood disorders are most likely a result of interactions among various chemicals, including neurotransmitters and hormones.

Brain pathways implicated in the pathophysiology of bipolar disorder are located in subregions of the prefrontal cortex (PFC) and medial temporal lobe (MTL). Dysregulation in the neurocircuits surrounding these areas has been viewed through functional imaging (e.g., positron emission tomography [PET] scans, magnetic resonance imaging [MRI]). Neuroimaging studies reveal structural and functional brain changes in people with bipolar disorder. Some structural changes seem to cause the disorder, and some seem to be *caused by* the disorder. For example, prefrontal cortical changes are evident in the early stages of the illness whereas lateral ventricle abnormalities develop with repeated episodes of mania and/or depression (Strakowski, 2005). Functional imaging also reveals differences in the anterior limbic regions of the brain, which are associated with emotion, motivation, memory, and fear—the areas most deeply affected by bipolar disorder (Bora et al., 2011).

Neuroendocrine

The hypothalamic-pituitary-thyroid-adrenal (HPTA) axis has been closely scrutinized in people with mood disorders. Hypothyroidism is known to be associated with depressed moods and is seen in some patients experiencing rapid cycling. In patients with treatment-resistant bipolar disorder, a high-dose thyroxine may be considered (Chakrabarti, 2011).

Psychological Factors

Although there is increasing evidence for genetic and biological vulnerabilities in the etiology of the mood disorders, psychological factors may play a role in precipitating manic episodes for many individuals. In the absence of severe stressful events, it is possible that a person with a genetic predisposition and a neurochemical imbalance may never experience symptoms of bipolar disorder; however, once the disease has been triggered by an event that is perceived as stressful—loss of a relationship, financial difficulties, failing an exam, being accepted to a highly desirable graduate school—it no longer requires environmental stress to continue.

Environmental Factors

Bipolar disorder is a worldwide problem that generally affects all races and ethnic groups equally, but some evidence suggests that bipolar disorders may be more prevalent in upper socioeconomic classes. The exact reason for this is unclear; however, persons with bipolar disorders appear to achieve higher levels of education and higher occupational status than individuals with unipolar depression. The educational levels of individuals with unipolar depressive disorders, on the other hand, appear to be no different from those of individuals with no symptoms of depression within the same socioeconomic class. Also, the proportion of patients with bipolar disorders among creative writers, artists, highly educated men and women, and professionals is higher than in the general population.

For children who have a genetic and biological risk of developing bipolar disorder, stressful family environments and adverse life events may result in increased vulnerability and more severe course of illness (Miklowitz & Chang, 2008).

APPLICATION OF THE NURSING PROCESS

ASSESSMENT

Individuals with bipolar disorder are often misdiagnosed or underdiagnosed. Early diagnosis and proper treatment can help people avoid:

- Suicide attempts
- Alcohol or substance abuse
- Marital or work problems
- Development of medical comorbidity

Figure 13-1 presents the Mood Disorder Questionnaire (MDQ). This is *not* a definitive diagnostic test; however, it is a helpful initial screening device.

General Assessment

The characteristics of mania discussed in the following sections are (1) mood, (2) behavior, (3) thought processes and speech patterns, and (4) cognitive function.

Mood

The euphoric mood associated with mania is unstable. During euphoria, the patient may state that he or she is experiencing an intense feeling of well-being, is "cheerful in a beautiful world," or is becoming "one with God." The overly joyous mood may seem out of proportion to what is going on, and cheerfulness may be inappropriate for the circumstances. This mood may change quickly to irritation and anger when the person is thwarted. The irritability and belligerence may be short-lived, or it may become the prominent feature of the manic phase of bipolar disorder.

People experiencing a manic state may laugh, joke, and talk in a continuous stream, with uninhibited familiarity. They

MOOD DISORDER QUESTIONNAIRE

Instructions: Please answer each question as best you can.

	Yes	No
1. Has there ever been a period of time when you were not your usual self and....		
you felt so good or so hyper that other people thought you were not your normal self or you were so hyper that you got into trouble?	○	○
you were so irritable that you shouted at people or started fights or arguments?	○	○
you felt much more self-confident than usual?	○	○
you got much less sleep than usual and found you didn't really miss it?	○	○
you were much more talkative or spoke much faster than usual?	○	○
thoughts raced through your head or you couldn't slow down your mind?	○	○
you were so easily distracted by things around you that you had trouble concentrating or staying on track?	○	○
you had much more energy than usual?	○	○
you were much more active or did many more things than usual?	○	○
you were much more social or outgoing than usual; for example, you telephoned friends in the middle of the night?	○	○
you were much more interested in sex than usual?	○	○
you did things that were unusual for you or that other people might have thought were excessive, foolish, or risky?	○	○
spending money got you or your family into trouble?	○	○
2. If you answered "Yes" to more than one of the above, have several of these ever happened during the same period of time?	○	○

3. How much of a problem did any of these cause you — like being unable to work; having family, money, or legal troubles; or getting into arguments or fights? Please select one response only.

○ No problem ○ Minor problem ○ Moderate problem ○ Serious problem

	Yes	No
4. Have any of your blood relatives (children, siblings, parents, grandparents, aunts, uncles) had manic-depressive illness or bipolar disorder?	○	○
5. Has a health care professional ever told you that you have manic-depressive illness or bipolar disorder?	○	○

Criteria for Results: Answering "Yes" to 7 or more of the events in question 1, answering "Yes" to question 2, and answering "Moderate problem" or "Serious problem" to question 3 is considered a positive screen result for bipolar disorder.

FIG 13-1 The Mood Disorder Questionnaire (MDQ). (From Hirschfeld, R., Williams, J., Spitzer, R., Calabrese, J., Flynn, L., Keck, P., . . . Zajecka, J. [2000]. Development and validation of a screening instrument for bipolar spectrum disorder: The Mood Disorder Questionnaire. *American Journal of Psychiatry,* 157[11], 1873-1875. Copyright © 2004 by Eli Lilly and Company.)

often demonstrate boundless enthusiasm, treat others with confidential friendliness, and incorporate everyone into their plans and activities. They know no strangers, and energy and self-confidence seem boundless.

Elaborate schemes to get rich and famous and acquire unlimited power may be frantically pursued, despite objections and realistic constraints. Excessive phone calls and e-mails are made, often to famous and influential people all over the world. Persons in the manic phase are busy during all hours of the day and night, furthering their grandiose plans and wild schemes. To the person experiencing mania, no aspirations are too high, and no distances are too far. No boundaries exist to curtail the elaborate schemes.

In the manic state, a person often gives away money, prized possessions, and expensive gifts. The person experiencing a manic episode may throw lavish parties, frequent expensive nightclubs and restaurants, and spend money freely on friends and strangers alike. This excessive spending, use of credit cards, and high living continue even in the face of bankruptcy. Intervention is often needed to prevent financial ruin.

As the clinical course progresses from hypomania to mania, sociability and euphoria are replaced by a stage of hostility, irritability, and paranoia. The following is a patient's description of the painful transition from hypomania to mania (Jamison, 1995b):

> At first when I'm high, it's tremendous . . . ideas are fast . . . like shooting stars you follow until brighter ones appear . . . all shyness disappears, the right words and gestures are suddenly there . . . uninteresting people, things become intensely interesting. Sensuality is pervasive; the desire to seduce and be seduced is irresistible. Your marrow is infused with unbelievable feelings of ease, power, well-being, omnipotence, euphoria . . . you can do anything . . . but somewhere this changes. . . .
>
> The fast ideas become too fast and there are far too many . . . overwhelming confusion replaces clarity . . . you stop keeping up with it—memory goes. Infectious humor ceases to amuse—your friends become frightened . . . everything now is against the grain . . . you are irritable, angry, frightened, uncontrollable, and trapped in the blackest caves of the mind—caves you never knew were there. It will never end. Madness carves its own reality.

Behavior

When persons experience hypomania, they have voracious appetites for social engagement, spending, and activity, even indiscriminate sex. Constant activity and a reduced need for sleep prevent proper rest. Although short periods of sleep are possible, some patients may not sleep for several days in a row. **This nonstop physical activity and the lack of sleep and food can lead to physical exhaustion and even death if not treated; it therefore constitutes an emergency.**

EVIDENCE-BASED PRACTICE

Sleep Disruption in the Manic Phase of Bipolar Disorder

Roybal, K., Theobold, D., Graham, A., DiNieri, J., Russo, S., Krishnan, V., . . . McClung, C. (2007). Mania-like behavior induced by disruption of *CLOCK*. *Proceedings of the National Academy of Sciences, USA, 104,* 6406-6411.

Problem

One of the most dramatic symptoms of bipolar disorder in the manic phase is sleep disruption. If you have ever stayed awake all night and tried to function the next day, you may have a partial appreciation for the thought impairment, decreased judgment, and emotional dysregulation experienced by people who have been awake for 3 nights. Researchers believe that a faulty circadian rhythm, the natural 24- to 25-hour sleep/wake cycle monitored by a body clock in the hypothalamus, may be to blame. This connection is strengthened by our knowledge that normal sleep/wake cycles are essential to mood stabilization and that sleep disruptions can trigger mania.

Purpose of Study

The purpose of this study was to examine the role of a specific gene in the disruption of circadian rhythms. This gene is the central transcriptional activator of molecular rhythms, or *Clock* gene.

Methods

Researchers mutated the *Clock* gene in mice that served in the study. Next, they implanted electrodes in the medial forebrain bundle of their brains, the area that allowed mice to give themselves pleasurable sensations. They then measured the degree of current, or reward, that the mice gave themselves.

Key Findings

- *Clock* mutant mice are similar to bipolar patients in a manic state in their increased preference for stimuli that are rewarding, including brain stimulation and cocaine.
- The experimental mice displayed other behaviors associated with mania, including less depressive behavior and decreased anxiety.
- Lithium treatment reverses manic-like behavior in *Clock* mutant mice.
- Once *Clock* mutant mice had their functional CLOCK restored, their abnormal behavior ceased.

Implications for Nursing

The study of molecular genetics holds great promise for how people are diagnosed and treated. At a personal level, understanding the mechanics of mania may lessen professional stigma (negative attitudes of health care workers) and even our own attitudes toward people experiencing mania. When you are dealing with someone who is hypertalkative, hypersexual, and constantly making requests, it is fairly easy to become irritated and even resentful. An increased understanding of the physiology behind the disorder can go a long way.

At a hands-on level, the importance of promoting an adaptive sleep/wake cycle in people with mood disorders, particularly people with mania, is highlighted by this study. Teaching aimed at understanding the importance of not "burning the midnight oil" (staying awake all night) is important for everyone but imperative for people with bipolar disorder. Furthermore, recognizing disturbed sleep patterns may aid patients in recognizing symptoms of impending mania.

When in full-blown mania, a person constantly goes from one activity, place, or project to another. Many projects may be started, but few if any are completed. Inactivity is impossible, even for the shortest period of time. Hyperactivity may range from mild, constant motion to frenetic, wild activity. Flowery and lengthy letters are written, and excessive phone calls are made. Individuals become involved in pleasurable activities that can have painful consequences. For example, spending large sums of money on frivolous items, giving money away indiscriminately, or making foolish business investments can leave an individual or family penniless. Sexual indiscretion can dissolve relationships and marriages and lead to sexually transmitted diseases. Religious preoccupation is a common symptom of mania.

Individuals experiencing mania may be manipulative, profane, fault finding, and adept at exploiting others' vulnerabilities. They constantly push limits. These behaviors often alienate family, friends, employers, health care providers, and others.

Modes of dress often reflect the person's grandiose yet tenuous grasp of reality. Dress may be described as outlandish, bizarre, colorful, and noticeably inappropriate. Makeup may be garish and overdone. People with mania are highly distractible. Concentration is poor, and individuals with mania go from one activity to another without completing anything. Judgment is poor. Impulsive marriages and divorces can take place.

People often emerge from a manic state startled and confused by the shambles of their lives. The following description conveys one patient's experience (Jamison, 1995b):

> *Now there are only others' recollections of your behavior—your bizarre, frenetic, aimless behavior—at least mania has the grace to dim memories of itself... now it's over, but is it?... Incredible feelings to sort through... Who is being too polite? Who knows what? What did I do? Why? And most hauntingly, will it, when will it, happen again? Medication to take, to resist, to resent, to forget... but always to take. Credit cards revoked... explanations at work... bad checks and apologies overdue... memory flashes of vague men (what did I do?)... friendships gone, a marriage ruined.*

Thought Processes and Speech Patterns

Flight of ideas is a nearly continuous flow of accelerated speech with abrupt changes from topic to topic that are usually based on understandable associations or plays on words. At times, the attentive listener can keep up with the flow of words, even though direction changes from moment to moment. Speech is rapid, verbose, and circumstantial (including minute and unnecessary details). When the condition is severe, speech may be disorganized and incoherent. The incessant talking often includes joking, puns, and teasing:

> How are you doing, kid, no kidding around, I'm going home . . . home sweet home . . . home is where the heart is, the heart of the matter is I want out and that ain't hay . . . hey, Doc . . . get me out of this place.

The content of speech is often sexually explicit and ranges from grossly inappropriate to vulgar. Themes in the communication of the individual with mania may revolve around extraordinary sexual prowess, brilliant business ability, or unparalleled artistic talents (e.g., writing, painting, and dancing). The person may actually have only average ability in these areas.

Speech is not only profuse but also loud, bellowing, or even screaming. One can hear the force and energy behind the rapid words. As mania escalates, the flight of ideas may give way to clang associations. **Clang associations** are the stringing together of words because of their rhyming sounds, without regard to their meaning:

> Cinema I and II, last row. Row, row, row your boat. Don't be a cutthroat. Cut your throat. Get your goat. Go out and vote. And so I wrote.

Grandiosity (inflated self-regard) is apparent in both the ideas expressed and the person's behavior. People with mania may exaggerate their achievements or importance, state that they know famous people, or believe they have great powers. The boast of exceptional powers and status can take delusional proportions during mania. Grandiose persecutory delusions are common. For example, people may think that God is speaking to them or that the FBI is out to stop them from saving the world. Sensory perceptions may become altered as the mania escalates, and hallucinations may occur; however, delusions and hallucinations are not present during hypomania.

Cognitive Function

The onset of bipolar disorder is often preceded by comparatively high cognitive function; however, there is growing evidence that about one third of patients with bipolar disorder display significant and persistent cognitive problems and difficulties in psychosocial areas. Cognitive deficits in bipolar disorder are milder but similar to those in patients with schizophrenia. Cognitive impairments are greater in bipolar I but are also present in bipolar II (Torrent, 2006).

The potential cognitive dysfunction among many people with bipolar disorder has specific clinical implications (Robinson, 2006):

- Cognitive function affects overall function.
- Cognitive deficits correlate with a greater number of manic episodes, history of psychosis, chronicity of illness, and poor functional outcome.
- Early diagnosis and treatment are crucial to prevent illness progression, cognitive deficits, and poor outcome.
- Medication selection should consider not only the efficacy of the drug in reducing mood symptoms but also the cognitive impact of the drug on the patient.

Self-Assessment

Witnessing mania can elicit numerous intense emotions in a nurse. The patient may use humor, manipulation, power struggles, or demanding behavior to prevent or minimize the staff's ability to set limits on and control dangerous behavior. People with mania have the ability to staff split, or divide the staff into either the good guys or the bad guys. "The nurse on the day shift is always late with my medication and never talks with me. You are the only one who seems to care." This divisive tactic may pit one staff member or group against another, undermining a unified front and consistent plan of care. Frequent staff meetings to deal with the behaviors of the patient and the nurses' responses to these behaviors can help minimize staff splitting and feelings of anger and isolation. Limit setting (e.g., lights out after 11 PM) is the main theme in treating a person in mania. **Consistency among staff is imperative if the limit setting is to be carried out effectively.**

The patient can become aggressively demanding, which often triggers frustration, worry, and exasperation in health care professionals. The behavior of a patient experiencing mania is often aimed at decreasing the effectiveness of staff control, which could be accomplished by getting involved in power plays. For example, the patient might taunt the staff by pointing out faults or oversights and drawing negative attention to one or more staff members. Usually, this is done in a loud and disruptive manner, which provokes staff to become defensive and thereby escalates the environmental tension and the patient's degree of mania.

If you are working with a patient experiencing mania, you may find yourself feeling helplessness, confusion, or even anger. Understanding, acknowledging, and sharing these responses and countertransference reactions will enhance your professional ability to care for the patient and perhaps promote your personal development as well. Collaborating with the multidisciplinary team, accessing supervision with your nursing faculty member, and sharing your experience with peers in post conference may be helpful, perhaps essential.

ASSESSMENT GUIDELINES

Bipolar Disorder

1. Assess whether the patient is a danger to self and others:
   - Patients experiencing mania can exhaust themselves to the point of death.
   - Patients may not eat or sleep, often for days at a time.
   - Poor impulse control may result in harm to others or self.
   - Uncontrolled spending may occur.
2. Assess the need for protection from uninhibited behaviors. External control may be needed to protect the patient from such consequences as bankruptcy, because patients experiencing mania may give away all of their money or possessions.
3. Assess the need for hospitalization to safeguard and stabilize the patient.
4. Assess medical status. A thorough medical examination helps to determine whether mania is primary (a mood disorder—bipolar disorder or cyclothymic disorder) or secondary to another condition.
   - Mania may be secondary to a general medical condition.
   - Mania may be substance-induced (caused by use or abuse of a drug or substance or by toxin exposure).
5. Assess for any coexisting medical condition or other situation that warrants special intervention (e.g., substance abuse, anxiety disorder, legal or financial crises).
6. Assess the patient's and family's understanding of bipolar disorder, knowledge of medications, and knowledge of support groups and organizations that provide information on bipolar disorder.

DIAGNOSIS

A primary consideration for a patient in acute mania is the prevention of exhaustion and death from cardiac collapse. Because of the patient's poor judgment, excessive and constant motor activity, probable dehydration, and difficulty evaluating reality, *risk for injury* is a likely and appropriate diagnosis. Table 13-1 lists potential nursing diagnoses for bipolar disorders.

OUTCOMES IDENTIFICATION

Table 13-1 lists associated outcomes for bipolar disorders. Specific outcome criteria will be based on which of the three phases of the illness the patient is experiencing.

Acute Phase

The primary outcome of the **acute phase** is injury prevention. Outcomes in the acute phase reflect both physiological and psychiatric issues. For example, the patient will:

- Be well hydrated.
- Maintain stable cardiac status.
- Maintain/obtain tissue integrity.
- Get sufficient sleep and rest.
- Demonstrate thought self-control.
- Make no attempt at self-harm.

Continuation Phase

The **continuation phase** lasts for 4 to 9 months. Although the overall outcome of this phase is relapse prevention, many other outcomes must be accomplished to achieve relapse prevention. These outcomes include the following:

- Psychoeducational classes for patient and family related to:
  - Knowledge of disease process
  - Knowledge of medication
  - Consequences of substance addictions for predicting future relapse
  - Knowledge of early signs and symptoms of relapse
- Support groups or therapy (cognitive-behavioral, interpersonal)
- Communication and problem-solving skills training

Maintenance Phase

The overall outcomes for the **maintenance phase** continue to focus on prevention of relapse and limitation of the severity and duration of future episodes.

- Participation in learning interpersonal strategies related to work, interpersonal, and family problems
- Participation in psychotherapy, group, or other ongoing supportive therapy modality

PLANNING

Planning care for an individual with bipolar disorder usually is geared toward the particular phase of mania the patient is in (acute, continuation, or maintenance) as well as any other co-occurring issues identified in the assessment (e.g., risk of suicide, risk of violence to person or property, family crisis, legal crises, substance abuse, risk-taking behaviors).

TABLE 13-1 SIGNS AND SYMPTOMS, NURSING DIAGNOSES, AND OUTCOMES FOR BIPOLAR DISORDERS

SIGNS AND SYMPTOMS	NURSING DIAGNOSES	OUTCOMES
Hyperactivity, locomotion into unauthorized spaces, pacing, poor judgment	*Wandering* *Risk for injury*	Remains in secure area when unaccompanied, can be redirected from unsafe activities, free from injury
Loud, profane, hostile, combative, aggressive, demanding behaviors	*Risk for other-directed violence*	Refrains from harming others, controls impulses, avoids violating others' space
Anxiety, agitation, inability to concentrate, restlessness, prolonged periods of time without sleep	*Sleep deprivation*	Sleeps 5-8 hours a night, reports feeling rejuvenated after sleep
Poor reality testing, gradiosity, denial of problems, difficulty organizing and attending to information, poor concentration, inability to meet basic needs	*Defensive coping* *Ineffective coping*	Reports an increase in concentration, refrains from manipulative behavior, uses effective coping strategies
Minimal nutritional intake, poor hygiene, clothing unclean	*Self-care deficit (feeding, bathing, dressing)*	Returns to precrisis level of care: Completes meals, tends to hygiene, dresses in clean clothing
Giving away of valuables, neglect of family, impulsive major life changes (divorce, career changes), stress and frustration of family members	*Interrupted family processes* *Caregiver role strain*	Family obtains adequate resources to meet the needs of members; family routine is reestablished
Pressured speech, flight of ideas, going from one person or event to another, annoyance or taunting of others, loud and crass speech, provocative behaviors	*Impaired verbal communication* *Impaired social interaction*	Initiates and maintains goal-directed and mutually satisfying verbal exchanges

Herdman, T.H. (Ed.). *Nursing diagnoses—Definitions and classification 2012-2014*. Copyright © 2012, 1994-2012 by NANDA International. Used by arrangement with John Wiley & Sons Limited.

Acute Phase

During the acute phase, planning focuses on medically stabilizing the patient while maintaining safety, and the hospital is usually the safest environment for accomplishing this (Case Study and Nursing Care Plan 13-1). Nursing care is geared toward managing medications, decreasing physical activity, increasing food and fluid intake, ensuring at least 4 to 6 hours of sleep per night, alleviating any bowel or bladder problems, and intervening so that self-care needs are met. Some patients may require seclusion or electroconvulsive therapy (ECT).

Continuation Phase

During the continuation phase, planning focuses on maintaining adherence to the medication regimen and prevention of relapse. Interventions are planned in accordance with the assessment data regarding the patient's interpersonal and stress-reduction skills, cognitive functioning, employment status, substance-related problems, and social support systems. During this time, psychoeducational teaching is necessary for the patient and family. The need for referrals to community programs, groups, and support for any co-occurring disorders or problems (e.g., substance abuse, family problems, legal issues, and financial crises) is evaluated.

Evaluation of the need for communication skills training and problem-solving skills training is also an important consideration. People with bipolar disorders often have interpersonal and emotional problems that affect their work, family, and social lives. Residual problems resulting from reckless, violent, withdrawn, or bizarre behavior that may have occurred during a manic episode often leave lives shattered and family and friends hurt and distant. For some patients, cognitive-behavioral therapy (in addition to medication management) is useful to address these issues although the focus of psychotherapeutic treatment will vary over time for each individual.

Maintenance Phase

During the maintenance phase, planning focuses on preventing relapse and limiting the severity and duration of future episodes. Patients with bipolar disorders require medications over long periods of time or even an entire lifetime. Psychotherapy, support groups, psychoeducational groups, and periodic evaluations help patients maintain their family, social, and occupational lives.

IMPLEMENTATION

Patients with bipolar disorders are often ambivalent about treatment. Only 39% of people experiencing symptoms of bipolar disorder seek treatment within the first year, and the median delay of treatment is 6 years (Wang, 2005). Patients may minimize the destructive consequences of their behaviors or deny the seriousness of the disease, and some are reluctant to give up the increased energy, euphoria, and heightened sense of self-esteem of hypomania.

Unfortunately, nonadherence to the regimen of mood-stabilizing medication is a major cause of relapse, so establishing a therapeutic alliance with the individual with bipolar disorder is crucial.

13-1 CASE STUDY AND NURSING CARE PLAN

Mania

Jasmine is brought to the emergency department after being found on the highway shortly after her car broke down. She is dressed in a long red dress, a blue and orange scarf, many long chains, and a yellow and green turban. The police report that when they came to her aid, she told them she was "driving to fame and fortune." She appeared overly cheerful and was constantly talking, laughing, and making jokes. At the same time, she paced up and down beside the car, sometimes tweaking the cheek of one of the policemen. She was coy and flirtatious with the police officers, saying at one point, "Boys in blue are fun to do."

When she reached into the car and started drinking from an open bottle of bourbon, the police decided that her behavior and general condition might result in harm to herself or others. When they explained to Jasmine that they wanted to take her to the hospital for a general checkup, her jovial mood turned to anger and rage, yet minutes after getting into the police car, she was singing "Rolling in the Deep."

In the emergency department a psychiatrist sees Jasmine, and her sister is called. The sister states that Jasmine stopped taking her lithium about five weeks ago and has become more and more agitated and out of control. She reports that Jasmine has not eaten in days, has stayed up all night calling friends and strangers all over the country, and finally fled the house when the sister called an ambulance to take her to the hospital. The psychiatrist contacts Jasmine's physician, and her previous history and medical management are discussed. She is hospitalized, and lithium therapy is restarted. It is hoped that medications and a controlled environment will prevent further escalation of the manic state and prevent possible exhaustion and cardiac collapse.

Self-Assessment

Jeff has worked as a registered nurse on the psychiatric unit for three years. He has learned to deal with many of the challenging behaviors associated with the mania of bipolar disorder. For example, he no longer takes verbal insults personally. He is also better able to recognize and set limits on some of the tactics used by the patient experiencing mania to split the staff. The staff on this unit work closely with one another, making the atmosphere positive and supportive.

The only aspects of Ms. Klein's behavior that Jeff finds challenging are the sexual advances and loud sexual comments she makes. When he discusses this with the unit coordinator, they decide that two nurses should provide care for Ms. Klein. A female nurse will spend time with her in her room, and Jeff will spend time with her in quiet areas on the unit. It is decided that neither Jeff nor any male staff member will be alone with Ms. Klein in her room at any time. Jeff will ask for relief if Ms. Klein's sexual remarks and acting-out behaviors become too much to take.

Assessment

Objective Data

Little if anything to eat for days
Little if any sleep for days
History of mania
History of lithium maintenance
Constant physical activity: unable to sit
Loud and distracting
Angry when wishes are curtailed
Flight of ideas
Dress loud and inappropriate
Suggestive remarks with sexual themes: calls nurse "lover"
Behavior that some patients find amusing
Remarks that suggest grandiose thinking
Poor judgment

Subjective Data

"Driving myself to fame and fortune."
"I'm untouchable . . . I'll get the FBI to set me free."
"Let me be . . . set me free, lover."

Diagnosis

1. *Risk for injury* related to dehydration and faulty judgment, as evidenced by inability to meet own physiological needs and set limits on own behavior
   - Has not slept for days
   - Has not consumed food or fluids for days
   - Engages in constant physical activity and is unable to sit
2. *Defensive coping* related to biochemical changes, as evidenced by change in usual communication patterns
   - Loud and distracting
   - Suggestive remarks with sexual themes
   - Behavior some patients find amusing
   - Comments suggest grandiose thinking
   - Flight of ideas
   - Loud, hostile, and sexual remarks to other patients

Outcomes Identification

Physical status will remain stable during manic phase.

Planning

The nurse plans interventions that will help de-escalate Ms. Klein's activity to minimize potential physical injury (dehydration, cardiac instability) through the use of medication and provision of a nonstimulating environment.

Implementation

Jeff makes the following nursing care plan.

13-1 CASE STUDY AND NURSING CARE PLAN—cont'd

Mania

SHORT-TERM GOAL	INTERVENTION	RATIONALE	EVALUATION
1. Patient will be well-hydrated, as evidenced by good skin turgor and normal urinary output and specific gravity, within 24 hours.	1a. Give haloperidol (Haldol) intramuscularly immediately and as ordered.	1a. Continuous physical activity and lack of fluids can eventually lead to cardiac collapse and death.	**GOAL MET** After 3 hours, patient takes small amounts of fluid (2-4 oz per hour). After 5 hours, patient starts taking 8 oz per hour with a lot of reminding and encouragement. After 24 hours, urine specific gravity is within normal limits.
	1b. Check vital signs frequently (every 1-2 hours).	1b. Cardiac status is monitored.	
	1c. Place patient in private or quiet room (whenever possible).	1c. Environmental stimuli are reduced—escalation of mania and distractibility is minimized.	
	1d. Stay with patient and divert patient away from stimulating situations.	1d. Nurse's presence provides support. Ability to interact with others is temporarily impaired.	
	1e. Offer high-calorie, high-protein drink (8 oz) every hour in quiet area.	1e. Proper hydration is mandatory for maintenance of cardiac status.	
	1f. Frequently remind patient to drink: "Take two more sips."	1f. Patient's concentration is poor; she is easily distracted.	
	1g. Offer finger food frequently in quiet area.	1g. Patient is unable to sit; snacks she can eat while pacing are more likely to be consumed.	
	1h. Maintain record of intake and output.	1h. Such a record allows staff to make accurate nutritional assessment for patient's safety.	
	1i. Weigh patient daily.	1i. Monitoring of nutritional status is necessary.	
2. Patient will sleep or rest 3 hours during the first night in the hospital with aid of medication and nursing interventions.	2a. Continue to direct patient to areas of minimal activity.	2a. Lower levels of stimulation can decrease excitability.	Patient is awake most of the first night. Sleeps for 2 hours from 4 to 6 AM. Patient is able to rest on the second day for short periods and engage in quiet activities for short periods (5-10 minutes).
	2b. When possible, try to direct energy into productive and calming activities (e.g., pacing to slow, soft music; slow exercise; drawing alone; or writing in quiet area).	2b. Directing patient to paced, nonstimulating activities can help minimize excitability.	
	2c. Encourage short rest periods throughout the day (e.g., 3-5 minutes every hour) when possible.	2c. Patient may be unaware of feelings of fatigue. Can collapse from exhaustion if hyperactivity continues without periods of rest.	
	2d. Patient should drink decaffeinated drinks only— decaffeinated coffee, tea, or colas.	2d. Caffeine is a central nervous system stimulant that inhibits needed rest or sleep.	
	2e. Provide nursing measures at bedtime that promote sleep—warm milk, soft music.	2e. Such measures promote nonstimulating and relaxing mood.	
3. Patient's blood pressure (BP) and pulse (P) will be within normal limits within 24 hours with the aid of medication and nursing interventions.	3a. Continue to monitor BP and P frequently throughout the day (every 30 minutes).	3a. Physical condition is presently a great strain on patient's heart.	**GOAL MET** Baseline measures on unit are not obtained because of hyperactive behavior. Information from family physician states that baseline BP is 130/90 mm Hg and baseline P is 88 beats per minute. BP at end of 24 hours is 130/70 mm Hg; P is 80 beats per minute.
	3b. Keep staff informed by verbal and written reports of baseline vital signs and patient progress.	3b. Alerting all staff regarding patient's status can increase medical intervention if a change in status occurs.	

Evaluation

After 2 days, the medical staff think that Ms. Klein's physical status is stable. Her vital signs are within normal limits, she is consuming sufficient fluids, and her urinary output is normal. Although her hyperactivity persists, it does so to a lesser degree; she is able to get periods of rest during the day and is sleeping 3 to 4 hours during the night.

Ms. Klein's hyperactivity continues to be a challenge to the nurses; however, she is able to participate in some activities that require gross motor movement. These activities are useful in channeling some of her aggressive energy. Shortly after her arrival on the unit, Ms. Klein starts a fight with another patient, but seclusion is avoided because she is able to refrain from further violent episodes as a result of medication and nursing interventions. She can be directed toward solitary activities, which channel some of her energies, at least for short periods.

As the effect of the drugs progresses, Ms. Klein's activity level decreases, and by discharge, she is able to discuss issues of concern with the nurse and make some useful decisions about her future. She is to come for follow-up at the community center and agrees to join a family psychoeducational group for patients with bipolar disorder and their families, which she will attend with her sister.

Acute Phase

Depressive Episodes

Depressive episodes of bipolar disorder have the same symptoms and risks as major depression (refer to Chapter 14) although they are often more intense. Hospitalization may be required if suicidal ideation, psychosis, or catatonia is present. Lithium and lamotrigine (Lamictal) are the first line of treatment for a person with bipolar disorder experiencing an acute depressive episode. Treatment with antidepressants is not recommended (particularly for bipolar I disorder) since the patient's central nervous system (CNS) may become overactive, and antidepressants may result in hypomania or mania. Patients who experience depression while taking maintenance levels of medications may benefit from increased doses of the original drugs. When depressive episodes have psychotic features, a second-generation antipsychotic may be added to the medication regimen.

Manic Episodes

Hospitalization provides safety for a patient experiencing acute mania (bipolar I disorder), imposes external controls on destructive behaviors, and provides for medication stabilization. There are unique approaches to communicating with and maintaining the safety of the patient during the hospitalization period (Table 13-2). Staff members continuously set limits in a firm, nonthreatening, and neutral manner to prevent further escalation of mania and provide safe boundaries for the patient and others.

Continuation Phase

The continuation phase is crucial for patients and their families. The outcome for this phase is prevention of relapse, and community resources are chosen based on the needs of the patient, the appropriateness of the referral, and the availability of resources. Frequently, a case manager evaluates appropriate follow-up care for patients and their families.

Medication adherence during this phase is perhaps the most important treatment outcome. This follow-up is frequently handled in a mental health center; however, adherence to the medication regimen is also addressed in day hospitals and psychiatric home-care visits. Some patients may attend day hospitals if they are not too excitable and are able to tolerate a certain level of stimuli. In addition to medication management, day hospitals

TABLE 13-2 INTERVENTIONS FOR THE PATIENT IN ACUTE MANIA

INTERVENTION	RATIONALE
Communication	
Use firm and calm approach: "John, come with me. Eat this sandwich."	Structure and control are provided for patient who is out of control. Feelings of security can result: "Someone is in control."
Use short and concise explanations or statements.	Short attention span limits comprehension to small bits of information.
Remain neutral; avoid power struggles and value judgments.	Patient can use inconsistencies and value judgments as justification for arguing and escalating mania.
Be consistent in approach and expectations.	Consistent limits and expectations minimize potential for patient's manipulation of staff.
Have frequent staff meetings to plan consistent approaches and set agreed-on limits.	Consistency of all staff is needed to maintain controls and minimize manipulation by patient.
With other staff, decide on limits and tell patient in simple, concrete terms with consequences. Example: "John, do not yell at or hit Peter. If you cannot control yourself, we will help you." Or "The seclusion room will help you feel less out of control and prevent harm to yourself and others."	Clear expectations help patient experience outside controls, as well as understand reasons for medication, seclusion, or restraints (if he or she is not able to control behaviors).
Hear and act on legitimate complaints.	Underlying feelings of helplessness are reduced, and acting-out behaviors are minimized.
Firmly redirect energy into more appropriate and constructive channels.	Distractibility is the nurse's most effective tool with the patient experiencing mania.
Structure in a Safe Milieu	
Maintain low level of stimuli in patient's environment (e.g., away from bright lights, loud noises, and people).	Escalation of anxiety can be decreased.
Provide structured solitary activities with nurse or aide.	Structure provides security and focus.
Provide frequent high-calorie fluids.	Serious dehydration is prevented.
Provide frequent rest periods.	Exhaustion is prevented.
Redirect violent behavior.	Physical exercise can decrease tension and provide focus.
When warranted in acute mania, use phenothiazines and seclusion to minimize physical harm.	Exhaustion and death can result from dehydration, lack of sleep, and constant physical activity.
Observe for signs of lithium toxicity.	There is a small margin of safety between therapeutic and toxic doses.
Protect patient from giving away money and possessions. Hold valuables in hospital safe until rational judgment returns.	Patient's "generosity" is a manic defense that is consistent with irrational, grandiose thinking.

TABLE 13-2 INTERVENTIONS FOR THE PATIENT IN ACUTE MANIA—cont'd

INTERVENTION	RATIONALE
Physiological Safety: Self-Care Needs	
Nutrition	
Monitor intake, output, and vital signs.	Adequate fluid and caloric intake are ensured; development of dehydration and cardiac collapse is minimized.
Offer frequent, high-calorie protein drinks and finger foods (e.g., sandwiches, fruit, milkshakes).	Constant fluid and calorie replacement are needed. Patient may be too active to sit at meals. Finger foods allow "eating on the run."
Frequently remind patient to eat. "Tom, finish your milkshake." "Sally, eat this banana."	The patient experiencing mania is unaware of bodily needs and is easily distracted. Needs supervision to eat.
Sleep	
Encourage frequent rest periods during the day.	Lack of sleep can lead to exhaustion and death.
Keep patient in areas of low stimulation.	Relaxation is promoted, and manic behavior is minimized.
At night, provide warm baths, soothing music, and medication when indicated. Avoid giving patient caffeine.	Relaxation, rest, and sleep are promoted.
Hygiene	
Supervise choice of clothes; minimize flamboyant and bizarre dress (e.g., garish stripes or plaids and loud, unmatching colors).	The potential is decreased for ridicule, which lowers self-esteem and increases the need for manic defense. The patient is helped to maintain dignity.
Give simple step-by-step reminders for hygiene and dress. "Here is your razor. Shave the left side . . . now the right side. Here is your toothbrush. Put the toothpaste on the brush."	Distractibility and poor concentration are countered through simple, concrete instructions.
Elimination	
Monitor bowel habits; offer fluids and foods that are high in fiber. Evaluate need for laxative. Encourage patient to go to the bathroom.	Fecal impaction resulting from dehydration and decreased peristalsis is prevented.

offer structure, decrease social isolation, and help patients channel their time and energy. If a patient is homebound, psychiatric home care is the appropriate modality for follow-up care.

Maintenance Phase

The goal of the maintenance phase is to prevent recurrence of an episode of bipolar disorder. The community resources cited earlier are helpful, and patients and their families often greatly benefit from mutual support and self-help groups that will be discussed later in this chapter.

Psychopharmacological Interventions

Individuals with bipolar disorder often require multiple medications. For severe manic episodes, lithium or valproate (Depakote) and a second-generation antipsychotic such as olanzapine (Zyprexa) or risperidone (Risperdal) are recommended. Individuals experiencing less severe symptoms may be given only one of these. There may be times when a benzodiazepine antianxiety agent can help reduce agitation or anxiety. Antidepressants that may have been prescribed previously are often tapered and possibly discontinued to reduce mania or hypomania.

Lithium Carbonate

The chemical name for **lithium carbonate** is $LiCO_3$, although you may see it abbreviated as $Li+$. Lithium is effective in the treatment of bipolar I acute and recurrent manic and depressive episodes. Lithium inhibits about 80% of acute manic and hypomanic episodes within 10 to 21 days (Sadock & Sadock). Lithium is less effective in people with mixed mania (elation and depression), those with rapid cycling, and those with atypical features.

Indications. Lithium is particularly effective in reducing the following:

- Elation, grandiosity, and expansiveness
- Flight of ideas
- Irritability and manipulation
- Anxiety

To a lesser extent, lithium controls the following:

- Insomnia
- Psychomotor agitation
- Threatening or assaultive behavior
- Distractibility
- Hypersexuality
- Paranoia

Lithium must reach therapeutic levels in the patient's blood to be effective. This usually takes 7 to 14 days, or longer for some patients. An antipsychotic or benzodiazepine can be used to prevent exhaustion, coronary collapse, and death until lithium reaches therapeutic levels. Antipsychotics act promptly to slow speech, inhibit aggression, and decrease psychomotor activity. As lithium becomes effective in reducing manic behavior, the antipsychotic drugs are usually discontinued. Although lithium is an effective intervention for treating the acute manic phase of a bipolar disorder, it is not a cure. Many patients receive lithium for maintenance indefinitely and experience manic and depressive episodes if the drug is discontinued.

Actress Patty Duke describes her response to lithium after years of alternating depression, elation, and bad choices (Moore, 2008):

> "Lithium saved my life. After just a few weeks on the drug, death-based thoughts were no longer the first I had when I got up and last when I went to bed. The nightmare that had spanned 30 years was over. I'm not a Stepford wife; I still feel the exultation and sadness that any person feels. I'm just not required to feel them 10 times as long or as intensively as I used to."

Therapeutic and Toxic Levels. Trade names for lithium carbonate include Lithane, Eskalith, and Lithonate. During the active phase, 300 mg to 600 mg is given 2 or 3 times a day by mouth to reach a clear therapeutic result or a lithium level of 0.8 to 1.4 mEq/L. The maintenance blood levels should range between 0.4 and 1.3 mEq/L; however, a level of 0.6 mEq/L may be effective for many. To avoid serious toxicity, lithium levels should not exceed 1.5 mEq/L (Lehne, 2007). At serum levels above 1.5 mEq/L, early signs of toxicity can occur; at 1.5 to 2.0 mEq/L, advanced signs of toxicity may be seen; at 2.0 to 2.5 mEq/L or above, severe lithium toxicity and death can occur, and emergency measures should be taken immediately. Gastric lavage and treatment with urea, mannitol, and aminophylline can hasten lithium excretion. Hemodialysis may also be necessary in extreme cases.

A small increment exists between the therapeutic and toxic levels of lithium. Lithium levels should be measured at least 5 days after beginning lithium therapy and after any dosage change, until the therapeutic level has been reached (Perlis, 2008). After therapeutic levels have been reached, blood levels are determined every month. After 6 months to a year of stability, measurement of blood levels every 3 months may suffice. Blood should be drawn in the morning, 8 to 12 hours after the last dose of lithium is taken. Table 13-3 details expected side effects of lithium, signs of lithium toxicity, and interventions for both.

For older adult patients, the principle of **start low and go slow** still applies. Levels are often monitored every 3 or 4 days. As mentioned earlier, toxic effects are usually associated with lithium levels of 2.0 mEq/L or higher although they can occur at much lower levels (even within a therapeutic range).

Maintenance Therapy. Some clinicians suggest that patients with bipolar disorder need to be given lithium for 9 to 12 months, and some patients may need lifelong lithium maintenance to prevent further relapses. Many patients respond well to lower dosages during maintenance or prophylactic lithium therapy.

Lithium is unquestionably effective in preventing both manic and depressive episodes in patients with bipolar disorder; however, complete suppression occurs in only 50% of patients or fewer, even with adherence to the maintenance therapy regimen. The patient and family therefore should be given careful instructions about (1) the purpose and requirements of lithium therapy,

TABLE 13-3 LITHIUM SIDE EFFECTS AND SIGNS OF LITHIUM TOXICITY

LEVEL	SIGNS	INTERVENTIONS
Expected Side Effects		
0.4-1.0 mEq/L (therapeutic level)	Fine hand tremor, polyuria, and mild thirst Mild nausea and general discomfort Weight gain	Symptoms may persist throughout therapy. Symptoms often subside during treatment. Weight gain may be helped with diet, exercise, and nutritional management.
Early Signs of Toxicity		
1.5 mEq/L	Nausea, vomiting, diarrhea, thirst, polyuria, lethargy, slurred speech, muscle weakness, and fine hand tremor	Medication should be withheld, blood lithium levels measured, and dosage reevaluated.
Advanced Signs of Toxicity		
1.5-2.0 mEq/L	Coarse hand tremor, persistent gastrointestinal upset, mental confusion, muscle hyperirritability, electroencephalographic changes, incoordination, sedation	Interventions outlined above or below should be used, depending on severity of circumstances.
Severe Toxicity		
2.0-2.5 mEq/L	Ataxia, giddiness, serious electroencephalographic changes, blurred vision, clonic movements, large output of dilute urine, seizures, stupor, severe hypotension, coma. Death is usually secondary to pulmonary complications.	Hospitalization is indicated. The drug is stopped, and excretion is hastened. If patient is alert, an emetic is administered.
>2.5 mEq/L	Convulsions, oliguria, and death can occur	In addition to the interventions above, hemodialysis may be used in severe cases.

Data from Lehne, R. A. (2007). *Pharmacology for nursing care* (4th ed., p. 357). Philadelphia, PA: Saunders; Lieberman, J. A., & Tasman, A. (2000). *Psychiatric drugs.* St. Louis, MO: Saunders.

(2) its adverse effects, (3) its toxic effects and complications, and (4) situations in which the physician should be contacted. The patient and family should also be advised that suddenly stopping lithium can lead to relapse and recurrence of mania. Health care providers must stress to patients and their families the importance of discontinuing maintenance therapy gradually. Box 13-1 outlines patient and family teaching regarding lithium therapy.

Patients need to know that **two major long-term risks of lithium therapy are hypothyroidism and impairment of the kidney's ability to concentrate urine;** therefore, a person receiving lithium therapy must have periodic follow-ups to assess thyroid and renal function.

Contraindications. Before lithium is administered, a medical evaluation is performed to assess the patient's ability to tolerate the drug. In particular, baseline physical and laboratory examinations should include assessment of renal function; determination of thyroid status, including levels of thyroxine and thyroid-stimulating hormone; and evaluation for dementia or neurological disorders, which presage a poor response to lithium. Other clinical and laboratory assessments, including an electrocardiogram, are performed as needed, depending on the individual's physical condition.

Lithium therapy is generally contraindicated in patients with cardiovascular disease, brain damage, renal disease, thyroid disease, or myasthenia gravis. Whenever possible, lithium is not given to women who are pregnant because it may harm the fetus. The fear of becoming pregnant and the wish to become pregnant are both major concerns for many women taking lithium. Lithium use is also contraindicated in mothers who are breast-feeding and in children younger than 12 years of age.

BOX 13-1 PATIENT AND FAMILY TEACHING: LITHIUM THERAPY

The patient and the patient's family should receive the following teaching, be encouraged to ask questions, and be given the material in written form as well.

- Lithium treats your current emotional problem and also helps prevent relapse; therefore, it is important to continue taking the drug after the current episode is over.
- Because therapeutic and toxic dosage ranges are so close, it is important to monitor lithium blood levels very closely—more frequently at first, then once every several months after that.
- Lithium is not addictive.
- It is important to eat a normal diet with normal salt and fluid intake (1500-3000 mL/day or six 12-oz glasses of fluid). Lithium decreases sodium reabsorption in the kidneys, which could lead to a deficiency of sodium. A low sodium intake leads to a relative increase in lithium retention, which could produce toxicity.
- You should stop taking lithium if you have excessive diarrhea, vomiting, or sweating. All of these symptoms can lead to dehydration. Dehydration can raise lithium levels in the blood to toxic levels. **Inform your physician if you have any of these problems.**
- Do not take diuretics (water pills) while you are taking lithium.
- Lithium is irritating to the lining of your stomach. Take lithium with meals.
- It is important to have your kidneys and thyroid checked periodically, especially if you are taking lithium over a long period. Talk to your doctor about this follow-up.
- Don't take any over-the-counter medicines without checking first with your doctor.
- If you find that you are gaining a lot of weight, you may need to talk this over with your doctor or nutritionist.
- Many self-help groups are available to provide support for people with bipolar disorder and their families. The local self-help group is (give name and telephone number).
- You can find out more information by calling (give name and telephone number).
- Keep a list of side effects and toxic effects handy, along with the name and number of a contact person (see Table 13-3).
- If lithium is to be discontinued, your dosage will be tapered gradually to minimize the risk of relapse.

Anticonvulsant Drugs

Researchers have hypothesized that mood instability could be viewed much the same as epilepsy and that a chain reaction of sensitivity, or *kindling*, was responsible for the worsening of bipolar symptoms over time (Bender & Alloy, 2011). This hypothesis led to the use of carbamazepine and valproate as a treatment for mania and the incorporation of anticonvulsant therapy. Subsequent research did not support the kindling theory, however. It is likely that symptom improvement for bipolar disorder is based on a different mechanism of action than seizure prevention.

Three **anticonvulsant drugs** have demonstrated efficacy and been approved for the treatment of mood disorders: valproate (Depakote), carbamazepine (Tegretol), and lamotrigine (Lamictal). Anticonvulsant drugs are thought to be:

- Superior for continuously cycling patients
- More effective when there is no family history of bipolar disease
- Effective at dampening affective swings in schizoaffective patients
- Effective at diminishing impulsive and aggressive behavior in some nonpsychotic patients
- Helpful in cases of alcohol and benzodiazepine withdrawal
- Beneficial in controlling mania (within 2 weeks) and depression (within 3 weeks or longer)

Valproate. Valproate (available as divalproex sodium [Depakote] and valproic acid [Depakene]) is useful in treating lithium nonresponders who are in acute mania, experience rapid cycles, are in dysphoric mania, or have not responded to carbamazepine. Valproate is also helpful in preventing future manic episodes. It is important to monitor liver function and platelet count periodically although serious complications are rare.

Carbamazepine. Some patients with treatment-resistant bipolar disorder improve after taking carbamazepine (Tegretol) and lithium, or carbamazepine and an antipsychotic. Carbamazepine seems to work better in patients with rapid cycling and in severely paranoid, angry, patients experiencing manias than in euphoric, overactive, overfriendly patients experiencing manias. It is also thought to be more effective in dysphoric patients experiencing manias.

As with valproate, liver function and platelet count should be monitored periodically. Blood levels of carbamazepine should be monitored at least weekly for the first 8 weeks of treatment, because the drug can increase levels of liver enzymes that can speed its own metabolism. In some instances, this can cause bone-marrow suppression and liver inflammation.

Lamotrigine. Lamotrigine (Lamictal) is a first-line treatment for bipolar depression and is approved for acute and maintenance therapy. Lamotrigine is generally well tolerated, but there is one serious but rare dermatological reaction: a potentially life-threatening rash. Patients should be instructed to seek immediate medical attention if a rash appears although most are likely benign.

Antianxiety Drugs

Clonazepam (Klonopin) and lorazepam (Ativan) are antianxiety (anxiolytic) drugs useful in the treatment of acute mania in some patients who are resistant to other treatments. These drugs are also effective in managing the psychomotor agitation seen in mania. They should be avoided, however, in patients with a history of substance abuse.

Second-Generation Antipsychotics

In addition to showing sedative properties during the early phase of treatment (help with insomnia, anxiety, agitation), the second-generation antipsychotics seem to have mood-stabilizing properties. Most evidence supports the use of olanzapine (Zyprexa) or risperidone (Risperdal).

Table 13-4 provides an overview of drugs used for bipolar disorder. It identifies drugs with U.S. Food and Drug Administration (FDA, 2012) approval for bipolar disorder and also drugs that are commonly prescribed "off label" even though they are not specifically approved. Additionally, American Psychiatric Association (2008) pharmacological recommendations for management of bipolar depression, mania, and maintenance are described.

Integrative Therapy

A few generations ago, children actively resisted a nightly dose of cod liver oil that mothers swore by as a method to prevent constipation. While the foul-tasting, evil-smelling liquid undoubtedly helped win that particular battle, it may have had other benefits as well. Cod liver oil is rich in omega-3 fatty acids, which have drawn increasing attention as being important in mood regulation. Fish oil is the target of this attention. It contains two omega-3 fatty acids, eicosapentaenoic acid (EPA) and docosahexaenoic acid (DHA), which are important in CNS functioning. EPA seems to be particularly important to behavior and mood.

The interest in these particular fatty acids developed as research began to suggest that people who live in areas with low seafood consumption (especially coldwater seafood) exhibited higher rates of depression and bipolar disorder. This led researchers to explore the influence of omega-3 fatty acids as protective for bipolar disorder (Parker, 2006). Alternative treatments are especially attractive for the depressive phase of the disorder, since drugs that are normally used to treat depression can catapult a person into a dangerous manic episode.

The jury is still out on the absolute benefits of either eating more fish or taking fish oil supplements (delivered in non—fishy-tasting gel capsules). In a review of published trials, one group of researchers was unable to come up with clear support for increasing dietary intake of omega-3 fatty acids (Appleton, 2006). But Kidd (2007) conducted another large-scale analysis of current research and concluded just the opposite: that multiple studies support the benefits of fish oil for the mood swings of bipolar disorder. What seems to be clear is that the real benefit of omega-3 fatty acids is in their ability to reduce the depression associated with bipolar disorder (Sarris et al., 2012).

CONSIDERING CULTURE

Racial Influence on the Diagnosis and Treatment of Bipolar Disorder

Imagine that Jason, a 28-year-old, Caucasian male, arrives at a community mental health center complaining of an inability to sleep. His speech is rapid, he paces, and he talks about the inability of the mayor to cleanse the sewers of chlorine gas. He jumps from topic to topic but seems to always return to his family being Russian rulers in exile. After some amount of deliberation, the nurse practitioner tentatively diagnoses him as having bipolar disorder, manic phase, and prescribes a mood stabilizer, lithium, and an antipsychotic, Zyprexa.

Shortly after that, George, a 32-year-old, African American male, arrives at the center. He is irritated that his wife threw him out for running up their credit card debt, being involved with another woman, and keeping her awake at night with loud music and incessant talking. George says that he is superhuman and no longer needs to eat or sleep. During the assessment, he wrings his hands, jumps up from his chair, and looks nervously around the room as if he is afraid or is hearing something. After further assessment, the nurse practitioner diagnoses him with a psychotic disorder (with a need to rule out schizophrenia) and prescribes Zyprexa.

What's the big difference between the patients? It is probably not their symptoms but quite likely their races. Research demonstrates that African Americans are far more likely to receive a diagnosis of schizophrenia than bipolar disorder (Haeri et al., 2011). Furthermore, even when bipolar disorder is diagnosed, African Americans are less like to receive lithium treatment and are far more likely to be prescribed antipsychotics (Kilbourne & Pincus, 2006). Implications of this study and many others are that bipolar disorder is not being treated uniformly among different races and that patients are suffering needlessly when cost-effective pharmacotherapy is available (lithium is far less expensive than either second-generation antipsychotic agents or mood stabilizers).

Haeri, S., Williams, J., Kopeykina, I., Johnson, J., Newmark, A., Cohen, L., & Galynker, I. (2011). Disparities in diagnosis of bipolar disorder in individuals of African and European descent. *Journal of Psychiatric Practice, 17*(6), 394-403; Kilbourne, A. M., & Pincus, H. A. (2006). Brief reports: Patterns of psychotropic medication use by race among veterans with bipolar disorder. *Psychiatric Services, 57*(1), 123-126.

TABLE 13-4 **DRUGS USED WITH FDA APPROVAL AND OFF-LABEL FOR THE TREATMENT OF BIPOLAR DISORDER**

GENERIC (TRADE)	FDA APPROVAL	OFF-LABEL	AMERICAN PSYCHIATRIC ASSOCIATION (APA) RECOMMENDATIONS
Lithium (Eskalith, Eskalith CR, Lithobid)	Acute mania Maintenance	Depression	A first line for bipolar depression Recommended for acute mania A first line of maintenance treatment of bipolar disorder
Anticonvulsants			
Divalproex sodium delayed release (Depakote), extended release (Depakote ER)	Acute mania	Depression Maintenance	
Valproate sodium injectable (Depacon)	Acute mania		
Valproic acid (Depakene) delayed release (Stavzor)	Acute mania	Depression Maintenance	A first line of maintenance treatment of bipolar disorder, often replacing lithium as drug of choice
Carbamazepine (Tegretol, Tegretol XR, Carbatrol, Equetro)	Acute mania and mixed episodes (Equetro)	Depression Maintenance	Recommended for maintenance treatment of bipolar disorder
Gabapentin (Neurotin)		Maintenance	
Lamotrigine (Lamictal)	Maintenance	Depression Acute mania	A first line for bipolar depression
Oxcarbazepine (Trileptal)		Depression Acute mania Maintenance	Recommended for maintenance treatment of bipolar disorder
Topiramate (Topamax)		Maintenance	
Antipsychotics			
Aripiprazole (Abilify)	Mania Maintenance from ages 10+	Depression	As monotherapy or adjunct to lithium or valproic acid
Asenapine (Saphris)	Mania Mixed		As monotherapy or adjunct with lithium or valproate
Clozapine (Clozaril)		Maintenance	
Olanzapine (Zyprexa)	Mania Mixed episodes Maintenance	Depression	Recommended for acute mania As monotherapy or adjunct with lithium or valproate
Olanzapine-fluoxetine combination (Symbyax)	Depression	Maintenance	
Quetiapine fumarate (Seroquel, Seroquel XR)	Depression Mania Mixed Maintenance		As monotherapy or adjunct with lithium or valproate
Risperidone (Risperdal), long-acting injectable (Risperdal Consta)	Mania Mixed Maintenance	Depression Maintenance	First-line treatment for severe mania
Ziprasidone (Geodon)	Mania Mixed Maintenance (Bipolar I)	Depression Maintenance	
Conventional Antipsychotics			
Chlorpromazine (Thorazine)	Mania	Maintenance	
Haloperidol (Haldol, Haldol Decanoate)		Mania Maintenance	
Thioridazine (Mellaril)		Mania Maintenance	
Trifluoperazine (Stelazine)		Mania Maintenance	

Continued

TABLE 13-4 **DRUGS USED WITH FDA APPROVAL AND OFF-LABEL FOR THE TREATMENT OF BIPOLAR DISORDER—cont'd**

GENERIC (TRADE)	FDA APPROVAL	OFF-LABEL	AMERICAN PSYCHIATRIC ASSOCIATION (APA) RECOMMENDATIONS
Antianxiety Agents			
Clonazepam (Klonopin)		Mania Maintenance	Recommended for agitation or severe symptoms
Antidepressants			
Maprotiline (Ludiomil)	Depression		

Data from Lehne, R.A. (2010). *Pharmacology for nursing care* (7th ed.). St. Louis, MO: Saunders; Howland, R.H. (2012). Drugs to treat bipolar disorder. *Journal of Psychosocial Nursing, 50*(6), 9-10.

Electroconvulsive Therapy

Electroconvulsive therapy (ECT) is used to subdue severe manic behavior, especially in patients with treatment-resistant mania and patients with rapid cycling (i.e., those who experience four or more episodes of illness a year). One promising research study used a monthly "maintenance" ECT for rapid cyclers with a positive response of significantly decreased episodes (Minnai et al., 2011). Depressive episodes—particularly those with severe, catatonic, or treatment-resistant depression—are an indication for this treatment and may be helpful for mania during pregnancy. ECT is effective for patients with bipolar disorder who have rapid cycling, for those with paranoid-destructive features (who often respond poorly to lithium therapy), and in acutely suicidal patients.

Teamwork and Safety

Staff work together to create a climate of teamwork and safety for patients who are at risk for self-harm during a depressive phase or at risk for self-harm or other harm during the acute phase. The whole treatment team is trained to recognize changes that may lead to unsafe behavior.

Control of hyperactivity during the acute phase almost always includes immediate treatment with an antipsychotic drug. When a patient is dangerously out of control, however, use of the seclusion room or restraints may also be indicated. The seclusion room provides comfort and relief to many patients who can no longer control their own behavior. Seclusion serves the following purposes:

- Reduces overwhelming environmental stimuli
- Protects a patient from injuring self, others, or staff
- Prevents destruction of personal property or property of others

Seclusion is warranted when documented data collected by the nursing and medical staff reflect the following points:

- Substantial risk of harm to others or self is clear.
- The patient is unable to control his or her actions.
- Problematic behavior has been sustained (continues or escalates despite other measures).
- Other measures have failed (e.g., setting limits beginning with verbal de-escalation or using chemical restraints).

The use of seclusion or restraints is associated with complex therapeutic, ethical, and legal issues. Most state laws prohibit the use of unnecessary physical restraint or isolation. Barring an emergency, the use of seclusion and restraints warrants the patient's consent; therefore, most hospitals have well-defined protocols for treatment with seclusion. Seclusion protocol includes a proper reporting procedure through the chain of command when a patient is to be secluded. For example, the use of seclusion and restraint is permitted only on the written order of a physician, which must be reviewed and rewritten every 24 hours. The order must include the type of restraint to be used. Only in an emergency may the charge nurse place a patient in seclusion or restraint; under these circumstances, a written physician's order must be obtained within a specified period of time (15 to 30 minutes).

Seclusion protocols also identify specific nursing responsibilities, such as how often the patient's behavior is to be observed and documented (e.g., every 15 minutes), how often the patient is to be offered food and fluids (e.g., every 30 to 60 minutes), and how often the patient is to be toileted (e.g., every 1 to 2 hours). Because phenothiazines are often administered to patients in seclusion, vital signs should be measured frequently (e.g., every 1 to 2 hours).

Careful and precise documentation is a legal necessity. The nurse documents the following:

- The behavior leading up to the seclusion or restraint
- The actions taken to provide the least restrictive alternative
- The time the patient was placed in seclusion
- Every 15 minutes, the patient's behavior, needs, nursing care, and vital signs
- The time and type of medications given and their effects on the patient

When a patient requires seclusion to prevent self-harm or violence toward others, it is ideal to have one nurse on each shift work with the patient on a continuous basis. Communication with a patient in seclusion is concrete and direct but also empathetic and limited to brief instructions. Patients need reassurance that seclusion is only a temporary measure and that they will be returned to the unit when their behavior is more controlled and they demonstrate the ability to safely be around others.

Frequent staff meetings regarding personal feelings are necessary to prevent using seclusion as a form of punishment or leaving a patient in seclusion for long periods of time without proper supervision. **Restraints and seclusion are never to be used as punishment or for the convenience of the staff.** Refer to Chapter 6 for a more detailed discussion of the legal implications of seclusion and restraints.

Support Groups

Patients with bipolar disorder, as well as their friends and families, benefit from forming mutual support groups, such as those sponsored by the Depression and Bipolar Support Alliance (DBSA), the National Alliance for the Mentally Ill (NAMI), the National Mental Health Association, and the Manic-Depressive Association.

Health Teaching and Health Promotion

Patients and families need information about bipolar illness, with particular emphasis on its chronic and highly recurrent nature. In addition, patients and families need to be taught the warning signs and symptoms of impending episodes. For example, changes in sleep patterns are especially important because they usually precede, accompany, or precipitate mania. Even a single night of unexplainable sleep loss can be taken as an early warning of impending mania. Health teaching stresses the importance of establishing regularity in sleep patterns, meals, exercise, and other activities. Box 13-2 lists health-teaching guidelines for patients with bipolar disorder and their families.

Mood stabilizers may cause weight gain and other metabolic disturbances such as altered metabolism of lipids and glucose (Fagiolini et al., 2008). These alterations increase the risk for diabetes, high blood pressure, dyslipidemia, cardiac problems, or all of these in combination (metabolic syndrome). Not only do these disturbances impair quality of life and life span, but they are also a major reason for nonadherence. Teaching aimed at weight reduction and management is essential to keeping patients physically healthy and emotionally stable.

Recovery concepts are particularly important for patients with bipolar disorder, who often have issues with adherence to treatment. The best method of addressing this problem is to follow a collaborative-care model in which responsibilities for treatment adherence are shared. In this model, patients are responsible for making it to appointments and openly communicating information, and the health care provider is responsible for keeping current on treatment methods and listening carefully as the patient shares perceptions. Through this sharing, treatment adherence becomes a self-managed responsibility.

BOX 13-2 PATIENT AND FAMILY TEACHING: BIPOLAR DISORDER

1. Patients with bipolar disorder and their families need to know:
   - The chronic and episodic nature of bipolar disorder
   - The fact that bipolar disorder is long term and that maintenance treatment therefore will require that one or more mood-stabilizing agents be taken for a long time
   - The expected side effects and toxic effects of the prescribed medication as well as whom to call and where to go in case of a toxic reaction
   - The signs and symptoms of relapse that may "come out of the blue"
   - The role of family members and others in preventing a full relapse
   - The phone numbers of emergency contact persons, which should be kept in an easily accessed place
2. The use of alcohol, drugs of abuse, even small amounts of caffeine, and over-the-counter medications can produce a relapse.
3. Good sleep hygiene is critical to stability. Frequently, the early symptom of a manic episode is lack of sleep. In some cases, mania may be averted by the use of sleep medications (e.g., temazepam [Restoril]).
4. Psychosocial strategies are important for dealing with work, interpersonal, and family problems; for lowering stress; for enhancing a sense of personal control; and for increasing community functioning.
5. Group and individual psychotherapy are invaluable for gaining insight and skills in relapse prevention, providing social support, increasing coping skills in interpersonal relations, improving adherence to the medication regimen, reducing functional morbidity, and decreasing rehospitalization.

Advanced Practice Interventions

When a patient with bipolar disorder is not experiencing acute mania, advanced practice registered nurses (APRNs) may use psychotherapy to help the patient cope more adaptively to stresses in the environment and decrease the risk of relapse. Specific approaches to psychotherapy include cognitive-behavioral therapy, family therapy, and interpersonal therapy. APRNs may also prescribe any of the medications used to treat bipolar disorders.

Psychotherapy

Pharmacotherapy and psychiatric management are essential in the treatment of acute manic attacks and during the continuation and maintenance phases of bipolar disorder. Individuals with bipolar disorder must deal with the psychosocial consequences of their past episodes and their vulnerability to experiencing future episodes. They also have to face the burden of long-term treatments that may involve unpleasant side effects. Many patients have strained interpersonal relationships, marriage and family problems, academic and occupational problems, and legal or other social difficulties. Psychotherapy can help them work through these difficulties, decrease some of the psychic distress, and increase self-esteem. Psychotherapeutic treatments can also help patients improve their functioning between episodes and attempt to decrease the frequency of future episodes.

Cognitive-behavioral therapy (CBT) is typically used as an adjunct to pharmacotherapy in many psychiatric disorders. It involves identifying maladaptive thoughts ("I am always going to be a loser") and behaviors ("I might as well drink") that may be barriers to a person's recovery and ongoing mood stability. It is also used for bipolar disorder in children. CBT focuses on adherence to the medication regimen, early detection and intervention for manic or depressive episodes, stress and lifestyle management, and the treatment of depression and comorbid conditions. Some research demonstrates that patients treated with cognitive therapy are more likely to take their medications as prescribed than are patients who do not participate in therapy, and psychotherapy results in greater adherence to the lithium regimen (Lam, 2003). Not everyone believes that CBT is helpful in bipolar disorder, however. Lynch and colleagues (2010) indicate that CBT is not an effective treatment for relapse rates in bipolar disorder.

A formalized psychotherapy called *interpersonal and social rhythm therapy* has been tested in combination with pharmacotherapy in randomized clinical trials as treatment for patients during the maintenance phase of bipolar illness. This therapy addresses the variables that relate to recurrence of symptoms, especially nonadherence with medication, stress management, and maintenance of social supports.

Often the patients receiving medication and therapy place more value on psychotherapy than do clinicians. A patient describes her feelings about drug therapy and psychotherapy as follows (Jamison, 1995b):

> I cannot imagine leading a normal life without lithium. From startings and stoppings of it, I now know it is an essential part of my sanity. Lithium prevents my seductive but disastrous highs, diminishes my depressions, clears out the weaving of my disordered thinking, slows me, gentles me out, keeps me in my relationships, in my career, out of a hospital, and in psychotherapy. It keeps me alive, too. But psychotherapy heals, it makes some sense of the confusion, it reins in the terrifying thoughts and feelings, it brings back hope and the possibility of learning from it all. Pills cannot, do not, ease one back into reality. They bring you back headlong, careening, and faster than can be endured at times. Psychotherapy is a sanctuary, it is a battleground, and it is where I have come to believe that someday I may be able to contend with all of this. No pill can help me deal with the problem of not wanting to take pills, but no amount of therapy alone can prevent my manias and depressions. I need both.

EVALUATION

Outcome criteria often dictate the frequency of evaluation of short-term and intermediate indicators. Are the patient's vital signs stable? Is he or she well-hydrated? Is the patient able to control personal behavior or respond to external controls? Is the patient able to sleep for 4 or 5 hours a night or take frequent, short rest periods during the day? Does the family have a clear understanding of the patient's disease and need for medication? Do the patient and family know which community agencies may help them?

If outcomes or related indicators are not achieved satisfactorily, the preventing factors are analyzed. Were the data incorrect or insufficient? Were nursing diagnoses inappropriate or outcomes unrealistic? Was intervention poorly planned? After the outcomes and care plan are reassessed, the plan is revised, if indicated. Longer-term outcomes include adherence to the medication regimen; resumption of functioning in the community; achievement of stability in family, work, and social relationships and in mood; and improved coping skills for reducing stress.

QUALITY IMPROVEMENT

As we look at the bigger picture of patient care we hope to find methods to improve care by examining outcomes data to improve the quality and safety of our care (Quality and Safety Education for Nurses, 2012). Quality of care for bipolar disorders is comprehensively addressed by the Standards for Bipolar Excellence Project (Centers for Quality Assessment and Improvement in Mental Health Care, 2007). This project provides 15 evidence-based performance measures regarding screening, assessment, treatment, and monitoring bipolar disorder and its care. Many valuable tools for research, teaching, and quality improvement are readily available:

- Screening for bipolar mania/hypomania
- Assessment for risk of suicide
- Assessment for substance use
- Use of antimanic agent in bipolar I disorder: manic phase
- Use of mood-stabilizing or antimanic agent in bipolar I disorder: depressed phase
- Avoidance of antidepressant monotherapy in bipolar I isorder
- Monitoring weight
- Monitoring for extrapyramidal symptoms
- Monitoring lithium serum levels
- Screening for hyperglycemia and hyperlipidemia when a second-generation antipsychotic is prescribed
- Providing condition-specific education/information
- Monitoring change in symptom complex
- Recommending adjunctive psychosocial interventions
- Monitoring change in level of functioning

The assessment forms used for monitoring care given to patients with bipolar disorder are available and quite interesting. You are encouraged to review some of the assessment forms listed above and consider how your patient might respond or try them out for yourself. They are available at http://www.cqaimh.org/stable.html.

KEY POINTS TO REMEMBER

- Biological factors appear to play a role in the etiology of the bipolar disorders. Strong genetic correlates have been revealed, especially through twin studies. Neurotransmitter (norepinephrine, dopamine, serotonin) excess and imbalance are also related to bipolar mood swings, which supports the existence of chemical influences. Neuroendocrine and neuroanatomical findings provide strong evidence for biological influences.
- Early detection of bipolar disorder can help diminish comorbid substance abuse, suicide, and decline in social and personal relationships and may help promote more positive outcomes. Unfortunately, bipolar disorder often goes unrecognized.
- Nurses assess the patient's level of mood (hypomania, acute mania), behavior, and thought processes and are alert to cognitive dysfunction.
- Analyzing the objective and subjective data helps the nurse formulate appropriate nursing diagnoses. Some of the nursing diagnoses appropriate for patients with mania are *risk for violence, defensive coping, ineffective coping,* and *situational low self-esteem.*
- During the acute phase of mania, physical needs often take priority and demand nursing interventions; therefore, *deficient fluid volume* and *imbalanced nutrition or elimination,* as well as *disturbed sleep pattern,* are usually addressed in the nursing plan.
- The diagnosis *interrupted family processes* is vital. Support groups, psychoeducation, and guidance for the family can greatly affect the patient's adherence to the medication regimen.
- Planning involves identifying the specific needs of the patient and family during the three phases of mania (acute,

continuation, and maintenance). Can the patient benefit from communication-skills training, improvement in coping skills, legal or financial counseling, or further psychoeducation? What community resources does the patient need at this time?

- Patients experiencing mania can be demanding and manipulative. The patient experiencing mania constantly interrupts activities and distracts groups with continuous physical motion and incessant joking and talking. The nurse sets limits in a firm, neutral manner and tailors communication techniques and interventions to maintain the patient's safety.
- Health care workers, family, and friends often feel angry and frustrated by the patient's disruptive behaviors. When these feelings are not examined and shared with others, the therapeutic potential of the staff is reduced, and feelings of confusion and helplessness remain.
- Antimanic medications are available. Lithium has a narrow therapeutic index, which necessitates thorough patient and family teaching and regular follow-up. Anticonvulsant drugs such as carbamazepine and valproic acid are useful, especially in treating people with disease refractory to lithium therapy. Anticonvulsant drugs are also useful in treating patients who need rapid de-escalation and do not respond to other treatment approaches.
- Antipsychotic agents may be used for their sedating and mood-stabilizing properties, especially during initial treatment.
- For some patients, ECT may be the most appropriate medical treatment.
- Patient and family teaching takes many forms and is most important in encouraging adherence to the medication regimen and reducing the risk of relapse.
- Evaluation includes examining the effectiveness of the nursing interventions, changing the outcomes as needed, and reassessing the nursing diagnoses. Evaluation is an ongoing process and is part of each of the other steps in the nursing process.

CRITICAL THINKING

1. Donald has a history of bipolar disorder and has been taking lithium for 4 months. During his clinic visit, he tells you that he does not think he will be taking his lithium anymore, because he feels great and is able to function well at his job and at home with his family. He tells you his wife agrees that he "has this thing licked."
   a. What are Donald's needs in terms of teaching?
   b. What are the needs of the family?
   c. Write a teaching plan or use an already constructed plan. Include the following issues with sound rationales for these teaching topics:
      - Use of alcohol, drugs, caffeine, over-the-counter medications
      - Need for sleep, hygiene
      - Types of community resources available
      - Signs and symptoms of relapse

   d. Role-play with a classmate how you can teach this family about bipolar illness and approach effective medication teaching, stressing the need for adherence and emphasizing those things that may threaten adherence.
   e. What referral information (websites, associations) can you give Donald and his family if they ask where they can access further information regarding this disease?

CHAPTER REVIEW

1. A major principle the nurse should observe when communicating with a patient experiencing elated mood is to:
   a. Use a calm, firm approach.
   b. Give expanded explanations.
   c. Make use of abstract concepts.
   d. Encourage lightheartedness and joking.
2. Nadia has been diagnosed with bipolar disorder. Which is an outcome for Nadia in the continuation of treatment phase of bipolar disorder?
   a. Patient will avoid involvement in self-help groups.
   b. Patient will adhere to medication regimen.
   c. Patient will demonstrate euphoric mood.
   d. Patient will maintain normal weight.
3. A medication teaching plan for a patient receiving lithium should include:
   a. Periodic monitoring of renal and thyroid function.
   b. Dietary teaching to restrict daily sodium intake.
   c. The importance of blood draws to monitor serum potassium level.
   d. Discontinuing the drug if weight gain and fine hand tremors are noticed.
4. Which symptom related to communication is likely to be present in a patient experiencing mania?
   a. Mutism
   b. Verbosity
   c. Poverty of ideas
   d. Confabulation
5. For assessment purposes, the nurse should identify the body system most at risk for decompensation during a severe manic episode as:
   a. Renal
   b. Cardiac
   c. Endocrine
   d. Pulmonary

Answers to Chapter Review
1. a; 2. b; 3. a; 4. b; 5. b.

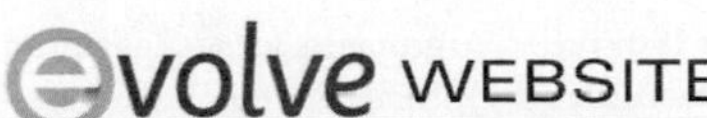

Visit the Evolve website for a posttest on the content in this chapter: http://evolve.elsevier.com/Varcarolis

Post-Test interactive review

REFERENCES

American Academy of Child and Adolescent Psychiatry. (2010). *Bipolar disorder center.* Retrieved from http://www.aacap.org/cs/bipolar_disorder_resource_center/more_on_bipolar_disorder.

Angst, J., Gamma, A., Bowden, C. L., Azorin, J. M., Perugi, G., Vieta, E., & Young, A. H. (2012). Diagnostic criteria for bipolarity based on an international sample of 5,635 patients with DSM-IV major depressive episodes. *European Archives of Psychiatry and Clinical Neuroscience, 262*(1), 3–11.

Appleton, K. M., Hayward, R. C., Gunnell, D., Peters, T. J., Rogers, P. J., Kessler, D., & Ness, A R. (2006). Effects of n-3 long-chain polyunsaturated fatty acids on depressed mood: Systematic review of published trials. *American Journal of Clinical Nutrition, 84,* 1308–1316.

American Psychiatric Association. (2013). *DSM-5 table of contents.* Retrieved from http://www.psychiatry.org/dsm5.

Baldesserini, R. J., Vazquez, G., & Tondo, L. (2011). Treatment of cyclothymic disorder: Commentary. *Psychotherapy and psychosomatics, 80,* 131–135.

Bauer, M., Beaulieu, S., Dunner, D. L., Lafer, B., & Kupka, R. (2008). Rapid cycling bipolar disorder—diagnostic concepts. *Bipolar Disorders, 10*(2), 153–162.

Baum, A. E., Akula, N., Cabanero, M., Cardona, I., Corona, W., Klemens, B., Schulze, T., Cichon, S., Reitschel, M., Nothen, M., & colleagues. (2008). A genome-wide association study implicates diacylglycerol kinase eta (DGKH) and several other genes in the etiology of bipolar disorder. *Molecular Psychiatry, 13,* 197–207.

Bender, R. E., & Alloy, L. B. (2011). Life stress and kindling in bipolar disorder: Review of the evidence and integration with emerging biopsychosocial theories. *Clinical Psychology Review, 31*(3), 383–398.

Birmaher, B., Axelson, D., Strober, M., Gill, M. K., Valeri, S., Chiappetta, L., Ryan, N., Leonard, H... Keller, M. (2006). Clinical course of children and adolescents with bipolar spectrum disorders. *Archives of General Psychiatry, 2,* 175–183.

Bora, E., Fornito, A., & Yucel, M. (2010). Voxelwise meta-analysis of gray matter abnormalities in bipolar disorder. *Biological Psychiatry, 67*(11), 1097–1105.

Bulechek, G. M., Butcher, H. K., Dochterman, J. M., & Wagner, C. (2013).*Nursing interventions classification (NIC)* (6th ed). St. Louis, MO: Mosby.

Burmeister, M., McInnis, M. G., & Zollner, S. (2008). Psychiatric genetics: Progress amid controversy. *Nature Reviews Genetics, 9,* 527–540.

Carpiniello, B., Lai, L., Pirarba, S., Sardu, C., Pinna, F. (2011). Impulsivity and aggressiveness in bipolar disorder with co-morbid borderline personality disorder. *Psychiatry Research, 188*(1), 40–44.

Chakrabarti, S. (2011). Thyroid functions and bipolar affective disorder. *Journal of Thyroid Research, 2011.* Article ID 306367. doi:10.4061/2011/306367.

Fagiolini, A., Chengappa, K. N., Soreca, I., & Chang, J. (2008). Bipolar disorder and the metabolic syndrome: Causal factors, psychiatric outcomes and economic burden. *CNS Drugs, 22,* 655–69.

Fiedorowicz, J. G., Endicott, J., Leon, A. C., Solomon, D.A., Keller, M. B., & Coryell, W. H. (2011). Subthreshold hypomanic symptoms in progression from unipolar major depression to bipolar disorder. *American Journal of Psychiatry, 168*(1), 40–48.

Gunderson, J. G., Weinberg, I., Daversa, M. T., Kueppenbender, K. D., Zanarini, M. C., Shea, M. T., ... Dyck, I. (2006). Descriptive and longitudinal observations on the relationship of borderline personality disorder and bipolar disorder. *American Journal of Psychiatry, 163,* 1173–1178.

Herdman, T.H. (Ed.) (2012). *NANDA international nursing diagnoses: Definitions and classification, 2012-2014.* Oxford, UK: Wiley-Blackwell.

Ivleva, E., Morris, D.W., Moates, A.F., Suppes, T., Thaker, G. K., & Tamminga, C.A. (2010). Genetics and intermediate phenotypes of the schizophrenia-bipolar disorder boundary. *Neuroscience and Biobehavioral Reviews, 34*(6), 897–921.

Jamison, K. R. (1995a). *Psychotherapy of bipolar patients.* Paper presented at the U.S. Psychiatric and Mental Health Congress, New York.

Jamison, K. R. (1995b). *An unquiet mind.* New York, NY: Knopf.

Kessler, R. C., Berglund, P. A., Demler, O., Jin, R., & Walters, E. E. (2005). Lifetime prevalence and age-of-onset distributions of *DSM-IV* disorders in the National Comorbidity Survey Replication (NCS-R). *Archives of General Psychiatry, 62,* 593–602.

Ketter, T. A. (2010). Diagnostic features, prevalence, and impact of bipolar disorder. *Journal of Clinical Psychiatry, 71*(6), e14.

Kidd, P. M. (2007). Omega-3 DHA and EPA for cognition, behavior, and mood: Clinical findings and structural-functional synergies with cell membrane phospholipids. *Alternative Medicine Review, 12*(3), 207–227.

Kilbourne, A. M., & Pincus, H. A. (2006). Patterns of psychotropic medication use by race among veterans with bipolar disorder. *Psychiatric Services, 57*(1), 123–126.

Lynch, D., Laws, K. R., & McKenna, P. J. (2010). Cognitive behavioural therapy for major psychiatric disorder: Does it really work? A meta-analytical review of well-controlled trials. *Psychological Medicine, 40,* 9–24.

Mazzarini, L., Colom, F., Pacchiarotti, I., Nivoli, A. M. A., Murru, A., Bonnin, C. M., Cruz, N., Sanchez-Moreno, J., Kotzalidis, G. D., & Girardi, P. (2010). Psychotic versus non-psychotic bipolar II disorder. *Journal of Affective Disorders, 126*(1), 55–60.

McClung, C. A. (2007). Circadian genes, rhythms, and the biology of mood disorders. *Pharmacology and Therapeutics, 114,* 222–232.

Merikangas, K. R., Akiskal, H. S., Angst, J., Greenberg, P. E., Hirschfeld, R. M., Petukhova, M., & Kessler, R. (2007). Lifetime and 12-month prevalence of bipolar spectrum disorder in the National Comorbidity Survey Replication. *Archives of General Psychiatry, 64,* 543–552.

Miklowitz, D. J., & Chang, K. D. (2008). Prevention of bipolar disorder in at-risk children: Theoretical assumptions and empirical foundations. *Development and Psychopathology, 20,* 881–897. doi: http://dx.doi.org/10.1017/S0954579408000424.

Minnai, G. P., Salis, P. G., Oppo, R., Loche, A. P., Scano, F., & Tondo, L. (2011). Effectiveness of maintenance electroconvulsive therapy in rapid-cycling bipolar disorder. *Journal of ECT, 27*(2), 123–126.

Moore, M. (2008). Patty Duke puts celebrity face on bipolar disorder. *Missoulian.* Retrieved from http://missoulian.com/articles/2008/10/11/news/local/news05.txt.

Moorhead, S., Johnson, M., Maas, M. L., & Swanson, E. (2013). *Nursing outcomes classification (NOC)* (5th ed.). St Louis, MO: Mosby.

Munk-Olsen, T., Lauresen, T. M., Meltzer-Brody, S., Mortensen, P. B., & Jones, I. (2012). Psychiatric disorders with postpartum onset: Possible early manifestations of bipolar affective disorders. *Archives of General Psychiatry, 69*(4), 428–434.

Parker, G., Gibson, N. A., Brotchie, H., Heruc, G., Rees, A., & Hadzi-Pavlovic, D. (2006). Omega-3 fatty acids and mood disorders. *The American Journal of Psychiatry, 163,* 969-978.

Robinson, L. J., Thompson, J. M., Gallagher, P., Goswami, U., Young, A., Ferrier, I., & Moore, P. B. (2006). A meta-analysis of cognitive deficits in euthymic patients with bipolar disorder. *Journal of Effective Disorders, 93,* 105–115.

Sadock , B. J., & Sadock, V. A. (2008). *Concise textbook of clinical psychiatry* (3rd ed.). Philadelphia, PA: Lippincott Williams & Wilkins.

Sarris, J., Mischoulon, D., & Schweitzer, I. (2012). Omega-3 for bipolar disorder: Meta-analyses of use in mania and bipolar depression. *Journal of Clinical Psychiatry, 73*(1), 81–86.

Sjoholm, L. K., Backlund, L., Cheteh, E. H., Ek, I.R., Frisen, L., Schalling, M., Osby, U., Lavebratt, C., & Nikamo, P. (2010). *CRY2* is associated with rapid cycling in bipolar disorder patients. *PLoS ONE, 5*(9): e12632. doi: 10.1371/journal.pone.0012632.

Smith, D. J., Griffiths, E., Kelly, M., Hood, K., Craddock, N., & Simpson, S. A. (2011). Unrecognized bipolar disorder in primary care patients with depression. *British Journal of Psychiatry, 199*(1), 49–56.

Strakowski, S. M., DelBello, M. P., & Adler, C. M. (2005). The functional neuroanatomy of bipolar disorder: A review of neuroimaging findings. *Molecular Psychiatry, 10,* 105–116.

Tondo, L., & Baldessarini, R. J. (2005). Suicidal risk in bipolar disorder. *Clinical Neuropsychiatry, 2,* 55–65.

Torrent, C., Sanchez-Moreno, J., Comes, M., Goikolea, J. M., Salamero, M., & Vieta, E. (2006). Cognitive impairment in bipolar II disorder. *The British Journal of Psychiatry, 189,* 254–259.

Van Meter, A., Youngstrom, E. A., Youngstrom, J. K., Feeny, N. C., & Findling, R. L. (2011). Examining the validity of cyclothymic disorder in a youth sample. *Journal of Affective Disorders, 132*(1), 55–63.

Vieta, E., & Suppes, T. (2008). Bipolar II disorder: Arguments for and against a distinct diagnostic entity. *Bipolar disorders, 10*(1), 163–178.

Wang, P. S., Berglund, P., Olfson, M., Pincus, H. A., Wells, K. B., & Kessler, R. C. (2005). Failure and delay in initial treatment contact after first onset of mental disorders in the National Comorbidity Survey Replication. *Archives of General Psychiatry, 62,* 603–613.

CHAPTER

14

Depressive Disorders

Mallie Kozy and Margaret Jordan Halter

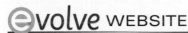

Visit the Evolve website for a pretest on the content in this chapter: http://evolve.elsevier.com/Varcarolis

Pre-Test interactive review

OBJECTIVES

1. Compare and contrast major depressive disorder and dysthymic disorder.
2. Explore disruptive mood dysregulation disorder and its impact on children.
3. Describe the symptoms of premenstrual dysphoric disorder.
4. Discuss the complex origins of depressive disorders.
5. Assess behaviors in a patient with depression in regard to each of the following areas: (a) affect, (b) thought processes, (c) feelings, (d) physical behavior, and (e) communication.
6. Formulate five nursing diagnoses for a patient with depression, and include outcome criteria.
7. Name unrealistic expectations a nurse may have while working with a patient with depression, and compare them to your own personal thoughts.
8. Role-play six principles of communication useful in working with patients with depression.
9. Evaluate the advantages of the selective serotonin reuptake inhibitors (SSRIs) over the tricyclic antidepressants (TCAs).
10. Explain the unique attributes of two of the unconventional antidepressants for use in specific circumstances.
11. Write a medication teaching plan for a patient taking a tricyclic antidepressant, including (a) adverse effects, (b) toxic reactions, and (c) other drugs that can trigger an adverse reaction.
12. Write a medication teaching plan for a patient taking a monoamine oxidase inhibitor, including foods and drugs that are contraindicated.
13. Write a nursing care plan incorporating the recovery model of mental health.
14. Discuss the use of electroconvulsive therapy (ECT) for depressive disorders.

KEY TERMS AND CONCEPTS

affect
anergia
anhedonia
bereavement exclusion
dysthymic disorder (DD)
electroconvulsive therapy (ECT)
hypersomnia
light therapy
major depressive disorder
mood disorders
psychomotor agitation
psychomotor retardation
selective serotonin reuptake inhibitors (SSRIs)
transcranial magnetic stimulation (TMS)
tricyclic antidepressants (TCAs)
vagus nerve stimulation (VNS)
vegetative signs of depression

To be a nurse is to work with patients with depression. Depression can exist along or in conjunction with other disorders and illnesses. Depression can present differently in different populations and different age groups, and depression can be manifested on a continuum from mild to severe. One thing is consistent—depression results in significant pain and suffering that disrupts social relationships, performance at school or on the job, and the ability for a person to live a full and happy life. Depression also has a negative impact on physical well-being and the course of other medical diagnoses. This chapter includes basic information and therapeutic tools that will facilitate the care of patients with depression.

CLINICAL PICTURE

According to the National Institute of Mental Health (NIMH, 2012b), **major depressive disorder** is one of the most common mental disorders, affecting approximately 13 million adults annually in the United States. Major depressive disorder, disruptive mood dysregulation disorder, dysthymic disorder, premenstrual dysphoric disorder, substance-induced depressive disorder, and depressive disorder not elsewhere classified are all disorders included in the category of depressive disorders in the *Diagnostic and Statistical Manual, fifth edition (DSM-5)* (American Psychiatric Association, 2013).

Major depressive disorder, or major depression, is characterized by a persistently depressed mood lasting for a minimum of two weeks. Children tend to be irritable rather than depressed. It may be a single episode or recurrent (more than one) episode. The depressed mood is accompanied by a lack of interest in previously pleasurable activity, also known as anhedonia (*an* "without" + *hedone* "pleasure"); fatigue; sleep disturbances; changes in appetite; feelings of hopelessness or worthlessness; persistent thoughts of death or suicide; an inability to concentrate or make decisions; and a change in physical activity (Wasserman, 2011).

While we tend to label anyone with a depressed mood as having depression, in actuality the diagnosis of major depression involves a cluster of symptoms. Not only does the patient have a depressed mood or anhedonia (inability to feel happy), but also additionally at least five of the other eight symptoms listed above. The patient will complain of problems with family members, friends or co-workers; fear of failing at school; or worries that his or her job performance has declined. In severe cases the patient may not be able to perform basic activities of daily living such as bathing, dressing, or preparing food.

Sleep disturbances might involve insomnia, or the inability to sleep. Sometimes people have trouble falling asleep; other times the patient may fall asleep quickly only to awaken after a few hours unable to return to sleep until it is time to get up for the day. Early morning awakening, known as terminal insomnia, is a red flag for depression. Sometimes the opposite can occur, and people are completely exhausted and sleep too much, as many as 12 to 16 hours a day. We refer to this symptom as hypersomnia.

Appetite changes also vary in individuals experiencing depression. Appetite loss is common, and sometimes patients can lose up to 5% of their body weight in less than a month. Other patients find they eat more often and complain of weight gain.

Feelings of guilt and worthlessness are sometimes hard to discern in patients with depression. As a nurse listens to a patient talk, he or she will hear phrases such as "I never seem to do anything right," "I was never a good parent," or "it's my fault that project at work failed." For a patient with major depression, these thoughts tend to occur over and over again and are difficult for the patient to stop. These thoughts can fuel the insomnia and the fatigue that accompanies depression.

Patients with depression will sometimes complain of an inability to think or make decisions. They will say that they can't concentrate at work, are easily distracted while they try to study, or they can't make up their mind what to wear or what to eat. For these patients, these difficulties represent a change in functioning. In some cases, especially for hospitalized patients, these symptoms can be severe. Some patients cannot concentrate long enough to complete tasks at work or attend class. Others find it so difficult to make decisions that they cannot get dressed or select, plan or prepare a meal.

Physical activity is also affected in major depression. Normally we think of depressed patients as having psychomotor retardation, a reduction in the amount of physical activity. This type of symptom results in less motor movement; patients tend to stay in bed or sit in one spot most of the day. When they do move, they move more slowly and posture is frequently stooped with the head down; however, patients with major depression may also have psychomotor agitation. When this occurs, the patient appears restless, changes position often, and may wring his or her hands and fidget. He or she also may pace up and down the hall. This is not goal-directed activity, and the patient does not feel energized. While many symptoms of major depression are subjective and must be described by the patient, psychomotor retardation and psychomotor agitation are visible signs to family members, friends, co-workers, and the nurse caring for the patient.

In depression a person can be abnormally preoccupied with death. This may be exhibited in the patient by fantasizing about his or her funeral or having recurring dreams about death. It is not uncommon for patients with depression to become suicidal. Suicidal thoughts may be relatively mild and fleeting. For other individuals, suicidal thoughts are quite serious or persistent and involve a plan. Suicidal thoughts, especially those in which the patient has a plan and the means to carry it out, represent an emergency requiring immediate intervention by the nurse (refer to Chapter 25) Suicidal thoughts are a major reason for hospitalization for patients with major depression.

Major depression can occur just once in a patient's lifetime or it can remit and recur. In bipolar disorder, patients may also experience depression that remits and recurs; however, patients with major depression differ from patients with bipolar disorder in that they experience no episodes of mania or hypomania (refer to Chapter 13).

Grief versus depression: People experiencing a significant loss can exhibit feelings and behaviors similar to depression. They may cry frequently, feel hopeless about the future, have disruptions in eating and sleeping, and lose pleasure in everyday activities. They may even temporarily lack interest in caring for themselves and neglect normal hygiene. At what point does grief become pathological, result in a diagnosis of depression and require intervention? This is a controversial question and one that is not easily answered.

Until recently, someone was not diagnosed with depression in the first two months following a significant loss. This was called a bereavement exclusion. There was a concern that the normal process of bereavement might be rendered pathological, resulting in a diagnostic label, unnecessary treatment and loss of dignity for the bereaved. Although controversial, a diagnosis of depression can now be given in the first two months following death of a loved one or other loss. The reason for the change is that grief, like other stressors, can result in depression. For some people, waiting two months for an official diagnosis of major depression may delay treatment and adversely affect prognosis. Further research and education about grief is needed in order to clarify diagnostic categories and prevent overdiagnosis of depression in the presence of grief (Shear et al., 2011).

Depressive disorders are classified according to symptoms or the situations under which they occur.

Disruptive mood dysregulation disorder relates to children between the ages of 6 and 18 and refers to situations in which a person has frequent temper tantrums resulting in verbal or behavioral outbursts out of proportion to the situation; in addition, others would describe the person's persistent mood between outbursts as irritable (Stringaris, 2011). A couple of things should be considered when considering whether the temper tantrums constitute disruptive mood dysregulation disorder. Temper tantrums are not unusual at certain developmental stages, and some other illnesses, such as autism, exhibit temper tantrums. For that reason, this diagnosis is given for the first time only to children between the ages of 6 and 18 who do not have other medical or mental health diagnoses that could account for the tantrums.

Dysthymic disorder occurs when feelings of depression persist consistently for at least two years. Children, adolescents, and adults may have this problem. The symptoms are difficult for the patient to live with and bring about social and occupational distress, but they are usually not severe enough to require hospitalization (Wasserman, 2011). Because the onset of dysthymic disorder is usually in teenage years, patients will frequently express that they have "always felt this way" and that being depressed seems like a normal way of functioning (NIMH, 2012b). It is not uncommon for people with this low-level depression to also have periods of full-blown major depressive episodes.

Premenstrual dysphoric disorder refers to a cluster of symptoms that occur in the last week prior to the onset of a woman's period. Symptoms include physical discomfort and emotional symptoms similar to major depression that are severe enough to interfere with the ability of a woman to work or interact with others. Symptoms decrease significantly or disappear with the onset of menstruation. The prevalence for Premenstrual Dysphoric Disorder is 2.5% to 5.5 % (Wasserman, 2011).

Substance-induced depressive disorder applies when symptoms of a major depressive episode arise as a result of prolonged drug or alcohol intoxication or as the result of withdrawal from drugs and alcohol. The person with this diagnosis would not experience depressive symptoms in the absence of drug or alcohol use or withdrawal (Niciu et al, 2009).

Depressive disorder associated with another medical condition can be the result of changes that are directly related to certain illnesses such as kidney failure, Parkinson's disease, and Alzheimer's disease however, the symptoms that result from medical diagnoses or that result from the use of certain medications are not considered major depressive disorder.

EPIDEMIOLOGY

Depression is the leading cause of disability in the United States. The most comprehensive statistics in the United States are from 2008. At that time the prevalence of depression was 6.7% for adults and 8.3% for children ages 12 to 17 (NIMH, 2012b). This means that at least 1 in every 20 people in the United States suffers from depression. This results in a significant loss of productivity (Beck et al., 2011) in addition to the more personal individual and family distress.

Because symptoms vary by age and circumstance, depression in children, until recently, has been underrecognized. We now know that even infants can display symptoms of depression (Jacobs & Taylor, 2009). With this understanding, we are just beginning to get a realistic view of the epidemiology of depression in children. Children and adolescents between 13 and 18 years of age have an 11.2% prevalence of depression, and 3.3% have a severe form of the illness (National Institute of Mental Health [NIMH], 2012a). If the first episode of depression occurs in childhood or adolescence, the likelihood of recurrence is high (Jacobs & Taylor, 2009), setting the stage for recurrent depression.

Although depression in older adults is common, it is *not* a normal result of aging. The risk of depression in the elderly increases as health deteriorates. It is estimated that about 1-5% of older adults living in the community have depression. This number rises to 11.5% of hospitalized older adults and 13.5% for those requiring home care (NIMH 2012a). Many older adults suffer from *subsyndromal depression,* in which they experience many, but not all, of the symptoms of a major depressive episode; these individuals have an increased risk of developing major depression. A disproportionate number of older adults with depression are likely to die by suicide (NIMH, 2012b). There are discrepancies in diagnosis and treatment along cultural and socioeconomic lines in older adults. For older adults, fewer African Americans (4.2%) are diagnosed with depression than whites (6.4%) or Hispanics (7.2%); however, only 63% of African American and Hispanic patients received treatment, while 73% of whites received treatment. Hispanic and African Americans are more likely to identify economic barriers to receiving treatment (NIMH, 2012a). Older individuals suffering from depression are at risk for being untreated, and this is especially true for minorities.

COMORBIDITY

A depressive syndrome frequently accompanies other psychiatric disorders, such as anxiety disorders, schizophrenia, substance abuse, eating disorders, and schizoaffective disorder. People with anxiety disorders (e.g., panic disorder, generalized anxiety disorder, obsessive-compulsive disorder) commonly have depression, as do people with personality disorders, particularly borderline personality disorder (Joska & Stein, 2008). The combination of anxiety and depression is perhaps one of the most common psychiatric presentations. Symptoms of anxiety occur in an average of 70% of cases of major depression. Some clinicians believe that mixed anxiety and depression should be a stand-alone diagnosis and be treated as a distinct entity.

The incidence of major depression greatly increases with the occurrence of a medical disorder, and people with chronic medical problems are at a higher risk for depression than those in the general population. Depression often develops secondary to a medical condition and may also be secondary to use of substances such as alcohol, cocaine, marijuana, heroin, and even anxiolytics and other prescription medications (Table 14-1). Depression can also be a consequence of bereavement and grief.

ETIOLOGY

Although many theories attempt to explain the cause of depression, many psychological, biological, and cultural variables make identification of any one cause difficult; furthermore, it is unlikely there is a single cause for depression. The high variability in symptom manifestation, response to treatment, and course of the illness supports the supposition that depression may result from a complex interaction of causes. For example, genetic predisposition to the illness combined with childhood stress may lead to significant changes in the central nervous system (CNS) that result in depression; however, there seem to be several common risk factors for depression, listed in Box 14-1 (Sadock & Sadock, 2008).

Biological Factors

Genetic

Twin studies consistently show that genetic factors play a role in the development of depressive disorders. Various studies reveal that the average concordance rate for mood disorders among monozygotic twins (twins sharing the same genetic material) is about 37%. That is, if one twin is affected, the second has a 37% chance of being affected as well (Joska & Stein, 2008). Increased heritability of mood disorders is associated with an earlier age of onset, greater rate of comorbidity, and increased risk of recurrent illness (Lahoff, 2010). It is likely that multiple genes are involved, each one having a small but substantial role in the

EVIDENCE-BASED PRACTICE

Depression in Adolescent Mothers

Meadows-Oliver, M., & Sadler, L. (2010). Depression among adolescent mothers enrolled in a high school parenting program. *Journal of Psychosocial Nursing, 48*(12), 34-41. doi: 10.3928/02793695-20100831-04.

Problem

The rate of depression in the general adolescent population has been reported at 7.5%. Among adolescent mothers, the rate is alarmingly high (between 46% and 54%). Depressive symptoms in adolescent mothers have been associated with negative outcomes for both the mother and her child. There is a need to better understand the presentation of depressive symptoms in adolescent mothers.

Purpose of the Study

The purpose of the study was to provide a descriptive analysis of the depressive symptoms of adolescent mothers who were participating in a larger study researching the transition to motherhood.

Methods

Mothers between the ages of 14 and 19 who were attending high school were recruited to participate in the study. The 45 volunteers completed the Beck Depression Inventory-II, a 21-item self-report questionnaire that measures symptoms of depression categorized into affective, cognitive, and somatic subdomains.

Key Findings

- One third (33%) of the participants were experiencing depressive symptoms.
- All of the mothers reported increased symptoms related to loss of energy, changes in sleep patterns, changes in appetite, and tiredness and fatigue.
- Adolescent mothers with children younger than 12 months reported depressive symptoms in 10 domains of the BDI-II. These domains included sadness, pessimism, guilty feelings, crying, agitation, loss of energy, changes in appetite and sleep patterns, fatigue, and loss of libido.
- Adolescent mothers with children older than 12 months reported increased depressive symptoms in four domains of the BDI-II. These domains included loss of energy, changes in sleeping patterns and appetite, and fatigue.

Implications for Nursing Practice

Adolescent mothers are at increased risk for depression. This risk has implications for improving the health and future of these adolescents by providing education and birth control to reduce pregnancy rates. Once a pregnancy and birth occur, both the mother and the child are at risk for a variety of problems, including physical and emotional neglect and abuse. Nurses are in an ideal situation to screen for depressive symptoms. Early detection in a variety of settings, such as pediatric offices or reproductive health services centers, can promote early treatment and better outcomes for both mothers and their children.

TABLE 14-1 DEPRESSION SECONDARY TO MEDICAL CONDITIONS AND SUBSTANCES/ MEDICATIONS

TYPE	DISORDERS
Medical Conditions	
Neurological	Epilepsies, Parkinson's disease, multiple sclerosis, Alzheimer's disease
Infectious or inflammatory	Neurosyphilis, AIDs
Cardiac disorders	Ischemic heart disease, cardiac failure, cardiomyopathies
Endocrine	Hypothyroidism, diabetes mellitus, vitamin deficiencies, parathyroid disorders
Inflammatory disorders	Collagen-vascular diseases, irritable bowel syndrome, chronic liver disorders
Neoplastic disorders	Central nervous system tumors, paraneoplastic syndromes
Substances/Medications	
Central nervous system depressants	Alcohol, barbiturates, benzodiazepines, clonidine
Central nervous system medications	Amantadine, bromocriptine, levodopa, phenothiazines, phenytoin
Psychostimulants	Amphetamines
Systemic medications	Corticosteroids, digoxin, diltiazem, enalapril, ethionamide, isotretinoin, mefloquine, methyldopa, metoclopramide, quinolones, reserpine, statins, thiazides, vincristine

From Joska, J. A., & Stein, D. J. (2008). Mood disorders. In R. E. Hales, S. C. Yudofsky, & G. O. Gabbard (Eds.), *Textbook of psychiatry* (5th ed., p. 464). Washington, DC: American Psychiatric Publishing.

BOX 14-1 PRIMARY RISK FACTORS FOR DEPRESSION

- Female gender
- Unmarried
- Low socioeconomic class
- Early childhood trauma
- The presence of a negative life event, especially loss and humiliation
- Family history of depression, especially in first-degree relatives
- Ineffective coping ability
- Postpartum time period
- Medical illness
- Absence of social support
- Alcohol or substance abuse

From Joska, J. A., & Stein, D. J. (2008). Mood disorders. In R. E. Hales, S. C. Yudofsky, & G. O. Gabbard (Eds.), *Textbook of psychiatry* (5th ed., pp. 457-504). Washington, DC: American Psychiatric Publishing

development and severity of depression. For instance, certain genetic markers seem to be related to depression when accompanied by early childhood maltreatment or a history of stressful life events (Smoller & Korf, 2008). In this case, there is no gene directly related to the development of the mood disorder; there is a genetic marker associated with depression in the context of stressful life events.

One of the more important aspects of understanding the role of genetics in relation to mental illness such as major depression may be in pharmacological treatments. Understanding genetic influences on the role of the transport of certain neurotransmitters, such as serotonin, across synapses will make it much easier to prescribe effective medical treatment of depression based on individual genetic patterns.

Biochemical

The brain is a highly complex organ that contains billions of neurons. There is much evidence to support the concept that many CNS neurotransmitter abnormalities may cause clinical depression. These neurotransmitter abnormalities may be the result of genetic or environmental factors or other medical conditions, such as cerebral infarction, Parkinson's disease, hypothyroidism, acquired immunodeficiency syndrome (AIDS), or drug use.

Two of the main neurotransmitters involved in mood are serotonin (5-hydroxytryptamine [5-HT]) and norepinephrine. Serotonin is an important regulator of sleep, appetite, and libido; therefore, serotonin-circuit dysfunction can result in sleep disturbances, decreased appetite, low sex drive, poor impulse control, and irritability (Joska & Stein, 2008). Norepinephrine modulates attention and behavior. It is stimulated by stressful situations, which may result in overuse and a deficiency of norepinephrine. A deficiency, an imbalance as compared to other neurotransmitters, or an impaired ability to use available norepinephrine can result in apathy, reduced responsiveness, or slowed psychomotor activity.

Research suggests that depression results from the dysregulation of a number of neurotransmitter systems beyond serotonin and norepinephrine. The dopamine, acetylcholine, and GABA systems are also believed to be involved in the pathophysiology of a major depressive episode (Sadock & Sadock, 2008). Glutamate is a common neurotransmitter with a number of different functions. Glutamate increases the ability of a nerve fiber to transmit information (NIMH, 2012d); therefore, a deficit in glutamate can interfere with normal neuron transmission in the areas of the brain that affect mood, attention, and cognition. Research is just beginning to understand the role of glutamate in depression.

Stressful life events, especially losses, seem to be a significant factor in the development of depression. Norepinephrine, serotonin, and acetylcholine play a role in stress regulation. When these neurotransmitters become overtaxed through stressful events, neurotransmitter depletion may occur. Research indicates that stress is associated with a reduction in **neurogenesis**, which is the ability of the brain to produce new brain cells. One of the antidepressants is associated with increasing these new cells (Anacker et al., 2011).

At this time, no single mechanism of depressant action has been found. The relationships among the serotonin, norepinephrine, dopamine, acetylcholine, GABA, and glutamate systems are complex and need further assessment and study; however, treatment with medication that helps regulate these neurotransmitters has proved empirically successful in the treatment of many patients. Figure 14-1 shows a positron emission tomographic (PET) scan of the brain of a woman with depression before and after taking medication. Refer to Chapter 3 for further discussion of brain imaging and depression.

Alterations in Hormonal Regulation

Although neuroendocrine findings are as yet inconclusive, the neuroendocrine characteristic most widely studied in relation to depression has been hyperactivity of the hypothalamic-pituitary-adrenal cortical axis. People with major depression have increased urine cortisol levels and elevated corticotrophin-releasing hormone (Joska & Stein, 2008). Dexamethasone, an exogenous steroid that suppresses cortisol, is used in the dexamethasone suppression test (DST) for depression. Results of this test are abnormal in about 50% of people with depression, which indicates hyperactivity of the hypothalamic-pituitary-adrenal cortical axis; however, the findings may also be abnormal in people with obsessive-compulsive disorder (OCD) and other medical conditions. Significantly, patients with major depression with psychotic features are among those with the highest rates of non suppression of cortisol on the dexamethasone suppression test.

Depression rates are almost equal for males and females in the years preceding puberty and in older adults; this has led to more research into the effect of hormones on depression in women. The results are inconclusive in humans; however, evidence is beginning to demonstrate a relationship with estrogen levels and neurological changes associated with depression. Recent studies have found that estradiol, a form of estrogen, affects receptors sensitive to serotonin in the areas of the brain responsible for mood in rats. Additional research has demonstrated that declines in the levels of estrogen around menstruation and menopause create changes in nerve structures in the brain, called dendritic pruning, that are associated with depression (Accortt et. al, 2008). As the relationships between sex hormones such as estrogen in women and testosterone in males are better understood, more effective therapies may be developed.

Inflammatory Processes

Inflammation is the body's natural defense to physical injury. There is growing evidence that inflammation may be the result of psychological injury as well. Researchers have focused in on two important blood components related to inflammation, C-reactive protein and interleukin-6. In young females with a history of adversity, depression is accompanied by elevations in these blood components, but not in children without a history of adversity (Miller & Cole, 2012). Adversity in life may compromise resilience and place children at risk for depression and other disorders.

While we do not believe that inflammation causes depression, research indicates that it does play a role (Krishnadas & Cavanagh, 2012). Support for this belief includes that about a third of people with major depression have elevated inflammatory biomarkers in the absence of a physical illness. Also, people who have inflammatory diseases have increased risk of major depression. Finally, people treated with cytokines to enhance immunity during cancer treatment develop major depression at a high rate.

Diathesis-Stress Model

The diathesis-stress model of depression takes into account the interplay between genetic and biological predisposition toward depression and life events. The physiological vulnerabilities such as genetic predispositions, biochemical makeup, and personality structure are referred to as a diathesis. The stress part of this model refers to the life events that impact individual

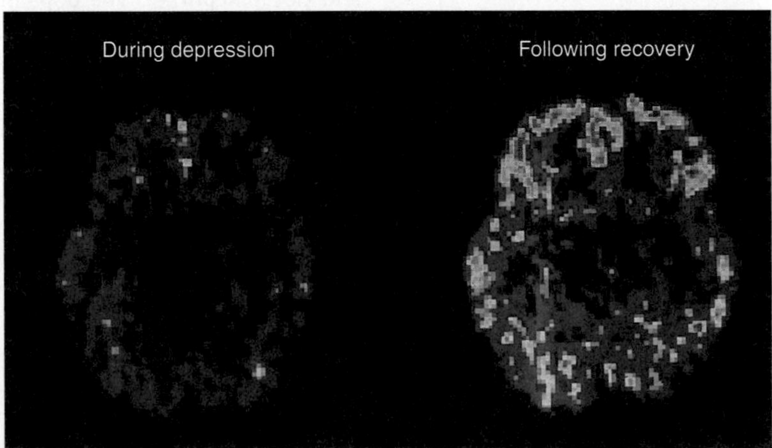

FIG 14-1 Positron emission tomographic (PET) scans of a 45-year-old woman with recurrent depression. The scan on the left was taken when the patient was on no medication and very depressed. The scan on the right was taken several months later when the patient was well, after she had been treated with medication for her depression. Note that her entire brain, particularly the left prefrontal cortex, is more active when she is well. (Courtesy Mark George, MD, Biological Psychiatry Branch, National Institute of Mental Health.)

vulnerabilities. This explains why two persons exposed to relatively similar events may respond differently. One person may demonstrate resilience and another may develop depression (Seriani, 2011).

Biochemically, the diathesis-stress model of depression is believed to work this way. Psychosocial stressors and interpersonal events trigger neurophysical and neurochemical changes in the brain. Early life trauma may result in long-term hyperactivity of the CNS corticotropin releasing factor (CRF) and norepinephrine systems, with a consequent neurotoxic effect on the hippocampus, which leads to overall neuronal loss. These changes could cause sensitization of the CRF circuits to even mild stress in adulthood, leading to an exaggerated stress response (Gillespie & Nemeroff, 2005).

Psychological Factors

Cognitive Theory

In cognitive theory, the underlying assumption is that a person's thoughts will result in emotions. If a person looks at life in a positive way, the person will experience positive emotions, but negative interpretation of life events can result in sorrow, anger, and hopelessness. Cognitive theorists believe that people may acquire a psychological predisposition to depression due to early life experiences. These experiences contribute to negative, illogical, and irrational thought processes that may remain dormant until they are activated during times of stress (Beck & Rush, 1995). Beck found that persons with depression process information in negative ways, even in the midst of positive factors. He believed that automatic, negative, repetitive, unintended, and not-readily-controllable thoughts perpetuate depression. Three assumptions constitute **Beck's cognitive triad**:

1. A negative, self-deprecating view of self
2. A pessimistic view of the world
3. The belief that negative reinforcement (or no validation for the self) will continue in the future

For a nursing student working with depressed patients, two things need to be understood. A patient will not immediately respond when the student offers a positive perspective to the patient. This may frustrate the student; however, the patient can learn over time to identify and disrupt the negative feedback loop that contributes to depression. Coming to realize that one has an ability to interpret life events in positive ways helps a person recognize that he or she has an element of control over emotions and therefore depression.

Learned Helplessness

An older but still plausible theory of depression is that of learned helplessness. Seligman (1973) stated that, although anxiety is the initial response to a stressful situation, it is replaced by depression if the person feels no control over the outcome of a situation. A person who believes that an undesired event is his or her fault and that nothing can be done to change it is prone to depression. The theory of learned helplessness has been used to explain the development of depression in certain social groups, such as older adults and people living in impoverished areas. Learned helplessness may best be explained as a subset of the cognitive theory of depression.

APPLICATION OF THE NURSING PROCESS

ASSESSMENT

There is a consensus that major depression goes unrecognized and underdiagnosed in the general population, but specifically in minority populations and in older adults. According to Louch (2009), less than half of depressed patients seek medical help. Of those who present for treatment only half are accurately diagnosed. Yet research suggests that early treatment for depression can result in improved outcomes. Nurses at both the generalist and advanced practice level are frequently in the position to screen and assess for signs of depression, facilitating early and appropriate treatment.

General Assessment

Assessment Tools

Numerous standardized depression-screening tools that help assess the type and severity of depression are available, including the Beck Depression Inventory, the Hamilton Depression Scale, the Zung Depression Scale, and the Geriatric Depression Scale. The Patient Health Questionnaire-9 (PHQ-9), a short inventory that highlights predominant symptoms seen in depression, is presented here because of its ease of use (Figure 14-2) in primary care and community settings. It is important to note that self-screening tools such as the PHQ-9 have been validated, meaning they screen for depression with 91% accuracy, providing a valuable tool for the nurse (Gilbody, Richards & Barkham, 2007). Use of these tools during multiple encounters with a patient also allows the nurse to follow changes in the patient's symptoms and depression severity over time.

The website www.depression-screening.org, sponsored by the National Mental Health Association (NMHA), enables people to take an online confidential screening test for depression and find reliable information on the illness (Live your life, 2009).

Assessment of Suicide Potential

The patient should always be evaluated for suicidal or homicidal ideation. About 15% of people with clinical depression commit suicide (Brendel et al., 2008). Risk for suicide in patients with major depression is increased in the presence of the following symptoms: severe hopelessness, overuse of alcohol, recent loss or separation, a history of past and serious suicide attempts, and acute suicidal ideation. Approaching initial suicide assessment might include the following statements or questions:

- You have said you are depressed. Tell me what that is like for you.
- When you feel depressed, what thoughts go through your mind?
- Have you gone so far as to think about taking your own life or hurting yourself in some way? Do you have a plan?
- Do you have the means to carry out your plan?
- Is there anything that would prevent you from carrying out your plan?

Refer to Chapter 25 for a detailed discussion of suicide, critical risk factors, warning signs, and strategies for suicide prevention. Also see Case Study and Nursing Care Plan 14-1.

14-1 CASE STUDY AND NURSING CARE PLAN

Depression

Ms. Glessner is a 35-year-old executive secretary. She has been divorced for 3 years and has two sons, 11 and 13 years old. She is brought into the emergency department (ED) by her neighbor. She has superficial slashes on her wrists and is bleeding. The neighbor shared that Ms. Glessner's sons are visiting their father for the summer. Ms. Glessner reports that she has been depressed for as long as she can remember, yet she has become more and more despondent since terminating a 2-year relationship with a married man 4 weeks ago. After this relationship ended, she became withdrawn and despondent. Ms. Glessner is about 20 pounds overweight, and her neighbor states that Ms. Glessner often stays awake late into the night, drinking by herself and watching television. She sleeps through most of the day on the weekends.

After receiving treatment in the ED, Ms. Glessner is seen by a psychiatrist. The initial diagnosis is dysthymic disorder with suicidal ideation. A decision is made to hospitalize her briefly for suicide observation and evaluation for appropriate treatment.

The nurse, Carrie, admits Ms. Glessner to the unit from the ED.

***Nurse:** Hello, Ms. Glessner, I'm Marcia Ward. I'll be your primary nurse.*

***Ms. Glessner:** Yeah . . . I don't need a nurse, a doctor, or anyone else. I just want to get away from this pain.*

***Nurse:** You want to get away from your pain?*

***Ms. Glessner:** I just said that, didn't I? Oh, what's the use? No one understands.*

***Nurse:** I would like to understand, Ms. Glessner.*

***Ms. Glessner:** Look at me. I'm fat . . . ugly . . . and no good to anyone. No one wants me.*

***Nurse:** Who doesn't want you?*

***Ms. Glessner:** My husband didn't want me . . . and now Jerry left me to go back to his wife.*

***Nurse:** You think because Jerry went back to his wife that no one else could care for you?*

***Ms. Glessner:** Well . . . he doesn't anyway.*

***Nurse:** Because he doesn't care, you believe that no one else cares about you?*

***Ms. Glessner:** Yes . . . .*

***Nurse:** Who do you care about?*

***Ms. Glessner:** No one . . . except my sons . . . . I do love my sons, even though I don't often show it.*

***Nurse:** Tell me more about your sons.*

Carrie continues to speak with Ms. Glessner. Ms. Glessner talks about her sons with some affect and apparent affection; however, she continues to state that she does not think of herself as worthwhile.

Self-Assessment

Carrie, a registered nurse, is aware that when patients have depression, they can be negative, think life is hopeless, and be hostile toward those who want to help. When Carrie was new to the unit, she withdrew from patients with depression and sought out patients who appeared more hopeful and appreciative of her efforts. The unit coordinator was supportive of Carrie when she was first on the unit. Carrie, along with other staff, went to in-service education sessions on working with patients with depression and was encouraged to speak up in staff meetings about the feelings many of these patients evoked in her. As a primary nurse, she was assigned a variety of patients. She found that as time went on, with the support of her peers and the opportunity to speak up at staff meetings, she was able to take what patients said less personally and not feel so responsible when patients did not respond as fast as she would like.

After 2 years, she had had the experience of seeing many patients who seemed hopeless and despondent upon admission respond well to nursing and medical interventions and go on to lead full and satisfying lives. This also made it easier for Carrie to understand that even though the patient with depression may think life is hopeless and may believe there is nothing in life to live for that change is always possible.

Assessment

Objective Data

- Slashed her wrists
- Recently broke off with boyfriend
- Has thought poorly of herself for 3 years since divorce
- Has two sons she cares about
- Is 20 pounds overweight
- Stays awake late at night, drinking by herself
- Has been withdrawn since divorce

Subjective Data

- "No one could ever love me."
- "I'm not good enough."
- "I just want to get rid of this pain."
- "I'm fat and ugly . . . no good to anyone."
- "I do love my sons, although I don't always show it."

Diagnosis

The nurse evaluates Ms. Glessner's strengths and weaknesses and decides to concentrate on two initial nursing diagnoses that seem to have the highest priority.

1. *Risk for suicide* related to separation from 2-year relationship, as evidenced by actual suicide attempt
   - Slashed her wrists
   - Recently broke off with boyfriend
   - Drinks at night by herself
   - Withdrawn for 3 years since divorce
2. *Situational low self-esteem* related to divorce and recent termination of love relationship, as evidenced by derogatory statements about self
   - "I'm not good enough."
   - "No one could ever love me."
   - "I'm fat and ugly . . . no good to anyone."
   - "I do love my sons, although I don't always show it."

Outcomes Identification

Patient refrains from attempting suicide.

Planning

Because Ms. Glessner is discharged after 48 hours, the issue of disturbance in self-esteem continues to be addressed in her therapy after discharge. Carrie later reviews the goals for her work with Ms. Glessner in the community.

Implementation

Ms. Glessner's plan of care is personalized as follows:

14-1 CASE STUDY AND NURSING CARE PLAN—cont'd

Depression

SHORT-TERM GOAL	INTERVENTION	RATIONALE	EVALUATION
1. Patient expresses at least one reason to live, and this is apparent by the second day of hospitalization.	1a. Observe patient every 15 minutes while she is suicidal. 1b. Remove all dangerous objects from patient.	1a, b. Patient safety is ensured. Impulsive self-harmful behavior is minimized.	**GOAL MET** By the end of the second day, Ms. Glessner states she really did not want to die, she just couldn't stand the loneliness in her life. She states that she loves her sons and would never want to hurt them.
	1c. Spend regularly scheduled periods of time with patient throughout the day.	1c. This interaction reinforces that patient is worthwhile and builds up experience to begin to relate better to nurse on one-to-one basis.	
	1d. Assist patient in evaluating both positive and negative aspects of her life.	1d. A depressed person is often unable to acknowledge any positive aspects of life unless they are pointed out by others.	
	1e. Encourage appropriate expression of angry feelings.	1e. Providing for expression of pent-up hostility in a safe environment can reinforce more adaptive methods of releasing tension and may minimize need to act out self-directed anger.	
	1f. Accept patient's negativism.	1f. Acceptance enhances feelings of self-worth.	
2. Patient will identify two outside supports she can call upon if she feels suicidal in the future.	2a. Explore usual coping behaviors.	2a. Behaviors that need reinforcing and new coping skills that need to be introduced can be identified.	**GOAL MET** By discharge, Ms. Glessner states that she is definitely going to try cognitive-behavioral therapy. She also discusses joining a women's support group that meets once a week in a neighboring town.
	2b. Assist patient in identifying members of her support system.	2b. Strengths and weaknesses in support available can be evaluated.	
	2c. Suggest a number of community-based support groups she might wish to discuss or visit (e.g., hotlines, support groups, women's groups).	2c. Patient needs to be aware of community supports to use them.	
	2d. Assist patient in identifying realistic alternatives she is willing to use.	2d. Unless patient is in agreement with any plan, she will be unable or unwilling to follow through in a crisis.	

Evaluation

During the course of her work with Carrie, Ms. Glessner decides to go to some meetings of Parents Without Partners. She states that she is looking forward to getting back to work and feels much more hopeful about her life. She has also lost 3 pounds while attending Weight Watchers. She states, "I need to get back into the world." Although Ms. Glessner still has negative thoughts about herself, she admits to feeling more hopeful and better about herself, and she has learned important tools to deal with her negative thoughts.

Key Assessment Findings

A depressed mood and anhedonia are the key symptoms in depression. Almost 97% of people with depression have **anergia** (lack of energy or physical passivity). **Anxiety**, a common symptom in depression, is seen in about 60% to 90% of patients with depression.

When people experience a depressive episode, their thinking is slow, and their memory and concentration are usually negatively affected. They also dwell on and exaggerate their perceived faults and failures and are unable to focus on their strengths and successes. A person with major depression may experience delusions of being punished for committing bad deeds or being a terrible person. Feelings of worthlessness, hopelessness, guilt, anger, and helplessness are common.

Psychomotor agitation may be evidenced by constant pacing and wringing of hands. The slowed movements of **psychomotor retardation**, however, are more common. Somatic complaints (headaches, malaise, backaches) are also common. **Vegetative signs of depression** (change in bowel movements and eating habits, sleep disturbances, and disinterest in sex) are usually

PATIENT HEALTH QUESTIONNAIRE-9 (PHQ-9)

Over the last 2 weeks, how often have you been bothered by any of the following problems?	**Not at all**	**Several days**	**More than half the days**	**Nearly every day**
1. Little interest or pleasure in doing things	0	1	2	3
2. Feeling down, depressed, or hopeless	0	1	2	3
3. Trouble falling or staying asleep, or sleeping too much	0	1	2	3
4. Feeling tired or having little energy	0	1	2	3
5. Poor appetite or overeating	0	1	2	3
6. Feeling bad about yourself — or that you are a failure or have let yourself or your family down	0	1	2	3
7. Trouble concentrating on things, such as reading the newspaper or watching television	0	1	2	3
8. Moving or speaking so slowly that other people could have noticed? Or the opposite — being so fidgety or restless that you have been moving around a lot more than usual	0	1	2	3
9. Thoughts that you would be better off dead or of hurting yourself in some way	0	1	2	3
	0 + ______	+ ______	+ ______	+ ______
			= Total score:	______

If you checked off any problems, how difficult have these problems made it for you to do your work, take care of things at home, or get along with other people?

Not difficult at all	**Somewhat difficult**	**Very difficult**	**Extremely difficult**
☐	☐	☐	☐

I confirm this information is accurate.	Patient's/Subject's initials:	Date:

A

PHQ-9 SCORING CARD FOR SEVERITY DETERMINATION

for health care professional use only

Scoring—add up all checked boxes on PHQ-9

Total Score	**Depression Severity**
0-4	None
5-9	Mild
10-14	Moderate
15-19	Moderately severe
20-27	Severe

B

FIG 14-2 A, Patient Health Questionnaire-9 (PHQ-9). **B,** Scoring the PHQ-9. (Copyright © 2005 by Pfizer, Inc. Developed by Drs. Robert L. Spitzer, Janet B. Williams, Kurt Kroenke, and colleagues.)

present. In primary care, people with major depression experience **chronic pain** at a rate of 66% and disabling pain at a rate of 41%, compared to 43% and 10%, respectively, of those who do not have depression (Arnow et al., 2006).

Areas to Assess

Affect

Affect is the outward representation of a person's internal state of being and is an objective finding based on the nurse's assessment. A person who has depression sees the world through gray-colored glasses. Posture is poor, and the patient may look older than the stated age. Facial expressions convey sadness and dejection, and the patient may have frequent bouts of weeping. Conversely, the patient may say that he or she feels numb or is unable to cry. Feelings of **hopelessness** and **despair** are readily reflected in the person's affect. For example, the patient may not make eye contact, may speak in a monotone, may show little or no facial expression (flat affect), and may make only yes or no responses. Frequent sighing is common.

Thought Processes

During a depressive episode, the person's ability to solve problems and think clearly is negatively affected. Judgment is poor, and indecisiveness is common. The individual may claim that the mind is slowing down. Memory and concentration are poor. Patients might complain of intrusive negative thoughts. Evidence of delusional thinking may also be seen in a person with major depression. Common statements of delusional thinking include, "I am responsible for Elvis Presley's death because I worked in a factory that made pill molds, and Elvis died from an overdose. I deserve to die."

Mood

Mood is the patient's subjective experience of sustained emotions or feelings. A person's mood can only be accurately assessed by asking the person how he or she feels. Feelings frequently reported by those with depression include anxiety, worthlessness, guilt, helplessness, hopelessness, and anger. Feelings of **worthlessness** range from feeling inadequate to having an unrealistically negative evaluation of self-worth. These feelings reflect the low self-esteem that is a painful partner to depression. Statements such as "I am no good" or "I'll never amount to anything" are common.

Feelings

Guilt is a common accompaniment to depression. A person may ruminate over present or past failings. In severe depression extreme guilt can assume psychotic proportions (see "Thought Processes" above).

Helplessness is demonstrated by a person's inability to solve problems in response to common concerns. In severe situations helplessness may be evidenced by the inability to carry out the simplest tasks (e.g., grooming, doing housework, working, caring for children) because they seem too difficult to accomplish. With feelings of helplessness come feelings of hopelessness, which are particularly correlated with suicidality (Beck et al., 2006). Even though most depressive episodes are time limited, people experiencing them believe things will never change. This feeling of utter hopelessness can lead people to view suicide as a way out of constant mental pain. **Hopelessness**, one of the core characteristics of depression and risk factors for suicide, is a combined cognitive and emotional state that includes the following attributes:

- Negative expectations for the future
- Loss of control over future outcomes
- Passive acceptance of the futility of planning to achieve goals
- Emotional negativism, as expressed in despair, despondency, or depression

Anger and **irritability** are natural outcomes of profound feelings of helplessness. Anger in depression is often expressed inappropriately through hurtful verbal attacks, physical aggression toward others, or destruction of property, and anger may be directed toward the self in the form of suicidal or otherwise self-destructive behaviors (e.g., alcohol abuse, substance abuse, overeating, smoking). These behaviors often reinforce feelings of low self-esteem and worthlessness.

Physical Behavior

Lethargy and fatigue may result in psychomotor retardation, in which movements are extremely slow, facial expressions are decreased, and gaze is fixed. The continuum of **psychomotor retardation** may range from slowed and difficult movements to complete inactivity and incontinence. **Psychomotor agitation**, in which patients constantly pace, bite their nails, smoke, tap their fingers, or engage in some other tension-relieving activity, may also be observed. At these times, patients commonly feel fidgety and unable to relax.

Grooming, dress, and personal hygiene may be markedly neglected. People who usually take pride in their appearance and dress may be poorly groomed and allow themselves to look shabby and unkempt. They may neglect to bathe, change clothes, or engage in other basic self-care activities.

Change in sleep patterns is a cardinal sign of depression. Often, people experience **insomnia**, wake frequently, and have a total reduction in sleep, especially deep-stage sleep (Sadock & Sadock, 2008). One of the hallmark symptoms of depression is waking at 3 or 4 AM and then staying awake or sleeping for only short periods. The light sleep of a person with depression tends to prolong the agony of depression over a 24-hour period. For some, sleep is increased (hypersomnia) and provides an escape from painful feelings. In any event, sleep is rarely restful or refreshing.

Changes in bowel habits are common. Constipation is seen most frequently in patients with psychomotor retardation. Diarrhea occurs less frequently, often in conjunction with psychomotor agitation or anxiety.

Interest in sex declines (loss of libido) during depression. Some men experience impotence, and a declining interest in sex often occurs among both men and women, which can further complicate marital and social relationships.

Vegetative signs of depression refer to alterations in those activities necessary to support physical life and growth (eating, sleeping, elimination, sex). For example, changes in eating patterns are common. About 60% to 70% of people with depression report having anorexia; however, overeating and weight gain may occur.

Communication

A person with depression may speak and comprehend very slowly. The lack of an immediate response by the patient to a remark does not necessarily mean the patient has not heard or chooses not to reply; the patient may need more time to comprehend what was said and then compose a reply. In extreme depression, however, a person may become mute.

Religious Beliefs and Spirituality

The role of religious beliefs and spirituality in depression is just beginning to be understood. Some of the recent research begins to shed light on this relationship. Miller and colleagues (2012) found that in a 20-year study of a cohort of 114 individuals at high risk for depression, spiritual beliefs and practices were associated with lower rates of depression and recurrence of depressive symptoms. Sreevani and Reddemma (2012) found that depression prevented individuals from engaging in the spiritual rituals, such as prayer and attendance at church, that helped in dealing with negative thoughts and other symptoms of depression. The authors concluded that efforts to support spirituality are beneficial in patients with depression.

Age Considerations

Assessment in Children and Adolescents

As children grow and develop, they may display a wide range of mood and behavior, making it easy to overlook signs of depression. The core symptoms of depression in children and adolescents are the same as for adults; namely, sadness and loss of pleasure. What differs is how these symptoms are displayed. For example, a very young child may cry, a school-age child might withdraw, and a teenager may become irritable in response to feeling sad or hopeless. In general, depressed children and adolescents may display increased irritability, negativity, isolation, and withdrawal along with a loss of energy (Lorberg & Prince 2010). Younger children may suddenly refuse to go to school while adolescents may engage in substance abuse or sexual promiscuity and be preoccupied with death or suicide. Depression in children and adolescents is frequently associated with anxiety and anger.

Assessment of Older Adults

It can be easy to overlook depression in older adults because they are more likely to complain of physical illness than emotional concerns. Older patients likely have comorbid physical issues, and it is difficult to ascertain whether fatigue, pain, and weakness are the result of an illness or depression (Cremens & Weichers, 2010). Patients and health care professionals may falsely believe that depression is a normal part of aging, but the nurse must assess older adults to see if the level of functioning represents a change from their normal patterns. The Geriatric Depression Scale is a tool that is both valid and reliable in screening for depression in the older adult (Sheikh & Yesavage, 1986); it can be helpful in determining suicidality in this population (Heisel et al, 2010).

Self-Assessment

Patients with depression often reject the advice, encouragement, and understanding of the nurse and others, and they often do not appear to respond to nursing interventions and seem resistant to change. When this occurs, the nurse may experience feelings of frustration, hopelessness, and annoyance. These problematic responses can be altered in the following ways:

- Recognizing any unrealistic expectations for yourself or the patient
- Identifying feelings that the patient may be experiencing
- Understanding the roles biology and genetics play in the precipitation and maintenance of a depressed mood

Feeling What the Patient Is Feeling

It is not uncommon for nurses and other health professionals to experience intense anxiety, frustration, annoyance, hopelessness, and helplessness while caring for individuals with depression; nurses empathetically sense what the patient is feeling. The novice nurse may interpret these emotions as personal reactions toward the patient with whom he or she is working; however, these feelings can be important diagnostic clues to the patient's experience. You can discuss feelings of annoyance, hopelessness, and helplessness with peers and supervisors to separate personal feelings from those originating with the patient. If personal feelings are not recognized, named, and examined, withdrawal by the nurse is likely to occur.

People instinctively avoid situations and persons that arouse feelings of frustration, annoyance, or intimidation. If the nurse also has unresolved feelings of anger and depression, the complexity of the situation is compounded. Nurses who work in psychiatric settings benefit from supervision. In this situation, supervision means an intentional sharing of personal feelings arising during contact with patients with a more experienced clinician. In the absence of structured supervision, sharing with peers can help minimize feelings of confusion, frustration, and isolation. Ultimately, supervision or peer support can increase the nurse's therapeutic potential and self-esteem while caring for individuals with depression.

ASSESSMENT GUIDELINES

Depression

1. Always evaluate the patient's risk of harm to self or others. Overt hostility is highly correlated with suicide (refer to Chapter 25).
2. Depression is a mood disorder that can be secondary to a host of medical or other psychiatric disorders as well as medications. A thorough medical and neurological examination helps determine if the depression is primary or secondary to another disorder. Essentially, evaluate whether:
   - The patient is psychotic.
   - The patient has taken drugs or alcohol.
   - Medical conditions are present.
   - The patient has a history of a comorbid psychiatric syndrome (eating disorder, borderline or anxiety disorder).
3. Assess the patient's history of depression and suicidality, and determine what happened and what worked and did not work.
4. Assess support systems, family, significant others, and the need for information and referrals.

DIAGNOSIS

Depression is a complex disorder, and individuals with depression have a variety of needs; therefore, nursing diagnoses are many. A high priority for the nurse is determining the risk of suicide, and the nursing diagnosis of *Risk for suicide* is always considered. Refer to Chapter 25 for assessment guidelines and interventions for suicidal individuals.

OUTCOMES IDENTIFICATION

The **recovery model** emphasizes that healing is possible and attainable for individuals with mental illnesses, including depression. Recovery is attained through partnerships between patients and health care providers who focus on the patient's strengths. Treatment goals are mutually developed based on the patient's personal needs and values, and interventions are evidenced-based. The recovery model is consistent with the focus on patient-centered care that has been identified as a key component of safe quality health care.

Major depressive disorder can be a recurrent and chronic illness. Care should be directed not only at resolution of the acute phase but also at long-term management. The nurse and the patient identify realistic outcome criteria and formulate concrete, measurable, short-term and long-term goals.

Table 14-2 identifies signs and symptoms commonly experienced in depression, offers potential nursing diagnoses, and suggests outcomes.

PLANNING

The planning of care for patients with depression is geared toward the patient's phase of depression, particular symptoms, and personal goals. At all times during the care of a person with

TABLE 14-2 SIGNS AND SYMPTOMS, NURSING DIAGNOSES, AND OUTCOMES FOR DEPRESSION

SIGNS AND SYMPTOMS	NURSING DIAGNOSES	OUTCOMES
Previous suicidal attempts, putting affairs in order, giving away prized possessions, suicidal ideation (has plan, ability to carry it out), overt or covert statements regarding killing self, feelings of worthlessness, hopelessness, helplessness	*Risk for self-directed violence* *Risk for suicide* *Risk for self-mutilation*	Expresses feelings, verbalizes suicidal ideas, refrains from suicide attempts, plans for the future.
Difficulty with simple tasks, inability to function at previous level, poor problem solving, poor cognitive functioning, verbalizations of inability to cope	*Ineffective coping*	Identifies ineffective and effective coping, uses support system, uses new coping strategies, engages in personal actions to manage stressors effectively
Dull/sad affect, no eye contact, preoccupation with own thoughts, seeks to be alone, uncommunicative, withdrawn, feels rejected and not good enough	*Social isolation*	Attends group meetings, interacts spontaneously with others, talks with the nurse in 1:1, demonstrates interest in engaging with family and others
Difficulty making decisions, poor concentration, inability to take action	*Decisional conflict*	Participates in health care decisions, makes judgments and chooses between alternatives.
Feelings of helplessness, hopelessness, powerlessness	*Hopelessness* *Powerlessness*	Expresses hope for a positive future, believes that personal actions impact outcomes, demonstrates optimism and describes plans for the future
Questioning meaning of life and existence, inability to participate in usual religious practices, conflict over spiritual beliefs, anger toward spiritual deity or religious representatives	*Spiritual distress* *Impaired religiosity* *Risk for impaired religiosity*	Shares feelings about spirituality and/or religious beliefs, expresses connection between self and spirituality and religious beliefs
Feelings of worthlessness, poor self-image, negative sense of self, self-negating verbalizations, feeling of being a failure, expressions of shame or guilt, hypersensitivity to slights or criticism	*Chronic low self-esteem* *Situational low self-esteem*	Identifies strengths, verbalizes self-acceptance, participates in groups, expresses a personal judgment of self-worth
Vegetative signs of depression: grooming and hygiene deficiencies, significantly reduced appetite, changes in sleeping, eating, elimination, sexual patterns	*Self-care deficit (bathing, hygiene, dressing, grooming)* *Self-neglect* *Disturbed sleep pattern* *Imbalanced nutrition: less than body requirements* *Constipation* *Sexual dysfunction*	Increases baseline personal care each day, reports adequate sleep, eating and elimination normalize, returns to a normal level of physiologic activity

depression, nurses and members of the health care team must be cognizant of the potential for suicide; assessment of risk for self-harm (or harm to others) is ongoing. A combination of therapy (cognitive, behavioral, or interpersonal) and psychopharmacology is an effective approach to the treatment of depression across all age groups.

Be aware that the vegetative signs of depression (changes in eating, sleeping, sexual satisfaction, etc.), as well as changes in concentration, activity level, social interaction, care for personal appearance, and so on, often need targeting. The planning of care for a patient with depression is based on the individual's symptoms and goals and attempts to encompass a variety of areas in the person's life. Safety is always the highest priority.

IMPLEMENTATION

There are three phases in treatment and recovery from major depression:

1. The **acute phase** (6 to 12 weeks) is directed at reduction of depressive symptoms and restoration of psychosocial and work function. Hospitalization may be required, and medication or other biological treatments may be initiated.
2. The **continuation phase** (4 to 9 months) is directed at prevention of relapse through pharmacotherapy, education, and depression-specific psychotherapy.
3. The **maintenance phase** (1 year or more) of treatment is directed at prevention of further episodes of depression. Depending on the risk factors for relapse, medication may be phased out or continued.

It is important to keep in mind that both the continuation and maintenance phases are geared toward maintaining the patient as a functional and contributing member of the community after recovery from the acute phase.

Counseling and Communication Techniques

Nurses often have great difficulty communicating with patients without talking; however, some patients with depression are so withdrawn that they are unwilling or unable to speak, and just sitting with them in silence may seem like a waste of time or be noticeably uncomfortable. As your anxiety increases, you may start daydreaming, feel bored, and believe that something "must be done now," and so on. It is important to be aware that this time can be meaningful, especially if you have a genuine interest in learning about and supporting the patient with depression.

It is difficult to say when a withdrawn patient will be able to respond, but certain techniques are known to be useful in guiding effective nursing interventions. Some communication techniques to use with a severely withdrawn patient are listed in Table 14-3. Counseling guidelines for use with patients with depression are offered in Table 14-4.

Health Teaching and Health Promotion

One basic premise of the recovery model of mental illness is that each individual controls his or her treatment based on individual goals. Within this model, health teaching is paramount because it allows patients to make informed choices. Health teaching is also an avenue for providing hope to the patient and should inform the patient that:

- Depression is an illness that is beyond a person's voluntary control.
- Although it is beyond voluntary control, depression can be managed through medication and lifestyle.
- Chronic illness management depends in large part on understanding personal signs and symptoms of relapse.
- Illness management depends on understanding the role of medication and possible medication side effects.
- Long-term management is best assured if the patient undergoes psychotherapy along with taking medication.
- Identifying and coping with the stress of interpersonal relationships—whether they are familial, social, or occupational—is key to stable illness management.

Including the family in discharge planning is also important and helps the patient in the following ways:

- Increases the family's understanding and acceptance of the family member with depression during the aftercare period
- Increases the patient's use of aftercare facilities in the community

CONSIDERING CULTURE

Depression in Female Latino Immigrants

Recent Latino immigrant women residing in the United States experience more depression than their white and African American counterparts. Latino women from South America or Central America are particularly vulnerable to depression, with rates running as high as 64% of the population. Some reasons for this include being separated from family and loved ones, fear of deportation, financial worries, and worry about loved ones left in their native country, especially children. Concerns for their children's safety and their children's loss of culture also contribute to depression.

Latinas' depressive symptoms frequently include stomach problems, lack of energy to perform household duties, mood swings, and sleep disturbances. They are aware of the fact that their stress and depression have a negative impact on their children. Latinas identify that mental health providers offer the best help for recovery for depression; however, they dislike the use of interpreters because they feel as if they are telling their secrets to two people, not just one.

Self-help activities for Latinas include distraction with hobbies, such as knitting, and engagement in spiritual activities, such as attending church and praying. Interventions, delivered in their own language and geared toward problem solving in the stressful areas identified above, are successful in reducing maternal depression and negative effects on their children. Language plays a big part in accessing treatment and coping with depression. Latinas benefit more from Spanish-speaking health care providers and religious services celebrated in Spanish.

Cowell, J., McNaughton, D., Ailey, S., Gross, D., & Fogg, L. (2009). Clinical trial outcomes of the Mexican American Problem Solving Program (MAPS). *Hispanic Health Care International, 7*(4), 178-189. doi: http://dx.doi.org/10.1891/1540-4153.7.4.178; Shattell, M., Villalba, J., Stokes, N., Hamilton, D., Foster, J., . . . Faulkner, C. (2009). Depression in Latinas residing in emerging Latino immigrant communities in the United States. *Hispanic Health Care International, 7*(4), 190-202.

TABLE 14-3 GUIDELINES FOR COMMUNICATION WITH SEVERELY WITHDRAWN PERSONS

INTERVENTION	RATIONALE
When a patient is mute, use the technique of making observations: "There are many new pictures on the wall." "You are wearing your new shoes."	When a patient is not ready to talk, direct questions can raise the patient's anxiety level and frustrate the nurse. Pointing to commonalities in the environment draws the patient into and reinforces reality.
Use simple, concrete words.	Slowed thinking and difficulty concentrating impair comprehension.
Allow time for the patient to respond.	Slowed thinking necessitates time to formulate a response.
Listen for covert messages, and ask about suicide plans.	People often experience relief and decrease in feelings of isolation when they share thoughts of suicide.
Avoid platitudes such as "Things will look up" or "Everyone gets down once in a while."	Platitudes tend to minimize the patient's feelings and can increase feelings of guilt and worthlessness, because the patient cannot "look up" or "snap out of it."

TABLE 14-4 GUIDELINES FOR COUNSELING PEOPLE WITH DEPRESSION

INTERVENTION	RATIONALE
Help the patient question underlying assumptions and beliefs and consider alternate explanations to problems.	Reconstructing a healthier and more hopeful attitude about the future can alter depressed mood.
Work with the patient to identify cognitive distortions that encourage negative self-appraisal. For example:	Cognitive distortions reinforce a negative, inaccurate perception of self and world.
a. Overgeneralizations	**a.** The patient takes one fact or event and makes a general rule out of it ("He always . . . "; "I never . . . ").
b. Self-blame	**b.** The patient consistently blames self for everything perceived as negative.
c. Mind reading	**c.** The patient assumes others don't like him or her, without any real evidence that assumptions are correct.
d. Discounting of positive attributes	**d.** The patient focuses on the negative.
Encourage activities that can raise self-esteem. Identify need for (a) problem-solving skills, (b) coping skills, and (c) assertiveness skills.	Many depressed people, especially women, are not taught a range of problem-solving and coping skills. Increasing social, family, and job skills can change negative self-assessment.
Encourage exercise, such as running and/or weight lifting.	Exercise can improve self-concept and potentially positively shift neurochemical balance.
Encourage formation of supportive relationships, such as through support groups, therapy, and peer support.	Such relationships reduce social isolation and enable the patient to work on personal goals and relationship needs.
Provide information referrals, when needed, for religious or spiritual information (e.g., readings, programs, tapes, community resources).	Spiritual and existential issues may be heightened during depressive episodes; many people find strength, support and comfort in spirituality or religion.

- Contributes to higher overall adjustment in the patient after discharge

Promotion of Self-Care Activities

In addition to feelings of hopelessness, despair, and physical discomfort, signs of physical neglect may be apparent. Nursing measures for improving physical well-being and promoting adequate self-care are initiated. Some effective interventions targeting physical needs in depression are listed in Table 14-5. Nurses in the community can work with family members to encourage a family member with depression to perform and maintain his or her self-care activities.

Teamwork and Safety

Safe, quality inpatient care requires the skills of a well-coordinated team. Treating a patient with depression will require the skills of not only the nurse and the physician but could also include a mental health technician, a pharmacist, a dietitian, a social worker, and the patient's family. All these people become members of the health care team, and the nurse must recognize each person's unique role and provide timely meaningful communication about the patient's condition.

Safety is a primary concern in all patient situations, but it becomes the most important issue facing the team that cares for people with depression who may be at high risk for suicide. Suicide precautions are usually instituted and include the removal of all harmful objects such as "sharps" (e.g. razors, scissors, and nail files), strangulation risks (e.g. belts), and medication that can be used to overdose. Some patients with severe depression may need to have someone check on them frequently, perhaps every 15 minutes, or even have 1:1 observation. A full discussion of inpatient safety measures is provided in Chapter 4.

Psychiatric care providers used to routinely institute no-harm contracts whereby patients agreed to a set of rules, such as "I will contact my nurse should I feel the urge to harm myself," and

TABLE 14-5 INTERVENTIONS TARGETING THE VEGETATIVE SIGNS OF DEPRESSION

INTERVENTION	RATIONALE
Nutrition (Anorexia)	
Offer small, high-calorie, and high-protein snacks frequently throughout the day and evening.	Low weight and poor nutrition render the patient susceptible to illness. Small, frequent snacks are more easily tolerated than large plates of food when the patient is anorexic.
Offer high-protein and high-calorie fluids frequently throughout the day and evening.	These fluids prevent dehydration and can minimize constipation.
When possible, encourage family or friends to remain with the patient during meals.	This strategy reinforces the idea that someone cares, can raise the patient's self-esteem, and can serve as an incentive to eat.
Ask the patient which foods or drinks he or she likes. Offer choices. Involve the dietitian.	The patient is more likely to eat the foods provided.
Weigh the patient weekly, and observe the patient's eating patterns.	Monitoring the patient's status gives the information needed for revision of the intervention.
Sleep (Insomnia)	
Provide periods of rest after activities.	Fatigue can intensify feelings of depression.
Encourage the patient to get up and dress and to stay out of bed during the day.	Minimizing sleep during the day increases the likelihood of sleep at night as well as the establishment of healthy routines.
Encourage the use of relaxation measures in the evening (e.g., tepid bath, warm milk).	These measures induce relaxation and sleep.
Reduce environmental and physical stimulants in the evening—provide decaffeinated coffee, soft lights, soft music, and quiet activities.	Decreasing caffeine and epinephrine levels increases the possibility of sleep.
Self-Care Deficits	
Encourage the use of toothbrush, washcloth, soap, makeup, shaving equipment, and so forth.	Being clean and well groomed can temporarily increase self-esteem.
When appropriate, give step-by-step reminders, such as, "Wash the right side of your face, now the left."	Slowed thinking and difficulty concentrating make organizing simple tasks difficult.
Elimination (Constipation)	
Monitor intake and output, especially bowel movements.	Many depressed patients are constipated. If the condition is not checked, fecal impaction can occur.
Offer foods high in fiber, and provide periods of exercise.	Roughage and exercise stimulate peristalsis and help evacuation of fecal material.
Encourage the intake of fluids.	Fluids help prevent constipation.
Evaluate the need for laxatives and enemas.	These measures prevent fecal impaction.

signed an informal contract on a daily basis. The logic behind this contract was that even that small agreement and connection with the staff could provide just enough support to prevent self-harm. Research (Garvey et al., 2009) indicates, however, that there is little empirical data to support the use of these contracts, no evidence to suggest that they help reduce suicide, and that contracting does not reduce legal liability.

Pharmacological Interventions

Because mood disorders are caused by problems with neurotransmitters, it follows that medications that alter brain chemistry are an important component in their treatment. Antidepressant therapy benefits about 80% of people with major depression (Mental Health America, 2008). It should be noted, however, that the combination of specific psychotherapies (e.g., CBT, IPT, behavioral) and antidepressant therapy is superior to either psychotherapy or psychopharmacological treatment alone (Depression: Treatment Guidelines, 2010).

Antidepressant Drugs

Antidepressant drugs can positively alter poor self-concept, degree of social withdrawal, vegetative signs of depression, and activity level. Target symptoms include the following:

- Sleep disturbance
- Appetite disturbance (decreased or increased)
- Fatigue
- Decreased sex drive
- Psychomotor retardation or agitation
- Diurnal variations in mood (often worse in the morning)
- Impaired concentration or forgetfulness
- **Anhedonia** (loss of ability to experience joy or pleasure in living)

A drawback of antidepressant drugs is that improvement in mood may take 1 to 3 weeks or longer. If a patient is acutely suicidal, electroconvulsive therapy (discussed in detail later in this chapter) can be a reliable and effective alternative for some.

The goal of antidepressant therapy is the complete remission of symptoms (Stahl, 2008). Often, the first antidepressant prescribed is not the one that will ultimately bring about remission; aggressive treatment helps in efficiently finding the proper treatment. An antidepressant adequate trial for the treatment of depression is 3 months. Individuals experiencing their first depressive episode are maintained on antidepressants for 6 to 9 months after symptoms of depression remit. Some people may have multiple episodes of depression or may have a chronic form and benefit from indefinite antidepressant therapy.

Antidepressants may precipitate a psychotic episode in a person with schizophrenia or a manic episode in a patient with bipolar disorder. Patients with bipolar disorder often receive a mood-stabilizing drug along with an antidepressant.

Choosing an Antidepressant. All antidepressants work to increase the availability of one or more of the neurotransmitters, serotonin, norepinephrine, and dopamine. All antidepressants have demonstrated similar efficacy in pharmaceutical trials; however, a variety of antidepressants or a combination of antidepressants may need to be tried before the most effective regimen is found for an individual patient, targeting individualized symptom manifestations and practical concerns. Each of the antidepressants has different adverse effects, costs, safety issues, and maintenance considerations. Selection of the appropriate antidepressant is based on the following considerations (Preston, Oneal &Talaga 2010):

- Symptom profile of the patient
- Side-effect profile (e.g., sexual dysfunction, weight gain)
- Ease of administration
- History of past response
- Safety and medical considerations

Table 14-6 provides an overview of antidepressants used in the United States.

Selective Serotonin Reuptake Inhibitors. The selective serotonin reuptake inhibitors (SSRIs) are recommended as first-line therapy for most types of depression. Essentially, the SSRIs selectively block the neuronal uptake of serotonin (e.g., 5-HT, 5-HT_1 receptors), which increases the availability of serotonin in the synaptic cleft. Refer to Chapter 3 for a more detailed discussion of how the SSRIs work.

SSRI antidepressant drugs have a relatively low side-effect profile compared with the older antidepressants (tricyclics—discussed later in this chapter); they do not create anticholinergic effects, dry mouth, blurred vision, or urinary retention, making it easier for patients to take these medications as prescribed. Consistent adherence to the medication regimen is a crucial step toward recovery or remission of symptoms. The SSRIs are effective in depression with anxiety features as well as depression with psychomotor agitation.

Because the SSRIs cause relatively few adverse effects and have low cardiotoxicity, they are less dangerous than older antidepressants when taken in overdose. The SSRIs, selective serotonin-norepinephrine reuptake inhibitors (SNRIs), and unconventional antidepressants have a low lethality risk in suicide attempts whereas the tricyclic antidepressants have a very high potential for lethality with overdose.

Indications. Because of the relatively low side-effect profile and relatively higher acceptance rate, SSRIs are frequently the first-line treatment in depression. The SSRIs have a broad base of clinical use. In addition to their use in treating depressive disorders, the SSRIs have been prescribed with success to treat some of the anxiety disorders—in particular obsessive-compulsive disorder and panic disorder. Fluoxetine has been found to be effective in treating some women who suffer from late-luteal-phase dysphoric disorder and bulimia nervosa.

Common adverse reactions. Agents that selectively enhance synaptic serotonin within the CNS may induce agitation, anxiety, sleep disturbance, tremor, sexual dysfunction (primarily anorgasmia), or tension headache. The effect of the SSRIs on sexual performance may be the most significant undesirable outcome reported by patients; however, nurses can help patients by educating them on ways to manage these side effects. Autonomic reactions (e.g., dry mouth, sweating, weight change, mild nausea, and loose bowel movements) may also be experienced with the SSRIs.

Potential toxic effects. One rare and life-threatening event associated with SSRIs is **serotonin syndrome**. This syndrome is thought to be related to over-activation of the central serotonin receptors caused by either too high a dose or interaction with other drugs. Symptoms include abdominal pain, diarrhea, sweating, fever, tachycardia, elevated blood pressure, altered mental state (delirium), myoclonus (muscle spasms), increased motor activity, irritability, hostility, and mood change. Severe manifestations can induce hyperpyrexia (excessively high fever), cardiovascular shock, or death. The risk of this syndrome seems to be greatest when an SSRI is administered in combination with a second serotonin-enhancing agent, such as a monoamine oxidase inhibitor (MAOI). A patient should discontinue all SSRIs for 2 to 5 weeks before starting an MAOI. Box 14-2 lists the signs and symptoms of serotonin syndrome and gives emergency treatment guidelines. Box 14-3 is a useful tool for patient and family teaching about the SSRIs.

Tricyclic Antidepressants. The tricyclic antidepressants (TCAs) inhibit the reuptake of norepinephrine and serotonin by the presynaptic neurons in the CNS, increasing the amount of time norepinephrine and serotonin are available to the postsynaptic receptors. This increase in norepinephrine and serotonin in the brain is believed to be responsible for mood elevations.

Indications. The sedative effects of the TCAs are attributed to the blockade of histamine receptors (Lehne, 2010). Patients must take therapeutic doses of TCAs for 10 to 14 days or longer before they begin to work; full effects may not be seen for 4 to 8 weeks. An effect on some symptoms of depression, such as insomnia and anorexia, may be noted earlier. Choosing a TCA for a patient is based on what has worked for the patient or a family member in the past and the drug's adverse effects.

A stimulating TCA, such as desipramine (Norpramin) or protriptyline (Vivactil), may be best for a patient who is lethargic and fatigued. If a more sedating effect is needed for agitation or restlessness, drugs such as amitriptyline (Elavil) and doxepin (Sinequan) may be more appropriate choices. Regardless of which TCA is given, the initial dose should always be low and increased gradually.

TABLE 14-6 DRUGS USED TO TREAT MAJOR DEPRESSION IN THE UNITED STATES

GENERIC (TRADE)	ACTION	NOTES	SIDE EFFECTS	WARNINGS
Selective Serotonin Reuptake Inhibitors (SSRIs)				
Citalopram (Celexa) Escitalopram (Lexapro) Fluoxetine (Prozac, Prozac Weekly) Fluvoxamine (Luvox) Paroxetine (Paxil) Sertraline (Zoloft)	Blocks the synaptic reuptake of serotonin	First line of treatment for major depression Some SSRIs activate and others sedate; choice depends on patient symptoms Risk of lethal overdose minimized with SSRIs	Agitation, insomnia, headache, nausea and vomiting, sexual dysfunction, and hyponatremia	Discontinuation syndrome—dizziness, insomnia, nervousness, irritability, nausea, and agitation—may occur with abrupt withdrawal (depending on half-life). Taper slowly.
Selective Serotonin Reuptake Inhibitor and Serotonin Receptor Agonist				
Vilazodone (Viibryd)	Main mechanism of action is blocking the synaptic reuptake of serotonin; also activates serotonin receptors	Has been reported to result in lower rates of sexual side effects and weight gain as compared to SSRIs	Diarrhea, nausea, headache	Withdrawal symptoms may occur if discontinued abruptly. Use with caution in pregnancy.
Serotonin Norepinephrine Reuptake Inhibitors (SNRIs)				
Desvenlafaxine (Pristiq)	Blocks the synaptic reuptake of serotonin and norepinephrine	A metabolite of venlafaxine	Nausea, headache, dizziness, insomnia, diarrhea, dry mouth, sweating, constipation	Neonates with in utero exposure have required respiratory support and tube feeding
Duloxetine (Cymbalta)	Blocks the synaptic reuptake of serotonin and norepinephrine	Cymbalta may be more effective than SSRIs in the treatment of severe depression	Nausea, dry mouth, insomnia, somnolence, constipation, reduced appetite, fatigue, sweating, blurred vision	May reduce pain associated with depression and is approved for fibromyalgia and pain of diabetic peripheral neuropathy.
Venlafaxine (Effexor, Effexor XR)	Blocks the synaptic reuptake of serotonin and norepinephrine	Effexor is a popular next-step strategy after trying SSRIs	Hypertension, nausea, insomnia, dry mouth, sedation, sweating, agitation, headache, sexual dysfunction	Monitor blood pressure, especially at higher doses and with a history of hypertension Discontinuation syndrome (see SSRIs above)
Serotonin Antagonists and Reuptake Inhibitors				
Nefazodone (formerly sold as Serzone)	Selective blockage of serotonin2 receptors and α1-adrenergic receptors	Lower risk of long-term weight gain than SSRIs or TCAs Lower risk of sexual side effects than SSRIs	Sedation, hepatotoxicity, dizziness, hypotension, paresthesias	Life-threatening liver failure is possible but rare Priapism of penis and clitoris is a rare but serious side effect
Trazodone (Desyrel, Oleptro)	Moderate blockade of 5-HT synaptic reuptake	Significant sedative effect. Helps with antidepressant-induced insomnia	Severe sedation, hypotension, nausea.	Priapism has been reported.
Norepinephrine Dopamine Reuptake Inhibitor (NDRI)				
Bupropion (Wellbutrin, also sold as Zyban for smoking cessation)	Blocks the synaptic reuptake of norepinephrine and dopamine	Stimulant action may reduce appetite May increase sexual desire Used as an aid to quit smoking	Agitation, insomnia, headache, nausea and vomiting, seizures (0.4%)	High doses increase seizure risk, especially in people who are predisposed to them

TABLE 14-6 DRUGS USED TO TREAT MAJOR DEPRESSION IN THE UNITED STATES—cont'd				
GENERIC (TRADE)	**ACTION**	**NOTES**	**SIDE EFFECTS**	**WARNINGS**
Norepinephrine and Serotonin Specific Antidepressant (NASSA)				
Mirtazapine (Remeron)	Blocks α1- adrenergic receptors that normally inhibit norepinephrine and serotonin	Antidepressant effects equal SSRIs and may occur faster	Weight gain/appetite stimulation, sedation, dizziness, headache; sexual dysfunction is rare	Drug-induced somnolence exaggerated by alcohol, benzodiazepines, and other CNS depressants
Tricyclic Antidepressants (TCAs)				
Amitriptyline (Elavil) Amoxapine (Asendin) Clomipramine (Anafranil) Desipramine (Norpramin) Doxepin (Adapin, Sinequan) Imipramine (Tofranil) Maprotiline (Ludiomil) Nortriptyline (Aventyl, Pamelor) Protriptyline (Vivactil) Trimipramine (Surmontil)	Inhibits the synaptic reuptake of serotonin and norepinephrine. Antagonizes adrenergic, histaminergic, muscarinic, and dopaminergic receptors	Therapeutic effects similar to SSRIs, but side effects are more prominent May work better in melancholic depression and in people with comorbid medical conditions Some therapeutic serum levels may be monitored	Dry mouth, constipation, urinary retention, blurred vision, hypotension, cardiac toxicity, sedation	Lethal in overdose Use cautiously in the elderly, with cardiac disorders, elevated intraocular pressure, urinary retention, hyperthyroidism, seizure disorders, and liver or kidney dysfunction.
Monoamine Oxidase Inhibitors (MAOIS)				
Isocarboxazid (Marplan) Phenelzine (Nardil) Selegiline Transdermal System Patch Tranylcypromine (Parnate)	Inhibits the enzyme monoamine oxidase, which normally breaks down neurotransmitters, including serotonin and norepinephrine	Efficacy similar to other antidepressants, but strict dietary (tyramine) restrictions and potential drug interactions make this drug class much less desirable	Insomnia, nausea, agitation, and confusion Hypertensive crisis	Contraindicated in people taking SSRIs, used cautiously in people taking TCAs Tyramine-rich food could bring about a hypertensive crisis Many other strong drug and dietary interactions

Data from Lehne, R. A. (2010). *Pharmacology for nursing care* (7th ed.). St. Louis, MO: Saunders; Citrome, L. (2012). Vilazodone for major depressive disorder. *International Journal of Clinical Practice, 66*(4), 356-68. doi: 10.1111/j.1742-1241.2011.02885.x.

Common adverse reactions. The chemical structure of the TCAs closely resembles that of antipsychotic medications, and the **anticholinergic** actions are similar (e.g., dry mouth, blurred vision, tachycardia, constipation, urinary retention, and esophageal reflux). These side effects are more common and more severe in patients taking antidepressants. They usually are not serious and are often transitory, but **urinary retention** and **severe constipation** warrant immediate medical attention. Weight gain is also a common complaint among people taking TCAs.

The α-adrenergic blockade of the TCAs can produce postural-orthostatic hypotension and tachycardia. Postural hypotension can lead to dizziness and increase the risk of falls. For this reason elderly patients on TCA must be monitored carefully for dizziness and falls.

Administering the total daily dose of TCA at night is beneficial for two reasons. First, most TCAs have sedative effects and thereby aid sleep. Second, the minor side effects occur while the individual is sleeping, which increases compliance with drug therapy.

Potential toxic effects. The most serious effects of the TCAs are cardiovascular: dysrhythmias, tachycardia, myocardial infarction, and heart block. Because the cardiac side effects are so serious, TCA use is considered a risk in older adults and patients with cardiac disease. Patients should have a thorough cardiac workup before beginning TCA therapy.

Adverse drug interactions. A few of the more common medications usually *not* given while TCAs are being used are monoamine oxidase inhibitors, phenothiazines, barbiturates, disulfiram (Antabuse), oral contraceptives (or other estrogen preparations),

BOX 14-2 SEROTONIN SYNDROME: SYMPTOMS AND INTERVENTIONS

Symptoms

- Hyperactivity or restlessness
- Tachycardia → cardiovascular shock
- Fever → hyperpyrexia
- Elevated blood pressure
- Altered mental states (delirium)
- Irrationality, mood swings, hostility
- Seizures → status epilepticus
- Myoclonus, incoordination, tonic rigidity
- Abdominal pain, diarrhea, bloating
- Apnea → death

Interventions

- Remove offending agent(s)
- Initiate symptomatic treatment:
  - Serotonin-receptor blockade with cyproheptadine, methysergide, propranolol
  - Cooling blankets, chlorpromazine for hyperthermia
  - Dantrolene, diazepam for muscle rigidity or rigors
  - Anticonvulsants
  - Artificial ventilation
  - Induction of paralysis

anticoagulants, some antihypertensives (clonidine, guanethidine, reserpine), benzodiazepines, and alcohol. A patient who is taking any of these medications along with a TCA should have medical clearance because some of the reactions can be fatal.

Contraindications. People who have recently had a myocardial infarction (or other cardiovascular problems), those with narrow-angle glaucoma or a history of seizures, and women who are pregnant should not be treated with TCAs, except with extreme caution and careful monitoring.

Patient and family teaching. Areas for the nurse to discuss when teaching patients and their families about TCA therapy are presented in Box 14-4.

Monoamine Oxidase Inhibitors. The enzyme monoamine oxidase is responsible for inactivating, or breaking down, certain monoamine neurotransmitters in the brain, such as norepinephrine, serotonin, dopamine, and tyramine. When a person ingests an MAOI, these amines do not get inactivated, and there is an increase of neurotransmitters available for synaptic release in the brain. The increase in norepinephrine, serotonin, and dopamine is the desired effect because it results in mood elevation. The increase in tyramine, on the other hand, poses a problem. When the level of tyramine concurrently increases, and it is not inactivated by monoamine oxidase, high blood pressure, hypertensive crisis, and eventually cerebrovascular accident can occur. Therefore, people taking these drugs must reduce or eliminate their intake of foods and drugs that contain high amounts of tyramine (Table 14-7 and Box 14-5).

Because people with depression are often lethargic, confused, and apathetic, adherence to strict dietary limitations may not be realistic. That is why MAOIs, although highly effective, are not often given as a first-line treatment.

BOX 14-3 PATIENT AND FAMILY TEACHING: SELECTIVE SEROTONIN REUPTAKE INHIBITORS (SSRIs)

- May cause sexual dysfunction or lack of sex drive. Inform nurse or primary care provider if this occurs.
- May cause insomnia, anxiety, and nervousness. Inform nurse or primary care provider if this occurs.
- May interact with other medications. Tell primary care provider about other medications patient is taking (e.g., digoxin, warfarin). SSRIs should not be taken within 14 days of the last dose of a monoamine oxidase inhibitor.
- No over-the-counter drug should be taken without first notifying primary care provider.
- Common side effects include fatigue, nausea, diarrhea, dry mouth, dizziness, tremor, and sexual dysfunction or lack of sex drive.
- Because of the potential for drowsiness and dizziness, patient should not drive or operate machinery until these side effects are ruled out.
- Alcohol should be avoided.
- Liver and renal function tests should be performed and blood counts checked periodically.
- Medication should not be discontinued abruptly. If side effects become bothersome, patient should ask primary care provider about changing to a different drug. Abrupt cessation can lead to serotonin withdrawal.
- Any of the following symptoms should be reported to the primary care provider immediately:
  - Increase in depression or suicidal thoughts
  - Rash or hives
  - Rapid heartbeat
  - Sore throat
  - Difficulty urinating
  - Fever, malaise
  - Anorexia and weight loss
  - Unusual bleeding
  - Initiation of hyperactive behavior
  - Severe headache

Indications. MAOIs are particularly effective for people with unconventional depression (characterized by mood reactivity, oversleeping, and overeating) as well as panic disorder, social phobia, generalized anxiety disorder, obsessive-compulsive disorder, posttraumatic stress disorder, and bulimia. The MAOIs commonly used in the United States at present are phenelzine (Nardil) and tranylcypromine sulfate (Parnate). Selegiline (Emsam), a newer MAOI delivered transdermally in a patch, does not seem to affect tyramine sensitivity.

Common adverse reactions. Some common and troublesome long-term side effects of the MAOIs are orthostatic hypotension, weight gain, edema, change in cardiac rate and rhythm, constipation, urinary hesitancy, sexual dysfunction, vertigo, overactivity, muscle twitching, hypomanic and manic behavior, insomnia, weakness, and fatigue.

Potential toxic effects. The most serious reaction to the MAOIs is an increase in blood pressure, with the possible development of intracranial hemorrhage, hyperpyrexia, convulsions, coma, and

BOX 14-4 PATIENT AND FAMILY TEACHING: TRICYCLIC ANTIDEPRESSANTS (TCAs)

- The patient and family should be told that mood elevation may take from 7 to 28 days. Up to 6 to 8 weeks may be required for the full effect to be reached and for major depressive symptoms to subside.
- The family should reinforce this frequently to the depressed family member because depressed people have trouble remembering and respond to ongoing reassurance.
- The patient should be reassured that drowsiness, dizziness, and hypotension usually subside after the first few weeks.
- When the patient starts taking TCAs, the patient should be cautioned to be careful working around machines, driving cars, and crossing streets because of possible altered reflexes, drowsiness, or dizziness.
- Alcohol can block the effects of antidepressants. The patient should be told to refrain from drinking.
- If possible, the patient should take the full dose at bedtime to reduce the experience of side effects during the day.
- If the patient forgets the bedtime dose (or the once-a-day dose), the patient should take the dose within 3 hours; otherwise, the patient should wait until the usual medication time the next day. The patient should not double the dose.
- Suddenly stopping TCAs can cause nausea, altered heartbeat, nightmares, and cold sweats in 2 to 4 days. The patient should call the primary care provider or take one dose of TCA until the primary care provider can be contacted.

BOX 14-5 DRUGS THAT CAN INTERACT WITH MONOAMINE OXIDASE INHIBITORS (MAOIs)

- Over-the-counter medications for colds, allergies, or congestion (any product containing ephedrine, phenylephrine hydrochloride, or phenylpropanolamine)
- Tricyclic antidepressants (imipramine, amitriptyline)
- Narcotics
- Antihypertensives (methyldopa, guanethidine, reserpine)
- Amine precursors (levodopa, l-tryptophan)
- Sedatives (alcohol, barbiturates, benzodiazepines)
- General anesthetics
- Stimulants (amphetamines, cocaine)

death; therefore, routine monitoring of blood pressure, especially during the first 6 weeks of treatment, is necessary.

Because many drugs, foods, and beverages can cause an increase in blood pressure in patients taking MAOIs, hypertensive crisis is a constant concern. The beginning of a hypertensive crisis usually occurs within a few hours of ingestion of the contraindicated substance. The crisis may begin with headaches, stiff or sore neck, palpitations, increase or decrease in heart rate (often associated with chest pain), nausea, vomiting, or increase in temperature (pyrexia). When a hypertensive crisis is suspected, immediate medical attention is crucial. Antihypertensive medications such as the calcium channel blocker nifedipine

TABLE 14-7 FOODS THAT CAN INTERACT WITH MONOAMINE OXIDASE INHIBITORS

FOODS THAT CONTAIN TYRAMINE

CATEGORY	UNSAFE FOODS (HIGH TYRAMINE CONTENT)	SAFE FOODS (LITTLE OR NO TYRAMINE)
Vegetables	Avocados, especially if overripe; fermented bean curd; fermented soybean; soybean paste	Most vegetables
Fruits	Figs, especially if overripe; bananas, in large amounts	Most fruits
Meats	Meats that are fermented, smoked, or otherwise aged; spoiled meats; liver, unless very fresh	Meats that are known to be fresh (exercise caution in restaurants; meats may not be fresh)
Sausages	Fermented varieties; bologna, pepperoni, salami, others	Nonfermented varieties
Fish	Dried or cured fish; fish that is fermented, smoked, or otherwise aged; spoiled fish	Fish that is known to be fresh; vacuum-packed fish, if eaten promptly or refrigerated only briefly after opening
Milk, milk products	Practically all cheeses	Milk, yogurt, cottage cheese, cream cheese
Foods with yeast	Yeast extract (e.g., Marmite, Bovril)	Baked goods that contain yeast
Beer, wine	Some imported beers, Chianti wines	Major domestic brands of beer; most wines
Other foods	Protein dietary supplements; soups (may contain protein extract); shrimp paste; soy sauce	

FOODS THAT CONTAIN OTHER VASOPRESSORS

FOOD	COMMENTS
Chocolate	Contains phenylethylamine, a pressor agent; large amounts can cause a reaction.
Fava beans	Contain dopamine, a pressor agent; reactions are most likely with overripe beans.
Ginseng	Headache, tremulousness, and mania-like reactions have occurred.
Caffeinated beverages	Caffeine is a weak pressor agent; large amounts may cause a reaction.

From Lehne, R. A. (2010). *Pharmacology for nursing* (7th ed.). (p. 351). Philadelphia, PA: Elsevier.

or an alpha-adrenergic blocker such as phentolamine may be given (Martinez et al., 2008). Pyrexia is treated with hypothermic blankets or ice packs.

Table 14-8 identifies common side effects and toxic effects of the MAOIs, and Box 14-6 can be used as an MAOI teaching guide for patients and their families.

Contraindications. The use of MAOIs may be contraindicated with each of the following:

- Cerebrovascular disease
- Hypertension and congestive heart failure
- Liver disease
- Consumption of foods containing tyramine, tryptophan, and dopamine (see Table 14-7)
- Use of certain medications (see Box 14-6)
- Recurrent or severe headaches
- Surgery in the previous 10 to 14 days
- Age younger than 16 years

Use of Antidepressants by Pregnant Women. Pharmaceutical use during pregnancy and lactation is always a concern, and a number of research studies have been done looking at fetal outcomes in pregnant women taking a range of antidepressants. Udechuku and colleagues (2010) reviewed studies of pregnancy outcomes in women taking antidepressants. The authors noted that the findings were mixed. There was a slight increase in the risk of preterm birth. Congenital malformations were noted in some studies of women taking MAOI and TCA and in women taking SSRI in the first trimester. Additional studies noted withdrawal symptoms of irritability and tremors in some neonates born to women taking SSRIs in the third trimester. In all cases the numbers of negative outcomes were very small, prompting the authors to conclude that antidepressants taken during pregnancy are relatively safe.

Women who suffer from depression while pregnant will need to be provided with current information and assisted in weighing the risks of taking medication against the benefits. There is much evidence documented that depression itself has a negative effect on birth outcomes. Preeclampsia, diabetes, hypertension have all been associated with maternal depression. Low birth weight, preterm birth, and small size for gestational age have been noted effects in infants born to depressed mothers. The severity of the symptoms and the degree to which depression interferes with the ability of the mother to care for herself and her unborn child need to be compared to the risk of taking medication. A nurse is in an excellent position to provide the patient with guidance and support during this process.

Use of Antidepressants by Children and Adolescents. In 2005, the U.S. Food and Drug Administration (FDA) (2004) issued a black-box warning for all antidepressants, alerting the public to the increased risk of suicidal thinking or attempts in children or adolescents taking antidepressants. Following the black-box warning, the number of prescriptions written for SSRIs for children and young adults decreased, but suicides in those age groups actually increased (Dudley et al., 2008). Dudley and colleagues concluded that the risk for suicide is greater in children and adolescents with depression who do not take antidepressants. To minimize the risk of suicide in persons taking antidepressants, close monitoring by health

TABLE 14-8 ADVERSE REACTIONS TO AND TOXIC EFFECTS OF MONOAMINE OXIDASE INHIBITORS

ADVERSE REACTIONS	COMMENTS
Hypotension Sedation, weakness, fatigue Insomnia Changes in cardiac rhythm Muscle cramps Anorgasmia or sexual impotence Urinary hesitancy or constipation Weight gain	Hypotension is an expected side effect of MAOIs. Orthostatic blood pressures should be taken—first lying down, then sitting or standing after 1-2 minutes. This may be a dangerous side effect, especially in older adults who may fall and sustain injuries as a result of dizziness from the blood pressure drop.
TOXIC EFFECTS	**COMMENTS**
Hypertensive crisis: Severe headache Tachycardia, palpitations Hypertension Nausea and vomiting	Patient should go to local emergency department immediately—blood pressure should be checked. One of the following may be given to lower blood pressure: 5 mg intravenous phentolamine (Regitine) or sublingual nifedipine to promote vasodilation Patients may be prescribed a 10 mg nifedipine capsule to carry in case of emergency

From Lehne, R.A. (2010). *Pharmacology for nursing care* (7th ed.). St. Louis, MO: Elsevier

BOX 14-6 PATIENT AND FAMILY TEACHING: MONOAMINE OXIDASE INHIBITORS (MAOIs)

- Tell the patient and family to avoid certain foods (especially those that are aged, cured, or ripened) and all medications (especially cold remedies) unless prescribed by and discussed with the patient's primary care provider (see Table 14-7 for specific food and drug restrictions).
- Give the patient a wallet card describing the MAOI regimen.
- Instruct the patient to avoid Chinese restaurants (sherry, brewer's yeast, and other contraindicated products may be used).
- Tell the patient to go to the emergency department immediately if he or she has a severe headache.
- Ideally, blood pressure should be monitored during the first 6 weeks of treatment (for both hypotensive and hypertensive effects).
- After the MAOI is stopped, instruct the patient that dietary and drug restrictions should be maintained for 14 days.

care professionals and patient/caregiver education are essential. Chapter 25 has a more detailed discussion of suicide risk factors and warning signs.

Use of Antidepressants by Older Adults. Polypharmacy and the normal metabolic processes of aging contribute to concerns about prescribing antidepressants for older adults. SSRIs are a first-line treatment for older adults, but the elderly have the potential for aggravated side effects. Starting doses are recommended to be half the lowest adult dose, with dose adjustments occurring no more frequently than every 7 days ("start low and go slow"). TCAs and MAOIs have side-effect profiles that are more dangerous for older adults, specifically cardiotoxicity with TCAs and hypotension with both classes. Any medication with a side effect of hypotension or sedation in older adults increases the risk of falls. Older adults should be cautioned against abrupt discontinuation of antidepressants because of the possibility of discontinuation syndrome, which causes anxiety, dysphoria, flulike symptoms, dizziness, excessive sweating, and insomnia (Akpafflong et al., 2008).

Electroconvulsive Therapy

Despite being a highly effective somatic (physical) treatment for psychiatric disorders, electroconvulsive therapy (ECT) has a bad reputation. This may be due to both historic misconceptions and even more contemporary media portrayals of patients being restrained on a gurney while having a full-blown seizure induced. Given the current sophistication of anesthetic and paralytic agents, ECT is actually not dramatic at all. Another possible reason for ECT's stigmatized status is that how it works remains a mystery (Stahl, 2008), although researchers have speculated as to its mechanism of action. It is likely that the seizure that is induced results in mobilization and activity of neurotransmitters.

Indications

ECT is used most commonly for depression. While as many as 50% of people taking antidepressants fail to achieve full remission, clinical trials of ECT report a rate of 70% to 90% remission (Welch, 2008). Suicidal thoughts respond to ECT in 80% of cases. Psychotic illnesses are the second most common indication for ECT. For drug-resistant patients, a combination of ECT and antipsychotic medication has resulted in sustained improvement about 80% of the time.

While medication is generally the first line of treatment for ease of use, according to Sadock and Sadock (2008), ECT may be a primary treatment in the following cases:

- When a patient is suicidal or homicidal and there is a need for a rapid, definitive response
- If previous medication trials have failed
- When there is marked agitation, marked vegetative symptoms, or catatonia
- For major depression with psychotic features or for pervasive hallucinations

ECT is useful in treating patients with major depression, especially when psychotic symptoms are present. Patients who have depression with marked psychomotor retardation and stupor also respond well. ECT is also indicated for manic patients whose conditions are resistant to treatment with lithium and antipsychotic drugs and for rapid cyclers. A **rapid cycler** is a patient with bipolar disorder who has many episodes of mood swings close together (four or more in 1 year). Persons with schizophrenia (especially catatonic), those with schizoaffective syndromes, psychotic patients who are pregnant, and patients with Parkinson's disease can also benefit from ECT.

ECT is not necessarily effective, however, in patients with Dysphoric Disorder, unconventional depression, personality disorders, drug dependence, or depression secondary to situational or social difficulties.

The usual course of ECT for a patient with depression is two or three treatments per week to a total of 6 to 12 treatments. Although no absolute contraindications to ECT exist, several conditions pose risks and require careful workup and management. Since the heart can be stressed at the onset of the seizure and for up to 10 minutes after, careful assessment and management in hypertension, congestive heart failure, cardiac arrhythmias, and other cardiac conditions is warranted (Welch, 2008). ECT also stresses the brain as a result of increased cerebral oxygen, blood flow, and intracranial pressure. Conditions such as brain tumors and subdural hematomas may increase the risk of using ECT. Providers of care and patients need to weigh the risk of continued disability or potential suicide from depression against ECT treatment risks.

Initiating Electroconvulsive Therapy

The procedure is explained to the patient, and informed consent is obtained if the patient is being treated voluntarily. For a patient treated involuntarily, permission may be obtained from the next of kin although in some states treatment must be court-ordered. The patient is usually given a general anesthetic to induce sleep (e.g., a short-acting barbiturate such as methohexital sodium [Brevital]) and a muscle-paralyzing agent (e.g., succinylcholine) to prevent muscle distress and fractures. These medications have revolutionized the comfort and safety of ECT. An electroencephalogram (EEG) monitors brain waves, and an electrocardiogram (ECG) monitors cardiac responses. Brief seizures (30 to 60+ seconds) are deliberately induced by an electrical current (as brief as 1 second) transmitted through electrodes attached to one or both sides of the head.

Potential Adverse Reactions

Patients wake about 15 minutes after the procedure. After awakening from ECT, the patient is often confused and disoriented for several hours. The nurse and family may need to orient the patient frequently during the course of treatment. Many patients state that they have memory deficits for the first few weeks after the course of treatment, but memory usually, although not always, recovers. ECT is not a permanent cure for depression, and maintenance treatment with antidepressants decreases the relapse rate. Maintenance ECT (once a week to once a month) may also help to decrease relapse rates for patients with recurrent depression or psychotic symptoms.

EVIDENCE-BASED PRACTICE

Electroconvulsive Therapy (ECT) and Older Adults

Amazon, J., McNeely, E., Lehr, S., & Marquardt, M. G. (2008). The decision-making process of older adults who elect to receive ECT. *Journal of Psychosocial Nursing, 46*(5), 45–52.

Problem

Electroconvulsive therapy (ECT) remains an effective treatment option for people experiencing late-life depression; however, the decision-making process of older adults opting for ECT remains largely misunderstood. Nurses must have a better understanding of this process in order to assist older adults as they make decisions about whether to have ECT.

Purpose of Study

The purpose of the study was to explore the decision-making process of older adults electing to receive ECT.

Methods

Seven older adults between the ages of 60 and 90 who had received ECT participated in this qualitative, exploratory phenomenological study. Each participant engaged in a 1-hour, in-depth interview in which they were asked to describe the process of deciding to receive ECT. The participants' responses were analyzed for common themes.

Key Findings

Four key themes that emerged were:

- Support from family, friends, and significant others
- Trust that the treatment would work
- Past experience with positive results from ECT, either for themselves or FOR a friend or acquaintance
- A sense of desperation for the need to get well

An overriding substantive theme involved the negative impact of the stigma of both mental illness and ECT. Participants feared what other people would think if knowledge of their ECT was made known.

Implications for Nursing Practice

In addition to providing education and information to older adults considering whether to receive ECT, psychiatric mental health nurses must also work to break through the stigma and discrimination or lack of support that these patients face.

Transcranial Magnetic Stimulation

Transcranial magnetic stimulation (TMS) is a noninvasive treatment modality that uses MRI-strength magnetic pulses to stimulate focal areas of the cerebral cortex. Mitchell and Loo (2006) analyzed 25 studies involving the use of TMS for patients with depression and concluded that benefits were statistically significant and treatment was safe. Ongoing research is needed to determine optimum treatment guidelines (frequency, intensity, and duration) and who would benefit most from this type of procedure. More recent studies show promise in using TMS as an alternative to antidepressants in pregnant women (Kim et al, 2011) and as an option in lieu of ECT (Keshtkar, Ghanizadeh, & Firoozabadi, 2011).

Indications

In 2008, the United States Food and Drug Administration (FDA) approved the use of TMS for patients who have been unresponsive to other methods of treatment for depression. A large-scale, multisite, randomized controlled trial reported that TMS is an effective stand-alone (without antidepressants) treatment (O'Reardon et al., 2010).

Initiating Transcranial Magnetic Stimulation

Outpatient treatment with TMS takes about 30 minutes and is typically ordered for 5 days a week for 4 to 6 weeks. Patients are awake and alert during the procedure. An electromagnet is placed on the patient's scalp, and short, magnetic pulses pass into the prefrontal cortex of the brain (Figure 14-3). These pulses are similar to those used by MRI scanners but are more focused. The pulses cause electrical charges to flow and induce neurons to fire or become active. During TMS, patients feel a slight tapping or knocking in the head, contraction of the scalp, and tightening of the jaws.

Potential Adverse Reactions

After the procedure, patients may experience a headache and lightheadedness. No neurological deficits or memory problems have been noted. Seizures are a rare complication of TMS; one research study that analyzed 10,000 treatment sessions reported no occurrence of seizures (Janicak et al., 2008). Most of the common side effects of TMS are mild and include scalp tingling and discomfort at the administration site.

Vagus Nerve Stimulation

The use of **vagus nerve stimulation (VNS)** originated as a treatment for epilepsy. Clinicians noted that while VNS decreased seizures, it also appeared to improve mood in a population that normally experiences increased rates of depression (Dougherty & Rauch, 2008). The theory behind VNS relates to the action of the vagus nerve, the longest cranial nerve, which extends from the brainstem to organs in the neck, chest, and abdomen. Researchers believe that electrical stimulation of the vagus nerve results in boosting the level of neurotransmitters, thereby improving mood and also improving the action of antidepressants (Stahl, 2008).

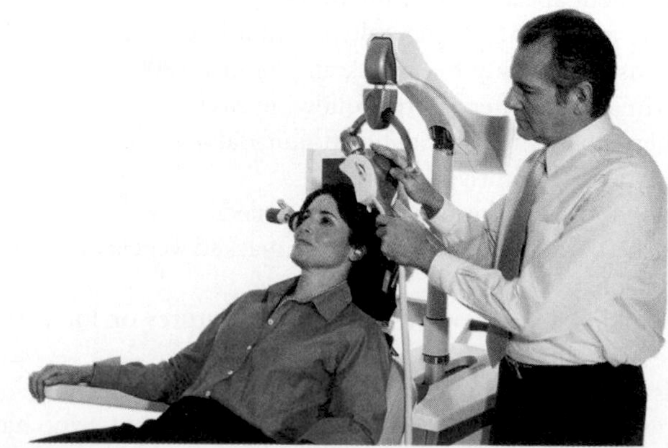

FIG 14-3 Transcranial magnetic stimulation. (Photo courtesy of Neuronetics.)

Indications

Nearly a decade after VNS was approved for use in Europe, the FDA granted approval for VNS use in the United States for treatment-resistant depression. The efficacy of VNS in treating depression is still being established. Other potential applications of VNS include anxiety, obesity, and pain (George et al., 2008).

Initiating Vagus Nerve Stimulation

The surgery to implant VNS is typically an outpatient procedure. A pacemaker-like device is implanted surgically into the left chest wall (Stahl, 2008). The device is connected to a thin, flexible wire that is threaded up and wrapped around the vagus nerve on the left side of the neck. After surgery, an infrared magnetic wand is held against the chest while a personal computer or personal digital assistant (PDA) is used to program the frequency of pulses. Pulses are usually delivered for 30 seconds, every 5 minutes, for 24 hours a day. Antidepressant action typically occurs in several weeks.

Potential Adverse Reactions

The implantation of VNS (Figure 14-4) is a surgical procedure, carrying with it the risks inherent in any surgical procedure (e.g., pain, infection, sensitivity to anesthesia). Side effects of active VNS therapy are due to the proximity of the lead on the vagus nerve, which is close to the laryngeal and pharyngeal branches of the left vagus nerve (Dougherty & Rauch, 2008). Voice alteration occurs in nearly 60% of patients. Other side effects include neck pain, cough, paresthesia, and dyspnea, which tend to decrease with time. The device can be temporarily turned off at any time by placing a special magnet over the implant. This may be especially helpful when engaging in public speaking or heavy exercise.

Deep Brain Stimulation

Deep brain stimulation (DBS) is a treatment whereby electrodes are surgically implanted into specific areas of the brain in order to stimulate those regions identified to be underactive in depression. DBS is a long-approved surgical treatment for Parkinson's disease but is just now being investigated as an effective treatment in depression (Fitzgerald, 2008). It differs from VNS in that electrodes are implanted directly into the brain to modify brain activity directly. While it is similar to VNS in that a device is implanted in the chest wall designed to provide electrical stimulation, DBS is more invasive and as such poses more of a risk, which includes the potential of intracranial hemorrhage. DBS is being evaluated primarily in regard to treatment-resistant major depression.

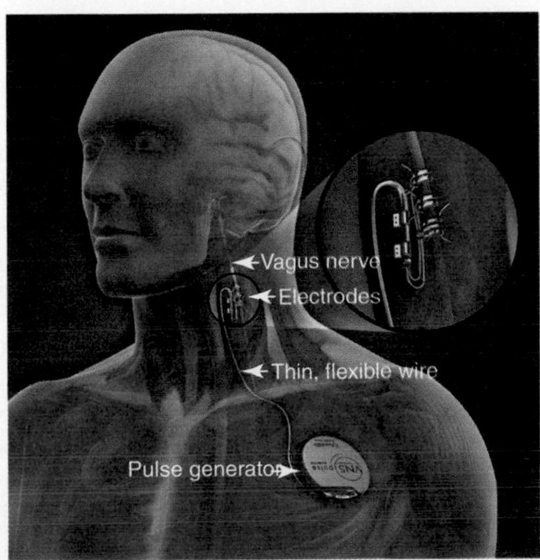

FIG 14-4 Vagus nerve stimulation. (Image courtesy of Cyberonics, Inc.)

Light Therapy

Light therapy has been researched for nearly 20 years and is accepted as a first-line treatment for seasonal affective disorder (SAD). People with SAD often live in regions in which there are marked seasonal differences in the amount of daylight, which is thought to disrupt melatonin production, circadian rhythms, or the ability to process dopamine and norepinephrine. Whatever the cause, the effect is a seasonal depression. Light therapy may also be useful as an adjunct in treating chronic major depressive disorder or dysphoric disorder with seasonal exacerbations (Lieverse et al, 2010).

Light therapy is thought to be effective because of the influence of light on melatonin. Melatonin is secreted by the pineal gland and is necessary for maintaining and shifting biological rhythms. Exposure to light suppresses the nocturnal secretion of melatonin, which seems to have a therapeutic effect on people with SAD (Harvard Medical School, 2008). Ideal treatment consists of 30 to 45 minutes of exposure daily to a 10,000-lux light source. Morning exposure is best; however, success has been reported when exposure occurs at other times of the day or in divided doses. Anecdotal reports suggest that increasing the available light by adding additional light sources may also help to elevate mood. For those affected by SAD, light therapy has been found to be as effective in reducing depressive symptoms as medications. Negative side effects include headache and jitteriness (Lakoski, 2010). Concerns about eye damage from light exposure have not been validated (Harvard Medical School, 2008).

St. John's Wort

St. John's wort *(Hypericum perforatum)* is a flower that can be processed into tea or tablets. It is thought to increase the amount of serotonin, norepinephrine, and dopamine in the brain, resulting in antidepressant effects. Studies of St. John's wort used in the treatment of depression offer mixed results. It has generally been found to be as effective as antidepressants in the treatment of mild to moderate depression, but usefulness in severe depression has not been established (Carpenter, 2011). Because St. John's wort is not regulated by the FDA, concentrations of the active ingredients may vary from preparation to preparation, which may account for some variation in research results. St. John's wort has the potential for adverse reactions when taken with other medications, and neither safety nor standardization of dose has been established; therefore, it should be used with caution during pregnancy or in children.

Exercise

Substantial evidence suggests that exercise can enhance mood and counteract symptoms of depression (Harris et al., 2006). Cripps (2008) reports that exercise has biological, social, and psychological effects on symptoms of depression. Research shows that exercise increases the availability of serotonin, which is typically low in depression. It has also been demonstrated to dampen the activity of the hypothalamic-pituitary-adrenocorticoid (HPA) axis, which is believed to be overly active in depression. People with depression who exercise regularly report feeling an elevated mood and greater happiness, and they become more socially involved. Additional benefits of exercise are that it is more easily accessed, less expensive, and results in fewer side effects than antidepressants.

Advanced Practice Interventions

The advanced practice nurse is qualified to provide psychotherapy, social skills training, and group therapy (American Psychiatric Nurses Association et al., 2007). In some states, nurses who have met appropriate educational standards may be certified to prescribe medication to treat depression.

Psychotherapy

Cognitive behavioral therapy (CBT), interpersonal therapy (IPT), time-limited focused psychotherapy, and behavioral therapy all are especially effective in the treatment of depression; however, only CBT and IPT demonstrate superiority in the maintenance phase. CBT helps people reconstruct their negative thought patterns and behaviors, leading to lasting mood improvements, whereas IPT focuses on working through personal relationships that may contribute to depression (Depression, 2010).

Group Therapy

Group therapy is a widespread modality for the treatment of depression; it increases the number of people who can receive treatment at a decreased cost per individual. Another advantage is that groups offer patients an opportunity to socialize and share common feelings and concerns, which decreases feelings of isolation, hopelessness, helplessness, and alienation. Therapy groups also provide a controlled environment in which patients can explore their patterns of interaction and response to others, which may contribute to or exacerbate their depression.

Future of Treatment

There is a great need for earlier detection, earlier intervention, prevention of progression, achievement of remission, and integration of neuroscience and behavioral science in the treatment of depression.

Healthy People 2020 (Mental Health and Mental Objectives, 2012) identified increasing screening for depression, increasing prevention efforts, and improving access to treatment in the national health goals. Particular emphasis is on:

- Improving screening for children and adolescents in a variety of health care and community settings
- Reducing the incidence of depressive episodes in children, adolescents, and adults
- Increasing mental health treatment to adults, children, and adolescents in primary care
- Increasing the number of patients with depression, both children and adults, who receive treatment

EVALUATION

Because each patient presents differently, outcome evaluation will be tailored to each patient's unique presentation; however, a patient with depression is usually admitted to an inpatient unit because of an inability to stay safe or to provide for basic needs. This means that when caring for a patient in the hospital, there will be some anticipated areas of evaluation. This will always include ongoing evaluation on the frequency and content of suicidal ideation. Are these thoughts still present? How frequently do they occur? Does the patient have a plan? Is the patient able to stop suicidal thoughts and formulate alternatives to suicidal thoughts? Is the patient able to eat? The nurse will check the patient's meal trays to see if the patient is maintaining an adequate intake. In an inpatient setting the nurse will also evaluate the patient's sleep pattern. Is the patient able to fall asleep? Stay asleep? Has the number of hours of sleep increased since admission? What about personal hygiene and grooming? Has the nurse objectively noticed improvement in the patient's appearance? If the depression is severe and the patient has demonstrated psychotic features, the nurse will ask about auditory hallucinations and evaluate for signs of delusions.

Outcomes relating to thought processes, self-esteem, and social interactions are frequently formulated because these areas are often problematic in people with depression. The nurse will ask the patient how he or she is feeling about himself or herself. How is she getting along with others, performing at school or managing at home? The nurse will evaluate if the patient gives a preponderance of negative answers or if the patient is able to identify positive aspects of his or her functioning.

If indicators have not been met, an analysis of the data, nursing diagnoses, goals, and planned nursing interventions is made. The care plan is reassessed and reformulated as necessary.

QUALITY IMPROVEMENT

National objectives for outcomes improvement related to major depressive disorder have been set by the Department of Health and Human Services in *Healthy People 2020* (Mental Health and Mental Objectives, 2012). National goals include increasing the percentage of individuals with major depressive disorder who receive treatment to 75% (up from 68% in 2008). Other goals involve increasing the number of physicians offices who routinely screen for depression. The Center for Quality Assessment and Improvement in Mental Health (CQAIMH, 2012) has links to reliable outcome measures for patients with major depression covering a variety of aspects of care that include treatment and screening.

Nurses caring for these patients should still be committed to improving outcomes within their own treatment settings. In order for quality improvement to be successful, nurses and other members of the health care team must try new approaches to improve various aspects of care (Goldberg, Pincus

& Ghinassi, 2006). The Center for Quality Assessment and Improvement in Mental Health (CQAIMH, 2012) has links to reliable outcome measures for patients with major depression, covering a variety of aspects of care that include treatment and screening. These tools are available at the CQAIMH website at http://www.cqaimh.org/index.html.

KEY POINTS TO REMEMBER

- Depression is the most common psychiatric disorder.
- There are a number of subtypes of depression and depressive clinical phenomena. The two primary depressive disorders are major depressive disorder (major depression) and dysthymic disorder (DD).
- The symptoms of major depression are usually severe enough to interfere with a person's social or occupational functioning. A person with major depression may or may not have psychotic symptoms, and the symptoms usually exhibited during an episode of major depression are different from the characteristics of the normal premorbid personality.
- The symptoms of CDD or DD are often chronic (lasting at least 2 years) and are considered mild to moderate. Usually a person's social or occupational functioning is not greatly impaired. The symptoms in a DD are often congruent with the person's usual pattern of functioning.
- Many theories exist about the cause of depression. The most accepted is psychophysiological theory; however, cognitive theory, learned helplessness theory, and the diathesis-stress theory help explain triggers to depression and maintenance of depressive thoughts and feelings.
- Nursing assessment includes the evaluation of affect, thought processes (especially suicidal thoughts), mood, feelings, physical behavior, communication, and religious beliefs and spirituality. The nurse also must be aware of the symptoms that may mask depression.
- Nursing diagnoses can be numerous. Individuals with depression are always evaluated for risk for suicide. Some other common nursing diagnoses are *Chronic low self-esteem, Imbalanced nutrition, Constipation, Disturbed sleep pattern, Ineffective coping,* and *Disabled family coping.*
- Working with people who have depression can evoke intense feelings of hopelessness and frustration in health care workers. Nurses must clarify expectations of themselves and their patients and sort personal feelings from those communicated by the patient via empathy. Peer supervision and individual supervision by an experienced nurse clinician, psychiatric social worker, or psychologist are useful in increasing therapeutic potential.
- Interventions with patients who have depression involve several approaches. Basic-level interventions include using specific principles of communication, planning activities of daily living, administering or participating in psychopharmacological therapy, maintaining a therapeutic environment, and teaching patients about the biochemical aspects of depression.
- Advanced practice interventions may include several short-term psychotherapies that are effective in the treatment of depression, including IPT, CBT, skills training (assertiveness and social skills), and some forms of group therapy.
- Depression is often overlooked in children, adolescents, and older adults because symptoms of depression are often mistaken for signs of normal development.
- Planning and interventions for patients with depression are based on the recovery model, which involves a therapeutic alliance with health care professionals in order to achieve outcomes based on individual patient needs and values.
- Evaluation is ongoing throughout the nursing process, and patients' outcomes are compared with the stated outcome criteria and short-term and intermediate indicators. The care plan is revised when indicators are not being met.

CRITICAL THINKING

1. You are spending time with Mr. Plotsky, who is undergoing a workup for depression. He hardly makes eye contact, slouches in his seat, and wears a blank but sad expression. Mr. Plotsky has had numerous bouts of major depression in the past and says to you, "This will be my last depression. I will never go through this again."
   - Since safety is the first concern, what are the appropriate questions to ask Mr. Plotsky at this time?
   - In terms of behaviors, thought processes, activities of daily living, and ability to function at work and home, give examples of the kinds of signs and symptoms you might find when assessing a patient with depression.
   - Mr. Plotsky tells you that he has been on every medication there is, but none has worked. He asks you about the herb St. John's wort. What should you tell him about its effectiveness for severe depression, interactions with other antidepressants, and regulatory status?
   - What might be some somatic options for a person who is resistant to antidepressant medications?
   - Mr. Plotsky asks what causes depression. In simple terms, how might you respond to his query?
   - Mr. Plotsky tells you that he has never tried therapy because he thinks it is for weaklings. What information could you give him about various therapeutic modalities that have proven effective for other patients with depression?
2. You are working with Ms. Folk, a 28-year-old with major depression on long-term antidepressant therapy. She asks you about the possibility of pregnancy while taking her SSRIs.
   - What are some of the things Ms. Folk might want to consider about taking antidepressants if she plans to get pregnant?
   - If she decides to stop taking her antidepressants, what are some things she might do to help manage her depression?

CHAPTER REVIEW

1. The nurse is caring for a patient who exhibits disorganized thinking and delusions. The patient repeatedly states, "I hear voices of aliens trying to contact me." The nurse should recognize this presentation as which type of major depressive disorder (major depression)?
   a. Seasonal Affective Disorder
   b. Dysthymic Disorder
   c. Premenstrual Dysphoric disorder
   d. Psychotic
2. A nurse is educating a patient about the causes of depression. Which statement lets the nurse know the patient understands the neurobiological theory of depression?
   a. "My depression is made worse because my marriage is stressful."

b. "Sometimes I believe that I can't help myself. That's why I get so depressed."
c. "I'm depressed because my parents were depressed."
d. "If I take these medications as prescribed, I should start to think clearly and feel energized."

3. The nurse is planning care for a patient with depression who will be discharged to home soon. What aspect of teaching should be the priority on the nurse's discharge plan of care?
   a. Pharmacological teaching
   b. Safety risk
   c. Awareness of symptoms that increase depression
   d. The need for interpersonal contact
4. The nurse is reviewing orders given for a patient with depression. Which order should the nurse question?
   a. A low starting dose of a tricyclic antidepressant
   b. An SSRI given initially with an MAOI
   c. Electroconvulsive therapy to treat suicidal thoughts
   d. Elavil to address the patient's agitation
5. A female patient tells the nurse that she would like to begin taking St. John's wort for depression. What teaching should the nurse provide?
   a. "St. John's wort should be taken several hours after your other antidepressant."
   b. "St. John's wort has generally been shown to be effective in treating depression."
   c. "This supplement is safe to take if you are pregnant."
   d. "St. John's wort is regulated by the FDA, so you can be assured of its safety."

Answers to Chapter Review
1. d; 2. d; 3. c; 4. b; 5. b.

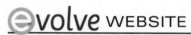

Visit the Evolve website for a posttest on the content in this chapter: http://evolve.elsevier.com/Varcarolis

Post-Test interactive review

REFERENCES

Accortt, E. E., Freeman, M. P., & Allen, J. J. (2008). Women and major depressive disorder: Clinical perspectives on causal pathways. *Journal of Women's Health, 17*, 1583–1590.

Akpafflong, M. J., Wilson-Lawson, M., & Kunik, M. E. (2008) Antidepressant-associated side effects in older adult depressed patients. *Geriatrics, 63*(4), 18–23.

American Psychiatric Association. (2013). *DSM-5 table of contents.* Retrieved from http://www.psychiatry.org/dsm5.

Arnow, B. A., Hunkeler, E. M., Blasey, C. M., Lee, J., Constantino, M. J., Fireman, B., . . . Hayward, C. (2006). Comorbid depression, chronic pain, and disability in primary care. *Psychosomatic Medicine, 68*, 262–268.

Beck, A., Crain, L., Solberg, L., Unutzer, J., Glasgow, R., Maciose, M., & Whitebird, R. (2011). Severity of depression and magnitude of productivity loss. *Annals of Family Medicine, 9*(4), 305–311.

Beck, A. T., Brown, G., Berchick, R. J., Stewart, B. L., & Steer, R. A. (2006). Relationship between hopelessness and ultimate suicide: A replication with psychiatric outpatients. *Focus, 4*, 291–296.

Beck, A. T., & Rush, A. J. (1995). Cognitive therapy. In H.I. Kaplan & B.J. Sadock (Eds.), *Comprehensive textbook of psychiatry/VI: Vol. 2* (pp. 1847–1856). Baltimore, MD: Williams & Wilkins.

Brendel, R. W., Lagomasino, I. T., Perlis, R. H., & Stern, T. A. (2008). The suicidal patient. In T.A. Stern, J.F. Rosenbaum, M. Fava, J. Biederman, & S.L. Rauch (Eds.), *Massachusetts General Hospital comprehensive clinical psychiatry* (pp. 733–745). St. Louis, MO: Mosby.

Bulechek, G. M., Butcher, H. K., Dochterman, J. M, & Wagner, C. M. (2013). *Nursing interventions classification (NIC)* (6th ed.). St. Louis, MO: Mosby.

Carpenter, D. (2011). St. John's wort and S-adenosyl Methionine as "natural" alternatives to conventional antidepressants in the era of the suicidality boxed warning: What is the evidence for clinically relevant benefit? *Alternative Medicine Health Review, 16*(1), 17–39.

Cowell, J., McNaughton, D., Ailey, S., Gross, D., & Fogg, L. (2009). Clinical trial outcomes of the Mexican American Problem Solving Program (MAPS). *Hispanic Health Care International, 7*(4), 178–189.

Cremens, M. C., & Wiechers, I. (2010). Care of the geriatric patient. In T. Stern, G. Fricchione, N. Cassem, M. Jellinek, J. Rosenbaum (Eds.), *Massachusetts General Hospital handbook of general hospital psychiatry* (6th ed.) Philadelphia, PA: Saunders.

Cripps, F. (2008). Exercise your mind: Physical activity as a therapeutic technique for depression. *International Journal of Therapy and Rehabilitation, 15*, 460–464.

Department of Health and Human Services. (2012). *Mental health and mental disorders.* Retrieved from http://www.healthypeople.gov/2020/topicsobjectives2020/objectiveslist.aspx?topicId=28.

Depression: The treatment and management of depression in adults. (2010). London, UK: National Collaborating Centre for Mental Health & The Royal College of Psychiatrists.

Dougherty, D. D., & Rauch, S. L. (2008). Neurotherapeutics. In T. A. Stern, J. F. Rosenbaum, M. Fava, J. Biederman, & S. L. Rauch (Eds.), *Massachusetts General Hospital comprehensive clinical psychiatry* (pp. 645–650). St. Louis, MO: Mosby.

Dudley, M., Hadzi-Pavlovic, D., Andrews, D., & Perich, T. (2008). New-generation antidepressants, suicide and depressed adolescents: How should clinicians respond to changing evidence? *The Australian and New Zealand Journal of Psychiatry, 42*, 456–466.

Fitzgerald, P. (2008). Brain stimulation techniques for the treatment of depression and other psychiatric disorders. *Australian Psychiatry, 16*(3), 183–190.

Garvey, K. A., Penn, J. V., Campbell, A. L., Esposito-Smythers, C., & Spirito, A. (2009). Contracting for safety with patients: Clinical practice and forensic implications. *Journal of the American Academy of Psychiatry Law, 37*(3), 363–370.

George, M. S., Nahas, Z. H., Borckardt, J. J., Anderson, B., & Foust, M. J. (2008). Nonpharmacological somatic treatments. In R.E. Hales, S.C. Yudofsky, & G.O. Gabbard (Eds.), *Textbook of psychiatry* (pp. 1133–1153). Washington, DC: American Psychiatric Publishing.

Gilbody, S., Richards, D., & Barkham, M. (2007). Diagnosing depression in primary care: UK validation of PHQ-9 and CORE-OM. *British Journal of General Practice, 57*, 650–652.

Greenberg, M., Pincus, H., & Ghinassi, F. (2006). Of treatment systems and depression: An overview of quality-improvement opportunities in hospital-based psychiatric care. *Harvard Review of Psychiatry, 14*(4), 195–203.

Harris, A. H., Cronkite, R., & Moos, R. (2006). Physical activity, exercise coping, and depression in a 10-year cohort study of depressed patients. *Journal of Affective Disorders, 93(1-3)*, 79–85.

Harvard Medical School. (2008). A *SAD* story: Light therapy and antidepressants help people who get depressed during the winter. *Harvard Health Letter*. Retrieved from http://www.health.harvard.edu/fhg/updates/Seasonal-affective-disorder.shtml.

Heisel, M., Duberstein, P., Lyness, J., & Feldman, M. (2010). Screening for suicide ideation among older primary care adults. *JABFM, 23*, 260–269.

Herdman, T. H. (Ed.), (2012). *NANDA international nursing diagnoses: Definitions and classification 2012–2014*. Oxford, UK: Wiley-Blackwell.

Jacobs, B., & Taylor, E. (2009). Depression in children and adolescents: A review. In H. S. Herman & M. Norman Maj (Eds.), *Depressive disorders*. Hoboken, NJ: Wiley.

Janicak, P. G., O'Reardon, J. P., Sampson, S. M., Husain, M. M., Lisanby, S. H., Rado, . . . Demitrack, M. A. (2008). Transcranial magnetic stimulation in the treatment of major depressive disorder: A comprehensive summary of safety experience from acute exposure, extended exposure, and during reintroduction treatment. *Journal of Clinical Psychiatry, 69*(2), 222–232.

Johnson, J. (2012). Quality improvement. In G. Sherwood & J. Barnsteiner (Eds.), *Quality and Safety in Nursing* (pp. 113-132). Ames, IA: Wiley-Blackwell.

Joska, J.A., & Stein, D.J. (2008). Mood disorders. In R.E. Hales, S.C. Yudofsky, & G.O. Gabbard (Eds.), *Textbook of psychiatry* (pp. 457–504). Washington, DC: American Psychiatric Publishing.

Keshtkar, M., Ghanizadeh, A., & Firoozabadi, A. (2011). Repetitive transcranial magnetic stimulation versus electroconvulsive therapy for the treatment of major depressive disorder, a randomized controlled clinical trial. *Journal of ECT, 27*(4), 310–314.

Kim, D., Epperson, N., Paré, E., Gonzalez, J., Parry, S., Thase, M., Cristancho, P., Sammel, M., & O'Reardon, J. (2011). An open label pilot study of transcranial magnetic stimulation for pregnant women with major depressive disorder. *Journal of Women's Health, 20*(2), 255–261.

Krishnadas, R., & Cavanagh, J. (2012). Depression: An inflammatory illness? *Journal of Neurology, Neurosurgery, and Psychiatry, 83*(5), 495–502.

Lahoff, F. W. (2010). Overview of the genetics of major depressive disorder. *Current Psychiatry Reports, 12*, 539–546.

Laskoski J. (2010). Is bright light therapy effective for improving depressive symptoms in adults with seasonal affective disorder (SAD)? *Internet Journal of Academic Physician Assistants, 7*(2) Retrieved from http://www.ispub.com/journal/the-internet-journal-of-academic-physician-assistants/volume-7-number-2/is-bright-light-therapy-effective-for-improving-depressive-symptoms-in-adults-with-seasonal-affective-disorder-sad.html#sthash.9rRO9oSA.dpbs.

Lehne, R. A. (2010). *Pharmacology for nursing care* (7th ed.). St. Louis, MO: Saunders.

Lieverse, R., Van Someren, E., Nielen, M., Uitdehaag, B., Smit, J., & Hoogendijk W. (2011). Bright light treatment in elderly patients with nonseasonal major depressive disorder: A randomized placebo-controlled trial. *Archives of General Psychiatry, 68*(1), 61–70.

Live your life well (2009). Retrieved from http://www.mentalhealthamerica.net/llw/depression_screen.cfm.

Lorberg, B., & Prince, J. (2010). Psychopharmacological management of children and adolescents. In T. Stern, G. Fricchione, N. Cassem, M. Jellinek, & J. Rosenbaum (Eds.), *Massachusetts General Hospital handbook of general hospital psychiatry* (6th ed.). Philadelphia, PA: Saunders.

Louch, P. (2009). Diagnosing and treating depression. *Practice Nurse, 37*(10), 42–48.

Martinez, M., Marangell, L. B., & Martinez, J. M. (2008). Psychopharmacology. In R. E. Hales, S. C. Yudofsky, & G. O. Gabbard (Eds.), *Textbook of psychiatry* (pp. 1073). Arlington, VA: American Psychiatric Publishing.

Meadows-Oliver, M., & Sadler, L. (2010). Depression among adolescent mothers enrolled in a high school parenting program. *Journal of Pyschosocial Nursing, 48*(12), 34–41.

Mental Health and Mental Objectives. (2012). *Healthy people 2020*. Washington, DC: U.S. Department of Health and Human Services.

Miller, G. E., & Cole, S. W. (2012). Clustering of depression and inflammation in adolescents previously exposed to childhood adversity. *Biological Psychiatry, 72*(1), 34–40.

Miller, L., Wickramaratne, P., Gameroff, M., Sage, M., Tenke, C., & Weissman, M. (2012). Religiosity and major depression in adults at high risk: A ten-year prospective study. *American Journal of Psychiatry, 69*(1), 89–94.

Moorhead, S., Johnson, M., Maas, M. L., & Swanson, E. (2013). *Nursing outcomes classification (NOC)* (5th ed.). St. Louis, MO: Mosby.

National Institute of Mental Health. (2012a). *Ethnic disparities persist in depression diagnosis and treatment among older Americans*. Retrieved from http://www.nimh.nih.gov/science-news/2012/ethnic-disparities-persist-in-depression-diagnosis-and-treatment-among-older-americans.shtml.

National Institute of Mental Health. (2012b). *Major depressive disorder among adults*. Retrieved from http://www.nimh.nih.gov/statistics/1MAJOR DEPRESSIVE DISORDER_ADULT.shtml.

National Institute of Mental Health. (2012c). *Older adults: Depression and suicide facts (fact sheet)*. Retrieved from http://www.nimh.nih.gov/health/publications/older-adults-depression-and-suicide-facts-fact-sheet/index.shtml#part-of-aging.

National Institute of Mental Health. (2012d). *Brain basics*. Retrieved from http://www.nimh.nih.gov/educational-resources/brain-basics/brain-basics.shtml#Brain-Basics-in-Real-Life.

Nemeroff, C. F., & Nemeroff, C. B. (2007). Corticotropin-releasing factor and the psychobiology of early-life stress. *Current directions in psychological science, 16*(2), 85–89.

Niciu, M., Chan, G., Gelernter, J., Arias, A., Douglas, K., Weiss, R., . . . Kranzler, H. (2009). Subtypes of major depression in substance dependence. *Addiction, 104*, 1700–1709.

O'Reardon, J., Altinay, M., & Christancho, P. (2010). Transcranial magnetic stimulation: A new treatment option for major depression. *Psychiatric Times, 27*(9), 26–29.

Pilkington, K., Rampes, H., & Richardson, J. (2006). Complementary medicine for depression. *Expert Review of Neurotherapeutics, 6*, 1741–1751.

Preston, J., O'Neal, J., & Talaga, M. (2010). *Handbook of clinical psychopharmaocology* (6th ed.). Oakland, CA: New Harbinger.

Randlov, C., Mehlsen, J., Thomsen, C. F., Hedman, C., Von Fircks, H., & Winther, K. (2006). The efficacy of St. John's wort in patients with minor depressive symptoms or dysthymia—A double-blind placebo-controlled study. *Phytomedicine, 13(4)*, 215–221.

Sadock, V.A., & Sadock, B. (2008). *Concise textbook of clinical psychiatry* (3rd ed.). Philadelphia, PA: Lippincott, Williams, and Wilkins.

Seligman, M. E. (1973). Fall into hopelessness. *Psychology Today, 43*(7), 43–48.

Seriani, D. (2011). *Living with depression*. Lanham, MD: Rowman and Littlefield.

Shattell, M., Villalba, J., Stokes, N., Hamilton, D., Foster, J., Petrini, R., . . . Faulkner, C. (2009). Depression in Latinas residing in emerging Latino immigrant communities in the United States. *Hispanic Health Care International, 7*(4), 190–202.

Shear, M., Simon, N., Wall, M., Zisook, S., Neimeyer, R., Duan, N., . . . Keshaviah, A. (2011). Complicated grief and related bereavement issues for DSM-5. *Depression and Anxiety, 28*, 103–117.

Sheikh, J., & Yesavage, J. (1986). Geriatric Depression Scale (GDS): Recent evidence and development of a shorter version. *Clinical Gerontologist, 5*(1–2), 165–173.

Simon, N. M., & Rosenbaum, J. F. (2003). *Anxiety and depression comorbidity: Implications and intervention*. Retrieved from http://www.medscape.com/viewarticle/451325.

Smoller, J., & Korf, B. (2008). The road ahead. In J. Smoller, B. Sheidley, & M. Tsuang (Eds.), *Psychiatric genetics* (pp. 277–304). Arlington, VA: American Psychiatric Association.

Sreevani, R., & Reddemma, K. (2012). Depression and spirituality—a qualitative approach. *International Journal of Nursing Education, 4*(1), 90–93.

Stahl, S. M. (2008). *Stahl's essential pharmacology* (3rd ed.). Cambridge, UK: Cambirdge University Press.

Stringaris, A. (2011). Irritability in children and adolescents: A challenge for the DSM-5. *European Child and Adolescent Psychiatry, 20*, 61–66.

Udechuku, A., Nguyen, T., Hill, R., & Szego, K. (2010). Antidepressants in pregnancy: A systematic review. *Australian & New Zealand Journal of Psychiatry, 44*, 978–996.

U.S. Food and Drug Administration, Center for Drug Evaluation and Research (2004). *Worsening depression and suicidality in patients being treated with antidepressant medications*. Retrieved from http://www.fda.gov/cder/drug/antidepressants/AntidepressantsPHA.htm.

Wasserman, D. (2011). *Depression*. New York: Oxford University Press.

Welch, C.A. (2008). Electroconvulsive therapy. In T. A. Stern, J. F. Rosenbaum, M. Fava, J. Biederman, & S. L. Rauch (Eds.), *Massachusetts General Hospital comprehensive clinical psychiatry* (pp. 635–644). St. Louis, MO: Mosby.

CHAPTER 15

Anxiety and Obsessive-Compulsive Related Disorders

Margaret Jordan Halter and Elizabeth M. Varcarolis

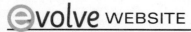

Visit the Evolve website for a pretest on the content in this chapter: http://evolve.elsevier.com/Varcarolis

Pre-Test interactive review

OBJECTIVES

1. Compare and contrast the four levels of anxiety in relation to perceptual field, ability to problem solve, and physical and other defining characteristics.
2. Identify defense mechanisms and consider one adaptive and one maladaptive (if any) use of each.
3. Describe clinical manifestations of each anxiety and obsessive-compulsive disorder.
4. Identify genetic, biological, psychological, and cultural factors that may contribute to anxiety and obsessive-compulsive disorders.
5. Describe feelings that may be experienced by nurses caring for patients with anxiety and obsessive-compulsive disorders.
6. Formulate four appropriate nursing diagnoses that can be used in treating a person with anxiety and obsessive-compulsive disorders.
7. Propose realistic outcome criteria for a patient with (a) generalized anxiety disorder, (b) panic disorder, and (c) obsessive-compulsive disorder.
8. Describe five basic nursing interventions used for patients with anxiety and obsessive-compulsive disorders.
9. Discuss four classes of medications appropriate for anxiety and obsessive-compulsive disorders.
10. Describe advanced-practice and basic-level interventions for anxiety and obsessive-compulsive disorders.

KEY TERMS AND CONCEPTS

agoraphobia
antianxiety (anxiolytic) drugs
anxiety
body dysmorphic disorder
defense mechanisms
fear
generalized anxiety disorder
hair pulling disorder
hoarding disorder
mild anxiety
moderate anxiety
obsessive-compulsive disorder
panic
panic disorder
separation anxiety disorder
severe anxiety
skin picking disorder
social anxiety disorder
specific phobias

For most people, anxiety is a part of everyday life. "I felt really nervous when I couldn't find a parking space right before my final exam; I know I would have done better if that hadn't happened." For some people, however, anxiety-related symptoms become severely debilitating and interfere with normal functioning. "Today I got so worried I wouldn't find a parking space before the final exam, I stayed home." Imagine being so incapacitated by anxiety that you live in dread of germs to the point where hand washing has become the focal point of your day. In this chapter, we will examine the concept of anxiety, defenses against anxiety, and an overview of anxiety and obsessive-compulsive disorders and their treatment.

ANXIETY

Anxiety is a universal human experience and is the most basic of emotions. It can be defined as a feeling of apprehension, uneasiness, uncertainty, or dread resulting from a real or perceived threat. Fear is a reaction to a specific danger, whereas anxiety is a vague sense of dread related to an unspecified or unknown danger; however, the body physiologically reacts in similar ways to both anxiety and fear. Another important distinction between anxiety and fear is that anxiety affects us at a deeper level. It invades the central core of the personality and erodes feelings of self-esteem and personal worth.

Dysfunctional behavior is often a defense against anxiety. When behavior is recognized as dysfunctional, nurses can initiate interventions to reduce anxiety. As anxiety decreases, dysfunctional behavior will frequently decrease, and vice versa.

Normal anxiety is a healthy reaction necessary for survival. It provides the energy needed to carry out the tasks involved in living and striving toward goals. Anxiety motivates people to make and survive change. It prompts constructive behaviors, such as studying for an examination, being on time for a job interview, preparing for a presentation, and working toward a promotion.

An understanding of the levels and defensive patterns used in response to anxiety is basic to psychiatric mental health nursing care. This understanding is essential for assessing and planning interventions to lower a patient's level of anxiety (as well as one's own) effectively. With practice, you will become skilled at identifying levels of anxiety, understanding the defenses used to alleviate anxiety, and evaluating the possible stressors that contribute to increased levels of anxiety.

LEVELS OF ANXIETY

As discussed in Chapter 2, Hildegard Peplau had a profound role in shaping the specialty of psychiatric mental health nursing. She identified anxiety as one of the most important concepts and developed an anxiety model that consists of four levels: mild, moderate, severe, and panic (Peplau, 1968). The boundaries between these levels are not distinct, and the behaviors and characteristics of individuals experiencing anxiety can and often do overlap. Identification of the specific level of anxiety is essential because interventions are based on the *degree* of the patient's anxiety.

Mild Anxiety

Mild anxiety occurs in the normal experience of everyday living and allows an individual to perceive reality in sharp focus. A person experiencing a mild level of anxiety sees, hears, and grasps more information, and problem solving becomes more effective. Physical symptoms may include slight discomfort, restlessness, irritability, or mild tension-relieving behaviors (e.g., nail biting, foot or finger tapping, fidgeting).

Moderate Anxiety

As anxiety increases, the perceptual field narrows, and some details are excluded from observation. The person experiencing moderate anxiety sees, hears, and grasps less information and may demonstrate **selective inattention**, in which only certain things in the environment are seen or heard unless they are pointed out. The ability to think clearly is hampered, but learning and problem solving can still take place although not at an optimal level. Sympathetic nervous system symptoms begin to kick in. The individual may experience tension, pounding heart, increased pulse and respiratory rate, perspiration, and mild somatic symptoms (e.g., gastric discomfort, headache, urinary urgency). Voice tremors and shaking may be noticed. Mild or moderate anxiety levels can be constructive because anxiety may be a signal that something in the person's life needs attention or is dangerous (see the Case Study and Nursing Care Plan for moderate anxiety on the Evolve website).

Severe Anxiety

The perceptual field of a person experiencing severe anxiety is greatly reduced. A person with severe anxiety may focus on one particular detail or many scattered details and have difficulty noticing what is going on in the environment, even when another points it out. Learning and problem solving are not possible at this level, and the person may be dazed and confused. Behavior is automatic and aimed at reducing or relieving anxiety. Somatic symptoms (e.g., headache, nausea, dizziness, insomnia) often increase; trembling and a pounding heart are common, and the person may experience hyperventilation and a sense of impending doom or dread (see Case Study and Nursing Care Plan 15-1).

Panic

Panic is the most extreme level of anxiety and results in markedly disturbed behavior. Someone in a state of panic is unable to process what is going on in the environment and may lose touch with reality. The behavior that results may be manifested as pacing, running, shouting, screaming, or withdrawal. Hallucinations, or false sensory perceptions (e.g., seeing people or objects not really there), may be experienced. Physical behavior may become erratic, uncoordinated, and impulsive. Automatic behaviors are used to reduce and relieve anxiety although such efforts may be ineffective. Acute panic may lead to exhaustion.

Review Table 15-1, which distinguishes among the levels of anxiety in regard to their (1) effects on perceptual field, (2) effects on problem solving, and (3) physical and other defining characteristics.

15-1 CASE STUDY AND NURSING CARE PLAN

Severe Level of Anxiety

The following case study describes a man experiencing a severe level of acute anxiety. See if you can match his signs and symptoms with those in Table 15-1.

Matt Michaels, a 63-year-old man, comes into the emergency department (ED) with his wife, Anne, who has taken an overdose of sleeping pills and antidepressant medications. Ten years earlier, Anne's mother died, and since that time she has suffered several episodes of severe depression with suicide attempts. She has needed hospitalization during these episodes. Anne Michaels had been released from the hospital 2 weeks earlier after treatment for depression and threatened suicide.

Matt has a long-established routine of giving his wife her antidepressant medications in the morning and her sleeping medication at night and keeping the bottles hidden when he is not at home. Today he had forgotten to hide the medications before he went to work. His wife had taken the remaining pills from both bottles with large quantities of alcohol. When Matt returned home for lunch, Anne was comatose. In the ED, Anne suffers cardiac arrest and is taken to the intensive care unit (ICU).

Matt is very jittery. He moves about the room aimlessly. He drops his hat, a medication card, and his keys. His hands are trembling, and he looks around the room, bewildered. He appears unable to focus on any one thing. He says over and over, in a loud, high-pitched voice, "Why didn't I hide the bottles?" He is wringing his hands and begins stomping his feet, saying, "It's all my fault. Everything is falling apart."

Other people in the waiting room appear distracted and alarmed by his behavior. Matt seems to be oblivious to his surroundings.

Assessment

Gabriel Brown, the psychiatric nurse clinician working in the ED, comes into the waiting room and assesses Matt's behavior as indicative of a severe anxiety level. After talking with Matt briefly, Gabriel believes nursing intervention is indicated. Gabriel bases his conclusion on the following assessment of the patient:

Objective Data

- Unable to focus on anything
- Engaging in purposeless activity (walking around aimlessly)
- Oblivious to his surroundings
- Showing unproductive relief behavior (stomping, wringing hands, dropping things)

Subjective Data

"Everything is falling apart."
"Why didn't I hide the bottles?"
"It's all my fault."

Diagnosis

- *Anxiety (severe)* related to the patient's perception of responsibility for his wife's coma and possible death, as evidenced by inability to focus, confusion, and the feeling that "everything is falling apart"

Outcomes Identification

Patient will demonstrate control of the anxiety response*

Planning

Gabriel thinks that if he can lower Matt's anxiety to a moderate level, he can work with Matt to get a clear picture of his situation and place the events in a more realistic perspective. He also thinks Matt needs to talk to someone and share some of his pain and confusion to help sort out his feelings. Gabriel identifies two short-term goals:

1. Patient's anxiety will decrease from severe to moderate by 4 PM.
2. Patient will verbalize his feelings and a need for assistance by 4 PM.

Implementation

Gabriel takes Matt to a quiet room in the back of the ED. He introduces himself to Matt and comments that he notices that Matt is upset. He says, "I will stay with you." At first, Matt finds it difficult to sit down and continues pacing around the room. Gabriel sits quietly and calmly while listening to Matt's self-recriminations. He attends carefully to what Matt is saying—and what he is not saying—to identify themes.

After a while, Matt becomes calmer and is able to sit next to Gabriel. Gabriel offers him orange juice, which he accepts and holds tightly.

Gabriel speaks calmly, using simple, clear statements. He uses communication tools that are helpful to Matt in sorting out his feelings and naming them.

DIALOGUE	THERAPEUTIC TOOL/COMMENT
Matt: Yes . . . yes . . . I forgot to hide the bottles. She usually tells me when she feels bad. Why didn't she tell me?	
Nurse: You think that if she had told you she wanted to kill herself, you would have hidden the pills?	Gabriel asks for clarification of Matt's thinking.
Matt: Yes, if I had only known, this wouldn't have happened.	
Nurse: It sounds as if you believe you should have known what your wife was thinking without her telling you.	Here Gabriel clarifies Matt's expectations that he should be able to read his wife's mind.
Matt: Well . . . yes . . . when you put it that way . . . I just don't know what I'll do if she dies.	

When Gabriel thinks that Matt has discussed his feelings of guilt sufficiently, he asks Matt to clarify his thinking about his wife's behavior. Matt is able to place his feelings of guilt in a more realistic perspective. Next, Gabriel brings up another issue—the question of whether Matt's wife will live or die.

DIALOGUE	THERAPEUTIC TOOL/COMMENT
Nurse: You said that if your wife dies, you don't know what you will do.	Gabriel reflects Matt's feelings back to him.
Matt: Oh, God (begins to cry); I can't live without her . . . she's all I have in the world.	
Silence	
Nurse: She means a great deal to you.	Gabriel reflects Matt's feelings back to him.
Matt: Everything. Since her mother died, we are each other's only family.	
Nurse: What would it mean to you if your wife died?	Gabriel asks Matt to evaluate his feelings about his wife.
Matt: I couldn't live by myself, alone. I couldn't stand it. (Starts to cry again.)	
Nurse: It sounds as if being alone is very frightening to you.	Gabriel restates in clear terms Matt's experience and feelings.
Matt: Yes . . . I don't know how I'd manage by myself.	
Nurse: A change like that could take time to adjust to.	Gabriel validates that if Matt's wife died, it would be very painful. At the same time, he implies hope that Matt could work through the death in time.
Matt: Yes . . . it would be very hard.	

*The expected outcome will be evaluated on a 5-point Likert scale ranging from 1 (never demonstrated) to 5 (consistently demonstrated).

15-1 CASE STUDY AND NURSING CARE PLAN—cont'd

Severe Level of Anxiety

Again, Gabriel gives Matt a chance to sort out his feelings and fears. Gabriel helps him focus on the reality that his wife may die and encourages him to express fears related to her possible death. After a while, Gabriel offers to go up to the ICU with Matt to see how his wife is doing. When they arrive at the ICU, although Anne is still comatose, her condition has stabilized, and she is breathing on her own.

After his arrival at the ICU, Matt starts to worry about whether he remembered to lock the door at home. Gabriel suggests that he call neighbors and ask them to check the door. At this time, Matt is able to focus on everyday things. Gabriel makes arrangements to see Matt the next day when he comes in to visit his wife.

The next day, Anne has regained consciousness. She is discharged 1 week later. At the time of discharge, Matt and Anne Michaels are considering family therapy with the psychiatric nurse clinician once a week in the outpatient department.

Evaluation

The first short-term goal is to lower anxiety from severe to moderate. Gabriel can see that Matt has become more visibly calm. His trembling, wringing of hands, and stomping of feet have ceased, and he is able to focus on his thoughts and feelings with Gabriel's help.

The second short-term goal established for Matt is that he will verbalize his feelings and his need for assistance. Matt is able to identify and discuss with Gabriel his feelings of guilt and fear of being left alone in the world if his wife should die. Both of these feelings are overwhelming him. He is also able to state that he needs assistance in coping with these feelings in order to make tentative plans for the future.

TABLE 15-1 LEVELS OF ANXIETY

MILD	MODERATE	SEVERE	PANIC
Perceptual Field			
Heightened perceptual field	Narrowed perceptual field; grasps less of what is going on	Greatly reduced and distorted perceptual field	Unable to attend to the environment
Focus is flexible and is aware of the anxiety	Focuses on the source of the anxiety; less able to pay attention.	Focuses on details or one specific detail Attention is scattered	Focus is lost; may feel unreal (depersonalization) or that the world is unreal (derealization)
Ability to Problem Solve			
Able to work effectively toward a goal and examine alternatives	Able to solve problems but not at optimal ability	Problem solving feels impossible. Unable to see connections between events or details	Completely unable to process what is happening; disorganized or irrational reasoning
Mild and moderate levels of anxiety can alert the person that something is wrong and can stimulate appropriate action.		Severe and panic levels of anxiety prevent problem solving. Unproductive relief behaviors perpetuate a vicious cycle.	
Physical or Other Characteristics			
Slight discomfort Attention-seeking behavior Restlessness Easily startled Irritability or impatience Mild tension-relieving behavior (foot or finger tapping, lip chewing, fidgeting)	Voice tremors Change in voice pitch Poor concentration Shakiness Somatic complaints, (urinary frequency, headache, backache, insomnia) Increased respiration, pulse, and muscle tension More tension-relieving behavior (pacing, banging of hands on table)	Feelings of dread Confusion Purposeless activity Sense of impending doom More intense somatic complaints (chest discomfort, dizziness, nausea, sleeplessness) Diaphoresis (sweating) Withdrawal Loud and rapid speech Threats and demands	Experience of terror Immobility or severe hyperactivity or flight Unintelligible communication or inability to speak Somatic complaints increase (numbness or tingling, shortness of breath, dizziness, chest pain, nausea, trembling, chills, overheating, palpitations) Severe withdrawal Hallucinations or delusions; likely out of touch with reality

DEFENSES AGAINST ANXIETY

Sigmund Freud and his daughter, Anna Freud, outlined most of the defense mechanisms we recognize today. **Defense mechanisms** are automatic coping styles that protect people from anxiety and maintain self-image by blocking feelings, conflicts, and memories. Although they operate all the time, defense mechanisms are not always apparent to the individual using them.

Adaptive use of defense mechanisms helps people lower anxiety to achieve goals in acceptable ways. Maladaptive use of defense mechanisms occurs when one or several are used in excess, particularly in the overuse of immature defenses. Figure 15-1 operationally defines anxiety and shows how defenses come into play.

With the exception of sublimation and altruism, which are always healthy coping mechanisms, most defense mechanisms

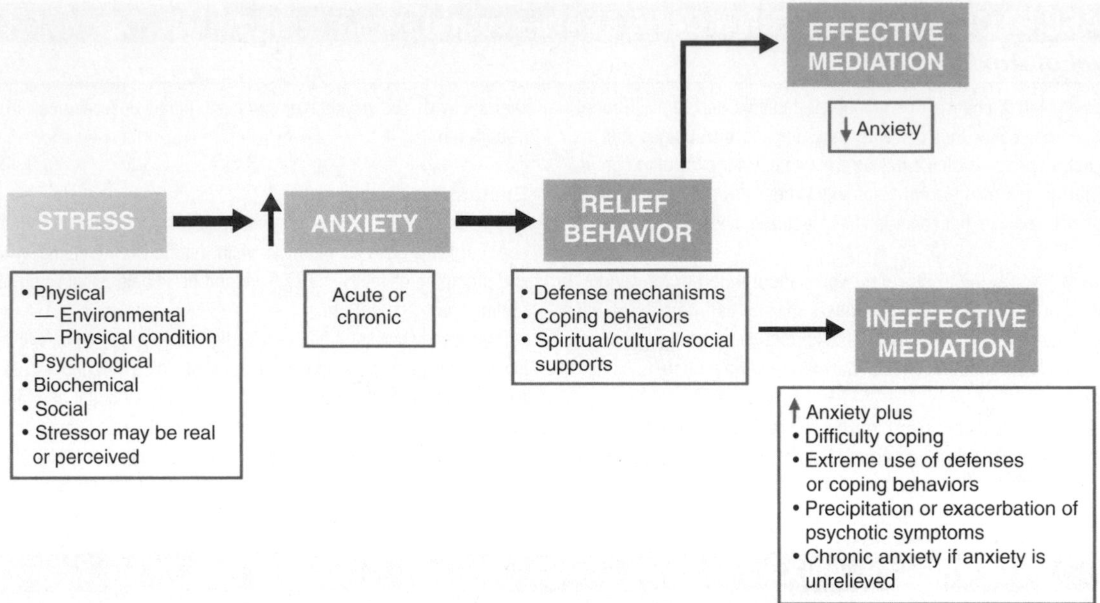

FIG 15-1 Anxiety operationally defined.

can be used in both healthy and unhealthy ways. Most people use a variety of defense mechanisms but not always at the same level. Keep in mind that evaluating whether the use of defense mechanisms is adaptive or maladaptive is determined for the most part by their *frequency*, *intensity*, and *duration* of use. Table 15-2 describes defense mechanisms and their adaptive and maladaptive uses.

ANXIETY DISORDERS

Individuals with anxiety disorders use rigid, repetitive, and ineffective behaviors to try to control their anxiety. The common element of such disorders is that those affected experience a degree of anxiety so high that it interferes with personal, occupational, or social functioning. The presence of chronic anxiety disorders may increase the rate of cardiovascular system-related deaths. Anxiety disorders tend to be persistent and often disabling. Chapter 10 offers a more complete description of the debilitating effects of chronic stress and resultant anxiety.

CLINICAL PICTURE

According to the American Psychiatric Association (2013), the term *anxiety disorder* refers to a number of disorders, including:

- Separation Anxiety Disorder
- Panic Disorder
- Agoraphobia
- Specific Phobia
- Social Anxiety Disorder (Social Phobia)
- Generalized Anxiety Disorder

In a closely related set of disorders anxiety results in abnormal selective overattention, or obsessions. These obsessive-compulsive and related disorders include the following:

- Obsessive-Compulsive Disorder
- Body Dysmorphic Disorder
- Hoarding Disorder
- Hair Pulling and Skin Picking Disorder

Separation Anxiety Disorder

Separation anxiety is a normal part of infant development; it begins around 8 months of age, peaks around 18 months, and begins to decline after that. People with **separation anxiety disorder** exhibit *developmentally inappropriate* levels of concern over being away from a significant other (Bostic & Prince, 2010). There may also be fear that something horrible will happen to the other person and that it will result in permanent separation. The anxiety is so intense that it distracts sufferers from their normal activities, causes sleep disruptions and nightmares without the significant other close by, and is often manifested in physical symptoms such as gastrointestinal disturbances and headaches.

This problem is typically diagnosed prior to the age of 18 after about a month of symptoms. Separation anxiety may develop after a significant stress, such as the death of a relative or pet, an illness, a move or change in schools, or a physical or sexual assault (Ursano et al., 2011).

Recently, clinicians have begun to recognize an adult form of separation anxiety disorder that may begin either in childhood or in adulthood. Those who are the subject of the attachment—a parent, a spouse, a child, or a friend—may grow weary of the constant neediness and clinginess. In fact, adults with this disorder often have extreme difficulties in romantic relationships and are more likely to be unmarried (Nichols, 2009). Characteristics of adult separation anxiety disorder include harm avoidance, worry, shyness, uncertainty, fatigability, and a lack of self-direction (Mertol & Alkin, 2012). It is accompanied by a significant level of discomfort and disability that impairs social and occupational functioning and does not respond well to the most popular type of psychotherapy, cognitive-behavioral therapy.

TABLE 15-2 ADAPTIVE AND MALADAPTIVE USES OF DEFENSE MECHANISMS

DEFENSE MECHANISM	ADAPTIVE USE	MALADAPTIVE USE
Compensation is used to counterbalance perceived deficiencies by emphasizing strengths.	A shorter-than-average man becomes assertively verbal and excels in business.	An individual drinks alcohol when self-esteem is low to temporarily diffuse discomfort.
Conversion is the unconscious transformation of anxiety into a physical symptom with no organic cause.	No example. Almost always a pathological defense	A man becomes blind after seeing his wife flirt with other men.
Denial involves escaping unpleasant, anxiety-causing thoughts, feelings, wishes, or needs by ignoring their existence.	A man reacts to the death of a loved one by saying "No, I don't believe you" to initially protect himself from the overwhelming news.	A woman whose husband died 3 years earlier still keeps his clothes in the closet and talks about him in the present tense.
Displacement is the transference of emotions associated with a particular person, object, or situation to another nonthreatening person, object, or situation.	A child yells at his teddy bear after being picked on by the school bully.	A child who is unable to acknowledge fear of his father becomes fearful of animals.
Dissociation is a disruption in consciousness, memory, identity, or perception of the environment that results in compartmentalizing uncomfortable or unpleasant aspects of oneself.	An art student is able to mentally separate herself from the noisy environment as she becomes absorbed in her work.	As the result of an abusive childhood and the need to separate from its realities, a woman finds herself perpetually disconnected from reality.
Identification is attributing to oneself the characteristics of another person or group. This may be done consciously or unconsciously.	An 8-year-old girl dresses up like her teacher and puts together a pretend classroom for her friends.	A young boy thinks a neighborhood pimp with money and drugs is someone to look up to.
Intellectualization is a process in which events are analyzed based on remote, cold facts and without passion, rather than incorporating feeling and emotion into the processing.	Despite the fact that a man has lost his farm to a tornado, he analyzes his options and leads his child to safety.	A man responds to the death of his wife by focusing on the details of day care and operating the household, rather than processing the grief with his children.
Projection refers to the unconscious rejection of emotionally unacceptable features and attributing them to others.	No example. This is considered an immature defense mechanism	A woman who has repressed an attraction toward other women refuses to socialize. She fears another woman will make homosexual advances toward her.
Rationalization consists of justifying illogical or unreasonable ideas, actions, or feelings by developing acceptable explanations that satisfy the teller as well as the listener.	An employee says, "I didn't get the raise because the boss doesn't like me."	A man who thinks his son was fathered by another man excuses his malicious treatment of the boy by saying, "He is lazy and disobedient," when that is not the case
Reaction formation is when unacceptable feelings or behaviors are controlled and kept out of awareness by developing the opposite behavior or emotion.	A recovering alcoholic constantly talks about the evils of drinking.	A woman who has an unconscious hostility toward her daughter is overprotective and hovers over her to protect her from harm, interfering with her normal growth and development.
Regression is reverting to an earlier, more primitive and childlike pattern of behavior that may or may not have been previously exhibited.	A 4-year-old boy with a new baby brother temporarily starts sucking his thumb and wanting a bottle.	A man who loses a promotion starts complaining to others, hands in sloppy work, misses appointments, and comes in late for meetings.
Repression is an *unconscious* exclusion of unpleasant or unwanted experiences, emotions, or ideas from conscious awareness.	A man forgets his wife's birthday after a marital fight.	A woman is unable to enjoy sex after having pushed out of awareness a traumatic sexual incident from childhood.
Splitting is the inability to integrate the positive and negative qualities of oneself or others into a cohesive image.	No example. Almost always a pathological defense	A 26-year-old woman initially values her acquaintances yet invariably becomes disillusioned when they turn out to have flaws.
Sublimation is an unconscious process of substituting mature and socially acceptable activity for immature and unacceptable impulses.	A woman who is angry with her boss writes a short story about a heroic woman.	The use of sublimation is always constructive.
Suppression is the *conscious* denial of a disturbing situation or feeling. For example, Jessica has been studying for the state board examination for a week solid. She says, "I won't worry about paying my rent until after my exam tomorrow."	A businessman who is preparing to make an important speech is told by his wife that morning that she wants a divorce. Although visibly upset, he puts the incident aside until after his speech, when he can give the matter his total concentration.	A woman who feels a lump in her breast shortly before leaving for a 3-week vacation puts the information in the back of her mind until after returning from her vacation.
Undoing is most commonly seen in children. It is when a person makes up for an act or communication.	After flirting with her male secretary, a woman brings her husband tickets to a concert he wants to see.	A man with rigid, moralistic beliefs and repressed sexuality is driven to wash his hands to gain composure when around attractive women.

Panic Disorders

Panic attacks are the key feature of panic disorder. A **panic attack** is the sudden onset of extreme apprehension or fear, usually associated with feelings of impending doom. The feelings of terror present during a panic attack are so severe that normal functioning is suspended, the perceptual field is severely limited, and misinterpretation of reality may occur. People experiencing panic attacks may believe they are losing their minds or having a heart attack. Uncomfortable physical symptoms such as palpitations, chest pain, breathing difficulties, nausea, and feelings of choking, chills, and hot flashes may occur. Typically, panic attacks come "out of the blue" (i.e., suddenly and not necessarily in response to stress), are extremely intense, last a matter of minutes, and then subside.

Unpredictability is a key aspect of panic disorder in children and adolescents. The attacks of panic seem to come out of nowhere, last about 10 minutes, and then subside. During the attack the young person has much the same symptoms as adults, but is often less able to articulate the psychological aspects, such as fear. They may become avoidant of situations where help is not available, may develop feelings of hopelessness in controlling these attacks, and may become depressed. Alcohol or substance abuse is not uncommon in adolescents with this disorder.

People who experience these attacks begin to "fear the fear" and become so preoccupied about future episodes of panic that they avoid what could be pleasurable and adaptive activities, experiences, and obligations. Table 15-3 outlines a generic nursing care plan for panic disorder, and the Evidence-Based Practice box provides additional information.

Agoraphobia

Agoraphobia is intense, excessive anxiety or fear about being in places or situations from which escape might be difficult or embarrassing or in which help might not be available. The feared places are avoided in an effort to control anxiety. Examples of situations that are commonly avoided by patients with agoraphobia are being alone outside; being alone at home; traveling in a car, bus, or airplane; being on a bridge; and riding in an elevator. These situations may be made more tolerable with the addition of a friend. Avoidance behaviors

TABLE 15-3 GENERIC CARE PLAN FOR PANIC DISORDER

Nursing diagnosis: Severe anxiety as evidenced by sudden onset of fear of impending doom or dying, increased pulse and respirations, shortness of breath, possible chest pain, dizziness, and abdominal distress.

Outcome criteria: Panic attacks will become less intense and time between episodes will lengthen so that patient can function comfortably at the usual level.

SHORT-TERM GOAL	INTERVENTION	RATIONALE
1. Patient's anxiety will decrease to moderate by (date).	1a. If hyperventilation occurs, instruct patient to take slow, deep breaths. Breathing with the patient may be helpful.	1a. Focus is shifted away from distressing symptoms.
	1b. Keep expectations minimal and simple.	1b. Anxiety limits ability to attend to complex tasks.
2. Patient will gain mastery over panic episodes by (date).	2a. Help patient connect feelings before attack with onset of attack: "What were you thinking about just before the attack?" "Can you identify what you were feeling just before the attack?"	2a. Physiological symptoms of anxiety usually appear first as the result of a stressor. They are immediately followed by automatic thoughts, such as "I'm dying" or "I'm going crazy," which are distorted assessments.
	2b. Help patient recognize symptoms as resulting from anxiety, not from a catastrophic physical problem. Examples: Explain physical symptoms of anxiety. Discuss the fact that anxiety causes sensations similar to those of physical events, such as a heart attack.	2b. Factual information and alternative interpretations can help patient recognize distortions in thought.
	2c. Identify effective therapies for panic episodes.	2c. Cognitive-behavioral treatment is highly effective. Antianxiety medication is appropriate.
	2d. Teach patient abdominal breathing to be immediately used when anxiety is detected.	2d. Breathing exercises break the cycle of escalating symptoms of anxiety.
	2e. Teach patient to use positive self-talk, such as "I can control my anxiety."	2e. Cognitive restructuring is an effective way to replace negative self-talk.
	2f. Teach patient and family about any medication ordered for patient's panic attacks.	2f. Patient and family need to know what the medication can do, what the side effects and toxic effects are, and whom to call if untoward reactions occur.

EVIDENCE-BASED PRACTICE

Using Exercise to Reduce Panic Attack Severity

Stoy, M., Graetz, B., Scheel, M., Wittmann, A., Gallinat, J., Lang, U.E., Dimeo, F., & Hellweg, R. (2010). Acute exercise ameliorates reduced brain-derived neurotrophic factor in patients with panic disorder. *Psychoneuroendocrinology, 35*(3), 364-368.

Problem

Panic attacks are terrifying and are accompanied by palpitations and feeling sweaty, faint, and weak. They may lead to disability and complete avoidance of normal activities. Medications and cognitive therapy are useful in the treatment of this disorder; the discovery of other natural treatments would be beneficial to sufferers.

Purpose of Study

Neurotrophin brain-derived neurotrophic factor (BDNF) is associated with anxiolytic (anxiety reduction) activity and is increased through exercise. The researchers wanted to see if exercise would improve symptoms of panic disorder.

Methods

Twelve patients with panic disorder were matched with 12 healthy control subjects. Serum samples for BDNF analyses were taken before and after either 30 minutes of exercise or 30 minutes of quiet rest. The two conditions were separated by 1 week, and the order of the exercise and rest was done randomly.

Key Findings

Prior to the experiment, increased anxiety was associated with reduced BDNF concentrations in all subjects, but for patients with panic disorder the BDNF concentration was significantly reduced. After 30 minutes of exercise there was a significant increase in BDNF concentrations for patients with panic disorder. For the control subjects, the increase in BDNF was not significant.

Implications for Nursing Practice

Nurses know that 30 minutes of exercise is good for almost anyone. For those who suffer from the overwhelming anxiety of panic disorder, this therapeutic exercise may be essential. Nurses can promote a prescription of daily exercise and can advocate for such equipment as treadmills and stationary bicycles to be included in designs of psychiatric facilities.

can be debilitating and life constricting. Consider the effect on a father whose agoraphobia renders him unable to leave home and prevents him from seeing his child's high school graduation or the businesswoman whose avoidance of flying prevents her from attending distant business conferences.

Specific Phobias

A **specific phobia** is a persistent, irrational fear of a specific object, activity, or situation that leads to a desire for avoidance, or actual avoidance of the object, activity, or situation. Specific phobias are characterized by the experience of high levels of anxiety or fear in response to specific objects or situations, such as dogs, spiders, heights, storms, water, blood, closed spaces, tunnels, and bridges.

Characteristically, phobic individuals experience overwhelming and crippling anxiety when faced with the object or situation provoking the phobic response. Daily functioning is compromised, and phobic people go to great lengths to avoid the feared object or situation. A phobic person may not be able to think about or visualize the object or situation without becoming severely anxious. The life of a phobic person becomes more restricted as activities are given up so that the phobic object can be avoided. All too frequently, complications ensue when sufferers try to decrease anxiety through self-medication with alcohol or drugs.

Consider the case of Daniel, who developed a profound fear of elevators after being trapped in one for 3 hours during a power outage. As his fear and anxiety intensified, it became necessary for him to use only stairs or escalators. He obsesses about the possibility that he will be forced to use an elevator in social situations and avoids attending events where this may occur. It has reached a point where even going inside closets or small storage rooms is unbearable. This fear of enclosed spaces is called claustrophobia. Other common phobias are listed in Table 15-4.

Social Anxiety Disorder

Social anxiety disorder, also called *social phobia*, is characterized by severe anxiety or fear provoked by exposure to a social or a performance situation that could be evaluated negatively by others. Situations that trigger this distress include fear of saying something that sounds foolish in public, not being able to answer questions in a classroom, looking awkward while eating or drinking in public, and performing badly on stage. Whenever possible, people with social anxiety disorder avoid these social situations; if they are unable to avoid them, they endure the situation with intense anxiety and emotional distress.

Small children with this disorder may be mute, nervous, and hide behind their parents. Older children and adolescents may be paralyzed by fear of speaking in class or interacting with other children; the worry over saying the wrong thing or being

TABLE 15-4 CLINICAL NAMES FOR COMMON PHOBIAS

CLINICAL NAME	FEARED OBJECT OR SITUATION
Acrophobia	Heights
Agoraphobia	Open spaces
Astraphobia	Electrical storms
Claustrophobia	Closed spaces
Glossophobia	Talking
Hematophobia	Blood
Hydrophobia	Water
Monophobia	Being alone
Mysophobia	Germs or dirt
Nyctophobia	Darkness
Pyrophobia	Fire
Xenophobia	Strangers
Zoophobia	Animals

criticized immobilizes them. Conversely, younger people may act out to compensate for this fear making an accurate diagnosis more difficult. This anxiety often results in physical complaints to avoid social situations, particularly school.

Fear of public speaking is the most common manifestation of social anxiety disorder. Interestingly, this disorder has afflicted famous singers and actors such as Barbra Streisand and Sir Laurence Olivier, both of whom were terrified that they might forget the words to songs and scripts.

Generalized Anxiety Disorder

The key pathological feature of **generalized anxiety disorder** is excessive worry (Newman & Llera, 2011). Children, teens, and adults may experience this worry, which is out of proportion to the true impact of events or situations. Persons with generalized anxiety disorder anticipate disaster and are restless, irritable, and experience muscle tension. Decision making is difficult due to poor concentration and dread of making a mistake.

Common worries in generalized anxiety disorder are inadequacy in interpersonal relationships, job responsibilities, finances, and health of family members. Because of this worry, huge amounts of time are spent in preparing for activities. Putting things off and avoidance are key symptoms and may result in lateness or absence from school or employment, and overall social isolation. Family members and friends are overtaxed as the person with this disorder seeks continual reassurance and perseverates about meaningless details.

Sleep disturbance is common because the individual worries about the day's events and real or imagined mistakes, reviews past problems, and anticipates future difficulties. Fatigue is a noticeable side effect of this sleep deprivation. Refer to Table 15-5 for a generic care plan for generalized anxiety disorder.

TABLE 15-5 GENERIC CARE PLAN FOR GENERALIZED ANXIETY DISORDER

Nursing diagnosis: Ineffective coping related to persistent anxiety, fatigue, difficulty concentrating
Outcome criteria: Patient will maintain role performance.

SHORT-TERM GOAL	INTERVENTION	RATIONALE
1. Patient will state that immediate distress is relieved by end of session.	1a. Stay with patient.	1a. Conveys acceptance and ability to give help.
	1b. Speak slowly and calmly.	1b. Conveys calm and promotes security.
	1c. Use short, simple sentences.	1c. Promotes comprehension.
	1d. Assure patient that you are in control and can assist him or her.	1d. Counters feeling of loss of control that accompanies severe anxiety.
	1e. Give brief directions.	1e. Reduces indecision. Conveys belief that patient can respond in a healthy manner.
	1f. Decrease excessive stimuli; provide quiet environment.	1f. Reduces need to focus on diverse stimuli. Promotes ability to concentrate.
	1g. After assessing level of anxiety, administer appropriate dose of antianxiety agent if warranted.	1g. Reduces anxiety and allows patient to use coping skills.
	1h. Monitor and control own feelings.	1h. Anxiety is transmissible. Displays of negative emotion can cause patient anxiety.
2. Patient will be able to identify source of anxiety by (date).	2a. Encourage patient to discuss preceding events.	2a. Promotes future change through identification of stressors.
	2b. Link patient's behavior to feelings.	2b. Promotes self-awareness.
	2c. Teach a cognitive therapy principle: Anxiety is the result of automatic thinking with a dysfunctional appraisal of a situation.	2c. Provides a basis for behavioral change.
	2d. Ask questions that clarify and dispute illogical thinking: "What evidence do you have?" "Explain the logic in that." "Are you basing that conclusion on fact or feeling?" "What's the worst thing that could happen?"	2d. Helps promote accurate cognition.
	2e. Have patient give an alternative interpretation.	2e. Broadens perspective. Helps patient think in a new way about problem or symptom.
3. Patient will identify strengths and coping skills by (date).	3a. Provides awareness of self as individual with some ability to cope.	3a. Identify what has provided relief in the past.
	3b. Have patient write assessment of strengths.	3b. Increases self-acceptance.
	3c. Reframe situation in ways that are positive.	3c. Provides a new perspective and converts distorted thinking.

TABLE 15-6 COMMON MEDICAL CAUSES OF ANXIETY

SYSTEM	DISORDERS
Respiratory	Chronic obstructive pulmonary disease
	Pulmonary embolism
	Asthma
	Hypoxia
	Pulmonary edema
Cardiovascular	Angina pectoris
	Arrhythmias
	Congestive heart failure
	Hypertension
	Hypotension
	Mitral valve prolapse
Endocrine	Hyperthyroidism
	Hypoglycemia
	Pheochromocytoma
	Carcinoid syndrome
	Hypercortisolism
Neurological	Delirium
	Essential tremor
	Complex partial seizures
	Parkinson's disease
	Akathisia
	Otoneurological disorders
	Postconcussion syndrome
Metabolic	Hypercalcemia
	Hyperkalemia
	Hyponatremia
	Porphyria

Other Anxiety Disorders

Substance-induced anxiety disorder is characterized by symptoms of anxiety, panic attacks, obsessions, and compulsions that develop with the use of a substance (e.g., alcohol, cocaine, heroin, hallucinogens).

In **anxiety due to a medical condition**, the individual's symptoms of anxiety are a direct physiological result of a medical condition, such as hyperthyroidism, pulmonary embolism, or cardiac dysrhythmias. To determine whether the anxiety symptoms are due to a medical condition, a careful and comprehensive assessment of multiple factors is necessary. Refer to Table 15-6 for a list of medical disorders that may contribute to anxiety symptoms.

OBSESSIVE-COMPULSIVE DISORDERS

Obsessive-compulsive disorders are a group of related disorders that all have obsessive-compulsive characteristics. **Obsessions** are defined as thoughts, impulses, or images that persist and recur, so that they cannot be dismissed from the mind even though the individual attempts to do so. Obsessions often seem senseless to the individual who experiences them (ego-dystonic), and their presence causes severe anxiety.

Compulsions are ritualistic behaviors an individual feels driven to perform in an attempt to reduce anxiety or prevent an imagined calamity. Performing the compulsive act temporarily reduces anxiety, but because the relief is only temporary, the compulsive act must be repeated again and again.

Although obsessions and compulsions can exist independently of each other, they most often occur together. Examples of common obsessions and compulsions are given in Table 15-7.

Obsessive-Compulsive Disorder

Obsessive-compulsive behavior exists along a continuum. Most sufferers may experience mildly obsessive-compulsive behavior such as nagging doubts as to whether a door is locked or the stove is turned off. These doubts require the person to go back to check the door or stove. Mild compulsions about timeliness, orderliness, and reliability are valued traits in U.S. society.

At the pathological end of the continuum is **obsessive-compulsive disorder** with symptoms that occur on a daily basis and may involve issues of sexuality, violence, contamination, illness, or death. Pathological obsessions or compulsions cause marked distress to individuals, who often feel humiliation and shame regarding these behaviors. The rituals are time-consuming and interfere with normal routines, social activities, and relationships with others. Severe obsessive-compulsive disorder occupies so much of the individual's mental processes that the performance of cognitive tasks is impaired. English soccer player David Beckham has shared his struggle with obsessive-compulsive disorder. He has a compulsion to count his clothes and line his magazines up in a straight line.

About a third of adult cases begin in childhood and can be present as early as age 3 (Bostic & Prince, 2010). Younger children are often preoccupied with turning off lights or locking doors and windows, while older children and adolescents tend to focus on contamination. Young people experience shame and helplessness as their rituals interfere with their ability to form relationships and attend school. See the Case Study and Nursing Care Plan for obsessive-compulsive disorder on the Evolve website.

Body Dysmorphic Disorder

Body dysmorphic disorder was first described over a century ago and continues to be a challenge to treat. Patients with body dysmorphic disorder are commonly seen in community, psychiatric, cosmetic surgery, and dermatological settings. Although patients usually have a normal appearance, their preoccupation with an imagined defective body part results in obsessional thinking and compulsive behavior, such as mirror checking and camouflaging. In body dysmorphic disorder levels of insight vary; people may be well aware that their thoughts are distorted, or they may be completely sure about existence of the defect.

False assumptions about the importance of appearance, fear of rejection by others, perfectionism, and conviction of being disfigured lead to overwhelming emotions of disgust, shame, and depression (Stangier, 2008). Patients frequently are concerned with their skin, hair, nose, stomach, teeth, weight,

TABLE 15-7 COMMON OBSESSIONS AND COMPULSIONS

TYPE OF OBSESSION	EXAMPLE	ACCOMPANYING COMPULSION
Losing control and religious concerns	A middle-age man worries, "If I go to church, what will stop me from blurting out obscenities?"	Despite his desire to attend services, has not gone to church in two years.
Harm	"If I don't turn the light switch off, the room will catch on fire, and my mom will die while I am at school," worries a 9-year-old girl.	Returns to her room four times before school, checks that the light is turned off, and taps the four sides of the light switch.
Unwanted sexual thoughts	A young man has a recurrent thought: "What if I get a sexually transmitted disease from a prostitute during sleepwalking?"	Ritualistically locks the doors of the house with a key each night and hides his wallet.
Perfectionism	"My work is never second best," proclaims an administrative assistant.	Gets to work early, leaves work late, never has a messy desk, always completes tasks.
Violence	A man repeatedly has the thought "I should kill her" when he sees a blonde woman.	Abruptly turns head away from women and squints eyes to try to avoid seeing blondes.
Contamination	A woman ruminates, "Everything is covered in germs."	Avoids touching all objects; scrubs hands if forced to touch any object.
Superstitions	"All lists need to end in an even number," thinks a college professor.	Adds or deletes items from tests, agendas, and other numbered items.

and breasts/chest. In one study, men were more likely to be concerned with the appearance of their genitals and body build (90% of men thought they were too small and/or inadequately muscular), and women were found to be more focused on the appearance of their skin, stomach, weight, breasts, buttocks, thighs, legs, hips, and toes (Phillips, Menard, & Fay, 2006). Often the patient keeps the disorder secret for many years and does not respond to reassurance. The disorder is chronic, and response to treatment is limited.

Hoarding Disorder

Have you ever reached the point where there is just too much clutter in your closet, and you proceed to sort through it and make stacks of Keep, Give Away, and Donate? You probably have, and for most of us this is not a painful experience. For those individuals with **hoarding disorder**, however, this could have been extremely distressing. In fact, the accumulation of belongings that may have little or no value is an obsession that prevents some people from leading normal lives. Belongings literally fill every available surface and area in their residences, and guests can (or will) no longer visit. The problem may progress to the point where the home is nearly uninhabitable due to unsafe and unsanitary conditions. Individuals who hoard may or may not be aware of the problem and how the quest to collect has consumed their lives and alienated others.

It is difficult to determine the age of onset for this disorder since children do not have the same means to add to their collections as adults do. Also, while more women are treated for hoarding disorder, it is likely that men are affected at much the same rate but do not seek treatment for this problem.

Hair Pulling and Skin Picking Disorders

Hair pulling disorder, or *trichotillomania*, and **skin picking disorder**, or *dermotillomania*, are two distressing problems that may result in varying degrees of disability, social stigma, and altered appearance. Both of the activities are irresistible to the individual who typically tries to hide the activity. These disorders have been linked to symptoms of obsessive-compulsive disorder. It occurs more often in children than adults and may begin as early as 1 year of age.

Hair pulling may be one of the oldest recorded psychiatric problems, and the phrase "I was so annoyed that I wanted to pull my hair out" attests to the anxiety-related component of the disorder. Typically, it is the hair of the head, but it may come from anywhere on the body, including eyebrows, eyelashes, pubic areas, axilla, and limbs. The amount of hair removed ranges from small patches to complete baldness. For some, the pain of hair pulling results in anxiety reduction, similar to those who engage in cutting. Most (about 75%) may be unaware of the behavior until they notice a wad of it close by (Hollander et al., 2011). The disorder may begin in childhood, adolescence, or even adulthood and may last weeks to decades. Trichophagia, or secretly swallowing the hair, is common in this disorder and may lead to hair masses, or trichobezoar, in the gastrointestinal system, masses that can be fatal. Incidentally, the masses are also referred to as the Rapunzel syndrome.

Skin picking disorder, or *dermotillomania*, is typically confined to the face, although other areas of the body may be targeted. As with hair pulling, the individual may engage in skin picking as a means to deal with stress and relieve anxiety, while others may engage in this activity without thinking about it. Most people occasionally pick at their skin, nails, and scabs; however, people with skin picking disorder damage their skin. Fingers and fingernails are the usual implements, but biting, nail cutters, and tweezers are also used. The most common areas of focus are the face, head, cuticles, back, arms and legs, and hands and feet. Complications include pain, sores, scars, and infections.

Other Compulsive Disorders

Substance-induced obsessive-compulsive and related disorders are characterized by obsessions and compulsions that develop with the use of a substance or within a month of stopping use of the substance. Drugs used to treat the movement disorders in Parkinson's disease have been reported to cause obsessions with gambling, irresistible urges for sex, and out-of-control spending (Ahlskog, 2011). This diagnosis is based on a thorough history, physical examination, and laboratory findings.

In **obsessive-compulsive or related disorders due to a medical condition**, the individual's symptoms of obsessions and compulsions are a direct physiological result of a medical condition, such as a postencephalatic syndrome, postanoxic event, traumatic brain injury, Huntington's disease, seizures, and cerebral infarctions (First & Tasman, 2011). To determine whether the symptoms are due to a medical condition, a careful and comprehensive assessment of multiple factors is necessary. Evidence must be present in the history, physical examination, or laboratory findings for this diagnosis.

EPIDEMIOLOGY

Anxiety disorders are the most common form of psychiatric disorders in the United States. They affect up to 40 million adults, or about 18% of the population aged 18 and older (Kessler, Chiu et al., 2005). Nearly three quarters of those with an anxiety disorder will have their first episode by age 21.5 (Kessler, Berglund et al., 2005). People with anxiety disorders frequently seek health care services for relief of physical symptoms, at a cost of approximately $22 billion per year. Women are affected more frequently than men. Table 15-8 lists the 1-year prevalence rates (those who are affected within any given year) for specific anxiety and obsessive-compulsive disorders in the United States.

Obsessive-compulsive disorder has an average age of onset of 19, a one-year prevalence rate of 1%, and about 50% of cases are considered to be severe (Kessler, Berglund et al., 2005). Body dysmorphic disorder is thought to occur in about 2.4% of the population, somewhat more frequently in women, and rates may be as high as 15% for those undergoing plastic surgery (Haas et al., 2008). Although hoarding disorders become more evident as people age and symptoms become more severe, they tend to begin in early adolescence. Hoarding compulsions affect about 2% to 5% of the population, and slightly more men than women are afflicted (Otte & Steketee, 2011). It is difficult to identify the rate of hair pulling and skin picking disorders since people do not often seek help or may attempt to hide the condition; it is estimated to have a lifetime prevalence of 1%.

COMORBIDITY

Clinicians and researchers have clearly shown that anxiety disorders frequently co-occur with other psychiatric problems. Several studies suggest that other psychiatric disorders coexist about 90% of the time in people with generalized anxiety or panic disorder and about 84% of the time in those with agoraphobia (Sadock & Sadock, 2008). Anxiety disorders are comorbid with major depression at a rate of 60%; in this type of comorbidity,

TABLE 15-8 ONE-YEAR PREVALENCE OF ANXIETY AND OBSESSIVE-COMPULSIVE DISORDERS IN ADULTS

DISORDER	PREVALENCE % ADOLESCENTS (AGES 13-17)	PREVALENCE % ADULTS	AGE OF ONSET	GENDER PREDILECTION
Separation anxiety	1.6	1.9	80% develop by age 30	One and a half times more frequent in women
Panic	1.9	2.7	Median age of onset 24 years	Two times more frequent in women
Agoraphobia	1.8	0.8	Median age of onset 20 years	Two times more frequent in women
Specific phobias	15.8	8.5	Median age of onset 7 years	Two times more frequent in women
Social anxiety	8.2	6.8	Median age of onset 13 years	Equal prevalence in men and women
Generalized anxiety	1.1	3.1	Median age of onset 31 years	Two times more frequent in women
Obsessive-compulsive	—	1	Median age of onset 15 years (boys before girls)	Equal prevalence in men and women
Hoarding	—	14	Uncertain	Uncertain

Data from Kessler, R.C., Chiu, W.T., Demler, O, & Walters, E.E. (2005). Prevalence, severity, and comorbidity of twelve-month DSM-IV disorders in the National Comorbidity Survey Replication (NCS-R). *Archives of General Psychiatry, 62,* 617-627; Kessler, R.C., Berglund, P. A., Demler O., Jin, R., & Walters, E.E. (2005). Lifetime prevalence and age-of-onset distributions of DSM-IV disorders in the National Comorbidity Survey Replication (NCS-R). *Archives of General Psychiatry, 62,* 593-602; Ruscio, A.M., Stein, D.J., Chiu, W.T., & Kessler, R.C. (2010). The epidemiology of obsessive-compulsive disorder in the national comorbidity survey replication. *Molecular Psychiatry, 15*(1), 53-63. doi: 10.1038/mp.2008.94.

anxiety symptoms tend to happen before depressive symptoms. In fact, treatments for both disorders are similar. This similarity leads to speculation that genetically anxiety and depression may be two sides of the same coin and not distinct disorders.

ETIOLOGY

There is no longer any doubt that biological factors predispose some individuals to pathological anxiety states (e.g., phobias, panic attacks). By the same token, traumatic life events, psychosocial factors, and sociocultural factors are also etiologically significant.

Biological Factors

Genetic

Numerous studies substantiate that anxiety disorders tend to cluster in families. Genetic variants have been identified that are associated with increased risk for anxiety (Serretti & Chiesa, 2010). Nearly half of people with panic disorders have a relative who is also affected (Sadock & Sadock, 2008). Twin studies demonstrate the existence of a genetic component to both panic disorder and obsessive-compulsive disorder. First-degree biological relatives of those with obsessive-compulsive disorder or phobias have a higher frequency of these disorders than exists in the general population.

Neurobiological

The amygdala plays a role in anxiety disorders. The amygdala alerts the brain to the presence of danger and brings about fear or anxiety to preserve the system. Memories with emotional significance are stored in the amygdala and have been implicated in phobic responses such as fears of snakes, heights, or open spaces.

Certain anatomic pathways (the limbic system) provide the transmission structure for the electrical impulses that occur when anxiety-related responses are sent or received. Neurons release chemicals (neurotransmitters) that convey these messages. The neurochemicals that regulate anxiety include epinephrine, norepinephrine, dopamine, serotonin, and gamma-aminobutyric acid (GABA).

GABA, an inhibitory neurotransmitter that puts a brake on excitatory neurotransmitters, is the common focus of pharmacological therapy for anxiety symptoms. It is believed that people with too little GABA may suffer from anxiety disorder. Since GABA is indirectly inhibited by benzodiazepine receptors, the binding of benzodiazepine medications to these receptors facilitates the action of GABA.

Children have developed obsessive-compulsive disorder after going through a strep infection that results in a condition called Pediatric Acute-onset Neuropsychiatric Syndrome (PANS). Compulsive behaviors and eating disorders have been known to develop dramatically after suffering from this bacterial infection (National Institute of Mental Health, 2012).

Psychological Theories

Psychodynamic theories explaining the development of anxiety disorders suggest that unconscious childhood conflicts are the basis for future symptom development. Sigmund Freud posited that anxiety results when threatening repressed ideas or emotions are close to breaking through from the unconscious mind into the aware and conscious mind. Freud also suggested that ego-defense mechanisms are used to keep anxiety at manageable levels (refer to Chapter 2). The use of defense mechanisms may result in overuse of behavior that is not wholly adaptive because of its rigidity and repetitive nature.

Harry Stack Sullivan (1953) believed that anxiety is linked to the emotional distress caused when early needs go unmet or disapproval is experienced (**interpersonal theory**). He also suggested that anxiety is "contagious," being transmitted to the infant from the mother or caregiver. Thus, the anxiety felt early in life becomes the prototype for anxiety responses when unpleasant events occur later in life.

Behavioral theories suggest that anxiety is a learned response to specific environmental stimuli (classical conditioning). An example of classical conditioning is a boy who is anxious in the presence of his abusive mother; he then generalizes this anxiety as a response to all women. Conditioning can be reversed through the influence of safe and loving female friends and significant others. The social learning model suggests that anxiety is learned through the modeling of parents or peers. For example, a mother who is fearful of thunder and lightning and hides in closets during storms may transmit her anxiety to her children, who continue to model her behavior into adult life. Such individuals can unlearn this behavior by observing others who react normally to a storm by lighting candles and telling stories.

Cognitive theorists believe that anxiety disorders are caused by distortions in an individual's thoughts and perceptions. Because individuals with such distortions exaggerate any mistake and believe that they will have catastrophic results, they experience acute anxiety. People who tend to perceive events and situations as being potentially dangerous may be overly responsive and become anxious or even experience panic attacks.

Cultural Considerations

Reliable data on the incidence of anxiety disorders are sparse, but sociocultural variation in symptoms of anxiety disorders has been noted. In some cultures, individuals express anxiety through somatic symptoms whereas in other cultures, cognitive symptoms predominate. Panic attacks in Latin Americans and Northern Europeans often involve sensations of choking, smothering, numbness, or tingling as well as fear of dying. In other cultural groups, panic attacks involve fear of magic or witchcraft. Social anxiety in Japanese and Korean cultures may relate to beliefs that the individual's blushing, eye contact, or body odor is offensive to others.

The Considering Culture box discusses factors relevant to one anxiety disorder (ataque de nervios) primarily experienced by people from Hispanic cultures. Also refer to Chapter 5 for more discussion of cultural issues.

CONSIDERING CULTURE

Attack of the Nerves in Hispanic People

Technology and the commonplace of travel have resulted in a "smaller" world. Psychiatric mental health nurses in the United States will be exposed to culture-bound syndromes with which they are unfamiliar. One example of a culture-bound syndrome is that of ataque de nervios, or in English, "attack of the nerves." This is a disorder found primarily among Hispanic populations in response to stressful events, such as a death, acute family discord, or witnessing an accident. Symptoms are dramatic, and people afflicted by ataque de nervios exhibit sudden trembling, faintness, palpitations, out-of-control shouting, heat that moves from the chest to head, and seizure like activities. After the episode, the affected individual often has little memory of it. This disorder is more common in socially disadvantaged females with less than a high school education.

What do these symptoms sound like to you? Some clinicians and researchers believe that it is closely related to an anxiety disorder and could even be a form of panic attack. Unlike persons who have panic attacks, however, individuals with this disorder are responding to a precipitating event, and they do not typically experience fear or apprehension prior to the attack.

Stern, T.A., Fricchione, G.L., Cassem, N.H., Jellinek, M.S. & Rosenbaum, J.F. (2010). *Massachusetts General Hospital handbook of general hospital psychiatry* (6th ed.). Philadelphia, PA: Saunders; Razzouk, D., Nogueira, B., & de Jesus Mari, J. (2011). The contribution of Latin American and Caribbean studies on culture-bound syndromes for the revision of the ICD-10: Key findings from a work in progress. *Revista Brasileira de Psiquiatria, 33*(1).

APPLICATION OF THE NURSING PROCESS

ASSESSMENT

General Assessment

People with anxiety and obsessive-compulsive disorders rarely need hospitalization unless they are suicidal or have compulsions that cause injury (cutting self, infected sores from picking). Most of these patients are encountered incidentally in a variety of community settings. A common example is someone taken to an emergency department to rule out a heart attack when in fact the individual is experiencing a panic attack. It is essential to determine whether the anxiety is the primary problem, as in an anxiety disorder, or secondary to another source (medical condition or substance).

Your assessment should be *patient-centered* in order to be helpful or meaningful. First and foremost is the recognition that the patient is the expert when it comes to his own illness. Elicit information about what has helped in the past; identify expectations for the patient's personal participation in care and for the family or significant other's participation in care. Assess for specific cultural, ethnic, and social backgrounds that may impact the care that you and the patient plan.

Objectively, there are a variety of scales available to measure anxiety and anxiety-related symptoms, and most are available online. The Yale-Brown Obsessive Compulsive Scale measures severity of compulsive behavior. The Hoarding Scale Self-Report often measures hoarding; phobias are measured on the Fear Questionnaire; panic symptoms are measured on the Panic Disorder Severity Scale. The Hamilton Rating Scale for Anxiety is a popular tool in measuring anxiety (Table 15-9). High scores may indicate generalized anxiety disorder or panic disorder although it is important to note that high anxiety scores may also be a symptom of major depressive disorder. See how you rate on this tool. Keep in mind that although The Hamilton Rating Scale highlights important areas in the assessment of anxiety, it is intended for use by experienced clinicians as a guide for planning care and not as a method of self-diagnosis.

Self-Assessment

As a nurse working with an individual with an anxiety or obsessive-compulsive disorder, you may have feelings of frustration, especially if it seems that their symptoms are a matter of choice or under personal control. The rituals of the patient with obsessive-compulsive disorder may seriously slow your ability to complete certain nursing tasks within the usual time. How do you respond to a person with a phobia who acknowledges that the fear is exaggerated and unrealistic yet continues to practice avoidant behavior? Behavioral change is often accomplished slowly. The process of recovery is very different from that seen in a patient with an infection, who might be given antibiotics and demonstrate improvement in 24 hours. Staging outcomes in small, attainable steps can help prevent you from feeling overwhelmed by the patient's slow progress and help the patient gain a sense of control.

DIAGNOSIS

The North American Nursing Diagnosis Association International (Herdman, 2012) provides many nursing diagnoses that can be considered for patients with anxiety disorders and obsessive-compulsive disorders. The "related-to" component will vary with the individual patient.

ASSESSMENT GUIDELINES

Anxiety and Obsessive-Compulsive Disorders

1. Ensure that a sound physical and neurological examination is performed to help determine whether the anxiety is primary or secondary to another psychiatric disorder, medical condition, or substance use.
2. Determine current level of anxiety (mild, moderate, severe, or panic).
3. Assess for potential for self-harm and suicide; persons suffering from high levels of intractable anxiety may become desperate and attempt suicide.
4. Perform a psychosocial assessment. Always ask the person, "What is going on in your life that may be contributing to your anxiety?" The patient may identify a problem (stressful marriage, recent loss, stressful job, or school situation) that should be addressed by counseling.

TABLE 15-9 HAMILTON RATING SCALE FOR ANXIETY

Max Hamilton designed this scale to help clinicians gather information about anxiety states. The symptom inventory provides scaled information that classifies anxiety behaviors and assists the clinician in targeting behaviors and achieving outcome measures. Provide a rating for each indicator based on the following scale: 0 = none; 1 = mild; 2 = moderate; 3 = disabling; 4 = severe, grossly disabling.

ITEM	SYMPTOMS	RATING
1. Anxious mood	Worries, anticipation of the worst, fearful anticipation, irritability	________
2. Tension	Feelings of tension, fatigability, startle response, moved to tears easily, trembling, feelings of restlessness, inability to relax	________
3. Fear	Fearful of dark, strangers, being left alone, animals, traffic, crowds	________
4. Insomnia	Difficulty in falling asleep, broken sleep, unsatisfying sleep and fatigue on waking, dreams, nightmares, night terrors	________
5. Intellectual (cognitive) manifestations	Difficulty in concentration, poor memory	________
6. Depressed mood swings	Loss of interest, lack of pleasure in hobbies, depression, early waking, diurnal	________
7. Somatic (sensory) symptoms	Tinnitus, blurring of vision, hot and cold flashes, feelings of weakness, picking sensation	________
8. Somatic (muscular) symptoms	Pains and aches, twitching, stiffness, myoclonic jerks, grinding of teeth, unsteady voice, increased muscular tone	________
9. Cardiovascular symptoms	Tachycardia, palpitations, skipped beats, pain in chest, throbbing of vessels, fainting feelings	________
10. Respiratory symptoms	Pressure or constriction in chest, choking feelings, sighing, dyspnea	________
11. Gastrointestinal symptoms	Difficulty in swallowing, flatulence, abdominal pain, burning sensations, abdominal fullness, nausea, vomiting, borborygmi, looseness of bowels, loss of weight, constipation	________
12. Genitourinary symptoms	Frequency of micturition, urgency of micturition, amenorrhea, menorrhagia, development of frigidity, premature ejaculation, loss of libido, impotence	________
13. Autonomic symptoms	Dry mouth, flushing, pallor, tendency to sweat, giddiness, tension headache, raising of hair	
14. Behavior at interview	Fidgeting, restlessness or pacing, tremor of hands, furrowed brow, strained face, sighing or rapid respiration, facial pallor, swallowing, belching, brisk tendon jerks, dilated pupils, exophthalmos	________

Scoring:
14-17 = Mild anxiety
18-24 = Moderate anxiety
25-30 = Severe anxiety

Adapted from Hamilton, M. (1959). The assessment of anxiety states by rating. *British Journal of Medical Psychology, 32*, 50-55.

OUTCOMES IDENTIFICATION

The *Nursing Outcomes Classification (NOC)* identifies desired outcomes for patients with anxiety-related or obsessive-compulsive disorders (Moorhead et al., 2013). Outcomes are linked with signs and symptoms and nursing diagnoses in Table 15-10.

PLANNING

Anxiety and obsessive-compulsive disorders are encountered in all health care settings. Nurses care for people with concurrent anxiety disorders in medical-surgical units as well as in homes, day programs, and clinics. Usually patients with these disorders do not require admission to inpatient psychiatric units, and planning for their care may involve selecting interventions that can be implemented in a community setting.

Whenever possible, the patient should be encouraged to participate actively in planning. By sharing decision making with the patient, you can increase the likelihood that positive outcomes will be attained. Shared planning is especially appropriate for someone with mild or moderate anxiety. When experiencing severe levels of anxiety, a patient may be unable to participate in planning, and the nurse may be required to take a more directive role.

IMPLEMENTATION

When working with patients with anxiety and obsessive-compulsive disorders, you must first determine what level of

TABLE 15-10 SIGNS AND SYMPTOMS, NURSING DIAGNOSES, AND OUTCOMES FOR ANXIETY-RELATED DISORDERS

SIGNS AND SYMPTOMS	NURSING DIAGNOSES	OUTCOMES
Separation from significant other, concern that a panic attack will occur, exposure to phobic object or situation, presence of obsessive thoughts, fear of panic attacks, preoccupation with perceived physical flaws, apprehension about losing prized possessions, pulling hair or picking skin	*Anxiety (moderate, severe, panic)*	Monitors intensity of anxiety, uses relaxation techniques, decreases environmental stimuli as needed, controls anxiety response, maintains role performance
Unable to attend social functions or take employment, anxiety interferes with the ability to work, avoidance behaviors (phobia, agoraphobia), inordinate time taken for obsession and compulsions	*Ineffective coping*	Identifies ineffective coping patterns, asks for assistance, seeks information about illness and treatment, identifies multiple coping strategies, modifies lifestyle as needed
Exaggerated negative perception of physical appearance, ashamed of the appearance of the house due to hoarding activity, believes that others are disgusted with his appearance, embarrassment about the hair or skin condition	*Chronic low self-esteem*	Verbalizes self-acceptance, communicates openly, increases confidence, describes a positive sense of self-worth
Skin excoriation related to rituals of excessive washing, excessive picking at the skin, or pulling hair out	*Self-mutilation*	Identifies feelings that lead to impulsive actions, practices self-restraint of compulsive behaviors

From Herdman, T.H. (Ed.) *Nursing diagnoses—Definitions and classification 2012-2014.* Copyright © 2012, 1994-2012 by NANDA International. Used by arrangement with John Wiley & Sons Limited; Moorhead, S., Johnson, M., Maas, M.L., & Swanson, E. (2013). *Nursing outcomes classification (NOC)* (5th ed.). St Louis, MO: Mosby.

anxiety they are experiencing. A general framework for anxiety interventions can then be built on a solid foundation of understanding.

Mild to Moderate Levels of Anxiety

A person experiencing a mild to moderate level of anxiety is still able to solve problems; however, the ability to concentrate decreases as anxiety increases. A patient can be helped to focus and solve problems when you use specific nursing communication techniques, such as asking open-ended questions, giving broad openings, and exploring and seeking clarification. Closing off topics of communication and bringing up irrelevant topics can increase a person's anxiety, making the *nurse*, not the *patient*, feel better.

Reducing the patient's anxiety level and preventing escalation to more distressing levels can be aided by providing a calm presence, recognizing the anxious person's distress, and being willing to listen. Evaluation of effective past coping mechanisms is also useful. Often, you can help the patient consider alternatives to problem situations and offer activities that may temporarily relieve feelings of inner tension. Table 15-11 identifies interventions useful in assisting people experiencing mild to moderate levels of anxiety.

Severe to Panic Levels of Anxiety

A person experiencing a severe to panic level of anxiety is unable to solve problems and may have a poor grasp of what is happening in the environment. Unproductive relief behaviors may take over, and the person may not be in control of his or her actions. Extreme regression and running about aimlessly are behavioral manifestations of a person's intense psychic pain.

Appropriate nursing interventions are to provide for the safety of the patient and others and to meet physical needs (e.g., fluids, rest) to prevent exhaustion. Anxiety-reduction measures may take the form of removing the person to a quiet environment with minimal stimulation and providing gross motor activities to drain some of the tension. The use of medications may have to be considered, but both medications and restraints should be used only after other more personal and less-restrictive interventions have failed to decrease anxiety to safer levels. Although a patient's communication may be scattered and disjointed, feeling understood can decrease the overwhelming sense of isolation and reduce anxiety.

Because individuals experiencing severe to panic levels of anxiety are unable to solve problems, the techniques suggested for communicating with persons with mild to moderate levels of anxiety may not be effective at more severe levels. Patients experiencing severe to panic anxiety levels are out of control, so they need to know they are safe from their own impulses. Firm, short, and simple statements are useful. Reinforcing commonalities in the environment and pointing out reality when there are distortions can also be useful interventions for severely anxious persons. Table 15-12 suggests some basic nursing interventions for patients with severe to panic levels of anxiety.

Anxiety management and reduction are primary concerns when working with patients who have anxiety and obsessive-compulsive disorders, but they may have a variety of other needs. When developing a plan of care, the psychiatric mental health nurse can utilize the *Psychiatric-Mental Health Nursing: Scope*

TABLE 15-11 INTERVENTIONS FOR MILD TO MODERATE LEVELS OF ANXIETY

Nursing diagnosis: Anxiety (moderate) related to situational event or psychological stress, as evidenced by increase in vital signs, moderate discomfort, narrowing of perceptual field, and selective inattention

INTERVENTION	RATIONALE
Help the patient identify anxiety. "Are you comfortable right now?"	It is important to validate observations with the patient, name the anxiety, and start to work with the patient to lower anxiety.
Anticipate anxiety-provoking situations.	Escalation of anxiety to a more disorganizing level is prevented.
Use nonverbal language to demonstrate interest (e.g., lean forward, maintain eye contact, nod your head).	Verbal and nonverbal messages should be consistent. The presence of an interested person provides a stabilizing focus.
Encourage the patient to talk about his or her feelings and concerns.	When concerns are stated aloud, problems can be discussed and feelings of isolation decreased.
Avoid closing off avenues of communication that are important for the patient. Focus on the patient's concerns.	When staff anxiety increases, changing the topic or offering advice is common but leaves the person isolated.
Ask questions to clarify what is being said. "I'm not sure what you mean. Give me an example."	Increased anxiety results in scattering of thoughts. Clarifying helps the patient identify thoughts and feelings.
Help the patient identify thoughts or feelings before the onset of anxiety. "What were you thinking right before you started to feel anxious?"	The patient is assisted in identifying thoughts and feelings, and problem solving is facilitated.
Encourage problem solving with the patient.*	Encouraging patients to explore alternatives increases sense of control and decreases anxiety.
Assist in developing alternative solutions to a problem through role play or modeling behaviors.	The patient is encouraged to try out alternative behaviors and solutions.
Explore behaviors that have worked to relieve anxiety in the past.	The patient is encouraged to mobilize successful coping mechanisms and strengths.
Provide outlets for working off excess energy (e.g., walking, playing ping-pong, dancing, exercising).	Physical activity can provide relief of built-up tension, increase muscle tone, and increase endorphin levels.

*Patients experiencing mild to moderate anxiety levels can problem solve.

and Standards of Practice (American Nurses Association [ANA] et al., 2007). The *Nursing Interventions Classification (NIC)* offers pertinent interventions in the behavioral and safety domains (Bulechek et al., 2013). Refer to Box 15-1 for potential nursing interventions for patients experiencing anxiety.

Guidelines for basic nursing interventions are:

1. Identify community resources that can offer the patient specialized treatment proven to be highly effective for people with a variety of anxiety disorders.
2. Identify community support groups for people with specific anxiety disorders and their families.
3. Use counseling, milieu therapy, promotion of self-care activities, and psychobiological and health teaching interventions as appropriate.

Counseling

Basic-level psychiatric mental health nurses use counseling to reduce anxiety, enhance coping and communication skills, and intervene in crises. When patients request or prefer to use integrative therapies, the nurse performs assessment and teaching as appropriate.

Teamwork and Safety

As mentioned earlier, most patients who demonstrate anxiety disorders can be treated successfully as outpatients. Hospital admission is necessary only if severe anxiety or symptoms interfere with the individual's health or if the individual is suicidal. When hospitalization is necessary, the health care team can be especially effective by:

- Collaborating to develop a multidisciplinary treatment plan to address goals, interventions, and outcomes that includes the patient's input.
- Evaluating and refining the plan of care at regular intervals.
- Documenting the plan and other essential communication electronically through an interactive and secure system.
- Identifying specific members of the treatment team to be responsible for carrying out specific actions of the plan.
- Maximizing safety through the provision of calm and consistent care.
- Stressing the value of unconditional positive regard.
- Maintaining a safe environment with an atmosphere of low-level stimulation.
- Providing ongoing education and training for the team to recognize escalating or problematic behaviors.

Promotion of Self-Care Activities

Respecting the patients' preferences for how involved they are in self-care, while recognizing that they may require more or less guidance depending on their level of ability, is a fine balance. Including the patient in decisions about his or her own care is always essential whenever possible. Patients with anxiety and obsessive-compulsive disorders are usually able to meet their own basic physical needs. Self-care activities that are most likely to be affected are discussed in the following sections.

TABLE 15-12 INTERVENTIONS FOR SEVERE TO PANIC LEVELS OF ANXIETY

Nursing diagnosis: Anxiety (severe, panic) related to severe threat (biochemical, environmental, psychosocial), as evidenced by verbal or physical acting out, extreme immobility, sense of impending doom, inability to differentiate reality (possible hallucinations or delusions), and inability to problem solve

INTERVENTION	RATIONALE
Maintain a calm manner.	Anxiety is communicated interpersonally. The quiet calm of the nurse can serve to calm the patient. The presence of anxiety can escalate anxiety in the patient.
Always remain with the person experiencing an acute severe to panic level of anxiety.	Alone with immense anxiety, a person feels abandoned. A caring face may be the patient's only contact with reality when confusion becomes overwhelming.
Minimize environmental stimuli. Move to a quieter setting, and stay with the patient.	Helps minimize further escalation of patient's anxiety.
Use clear and simple statements and repetition.	A person experiencing a severe to panic level of anxiety has difficulty concentrating and processing information.
Use a low-pitched voice; speak slowly.	A high-pitched voice can convey anxiety. Low pitch can decrease anxiety.
Reinforce reality if distortions occur (e.g., seeing objects that are not there or hearing voices when no one is present).	Anxiety can be reduced by focusing on and validating what is going on in the environment.
Listen for themes in communication.	In severe to panic levels of anxiety, verbal communication themes may be the only indication of the patient's thoughts or feelings.
Attend to physical and safety needs when necessary (e.g., need for warmth, fluids, elimination, pain relief, family contact).	High levels of anxiety may obscure the patient's awareness of physical needs.
Because safety is an overall goal, physical limits may need to be set. Speak in a firm, authoritative voice: "You may not hit anyone here. If you can't control yourself, we will help you."	A person who is out of control is often terrorized. Staff must offer the patient and others protection from destructive and self-destructive impulses.
Provide opportunities for exercise (e.g., walk with nurse, punching bag, ping-pong game).	Physical activity helps channel and dissipate tension and may temporarily lower anxiety.
When a person is constantly moving or pacing, offer high-calorie fluids.	Dehydration and exhaustion must be prevented.
Assess need for medication or seclusion after other interventions have been tried and have been unsuccessful.	Exhaustion and physical harm to self and others must be prevented.

BOX 15-1 NIC INTERVENTIONS FOR ANXIETY DISORDERS

Coping Enhancement

Definition: Assisting a patient to adapt to perceived stressors, changes, or threats that interfere with meeting life demands and roles

Activities:*

Provide an atmosphere of acceptance.

Encourage verbalization of feelings, perceptions, and fears.

Acknowledge the patient's spiritual/cultural background.

Discourage decision making when the patient is under severe stress.

Hope Instillation

Definition: Enhancing the belief in one's capacity to initiate and sustain actions

Activities:*

Assist the patient to identify areas of hope in life.

Demonstrate hope by recognizing the patient's intrinsic worth and viewing the patient's illness as only one facet of the individual.

Avoid masking the truth.

Help the patient expand spiritual self.

Self-Esteem Enhancement

Definition: Assisting a patient to increase his or her personal judgment of self-worth

Activities:*

Make positive statements about the patient.

Monitor frequency of self-negating verbalizations.

Explore previous achievements.

Explore reasons for self-criticism or guilt.

Relaxation Therapy

Definition: Use of techniques to encourage and elicit relaxation for the purpose of decreasing undesirable signs and symptoms such as pain, muscle tension, or anxiety

Activities:*

Demonstrate and practice the relaxation technique with the patient.

Provide written information about preparing and engaging in relaxation techniques.

Anticipate the need for the use of relaxation.

Evaluate and document the response to relaxation therapy.

*Partial list.

From Bulechek, G. M., Butcher, H. K., Dochterman, J. M., & Wagner, C. (2013). *Nursing interventions classification (NIC)* (6th ed). St. Louis, MO: Mosby.

Nutrition and Fluid Intake

Patients who engage in ritualistic behaviors may be too involved with their rituals to take time to eat and drink. Some phobic patients may be so afraid of germs that they cannot eat. In general, nutritious diets with snacks should be provided. Hoarders may have created an environment that is so dysfunctional that normal intake may be impossible. Adequate intake should be firmly encouraged, but a power struggle should be avoided. Weighing patients frequently (e.g., three times a week) is useful in assessing nutrition.

Personal Hygiene and Grooming

Some patients, especially those with obsessive-compulsive disorder and phobias, may be excessively neat and engage in time-consuming rituals associated with bathing and dressing. Hygiene, dressing, and grooming may take several hours. Maintenance of skin integrity may become a problem when the rituals involve excessive washing and skin becomes excoriated and infected. Assessment of skin integrity is also a concern for individuals who pull their hair or pick at their skin.

Some patients with anxiety and obsessive-compulsive disorders are indecisive about bathing or about what clothing should be worn. For the latter, limiting choices to two outfits is helpful. In the event of severe indecisiveness, simply presenting the patient with the clothing to be worn may be necessary. You may also need to remain with the patient to give simple directions: "Put on your shirt. Now put on your slacks." Matter-of-fact support is effective in assisting patients to independently perform as much of a task as possible. Encourage patients to express thoughts and feelings about self-care. This communication can provide a basis for later health teaching or for ongoing dialogue about the patient's abilities.

Elimination

Patients with obsessive-compulsive disorder may be so involved with the performance of rituals that they may suppress the urge to void and defecate. Constipation and urinary tract infections may result. Interventions may include creating a regular schedule for taking the patient to the bathroom.

Sleep

Patients experiencing anxiety and obsessive-compulsive disorders frequently have difficulty sleeping, particularly in falling asleep. Patients with generalized anxiety disorder often experience sleep disturbance from nightmares. Separation anxiety disorder may create such profound psychic disturbance that sleep seems impossible. Patients may perform rituals to the exclusion of resting and sleeping, and physical exhaustion may occur. Teaching patients how to discover ways to promote sleep (e.g., warm bath, warm milk, and relaxing music) and monitoring sleep through a sleep record are useful interventions. Chapter 19 offers an in-depth discussion of sleep disturbances.

Pharmacological Interventions

Several classes of medications have been found to be effective in the treatment of anxiety disorders. Table 15-13 identifies medications approved by the U.S. Food and Drug Administration (FDA) for the treatment of anxiety, as well as medications that do not have specific approval but are commonly used "off-label" for anxiety disorders. Refer to Chapter 3 for a more detailed explanation of the actions of psychotropic medications.

There are no medications with FDA approval for children with anxiety disorders (Bostic & Prince, 2010); however, medications approved for other age groups are often prescribed. Selective serotonin reuptake inhibitors (SSRIs) are being used for generalized anxiety disorder, panic disorder, and social anxiety disorder with good results. For children with obsessive-compulsive and related disorders, SSRIs are also often used; a tricyclic antidepressant, clomipramine (Anafranil), is also used as a pharmacological treatment.

Antidepressants

Selective serotonin reuptake inhibitors (SSRIs) are considered the first line of defense in most anxiety and obsessive-compulsive related disorders. These SSRIs include paroxetine (Paxil), fluoxetine (Prozac), escitalopram (Lexapro), fluvoxamine (Luvox), and sertraline (Zoloft). Some of these antidepressants exert more of an "activating" effect than others and may actually increase anxiety. Sertraline (Zoloft) and paroxetine (Paxil) seem to have a more calming effect than the other SSRIs. Antidepressants have the secondary benefit of treating comorbid depressive disorders.

Venlafaxine (Effexor) is a serotonin-norepinephrine reuptake inhibitor (SNRI) that is quite successful in the treatment of several anxiety disorders. Another SNRI, Duloxetine (Cymbalta), is effective in the treatment of generalized anxiety disorder.

Monoamine oxidase inhibitors (MAOIs) are reserved for treatment-resistant conditions because of the risk of life-threatening hypertensive crisis if the patient does not follow dietary restrictions (patients cannot eat foods containing tyramine and must be given specific dietary instructions). The risk of hypertensive crisis also makes the use of MAOIs contraindicated in patients with comorbid substance abuse.

Antianxiety Drugs

Antianxiety (anxiolytic) drugs are often used to treat the somatic and psychological symptoms of anxiety disorders. When moderate or severe anxiety is reduced, patients are better able to participate in treatment of their underlying problems. Benzodiazepines are most commonly used because they have a quick onset of action; however, due to the potential for dependence, these medications ideally should be used for short periods, only until other medications or treatments reduce symptoms. An important nursing intervention is to monitor for side effects of the benzodiazepines, including sedation, ataxia, and decreased cognitive function. Benzodiazepines are not recommended for patients with a known substance abuse problem and should not be given to women during pregnancy or breastfeeding. Box 15-2 gives other important information for patient teaching.

BOX 15-2 PATIENT AND FAMILY TEACHING: ANTIANXIETY MEDICATIONS

1. Caution the patient:
   Not to change dose or frequency of medicating without prior approval of the prescriber.
   That these medications may make it unsafe to handle mechanical equipment (e.g., cars, saws, and machinery).
   Not to drink alcoholic beverages or take other antianxiety drugs, because depressant effects of both will be potentiated.
   To avoid drinking beverages containing caffeine because they decrease the desired effects of the drug.
2. Recommend that the patient taking benzodiazepines avoid becoming pregnant because these drugs increase the risk of congenital anomalies.
3. Advise the patient to discuss breast-feeding with care provider since these drugs are excreted in the milk and would have adverse effects on the infant.
4. Teach a patient who is taking monoamine oxidase inhibitors about the details of a tyramine-restricted diet (refer to Chapter 3).
5. Teach the patient that:
   Cessation of benzodiazepine use after 3 to 4 months of daily use may cause withdrawal symptoms such as insomnia, irritability, nervousness, dry mouth, tremors, convulsions, and confusion.
   Medications should be taken with or shortly after meals or snacks to reduce gastrointestinal discomfort.
   Drug interactions can occur: Antacids may delay absorption; cimetidine interferes with metabolism of benzodiazepines, causing increased sedation; central nervous system depressants, such as alcohol and barbiturates, cause increased sedation; serum phenytoin concentration may build up because of decreased metabolism.

TABLE 15-13 DRUGS USED WITH FDA APPROVAL AND AS OFF-LABEL USE FOR THE TREATMENT OF GENERALIZED ANXIETY, OBSESSIVE-COMPULSIVE, PANIC, AND SOCIAL ANXIETY DISORDERS

GENERIC (TRADE)	FDA-APPROVED USES	OFF-LABEL USES
Antidepressants		
Selective Serotonin Reuptake Inhibitors		
Citalopram (Celexa)		Generalized anxiety disorder Obsessive-compulsive disorder Panic disorder Social anxiety disorder
Escitalopram (Lexapro)	Generalized anxiety disorder	Obsessive-compulsive disorder Panic disorder Social anxiety disorder
Fluoxetine (Prozac)	Obsessive-compulsive disorder Panic disorder	Generalized anxiety disorder Social anxiety disorder
Fluvoxamine (Luvox)	Obsessive-compulsive disorder Social anxiety disorder	Panic disorder Generalized anxiety disorder
Paroxetine (Paxil)	Generalized anxiety disorder Obsessive-compulsive disorder Panic disorder Social anxiety disorder	
Sertraline (Zoloft)	Obsessive-compulsive disorder Panic disorder Social anxiety disorder	Generalized anxiety disorder
Vilazodone (Viibryd)*	Generalized anxiety disorder	
Selective Serotonin Norepinephrine Reuptake Inhibitors		
Duloxetine (Cymbalta)	Generalized anxiety disorder	Obsessive-compulsive disorder Panic disorder Social anxiety disorder
Milnacipran (Savella)		Generalized anxiety disorder Obsessive-compulsive disorder Panic disorder Social anxiety disorder
Venlafaxine (Effexor)	Generalized anxiety disorder Panic disorder Social anxiety disorder	Obsessive-compulsive disorder
Tetracyclics/Tricyclics		
Amitriptyline (Elavil)		Generalized anxiety disorder Panic disorder
Amoxapine (Asendin)		Generalized anxiety disorder Panic disorder

*Dual action selective serotonin reuptake inhibitor and serotonin 1A receptor partial agonist.

Data from Howland, R.H. (2012). Drugs to treat anxiety disorders. *Journal of Psychosocial and Mental Health Services, 50*(5), 1-2; Stahl, S. M. (2006). *Essential psychopharmacology: The prescriber's guide* (Revised and updated ed.). New York, NY: Cambridge; Lehne, R.E. (2010). *Pharmacology for nursing care* (7th ed.). St Louis, MO: Elsevier.

Continued

TABLE 15-13 DRUGS USED WITH FDA APPROVAL AND AS OFF-LABEL USE FOR THE TREATMENT OF GENERALIZED ANXIETY, OBSESSIVE-COMPULSIVE, PANIC, AND SOCIAL ANXIETY DISORDERS—cont'd

GENERIC (TRADE)	FDA-APPROVED USES	OFF-LABEL USES
Clomipramine (Anafranil)	Obsessive-compulsive disorder	Generalized anxiety disorder Panic disorder Social anxiety disorder
Desipramine (Norpramin)		Generalized anxiety disorder Panic disorder
Doxepin (Adapin, Sinequan)		Generalized anxiety disorder Panic disorder Social anxiety disorder
Imipramine (Tofranil)		Generalized anxiety disorder Panic disorder Social anxiety disorder
Maprotiline (Ludiomil)		Generalized anxiety disorder Panic disorder
Mirtazapine (Remeron)		Generalized anxiety disorder Obsessive-compulsive disorder Panic disorder
Nortriptyline (Aventyl, Pamelor)		Generalized anxiety disorder Panic disorder
Trazodone (Desyrel)		Generalized anxiety disorder
Trimipramine (Surmontil)		Generalized anxiety disorder Panic disorder
Monoamine Oxidase Inhibitors		
Isocarboxazid (Marplan)		Panic disorder Social anxiety disorder
Phenelzine (Nardil)		Generalized anxiety disorder Panic disorder Social anxiety disorder
Tranylcypromine (Parnate)		Generalized anxiety disorder Panic disorder Social anxiety disorder
Antianxiety Agents		
Benzodiazepines		
Alprazolam (Xanax)	Generalized anxiety disorder Panic disorder	Social anxiety disorder
Buspirone (BuSpar)	Generalized anxiety disorder	Obsessive-compulsive disorder Panic disorder Social anxiety disorder
Chlordiazepoxide (Librium)	Generalized anxiety disorder	Panic disorder Social anxiety disorder
Clonazepam (Klonopin)	Panic disorder	Generalized anxiety disorder Social anxiety disorder
Clorazepate (Tranxene)	Generalized anxiety disorder	Panic disorder Social anxiety disorder
Diazepam (Valium)	Generalized anxiety disorder	Panic disorder Social anxiety disorder
Halazepam (Paxipam)	Generalized anxiety disorder	
Lorazepam (Ativan)	Generalized anxiety disorder	Panic disorder Social anxiety disorder
Oxazepam (Serax)	Generalized anxiety disorder	Panic disorder Social anxiety disorder
Antipsychotics		
Chlorpromazine (Thorazine)		Generalized anxiety disorder
Fluphenazine (Prolixin)		Obsessive-compulsive disorder
Haloperidol (Haldol)		Obsessive-compulsive disorder
Olanzapine (Zyprexa)		Generalized anxiety disorder Obsessive-compulsive disorder
Quetiapine (Seroquel)		Generalized anxiety disorder
Risperidone (Risperdal)		Obsessive-compulsive disorder
Trifluoperazine (Stelazine)	Generalized anxiety disorder	
Anticonvulsants		
Carbamazepine (Tegretol)		Generalized anxiety disorder
Divalproex sodium (Depakote)		Generalized anxiety disorder
Gabapentin (Neurontin)		Generalized anxiety disorder Social anxiety disorder
Pregabalin (Lyrica)		Generalized anxiety disorder
Tiagabine (Gabitril)		Generalized anxiety disorder
Other Classes		
Diphenhydramine (Benadryl)		Generalized anxiety disorder
Hydroxyzine (Atarax, Vistaril)		Generalized anxiety disorder
Propranolol (Inderal)		Generalized anxiety disorder Panic disorder Social anxiety disorder

Buspirone (BuSpar) is an alternative antianxiety medication that does not cause dependence, but 2 to 4 weeks are required for it to reach full effects. The drug may be used for long-term treatment and should be taken regularly.

Other Classes of Medications

Other classes of medications sometimes used to treat anxiety disorders include β-blockers, antihistamines, and anticonvulsants. These agents are often added if the first course of treatment is ineffective. β-blockers block the nerves that stimulate the heart to beat faster and have been used to treat social anxiety disorder. Anticonvulsants have shown some benefit in the management of generalized anxiety disorder and social anxiety disorder (Howland, 2012). Antihistamines are a safe, nonaddictive alternative to benzodiazepines to lower anxiety levels and again are helpful in treating patients with substance use problems.

Another therapeutic strategy may come in a most unusual form. D-cycloserine is an antibiotic used to treat tuberculosis that has also been demonstrated to enhance learning. D-cycloserine binds with N-methyl-D-aspartate (NMDA) receptors in the area of the brain that mediates fears and phobic responses, the amygdala, and may help patients *unlearn* fear responses more quickly (Stahl, 2008). Administration of this drug while undergoing cognitive-behavioral therapy actually promotes fear extinction, not just fear conditioning, in phobic individuals. It has also been useful when combined with cognitive-behavioral therapy in the treatment of panic disorder and social anxiety disorder (Otto et al., 2010; Hofmann et al., 2006).

Psychobiological Interventions

Besides medication, there are few biological interventions available to disrupt the course of the anxiety and anxiety-related disorders. One controversial surgical treatment being used for obsessive-compulsive disorder is deep brain stimulation for those 10% of individuals who do not respond to usual treatment (Denys et al., 2010). Only about 50 people in the United States have had the procedure so far. Electrodes are surgically placed in the subthalamic nucleus of the brain; then an implanted pulse generator activates a low-dose current for a specified period of time (several months in some cases). Researchers have reported a decrease of 35% on a measurement of obsessive-compulsive symptoms. This treatment has come under the scrutiny of some members of the medical community who believe that the Food and Drug Administration's approval was premature and that full-scale clinical trials should be done (Fins et al., 2011). Infection and cerebral hemorrhage have been reported, and this therapy will continue to be investigated.

Integrative Therapy

Chapter 35 identifies a number of complementary practices or integrative therapies that people use to cope with stress in their lives. Herbal therapy and dietary supplements are commonly used, yet they are not subject to the same rigorous testing as prescription medications. Also, herbs and dietary supplements may not be uniformly prepared or dosed, and there is no guarantee of bioequivalence of the active compound among preparations. Problems that can occur with the use of psychotropic herbs include toxic side effects and herb-drug interactions. Nurses and other health care providers do well to improve their knowledge of these products so that discussions with their patients provide informed and reliable information.

One example is kava, which is derived from the roots of *Piper methysticum,* a South American plant, and is used as a sedative with antianxiety effects. Prior to seeking professional care, people with anxiety disorders may try kava in the belief that herbs are safer than medications, but it has a dark side. In 2010 the Food and Drug Administration issued a warning regarding its risk of liver damage. Kava is known to dramatically inhibit a liver enzyme (P450) necessary for the metabolism of many medications. This inhibition could result in liver failure, especially when taken along with alcohol or other medications such as central nervous system depressants (antianxiety agents fall into this category).

Health Teaching

Health teaching is a significant nursing intervention for patients with anxiety disorders. Patients may conceal symptoms for years before seeking treatment and often come to the attention of health care providers during a co-occurring problem. Persons with panic disorder and generalized anxiety disorder seem more motivated than those with other anxiety disorders to get treatment; most seek help during the first year of symptoms (Wang et al., 2005).

Teaching about the specific disorder and available effective treatments is a major step to improving the quality of life for those with anxiety disorders. Whether in a community or hospital setting, nurses can teach patients about signs and symptoms of anxiety disorders, presumed causes or risk factors (especially substance abuse), medications, the use of relaxation techniques, and the benefits of psychotherapy.

Advanced Practice Interventions

Advanced practice nurses use several cognitive and behavioral treatment approaches, including relaxation training, modeling, systematic desensitization, flooding, response prevention, and thought stopping.

Cognitive Therapy

Cognitive therapy is based on the belief that patients make errors in thinking that lead to mistaken negative beliefs about self and others. For example, "I have to be perfect or my boyfriend will not love me." Through a process called **cognitive restructuring**, the therapist helps the patient (1) identify automatic negative beliefs that cause anxiety, (2) explore the basis for these thoughts, (3) reevaluate the situation realistically, and (4) replace negative self-talk with supportive ideas.

Behavioral Therapy

There are currently several forms of **behavioral therapy**, which involve teaching and physical practice of activities to decrease anxious or avoidant behavior:

- **Relaxation training:** Relaxation exercises for breathing or muscle groups are taught. The relaxation response is the opposite of the stress response and results in a reduced heart rate and breathing and relaxed muscles. Refer to Chapter 10 for a description of different approaches to relaxation training.
- **Modeling:** The therapist or significant other acts as a role model to demonstrate appropriate behavior in a feared situation, and then the patient imitates it. For example, the role model rides in an elevator with a claustrophobic patient.
- **Systematic desensitization:** The patient is gradually introduced to a feared object or experience through a series of steps, from the least frightening to the most frightening (graduated exposure). The patient is taught to use a relaxation technique at each step when anxiety becomes overwhelming. For example, a patient with agoraphobia would start with opening the door to the house to go out on the steps and advance to attending a movie in a theater. The therapist may start with imagined situations in the office before moving on to in vivo (live) exposures.
- **Flooding:** Unlike systematic desensitization, this method exposes the patient to a large amount of an undesirable stimulus in an effort to extinguish the anxiety response. The patient learns through prolonged exposure that survival is possible and that anxiety diminishes spontaneously. For example, an obsessive patient who usually touches objects with a paper towel may be forced to touch objects with a bare hand for 1 hour. By the end of that period, the anxiety level is lower.
- **Response prevention:** This method is used for compulsive behavior. The therapist does not allow the patient to perform the compulsive ritual (e.g., hand washing), and the patient learns that anxiety does subside even when the ritual is not completed. After trying this in the office, the patient learns to set time limits at home to gradually lengthen the time between rituals until the urge fades away.
- **Thought stopping:** Through this technique a negative thought or obsession is interrupted. The patient may be instructed to say "Stop!" out loud when the idea comes to mind or to snap a rubber band worn on the wrist. This distraction briefly blocks the automatic undesirable thought and cues the patient to select an alternative, more positive idea. (After learning the exercise, the patient gives the command silently.)

Cognitive-Behavioral Therapy

Cognitive-behavioral therapy combines cognitive therapy with specific behavioral therapies to reduce the anxiety response. Cognitive-behavioral therapy includes cognitive restructuring, psychoeducation, breath restraining and muscle relaxation, teaching of self-monitoring for panic and other symptoms, and in vivo (real life) exposure to feared objects or situations.

EVALUATION

Identified outcomes serve as the basis for evaluation. In general, evaluation of outcomes for patients with anxiety and obsessive-compulsive disorders deals with questions such as the following:

- Is the patient experiencing a reduced level of anxiety?
- Does the patient recognize symptoms as anxiety-related?
- Does the patient continue to display signs and symptoms such as obsessions, compulsions, phobias, worrying, or other symptoms of anxiety disorders? If still present, are they more or less frequent? More or less intense?
- Is the patient able to use newly learned behaviors to manage anxiety?
- Does the patient adequately perform self-care activities?
- Can the patient maintain satisfying interpersonal relations?
- Is the patient able to assume usual roles?

QUALITY IMPROVEMENT

This chapter focused on the problem of anxiety disorders and addressed the care for this group of patients. As much as possible this care is evidence-based, yet the provision of psychiatric care (like general medical care) is also based on tradition. Unfortunately, this care is not always adequate. Quality improvement attempts to quantitatively measure severity of disorders, develop outcomes and guidelines for care, and monitor patients' progress. In primary care (where most people get their mental health care) evidence-based practice guidelines result in practitioners more confident in their skills and more likely to treat anxiety (Smolders et al., 2010). Evidence-based treatment includes using cognitive-behavioral therapy, using appropriate medication, and following up with patients. Primary care providers may need expert support to provide this care (Roy-Byrne et al., 2010).

A variety of instruments are used in quality improvement initiatives for psychiatric disorders. A simple tool for measuring quality improvement for anxiety care is the Clinical Global Impression-Severity (CGI-S) Scale for inpatient, outpatient, or primary care. It asks the clinician to rate the severity of illness on a seven-point continuum from normal-not ill to among the most extremely ill. Versteeg and colleagues (2012) developed the following outcomes for use with the tool:

- At least 80% of patients with anxiety disorders are monitored every 6 weeks with the CGI-S scale.
- After 6 months of treatment, 50% of patients with severe anxiety disorders will score less than three on the CGI-S.

Nurses are at the forefront in gathering information to improve the quality of care in all settings. Understanding anxiety disorders and their treatment is more fully accomplished when we consider the seriousness and importance of continuous quality improvement in improving care.

KEY POINTS TO REMEMBER

- Anxiety has an unknown or unrecognized source whereas fear is a reaction to a specific threat.
- Peplau operationally defined four levels of anxiety (mild, moderate, severe, and panic). The patient's perceptual field, ability to learn, and physical and other characteristics are different at each level.
- Defenses against anxiety can be adaptive or maladaptive and in a hierarchy from healthy to intermediate to immature.
- Anxiety disorders are the most common psychiatric disorders in the United States and frequently co-occur with depression or substance abuse.
- Another closely related set of disorders is obsessions, in which anxiety results in abnormal selective overattention.
- Research has identified biological, psychological, and environmental factors in the etiology of anxiety and obsessive-compulsive disorders.
- Patients with anxiety and obsessive-compulsive disorders suffer from debilitating anxiety, panic attacks, irrational fears, excessive worrying, uncontrollable rituals, or severe reactions to stress.
- Embarrassment and shame often prevent people from seeking psychiatric help. Instead, they may go to primary care providers with multiple somatic complaints.
- Psychiatric treatment is effective for anxiety and obsessive-compulsive disorders.
- Basic-level nursing interventions include counseling, milieu therapy, promotion of self-care activities, psychobiological intervention, and health teaching.
- Understanding the levels of anxiety will help in planning basic care, including how much direction your patient will need, what precautions should be taken to prevent harm, and how able your patient is to learn.
- Advanced practice nursing interventions include behavioral and cognitive-behavioral therapies.
- Quality improvement initiatives will help to measure severity of symptoms and to establish interventions that are evidence based rather than tradition based.

CRITICAL THINKING

1. Corey is a senior in college and is taking his final examinations for an engineering course. The professor catches him copying from the examination of his willing partner, Katie, and takes his exam away. Corey's heart immediately begins to pound, his pulse and respiration rates increase, and he has to wipe perspiration from his hands and face several times. He feels like he may vomit and has a throbbing in his head.

   After the examination, he approaches the professor, but has difficulty focusing; when he starts to speak, his voice trembles. Corey says that Katie suggested that cheating is no big deal, that he needed to do it to be competitive, and that it was done all the time. Corey goes on to say that this "silly exam" doesn't mean anything anyway, that he already passed the important courses. He tells the professor, "I thought you were the greatest, and now I see that you're a fool."

   The professor remains calm and explains that regardless of Corey's thoughts on this matter, he was, in fact, caught cheating, and he will have to take responsibility for his actions. The professor will refer Corey to the disciplinary board. When Corey realizes how serious this incident is, he flips out and yells at the professor and calls him offensive names. Another professor walking past the classroom witnesses this encounter.

   a. Identify the level of anxiety Corey was experiencing once he was caught cheating, and describe the signs and symptoms that helped you determine this level.
   b. Identify and define five defense mechanisms Corey used to lessen his anxiety.

   Given the circumstances once Corey was caught, how could he have reacted using healthier coping defenses in a manner that would have reflected more self-responsibility?
2. Tiffany, a teenager with obsessive-compulsive disorder, washes her hands until they are cracked and bleeding. Your nursing goal is to promote healing of her hands. What interventions will you plan?
3. This is Logan's third emergency department visit in a week. He is experiencing severe anxiety accompanied by many physical symptoms. He clings to you, desperately crying, "Help me! Help me! Don't let me die!" Diagnostic tests have ruled out a physical disorder. The patient outcome has been identified as "Patient's anxiety level will be reduced to moderate/mild within one hour."
   a. What interventions should you use? Be comprehensive in your approach.
   b. Logan is given an appointment at the anxiety disorders clinic. How will you explain the importance of keeping the clinic appointment? Are there any factors you would have to consider while providing patient education?
4. Liz is a patient with generalized anxiety disorder. She has a history of substance abuse and is now a recovering alcoholic. During a clinic visit, she tells you she plans to ask the psychiatrist to prescribe diazepam (Valium) to use when she feels anxious. She asks whether you think this is a good idea. How would you respond? What action could you take?

CHAPTER REVIEW

1. Which of the following statements are correct regarding obsessive-compulsive disorder (OCD)? *Select all that apply.*
   a. Obsessions are repetitive thoughts, whereas compulsions are ritualistic behaviors.
   b. OCD symptoms can start as early as 3 years of age.
   c. OCD patients often have difficulty sleeping.
   d. Schizophrenia often occurs comorbidly with OCD.
   e. There is a tool (scale) to measure compulsive behaviors.
   f. Patients diagnosed with OCD are at higher risk for suicide than patients with depression.
2. Since learning that he will have a trial pass to a new group home tomorrow, Luke's usual behavior has changed. He has started to pace, has become distracted, and is breathing rapidly. He has trouble focusing on anything other than the group home issue and complains that he suddenly feels nauseated. Which initial nursing response is most appropriate for Luke's level of anxiety?
   a. "You seem anxious. Would you like to talk about how you are feeling?"
   b. "If you do not calm down, I will have to give you prn medicine to help you."
   c. "Luke, slow down. Listen to me. You are safe. Take a deep breath, and let's go to a quieter place."
   d. "We can delay the visit to the group home if that would help you calm down."
3. Michael seems to be angry when his family fails to visit him in the hospital as promised. However, he tells you that he is fine and that the visit wasn't important to him. When you suggest that perhaps he might be disappointed or even a little angry that the family has again let him down, the patient responds that it is his family that is angry, not him, or else they would have visited. What defense mechanism(s) is this patient using to deal with his feelings? *Select all that apply.*
   a. Rationalization
   b. Projection
   c. Regression
   d. Denial
   e. Dissociation
4. A variety of medications are used in the treatment of severe anxiety disorders. Which class of medication used to treat anxiety is potentially addictive?
   a. Selective serotonin reuptake inhibitors (SSRIs)
   b. β-blockers
   c. Antihistamines
   d. Buspirone
   e. Benzodiazepines
5. A disorder in which one experiences fear of being in places or situations from which escape might be difficult or embarrassing or in which help might not be available if a panic attack occurs is called ________________.

Answers to Chapter Review
1. a, b, c, e; 2. c; 3. a, b, d; 4. e; 5. agoraphobia.

evolve WEBSITE

Visit the Evolve website for a posttest on the content in this chapter: http://evolve.elsevier.com/Varcarolis

Post-Test interactive review

REFERENCES

Ahlskog, J.E. (2011). Pathological behaviors provoked by dopamine agonist therapy of Parkinson's disease. *Physiology and Behavior, 104*(1), 168–172.

American Nurses Association, American Psychiatric Nurses Association, & International Society of Psychiatric-Mental Health Nurses. (2007). *Psychiatric-mental health nursing: Scope and standards of practice.* Silver Spring, MD: NurseBooks.org.

American Psychiatric Association. (2013). *DSM-5 table of contents.* Retrieved from http://www.psychiatry.org/dsm5.

Bostic, J. Q., & Prince, J. B. (2010). Child and adolescent psychiatric disorders. In T. A. Stern, G. L. Fricchione, N. H. Cassem, M. S. Jellinek, & J. F. Rosenbaum (Eds.), *Massachusetts General Hospital handbook of general hospital psychiatry* (6th ed.) (pp. 937-959). Philadelphia, PA: Saunders

Bulechek, G. M., Butcher, H. K., Dochterman, J. M., & Wagner, C. (2013). *Nursing interventions classification (NIC)* (6th ed). St. Louis, MO: Mosby.

Denys, D., Mantione, M., Figee, M., van den Munchkhoff, P., Koerselman, F., Westenberg, H., et al. (2010). Deep brain stimulation of the nucleus accumbens for treatment-refractory obsessive-compulsive disorder. *Archives of General Psychiatry, 67*(10), 1061–1068. doi:10.1001/archgenpsychistry.2010.122.

Fins, J. J., Mayberg, H. S., Nuttin, B., Kubu, C. S., Galert, T., Sturm, V., et al. (2011). Misuse of the FDA's humanitarian device exemption in deep brain stimulation for obsessive-compulsive disorder. *Health Affairs, 30*(2), 302–311. doi:10.1377/hlthaff.2010.0157.

First, M. B., & Tasman, A. (2011). *Clinical guide to the diagnosis and treatment of mental disorders* (2nd ed.). West Sussex, UK: Wiley.

Haas, C. F., Champion, A., & Secor, D. (2008). Motivating factors for seeking cosmetic surgery: A synthesis of the literature. *Plastic Surgical Nursing, 28*(4), 177–82.

Herdman, T.H. (Ed.). (2012). *NANDA International Nursing Diagnoses: Definitions and Classification, 2012–2014.* Oxford, UK: Wiley Blackwell.

Hofmann, S. G., Meuret, A. E., Smits, J. A. J., Simon, N. M., Pollack, M. H., Eisenmenger, K., et al. (2006). Augmentation of exposure therapy with d-cycloserine for social anxiety disorder. *Archives of General Psychiatry, 63,* 298–304.

Hollander, E., Berlin, H. A., & Stein, D. J. (2011). Impulse-control disorders not elsewhere classified. In R. E. Hales, S. C. Yudofsky, & G. O. Gabbard (Eds.), *Essentials of psychiatry* (3rd ed.) (pp. 271-292). Washington, DC: American Psychiatric Publishing.

Howland, R. H. (2012). Drugs to treat anxiety disorders. *Journal of Psychosocial and Mental Health Services, 50*(5), 1–2.

Kessler, R. C., Chiu, W. T., Demler, O., & Walters, E. E. (2005). Prevalence, severity, and comorbidity of twelve-month *DSM-IV* disorders in the National Comorbidity Survey Replication (NCS-R). *Archives of General Psychiatry, 62,* 617–627.

Kessler, R. C., Berglund, P. A., Demler, O., Jin, R., & Walters, E. E. (2005). Lifetime prevalence and age-of-onset distributions of *DSM-IV* disorders in the National Comorbidity Survey Replication (NCS-R). *Archives of General Psychiatry, 62*(6), 593–602.

Mertol, S., & Alkin, T. (2012). Temperament and character dimensions of patients with adult separation anxiety disorder. *Journal of Affective Disorders, 139*(2) 199–203. doi:10.1016/j.jad.2012.02.034.

Moorhead, S., Johnson, M., Maas, M., & Swanson, E. (2013). *Nursing outcomes classification (NOC)* (5th ed.). St. Louis, MO: Mosby.

National Institute of Mental Health. (2012). *A PANDAS study is currently recruiting patients*. Retrieved from http://intramural.nimh.nih.gov/pdn/web.htm.

Newman, M. G., & Llera, S. J. (2011). A novel theory of experiential avoidance in generalized anxiety disorder: A review and synthesis of research supporting a contrast avoidance model of worry. *Clinical Psychology Review, 31*(3), 371–82.

Nichols, M. (2009). Adult separation anxiety disorder. *Anxiety, panic, and health*. Retrieved from http://anxietypanichealth.com/reference/separation-anxiety-disorder-adult/.

Otte, S., & Steketee, G. (2011). Psychiatric issues in hoarding: Strategies for diagnosing and treating symptoms of hoarding. *Psychiatric Times*. Retrieved from http://www.psychiatrictimes.com/bipolar-disorder/content/article/10168/1932177.

Otto, M. W., Tolin, D. F., Simon, N. M., Pearlson, G. D., Basden, S., Meunier, S. A., et al. (2010). Efficacy of d-cycloserine for enhancing responses to cognitive-behavior therapy for panic disorder. *Biological Psychiatry, 67*(4), 365–370.

Peplau, H. E. (1968). A working definition of anxiety. In S. F. Burd & M. A. Marshall (Eds.), *Some clinical approaches to psychiatric nursing* (pp. 323-327). New York, NY: Macmillan.

Phillips, K. A., Menard, W., & Fay, C. (2006). Gender similarities and differences in 200 individuals with body dysmorphic disorder. *Comprehensive Psychiatry, 46*, 77–87.

Roy-Byrne, P., Craske, M. G., Sullivan, G., Rose, R. D., Edlund, M. J., Lang, A. J., et al. (2010). Delivery of evidence-based treatment for multiple anxiety disorders in primary care: A randomized controlled trial. *Journal of the American Medical Association, 303*(19), 1921–1928.

Sadock, B. J., & Sadock, V. A. (2008). *Kaplan and Sadock's concise textbook of clinical psychiatry* (3rd ed.). Philadelphia, PA: Lippincott.

Serretti, A., & Chiesa, A. (2012). The challenges of uncovering the genetics of anxiety. *Acta Psychiatrica Scandinavica, 125*(3), 185–186. doi:10.1111/j.1600–0447.2011.01765.x.

Smolders, M., Laurant, M., Verhaak, P., Prins, M., van Marwijk, H., Penninx, B., et al. (2010). Which physician and practice characteristics are associated with adherence to evidence-based guidelines for depressive and anxiety disorders? *Medical Care, 48*(3), 240–248.

Stahl, S. M. (2008). *Stahl's essential psychopharmacology* (3rd ed.). Cambridge, UK: Cambridge University Press.

Stangier, U., Adam-Schwebe, S., Muller, T., & Wolter, M. (2008). Discrimination of facial appearance stimuli in body dysmorphic disorder. *Journal of Abnormal Psychology, 117*(2), 435–443. doi:10.1037/0021-843X.117.2.435.

Stern, T. A., Fricchione, G. L., Cassem, N. H., Jellinek, M. S., & Rosenbaum, J. F. (2010). *Massachusetts General Hospital handbook of general hospital psychiatry* (6th ed.). Philadelphia, PA: Saunders.

Sullivan, H. S. (1953). *The interpersonal theory of psychiatry*. New York, NY: W. W. Norton.

Versteeg, M. H., Laurant, M. G. H., Franx, G. C., Jacobs, A. J., & Wensing, M. J. P. (2012). Factors associated with the quality improvement collaboratives in mental health care: An exploratory study. *Implementation Science, 7*(1). Retrieved from http://www.implementationscience.com/content/7/1/1.

Ursano, A. M., Kartheiser, P. H., & Barnhill, L. J. (2011). Disorders usually first diagnosed in infancy, childhood, or adolescence. In R. E. Hales, S. C. Yudofsky, & G. O. Gabbard (Eds.), *Essentials of psychiatry* (3rd ed.) (pp. 325-382). Washington, DC: American Psychiatric Publishing.

Wang, P. S., Berglund, P., Olfson, M., Pincus, H. A., Wells, K. B., & Kessler, R.C. (2005). Failure and delay in initial treatment contact after first onset of mental disorders in the national comorbidity survey replication. *Archives of General Psychiatry, 62*, 603–613.

CHAPTER

16

Trauma, Stressor-Related, and Dissociative Disorders

Kathleen Wheeler

evolve WEBSITE

Visit the Evolve website for a pretest on the content in this chapter: http://evolve.elsevier.com/Varcarolis

Pre-Test interactive review

OBJECTIVES

1. Describe clinical manifestations of each disorder covered under the general umbrella of trauma-related and dissociative disorders.
2. Describe the symptoms, epidemiology, comorbidity, and etiology of trauma-related disorders in children.
3. Discuss at least five of the neurobiological changes that occur with trauma.
4. Apply the nursing process to the care of children who are experiencing trauma-related disorders.
5. Differentiate between the symptoms of posttraumatic stress, acute stress, and adjustment disorders in adults.
6. Describe the symptoms, epidemiology, comorbidity, and etiology of trauma-related disorders in adults.
7. Discuss how to deal with common reactions the nurse may experience while working with a patient who has suffered trauma.
8. Apply the nursing process to trauma-related disorders in adults.
9. Develop a teaching plan for a patient who suffers from posttraumatic stress disorder.
10. Identify dissociative disorders, including depersonalization/derealization disorder, dissociative amnesia, and dissociative identity disorder
11. Create a nursing care plan incorporating evidence-based interventions for symptoms of dissociation, including flashbacks, amnesia, and impaired self-care.
12. Role-play intervening with a patient who is experiencing a flashback.

KEY TERMS AND CONCEPTS

acute stress disorder
adjustment disorder
alternate personality (alter)
debriefing
depersonalization
derealization
disinhibited social engagement disorder
dissociation
dissociative amnesia
dissociative fugue
dissociative identity disorder
eye movement desensitization and reprocessing
flashbacks
hypervigilance
neuroplasticity
posttraumatic stress disorder (PTSD)
reactive attachment disorder
resilience
trauma-informed care
window of tolerance

Traumatic life events are associated with a wide range of psychiatric and other medical disorders. Traumatic events are not always as extraordinary as war and may be as common as interpersonal trauma, sexual abuse, physical abuse, severe neglect, emotional abuse, repeated abandonment, or sudden and traumatic loss in childhood, adolescence, or adulthood (Huckshorn, 2012).

Our understanding of the long-term physiological and psychological effects of trauma has expanded, and effective treatments are available; however, people who need these treatments do not always get the care that they need. Integrating **trauma-informed care** into all health care settings, both behavioral and medical, can reduce or ameliorate (improve) the effects of trauma and prevent the pervasive and damaging psychological and physical consequences of trauma.

Many psychiatric disorders have trauma as a precipitant. According to the American Psychiatric Association (APA) (2013), disorders included under the trauma umbrella include posttraumatic stress disorder (PTSD), reactive attachment disorder, disinhibited social engagement disorder, acute stress disorder, and adjustment disorders. This chapter begins with trauma-related disorders in children and then discusses adult trauma-related disorders.

The last part of the chapter addresses dissociative disorders (APA, 2013). Dissociative disorders are also related to trauma; they include depersonalization/derealization disorder, dissociative amnesia, and dissociative identity disorder.

TRAUMA-RELATED DISORDERS IN CHILDREN

Tragically, children are exposed to many traumatic events without the strength or coping skills to adequately defend themselves. Abuse, interpersonal violence, automobile accidents, natural disasters, war, medical procedures, and illnesses are all traumatizing incidents. Children who have been abused and neglected by their caretakers and other adults are at great risk for developing emotional, intellectual, and social handicaps as a result of their traumatic experiences (U.S. Department of Health and Human Services, 2008).

According to the National Child Abuse and Neglect Data System (2010), nearly 700,000 children were victims of abuse and neglect in 2010. Neglect is the most prevalent form of child abuse in the United States. Of those children who died from abuse and neglect, about 68% were due to neglect, 45% from physical abuse *and* neglect, and 26% as a result of multiple types of abuse. In addition, more than 1% of cases involved sexual abuse. These statistics reflect known cases of abuse; there is little doubt that far more children suffer abuse and neglect than are reported to child protective services agencies.

Sexual abuse of a child is a particularly reprehensible act. Sexual abuse ranges from forcing a child to observe lewd acts, to fondling, and all the way to sexual intercourse. All instances of sexual abuse are devastating to a child who lacks the mental capacity or emotional maturation to consent to this type of a relationship. Children who are starved for affection may be particularly vulnerable and confused by this attention.

Witnessing violence is traumatizing and a well-documented risk factor for many mental health problems, including depression, anxiety, PTSD, aggressive and delinquent behavior, drug use, academic failure, and low self-esteem (Farrell et al., 2007). Children who have been abused are at risk for abusing others as well as developing dysfunctional patterns in close interpersonal relationships.

Other traumatic events for children include invasive medical procedures and critical life-threatening illnesses. It is thought that the younger the child, the more seriously ill, and the more invasive the procedure, the more likely the child will develop PTSD. Research has found that those children who have survived cancer have four times the risk of developing PTSD than their siblings (Stuber et al., 2010).

CLINICAL PICTURE

Posttraumatic stress disorder (PTSD) in preschool children may manifest as a reduction in play, repetitive play that includes aspects of the traumatic event, social withdrawal, and negative emotions such as fear, guilt, anger, horror, sadness, shame, or confusion. Children may blame themselves for the traumatic event and manifest persistent negative thoughts about themselves such as: "I am a bad person." In addition there may be a feeling of detachment or estrangement from others and diminished interest or participation in significant activities. Often there is irritability, aggressive or self-destructive behavior, sleep disturbances, problems concentrating, and hypervigilance.

Children also may suffer relationship trauma from a grossly inadequate caregiving environment that may result in one of two extremes: severe emotional inhibition or indiscriminately social behaviors. These disorders are termed **reactive attachment disorder** and **disinhibited social engagement disorder**, respectfully. Children with reactive attachment disorder have a consistent pattern of inhibited, emotionally withdrawn behavior, and the child rarely directs attachment behaviors toward any adult caregivers. This problem is caused by a lack of bonding experiences with a primary caregiver by the age of eight months. Another response to inadequate parenting is manifested in disinhibited social engagement disorder. These children demonstrate no normal fear of strangers, seem unfazed in response to separation from a primary caregiver, and are usually willing to go off with people who are unknown to them.

EPIDEMIOLOGY

Studies estimate that about the same percentage of boys as girls experience at least one traumatic event: 15% to 43% (U.S. Department of Veterans Affairs, 2010b). Of these children and adolescents who experience trauma, 3% to 15% of girls and 1% to 6% of boys have diagnosable PTSD. Nearly 100% of children who witness their parent's murder or sexual assault will develop PTSD. Other alarming statistical relationships with PTSD are for children who are sexually abused (90%), exposed to a shooting at school (77%), and who see community violence in urban settings (35%).

Reactive attachment disorder and disinhibited social engagement disorder are rare. The rates of these problems have been estimated at 1% of all children under the age of 5.

COMORBIDITY

Comorbidities increase the child's vulnerability to developing or exacerbating (making worse) PTSD symptoms. Children and adolescents who have suffered toxic stress and trauma often meet the criteria for more than one diagnostic category. Even if a child does not have sufficient symptoms for a diagnosis of PTSD, he or she can still suffer from overwhelming nightmares or difficulties with trust, phobias, somatic problems, impulse control, and identity issues. Learning and attention problems, behavioral problems, sleep disorders, depression, suicide attempts, dissociation, and substance-abuse problems are all significant comorbidities (National Institute on Drug Abuse, 2011; Friedman et al., 2011a, 2011b). These comorbidities cause these injured children to be subjected to an endless cycle of medications, punishments, and inadequate responses that revictimize and stigmatize the child.

ETIOLOGY

Biological Factors

Genetic

Genetic variability is thought to play a role in stress reactivity, and epigenetic factors modulate the expression of genotype. Research on animals and humans has found that prenatal exposure to maternal stress can influence later responses to stress in the offspring (Darnaudery & Maccari, 2008). Also, early adversity has been found to alter the DNA in the brain through a process called methylation (Weaver et al., 2010). Methyl groups are attached to genes that govern the production of stress hormone receptors in the brain. This in turn prevents the brain from regulating its response to stress. Parental nurturing may mediate this response, but in the absence of nurturing, these children have difficulties with attention and following directions, are more likely to engage in high-risk behavior as teenagers, and show increased aggression, impulsivity, weakened cognition, and an inability to discriminate between real and imagined threats as adults.

Neurobiological

The most rapid phase of brain development occurs during the first 5 years of life, and a person is particularly vulnerable to adverse events during these years. The right hemisphere develops first and is involved in processing social-emotional information, promoting attachment functions, regulating body functions, and supporting the individual in coping with stress.Since the right brain develops first and is involved with developing templates for relationships and regulation of emotion and bodily function, early attachment relationships are particularly important for healthy development and lifelong health.

It is only in the context of attachments that regulatory functions develop in the child. Through day-to-day interactions with a caring person, the child develops adaptive coping strategies that are fundamental in regulating physical and emotional processes. Neural connections between the limbic system and prefrontal cortex are established between 10 and 18 months of age, and these neural pathways play a crucial role in modulating arousal and emotional regulation.

Normally, information from the environment is taken in through our senses, matched against previous experiences, and processed adaptively. Experiences are integrated into adaptive memory neural networks in a way that allows for connection with other memory networks. In a normal stress response, the hyperarousal in the sympathetic system is balanced by the parasympathetic system. Neuronal circuits connect the amygdala to the prefrontal lobe in the cortex that serves as the translator of the emotion so that amygdala activation can be modulated. The prefrontal association area keeps track of where information has been stored in long-term memory and is responsible for retrieving and then integrating memories with sensory input for decision making.

Trauma, however, causes a dysregulation that disrupts the integration of these neural networks. The more intense the arousal, the less likely it is that the experience will be processed (Bergmann, 2012). It is thought that the more helpless and less in control of the situation the person feels, the more vulnerable to pathophysiological changes he or she is.

Following exposure to violence and trauma, the parasympathetic response triggers a hypoaroused state with dysregulation of the hypothalamic pituitary adrenal axis resulting in **dissociation**. Dissociation is a disconnection of thoughts, emotions, sensations, and behaviors connected with a memory, with some dissociation considered a normal experience for most people, such as when we "space out" during a movie or when driving; however, severe dissociation or "mindflight" occurs for those who have suffered significant trauma (Boon et al., 2012). The episodic failure of dissociation causes intrusive symptoms such as flashbacks, thus dysregulating cortisol, resulting in either too much or too little cortisol.

Polyvagal theory posits that the autonomic nervous system is not limited to a fight-or-flight response to threat and actually consists of three different responses (Porges, 2011). The sympathetic and parasympathetic systems are governed by the tenth cranial nerve, or vagus nerve, that sends and receives information between the body and the brain through two major vagus nerves, ventral and dorsal, with two branches, myelinated and unmyelinated. Responses are as follows:

1. Myelinated ventral vagal responses are activated during social or intellectual engagement when the individual is "on," in a state of pleasant, not overwhelming, arousal. This state serves as a gentle brake by inhibiting sympathetic responses of the autonomic system.
2. Unmyelinated ventral vagus responses are activated when we perceive a threat. The attending sympathetic arousal symptoms of rapid heart rate and rapid respiration prepare the person for fight-or-flight responses. After many hours, days, or months the body cannot sustain this state.
3. The third response is the dorsal vagal response that occurs to dampen down the sympathetic nervous system. This is a parasympathetic response, with the heart rate and respiration slowing down and a decrease in blood pressure. Animals in the wild illustrate the ultimate dorsal vagal shutdown by playing dead when extremely threatened.

Subjectively, the person may just want to sleep or escape through mind-numbing activities and stay in this hypoaroused or depressed state and/or alternate with a hyperaroused or

EVIDENCE-BASED PRACTICE

Traumatic Stress Responses among Nurses

Buurman, B. M., Mank, A.P.M., Beijer, H.J.M., & Olff, M. (2011). Coping with serious events at work: A study of traumatic stress among nurses. *Journal of the American Psychiatric Nurses Association, 17*, 321-329.

Problem

Nurses frequently encounter traumatic events and experience chronic stress in the workplace that can lead to PTSD and burnout. Events that are traumatic include aggression among themselves as well as witnessing the pain, suffering, and death of others. These serious events involve helplessness, fear, or horror that can lead to PTSD while chronic interpersonal stressors at work often lead to burnout.

Purpose of Study

The purpose of this study was to describe the nature and number of serious events nurses encounter and their coping and reactions and to investigate which factors were related to traumatic stress after a serious event.

Methods

Nurses ($n = 69$) at a large university hospital in Amsterdam were asked to complete two questionnaires, the Utrecht Coping List and the List of Serious Events and Traumatic Stress in Nursing.

Key Findings

- 98% of nurses reported traumatic stress with a mean of 8 serious events experienced in the past 5 years.
- Active coping decreased the risk of experiencing traumatic stress while comforting cognition and social support increased the likelihood of appraising a serious event as traumatic.

Implications for Nursing Practice

Many nurses experience traumatic stress. Nurses need additional help particularly after events that threaten their physical integrity. More experienced nurses had more reactions after patients' deaths, perhaps because of cumulative trauma. Thus, experienced nurses are particularly vulnerable for developing PTSD and burnout. Interventions should be initiated consistently after traumatic events, and future research is warranted in order to determine what interventions are most effective in preventing PTSD and burnout.

anxious state. This theory provides an explanation of why many people with PTSD also suffer from depression.

Psychological Factors

Attachment Theory

A psychological theory that has important implications for trauma-related disorders is that of attachment theory. This theory describes the importance and dynamics of the early relationship between the infant and the caretaker based on the early work of Bowlby (1988). Attachment patterns or schemas are formed early in life through interaction and experiences with caregivers, and this relationship is embedded in implicit emotional and somatic memories. Research has demonstrated that these templates or patterns of attachment persist into adulthood. These schemas were studied and classified for young children and include secure, avoidant, ambivalent, and disorganized attachment styles (Ainsworth, 1967).

Environmental Factors

To a greater degree than adults, children are dependent on others. It is this dependency in tandem with the **neuroplasticity** (malleability) of the developing brain that can increase vulnerability to adverse life experiences. External factors in the environment can either support or put stress on children and adolescents and shape development. Young persons are vulnerable in an environment in which systems (e.g., schools, court systems) and adults (e.g., parents, counselors) have power and control. Parents model behavior and provide the child with a view of the world. If parents are abusive, rejecting, or overly controlling, the child may suffer detrimental effects during the period of development when the trauma occurs. Most children, however, who suffer a traumatic and stressful event do develop normally.

Poverty, parental substance abuse, and exposure to violence have received increasing attention and place minority children at greater risk for trauma and stress. Pervasive and persistent economic, racial, and ethnic disparities are called the "millennial morbidities" (Shonkoff & Garner, 2012). A review of 58 studies found that racial and ethnic disparities in children's health are worsening (Flores, 2010). Differences in cultural expectations, presence of stresses, and lack of support by the dominant culture may have profound effects and increase the risk of mental, emotional, and academic problems. Family stability may provide cushioning effects in the face of poverty and adversity. Working with children and adolescents from diverse backgrounds requires an increased awareness of one's own biases and of the patient's needs.

The term **resilience** refers to positive adaptation, or the ability to maintain or regain mental health despite adversity. Studies have shown that factors that enhance resilience include the presence of supportive relationships and attachments as well as the avoidance of frequent and prolonged stress (Herrman et al., 2011). Children brought up in a chaotic or non-nurturing environment suffer neurological consequences that are long-lasting and difficult to remediate (Shonkoff & Garner, 2012). Toxic stress and adverse childhood experiences have been found to result in lifelong consequences for both psychological and physical health (Shonkoff, 2010). Trauma in early childhood also plays a role in the intergenerational transmission of disparities in health outcomes. The nurse's role is to identify and foster qualities to keep at-risk children from developing emotional problems.

Attachment at its most basic level ensures survival of the species. Lack of attachment is counter to such a basic drive. Tizard (1977) conducted one of the best-known early studies related to attachment disorder. Children in this study were abandoned by their parents and lived in an institutional setting. They were provided with play areas, books, and basic needs. What they were not provided with was an adequate ratio of caregivers to children, and caregivers were instructed not to form attachments with the children. After 4 years, eight of the 26 children managed to somehow form attachment with caregivers, eight of the children became emotionally unresponsive, and 10 of the children became indiscriminately social and attention-seeking. The latter two groups coincide with the attachment disorders discussed in this section.

APPLICATION OF THE NURSING PROCESS

ASSESSMENT

A child or adolescent with a trauma or stressor-related disorder is one whose development may be delayed if adequate assessment, diagnosis, and treatment are not available. It is important for nurses working in school, community settings, and juvenile detention to assess for PTSD and the safety of the environment for young people who have been traumatized or experienced abuse and a history of violence.

The type of data collected to assess the child depends on the setting, the severity of the presenting problem, and the availability of resources; however, assessment is an ongoing process throughout treatment. Methods of collecting data include interviewing, screening, testing (neurological, psychological, intelligence), observing, and interacting with the child or adolescent. Histories are taken from multiple sources, including parents, other caregivers, the child or adolescent, and other adults, such as teachers, when possible. A genogram can document family composition, history, and relationships (refer to Chapter 34). How do family members interact and is the family reinforcing unhealthy behaviors?

Assessment of the mental status of children is similar to that of adults. It provides information about the child's state at the time of the examination and identifies problems with thinking, feeling, and behaving. Broad categories to assess include safety, general appearance, socialization, activity level, speech, coordination and motor function, affect, manner of relating, intellectual function, thought processes and content, and characteristics of play. The observation-interaction part of a mental health assessment begins with a semistructured interview in which the nurse asks the young person about the home environment, parents, and siblings and about the school environment, teachers, and peers. In this format, the child is free to describe current problems and give information about his or her developmental history. Play activities, such as games, drawings, and puppets, are used for younger children who cannot respond to a direct approach. The initial interview is key to observing interactions among the child, caregiver, and siblings (if available) and to building trust and rapport.

Essential symptom assessment data includes sudden state changes such as uncontrollable rage, somatic symptoms, posttraumatic symptoms (e.g., nightmares, night terrors, disturbing hallucinations, intrusive traumatic thoughts and memories, re-experiencing or flashbacks, traumatic re-enactments, and self-injurious behaviors), and negative symptoms such as numbing and avoidance. Somatic symptoms may manifest as headaches, stomachaches or pain; memory problems include amnesia, forgetfulness, difficulty concentrating, or trance states. The child may disturbingly re-enact the trauma in play. Children may be distracted by intrusive thoughts or flashbacks. Comorbid conditions should be assessed.

Specific assessment tools may include instruments such as the Child Dissociative Checklist (Putnam, Helmers, & Trickett, 1993), Trauma Symptoms Checklist for Children (Briere, 1996), and the Child Sexual Behavior Inventory (Friedrich et al., 2001). For those children who are thought to suffer from an attachment disorder, the Disturbances of Attachment interview may be administered (Smyke & Zeanah, 1999). Although a licensed mental health practitioner, such as the advanced practice psychiatric nurse or psychologist, usually gives these assessment tools, parents and teachers can complete structured questionnaires and behavior checklists.

Developmental Assessment

Developmental testing should also be conducted for young children since significant developmental delays may be present. The developmental assessment provides information about the child or adolescent's maturational level. Is the child behaving and functioning at his or her chronological age, or are there areas where the child lags behind the norms and peers? These data are then reviewed in relation to the child's chronological age to identify developmental strengths or deficits. The Denver II Developmental Screening Test for infants and children up to 6 years of age is a popular assessment tool (Frankenburg et al., 1992). For adolescents, tools may be tailored to specific areas of assessment, such as neuropsychological, physical, hormonal, and biochemical. Some computer-based screening tools for children and adolescents are used in primary care settings to gather sensitive information; these tools will provide privacy while the child is waiting to be seen (Johnson & Newland, 2012).

Abnormal findings in the developmental and mental status assessments may be temporary. The nurse working with parents may handle stress-related behaviors or minor regressions; however, as young people develop maladaptive coping behaviors and use these behaviors over time, they are at risk of developing many psychiatric disorders. Serious psychopathology requires evaluation by an advanced practice nurse in collaboration with clinicians from other child and adolescent mental health and pediatric disciplines.

DIAGNOSIS

After a comprehensive trauma assessment, two priority nursing diagnoses are applicable (Herdman, 2012). The first is *risk for impaired parent/child attachment*. This is defined as the risk for disruption of the interactive process between parent/significant other and child that fosters the development of a protective and nurturing reciprocal relationship. Risk factors include:

- Anxiety associated with the parent role
- Ill infant/child who is unable to effectively initiate parental contact due to altered behavioral organization
- Inability of parents to meet personal needs
- Parental conflict due to altered behavior
- Substance abuse
- Separation

Another nursing diagnosis is *risk of delayed development*. It is defined as at risk for delay of 25% or more in one or more of the areas of social or self-regulatory behavior, or in cognitive, language, gross or fine motor skills. Risk factors include:

- Substance abuse
- Failure to thrive

- Unstable home
- Unwanted pregnancy
- Poverty

OUTCOMES IDENTIFICATION

A child with a trauma-related disorder is at risk for developmental and regulatory disorders. A number of outcomes have been identified related to the nursing diagnoses listed above (Moorhead et al., 2013). An overall attachment outcome would be for the parent and infant/child to demonstrate an enduring affectionate bond. In regard to development, general outcomes would pertain to meeting age-appropriate milestones.

IMPLEMENTATION

Nurses and other licensed health care providers are mandated by law to report all instances of suspected abuse of a minor child to the local child protective services. The overall treatment plan for trauma includes psychobiological, psychological and family goals within a staged treatment protocol.

The staged model of treatment for trauma includes the following:

Stage 1: Providing safety and stabilization through creating a safe, predictable environment; stopping self-destructive behaviors; providing education about trauma and its effects.

Stage 2: Reducing arousal and regulating emotion through symptom reduction and memory work through reducing arousal; finding comfort from others; tolerating affect; integrating disavowed emotions and accepting ambivalence; overcoming avoidance; improving attention and decreasing dissociation; working with memories; and transforming memories.

Stage 3: Developmental skills catch up through enhancing problem-solving skills; nurturing self-awareness; social skills training; and developing a value system. Interventions in this phase should focus on teaching coping skills to deal with trauma, supporting efforts to achieve socially appropriate goals, and facilitating development of and integration into healthy social support systems.

Treatment strategies for the traumatized child are designed to modulate arousal so that the child is helped to stay within a window of tolerance. The window of tolerance is a term that means a balance between sympathetic and parasympathetic arousal (Porges, 2011). Traumatized children have difficulty shifting their emotional and physiological state to accommodate different environments and social contexts. They alternate between hyperarousal (anxiety, fear, hyperactivity, aggression) and hypoarousal (withdrawal, isolation, numbness). Increasing the child's ability to self-regulate through specific strategies designed to mediate these arousal states while providing a nurturing safe environment supports a sense of well-being, competency and mastery.

Interventions

Since the child with trauma has suffered significant disconnection and fragmentation of relationships with self and others, the most important healing ingredient is that of relationship and connection to others. Connection, caring, and management of the patient's anxiety are essential to provide the foundation so that integration is possible. Box 16-1 identifies interventions appropriate for a child who has suffered a specific trauma.

Interventions for the traumatized child are used in a variety of settings: inpatient, residential, outpatient, day treatment, outreach programs in schools, and home visits. Many of the modalities can encompass activities of daily living, learning activities, multiple forms of play and recreational activities, and interactions with adults and peers.

Adjunctive therapies include family therapy, group therapy, play therapy, mutual storytelling, therapeutic games, bibliotherapy, therapeutic drawing, and mindfulness exercises. The family is seen as critical in helping a child recover from trauma, with family counseling a key component of treatment. Educating the child and family is essential and helps to absolve the child of blame.

Often, traumatized children feel responsible for what happened to them and are frightened by flashbacks, amnesia, or hallucinations that may be due to trauma. For example, a child may use an imaginary friend as a coping mechanism and not understand that this was adaptive at the time and that this is really a part of the self and not a separate person. In such a case, explain to the child that sometimes when really bad things happen, our brain helps us by forgetting and creating special parts of ourselves. If the trauma was chronic and severe, ongoing, or intermittent, treatment may be needed, and it is important to explain to the family and child the process of recovery.

In addition to teaching about the recovery process and normalizing the experiences, traumatized children need to learn strategies to regulate emotion and arousal levels. Teaching deep breathing techniques and mindfulness techniques helps to decrease arousal levels and restore natural rhythms. Soothing strategies that redirect behavior might also include warm baths, singing, distraction, listening to music, guided imagery, and using a low, calming voice. These strategies help the child to manage feelings. Talking about feelings and helping the child to identify emotions is essential, and teaching the family how to set limits without being punitive helps the child to feel in control.

BOX 16-1 TRAUMA INTERVENTIONS FOR A CHILD WITH PTSD

Definition: Use of an interactive helping process to resolve a trauma experienced by a child

Establish trust and safety in the therapeutic relationship.

Use developmentally appropriate language to explore feelings.

Teach relaxation techniques before trauma exploration to restore a sense of control over thoughts and feelings.

Help the child to identify and cope with feelings through the use of art and play to promote expression.

Involve the parents or appropriate caretakers in 1:1s unless they are the cause of the trauma.

Educate the child and parents about the grief process and response to the trauma.

Assist parents in resolving their own emotional distress about the trauma.

Coordinate with social work for protections as indicated.

Bulechek, G.M., Butcher, H.K., Dochterman, J.M., & Wagner, C. (2013). *Nursing interventions classification (NIC)* (6th ed.). St. Louis, MO: Mosby.

Advanced Practice Interventions

International guidelines recommend the use of cognitive-behavioral therapy (CBT) and eye movement desensitization and reprocessing (EMDR) as first-line treatments for the treatment of traumatized children (National Institute for Health and Clinical Excellence, 2005). CBT uses a range of strategies such as psychoeducation, behavior modification, cognitive therapy, exposure therapy, and stress management to help the child manage behavior and change maladaptive beliefs and thoughts.

EMDR is an innovative evidence-based therapy used to treat children and adults (Fleming, 2012). EMDR processes traumatic memories though a specific eight-phase protocol that allows the person to think about the traumatic event while attending to other stimulation, such as eye movements, audio tones, or tapping. Some believe that it works by causing neurological and physiological changes that help to process and integrate traumatic memories. Specific protocols have been developed for the treatment of children, and even if the child does not remember what happened, EMDR can be helpful. As a licensed mental health provider, advanced practice psychiatric nurses can become certified to use EMDR through additional training.

Psychopharmacology

Medicating children works best when combined with another treatment such as EMDR or cognitive-behavioral therapy. Medications that target specific symptoms or comorbidities such as attention deficit hyperactivity disorder (ADHD) or depression can enhance the child or adolescent's potential for growth and may make a real difference in a family's ability to cope and quality of life.

EVALUATION

Treatment is effective when:

1. The child's safety has been maintained.
2. Anxiety has been reduced, and stress is handled adaptively.
3. Emotions and behavior are appropriate for the situation.
4. The child achieves normal developmental milestones for his or her chronological age.
5. The child is able to seek out adults for nurturance and help when needed.

TRAUMA-RELATED DISORDERS IN ADULTS

POSTTRAUMATIC STRESS DISORDER

As in children, posttraumatic stress disorder (PTSD) in adults is characterized by persistent re-experiencing of a highly traumatic event that involves actual or threatened death or serious injury to self or others, to which the individual responded with intense fear, helplessness, or horror. PTSD may occur after any traumatic event that is outside the range of usual experience. Examples are military combat; detention as a prisoner of war; natural disasters, such as floods, tornadoes, and earthquakes; human disasters, such as plane and train accidents; crime-related events, such as bombing, assault, mugging, rape, and being taken hostage; or diagnosis of a life-threatening illness. PTSD symptoms can begin after a month from exposure, but a delay of months or years is not uncommon.

As in children, the major features of PTSD include the following: (1) Re-experiencing of the trauma through recurrent intrusive recollections of the event, dreams about the event, and flashbacks—dissociative experiences during which the event is relived, and the person behaves as though he or she is experiencing the event at that time, (2) **Avoidance** of stimuli associated with the trauma, causing the individual to avoid talking about the event or avoid activities, people, or places that arouse memories of the trauma, accompanied by feelings of detachment, emptiness, and numbing, (3) Persistent symptoms of increased arousal, as evidenced by irritability, difficulty sleeping, difficulty concentrating, hypervigilance, or exaggerated startle response, and (4) **Alterations in mood**, such as chronic depression (Friedman et al., 2011).

The flashbacks and hypervigilance of PTSD can be terrifying. When the person recalls a traumatic memory, physiological reactions (e.g., sensation of terror in the stomach, heart palpitations, muscles tensing) occur. The person often does not know where these sensations are coming from and attributes them to present circumstances, and the past becomes the present. Because of the changes in the brain, the individual can fluctuate radically from moments of overstimulation and anxiety to moments of complete shutdown and depression. Just when the person feels at rest, as while asleep, intrusive flashbacks occur. Victims who suffer from PTSD begin to feel permanently damaged and often hate themselves for feeling so needy and helpless.

EPIDEMIOLOGY

Epidemiological studies confirm that most, 55% to 90%, people have experienced at least one traumatic event in their lifetimes, with an average of five traumatic events reported per person (Centers for Disease Control and Prevention, 2010). An individual's response and the long-term sequelae of a disturbing event is highly individualistic and depends on a multitude of factors, such as the person's age, developmental stage, coping skills, support system, cognitive deficits, preexisting neural physiology, and the nature of the trauma.

Following a traumatic event, nearly 8% of people will develop PTSD (Kessler et al., 1995), with some populations particularly vulnerable. The lifetime prevalence for PTSD is 3.5% of the adult population in the United States with more than a third of these cases classified as severe (National Institute of Mental Health, 2011). The average age of onset is 23 years old, with women more than twice as likely as men (10% vs. 4%) to develop PTSD. This is thought to be due to the greater incidence of sexual assault on women and also the higher likelihood for women to have a past mental health problem such as anxiety and depression, which may make them more vulnerable to response to a traumatic event (National Center for PTSD, 2011).

COMORBIDITY

The more adverse childhood experiences (ACE) experienced, the more both medical and mental illness occurs later as adults. Also, while short-term dissociation may actually be adaptive during a distressing event, the tendency toward persistent dissociation may be another significant risk factor (Bryant et al., 2011). Consequences of ACE include obesity, sexually transmitted diseases, alcoholism, severe and persistent mental illness, psychosis, substance abuse, eating disorders, sleep disorders, dissociative disorders, anxiety, and depression (Felitti et al., 1998).

Comorbidities for adults with PTSD include depression, anxiety disorders, sleep disorders, and dissociative disorders (Friedman et al., 2011a, 2011b). Often substances are used to try to manage the feelings and symptoms. Individuals with PTSD are sad, anhedonic, aggressive, angry, guilty, dissociative, and abuse substances. Difficulty with interpersonal, social, or occupational relationships nearly always accompanies PTSD, and trust is a common issue of concern. Common presenting symptoms include chronic pain, migraines, vague somatic complaints, intoxications, anxiety or depression, irritability, avoidance, anger or nonadherence, self-risk behavior, threatening or aggressive behavior, dissociative symptoms, or a change in functioning. Spousal abuse may be associated with hypervigilance and irritability, and chemical abuse may begin as an attempt to self-medicate to relieve anxiety.

ETIOLOGY

See earlier discussion on biological factors in trauma-related disorders for children.

APPLICATION OF THE NURSING PROCESS

ASSESSMENT

Screening tools for PTSD in adults include the Primary Care PTSD Screen (PC-PTSD) (Prins et al., 2003) and the PTSD Checklist (PCL) (Lang & Stein, 2005). A more comprehensive assessment is indicated for those who initially screen positive. Additional history about the time of onset, frequency, course, severity, level of distress, and degree of functional impairment is important. Further assessment for suicidal or violent ideation, family and social supports, insomnia, social withdrawal, functional impairment, current life stressors, medication, past medical and psychiatric history, and a Mental Status Exam are indicated (refer to Chapter 7). The diagnosis of PTSD involves a comprehensive clinical interview that assesses all symptoms collectively.

DIAGNOSIS

Nursing diagnoses include the following:

- Anxiety (moderate, severe, panic)
- Ineffective coping
- Social isolation
- Insomnia
- Sleep deprivation
- Hopelessness
- Chronic low self-esteem
- Self-care deficit

OUTCOMES IDENTIFICATION

Outcomes for trauma-related disorders for adults include the following:

1. The person is able to manage anxiety as demonstrated by use of relaxation techniques, adequate sleep, and ability to maintain role or work requirements.
2. Enhanced self-esteem as demonstrated by maintenance of grooming/hygiene, maintenance of eye contact, positive statements about self, and acceptance of self-limitations.
3. Enhanced ability to cope as demonstrated by decrease in physical symptoms, ability to ask for help, and seeks information about treatment.

IMPLEMENTATION

A stage model of treatment as previously described for children is the standard for trauma treatment for adults as well. A primary consideration for caring for the person with PTSD is establishing a therapeutic relationship through nonjudgmental acceptance and empathy. In this context, the nurse assists the person in managing their arousal level. The latter can be accomplished through providing a safe, predictable environment; teaching strategies to manage anxiety such as deep breathing, imagery, and mindfulness exercises; connecting the person to support groups, family, and friends; and encouraging a narrative of the event and the meaning of the event to the person. The person often feels guilty and responsible for the event, and the nurse, as a witness through listening and reflecting back to the person their concerns, can gently suggest that the person was not responsible for what happened. Through sharing his or her experience, the patient can begin to heal and integrate what happened into his or her life.

Psychoeducation

Educating the person and family about PTSD is important to normalize the situation, because often the person feels as if he or she is going crazy and does not understand that theirs is a normal reaction to an abnormal event. Initial education should include reassurance that reactions to trauma are common and that these reactions do not indicate personal failure or weakness. Patients may be told that a significant trauma occurred and that the distressing symptoms are a consequence of an overwhelming event. Also, the patient and his or her family should be informed of the many ways that trauma can present, such as interpersonal problems with family and friends, occupational problems, and/or substance-use disorders and problems with alcohol use. In addition, strategies to improve coping, enhance self-care, and facilitate recognition of problems are essential, as are instructions in relaxation techniques and in the avoidance of caffeine and alcohol. All patients should be informed of effective treatment options for PTSD and referred to an experienced licensed mental health practitioner.

Psychopharmacology

Initial medication may include a selective serotonin reuptake inhibitor (SSRI) such as fluoxetine (Prozac), paroxetine (Paxil), or sertraline (Zoloft), or a serotonin norepinephrine reuptake inhibitor (SNRI) such as venlafaxine (Effexor) to decrease anxiety

16-1 CASE STUDY AND NURSING PLAN

A distraught wife brings Mr. Blake, 46, to the emergency department after she finds him writing a suicide note and planning to shoot himself in the woods with a handgun. Mr. Blake is subdued, shows minimal affect, and his breath has the distinct odor of alcohol. When asked about suicidal thoughts, he states that he is worthless and that his wife and family would be better off if he were dead. He refuses to contract for safety. The decision is made to hospitalize him to protect him from danger to himself.

Mr. Blake's wife provides further history. Her husband is a construction contractor who served in the U.S. National Guard during the Iraq War. He lost half his squad from a roadside bombing, narrowly escaping with his life. He walks with a permanent limp due to the attack. Upon returning home, he showed no signs of anxiety and refused offers of crisis treatment, stating, "I was in a war; I can handle stress." But six months later, Mrs. Blake noticed that her husband had trouble sleeping, his mood was irritable or withdrawn, he avoided news reports on television, and he started to drink daily. He complained of nightmares but would not talk to her about his fears. He only agreed to go to his primary care nurse practitioner to request sleeping medication.

Mr. Blake was admitted to the psychiatric unit and his care assigned to Ms. Dawson, a registered nurse. She observes that Mr. Blake is quiet and passive as he is oriented to the unit but that he looks around vigilantly and is easily startled by sounds on the unit.

Self-Assessment

Ms. Dawson is a registered nurse with an associate degree and 3 years of experience on this unit. Initially she feels sympathy for Mr. Blake, and he reminds her of her Uncle James, who served in Vietnam. She is concerned because his suicide plan was lethal and he is guarded in his speech, not revealing his thoughts or feelings. She realizes that as she implements suicide precautions, she must demonstrate an attitude of hope and acceptance to encourage him to develop trust. Also, she must stay neutral and not convey any pity or sympathy.

Assessment

Screening tools include the Primary Care PTSD Screen (PC-PTSD) (Veteran Affairs/Department of Defense, 2012), Impact of Events Scale (IES) (Horowitz et al., 1979) (Box 16-2), Impact of Events Scale-Revised (IES-R) (Weiss & Marmar, 1997), and the PTSD Checklist (PCL) (Lang & Stein, 2005). A more comprehensive assessment is indicated for those who initially screen positive. Additional history about the time of onset, frequency, course, severity, level of distress, and degree of functional impairment is important. Further assessment for suicidal or violent ideation, family and social supports, insomnia, social withdrawal, functional impairment, current life stressors, medication, past medical and psychiatric history, and a Mental Status Exam are indicated (refer to Chapter 7). The diagnosis of PTSD involves a comprehensive clinical interview that assesses all symptoms collectively.

OBJECTIVE DATA	SUBJECTIVE DATA
Sleep difficulty, nightmares	"I don't deserve to live; I should have died with the others."
Hypervigilance	"You can't stop me."
Alcohol use	
Irritability	
Withdrawn mood	
Constricted/reduced range of affect	
Feels estranged from wife and children	
Avoidance of news coverage with potential for emergency reports	
Refusal of treatment and safety contract	
Plan for suicide	

Diagnosis

The initial plan is to maintain safety for Mr. Blake while encouraging him to express feelings and recognize that his situation is not hopeless. His nursing diagnosis is: *Risk for suicide as evidenced by suicidal plan and verbalization of intent.*

Outcomes Identification

Patient will consistently refrain from attempting suicide.

Planning

The initial plan is to maintain safety for Mr. Blake while encouraging him to express feelings and recognize that his situation is not hopeless.

Implementation

Mr. Blake's plan of care is personalized as follows:

SHORT-TERM GOAL	INTERVENTION	RATIONALE	EVALUATION
1. Patient will speak to staff whenever experiencing self-destructive thoughts.	**1a.** Administer medications with mouth checks. **1b.** Provide ongoing surveillance of patient and environment. **1c.** Contract for "no self-harm" for specified periods. **1d.** Use direct, nonjudgmental approach in discussing suicide. **1e.** Provide illness teaching regarding PTSD.	**1a.** Addresses risk of hiding medications. **1b.** Provides one-to-one monitoring for safety. **1c.** Encourages increased self-control. **1d.** Shows acceptance of patient's situation with respect. **1e.** Offers reality of treatment.	**GOAL MET** After 8 hours, patient contracts for safety every shift and starts to discuss feelings of self-harm.
2. Patient will express feelings by the third day of hospitalization.	**2a.** Interact with patient at regular intervals to convey caring and openness and to provide an opportunity to talk. **2b.** Use silence and listening to encourage expression of feelings. **2c.** Be open to expressions of loneliness and powerlessness. **2d.** Share observations or thoughts about patient's behavior or response.	**2a.** Encourages development of trust. **2b.** Shows positive expectation that patient will respond. **2c.** Allows patient to voice these uncomfortable feelings. **2d.** Directs attention to here-and-now treatment situation.	**GOAL MET** By second day, patient occasionally answers questions about feelings and admits to anger and grief.

16-1 CASE STUDY AND NURSING PLAN—cont'd

SHORT-TERM GOAL	INTERVENTION	RATIONALE	EVALUATION
3. Patient will express will to live by discharge from unit.	**3a.** Listen to expressions of grief. **3b.** Encourage patient to identify own strengths and abilities. **3c.** Explore with patient previous methods of dealing with life problems. **3d.** Assist in identifying available support systems. **3e.** Refer to spiritual advisor of individual's choice.	**3a.** Supports patient, communicating that such feelings are natural. **3b.** Affirms patient's worth and potential to survive. **3c.** Reinforces patient's past coping skills and ability to problem solve now. **3d.** Addresses fact that anxiety has narrowed patient's perspective, distorting reality about loved ones. **3e.** Allows opportunity to explore spiritual values and self-worth.	**GOAL MET** By third day, patient becomes tearful and states that he does not want to hurt his wife and daughter.

Evaluation

See individual outcomes and evaluation within the care plan.

and depressive symptoms. Tricyclic antidepressants (TCAs) or mirtazapine (Remeron) may be prescribed if SSRIs or SNRIs are not tolerated or do not work. Clonidine (Catapress) and prazosin (Minipress) are centrally acting alpha agonists used for the hyperarousal and intrusive symptoms; propranolol (Inderol), a beta-blocker, is used for hyperarousal and panic. The most-difficult-to-tolerate side effect of these medications is hypotension (U.S. Department of Veterans Affairs, 2010a).

Advanced Practice Interventions

Evidence-based treatments for PTSD include trauma-focused psychotherapy that may include components of exposure and/or cognitive restructuring and EMDR. These modalities are often combined with anxiety management/stress reduction that focuses on alleviation of symptoms. Other helpful strategies include brief psychodynamic psychotherapy, imagery, relaxation techniques, hypnosis, and group therapy. Refer to Chapter 2 for more information about these therapies.

EVALUATION

Treatment is effective when:

1. The patient recognizes symptoms as related to the trauma.
2. The patient is able to use newly learned strategies to manage anxiety.
3. The patient experiences no flashbacks or intrusive thoughts about the traumatic event.
4. The patient is able to sleep adequately without nightmares.
5. The patient can assume usual roles and maintains satisfying interpersonal relationships.
   (See Case Study and Nursing Care Plan 16-1.)

ACUTE STRESS DISORDER

Acute stress disorder (ASD) may develop after exposure to a highly traumatic event, such as those listed in the prior section on PTSD. To be diagnosed with acute stress disorder, the individual must display eight out of the following 14 symptoms either during or after the traumatic event, including a subjective sense of numbing; derealization (a sense of unreality related to the environment); inability to remember at least one important aspect of the event; intrusive distressing memories of the event; recurrent distressing dreams; feeling as if the event is recurring; intense prolonged distress or physiological reactivity; avoidance of thoughts or feelings about the event; sleep disturbances; hypervigilance; irritable, angry or aggressive behavior; exaggerated startle response; and agitation or restlessness (Bryant et al., 2011). ASD is diagnosed from 3 days to 1 month after the traumatic event.

VIGNETTE

Olivia, a 22-year-old college student, is sexually assaulted by a family acquaintance. After being brought into the emergency department by a friend, she describes feeling detached from her body and being unaware of her surroundings during the assault, "as though it took place in a vacuum." She displays virtually no affect (i.e., she does not cry or appear anxious, angry, or sad). Olivia finds it difficult to concentrate on the examiner's questions. After a week, Olivia still feels as though her mind is detached from her body; she reports having difficulty sleeping, not being able to concentrate, and startling whenever anyone touches her.

DIAGNOSIS

A possible appropriate nursing diagnosis for a patient with ASD (NANDA, 2012) is *posttrauma syndrome* as manifested by:

- aggression
- headaches
- intrusive dreams
- irritability
- anxiety

Related to:

- serious automobile accident
- serious injury to loved one
- disaster
- abuse

BOX 16-2 IMPACT OF EVENTS SCALE

On (date) ________ you experienced a motor vehicle accident. Below is a list of comments made by people after stressful life events. Please check each item, indicating how frequently these comments were true for you DURING THE PAST SEVEN DAYS. If they did not occur during that time, please mark the "not at all" column.

1. I thought about it when I didn't mean to.
   - Not at all
   - Rarely
   - Sometimes
   - Often
2. I avoided letting myself get upset when I thought about it or was reminded of it.
   - Not at all
   - Rarely
   - Sometimes
   - Often
3. I tried to remove it from memory
   - Not at all
   - Rarely
   - Sometimes
   - Often
4. I had trouble falling asleep or staying asleep, because pictures or thoughts about it came into my mind.
   - Not at all
   - Rarely
   - Sometimes
   - Often
5. I had waves of strong feelings about it.
   - Not at all
   - Rarely
   - Sometimes
   - Often
6. I had dreams about it.
   - Not at all
   - Rarely
   - Sometimes
   - Often
7. I stayed away from reminders of it.
   - Not at all
   - Rarely
   - Sometimes
   - Often
8. I felt as if it hadn't happened or it wasn't real.
   - Not at all
   - Rarely
   - Sometimes
   - Often
9. I tried not to talk about it.
   - Not at all
   - Rarely
   - Sometimes
   - Often
10. Pictures about it popped into my mind.
    - Not at all
    - Rarely
    - Sometimes
    - Often
11. Other things kept making me think about it.
    - Not at all
    - Rarely
    - Sometimes
    - Often
12. I was aware that I still had a lot of feelings about it, but I didn't deal with them.
    - Not at all
    - Rarely
    - Sometimes
    - Often
13. I tried not to think about it.
    - Not at all
    - Rarely
    - Sometimes
    - Often
14. Any reminder brought back feelings about it.
    - Not at all
    - Rarely
    - Sometimes
    - Often
15. My feelings about it were kind of numb.
    - Not at all
    - Rarely
    - Sometimes
    - Often

OUTCOMES IDENTIFICATION

A general outcome may relate to aggression. The patient will practice self-restraint of assaultive, combative, or destructive behaviors toward others. For anxiety, a general outcome may be that the patient's anxiety level be maintained at a level of mild to moderate.

IMPLEMENTATION

The nurse's role in caring for a patient with ASD involves primarily establishing a therapeutic relationship with the person, helping the person to problem solve, connecting the person to supports such as family and friends, educating about ASD, coordination of care through collaboration with others, ensuring and maintaining safety, and monitoring response and/or adherence to treatment.

There are few studies that evaluate the efficacy of treatments for ASD. Historically, critical incident stress debriefing (CISD) was widely used for those who had suffered from acute trauma. Typically **debriefing** occurs within 12 to 48 hours after the traumatic event and is often offered as a group intervention. Group members receive information on the facts of the event and psychological consequences of trauma and the possible ways of coping, and they exchange the details of the incident. Research on CISD has not supported its efficacy as an intervention after a traumatic event. In fact, several studies have found a higher incidence of PTSD for those who received CISD (Bisson & Andrew, 2007).

Advanced Practice Interventions

Cognitive-behavioral therapy (CBT) has been found to be effective in reducing the subsequent development of PTSD for people with ASD (Bryant et al., 2003). Other promising new therapies for ASD include specialized protocols for EMDR; the EMDR Protocol for Recent Critical Incidents (EMDR-PRECI) (Jarero, Artigas, & Luber, 2011), the Recent Event Protocol (Luber, 2009), and the Recent Traumatic Episode Protocol (R-TEP) (Shapiro & Laub, 2008).

EVALUATION

See the Evaluation section for PTSD above.

ADJUSTMENT DISORDER

What may considered to be a milder, less specific version of ASD and PTSD is **adjustment disorder**. Like ASD and PTSD, it is precipitated by a stressful event; however, the event—including retirement, chronic illness, or a breakup—may not be as severe and may not be considered a traumatic event (Strain & Friedman, 2011). This problem may be diagnosed immediately or within 3 months of exposure. The hallmarks of adjustment disorder are cognitive, emotional, and behavioral symptoms that negatively impact functioning. Responses to the stressful event may include combinations of depression, anxiety, and conduct disturbances.

Symptoms of adjustment disorder run the gamut of all forms of distress, including guilt, depression, anxiety, and anger. These feelings may be combined with other manifestations of distress, including physical complaints, social withdrawal, or work or academic inhibition. Quality of life scores are higher with adjustment disorder than for major depression but lower than for people without any disorder (Fernandez et al., 2012).

There is a type of adjustment disorder that addresses the needs of those who have lost a loved one within the past 12 months—a sort of complicated grief (Strain & Friedman, 2011). This type of adjustment disorder is manifested by intense yearning/longing for the deceased and intense sorrow and emotional pain or preoccupation with the deceased or the circumstances of the death. In addition, the person may feel anger, a diminished sense of self, emptiness, and/or difficulty in relationships or in planning future activities. This may be in accordance with cultural norms.

The prevalence of adjustment disorder has been estimated at about 3% of the population (Fernandez et al., 2012). Treatment of adjustment disorder is not uniform due to the lack of specificity of the problem; practitioners tend not to recognize this disorder. Symptoms are generally treated with antidepressants (Casey & Doherty, 2012).

DISSOCIATIVE DISORDERS

Dissociative disorders occur after significant adverse experiences/traumas, and individuals respond to stress with a severe interruption of consciousness. Dissociation is an unconscious defense mechanism that protects the individual against overwhelming anxiety through an emotional separation; however, this separation results in disturbances in memory, consciousness, self-identity, and perception.

Patients with dissociative disorders have intact reality testing; that is, although the person may have flashbacks or images, these are triggered by current events, relate to the past trauma, and are not delusions or hallucinations. Mild, fleeting dissociative experiences are relatively common to all of us; for example, we say we are on "automatic pilot" when we drive home from work and cannot recall the last 15 minutes before reaching the house.

These common experiences are distinctly different from the processes of pathological dissociation. Dissociation is involuntary and results in failure of the normal control over a person's mental processes and normal integration of conscious awareness (Spiegel et al., 2011). Dimensions of a memory that should be linked are not and are fragmented. For example, a person may be aware of a sound or smell, but these sensations would not be linked to the actual event itself, leaving the person fearful and/or confused. In addition, the person may re-enact, as well as re-experience, trauma without consciously knowing why.

Symptoms of dissociation may be either positive or negative. Positive symptoms refer to unwanted additions to mental activity such as flashbacks; negative symptoms refer to deficits such as memory problems or the ability to sense or control different parts of the body. It is thought that dissociation decreases the immediate subjective distress of the trauma and also continues to protect the individual from full awareness of the disturbing event.

Dissociation can be seen as somewhat protective for a child so that he or she can continue to be attached to caretakers who are abusive or neglectful. This highlights the importance of attachments and relationships in allowing the child to grow socially, intellectually, and cognitively. If abuse or neglect has occurred, these memories become compartmentalized and often do not intrude into awareness until later in life when the person is in a stressful situation. Dissociative disorders include: (1) depersonalization/derealization disorder, (2) dissociative amnesia, and (3) dissociative identity disorder.

EPIDEMIOLOGY

Although mental health providers in the United States believe that dissociative disorders are rare, research studies worldwide dispute this notion and have found that the prevalence of dissociative disorders (DD) occurring at some time during a person's life in the United States is thought to be fairly high with a range from 2% to 10% (International Society for the Study of Trauma and Dissociation (ISSTD), 2012).

Depersonalization disorder ranges from about 1% to 3%, which is comparable to other disorders such as schizophrenia, bipolar disorder, and obsessive-compulsive disorder (Spiegel et al., 2011). Dissociative amnesia is also fairly common with a prevalence of about 2% to 7%. Dissociative identity disorder was formerly called multiple personality disorder, and a requirement for this diagnosis was the presence of alternate identities. Since switching from one personality to another happens infrequently, many people with this disorder are not properly diagnosed and often are misdiagnosed as having a psychotic disorder such as schizophrenia.

Anyone may experience a transient or temporary depersonalization. An actual depersonalization disorder is more severe and is found in both adolescents and adults, often in response to acute stress. Patients with this disorder usually seek treatment for another problem such as anxiety or depression. Dissociative amnesia may occur in any age group from children to adults. The amnesia is often related to trauma, and memory returns spontaneously after the individual is removed from the stressful situation (ISSTD, 2012). Dissociative identity disorder may occur at any age but is diagnosed three to nine times more frequently in adult females than in adult males. There is usually a childhood history of severe physical or sexual abuse.

COMORBIDITY

Comorbidity is common with dissociative disorders. Depression, panic attacks, eating disorders, PTSD, somatoform symptoms, eating disorders, obsessive-compulsive disorder (OCD), reactive attachment disorder (RAD), attention deficit disorder (ADD) with or without hyperactivity, personality disorders such as borderline personality disorder, and substance-use disorders, as well as sexual and sleep disorders, commonly co-occur with all of the dissociative disorders (ISSTD, 2012). In addition, dissociative amnesia may be comorbid with conversion disorder or a personality disorder. Dissociative fugue, a type of dissociative amnesia, may co-occur with PTSD. Depersonalization and derealization also occur in hypochondriasis, mood and anxiety disorders, OCD, and schizophrenia (Spiegel et al., 2011).

ETIOLOGY

Childhood physical, sexual, or emotional abuse and other traumatic life events are associated with adults experiencing dissociative symptoms. Dissociative symptoms, or "mind-flight," actually reduce disturbing feelings and protect the person from full awareness of the trauma.

Biological Factors

Genetic

Although genetic variability is thought to play a role in stress reactivity, dissociation is thought to be largely due to extreme stress or environmental factors.

Neurobiological

Research suggests that the limbic system is involved in the development of dissociative disorders. Animal studies show that early, prolonged detachment from the caretaker negatively affects the development of the limbic system. Traumatic memories are processed in the limbic system, and the hippocampus stores this information. Individuals with DDs have increased activation of the orbital frontal cortex that inhibits activation of the amygdala and insular cortex as well as the hippocampal areas (Spiegel et al., 2011).

Psychological Factors

One of the most primitive ego defense mechanisms is dissociation. The theory of structural dissociation of the personality proposes that patients with complex trauma have different parts of their personality, the apparently normal part and the emotional part, that are not fully integrated with each other (Steele et al., 2005). Each part has its own responses, feelings, thoughts, perceptions, physical sensations, and behaviors. These different parts may not be aware of each other, with only one dominant personality operating depending on the situation and circumstance of the moment.

Environmental Factors

Dissociative disorders are responses to acute overwhelming trauma and as such are due to environmental factors. These may include any experience that is overwhelming to the person such as a motor vehicle accident, combat, emotional/verbal abuse, incest, neglectful or abusive caregivers, imprisonment, and many other types of traumatic events

Cultural Considerations

Certain culture-bound disorders exist in which there is a high level of activity, a trancelike state, and running or fleeing, followed by exhaustion, sleep, and amnesia regarding the episode. These syndromes include *piblokto*, seen in native people of the Arctic, *frenzy* witchcraft among the Navajo, and *amok* among Western Pacific natives. These syndromes, if observed in individuals native to the corresponding geographical areas, should be differentiated from dissociative disorders.

CONSIDERING CULTURE

Culture and Acute Stress Disorder

Panic attacks often occur during acute stress reactions, and there are culturally specific features in the way these symptoms manifest. For example, *ataques de nervios* have been documented in Dominican and Puerto Rican people, which have shown that although this construct overlaps with panic, it is not identical. Whereas *ataques de nervios* share features with panic attacks (fear of losing control, dizziness, fear of dying), there are other features not included in the official definition of panic attacks (e.g., screaming, striking out). Much work on *ataques de nervios* has focused on the overlap between it and panic disorder; however, the relevant issue for ASD is the breadth of description of acute reactions of panic attacks that does not limit it to strict panic disorder-type attacks.

Similarly, there has been much work done on panic attacks among Cambodians *(khya'l)*, which involves a perception that a "wind" can enter the body in the diaphragm and rise through the body and cause a range of symptoms, including shortness of breath, tinnitus, dizziness, soreness in the neck, and catastrophic fears for one's well-being. Rather than specifying the exact nature of the panic symptoms associated with Cambodian reactions, it is sufficient to note that culturally specific descriptions of panic should be applied to ASD because variations of panic attacks or panic symptoms (as distinct from panic disorder) are common in the acute phase after trauma.

Bryant, R., Friedman, M., Spiegel, D., Ursano, R., & Strain, J. (2011). A review of Acute Stress Disorder in DSM-V. *Depression and Anxiety, 28,* 809.

DEPERSONALIZATION/DEREALIZATION DISORDER

In depersonalization the focus is on oneself. It is an extremely uncomfortable feeling of being an observer of one's own body or mental processes. In derealization the focus is on the outside world. It is the recurring feeling that one's surroundings are unreal or distant. The person may feel mechanical, dreamy, or detached from the body. Some people suffer episodes of these problems that come and go, while others have episodes that begin with stressors and eventually become constant. Patients describe these experiences as very distressing.

> **VIGNETTE**
> Elizabeth, a 42-year-old executive, gasps as she looks in the mirror. She can't believe the changes in her appearance. She thinks that her body looks wavy and out of focus. She says that it feels as though she is floating in a fog and her feet are not actually touching the ground. "I wonder if I am really awake or if my life is a dream." As she is admitted to the stress-management unit, Elizabeth confides to the nurse that her son has recently been charged with insider trading in the stock market and that he may be facing a lengthy jail sentence.

DISSOCIATIVE AMNESIA

Dissociative amnesia is marked by the inability to recall important personal information, often of a traumatic or stressful nature; this lack of memory is too pervasive to be explained by ordinary forgetfulness. In dissociative amnesia, autobiographical memory is available but is not accessible. In contrast, a patient with generalized amnesia is unable to recall information about his or her entire lifetime. The amnesia may also be localized (the patient is unable to remember all events in a certain period) or selective (the patient is able to recall some but not all events in a certain period).

A subtype of dissociative amnesia is dissociative fugue, which is characterized by sudden, unexpected travel away from the customary locale and inability to recall one's identity and information about some or all of the past. In rare cases, an individual with dissociative fugue assumes a whole new identity. During a fugue state, individuals tend to lead rather simple lives, rarely calling attention to themselves. After a few weeks to a few months, they may remember their former identities and then become amnesic for the time spent in the fugue state. Usually a dissociative fugue is precipitated by a traumatic event.

> **VIGNETTE**
> A young woman found wandering in a Florida park is partly dressed and poorly nourished. She has no knowledge of who she is. Her parents identify her two 2 weeks later when she appears in an interview on a national television show. She had just broken up with her boyfriend of 3 years.

DISSOCIATIVE IDENTITY DISORDER

The essential feature of dissociative identity disorder is the presence of two or more distinct personality states that recurrently take control of behavior. Each alternate personality (alter) has its own pattern of perceiving, relating to, and thinking about the self and the environment. It is believed that severe sexual, physical, or psychological trauma in childhood predisposes an individual to the development of dissociative identity disorder.

Dissociative identity disorder appears to be associated with at least two dissociative identity states: one is a state or personality that functions on a daily basis and blocks access and responses to traumatic memories, and another state (also referred to as an alter state) is fixated on traumatic memories. There is evidence of different regional cerebral blood flow patterns and autonomic and subjective reactions during each of these physiological states when the individual is exposed to trauma-related stimuli (Reinders et al., 2006).

Each alter is a complex unit with its own memories, behavioral patterns, and social relationships that dictate how the person acts when that personality is dominant. Often the original or primary personality is religious and moralistic, and the alters are pleasure-seeking and nonconforming. The alter personalities may behave as individuals of a different sex, race, or religion. The dominant hand and the voice may also be different; intelligence and electroencephalographic findings may also be altered.

Typical cognitive distortions include the insistence that alternate personalities inhabit separate bodies and are unaffected by the actions of one another. The primary personality or host is usually not aware of the alters and is perplexed by lost time and unexplained events. Experiences such as finding unfamiliar clothing in the closet, being called a different name by a stranger, or not having childhood memories are characteristic of dissociative identity disorder. Alters may be aware of the existence of each other to some degree. Transition from one personality to another (switching) occurs during times of stress and may range from a dramatic to a barely noticeable event. Some patients experience the transition when awakening. Shifts may last from minutes to months, although shorter periods are more common.

Several movies and TV shows that demonstrate actual case studies of individuals diagnosed with dissociative identity disorder have been produced, including *Sybil* (1976), *The Three Faces of Eve* (1957), *Fight Club* (1999), *Me, Myself and Irene* (2000), and the television series *The United States of Tara.*

APPLICATION OF THE NURSING PROCESS

ASSESSMENT

For a diagnosis of dissociative disorder to be made, medical and neurological illnesses, substance use, and other coexisting psychiatric disorders must be ruled out as the cause of the patient's symptoms. The assessment should include objective data from physical examination, electroencephalography, imaging studies, and specific questions to identify dissociative symptoms.

Scales have been developed to assess dissociation, including the Dissociative Experience Scale (DES) (Bernstein & Putnam, 1986), the Somatoform Questionnaire (SDQ) (Nijenhuis et al., 2012) (available from http://www.enijenhuis.nl/sdq.html), and the Dissociative Disorders Interview Schedule (DDIS) (Ross et al., 1989). The latter can be downloaded for free from http://www.rossinst.com

These assessment tools are important because a psychiatric interview will often miss the presence of dissociation. By definition, dissociative periods involve lapses of memory that a person may not even be aware of, and patients with dissociative disorders do not know what they do not know. Specific information about identity, memory, consciousness, life events, mood, suicide risk, and the impact of the disorder on the patient and the family are important dimensions to assess.

Assessing patients' ability to identify themselves requires more than asking them to state their names. Changes in patient behavior, voice, and dress might signal the presence of an alternate personality. Referring to the self by another name or in the third person and using the word *we* instead of *I* are indications that the patient may have assumed a new identity. The nurse should consider the following when assessing memory:

1. Can the patient remember recent and past events?
2. Is the patient's memory clear and complete or partial and fuzzy?
3. Is the patient aware of gaps in memory, such as lack of memory for events such as a graduation or a wedding?
4. Do the patient's memories place the self with a family, in school, or in an occupation?
   Patients with amnesia and fugue may be disoriented with regard to time and place as well as person.
5. Does the patient ever lose time or have blackouts?
6. Does the patient ever find herself or himself in places with no idea how she or he got there?

History

The nurse must gather information about events in the person's life. Has the patient sustained a recent injury, such as a concussion? Does the patient have a history of epilepsy, especially temporal lobe epilepsy? Does the patient have a history of early trauma, such as physical, mental, or sexual abuse? If dissociative identity disorder is suspected, pertinent questions include the following:

1. Have you ever found yourself wearing clothes you cannot remember buying?
2. Have you ever had strange persons greet and talk to you as though they were old friends?
3. Does your ability to engage in things such as athletics, artistic activities, or mechanical tasks seem to change?
4. Do you have differing sets of memories about childhood?

Mood

Is the individual depressed, anxious, or unconcerned? Many patients with dissociative identity disorder seek help when the primary personality is depressed. The nurse also observes for mood shifts. When alternate identities of dissociative identity disorder take control, their predominant moods may be different from that of the principal personality. If the alternate identities shift frequently, marked mood swings may be noted.

Impact on Patient and Family

In fugue states, individuals often function adequately in their new identities by choosing simple, undemanding occupations and having few intimate social interactions. Patients with amnesia, in contrast to those with fugue, may be more dysfunctional. Their perplexity often renders them unable to work, and their memory loss impairs normal relationships. Families often direct considerable attention toward the patient but may exhibit concern over having to assume roles that were once assigned to the patient.

Patients with dissociative identity disorder often have both family and work problems. Families find it difficult to accept the seemingly erratic behaviors of the patient. Employers dislike the lost time that may occur when alternate identities are in control. Patients with depersonalization disorder are often fearful that others may perceive their appearance as distorted and may avoid being seen in public. If they exhibit high anxiety, the family is likely to find it difficult to keep relationships stable.

Suicide Risk

Whenever a patient's life has been substantially disrupted, the patient may have thoughts of suicide. The nurse gathering data should be alert for expressions of hopelessness, helplessness, or worthlessness and for verbalization or other behavior of an alternate identity that indicates the intent to engage in self-destructive or self-mutilating behaviors.

Self-Assessment

It is natural to experience feelings of skepticism while caring for patients who are diagnosed with dissociative identity disorder. You may find it difficult to believe in the authenticity of the symptoms the patient is displaying. A sense of inadequacy may accompany the need to be ready to interact in a therapeutic way with whichever personality is in control at the moment; however, some nurses experience feelings of fascination and are caught up in the intrigue of caring for a patient with multiple identities.

Feelings of inadequacy can also arise when establishment of a trusting relationship occurs slowly. It is important to remember that the patient with a dissociative disorder has often experienced relationships in which trust was betrayed. When alters vie for control and attempt to embarrass or harm each other, crises are common, and nurses must be alert and ready to intervene. Preparing for the unexpected, including the possibility of a suicide attempt, means constant hypervigilance by staff, and such observational demands can eventually lead to great fatigue. Caring for a patient with dissociative disorder can generate anxiety in any of the following situations:

1. When a patient who has regained memory develops panic-level anxiety
2. When a patient becomes assaultive because of extreme confusion or panic-level anxiety
3. When a patient attempts self-harm by acting out against the primary personality or other personalities

If the patient manifesting symptoms of a dissociative disorder has been involved in the commission of a crime, the medical record is likely to be a court exhibit. You may experience concern over that fact or be angry if you believe the patient is faking illness to avoid being found guilty of the crime. Supervision should always be available for nursing staff and clinicians caring for a patient with a dissociative disorder. By discussing feelings and the plan of care with the treatment team or peers, the nurse can better ensure objective and appropriate care for the patient.

General guidelines for assessment of a patient with a dissociative disorder include:

1. Assess for a history of self-harm.
2. Evaluate level of anxiety and signs of dissociation.
3. Identify support systems through a psychosocial assessment.

DIAGNOSIS

The overall goal for dissociative disorder is the integration of personalities into a single personality. Nursing diagnoses relate to personal identity, role performance, and anxiety.

OUTCOMES IDENTIFICATION

Table 16-1 provides examples of signs and symptoms, suggestions for nursing diagnoses, and possible outcomes for dissociative disorders.

PLANNING

The setting and presenting problem influence the planning of nursing care for the patient with a dissociative disorder; however, a phase-oriented treatment model is recommended and includes the following (ISSTD, 2012):

Phase 1: Establishing safety, stabilization, and symptom reduction
Phase 2: Confronting, working through, and integrating traumatic memories
Phase 3: Identity integration and rehabilitation

The nurse will most often encounter the patient in times of crisis (i.e., when the patient is admitted to the hospital for suicidal or homicidal behavior). The care plan will focus on Phase 1 strategies to ensure safety and crisis intervention. The patient may also come for treatment of a comorbid depression or anxiety disorder in the community setting. Planning will address the presenting complaint with appropriate referrals for treatment of the dissociative disorder.

IMPLEMENTATION

Healing trauma can be thought of as a process of integration and linking neural networks that have become disconnected during an overwhelming event. Basic-level interventions are aimed at offering emotional presence during the recall of painful experiences, providing a sense of safety, and encouraging an optimal level of functioning. *NIC* topics that offer relevant interventions include *Anxiety reduction, Coping enhancement, Self-Awareness enhancement, Self-Esteem enhancement,* and *Emotional support.* Refer to Table 16-2 for examples of basic-level interventions.

Psychoeducation

Patients with dissociative disorders need to be educated about their illness and given ongoing instruction about coping skills and stress management. Normalizing experiences by explaining to the patient that his or her symptoms are adaptive responses to past overwhelming events is important. Often, the victim of childhood trauma feels as if he or she is a bad person and grows up with the false negative belief that the abuse was deserved punishment.

Teaching **grounding techniques** that bring the person's awareness to noticing real things in the present helps to counter dissociative episodes. Examples of grounding techniques can include the following: stomping one's feet on the ground, taking a shower, holding an ice cube, exercising, deep breathing, counting beads, or touching fabric or upholstery on a chair. Patients should also be taught to keep a daily journal to increase their awareness of feelings and to identify triggers to dissociation. If a patient has never written a journal, the nurse should suggest beginning with a 5- to 10-minute daily writing exercise.

Pharmacological Interventions

There are no specific medications for patients with dissociative disorders, but appropriate medications are often prescribed for the hyperarousal and intrusive symptoms that accompany

TABLE 16-1 SIGNS AND SYMPTOMS, NURSING DIAGNOSES, AND OUTCOMES FOR DISSOCIATIVE DISORDERS

SIGNS AND SYMPTOMS	NURSING DIAGNOSES	OUTCOMES
Amnesia or fugue related to a traumatic event; symptoms of depersonalization; feelings of unreality and/or body image distortions	*Disturbed personal identity*	Verbalizes clear sense of personal identity, perceives environment accurately, performs social roles well
Alterations in consciousness, memory, or identity, abuse of substances, disorganization or dysfunction in usual patterns of behavior (absence from work, withdrawal from relationships, changes in role function)	*Ineffective role performance*	Performs family, parental, intimate, community, and work roles adequately; reports comfort with role expectations
Feeling of being out of control of memory, behaviors, and awareness; inability to explain actions or behaviors when in altered state	*Anxiety self-control*	Monitors intensity of anxiety, eliminates precursors of anxiety, uses effective coping strategies, maintains role performance and relationships

From Herdman, T.H. (Ed.) *Nursing diagnoses—Definitions and classification 2012-2014.* Copyright © 2012, 1994-2012 by NANDA International. Used by arrangement with John Wiley & Sons Limited; Moorhead, S., Johnson, M., Maas, M.L., & Swanson, E. (2013). *Nursing outcomes classification (NOC)* (5th ed.). St Louis, MO: Mosby.

TABLE 16-2 **BASIC-LEVEL NURSING INTERVENTIONS FOR DISSOCIATIVE DISORDERS**

INTERVENTION	RATIONALE
Provide undemanding, simple routine.	Reduces anxiety
Ensure patient safety by providing safe, protected environment and frequent observation.	Sense of bewilderment may lead to inattention to safety needs; some alters may be thrill-seeking, violent, or careless
Confirm identity of patient and orientation to time and place.	Supports reality and promotes ego integrity
Encourage patient to do things for self and make decisions about routine tasks.	Enhances self-esteem by reducing sense of powerlessness and reduces secondary gain associated with dependence
Assist with major decision making until memory returns.	Lowers stress and prevents patient from having to live with the consequences of unwise decisions
Support patient during exploration of feelings surrounding the stressful event.	Helps lower the defense of dissociation used by patient to block awareness of the stressful event
Do not flood patient with data regarding past events.	Memory loss serves the purpose of preventing severe to panic levels of anxiety from overtaking and disorganizing the individual
Allow patient to progress at own pace as memory is recovered.	Prevents undue anxiety and resistance
Provide support through empathetic listening during disclosure of painful experiences.	Can be healing, while minimizing feelings of isolation
Teach patient grounding techniques such as taking a shower, deep breathing, touching fabric on chair, exercising or stomping feet.	Helps to keep the person in the present and decrease dissociation
Accept patient's expression of negative feelings.	Conveys permission to have negative or unacceptable feelings
Teach stress-reduction methods.	Provides alternatives for anxiety relief
If patient does not remember significant others, work with involved parties to reestablish relationships.	Helps patient experience satisfaction and relieves sense of isolation

PTSD and dissociation (ISSTD, 2012). These might include antidepressant medication, anxiolytics, and antipsychotics. Substance-use disorders and suicidal risk, which are common, must be assessed carefully in selecting safe and appropriate pharmacotherapy. In the acute setting, the nurse may witness dramatic memory retrieval in patients with dissociative amnesia or fugue after treatment with intravenous benzodiazepines.

Advanced Practice Interventions

Advanced practice nurses and other skilled licensed mental health professionals use cognitive-behavioral therapy, psychodynamic psychotherapy, exposure therapy, modified EMDR, hypnotherapy, neurofeedback, ego state therapies, somatic therapies, and medication to treat patients with dissociative disorders. Advanced training is needed to treat these patients effectively as such, and ongoing supervision for the therapist is suggested.

Somatic Therapy

Dissociation causes people to experience a distressing fragmentation of consciousness and a sense of separation from themselves. Disturbances of perception, sensation, autonomic regulation, and movement are common for those who have suffered significant trauma since trauma is often stored physically in the body. Verbal and bodily psychotherapies are seen as complementary by the discipline of Dance Movement Therapists in working with traumatized dissociative patients in emotional recovery (Koch & Harvey, 2012).

A specific type of somatic psychotherapy, sensorimotor psychotherapy, combines talking therapy with body-centered interventions and movement to address the dissociative symptoms inherent in trauma (Ogden et al., 2006). This type of therapy is integrated into phase-oriented trauma treatment to facilitate symptom reduction and stability, to integrate the traumatic memory, and to restore the person's ability to stay in the present moment. This therapy is based on the premise that the body, mind, emotions, and spirit are interrelated, and a change at one level results in changes in the others. Awareness, focusing on the present, and recognizing touch as a means of communicating are some of the principles of this therapy. During psychotherapy sessions, the patient is asked to describe physical sensations he or she is experiencing. The goal is to safely disarm the pathological defense mechanism of dissociation and replace it with other resources, especially body awareness and mindfulness.

EVALUATION

Overall, treatment effectiveness for dissociative identity disorder is "integration," coordinated functioning among alternate identities to promote optimal functioning (ISSTD, 2011). This occurs primarily through long-term psychotherapy.

In general, treatment for trauma-related disorders is considered successful when outcomes are met. In the final analysis, the evaluation is positive when:

1. Patient safety has been maintained.
2. Anxiety has been reduced, and the patient has returned to a functional state.
3. Integration of the fragmented memories has occurred.
4. New coping strategies have permitted the patient to function at a better level.
5. Stress is handled adaptively, without the use of dissociation.

KEY POINTS TO REMEMBER

- Childhood trauma changes the brain and can cause medical and psychological problems in adulthood.
- A phase model of treatment is most effective with safety and stabilization first.
- Evidenced-based treatments for trauma are EMDR and CBT.
- Understanding patients as traumatized changes the conversation from "What is wrong with this person?" to "What happened to this person?"
- Trauma fractures and fragments memory; healing involves connection and integration.
- Trauma is stored in the body and often manifests as physical symptoms.
- Dissociative disorders involve a disruption in consciousness with significant impairments in memory, identity, and perception of self.
- Assessment is especially important in clarifying the history and course of past symptoms as well as obtaining a complete picture of the current physical, mental, and safety status.
- Patients with dissociative disorders are often misdiagnosed with depression, schizophrenia, or borderline personality disorder.
- Psychotherapy is the treatment of choice for trauma, with medication prescribed only to ameliorate symptoms.
- Patients with trauma-related disorders are often treated on an outpatient basis except during a period of crisis such as suicidal risk.
- Crisis intervention is important for stabilization; referral for psychotherapy to attain sustained improvement in level of functioning is typically necessary.

CRITICAL THINKING EXERCISES

1. Jeanne is a 48-year-old woman with dissociative identity disorder who was admitted to the crisis unit for a short-term stay after a suicide threat. On the unit, she has repeated the statement that she will kill herself to get rid of "all the others," meaning her alters. Jeanne refuses to sign a "no harm" contract.
   a. How do you think that staff reacts to working with patients such as Jeanne?
   b. What do you believe needs to be done to protect Jeanne?
2. Steven is an 8-year-old child who was in a devastating earthquake and came to the outpatient clinic with his parents because he was having nightmares and trouble sleeping. How would you explain what is happening to Steven?
3. John, a 24-year-old young man, returned from the Iraqi war last month and has become increasingly irritable, isolated, and depressed. His wife says he does not want to go anywhere and won't leave his home for days at a time. In the interview with the nurse at the clinic, he indicates that he feels helpless and anxious and jumpy. Identify priorities in providing care for this patient, and develop a nursing care plan.

CHAPTER REVIEW

1. Nick, a construction worker, is on duty when a nearly completed wall suddenly falls, crushing a number of co-workers. Although badly shaken initially, he seemed to be coping well. About two weeks after the tragedy he begins to experience tremors, nightmares, and periods during which he feels numb or detached from his environment. He finds himself frequently thinking about the tragedy and feeling guilty that he was spared while many others died. Which statement about this situation is most accurate?
   a. Nick has acute stress disorder and will benefit from antianxiety medications.
   b. Nick is experiencing posttraumatic stress disorder (PTSD) and should be referred for outpatient treatment.
   c. Nick is experiencing anxiety and grief and should be monitored for PTSD symptoms.
   d. Nick is experiencing mild anxiety and a normal grief reaction; no intervention is needed.
2. You are caring for Susannah, a 29-year-old who has been diagnosed with dissociative identity disorder. She was recently hospitalized after coming to the emergency room with deep cuts on her arms with no memory of how this occurred. The priority nursing intervention for Susannah is:
   a. Assist in recovering memories of abuse.
   b. Maintain 1:1 observation.
   c. Teach coping skills and stress-management strategies.
   d. Refer for integrative therapy.
3. You are caring for Connor, an 8-year-old boy who has been diagnosed with reactive attachment disorder. Which of the following nursing outcomes would be the most appropriate to achieve?
   a. Increases ability to self-control and decreases impulsive behaviors.
   b. Avoids situations that trigger conflicts.
   c. Expresses complex thoughts.
   d. Writes or draws feelings in a journal.
4. Ashley is a 21-year-old college student who was sexually assaulted at a party. She was seen in the local emergency department and referred for counseling after being diagnosed by the provider on call as having acute stress disorder. Which of the following treatment modalities would you expect to see used in therapy with Ashley?
   a. Aversion therapy
   b. Stress-reduction therapy
   c. Cognitive-behavioral therapy
   d. Short-term classical analysis therapy
5. Jamie, age 24, has been diagnosed with a dissociative disorder following a traumatic event. Jamie's mother asks you, "Does this mean my daughter is now crazy?" Your best response would be:
   a. "People with dissociative disorders are out of touch with reality, so in that way, your daughter is now mentally ill. Don't worry. Treatment is available."
   b. "Jamie will most likely need long-term intensive in patient treatment to deal with her traumatic memories as well as to work through her delusions."
   c. "Most mental health providers are skeptical about dissociative disorders and aren't sure they truly exist. Jamie may be making up her symptoms as a cry for help."
   d. "Jamie is dealing with the anxiety associated with the trauma by separating herself from it. With treatment she can get back to her previous level of functioning."

Answers to Chapter Review
1. a; 2. b; 3. d; 4. c; 5. d.

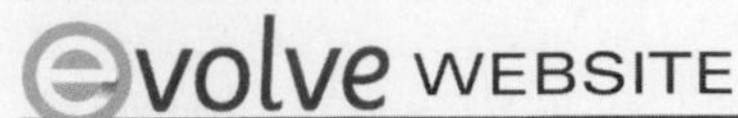

Visit the Evolve website for a posttest on the content in this chapter: http://evolve.elsevier.com/Varcarolis

Post-Test interactive review

REFERENCES

Ainsworth, M. D. (1967). *Infancy in Uganda.* Baltimore, MD: Johns Hopkins.

American Psychiatric Association. (2013). *DSM-5 table of contents.* Retrieved from http://www.psychiatry.org/dsm5.

Bergmann, U. (2012). *Neurobiological foundations for EMDR practice.* New York, NY: Springer.

Bernstein, E. M., & Putnam, F. W. (1986). Development, reliability, and validity of a dissociation scale. *Journal of Nervous and Mental Disease, 174*(12), 727–735.

Bisson, J., & Andrew, M. (2007). Psychological treatment of post-traumatic stress disorder (PTSD). *Cochrane Database of Systematic Reviews, 3.* Art. No.: CD003388. doi: 10.1002/14651858.CD003388.pub3.

Boon, S., Steele, K., & van der Hart, O. (2011). *Coping with trauma-related dissociation: Skills training for patients and therapists.* New York, NY: Norton.

Bowlby, J. (1988). *A secure base: Clinical applications of attachment theory.* London, UK: Routledge.

Briere, J. (1996). *The trauma symptom checklist for children.* Retrieved from http://www4.parinc.com/Products/Product.aspx?ProductID5TSCC.

Bryant, R. A., Moulds, M., Guthrie, R., & Nixon, R. D. (2003). Treating acute stress disorder following mild traumatic brain injury. *American Journal of Psychiatry, 160,* 585–587.

Bryant, R., Friedman, M., Spiegel, D., Ursano, R., & Strain, J. (2011). A review of acute stress disorder in DSM-V. *Depression and Anxiety, 28,* 802–817.

Bulechek, G. M., Butcher, H. K., Dochterman, J. M., & Wagner, C. (2013). *Nursing interventions classification (NIC)* (6th ed). St. Louis, MO: Mosby.

Buurman, B. M., Mank, A. P. M., Beijer, H. J. M., & Olff, M. (2011). Coping with serious events at work: A study of traumatic stress among nurses. *Journal of the American Psychiatric Nurses Association, 17*(5), 321–329.

Casey, P., & Doherty, A. (2012). Adjustment disorder: Implications for ICD-11 and DSM-5. *British Journal of Psychiatry, 201,* 90–92. doi: 10.1192/bjp.bp.112.110494.

Centers for Disease Control and Prevention. (2010). Adverse childhood experiences reported by adult—Five states, 2009. *Morbidity and Mortality Weekly Report, 59*(49), 1609–1613.

Darnaudéry, M., & Maccari, S. (2008). Epigenetic programming of the stress response in male and female rats by prenatal restraint stress. *Brain Research Review, 57*(2), 571–585.

Farrell, A., Erwin, E., Allison, K., Meyer, A., Sullivan, T., Camou, S., et al. (2007). Problematic situations in the lives of urban African American middle school students: A qualitative study. *Journal of Research on Adolescence, 17*(2), 413–454.

Felitti, V. J., Anda, R. F., Nordenberg, D., Williamson, D. F., Spitz, A. M., Edwards, V., et al. (1998). Relationship of childhood abuse and household dysfunction to many of the leading causes of death in adults: The adverse childhood experiences (ACE) study. *American Journal of Preventive Medicine, 14*(4), 245–258.

Fernández, A., Mendive, J. M., Salvador-Carulla, L., Rubio-Valera, M., Luciano, J. V., Pinto-Meza, A., et al. (2012). Adjustment disorders in primary care: Prevalence, recognition, and use of services. *British Journal of Psychiatry, 201,* 137–142.

Fleming, J. (2012). The effectiveness of eye movement desensitization and reprocessing in the treatment of traumatized children and youth. *Journal of EMDR Practice and Research, 6*(1), 16–24.

Flores, G. (2010). Committee on pediatric research. Technical report—Racial and ethnic disparities in the health and health care of children. *Pediatrics, 125*(4), e979-e1020. doi: 10.1542/peds.2010-0188.

Frankenburg, W. K., Dodds, J., Archer, P., Shapiro, H., & Bresnick, B. (1992). The Denver II: A major revision and restandardization of the Denver Developmental Screening test. *Pediatrics, 89*(1), 91–97.

Friedman, M. J., Resick, P., Bryant, R. A., & Brewin, C. (2011a). Considering PTSD for DSM-V. *Depression and Anxiety, 28*(9), 750–769.

Friedman, M. J., Resick, P. A., Bryant, R. A., Strain, J., Horowitz, M., & Spiegel, D. (2011b). Classification of trauma and stressor-related disorders in DSM-5. *Depression and Anxiety, 28*(9), 737–749.

Friedrich, W., Gerber, P., Koplin, B., Davis, M., Giese, J., Mykelebust, C., & Franckowiak, D. (2001). Multimodal assessment of dissociation in adolescents: Inpatients and juvenile sex offenders. *Sexual Abuse: Journal of Research and Treatment, 13,* 167–177.

Herdman, T. H. (Ed.). (2012). *NANDA international nursing diagnoses: Definitions and classifications, 2012-2014.* Oxford, UK: Wiley-Blackwell.

Herrman, H., Stewart, D., Diaz-Grandos, N., Berger, E., Jackson, B., & Yuen, T. (2011). What is resilience? *The Canadian Journal of Psychiatry,* 65(5), 258–265.

Horowitz, M., Wilner, N., & Alvarez, W. (1979). Impact of Event Scale: A measure of subjective stress. *Psychosomatic Medicine, 41,* 209–218.

Huckshorn, K. (2012). Trauma-informed care: A shift in thinking for service providers. *Webinar: Assessing for and addressing trauma in recovery-oriented practice.* Retrieved from http://www.dsgonline.com/rtp/webinars/1.25.2012.html.

International Society for the Study of Trauma and Dissociation. (2012). Guidelines for treating dissociative identity disorder in adults, 3rd rev. *Journal of Trauma and Dissociation, 12(2),* 115–187.

Jarero, I., Artigas, L., & Luber, M. (2011). The EMDR protocol for recent critical incidents: Application in a disaster mental health continuum of care context. *Journal of EMDR Practice and Research, 5*(3), 82–94.

Johnson, B. S., & Newland, J. A. (2012). Integration of physical and psychiatric assessment. In E. L. Yearwood, G. S. Pearson, & J. A. Newland (Eds.), *Child and adolescent behavioral health* (pp. 57–88). Ames, IA: John Wiley & Sons.

Kessler, R. C., Sonnega, A., Bromet, E., Hughes, M., & Nelson, C. (1995). Posttraumatic stress in the national comorbidity survey. *Archives of General Psychiatry, 52,* 1048–1060.

Koch, S. C., & Harvey, S. (2012). Dance/movement therapy with traumatized dissociative patients. In S. C. Koch, T. Fuchs, M. Summa & C. Muller (Eds.), *Body memory, methaphor and movement* (pp. 369–386). Philadelphia, PA: John Benjamins.

Lang, A., &,Stein, M. B. (2005). An abbreviated PTSD checklist for use as a screening instrument in primary care. *Behaviour Research and Therapy, 43,* 585–594.

Luber, M. (2009). *Eye movement desensitization and reprocessing scripted protocols: basics and special situations.* New York, NY: Springer.

Moorhead, S., Johnson, M., Maas, M. L., & Swanson, E. (Eds.). (2013). *Nursing outcome classification (NOC)* (5th ed.). St. Louis, MO: Mosby.

National Center for PTSD. (2011). *Research on women, trauma and PTSD.* Retrieved from http://www.ptsd.va.gov/professional/pages/women-trauma-ptsd.asp.

National Child Abuse and Neglect Data System (2010). *Child abuse and neglect statistics.* Retrieved from https://www.childwelfare.gov/can/statistics/.

National Institute for Health and Clinical Excellence (NICE). (2005). *Post traumatic stress disorder (PTSD): The management of adults and children in primary and secondary care.* London, UK: NICE.

National Institute on Drug Abuse. (2011). Research report series, Comorbidity: Addiction and other mental illnesses. Retrieved from http://drugabuse.gov/PDF/RRComorbidity.pdf.

National Institute of Mental Health. (2011). *Posttraumatic Stress Disorder among adults.* Retrieved from http://www.nimh.nih.gov/statistics/1AD_PTSD_ADULT.shtmla.

Nijenhuis, E. R. S., Spinhoven, P., Van Dyck, R., Van der Hart, O., & Vanderlinden, J. (1996). The development and the psychometric characteristics of the somatoform dissociation questionnaire (SDQ-20). *Journal of Mental and Nervous Disease, 184,* 688–694.

Ogden, P., Minton, K., & Pain, C. (2006). *Trauma and the body: a sensorimotor approach to psychotherapy*. New York, NY: Norton.

Porges, S. W. (2011). *The polyvagal theory*. New York, NY: W.W. Norton.

Prins, A., Ouimette, P., Kimerling, R., Cameron, R. P., Hugelshofer, D. S., Shaw-Hegwer, J., . . . Sheikh, J. I. (2003). The primary care PTSD screen (PC-PTSD): Development and operating characteristics. *Primary Care Psychiatry, 9*, 9–14.

Putnam, F. W., Helmers, K., & Trickett, P. K. (1993). Development, reliability, and validity of a child dissociation scale. *Child Abuse & Neglect, 17*, 731–742.

Reinders, A. A., Nijenhuis, E. R., Ouak, J., Korf, J., Haaksma, J., Paans, A.M., et al. (2006). Psychobiological characteristics of dissociative identity disorder: A symptom provocation study. *Biological Psychiatry, 60*(1), 730–740.

Ross, C. A., Heber, S., Norton, G. R., Anderson, D., Anderson, G., & Barchet, P. (1989). The Dissociative Disorders Interview Schedule: A structured interview. *Dissociation, 2*, 169–189.

Shapiro, E., & Laub, B. (2008). Early EMDR Intervention (EEI): A summary, a theoretical model, and the recent traumatic episode protocol (R-TEP). *Journal of EMDR Practice and Research, 2*(2), 79–96.

Shonkoff, J. P. (2010). Building a new bio-developmental framework to guide the future of early childhood policy. *Child Development, 81*(1), 357–367.

Shonkoff, J. P., & Garner, A. S. (2012). The lifelong effects of early childhood adversity and toxic stress. *Pediatrics, 129*(1), 232–246.

Smyke, A., & Zeanah, C. H. (1999). *Disturbances of attachment interview*. Unpublished manuscript.

Spiegel, D., Loewenstein, R., Lewis-Fernancdez, R., Sar, V., Simeon, D., Vermetten, E., et al. (2011). Dissociative disorders in DSM-5. *Depression and Anxiety, 28*, 824–852.

Steele, K., van der Hart, O., & Nijenjuis, E. (2005). Phase-oriented treatment of structural dissociation in complex traumatization: Overcoming trauma-related phobias. *Journal of Trauma and Dissociation, 6*(3), 11–53.

Strain, J. J., & Friedman, M. J. (2011). Considering adjustment disorders as stress response syndromes for DSM-5. *Depression and Anxiety, 28*(9), 818–823. doi: 10.1002/da.2078.

Stuber, M., Meeske, K., Krull, K., Leisenring, W., Stratton, K., Kazak, A., et al. (2010). Prevalence and predictors of posttraumatic stress disorder in adult survivors of childhood cancer. *Pediatrics, 125*(5), 1124–1134.

Tizard, B. (1977). *Adoption: A second chance*. London, UK: Open Books.

United States Department of Health and Human Services. (2008). *Reauthorization of the Child Abuse Protection and Treatment Act*. Retrieved from http://www.hhs.gov/asl/testify/2008/06/t20080626a.html.

United States Department of Veterans Affairs. (2010a). *Clinical practice guideline for the management of post-traumatic stress*. Retrieved from http://www.healthquality.va.gov.

United States Department of Veterans Affairs. (2010b). *PTSD in children and adolescents*. Retrieved from http://www.ptsd.va.gov/professional/pages/ptsd_in_children_and_adolescents_overview_for_professionals.asp.

United States Department of Veterans Affairs. (2012). *Primary care PTSD screen (PC-PTSD)*. Retrieved from http://www.ptsd.va.gov/professional/pages/assessments/pc-ptsd.asp.

Weaver, I., Meaney, M., & Szyf, M. (2006). Maternal care effects on the hippocampal transciptome and anxiety-mediated behaviors in the offspring that are reversible in adulthood. In *Proceedings of the National Academy of Sciences of the United States*. Retrieved from http://www.pnas.org/content/103/9/3480.full.

Zeanah, C. H. (2010). *Proposal to include child and adolescent age related manifestation and age related subtypes for PTSD in DSM-V*. Retrieved from http://www.dsm5.org/Proposed%20Revision%20Attachments/DSM-5%20Child%20PTSD%20Review%2012-22-08.pdf.

CHAPTER

17

Somatic Symptom Disorders

Lois Angelo and Faye J. Grund

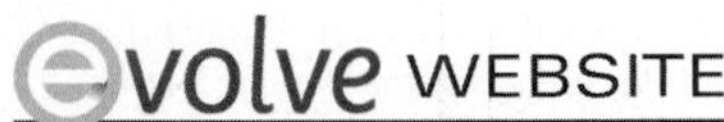

Visit the Evolve website for a pretest on the content in this chapter: http://evolve.elsevier.com/Varcarolis

Pre-Test interactive review

OBJECTIVES

1. Describe clinical manifestations of each of the somatic symptom disorders.
2. Discuss biological, psychological, behavioral, cognitive, environmental, and cultural factors influencing the onset and course of the somatic symptom disorders.
3. Analyze the impact of childhood trauma on adult somatic preoccupation.
4. Apply the nursing process to individuals with somatic symptom disorders.
5. Evaluate the importance of a assessing the patient's coping skills and strengths.
6. Describe five psychosocial interventions for the care of the patient who has a somatic symptom disorder.
7. Identify the role of the advanced practice psychiatric nurse in the primary care setting.
8. Discuss the problem of factitious disorders and their implications for care.
9. Define malingering as a distinct but related problem with which health care providers are faced.

KEY TERMS AND CONCEPTS

conversion disorder
factitious disorders
functional neurological disorder
holistic approach
illness anxiety disorder
la belle indifference
psychological factors affecting medical condition
secondary gain
somatic symptom disorder
somatization

Soma is the Greek word for "body," and somatization is the expression of psychological stress through physical symptoms. Instead of feeling anxiety, depression, or irritability, some individuals experience pain, paralysis, unexplained skin rashes, and other symptoms (Webb, 2010). Somatization disorders have been around for centuries and have disrupted countless lives; our understanding of the complexity of these disorders has only just begun (Hale & Reck, 2010). These disorders baffle both patients and health care providers. Patients worry that their problems are all in their heads and then worry that they will actually die (Dickson et al., 2009).

When psychiatric disorders are present along with general medical conditions, they may increase the likelihood of increased health care costs and length of stay. They also can negatively impact outcomes and increase morbidity and mortality. Anxiety, depression, and trauma exert a powerful influence on the mind and may lead to a variety of clinical conditions—both mental and physical. In somatic disorders, the primary focus is on physical manifestations of emotional states.

Somatic disorders demonstrate complex mind-body interactions that cause real distress to the patient, with significant impairment in social and occupational functioning. These conditions are relatively rare in the psychiatric setting, but the nurse may encounter patients with such disorders in the outpatient primary care office, in acute care general medical settings, or in specialized units.

This chapter helps to prepare nurses to utilize a holistic approach in nursing care so that they may address the multidimensional interplay of biological, psychological, and sociocultural needs and its effects on the somatization process. It is important for psychiatric mental health nurses who are caring for patients with physical illnesses and also essential for nurses who work outside of psychiatric settings to be aware of the influence of environment, stress, individual lifestyle, and coping skills of each patient. In the beginning of this chapter we will address all of the somatic disorders except for factitious disorder. This problem will be addressed separately at the end of this chapter.

CLINICAL PICTURE

According to the American Psychiatric Association (2013), the somatic disorders include the following:

- Somatic symptom disorder
- Illness anxiety disorder (previously hypochondriasis)
- Conversion disorder (functional neurological disorder)
- Psychological factors affecting medical condition
- Factitious disorder

Somatic Symptom Disorder

Somatic symptom disorder is characterized by a combination of distressing symptoms and an excessive or maladaptive response or associated health concerns without significant physical findings and medical diagnosis. Patients' suffering is authentic, and they typically experience a high level of functional impairment.

The predominance of women with somatization is significant. It has been proposed that women are more aware of their bodily sensations, have different health-seeking behaviors when faced with physical and psychological distress, and use more health care services than men (So, 2008). In particular, young women, aged 16 to 25, are more likely to receive a somatic diagnosis than men or older individuals (Huang & McCarron, 2011).

Symptoms may be initiated, exacerbated, or maintained by combinations of biological, psychological, and sociocultural factors. Somatic symptom disorder is difficult to distinguish from physical disorders with organic causes, and the patient's history is extremely important for accurate diagnosis. Often, the patient has a comorbid psychiatric disorder such as depression, anxiety, and/or a personality disorder.

There may be a high level of medical care utilization, which rarely alleviates the patient's concerns. Included in the most common symptoms for visits to primary care providers are chest pain, fatigue, dizziness, headache, swelling, back pain, shortness of breath, insomnia, abdominal pain, and numbness. They account for 40% of all visits to primary care providers; however, a biological cause for these symptoms is identified in only 26% of patients (Edwards et al., 2010). Health-related quality of life is frequently severely impaired, and patients appraise their bodily symptoms as unduly threatening, harmful, or troublesome, often fearing the worst about their health.

Some patients feel that their medical assessment and treatment have been inadequate. When the health care provider is unable to provide a clear diagnosis for discomfort, patients can feel discounted and misunderstood. These patients tend to be devalued, stigmatized, and told that the problem is only in their heads (Noyes et al., 2010).

Likewise, health care workers experience frustration in providing care for people who are not organically ill. Providers tend to use less patient-centered communication in comparison to patients with straightforward symptoms, even though somatic symptom visits are longer (Huang & McCarron, 2011). A "difficult" patient may receive a somatic diagnosis more readily than a "pleasant" patient, which could contribute to an inadequate workup. Studies show that the strongest predictor of misdiagnosing somatic disorders is the primary care provider's dissatisfaction with the clinical encounter (Huang & McCarron, 2011).

Illness Anxiety Disorder

Previously known as hypochondriasis, illness anxiety disorder results in the misinterpretation of physical sensations as evidence of a serious illness. Illness anxiety can be quite obsessive as thoughts about illness may be intrusive and hard to dismiss even when the patients realize their fears are unrealistic (MacDonald, 2011). People experience extreme worry and fear about the possibility of having a disease. Even normal bodily changes, such as a change in heart rate or abdominal cramps, can be seen as red flags for serious illness.

In response to these symptoms, primary care providers may suggest a consultation with a mental health professional, but the suggestion is typically refused. The course of the illness is chronic and relapsing, with symptoms becoming amplified during times of increased stress (Braun et al., 2010). Depression may play a role. Consider the case of a 72-year-old woman with illness anxiety who was treated with electroconvulsive therapy (ECT), a treatment most often used for depression. After one session her somatic complaints stopped abruptly. This patient's success with ECT may indicate that depressive symptoms may have been the catalyst for her symptoms, leading to the diagnosis of illness anxiety (Dols et al., 2012)

Overall, the illness anxiety patient uses about 41% to 78% more health care services per year, excluding laboratory tests and x-rays prescribed in primary care, than patients with well-defined medical conditions (Fink, 2010). As illness anxiety is so prevalent, it is important that clinicians achieve basic skills in treating and identifying this disorder. If patient health concerns are addressed at an early stage, repeated consultations, multiple trials of medications, and medical examinations may be prevented (Fink, 2010). Frequent exposure to media messages reminding us to seek regular medical screenings may also contribute to fears about health (MacDonald, 2011). Studies show a relationship between exposure to breast cancer coverage in television programs to heightened fear of breast cancer (Lemal & den Bulck, 2009).

Conversion Disorder

Conversion disorder (also known as functional neurological disorder) manifests itself as neurological symptoms in the absence of a neurological diagnosis (Feinstein, 2011). Conversion disorder is marked by the presence of deficits in voluntary motor or sensory functions, including paralysis, blindness, movement disorder, gait disorder, numbness, paresthesia (tingling or burning sensations), loss of vision or hearing, or episodes resembling epilepsy.

Conversion disorder is a clinical problem that requires the application of multiple perspectives—biological, psychological, and social—to fully understand the symptoms of individual patients. Patients with conversion disorder symptoms may be found to have "no neurological disorder" by the neurologist and "no psychiatric disorder" by the psychiatrist (Stone et al., 2010).

Conversion disorder is attributed to channeling of emotional conflicts or stressors into physical symptoms; however, some MRI studies suggest that patients with conversion disorder have an abnormal pattern of cerebral activation (Feinstein, 2011). Many patients show a lack of emotional concern about the symptoms (**la belle indifference**) although others are quite distressed. Imagine someone casually discussing sudden blindness. Care providers should assume there is an organic cause to the symptoms until physical pathology has been ruled out. Patients truly believe in the presence of the symptoms; they are not fabricated or under voluntary control.

Childhood physical or sexual abuse is common in patients with conversion disorder, and comorbid psychiatric conditions include depression, anxiety, posttraumatic stress disorder, other somatic disorders, and personality disorders. There are also cases in which a comorbid medical or neurological condition exists, and the conversion disorder is an exaggeration of the original problem (Nicholson et al, 2011).

The course of the disorder is related to its acuity. In cases with acute onset during stressful events, remission rate is high; in cases with a more gradual onset, the disorder is not readily treated. Cases generally remit by themselves 95% of the time (Sadock & Sadock, 2008). Recurrence is as high as 25%, often within the first year.

Psychological Factors Affecting Medical Condition

Both the medical and mental health communities recognize the interrelationships between psychiatric and medical comorbidities. Psychological factors may present a risk for medical disease, or they may magnify and/or adversely affect a medical condition. Studies in recent years have contributed to the growing body of evidence for links between mental disorders and cardiovascular disease; in particular, major depressive disorder is now seen as a risk factor in the occurrence of coronary heart disease (Charlson et al., 2011). Also, a link between a history of depression and cancer incidence has been postulated since the time of the ancient Greeks, with statistical evidence reported as early as 1893. A recent study on depression as a risk factor for the incidence of cancer, conducted between 1981 and 2005, showed a significant relationship between history of depression and risk of overall cancer (Gross et al., 2010)

Stress is certainly a psychological factor that can affect the disease process. Hans Selye (1956) was the first to introduce the concept of stress into the fields of medicine and physiology. Stress can lead to changes in physical and mental health in many ways. Cannon's identification of the fight-or-flight response (1914) and Selye's description of the general adaptation syndrome provided insight into the biological and molecular reactions to stressors in the sympathetic nervous system, the pituitary-adrenocortical axis, and the immune system. Extensive studies have left little doubt that psychosocial stress can affect the course and severity of illness (Table 17-1).

Chronic stressors cause components of the immune system to be affected in detrimental ways. Research in the field of psychoneuroimmunology has provided insights into the relationship between psychological and physiological health in human immunodeficiency virus (HIV) and other diseases (Temoshok et al., 2008). This research explains the negative impact of perceived stress on HIV disease progression, primarily as a function of immunosuppression mediated by elevated cortisol. Being able to reduce the stress response within this patient population is important because we can potentially positively affect not only the quality of life but also the illness trajectory of persons living with HIV. A variety of other medical disorders have been studied with regard to the effects of stress on the course of the illness. In fact, anyone experiencing a serious medical condition needs a variety of supports and may benefit from learning new coping skills.

VIGNETTE

Gerald is a 63-year-old real estate agent who was recently hospitalized for congestive heart failure. Because of insomnia, lack of appetite, and some anger problems toward his wife, his primary care provider refers him for a mental health consultation. Gerald complains of waking up at night obsessing about lack of funds for retirement, how his wife will survive if he dies soon, and if he will lose his job. He states, "I feel very scared, and I worry about my health and having to retire. I don't know where I would get the money to live or to pay for medical insurance if I get sick again. I am too old to start another career." These observations were reported to the nurse practitioner. After a thorough assessment and medical workup, it is determined that Gerald is experiencing depression and severe anxiety that precipitated increased symptoms of congestive heart failure. Gerald has responded well to couple therapy and a men's support group. His blood pressure has decreased, and his mood is improved.

Any abnormality in the structure of the brain or the function of the neurotransmitters can lead to a misinterpretation of ordinary events. For example, the brain may misunderstand (or amplify) a stimulus, identifying a minor gas pain as a serious abdominal injury (somatization); the brain may also overreact in its analysis of the stimulus, deciding that the same minor gas pain is a sign of colon cancer (illness anxiety).

Remember that research into anxiety disorders has demonstrated structural changes in the brain that may result from prolonged stress or trauma as well as imbalances in neurotransmitters. In the case of anxiety disorders, these abnormalities create altered feeling and thinking processes whereas the processes of perception and interpretation of bodily sensations are fairly intact. It is not known why some patients develop an anxiety disorder and others develop a somatic symptom disorder.

TABLE 17-1 COMMON MEDICAL CONDITIONS NEGATIVELY AFFECTED BY STRESS

MEDICAL CONDITION	INCIDENCE	GENETIC AND BIOLOGICAL CORRELATES	COMMON PRECIPITATING FACTORS	HOLISTIC THERAPIES IN ADDITION TO MEDICAL MANAGEMENT
Cardiovascular disease (e.g., coronary heart disease)	Rates higher in males until age 60 years Rates higher in white population than in African American population	Family history of cardiac disease a risk factor Other risk factors include hypertension, increased serum lipid levels, obesity, sedentary lifestyle, and cigarette smoking Psychosocial risk factors (stress, depression, loneliness) High anxiety risk in patient with prior cardiac events	Often, myocardial infarction occurs after sudden stress preceded by a period of losses, frustration, and disappointments	Relaxation training, stress management, group social support, and psychosocial intervention Support groups for type A personalities and type A modification helpful Anxiolytics (benzodiazepines) and antidepressants when indicated
Peptic ulcer (caused by *Helicobacter pylori* infection)	Occurs in 12% of men, 6% of women (more prevalent in industrialized societies)	Infection with *H. pylori* is associated with 95% to 99% of peptic ulcers Both peptic and duodenal ulcers cluster in families, but separately from each other	Periods of social tension and increased life stress After losses; often after menopause	Biofeedback can alter gastric acidity; cognitive-behavioral approaches are used to reduce stress (stress management)
Cancer	Men: most common in lung, prostate, colon, and rectum Women: most common in breast, uterus, colon, and rectum Death rate higher in men (especially African American men) than in women	Genetic evidence suggests dysfunction of cellular proliferation Familial patterns for breast cancer, colorectal cancer, stomach cancer, melanoma	Prolonged and intensive stress Stressful life events (e.g., separation from or loss of significant other 2 years before diagnosis) Feelings of hopelessness, helplessness, and despair (depression) may precede the diagnosis of cancer	Relaxation (e.g., meditation, autogenic training, self-hypnosis) Visualization Psychological counseling Support groups Massage therapy Stress management
Tension headache	Occurs in 80% of population when under stress Begins at end of workday or early evening		Associated with anxiety and depression	Psychotherapy usually prescribed for chronic tension headaches Learning to cope or avoiding tension-creating situations or people Relaxation techniques, stress management techniques, cognitive restructuring techniques
Essential hypertension	Rates higher in males until age 60 years	Family history of cardiac disease and hypertension a risk factor	Life changes and traumatic life events Stressful job (e.g., air traffic controller) Hypothesized to be found more in areas of social stress and conflict	Behavioral feedback, stress reduction techniques, meditation, yoga, hypnosis NOTE: pharmacological treatment considered primary for treatment of hypertension

ETIOLOGY

Somatizations are likely to be a complex biopsychosocial phenomenon, with many factors influencing the onset and course of the illness. A link between somatization and traumatic experiences is frequently reported (Aragona et al., 2010). Studies have also shown that patients with somatic disorders are more sensitive to negativity, less resilient in response to stress, and more prone to catastrophic thinking and negative interpretation to life events (Miller, 2009). There is increasing evidence that the behavior and mental health of primary caregivers and close family members play an important role in the development of somatization (Schulte &

Petermann, 2011). In early development, stress has been implicated as a triggering factor, most often stemming from parents and the pressure to perform. Somatization is often the "tip of the iceberg" that calls for attention to a psychiatric disorder necessitating mental health treatment. Unfortunately, many untreated children risk continuous somatization as adults (Silber, 2011).

Biological Factors

Somatic disorders tend to run in families, occurring in 10% to 20% of first-degree female relatives of women with somatization disorder (Sadock & Sadock, 2008). Twin studies show an increased risk of conversion disorder in monozygotic twin pairs. First-degree biological relatives of people with chronic pain disorder are more likely to have chronic pain, depressive disorder, and alcohol dependence.

Psychological Factors

Psychodynamic Theories

Psychoanalytic theorists believe that psychogenic complaints of pain, illness, or loss of physical function are related to repression of a conflict and/or unwelcome experiences (usually of an aggressive or sexual nature), and that transformation of anxiety into a physical symptom is symbolically related to the conflict (Nicholson et al., 2011).

For example, in conversion disorder, conversion symptoms allow a forbidden wish or urge to be partly expressed but sufficiently disguised so that the individual does not have to face the unacceptable wish. The symptoms also permit the individual to communicate a need for special treatment or consideration from others. Since the late 19th century, psychoanalytic theory has dominated medical thinking about conversion disorder. Neither psychiatry nor neurology has successfully tackled the challenge by Freud a century ago regarding what causes this "mysterious leap from mind to body" (Stone et al., 2010)

Illness anxiety disorder is considered by many clinicians to have psychodynamic origins. These clinicians suggest that anger, aggression, or hostility that had its source in past losses or disappointments is expressed as a need for help and concern from others. Other clinicians suggest that illness anxiety is a defense against guilt or low self-esteem. In the patient's view, the somatic symptoms often serve as deserved punishment.

Behavioral Theories

Behaviorists suggest that people with somatic symptoms learn methods of communicating helplessness and that these methods help the individuals to manipulate others to care for them. The symptoms become more intense when they are reinforced by attention from others. In the United States, primary care providers and nurses are taught to be attentive and responsive to a patient's reports of pain. Other reinforcers include avoiding activities the individual considers distasteful, obtaining financial benefit, or gaining some advantage in interpersonal relationships.

Cognitive Theories

Cognitive theorists believe that the patient with somatic symptoms focuses on body sensations, misinterprets their meaning, and may become excessively alarmed by them.

Environmental Factors

We know that adverse childhood events result in lifelong problems, including somatization disorders. The Adverse Childhood Experiences Study (ACE) (Fuller-Thomson et al., 2011) surveyed more than 16,000 adults and discovered that childhood trauma exposure accounted for negative outcomes across a variety of diagnoses in later life, including multiple somatic symptoms diabetes, heart disease, cancer, gastrointestinal conditions, and immune functioning. Childhood maltreatment has been associated with elevated levels of C-reactive protein, a biomarker of inflammation that may play a role in autoimmune diseases in adults 20 years later (Dube et al., 2009). The Evidence-Based Practice Box provides more information on the connection between childhood trauma and subsequent somatization.

EVIDENCED-BASED PRACTICE

Childhood Trauma and Somatic Preoccupation

Sansone, R., Wiederman, M., Tahir, N.A., & Buckner, V.R. (2009). A re-examination of childhood trauma and somatic preoccupation. *International Journal of Psychiatry in Clinical Practice, 13*(3), 227-231. doi: 10.1080/13651500802621551.

Problem

Studies of childhood abuse have typically concentrated in the area of psychological outcomes; however, a number of studies suggest that abuse in childhood is related to somatic preoccupation in adulthood. In past studies, each type of trauma was not examined for its individual contribution to adult somatic problems.

Purpose of Study

The aim of this study is to explore five types of childhood trauma—(1) physical, (2) sexual, (3) emotional, (4) witness to violence, and (5) physical neglect—to determine each type of trauma's unique contribution, if any, to somatic preoccupation in adulthood.

Methods

Participants were male and female outpatients (N= 36 males and 77 females), between the ages of 18 and 87 years, who were being seen for non-emergent medical care in an outpatient internal medicine setting located in a Midwestern, medium-sized city.

Participants were asked, "Prior to age 12, did you ever experience any of five types of trauma," with yes/no options.

Key Findings

- Physical and emotional abuse showed significant associated relationships with somatic preoccupation in adulthood.
- Sexual abuse, the witnessing of violence, and physical neglect were not associated with subsequent somatization.

Implications for Nursing Practice

Patients in general medical settings with high levels of somatic symptoms may have been victims of childhood abuse. An awareness of this association will facilitate more mental health assessments within the general physical exam and history. These individuals have a history of extreme discomfort and emotional distress. Compassion and empathy will go a long way in reducing their emotional and physical pain.

Cultural Considerations

The type and frequency of somatic symptoms vary across cultures. Burning hands and feet or the sensation of worms in the head or ants under the skin is more common in Africa and southern Asia than in North America. Alteration of consciousness with falling is a symptom commonly associated with culture-specific religious and healing rituals. Somatization disorder, which is rarely seen in men in the United States, is often reported in Greek and Puerto Rican men, which suggests that cultural customs may permit these men to use somatization as an acceptable approach to dealing with life stress. Somatization related to posttraumatic stress and depression was the most prevalent psychiatric symptom in North Korean defectors to South Korea (Kim et al., 2011)

West Indians (Caribbean) attribute somatic symptoms to chronic overwork and the irregularity of daily living, citing symptoms such as dizziness, fatigue, joint pain, and muscle tension. Patients from Korea may explain some distress as "hwa-byung," a syndrome of both somatic and depressive symptoms, commonly attributed to suppressed anger or rage (Edwards et al., 2010).

In some cultures, certain physical symptoms are believed to result from the casting of spells. Spellbound individuals often seek the help of traditional healers in addition to modern medical staff. The medical provider may diagnose a non–life-threatening somatic symptom disorder whereas the traditional healer may offer an entirely different explanation and prognosis. The individual may not show improvement until the traditional healer removes the spell.

In contemporary Western culture, there has been unprecedented growth and comfort in the past few decades; however, levels of health have not increased. Core values such as materialism, consumerism, and individualism may be damaging to individuals' sense of well-being and health, including a high incidence of somatization. A study of children reared in the United States from 1970 through the 1990s shows these adults as tolerant, confident, open-minded and ambitious, but also cynical, depressed, lonely, and anxious, characteristics that contribute to the development of somatic symptomatology (Carlisle & Hanlon, 2007).

Abraham Maslow in his "hierarchy of needs" theorizes that humans are inclined to shift attention to higher-level needs (social, intellectual, spiritual) once lower-level needs of food, shelter, and clothing are attained; however, Western consumer culture has become extremely adept at persuading people to remain fixated upon materialism, resisting movement to higher-level needs such as love, belonging, and respect for others (Schumaker, 2007). This current consumer culture of individualism with decreased interest in family/group needs negatively impacts supportive development of communities, socialization, and overall mental and physical health, including somatic responses of individuals.

In addition, somatization among the immigrant population in the United States in primary care is significantly related to traumatic events (see Considering Culture box). Immigrants frequently experience multiple traumatic events, both intentional and unintentional, in premigration as well as postmigration life. A study of asylum seekers reported 79% had experienced a traumatic event such as witnessing killings, being assaulted, or suffering torture and captivity. It is important for primary care providers evaluating immigrants to be aware of the possible link between somatization symptoms reported by the patient and undisclosed traumatic experiences (Aragona et al., 2010).

Patients across cultures with somatic symptoms often offer clues about their underlying concerns and want more emotional support from their health care provider in comparison to other patients, and they are most satisfied with their care when their health care provider shares their understanding of the presenting problems and treatment options (Edwards et al., 2010).

CONSIDERING CULTURE

Culture, Trauma, and Somatization in Primary Care

Immigrants and refugees, as well as patients from ethnic and racial minorities, frequently present to primary care clinicians with a spectrum of physical and psychological symptoms that often are best understood within the context of their cultural background and experiences.

Carlos is a 27-year-old male from El Salvador. He fled his native country after finding out that his name was on a death squad list for immediate execution. Nine months after his arrival in the United States, he learned his wife and children were assaulted, resulting in the death of his wife during an attempt to extract information about Carlos' whereabouts.

Shortly thereafter, Carlos presented to a primary care physician at a community clinic where he was referred from the emergency room of a local hospital. During the previous weeks, he had experienced multiple symptoms, including weakness (which caused him to be terminated from his temporary job), changes in sensation, abdominal pain, chest pain, insomnia, and weight loss. After extensive diagnostic studies, Carlos' primary care physician could find no physical cause for his symptoms.

Psychiatric consultation was then sought. Somatization was diagnosed. Low-dose antidepressant medication was instituted along with individual therapy. The psychiatrist coordinated follow-up with the primary care physician. Carlos grew more aware of the emotional factors that exacerbated his symptoms and developed new coping strategies. He joined a group of local Central American refugees, where he was encouraged to write and to recite poetry as a therapeutic tool. During the following months, his somatic symptoms gradually decreased.

Carlos and others like him have raised questions. First, how frequently does somatization rooted in trauma occur among people who seek primary care, and is it consistently noted in history taking? Second, do the health care plans and explanations given to patients have meaning in the context of their culture?

Waitzkin, H. (2009). Culture, communication, and somatization in health care. In D.E. Brashers & D. Goldsmith (Eds.), *Communicating to manage health and illness* (p. 114). New York and London: Routledge.

APPLICATION OF THE NURSING PROCESS

ASSESSMENT

Assessment of patients with somatization disorders is a complex process that requires careful and complete documentation. This section outlines several areas that are important in the assessment of a patient with a suspected somatization disorder.

ASSESSMENT GUIDELINES

Somatization Disorders

1. Assess for nature, location, onset, characteristics, and duration of the symptom(s).
2. Explore past history of adverse childhood events.
3. Identify symptoms of anxiety, depression, and past trauma that may be contributing to somatic symptoms and ability to meet basic physical, and safety/security needs.
4. Determine current quality of life, social support, and coping skills, including spirituality.
5. Identify any secondary gain that the patient is experiencing from symptom(s).
6. Explore the patient's cognitive style and ability to communicate feelings and needs.
7. Assess current psychosocial and biological needs, including overuse/dependence on medication.

Assessment should begin with collection of data about the nature, location, onset, character, and duration of the symptom or symptoms. A thorough medical and psychosocial history is also essential. Assessment of nutrition, fluid balance, and elimination needs should be a high priority as patients with somatization disorders often complain of gastrointestinal distress, diarrhea, constipation, and anorexia.

A useful assessment tool to understand the degree of somatization is the Patient Health Questionnaire-15 (PHQ), a somatic symptom severity scale for the purpose of diagnosis (Figure 17-1). The questionnaire inquires about 15 somatic symptoms that account for more than 90% of physical complaints reported in the primary care setting by asking patients to rate severity of symptoms during the previous 4 days on a 3-point scale. Those symptoms are stomach pain, back pain,

During the past four (4) days, how much have you been bothered by....				
		Not bothered at all	**Bothered a little**	**Bothered a lot**
1.	Stomach pain	0	1	2
2.	Back pain	0	1	2
3.	Pain in your arms, legs, or joints	0	1	2
4.	Menstrual cramps or other problems with your periods (women)	0	1	2
5.	Headaches	0	1	2
6.	Chest pain	0	1	2
7.	Dizziness	0	1	2
8.	Fainting spells	0	1	2
9.	Feeling your heart pound or race	0	1	2
10.	Shortness of breath	0	1	2
11.	Pain or problems during sexual intercourse	0	1	2
12.	Constipation, loose bowels, or diarrhea	0	1	2
13.	Nausea, gas, or indigestion	0	1	2
14.	Feeling tired or having no energy	0	1	2
15.	Trouble sleeping	0	1	2

FIG 17-1 PHQ Somatic Symptom Short Form (PHQ-SSS). Scores of 5 or less indicate mild somatization, scores of 10 or less indicate moderate somatization, and and scores 15 or more are considered severe indications of somatization. (Adapted from Spitzer, R.L., Williams, J.B.W., & Kroenke, K. [2010]. The patient health questionnaire somatic, anxiety, and depressive symptom scales: A systematic review. *General Hospital Psychiatry, 32*[4], 345-359.)

headache, chest pain, dizziness, fainting, palpitations, shortness of breath, bowel complaints, nausea, fatigue, sleep problems, pain in joints/limbs, menstrual pain, and problems during sexual intercourse (Korber et al., 2011).

In addition, information should be sought about patients' ability to meet their own basic needs. Rest, comfort, activity, and hygiene needs may be altered as a result of patient problems such as fatigue, weakness, insomnia, muscle tension, pain, and avoidance of diversional activity. Safety and security needs may be threatened by patient experiences of blindness, deafness, loss of balance and falling, and anesthesia of various parts of the body.

During assessment, it is important to determine whether symptoms are under the patient's voluntary control. Somatic symptoms *are not under the individual's voluntary control.* Although the relationship between symptoms and interpersonal conflicts may be obvious to others, the patient cannot see it.

Symptom reporting will vary depending upon the disorder. Patients with conversion disorder may matter-of-factly report having a sudden loss in function of a body part: "I woke up this morning and couldn't move my arm." In contrast, patients with somatic symptom disorder and illness anxiety disorder usually discuss their symptoms in dramatic terms. They may use colorful metaphors and exaggerations: "The pain was searing, like a hot sword drawn across my forehead." "My symptoms are so rare that I've stumped hundreds of doctors."

Psychosocial Factors

Psychosocial factors are relevant to somatic symptoms, and the way a person thinks and feels can have a profound effect on patient progress. Struggling with distress evokes a range of difficult emotions such as fear, anger, sadness, confusion, and guilt. Patients may feel overwhelmed and alone while friends and family members may feel helpless and at a loss emotionally. How can a health care worker know what a patient thinks or feels unless the patient's psychosocial situation is assessed?

The following are some highlights that can help the nurse plan necessary interventions. When working with a somatic patient, it is important to assess/determine if the person has:

- Someone who can share his or her concerns and who cares for him or her
- Friends and supports in the community and/or involvement in individual therapy
- Any coexisting conditions that could negatively affect healthy adaptation or ability to heal (e.g., anxiety, depression, personality disorder, posttraumatic stress disorder, or substance abuse and other compulsive behaviors)
- Risky health behaviors (e.g., sedentary lifestyle, smoking, engaging in unsafe sex practices, and/or abusing alcohol or drugs)
- A cultural view of health and illness that helps or impedes the process of seeking adequate care (e.g., resilience, communication skills, assertiveness)

Table 17-2 provides an outline for a psychosocial assessment of a patient with a medical condition. A psychosocial assessment is performed in tandem with a thorough physical workup and mental status examination.

Coping Skills

Assessing how a patient has dealt with adversity in the past provides information about coping skills available for use now and in the future. Health care workers can also support the patient in gaining additional coping skills that may help an individual better manage a healthier lifestyle.

Spirituality and Religion

Nurses and other health care workers are becoming increasingly aware of the role spirituality or religion plays in many patients' lives and its importance as a source of peace. Support from a priest, pastor, rabbi, or other religious leader may be indicated, especially in a case of spiritual distress. Beliefs and practices are forces that promote resilience; the practice of healthy coping depends upon the capacity to create meaning from life experiences.

Secondary Gains

The nurse tries to identify secondary gains the patient may be receiving from the symptoms. **Secondary gains** are those benefits derived from the symptoms alone; for example, in the sick role, the patient is not able to perform the usual family, work, and social functions and receives extra attention from loved ones. If a patient derives personal benefit from the symptoms, giving up the symptoms is more difficult. The clinician works with the patient to achieve the same benefits through healthier avenues, such as learning to communicate more adaptively and connect with others. One approach to identifying the presence of secondary gains is to ask the patient questions such as:

- What are you unable to do now that you used to be able to do?
- How has this problem affected your life?

Cognitive Style

In general, patients with these disorders may misinterpret physical stimuli and distort reality regarding their symptoms. Sensations a normal individual would interpret as a headache might suggest a brain tumor to a patient with illness anxiety.

Ability to Communicate Feelings and Emotional Needs

Patients with somatic disorders have difficulty communicating their emotional needs. Although they are able to describe their physical symptoms, they frequently do not verbalize feelings, especially those related to anger, guilt, and dependence. The somatic symptom may be the patient's chief means of communicating emotional needs. Psychogenic blindness or hearing loss may represent the symbolic statement "I can't face this knowledge." For example, after a woman overheard friends discussing her husband's sexual infidelity, she developed total deafness.

Dependence on Medication

Individuals experiencing many somatic complaints often become dependent on medication to relieve pain or anxiety or to induce

TABLE 17-2 PSYCHOSOCIAL ASSESSMENT OF PATIENTS WITH MEDICAL CONDITIONS

AREAS TO ASSESS	SPECIFIC QUESTIONS TO ASK
Social Supports and Cultural Issues	
Family	What were the effects of the patient's illness, treatments, and recovery on the family in the past?
Friends	Who can the patient share painful feelings with?
	Does the patient have friends to joke and laugh with?
	Are there people the patient believes would stand by him or her?
Religious or spiritual beliefs	Does the patient find comfort and support in spiritual practices?
	Is the patient a member of a spiritual or religious group in the community (church, temple, other place of worship)?
	Does the patient find inner peace and strength in religious or spiritual practices?
	The following statements may be used in performing a spiritual assessment of a patient:
	I [often/sometimes/seldom] believe that life has value, meaning, and direction.
	I [often/sometimes/seldom] feel a connection with the universe.
	I [often/sometimes/seldom] believe in a power greater than myself.
	I [often/sometimes/seldom] believe that my actions make a difference.
	I [often/sometimes/seldom] believe that my actions express my true self.
Cultural beliefs	Does the patient use specific culture-oriented treatments or remedies for his or her condition?
	Do the patient's cultural beliefs allow for adequate treatment by Western medical standards?
Work	Are there colleagues at work the patient can count on for support?
Concurrent Physical Conditions Affecting Psychosocial Well-Being	
Physical pain	Is the patient in pain?
	How does the patient cope with it?
	Is the pain disabling?
	Are there pain-reducing techniques that might help?
Major illness	Does the patient have a co-occurring major illness that will negatively affect his or her current condition?
	Is the patient undergoing treatments that are affecting daily life more than expected?
	Are there interventions that would help the patient better cope with the sequelae of the illness and treatments?
	Has the patient been hospitalized in the past?
	How many times?
	For what?
	How did the patient cope?
Addictions and mental health	Does the patient have a co-occurring mental health problem (depression, anxiety, compulsions)?
	Has the patient suffered a mental disease in the past?
	Does the patient participate in any compulsive behavior (e.g., smoking, overworking, excessive spending, gambling, cybersex)?
	Does the patient abuse substances (alcohol, drugs [illicit, over the counter, prescription])?

sleep. Primary care providers prescribe anxiolytic agents for patients who seem highly anxious and concerned about their symptoms. Patients often return to the primary care provider for prescription renewal or seek treatment from numerous primary care providers. It is important that the nurse assess the type and amount of medications being used.

Self-Assessment

Nurses and other health care workers often find work with patients with somatization disorders to be difficult and unsatisfying. When a physiological basis for the patient's symptoms is absent, you may wonder why this patient is taking up valuable time that might better be spent on a "sick" patient. You may feel resentment or anger toward such a patient. Negative feelings occur whether the patient is being cared for in a medical setting—whose staff tend to feel more comfortable working with patients who have physical illnesses—or by psychiatric staff, who tend to prefer working with disorders of emotion or thought.

It is helpful to remember that the symptom the patient is experiencing feels *real* to him or her, even though the objective data may not support a physiological basis for it. It is important for clinicians not to convey by word or body language their own frustration about the difficult and time-consuming task they are facing with somatic disorder. Clinicians should also avoid the temptation to perform unnecessary, repetitive, or extensive testing in an attempt to demonstrate to the patient and/or family that the presenting complaint is of somatic origin (Silber, 2011).

Anger may also arise when staff members find themselves dealing with a patient who uses somatic symptoms to manipulate the environment and the people within it. Feelings of helplessness over being unable to make a patient realize his or her symptoms have no organic basis can be a source of frustration. Patients who use somatization exhibit remarkable resistance to change. They cling to unrealistic beliefs about the origin of the somatic symptoms, despite objective evidence to the contrary. As you plan the care of this patient, a useful strategy is to set goals with staged outcomes (i.e., small, attainable steps) to offset feelings of helplessness or ineffectuality.

It is helpful for health care workers, no matter the setting, to discuss responses to these patients in conferences with other health care members to allow for expression of feelings and, ultimately, to provide for consistent care.

NURSING DIAGNOSIS

Patients with somatic disorders present various nursing problems. *Ineffective coping* is frequently diagnosed. Other potential nursing diagnoses include anxiety, risk for loneliness, powerlessness, hopelessness, social isolation, pain, altered family processes, and risk for suicide (Ackley & Ladwig, 2011).

OUTCOMES IDENTIFICATION

Because shared decision making promotes goal attainment, the patient should participate in identifying desired outcomes. Outcome criteria must be realistic and attainable. Structuring outcomes in small steps helps the patient see concrete evidence of progress. Table 17-3 describes signs and symptoms, potential nursing diagnoses, and outcomes for somatization disorders.

IMPLEMENTATION

Because patients are seldom admitted to psychiatric care settings specifically for treatment of somatic disorders, long-term interventions usually take place on an outpatient basis. Short-term planning may be initiated if the patient is admitted to a medical-surgical unit. Such a stay is usually short, and discharge will occur as soon as diagnostic tests are completed and negative results are received.

Patients who somatize often do not mention psychological symptoms and attribute their symptoms to physical problems when consulting their health care providers. Somatization is common in primary care, but providers are not confident in managing it and often prescribe unnecessary interventions (Walters et al., 2007). As high comorbidities between somatic disorders and major depression and anxiety are common in primary care, it is essential that an integrated model of care/interventions exists between mental health and medical clinicians (Steinbrecher et al., 2011).

Initially, nursing interventions should focus on establishing a helping relationship with the patient. The therapeutic relationship is vital to the success of the care plan, given (1) the patient's resistance to the concept that no physical cause for the symptom exists and (2) the patient's tendency to go from caregiver to caregiver.

To be successful, therapeutic interventions must address ways to help the patient get needs met without resorting to somatization. The secondary gains derived from illness behaviors become less important to the patient when underlying needs can be met directly. A specific treatment approach for somatization is provided in Box 17-1.

Given that multiple health care providers are often involved in the management of this disorder, good communication among treating clinicians is required to maintain a consistent approach (Feinstein, 2011). In an ideal situation, a multidisciplinary team of caretakers, including an advanced practice nurse who provides consultation to nurses outside of

TABLE 17-3 SIGNS AND SYMPTOMS, NURSING DIAGNOSES, AND OUTCOMES FOR SOMATIZATION DISORDERS

SIGNS AND SYMPTOMS	NURSING DIAGNOSES	OUTCOMES
Inability to meet occupational, family, or social responsibilities because of symptoms; inability to participate in usual community activities or friendships because of psychogenic symptoms	*Ineffective coping* *Ineffective role performance* *Altered family processes*	Identifies effective coping patterns, verbalizes sense of control, uses support system, family obtains resources to cope with symptoms
Presence of secondary gains by adoption of sick role,	*Pain, acute or chronic*	Recognizes associated symptoms of pain, reports pain control
Absence of supportive significant other(s), friends and family alienated by physical obsessions	*Social isolation* *Risk for loneliness*	Willing to call on others for assistance, develops a confidant relationship, feels a sense of belonging
Chronic pain, inability to control symptoms; negative self-evaluation, feeling useless, not feeling valued by significant others; dependence on pain relievers	*Risk for suicide* *Chronic low self-esteem* *Powerlessness* *Hopelessness*	Refrains from attempting suicide, verbalizes positive regard for self, maintains grooming and hygiene, describes self as successful; strong beliefs that decisions and actions control health outcomes

From Herdman, T.H. (Ed.) *Nursing diagnoses—Definitions and classification 2012-2014*. Copyright © 2012, 1994-2012 by NANDA International. Used by arrangement with John Wiley & Sons Limited; Moorhead, S., Johnson, M., Maas, M.L., & Swanson, E. (2013). *Nursing outcomes classification (NOC)* (5th ed.). St Louis, MO: Mosby.

BOX 17-1 REATTRIBUTION TREATMENT TO LINK PHYSICAL COMPLAINTS AND PSYCHOLOGICAL DISTRESS

Reattribution treatment is a structured intervention designed to provide a simple explanation of somatic symptoms to patients. Reattribution skills from the health care provider help the patient feel understood and help the patient make the link between physical complaints and psychological distress.

The four stages of reattribution are:

Stage 1: Feeling Understood
Empathetic listening skills are used in taking the history of physical, emotional, and psychosocial factors of the presenting symptoms, including patient beliefs and perceptions of the causality of illness, when is it worse, and what helps. This stage includes a brief, focused physical exam.

Stage 2: Broadening the Agenda
The care provider gives feedback and implications of assessment findings, and acknowledges the patient's distress.

Stage 3: Making the Link
The care provider uses patient cues to give an empowering explanation of the symptoms. For example, "You may have a heightened sensitivity to particular stressors that is affected by genetics, your personal experiences, and the environment" is a patient-centered comment that removes any sense of blame from the patient (Fuller-Thomson et al., 2011).

Stage 4: Negotiating Further Treatment
The provider and the patient create a treatment plan that includes regular follow-up visits.

Walters, P., Tylee, A., Fisher, J., & Goldberg, D. (2007). Teaching junior doctors to manage patients who somatise: Is it possible in an afternoon? *Medical Education, 41*, 995-1001.

HEALTH POLICY

Primary Care and Mental Health Services: A Call for Integration

Of approximately 25% to 50% of symptoms seen in primary health care, there is no evidence of physical disease (Van Ravenzwaaij et al., 2010). The high prevalence of behavioral health problems and the interrelated nature of mental and physical treatment have led the Institutes of Medicine (IOM) to call for integration of behavioral and physical care. A critical component of the Patient Protection and Affordable Care Act (National Prevention Council, 2010) is to identify and integrate mental health needs into primary care settings as a top priority.

One of the many advantages for integrating mental health services into primary health care includes less stigmatization. Because primary health care services are not associated with any specific health conditions, stigma is reduced when seeking mental health care from a primary health care provider, making this level of care far more acceptable, and therefore accessible, for most users and families (WHO, 2007). Psychiatric-mental health nurses can bring a strong perspective in managing both physical and mental health needs in integrated care settings.

National Prevention Council. (2011). *National prevention strategy.* Retrieved from http://www.healthcare.gov/prevention/nphpphc/strategy/report.pdf; Van Ravenzwaaij, J., Hartman, T.C., Ravesteijn, H., Eveleigh, R., Rijswijk, E., & Lucassen, P. (2010). Explanatory models of medically unexplained symptoms: A qualitative analysis of the literature. *Mental Health in Family Medicine, 7*, 223-31; World Health Organization. (2007). Integrating mental health services into primary health care. *Mental Health Policy, Planning and Service Development Sheet.*

psychiatry, would be involved in the treatment of patients with somatization disorders. Using the data from the holistic assessment, nurse clinicians, along with a physician, are in a position to provide useful and effective interventions. A national movement and legislation that involve integrating care have gained strong support. A discussion of these policy initiatives is in the Health Policy box.

People who have distressing symptoms are vulnerable to a variety of psychosocial stresses. How they cope with these stresses may make the difference between living with an acceptable quality of life and giving in to despair, withdrawal, helplessness, or hopelessness. Nurses are in a position to assess and understand patients' psychosocial stressors, identify needed coping skills, and teach stress-management techniques. Nurses can play an important role not only in managing patients' immediate care but also in helping patients to improve their ability to cope and increase the quality of life during the course of somatic disorders.

Effective **coping skills** that can be taught are many and varied (e.g., assertiveness training, cognitive reframing, problem-solving skills, and social supports). Nurses are in key positions to assess, educate, or provide referrals to a patient to enable healthier ways of looking at and dealing with illness. Consider referring the patient for instruction in a variety of relaxation techniques, such as reiki, meditation, guided imagery, breathing exercises, and others, or teaching the patient some techniques yourself. Behavioral techniques are useful, and nurses with special training can offer their patients progressive muscle relaxation exercises or biofeedback. Relaxation techniques, stress management, and supportive education should be part of the care of the patient, regardless of the medical diagnosis.

The following interventions have all been shown to affect a patient's recovery positively:

- Educating the patient regarding specific treatments
- Referring the patient to community support groups (or systems)
- Teaching patients more effective coping skills that take into consideration patients' values, preferences, and lifestyle
- Focusing on a patient's strengths and reinforcing coping skills that work (e.g., prayerfulness, participation in hobbies, relaxation techniques)
- General recommendations for health care providers in working with patients with somatic symptoms include

six key elements for effective relationships and treatment (Kenny & Egan, 2011):

1. Provide continuity of care.
2. Avoid unnecessary tests and procedures.
3. Provide frequent, brief, and regular office visits.
4. Always conduct a physical exam.
5. Avoid making disparaging comments such as, "Your symptoms are all in your head."
6. Set reasonable therapeutic goals such as maintaining function despite ongoing pain.

Psychosocial Interventions

Nursing interventions for patients with somatization disorders generally take place in the home or clinic setting and entail helping the patient improve overall functioning through the development of effective coping strategies. The *Nursing Interventions Classification (NIC)* offers several categories pertinent to caring for patients with somatization disorders: *Assertiveness Training, Family Involvement Promotion, Limit Setting, Self-Awareness Enhancement,* and *Self-Esteem Enhancement* (Bulechek et al., 2013).

Promotion of Self-Care Activities

When somatization is present, the patient's ability to perform self-care activities may be impaired, and nursing intervention is necessary. In general, interventions involve the use of a matter-of-fact approach to support the highest level of self-care the patient is capable of. For patients manifesting paralysis, blindness, or severe fatigue, an effective nursing approach is to support patients while expecting them to feed, bathe, or groom themselves (e.g., the patient who demonstrates paralysis of an arm can be expected to eat using the other arm). To encourage the patient experiencing blindness to feed himself, he can be told at what numbers on an imaginary clock the food is located on the plate. These strategies are effective in reducing secondary gain.

Assertiveness training is often identified as appropriate teaching for patients with somatization disorders. Use of assertiveness techniques gives patients a direct means of getting needs met and thereby decreases the need for somatic symptoms. Teaching an exercise regimen, such as doing range-of-motion exercises for 15 to 20 minutes daily and taking regular walks, if possible, can help the patient feel in control, can increase endorphin levels, and may help decrease anxiety.

Table 17-4 provides basic-level interventions for somatization disorders.

Pharmacological Interventions

It is unclear whether medications are useful for treatment in all the somatization disorders. Certainly if there are underlying psychiatric diagnoses, appropriate utilization of medication is indicated and may result in the decrease of somatoform symptoms. The decision to medicate patients with a somatization disorder should weigh the benefits against the possibility that these patients may misuse their medication, taking it erratically and irregularly (Sadock & Sadock, 2008).

TABLE 17-4 BASIC-LEVEL INTERVENTIONS FOR SOMATIZATION DISORDERS

INTERVENTION	RATIONALE
Offer explanations and support during diagnostic testing.	Reduces anxiety while ruling out organic illness
After physical complaints have been investigated, avoid further reinforcement (e.g., do not take vital signs each time patient complains of palpitations).	Directs focus away from physical symptoms
Spend time with patient at times other than when patient summons nurse to voice physical complaint.	Rewards non–illness-related behaviors and encourages repetition of desired behavior
Observe and record frequency and intensity of somatic symptoms. (Patient or family can give information.)	Establishes a baseline and later enables evaluation of effectiveness of interventions
Do not imply that symptoms are not real.	Acknowledges that psychogenic symptoms are real to the patient
Shift focus from somatic complaints to feelings or to neutral topics.	Conveys interest in patient as a person rather than in patient's symptoms; reduces need to gain attention via symptoms
Assess secondary gains "physical illness" provides for patient (e.g., attention, increased dependency, and distraction from another problem).	Allows these needs to be met in healthier ways and thus minimizes secondary gains
Use matter-of-fact approach to patient exhibiting resistance or covert anger.	Avoids power struggles; demonstrates acceptance of anger and permits discussion of angry feelings
Have patient direct all requests to case manager.	Reduces manipulation
Help patient look at effect of illness behavior on others.	Encourages insight; can help improve intrafamily relationships
Show concern for patient while avoiding fostering dependency needs.	Shows respect for patient's feelings while minimizing secondary gains from "illness"
Reinforce patient's strengths and problem-solving abilities.	Contributes to positive self-esteem; helps patient realize that needs can be met without resorting to somatic symptoms
Teach assertive communication.	Provides patient with a positive means of getting needs met; reduces feelings of helplessness and need for manipulation
Teach patient stress-reduction techniques, such as meditation, relaxation, and mild physical exercise.	Provides alternate coping strategies; reduces need for medication

Tricyclic antidepressants (TCAs) and selective serotonin reuptake inhibitors (SSRIs) may be helpful in somatic disorders directly by reducing depressive symptoms and hence somatic responses, but also indirectly by affecting nerve circuits that affect not only mood but fatigue, pain perception, GI distress, and other somatic symptoms (Kroenke, 2007).

Medication trials with other antidepressants, including serotonin norepinephrine reuptake inhibitors (SNRIs)—venlafaxine (Effexor) and duloxetine (Cymbalta)—and a noradrenergic specific serotonergic antidepressant—mirtazapine (Remeron)—have been effective with somatic disorders, but further controlled trials are needed (Han et al., 2008; Garcia-Martin et al., 2012).

Patients may also benefit from short-term use of antianxiety medication, which must be monitored carefully because of the risk of dependence. The nurse may administer these medications in certain settings, but teaching patients and families about the medication is helpful in all settings.

Health Teaching and Health Promotion

Some patients who use somatization as a way of coping with anxiety have little formal education; therefore, teaching these patients basic information about bodily functions is often warranted. Pictures and charts can be helpful, and it is useful to review the same information with the family because their knowledge may also be faulty.

Case Management

Doctor shopping" is common among patients with somatization disorders. They go from physician to physician, clinic to clinic, or hospital to hospital, hoping to establish a physical basis for their distress. Repeated computed tomographic scans, magnetic resonance images, and other diagnostic tests are often documented in the medical record. Case management can help limit health care costs associated with such visits. The case manager can recommend to the primary care provider that the patient be scheduled for brief appointments every 4 to 6 weeks at set times, rather than on demand, and that laboratory tests be avoided unless they are absolutely necessary. The patient who establishes a relationship with the case manager often feels less anxiety because the patient has someone to contact and knows that someone is "in charge."

Advanced Practice Interventions

Advanced practice nurses may use various types of psychotherapy or consultation with the primary care provider in the treatment of somatization disorders. As nursing is a profession with a major focus on viewing the patient in a holistic way, the advanced practice nurse can lead the health care team in assessing each patient's unique biological, environmental, psychological, spiritual, and sociocultural needs to develop the most comprehensive, individualized plan of care to alleviate the distress of somatic symptoms.

Advanced practice nurses can practice cognitive behavioral therapy (CBT). It is the most consistently supported treatment for the full spectrum of somatic disorders. CBT helps patients to find ways to reframe their thoughts and gain control of their situation and break what can become a self-fulfilling cycle of pain, despair, and health-seeking behaviors (Kroenke, 2007). Refer to Chapter 2 for a more complete explanation of CBT. Table 17-5 provides a summary of advanced practice interventions.

Managing psychiatric symptoms and physical symptoms can be a challenge for general medical nurses. Advanced practice

TABLE 17-5 ADVANCED PRACTICE INTERVENTIONS FOR SOMATIZATION DISORDERS

DISORDER	COURSE	INTERVENTIONS
Somatic symptom disorder	Chronic and relapsing	Consistent primary care provider with regular patient visits, limited tests Group therapy Cognitive-behavioral therapy
Illness anxiety disorder	Chronic and relapsing, but 50% of patients improve	Cognitive-behavioral therapy Insight-oriented therapy Group therapy Psychopharmacological management for comorbid conditions Stress management
Conversion disorder	Usually acute onset; resolves quickly	Suggest that the conversion symptom will gradually improve Behavioral therapy Insight-oriented therapy Hypnosis Antianxiety drugs
Psychological factors affecting medical condition	Acute and chronic; variable resolution	Treat psychiatric symptoms Tailor treatment to address both the psychological symptom and the medical condition
Factitious disorder	Highly treatment-resistant	Confrontation is counterproductive Emphasis on management over cure Legal interventions may be necessary in the case of Munchausen by proxy

Braun, I.M., Greenberg, D. B., Smith, F.A., & Cassem, N. H. (2010). Functional somatic symptoms, deception syndromes, and somatoform disorders. In T. A. Stern, G.L. Fricchione, N.H. Cassem, M.S. Jellinek, & J. F. Rosenbaum, (Eds.), *Massachusetts General Hospital handbook of general hospital psychiatry* (6th ed., pp. 173-187). Philadelphia, PA: Saunders.

psychiatric nurses can bridge that gap. They function as consultants who assist other nurses in managing psychiatric symptoms and also as clinicians working directly to help the patient deal more effectively with physical and emotional problems. As a consultant, or liaison, the advanced practice psychiatric nurse first meets with the nurse who initiated the consultation and then reviews the medical records, talks with the physicians, and interviews the patient. After the patient interview, the liaison nurse discusses the assessment and suggestions with the referring nurse. If a psychiatric consultation is warranted, the psychiatric liaison nurse initiates the consultation by contacting the patient's physician. A case conference is sometimes needed to enhance communication and consistency in the care of a particular patient.

EVALUATION

Evaluation of patients with somatization disorders is a simple process when measurable behavioral outcomes have been written clearly and realistically. For these patients, you might often find that goals and outcomes are only partially met. Patients are likely to report the continuing presence of somatic symptoms, but they often say they are less concerned about the symptoms. Families frequently report relatively high satisfaction with outcomes, even without total eradication of the patient's symptoms.

FACTITIOUS DISORDERS

Whereas most somatic disorders are not under conscious control, people with a factitious disorder consciously pretend to be ill to get emotional needs met and attain the status of "patient" (Sadock & Sadock, 2008). The term *factitious* is derived from the Latin word meaning "artificial or contrived." Patients with this disorder artificially, deliberately, and dramatically fabricate symptoms or self-inflict injury, with the goal of assuming a sick role. The contrived illness may be physical or psychiatric. Examples of contrived illnesses include bleeding, fever, hypoglycemia, seizures, hallucinations, and even cancer and human immunodeficiency virus (HIV) (Braun et al., 2010). Factitious disorder results in disability and immeasurable costs to the health care system.

CLINICAL PICTURE

The patient may get admitted to the hospital through the emergency room, where he or she dramatically describes the illness using proper medical terminology and can be quite convincing. The patient is often reluctant for professionals to speak with family members, friends, or previous health care providers. Once admitted, the patient is frequently demanding and requests specific treatments and interventions. Negative test results are often followed by new or additional symptoms. If the health care team sets limits and does not follow through with requests, the patient may become angry and accuse the staff of incompetence and maltreatment.

An older term for factitious disorder is **Munchausen syndrome,** which was named after Baron Karl Friedrich Hieronymus von Münchausen (1720–1797), an 18th-century German cavalry officer with a reputation for fabricating exaggerated tales. Munchausen syndrome is notable for the way patients go from one primary care provider or hospital to another, seeking attention. The severity of the symptoms is evident in the aggressiveness of treatments by clinicians. Serious complications and sepsis may result from self-injections of toxins such as *E. coli.* Patients may have "criss-crossed" or "railroad-track" abdomens due to scars from numerous exploratory surgeries to investigate unexplained symptoms. In the extreme, amputations may even result from this disorder.

The most insidious form of factitious disorders is **factitious disorder imposed on another** (commonly called *Munchausen syndrome by proxy*), in which a caregiver deliberately feigns illness in a vulnerable dependent. People with this disorder do not do it in order to receive awards such as insurance money or other compensation. They do it for the purpose of the attention and excitement and to perpetuate the relationship with health care providers of that dependent. The caregiver frequently is a health care worker or someone with extensive knowledge of the health care system. The disorder results in unnecessary medical visits and sometimes-harmful medical procedures. Examples of this disorder include inducing premature delivery by rupturing the amniotic sac with a fingernail, infant apnea and sudden infant death, and introducing microorganisms into a child's wound. Falsification of illnesses results in extreme pain, surgical procedures, and even death of dependents.

Malingering

While not a specific mental disorder, **malingering** is mentioned here as a condition that is related to the factitious disorders. Malingering is a consciously motivated act to deceive based on the desire for material gain (Sadock & Sadock, 2008). It involves a process of fabricating an illness or exaggerating symptoms in order to become eligible for disability compensation, commit fraud against insurance companies, obtain prescription medications, evade military service, or receive a reduced prison sentence. Reported pains are vague and hard for clinicians to prove or disprove (e.g., back pain, headache, or toothache).

EPIDEMIOLOGY

Epidemiological studies estimate an incidence rate of 0.8-1.3%. Explanation for the low incidence rate includes the belief that a large number of cases are missed due to frequent denial of factitious disorder behaviors, the challenge to differentiate between real and feigned illness, and the fact that many patients often flee the health care setting (Hagglund, 2009). Factitious disorder, however, is thought to be more prevalent than previously recognized with suggestions that up to 6% of health care provider contacts may involve factitious disorder. This diagnosis should be considered in complicated patients, especially those with a history of emotional or physical distress, excessive dependence, and resistance to discharge (Williams, 2012).

17-1 CASE STUDY AND NURSING CARE PLAN

Somatic Symptom Disorder

Cara, age 49, a recently divorced mother of twin teenage daughters, works as copy editor for a local newspaper and has been trying to sell her house in order to downsize after her daughters graduate next year from high school. She has a 2-year history of numerous physical complaints—insomnia, fatigue, muscle aches, irritable bowel syndrome, and occasional paroxysmal arterial tachycardia (PAT)—and feels "nervous most of the time" and only leaves the house for work or to do grocery shopping. She attends work regularly but has no real social life as she is often "too tired to go out."

She has been referred to a variety of specialists, but there continues to be no evidence of organic origins of her pathophysiology. Today, she presented in the local emergency room with tachycardia in normal sinus rhythm and shortness of breath. All diagnostic tests were normal.

Cara agreed to attend an outpatient mental health intensive outpatient program three mornings each week. After attending IOP for 2 days, she has not made much progress and states concern about a possible job loss if she does not return to work as soon as possible. She states that she feels happy at times when at home but is very frustrated that her fatigue and physical symptoms are continuing. She states that nothing seems to help her and that her future looks bleak. Most staff have reported frustration that Cara is helpful with other patients but not actively engaged in working on any of her own issues, and she continually states that her mood is fine but her body is a "major problem."

Self-Assessment

Ms. Silverthorn is a registered nurse with a BSN degree and 3 years of experience in this intensive outpatient program. She recognizes her own mixed feelings toward Cara. On the one hand, the patient is interesting, talkative, and charming as she discusses her happy childhood. On the other hand, she is refusing to identify any psychological concerns and consistently prods staff to see if she can "graduate" from this program and go back to work. Staff members feel that Cara negates any of their interventions. Ms. Silverthorn realizes she has to carefully monitor her emotional reactions to Cara and adopt a persistent, matter-of-fact approach to encourage the patient to be more assertive, self-aware, and independent. Ms Silverthorn plans to actively support Cara in creating her discharge plan.

Assessment

Objective Data

- Results of all diagnostic tests are negative except it was determined through hormone testing that the patient is in perimenopause.
- Onset of symptoms coincides with her divorce and impending loss of daughters as their high school graduations are approaching.
- There is no prior history of somatic or psychiatric disorders.

Subjective Data

- "I don't know what I'm doing here with all of these mental patients."
- "Wouldn't you know, after all these tests now they tell me I am perimenopausal and that is probably what is causing all my problems."

Nursing Diagnoses

1. *Complicated grieving* related to loss of significant other and anticipatory losses of children and home as evidenced by multiple somatic symptoms, anxiety, and depressed mood
2. *Social isolation* related to fatigue/pain as evidenced by decreased contact and interaction with family and friends

Supporting Data

- Patient reports frequent fatigue and loss of social interests.
- Patient has difficulty communicating needs or emotions.
- Patient has minimal support system.
- Patient reports recent and impending losses with lack of emotion/concern.

Outcomes Identification

Long-term goal: Patient will identify and express emotions without physical symptoms.

Planning

The initial plan is to encourage Cara to explore feelings related to recent and impending losses and to develop a support system.

Implementation

The plan of care for Cara is personalized as follows:

SHORT-TERM GOAL	INTERVENTION	RATIONALE	EVALUATION
1. Patient will be safe from self-harm	1. Assess for suicidal ideation.	1. Suicidal ideation may occur in response to depression or hopelessness over medical conditions.	**GOAL MET**
2. Patient will identify levels of anxiety in at least three situations and encounters with IOP patients and staff.	2. Teach the patient techniques to identify and manage anxiety.	2. Identifying anxiety and anxiety reduction techniques helps to manage distress and provides patient with self-care behaviors, thereby enhancing self-esteem	**GOAL MET**
3. Patient will develop a contract in conjunction with staff to plan for behavior change.	3. Develop a relationship with the patient that includes a mutually agreed upon contract that details expected changes in behaviors.	3. A concrete means to keep track of patient actions will enhance self-direction and independent actions.	**GOAL MET**
4. Patient will seek support from staff and patients when feelings of anxiety become difficult to handle or physical symptoms increase.	4. Educate the patient about sharing feelings of loss with staff, friends, and family members.	4. Communication and expression of feelings with family and friends helps to alleviate stress and often provides a more supportive environment	**GOAL MET**
5. Patient will make a list with contacts and phone numbers of community resources of interest to her.	5. Assist in the identification of available support systems.	5. Clients are more successful with stressful life events if there is adequate support.	**GOAL MET**
6. Patient will utilize the therapeutic milieu to increase her ability to express feelings.	6. Support expression of feelings via the arts such as writing, music, and role-playing.	6. Various forms of artistic expression encourage promotion of feelings	**GOAL MET**

17-1 CASE STUDY AND NURSING CARE PLAN—cont'd

Somatic Symptom Disorder

SHORT-TERM GOAL	INTERVENTION	RATIONALE	EVALUATION
7. Patient will be active in unit activities	7. Assist the patient in identification of appropriate diversional activities.	7. Diversional activities assist the patient to be less attentive to inner turmoil. Activities that are of specific interest to the patient will be more likely to be utilized.	**GOAL MET**
8. Patient will challenge negative and self-defeating thoughts and replace them with positive thoughts.	8. Encourage the patient to use positive self-talk such as, "I can do this one step at a time," "Right now I need to stretch and breathe," and "I don't need to be perfect".	8. Cognitive techniques focus on changing behaviors and feelings by changing thoughts. Replacing negative thoughts with positive ones help to decreased anxiety.	**GOAL MET**

Evaluation

See individual outcomes and evaluation in the care plan.

Short-term goals met: After spending 3 weeks in the intensive outpatient mental health program, Cara developed a trusting relationship with one staff person and two patients. Ms. Silverthorn made several attempts to engage Cara in a discussion of feelings, losses, and conflicts to no avail until she arranged for a family meeting with Cara, her daughters, and her former husband. Cara was able to express her anxiety and occasional anger about the loss of her role as wife and the impending loss of her daughters when they attend college away from home. Her daughters expressed their concerns and emotions about leaving home as well. Cara's sister visited with her regularly and was able to provide support and to encourage Cara to reach out to her more often. Cara also became more active expressing her grief, particularly in the assertiveness and anger-management classes and actively sought out Ms. Silverthorn on three occasions to discuss her feelings. Cara felt the music group amazingly improved her mood, and she often played the piano, which she had not done in several years. Following discharge from the IOP, Cara decided to take piano lessons and also enrolled in some of her town's adult education classes. She is meeting more people in the community but states she hasn't really found a real friend there. Her daughters have been more eager to discuss their college goals with her and want to include her in plans to visit some colleges.

Long-term goal, partially met: Many of Cara's symptoms have decreased; in particular, there have been no further episodes of tachycardia and PAT. However, Cara states she is still hindered by some fatigue and muscle pain but much less than previously. She admits she has not really adhered closely to her exercise and healthy eating plan, and occasionally she still feels furious with herself for not coping as well as she would like in social situations. Cara feels that the assertiveness training was particularly helpful to her as she realized how her passivity and bottled-up anger could have contributed to her physical symptoms and distress. She states it is often bothersome but does try and take time each day to identify feelings of anxiety, depression, and anger regarding her recent losses. Cara will continue to see her nurse therapist weekly, work on assertiveness skills, identification and expression of feelings, and a healthier lifestyle.

Malingering is thought to be more common in men than in women (Raine, 2009). Among the criminal population, the rates may be as high as 10% to 20% (Sadock & Sadock, 2008). It is nearly impossible to determine the prevalence of malingering, owing to the concealment of its origins. Childhood neglect and abuse are thought to be causative. A childhood history of frequent illnesses, especially those that result in hospitalization, may also be present in people who develop this disorder (Braun et al., 2010).

COMORBIDITY

People with factitious disorders tend to complain of physiological problems although some patients may also try to convince clinicians that they have a psychiatric disorder. Patients may describe symptoms of depression, dissociation, conversion, and psychoses and seek treatment for these problems (Sadock & Sadock, 2008). According to some reports, substance abuse, borderline personality disorders, and sexual disorders are frequently present along with a normal to high intelligence quotient (IQ) and an intimate knowledge of the health care system (Ardesrani et al., 2009). Malingering is associated with antisocial, narcissistic, and borderline personality disorders.

ETIOLOGY

Biological Factors

Brain dysfunction has been identified as a possible source of the symptoms of factitious disorders (Sadock & Sadock, 2008). Specifically, impaired information processing has been suggested as causative. No other biological abnormalities have been proposed at this time.

Psychological Factors

It is difficult to determine or understand the psychological basis of these disorders because of the patients' intention to skew the facts. There is some evidence that persons with these disorders suffered abuse and neglect as children and may have been hospitalized more frequently than is typical (Sadock & Sadock, 2008). These hospitalizations may have been perceived as a refuge from a chaotic home life. It has also been suggested that patients with factitious disorders may have a masochistic side and feel a need to be punished through painful procedures.

APPLICATION OF THE NURSING PROCESS

ASSESSMENT AND DIAGNOSIS

Many of the principles of care for somatization disorders apply to factitious disorders. Often, determining if a patient's signs and symptoms are conscious or unconscious (i.e., whether they are a somatic disorder or a factitious disorder) is a challenge for clinicians, particularly those in the position to diagnose psychiatric disorders. Your role as a nurse, whether you work in psychiatry and mental health or any other setting, is to carefully assess the patient and document your care. A general principle in treating people with a factitious disorder is to avoid confrontation, which may result in the patient's defensiveness, elusiveness, or departure from the treatment facility.

Self-Assessment

Nurses who work with patients with factitious disorders—patients who intentionally and consciously feign illnesses—are often angry and resentful. After all, there are patients who really need care and have no control over how sick they are, and then there are patients with factitious disorders who are probably causing their own problems. These countertransference reactions should be acknowledged and can be addressed through discussions with other members of the treatment team and careful treatment planning. It is important to consider that factitious disorders may cause real problems that can be overlooked.

PLANNING AND IMPLEMENTATION

In cases of self-directed factitious disorder and particularly other-directed factitious disorder, the nurse must consider safety. Patients who may purposefully inflict damage to themselves or others must be carefully monitored, and suspicious activities should be reported to and discussed by the health care team. It is essential that the nurse share any information that may prevent a person or a vulnerable and unsuspecting child from undergoing unnecessary surgery or treatments.

EVALUATION

Evaluation with factitious disorders is positive when patient safety has been maintained, conflicts have been explored, new coping strategies have permitted the patient to function at a higher level, and stress is handled adaptively without the desire or need of the pretense of a physiological disorder.

KEY POINTS TO REMEMBER

- There is irrefutable evidence that adverse emotional conditions may precipitate and often increase the severity of physical symptoms. Likewise, physical illnesses are often accompanied by a spectrum of emotional responses.
- Somatization disorders are characterized by the presence of multiple, real physical symptoms, with or without an identifiable medical illness.
- Somatization disorders are believed to be responses to psychosocial stress although the patient often shows no insight in the potential stressors.
- The course of somatization disorders may be brief, with acute onset and spontaneous remission, or chronic, with a gradual onset and prolonged impairment.
- The nursing assessment is especially important in identifying symptoms of adverse childhood events, depression, anxiety, posttraumatic stress disorder, and substance abuse that are contributing to the somatic symptom disorder.
- Health care personnel in the medical and mental health communities recognize the need for integrated, holistic interventions to target both the psychological and medical problems of a patient to increase adherence to the care regimen, maximize quality of life, promote healing, and minimize escalating health care costs.
- The advanced practice nurse is in a key position to assist other health care personnel to view patients in an integrated, holistic approach in both inpatient and outpatient settings.
- Factitious disorders, in contrast to other somatic disorders, are under conscious control. Nurses are challenged to provide care for persons who are feigning disorders when there are others with real illnesses who need their time.

CRITICAL THINKING

1. A patient with suspected somatization disorder has been admitted to the medical-surgical unit after an episode of chest pain with possible electrocardiographic changes. While on the unit, she frequently complains of palpitations, asks the nurse to check her vital signs, and begs staff to stay with her. Some nurses take her pulse and blood pressure when she asks. Others evade her requests. Most of the staff tries to avoid spending time with her.
   a. Consider why staff wish to avoid her. How would you feel as a nurse in this situation?
   b. Design interventions to cope with the patient's behaviors. Give rationales for your interventions.
2. Maria Valdez is a 45-year-old who has learned that she is HIV-positive. She is asymptomatic, has a normal physical examination, and all routine laboratory tests are normal. Her CD4 cell count is 325 cells per cubic millimeter, and her plasma HIV-1 RNA level is 60,000 copies per milliliter (both confirmed on repeated testing).

   She and her ex-husband have been divorced for years but maintain good relationships. Maria has a supportive extended family, church community, and neighbors. She has a full-time job and several committed friends that she grew up with. Maria has been seeing her current boyfriend for 2 years; however, she was not aware that he was engaging in unprotected sex outside of their relationship.

   Maria is distraught. "How can I live with myself? I am a disgrace to my children and family." Within several weeks, Maria returns to work and starts to assume more daily household responsibilities. When she is encouraged to talk about her feelings and see a therapist, Maria states, "I will be able to do everything I did before. I feel healthy." The nurse has several concerns, including Maria's focus on self-care, acceptance and understanding of her HIV-positive status, and her willingness to disclose her status to sexual/intimate partners.
   a. How would you evaluate Maria's social support system?
   b. What other information would you like to know about her situation that might help your assessment?
   c. What do you need to know about her cultural beliefs about illness?
   d. What recommendations or referrals could you make for her? How would you approach these recommendations?
   e. From what you know about Maria, identify the strengths she has that you would support and encourage.

CHAPTER REVIEW

1. The information that is least relevant when assessing a patient with a suspected somatization disorder is:
   a. Understanding coping mechanisms.
   b. Results of diagnostic workups.
   c. Limitations in activities of daily living.
   d. Potential for violence.
2. A suitable outcome criterion for the nursing diagnosis *Ineffective coping* related to dependence on pain relievers to treat chronic pain of psychological origin is:
   a. Patient will participate in self-care with optimal participation.
   b. Patient will learn and practice effective coping skills.
   c. Patient will demonstrate improved self-esteem as evidenced by focusing less on weaknesses.
   d. Patient will replace demanding, manipulative behaviors with more socially acceptable behavior.
3. You are caring for Yolanda, a 67-year-old patient who has been receiving hemodialysis for 3 months. Yolanda reports that she feels angry whenever it is time for her dialysis treatment. You attribute this to:
   a. Organic changes in Yolanda's brain.
   b. A flaw in Yolanda's personality.
   c. A normal response to grief and loss.
   d. Denial of the reality of a poor prognosis.
4. Lucas is a nurse on a medical floor caring for Kelly, a 48-year-old patient with newly diagnosed type 2 diabetes. He realizes that depression is a complicating factor in the patient's adjustment to her new diagnosis. What problem has the most potential to arise?
   a. Development of agoraphobia
   b. Treatment nonadherence
   c. Frequent hypoglycemic reactions
   d. Sleeping rather than checking blood sugar
5. You are caring for Aaron, a 38-year-old patient diagnosed with somatic symptom disorder. When interacting with you, Aaron continues to focus on his severe headaches. In planning care for Aaron, which of the following interventions would be appropriate?
   a. Call for a family meeting with Aaron in attendance to confront Aaron regarding his diagnosis.
   b. Educate Aaron on alternative therapies to deal with pain.
   c. Improve reality testing by telling Aaron that you do not believe that the headaches are real.
   d. Shift focus from Aaron's somatic concerns to feelings and effective coping skills.

Answers to Chapter Review
1. d; 2. b; 3. c; 4. b; 5. d.

evolve WEBSITE

Visit the Evolve website for a posttest on the content in this chapter: http://evolve.elsevier.com/Varcarolis

Post-Test interactive review

REFERENCES

Ackley, B.J., & Ladwig, G.B. (2011). *Nursing diagnosis handbook: An evidence-based guide to planning care* (9th ed.). St. Louis, MO: Mosby/Elsevier.

American Psychiatric Association. (2013). *DSM-5 table of contents.* Retrieved from http://www.psychiatry.org/dsm5.

Aragona, M., Catino, E., Pucci, D., Carrer, S., Colosimo, F., Lafuente, M., et al. (2010). The relationship between somatization and posttraumatic symptoms among immigrants receiving primary care services. *Journal of Traumatic Stress, 23*(5), 615–622.

Ardesrani, S. M. S., Zairoddin, A. R., Shahpouri, H. R., & Mousavi, S. S. (2009). Comorbidity of factitious disorders and intellectual disability: A case report. *Iranian Journal of Psychiatry and Behavioral Sciences, 3*(2), 44–46.

Braun, I. M., Greenberg, D. M., Smith, F. A., & Cassem, N. H. (2010). Functional somatic symptoms and somatoform disorders. In T. A. Stern, J. F. Rosenbaum, M. Fava, J. Biederman, & S. L. Rauch (Eds.), *Massachusetts General Hospital handbook of general hospital psychiatry* (6th ed., pp. 173–188). Philadelphia, PA: Saunders.

Bulechek, G. M., Butcher, H. K., Dochterman, J. M., & Wagner, C. (2013). *Nursing interventions classification (NIC)* (6th ed.). St. Louis, MO: Mosby.

Cannon, W.B. (1914). The emergency function of the adrenal medulla in pain and the major emotions. *American Journal of Physiology, 33*, 356–372.

Carlisle, S., & Hanlon, P. (2007). Well-being and consumer culture: A different kind of public health problem? *Health promotion international, 22*(3), 261–268.

Charlson, F. J., Stapelberg, N. J. C., Baxter, A. J., & Whiteford, H. A. (2011). Should global burden of disease estimates include depression as a risk factor for coronary heart disease? *BMC Medicine, 9*(47). doi:10.1186/1741-7015-9-47.

Dickson, B., Hay-Smith, E. J. C., & Dean, S. G. (2009). Demonised diagnosis: The influence of stigma on interdisciplinary rehabilitation of somatoform disorder. *New Zealand Journal of Physiotherapy, 37*(3), 115–121.

Dols, A., Rhebergen, D., Eikelenboom, P., & Stek, M. L. (2012). Hypochondriacal delusion in an elderly woman recovers quickly with electroconvulsive therapy. *Clinical and Practice, 2*(11), 21–22. doi:10.4081/cp.2012.ell

Dube, S., Fairweather, D., Pearson, W. S., Felitti, V. J., Anda, R. F., & Croft, J. B. (2009). Cumulative childhood stress and autoimmune diseases in adults. *Psychosomatic Medicine, 71*(2), 243–250.

Edwards, T., Stern, A., Clarke, D. D., Ivbijaro, G., & Kasney, L. M. (2010). The treatment of the patient with medically unexplained symptoms in primary care: A review of the literature. *Mental Health in Family Medicine, 7*, 209–21.

Feinstein, A. (2011). Conversion disorder: Advances in our understanding. *Canadian Medical Association Journal, 183*(8), 915–920. doi:10.1503/cmaj.110490

Fink, P. (2010). The outcome of health anxiety in primary care: A two-year follow up study on health care costs and self-rated health. *PloS ONE, 5*(3), e9873. doi: 10.1371/journal.pone.0009873.

Fuller-Thomson, E., Sulman, J., Brennenstuhl, S., & Merchant, M. (2011). Functional somatic syndromes and childhood physical abuse in women: Data from a representative community-based sample. *Journal of Aggression, Maltreatment and Trauma, 20*, 445–469.

Garcia-Martin, M. I., Miranda, V. E. M., & Soutullo, C.A. (2012). Duloxetine in the treatment of adolescents with somatoform disorders: A report of two cases. *Actas espanolas de psiquiatra, 20*(3), 165–168.

Gross, A., Gallo, J. J., & Eaton, W. W. (2010). Depression and cancer risk: 24 years of follow up of the Baltimore epidemiologic catchment area sample. *NIH Cancer Causes Control, 21*(2), 191–199.

Hagglund, L. (2009). Challenges in the treatment of factitious disorder: A case study. *Archives of Psychiatric Nursing, 23*(1), 58–64.

Hale, D., & Reck, A. (2010). Somatoform disorder: Understanding hypochondriasis and somatization. *Journal of Health Sciences and Practice, 1*(9), 1–7.

Han, C., Pae, C. U., Lee, B. H., Ko, Y. H., Masand, P. S., Patkar, A. A., et al. (2008). Venlafaxine versus mirtazapine in the treatment of undifferentiated somatoform disorder: A 12-week prospective, open-label, randomized, parallel-group trial. *Clinical Drug Investigation, 28*(4), 251–261.

Herdman, T. H. (Ed.). (2012). *NANDA International Nursing diagnoses: Definitions and classification*, 2012–2014. Oxford, UK: Wiley-Blackwell.

Huang, H., & McCarron, R. M. (2011). Medically unexplained symptoms: Evidence-based interventions. *Current Psychiatry, 10*(7), 17-31.

Kenny, M., & Egan, J. (2011). Somatization disorder: What clinicians need to know. *Psychologist, 37*(4), 93–96.

Kim, H. H., Lee, Y. J., Kim, H. K., Kim, J. E., Kim, S. J., Bae, S., et al. (2011). Prevalence and correlates of psychiatric symptoms in North Korean defectors. *Psychiatry Investigation, 8*(3), 179–185.

Korber, S., Frieser, D., Steinbrecher, N., & Hiller, W. (2011). Classification characteristics of Patient Health Questionnaire-15 screening for somatoform disorders in a primary care setting. *Journal of Psychosomatic Research, 71*, 142–147.

Kroenke, K. (2007). Efficacy of treatment of somatoform disorders: A review of randomized controlled trials. *Psychosomatic Medicine, 69*(9), 881–888.

Lemal, M., & den Bulck, J. V. (2009). Television news exposure is related to fear of breast cancer. *Preventative Medicine, 48*, 189–192.

MacDonald, P. (2011). Dealing with health anxiety. *Practice Nurse, 41*(16), 38.

Miller, M. (2009). Treating somatoform disorders. *Harvard Mental Health Letter*. Retrieved from http://www.health.harvard.edu/newsletters/harvard_mental_health_letter/2009/November.

National Prevention Council. (2011). *National prevention strategy*. Retrieved from http://www.healthcare.gov/prevention/nphpphc/strategy/report.pdf.

Nicholson, T., Stone, J., & Kanaan, R. A. A. (2011). Conversion disorder: A problematic diagnosis. *Journal of Neurology, Neurosurgery, and Psychiatry, 82*, 1267–1273.

Noyes, R., Longley, S. L., Langbehn, D. R., Stuart, S. P., & Kukoyi, O. A. (2010). Hypochondriacal symptoms associated with a less therapeutic physician-patient relationship. *Psychiatry, 73*(1), 57–69.

Raine, M. (2009). Helping advocates to understand the psychological diagnosis and assessment of malingering. *Psychiatry, Psychology, and Law, 16*(2), 322–328.

Schulte, I. E., & Petermann, F. (2011). Familial risk factors for the development of somatoform symptoms and disorders in children and adolescents: A systemic review. *Child Psychiatry and Human Development, 42*(5), 569–583.

Schumaker, J. F. (2007). *In search of happiness: Understanding an endangered state of mind*. Westport, CT: Praeger.

Selye, H. (1956). *The stress of life*. New York, NY: McGraw-Hill.

Silber, T. J. (2011). Somatization disorders: Diagnosis, treatment and prognosis. *Pediatrics in Review, 32*(2), 56–64.

So, J. (2008). Somatization as a cultural idiom of distress: Rethinking mind and body in a multicultural society. *Counseling Psychology Quarterly, 21*(2), 167–174. doi:10.1080/095150802066854.

Steinbrecher, N., Koerber, S., Frieser, D., & Hiller, W. (2011). The prevalence of medically unexplained symptoms in primary care. *Psychosomatics, 52*, 263–271. doi:10.1016/j.psym.2011.01.007.

Stone, J., Vuilleumier, P., & Friedman, J. H. (2010). Conversion disorder: Separating "how" from "why." *Neurology, 74*, 190–191.

Temoshok, L. R., Wald, R. L., Synowski, S., & Garzino-Demo, A. (2008). Coping as a multisystem construct associated with pathways medicating HIV-relevant immune function and disease progression. *Psychosomatic Medicine, 70*, 555–561.

Walters, P., Tylee, A., Fisher, J., & Goldberg, D. (2007). Teaching junior doctors to manage patients who somatise: Is it possible in an afternoon? *Medical Education, 41*, 995–1001.

Webb, T. (2010). Medically unexplained symptoms. *Therapy Today*, 21(3). Retrieved from http://www.therapytoday.net/article/15/49/categories/.

Williams, L. (2012). Factitious disorder in a psychogeriatric patient. *General Hospital Psychiatry, 34*(4), 5–6.

CHAPTER

18

Feeding, Eating, and Elimination Disorders

Carissa R. Enright

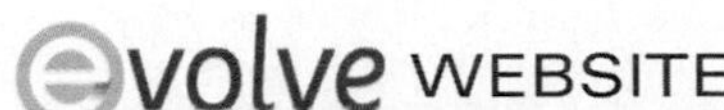

Visit the Evolve website for a pretest on the content in this chapter:
http://evolve.elsevier.com/Varcarolis

Pre-Test interactive review

OBJECTIVES

1. Compare and contrast the signs symptoms (clinical picture) of anorexia nervosa, bulimia nervosa, and binge-eating disorder.
2. Describe the biological, psychological, and environmental factors associated with eating disorders.
3. Apply the nursing process to patients with anorexia nervosa, patients with bulimia nervosa, and patients with binge-eating disorder.
4. Identify three life-threatening conditions, stated in terms of nursing diagnoses, for a patient with an eating disorder.
5. Identify two realistic outcome criteria for a patient with anorexia nervosa, a patient with bulimia nervosa, and a patient with binge-eating disorder.
6. Describe three feeding disorders usually seen in childhood, including pica, rumination disorder, and avoidant/restrictive food intake disorder.
7. Identify the elimination disorders, enuresis and encopresis.

KEY TERMS AND CONCEPTS

anorexia nervosa
binge eating disorder
bulimia nervosa
encopresis
enuresis
ideal body weight
pica
rumination

Of all the psychiatric disorders, eating disorders may be the most perplexing. The eating and sharing of food is usually pleasurable and culturally important. It is difficult for many of us to understand how people could starve themselves or induce vomiting and seem to have little regard for how it affects them physically and socially. Many theories of the etiology of these disorders have been postulated, but to date, the reasons behind the behavior are still a mystery that drives research.

In this chapter we begin with a general overview of eating disorders. Since there are no etiological or nursing care similarities, this chapter will give a detailed view of the nursing care of the eating disorders followed by a description of the feeding and elimination disorders.

CLINICAL PICTURE

The three main eating disorders are anorexia nervosa, bulimia nervosa, and binge eating disorder (American Psychiatric Association, 2013). Some behaviors do not meet the specifications for full-blown eating disorders but do cause problems with food intake. They are categorized under other specified feeding or eating disorder and unspecified feeding or eating disorder (Walsh & Sysko, 2009).

Individuals with **anorexia nervosa** refuse to maintain a minimally normal weight for height and express intense fear of gaining weight. The term *anorexia* is a misnomer, because loss of appetite is rare. Some people with anorexia nervosa restrict

BOX 18-1 CHARACTERISTICS OF EATING PROBLEMS

ANOREXIA NERVOSA

- Intense fear of weight gain
- Distorted body image
- Restricted calories with significantly low BMI
- Subtypes:
  - Restricting (no consistent bulimic features)
  - Binge/eating/purging type (primarily restriction, some bulimic behaviors)

BULIMIA NERVOSA

- Recurrent episodes of uncontrollable binging
- Inappropriate compensatory behaviors: vomiting, laxatives, diuretics, or exercise
- Self-image largely influenced by body image

BINGE EATING

- Recurrent episodes of uncontrollable binging without compensatory behaviors
- Binging episodes induce guilt, depression, embarrassment or disgust

their intake of food; others engage in binge eating and purging. Individuals with **bulimia nervosa** engage in repeated episodes of binge eating followed by inappropriate compensatory behaviors, such as self-induced vomiting; misuse of laxatives, diuretics, or other medications; fasting; or excessive exercise. These disorders are characterized by a significant disturbance in the perception of body shape and weight (Sysko et al., 2012). Individuals with **binge eating disorder** engage in repeated episodes of binge eating, after which they experience significant distress. These individuals do not regularly use the compensatory behaviors that are seen in patients with bulimia nervosa. Although individuals who start binge eating may be of normal weight, repeated bingeing inevitably causes obesity in this cohort. Box 18-1 identifies characteristics of anorexia nervosa, bulimia nervosa, binge eating, and other specified feeding and eating disorders.

Hospitalization for anorexia nervosa is often necessary due to the life-threatening effect that starvation has on the body. Inpatient treatment may be required for people with bulimia nervosa, especially if they have co-occurring depression and suicidal ideation. See criteria for hospitalization for these disorders in Box 18-2. People with binge eating disorder are not typically hospitalized for the eating disorder but may require psychiatric treatment for other disorders. Additionally, binge eating disorder results in a vast array of physical problems that often require inpatient treatment.

BOX 18-2 CRITERIA FOR HOSPITAL ADMISSION OF PATIENTS WITH EATING DISORDERS

Physical Criteria

- Weight loss over 30% over 6 months
- Rapid decline in weight
- Inability to gain weight with outpatient treatment
- Severe hypothermia due to loss of subcutaneous tissue or dehydration (temperature lower than 36° C or 96.8° F)
- Heart rate less than 40 beats per minute
- Systolic blood pressure less than 70 mm Hg
- Hypokalemia (less than 3 mEq/L) or other electrolyte disturbances not corrected by oral supplementation
- Electrocardiographic changes (especially arrhythmias)

Psychiatric Criteria

- Suicidal or severely out-of-control, self-mutilating behaviors
- Out-of-control use of laxatives, emetics, diuretics, or street drugs
- Failure to comply with treatment contract
- Severe depression
- Psychosis
- Family crisis or dysfunction

EPIDEMIOLOGY

For women, the lifetime incidence of anorexia nervosa, bulimia nervosa, and binge eating disorder is 0.9%, 1.5%, and 3.5%, respectively; and the lifetime incidence for men is 0.3%, 0.5%, and 2% (Hudson et al., 2007). It is extremely difficult to determine the specific number of people afflicted with eating disorders since fewer than half seek health care for their illness. With revised criteria for the eating disorders, these statistics can be expected to change in coming years. Most eating disorders begin in the early teens to mid-20s although they commonly occur following puberty, with bulimia occurring in later adolescence. Anorexia nervosa may start early (between ages 7 and 12), but bulimia nervosa is rarely seen in children younger than 12 years.

COMORBIDITY

Comorbidity for patients with eating disorders is more likely than not. (Treasure et al., 2010). In a replication of the National Comorbidity Survey, respondents with anorexia nervosa, bulimia nervosa, and binge eating disorder also met criteria for at least one of the core DSM IV disorders at rates of 56%, 94%, and 79%, respectively (Hudson et al., 2007).

In individuals 13 to 18 years of age, anorexia nervosa is associated with oppositional defiant disorder (Swanson et al., 2011). For this age group, bulimia and binge eating mood and anxiety disorders are strongly associated with mood and anxiety disorders.

Personality disorders occur more often in the eating-disordered population than the general population. In particular, obsessive-compulsive personality disorder represents only 8% of the general population but accounts for 22% of anorexia nervosa restricting type. Borderline personality disorder occurs in 6% of the general population but represents 25% of anorexia nervosa binge eating purging type and 28% of bulimia nervosa patients (Sansone & Sansone, 2011).

Overeating is frequently noted as a symptom of an affective disorder (e.g., atypical depression). Higher rates of affective and personality disorders are found among binge eaters. Binge eaters report a history of major depression and anxiety disorders significantly more often than non–binge eaters, with lifetime rates of 45.3% to 65.2% (Swanson et al., 2011).

ETIOLOGY

Childhood trauma and sexual abuse have been reported in 20% to 50% of patients with eating disorders, and those patients with reported abuse have poorer outcomes from treatment than those who don not. Physical neglect, emotional abuse, and sexual abuse have been found to be significant predictors for eating disorders (Kong & Bernstein, 2009).

The eating disorders—anorexia nervosa, bulimia nervosa, and binge eating disorder—are actually entities or syndromes and are not considered to be specific diseases. It is not known if they share a common cause and pathology; therefore, it may be more appropriate to conceptualize them as syndromes on the basis of the cluster of symptoms they present (Halmi, 2011). A number of theories attempt to explain eating disorders. Because binge eating disorder has been newly defined, little comparative research has been done to show how this pattern of eating is similar to the others in etiology or progression.

Biological Factors

Genetic

There is a strong genetic link for eating disorders. In fact, a literature search of relevant studies has suggested that the heritability of anorexia nervosa is 60% (Bienvenu et al., 2011). A genetic vulnerability may lead to poor affect and impulse control or to an underlying neurotransmitter dysfunction, but no single causative gene has been discovered to date. The most recent research suggests that there is a gene-environmental interaction that may be responsible for the prevalence of the eating disorders (Campbell et al., 2011).

Neurobiological

Research demonstrates that altered brain serotonin function contributes to dysregulation of appetite, mood, and impulse control in the eating disorders. These patients consistently exhibit personality traits of perfectionism, obsessive-compulsiveness, and dysphoric mood, all of which are modulated through serotonin pathways in the brain. Because these traits appear to begin in childhood—before the onset of actual eating-disorder symptoms—and persist into recovery, they are believed to contribute to a vulnerability to disordered eating (Kaye & Strober, 2009).

Tryptophan, an amino acid essential to serotonin synthesis, is only available through diet. A normal diet boosts serotonin in the brain and regulates mood. Temporary drops in dietary tryptophan may actually relieve symptoms of anxiety and dysphoria and provide a reward for caloric restriction; however, continued malnutrition will result in a physiological dysphoria. This cycle of temporary relief, followed by more dysphoria, sets up a positive feedback loop that reinforces the disordered eating behavior (Kaye et al., 2009). This dietary need for tryptophan may account for the fact that antidepressants that boost serotonin do not improve mood symptoms until after an underweight patient has been restored to 90% of optimal weight.

Newer brain imaging capabilities allow for better understanding of the etiological factors of anorexia nervosa. Much research has focused on the changes that occur in the brains of patients during the active phase of the eating disorder and after a period of recovery. Comparing brain images will help researchers to distinguish between the physiological effects of starvation and the pathology associated with the disorder (Kaye et al., 2009).

Psychological Factors

Because anorexia nervosa was observed primarily in girls approaching puberty, early psychoanalytic theories linked the symptoms to an unconscious aversion to sexuality. Throughout the 20th century many authors examined the family dynamics of these patients and concluded that a failure to separate from parents and a rebellion against the maternal bond explained the disordered eating behaviors. Further work by Bruch in the 1970s explored the symptoms as a defense against an overwhelming feeling of ineffectiveness and powerlessness. Even with these theories of unconscious processes, therapies based on this understanding have not made a major impact (Caparrotta & Ghaffari, 2006).

Currently, cognitive-behavioral theorists suggest that eating disorders are based on learned behavior that has positive reinforcement. For example, a mildly overweight 14-year-old has the flu and loses a little weight. She returns to school, and her friends say, "Wow, you look great." Now she purposefully strives to lose weight. When people say, "Wow, you look really skinny," she hears, "Wow, you look great." Her behavior is powerfully reinforced by these comments despite the fact that her health is at risk.

Family theorists maintain that eating disorders are a problem of the whole family, but research has not been able to determine any definitive family characteristics specific to the eating disorders. In general, family therapies focus on facilitating emotional communication and conflict resolution (le Grange et al., 2010).

Environmental Factors

Studies have shown that culture influences the development of self-concept and satisfaction with body size. The Western cultural ideal that equates feminine beauty to tall, thin models has received much attention in the media as an etiology for the eating disorders. However, research has not proven a direct relationship between social ideals portrayed in the media and the development of an eating disorder. It is known that peer behaviors and attitudes may contribute to the body dissatisfaction that all eating disordered patients feel (Eisenberg & Neumark-Sztainer, 2010; Ferguson et al., 2011).

The rate of obesity in the United States is at an alarming level, as 35.5% of adult women and 15% of 2- to 19-year-old girls are obese (Ogden et al., 2012). Record numbers of men and women are on diets to reduce body weight, but no study has been able to explain why only an estimated 0.3% to 3% of the population develops an eating disorder. Research has not proven a direct relationship between social ideals portrayed in the media and the development of an eating disorder; however, peer behaviors and attitudes may contribute to the body dissatisfaction that all eating-disordered patients feel (Eisenberg & Neumark-Sztainer, 2010; Ferguson et al., 2011).

EVIDENCE-BASED PRACTICE

Does Viewing Pro-Anorexia Websites Predict Development of an Eating Disorder?

Custers, K., & Van den Bulck, J. (2009). Viewership of pro-anorexia websites in seventh, ninth and eleventh graders. *European Eating Disorders Review, 17*(3), 214–219. doi: 10.1002/erv.910.

Problem

With the increased use of the Internet to find information, more adolescents are exposed to websites that promote behaviors common to anorexia nervosa, called "pro-ana" sites. Other studies have shown that children with eating disorders are known to visit these sites, but little is known about the overall characteristics of viewers of these sites.

Purpose of the Study

The purpose of this study was to identify the frequency of girls and boys viewing these sites and also to determine if there is a relationship between the attitudes of these viewers and known predictors of anorexia nervosa.

Methods

This qualitative study sampled 711 boys and girls enrolled in the seventh, ninth, and eleventh grades in a single, assembly-type testing session in Flanders, Belgium. The study included questions about how often they visited pro-ana websites and their attitudes toward the existence of these sites. There were also questions that measured the student's drive for thinness, perfectionism, body mass index, and perception of their own appearance. A logical regression was used to test the relationship between gender, grade, and attitude toward pro-ana sites with the actual prevalence of visiting these websites. Another analysis examined the correlation between prevalence of viewing these websites and the drive for thinness, perception of appearance, and perfectionism.

Key Findings

- Both girls and boys admit to visiting pro-ana websites.
- Only one fourth of the participants regard these websites as totally unacceptable.
- Girls who have visited pro-ana sites have a higher drive for thinness and perfectionism.
- Visiting pro-ana sites is significantly correlated with predictors of anorexia nervosa.

Implications for Nursing Practice

Visiting pro-anorexia websites is not without risks. They attract both boys and girls but are more often viewed by girls. These websites provide adolescents with a social support community that can reinforce attitudes and behaviors that are consistent with disordered eating patterns. Patients with anorexia nervosa often try to rationalize their food choices as a lifestyle and not a mental disorder with life-threatening consequences. It is more difficult to change this attitude when the online environment provides "evidence" for the truth of this belief.

ANOREXIA NERVOSA

APPLICATION OF THE NURSING PROCESS

ASSESSMENT

Anorexia nervosa is a serious psychiatric disorder. Box 18-3 lists several thoughts and behaviors associated with anorexia nervosa, and Table 18-1 identifies clinical signs and symptoms of anorexia nervosa along with their causes.

Eating disorders are serious and in extreme cases can lead to death. Box 18-4 identifies a number of medical complications that can occur in individuals with anorexia nervosa and the laboratory findings that may result. Because the eating

TABLE 18-1 POSSIBLE SIGNS AND SYMPTOMS OF ANOREXIA NERVOSA

CLINICAL PRESENTATION	CAUSE
Low weight	Caloric restriction, excessive exercising
Amenorrhea	Low weight
Yellow skin	Hypercarotenemia
Lanugo	Starvation
Cold extremities	Starvation
Peripheral edema	Hypoalbuminemia and refeeding
Muscle weakening	Starvation, electrolyte imbalance
Constipation	Starvation
Abnormal laboratory values (low triiodothyronine, thyroxine levels)	Starvation
Abnormal computed tomographic scans, electroencephalographic changes	Starvation
Cardiovascular abnormalities (hypotension, bradycardia, heart failure)	Starvation, dehydration
	Electrolyte imbalance
Impaired renal function	Dehydration
Hypokalemia (low potassium)	Starvation
Anemic pancytopenia	Starvation
Decreased bone density	Estrogen deficiency, low calcium intake

BOX 18-3 THOUGHTS AND BEHAVIORS ASSOCIATED WITH ANOREXIA NERVOSA

- Terror of gaining weight
- Preoccupation with thoughts of food
- View of self as fat even when emaciated
- Peculiar handling of food: cutting food into small bits
- Pushing pieces of food around plate
- Possible development of rigorous exercise regimen
- Possible self-induced vomiting, use of laxatives and diuretics
- Cognition so disturbed that individual judges self-worth by his or her weight

BOX 18-4 MEDICAL COMPLICATIONS OF ANOREXIA NERVOSA

- Bradycardia
- Orthostatic changes in pulse or blood pressure
- Cardiac arrhythmias
- Prolonged QT interval and ST-T wave abnormalities
- Peripheral neuropathy
- Acrocyanosis
- Symptomatic hypotension
- Leukopenia
- Lymphocytosis
- Carotenemia (elevated carotene levels in blood), which produces skin with yellow pallor
- Hypokalemic alkalosis (with self-induced vomiting or use of laxatives and diuretics)
- Elevated serum bicarbonate levels, hypochloremia, and hypokalemia
- Electrolyte imbalances, which lead to fatigue, weakness, and lethargy
- Osteoporosis, indicated by decrease in bone density
- Fatty degeneration of liver, indicated by elevation of serum enzyme levels
- Elevated cholesterol levels
- Amenorrhea
- Abnormal thyroid functioning
- Hematuria
- Proteinuria

Data from Halmi, K. A. (2008). Eating disorders: Anorexia nervosa, bulimia nervosa, and obesity. In R. E. Hales, S. C. Yudofsky, & G. O. Gabbard (Eds.), *Textbook of psychiatry* (5th ed., pp. 762, 769–770). Washington, DC: American Psychiatric Publishing.

behaviors in these conditions are so extreme, hospitalization may become necessary (often via the emergency department).

Fundamental to the care of individuals with eating disorders is establishing and maintaining a therapeutic alliance. This will take both time and diplomacy on the part of the nurse. In treating patients who have been sexually abused or who have otherwise been victims of boundary violations, it is critical that the nurse and other health care workers maintain and respect clear boundaries (Wright & Hacking, 2011).

General Assessment

Individuals with the binge-purge type of anorexia nervosa may present with severe electrolyte imbalance (as a result of purging) and enter the health care system through admission to an intensive care unit. The patient with the restricting type of anorexia will be severely underweight and may have growth of fine, downy hair (lanugo) on the face and back. The patient will also have mottled, cool skin on the extremities and low blood pressure, pulse, and temperature readings, consistent with a malnourished, dehydrated state (see Table 18-1).

As with any comprehensive psychiatric nursing assessment, a complete evaluation of biopsychosocial function is mandatory. The areas to be covered include the patient's:

- Perception of the problem
- Eating habits
- History of dieting
- Methods used to achieve weight control (restricting, purging, exercising)
- Value attached to a specific shape and weight
- Interpersonal and social functioning
- Mental status and physiological parameters

Self-Assessment

When caring for the patient with anorexia, you may find it difficult to appreciate the compelling force of the illness, incorrectly believing that weight restriction, bingeing, and purging are self-imposed. If we see such self-destructive behaviors as choices, it is only natural to blame the patient for any consequent health problems. The common personality traits of these patients—perfectionism, obsessive thoughts and actions relating to food, intense feelings of shame, people pleasing, and the need to have complete control over their therapy—pose additional challenges.

In your efforts to motivate such patients and take advantage of their decision to seek help and be healthier, take care not to allow encouragement to cross the line into authoritarianism and assumption of a parental role. A patient's terror at gaining weight and her or his resistance to clinical interventions may engender significant frustration in the nurse struggling to build a therapeutic relationship and be empathetic. Guard against any tendency to be coercive in your approach, and be aware that one of the primary goals of treatment—weight gain—is the very thing the patient fears. When patients appear to be resistant to change, it is helpful to acknowledge the constant struggle that so characterizes the treatment.

DIAGNOSIS

Imbalanced nutrition: less than body requirements is usually the most appropriate initial nursing diagnosis for individuals with anorexia and generates further nursing diagnoses. They include *Decreased cardiac output, Risk for injury* (electrolyte imbalance), and *Risk for imbalanced fluid volume* (which would have first priority when problems are addressed). Other nursing

ASSESSMENT GUIDELINES

Anorexia Nervosa

Determine whether:

1. The patient has a medical or psychiatric condition that warrants hospitalization (see Box 18-2).
2. A thorough physical examination with appropriate blood work has been done.
3. Other medical conditions have been ruled out.
4. The patient is amenable to receiving or compliant with appropriate therapeutic modalities.
5. The family and patient need further teaching or information regarding the patient's treatment plan (e.g., psychopharmacological interventions, behavioral therapy, cognitive therapy, family therapy, individual psychotherapy).
6. The patient and family desire to participate in a support group.
7. The patient and family have been provided referral to a support group.

diagnoses include *Disturbed body image, Ineffective coping, Chronic low self-esteem, and Powerlessness.*

OUTCOMES IDENTIFICATION

Outcomes are patient-centered and should always be developed in conjunction with the person diagnosed with anorexia nervosa or someone who can represent the person. To evaluate the effectiveness of treatment, outcome criteria are established to measure treatment results. The most important outcome is in the attainment of a safe weight. Table 18-2 identifies signs and symptoms commonly experienced with anorexia nervosa, offers potential nursing diagnoses, and suggests outcomes.

PLANNING

Planning is affected by the acuity of the patient's situation. When a patient with anorexia is experiencing extreme electrolyte imbalance or weighs below 75% of **ideal body weight**, the plan is to provide immediate medical stabilization, most likely in an inpatient unit. If a specialized eating-disorder unit is not available, hospitalization on a cardiac or medical unit is usually brief, providing only limited weight restoration and addressing only the acute complications (e.g., electrolyte imbalance and dysrhythmias) and acute psychiatric symptoms (e.g., significant depression). With the initiation of therapeutic nutrition, malnourished patients may need treatment on a medical unit, owing to **refeeding syndrome**, a potentially catastrophic treatment complication involving a metabolic alteration in serum electrolytes, vitamin deficiencies, and sodium retention (Kohn, et al., 2011)

Once a patient is medically stable, the plan addresses the issues underlying the eating disorder. These psychological issues are usually addressed on an outpatient basis. The plan of care will include individual, group, and family therapy as well as psychopharmacological therapy during different phases of the illness. The nature of the treatment is determined by the intensity of the symptoms—which may vary over time—and the experienced disruption in the patient's life.

Discharge planning is a critical component in treatment. Often, family members benefit from counseling. The discharge planning process must address living arrangements, school, work, the feasibility of independent financial status, applications for state and/or federal program assistance (if needed), and follow-up outpatient treatment.

IMPLEMENTATION

Acute Care

Typically, a patient with an eating disorder is admitted to the inpatient psychiatric facility in a crisis state. The initial focus depends on the results of a comprehensive assessment. Any acute psychiatric symptoms, such as suicidal ideation, are addressed immediately. The nurse is challenged to establish trust and monitor the eating pattern.

Psychosocial Interventions

After working through acute symptoms, the patient with anorexia begins a weight restoration program that allows for incremental weight gain. Based on the patient's height, a treatment goal is set at 90% of ideal body weight, the weight at which most women are able to menstruate.

As patients begin to re-feed, they ideally participate in the unit's milieu. In this setting, the patient should feel accepted and safe from judgmental evaluations. The focus should be on the eating behavior and underlying feelings of anxiety, dysphoria, low self-esteem, and lack of control. Discussions about physical appearance should be approached carefully because comments may be misinterpreted, as demonstrated in the first vignette on the next page.

TABLE 18-2 SIGNS AND SYMPTOMS, NURSING DIAGNOSES, AND OUTCOMES FOR ANOREXIA NERVOSA

SIGNS AND SYMPTOMS	NURSING DIAGNOSES	OUTCOMES
Emaciation, dehydration, arrhythmias, inadequate intake, dry skin, decreased blood pressure, decreased urine output, increased urine concentration, weakness	*Imbalanced nutrition: less than body requirements* *Decreased cardiac output* *Risk for injury (electrolyte imbalance)* *Risk for imbalanced fluid volume*	Nutrients are ingested and absorbed to meet metabolic needs; cardiac pump supports systemic perfusion pressure; electrolytes are in balance; fluids are in balance
Excessive self-monitoring, describes self as fat despite emaciation	*Disturbed body image*	Congruence between body reality, body ideal, and body presentation; satisfaction with body appearance
Destructive behavior toward self, poor concentration, inability to meet role expectations, inadequate problem solving	*Ineffective coping*	Demonstrates effective coping, reports decrease in stress, uses personal support system, uses effective coping strategies, reports increase in psychological comfort
Indecisive behavior, lack of eye contact, passive, reports feelings of shame, rejects positive feedback about self	*Chronic low self-esteem* *Powerlessness*	Verbalizes a positive level of confidence; makes informed life decisions, expresses independence with decision-making processes

From Herdman, T. H. (Ed.), (2012). *Nursing diagnoses—Definitions and classification 2012-2014.* Copyright © 2012, 1994-2012 by NANDA International. Used by arrangement with John Wiley & Sons Limited; Moorhead, S., Johnson, M., Maas, M. L., & Swanson, E. (2013). *Nursing outcomes classification (NOC)* (5th ed.). St. Louis, MO: Mosby.

VIGNETTE

Alicia, a 17-year-old cheerleader, did not come to treatment for weight loss until she fainted at a football game. She insisted that she only needed to "get more energy, not get fat." When the nurse pointed out that Alicia's ribs were clearly visible and that her backbone looked like a skeleton, Alicia grinned and said, "Thank you."

CONSIDERING CULTURE

Latinas' Paradoxical Body Images

The literature reports conflicting findings regarding Latinas' body image and body satisfaction. Some research has suggested that Latina women are more tolerant of a curvy body shape than are white women. However, another line of investigation argues that Latinas may actually face greater concerns regarding their body image with more fear of weight gain than their white counterparts. This study attempted to examine body satisfaction among a cohort of Latinas as well as their beliefs and attitudes regarding mainstream American cultural ideals. All the participants actually reported a preference for a body shape thinner than they actually considered themselves to have. However, they were also more accepting of a heavier, curvy body shape as a Latina ideal. Further study may help nurses understand the influence of cultural perceptions of body shape on patients' attitudes toward their own body image and their desire to maintain a healthy weight.

Viladrich, A., Yeh, M. C., Bruning, N., & Weiss, R. (2009). Do real women have curves? Paradoxical body image among Latinas in New York City. *Journal of Immigrant and Minority Health, 11*(1), 20–28.

Pharmacological Interventions

There are no drugs approved by the U.S. Food and Drug Administration (FDA) for the treatment of anorexia nervosa, and research does not support the use of pharmacological agents to treat the core symptoms (Treasure et al., 2010). The selective serotonin reuptake inhibitor (SSRI) fluoxetine (Prozac), however, has proven useful in reducing obsessive-compulsive behavior *after* the patient has reached a maintenance weight. Unconventional antipsychotic agents such as olanzapine (Zyprexa) may be helpful in improving mood and decreasing obsessive behaviors and resistance to weight gain (Treasure et al., 2010) but are not well accepted by patients who are frightened by the side effect of weight gain with this classification of drugs.

Integrative Medicine

Patients with eating disorder may benefit by a number of complementary alternative medicine therapies (Breuner, 2010). A comprehensive treatment plan can include the usual medical and nutritional interventions along with the beneficial effects of massage, biofeedback, acupuncture, or yoga to manage mood. It is also important that the nurse ask if patients are taking herbals, such as St. John's wort for depression, valerian for sleep, and chamomile for anxiety. Patients will need proper guidance and education to assist them when they choose to add these therapies to their recovery program.

Health Teaching and Health Promotion

Self-care activities are an important part of the treatment plan. These activities include learning more constructive coping skills, improving social skills, and developing problem-solving and decision-making skills. The skills become the focus of both therapy sessions and supervised food-shopping trips. As the patient approaches the goal weight, she or he is encouraged to expand the repertoire to include eating out in a restaurant, preparing a meal, and eating forbidden foods. The following vignette illustrates the need for supportive education.

VIGNETTE

A nursing assessment of a small group of three young women and one young man in a nutrition group finds that all the participants are very knowledgeable about the caloric value of common foods; as a group, they all avoid any "fatty" foods. The topic of fat-soluble vitamins and the consequences of vitamin deficiencies on the body was new information to all of the participants, and one of the young women started to cry, saying, "I had no idea I was doing that to my body." This show of emotion promoted a supportive interaction among the other group members as they shared their own stories of symptoms they could now identify as vitamin deficits.

Teamwork and Safety

Patients admitted to an inpatient unit designed to treat eating disorders participate in a combination of therapeutic modalities provided by a multidisciplinary team. These modalities are designed to normalize eating patterns and begin to address the medical, family, and social issues raised by the illness.

The milieu of an eating-disorder unit is purposefully organized to assist the patient in establishing more adaptive behavioral patterns, including normalization of eating. The highly structured environment includes precise meal times, adherence to the selected menu, observation during and after meals, and regularly scheduled weighing.

Close monitoring of patients includes monitoring all trips to the bathroom after eating to prevent self-induced vomiting.

VIGNETTE

A 20-year-old woman who primarily restricts her eating has also resorted to purging when her family forces her to eat. As part of her treatment plan on a general psychiatric unit, the dietitian ordered specific meals for her. She became visibly distressed after eating one of these meals and requested permission to go to the bathroom alone because she had "embarrassing gas." The nurse agreed to stand away from the bathroom door if the patient agreed not to flush the toilet until the nurse was able to inspect the contents; however, the patient flushed the toilet. The treatment team concluded that she broke the contract with the nurse and was not able to adhere to her prescribed treatment without additional structure. The treatment team established a new goal that she gain 2 pounds and an intervention that she wait 30 minutes after every meal before she was allowed supervised bathroom breaks.

18-1 CASE STUDY AND NURSING CARE PLAN

Anorexia Nervosa

Cynthia is a 20-year-old woman who is brought to the inpatient eating-disorders unit of a psychiatric research hospital by two older brothers, who support her on either side. She is profoundly weak, holding her head up with her hands.

Self-Assessment

Mindy Jacobs, RN, is assigned to care for Cynthia. Although Mindy is a young nurse, she has spent the last 3 years working on the eating-disorders unit. When she began working on the unit, she had difficulty with overidentifying with patients. During college, Mindy struggled with bulimia, but with treatment she has done well. She seeks guidance from her nursing supervisor and the multidisciplinary team. This support allows her to maintain appropriate boundaries while creating a therapeutic alliance with patients.

Assessment

Objective Data

- Height: 62 inches (5 feet 2 inches)
- Weight: 58 lb—50% of ideal body weight
- Blood pressure: 74/50 mm Hg
- Pulse: 54 beats per minute
- Anemic—hemoglobin: 9 g/dL
- Cachectic appearance, pale, with fine lanugo
- Sad facial expression
- Bruising on inside of each knee from sleeping on her side with knees touching

Subjective Data

- Denies being underweight: "I need treatment because I get fatigued so easily."
- "I check my legs every night. I'm so afraid of getting fat. I hate it if my legs touch each other."
- "I don't like to start anything until I know I can do it perfectly the first time. I wouldn't want anyone to see me make a mistake."
- Depressed mood.

Diagnosis

1. *Imbalanced nutrition: less than body requirements* related to restriction of caloric intake secondary to extreme fear of weight gain.
2. *Chronic low self-esteem* related to perception that others are always judging her.

Outcomes Identification

Patient will reach 75% of ideal weight (92 lb) by discharge.

Planning

The initial plan is to address Cynthia's unstable physiological state.

Implementation

Cynthia's care plan is personalized as follows:

SHORT-TERM GOAL	INTERVENTION	RATIONALE	EVALUATION
1. Patient will gain a minimum of 2 lb and a maximum of 3 lb weekly through inpatient stay.	1a. Acknowledge the emotional and physical difficulty patient is experiencing. Use patient's extreme fatigue to engage cooperation in the treatment plan.	1a. A first priority is to establish a therapeutic alliance.	**WEEK 1:** Patient increases caloric intake with liquid supplement only. Patient unable to eat solid food. Patient does not gain weight. Patient remains hypotensive, bradycardic, anemic (hemoglobin [HGB] = 9 g/dL).
	1b. Weigh patient daily for the first week, then three times a week. Patient should be weighed in bra and panties only. There should be no oral intake, including a drink of water, before the early-morning weigh-in.	1b. These measures ensure that weight is accurate.	**WEEK 2:** Patient gains 2 lb drinking liquid supplement—minimal solid food. Patient remains hypotensive, bradycardic (HGB = 10 g/dL).
	1c. Do not negotiate weight with patient or reweigh. Patient may choose not to look at the scale or request that she not be told the weight.	1c. Patient may try to control and sabotage treatment.	**WEEK 3:** Patient gains I lb drinking liquid supplement. Patient selects meal plan but is unable to eat most of solid food.
	1d. Measure vital signs tid until stable, then daily. Repeat ECG and laboratory tests until stable.	1d. As patient begins to increase in weight, cardiovascular status improves to within normal range, and monitoring is less frequent.	Patient's blood pressure (BP) = 84/60 mm Hg; pulse = 68 beats per minute, regular; HGB = 11 g/dL.
	1e. Provide a pleasant, calm atmosphere at mealtimes. Patient should be told the specific times and duration (usually a half hour) of meals.	1e. Mealtimes become episodes of high anxiety, and knowledge of regulations decreases tension in the milieu, particularly when patient has given up so much control by entering treatment.	**WEEKS 4-6:** Patient gains an average of 2.5 lb/wk. Patient samples more of solid food selected from meal plan. Patient's BP = 90/60 mm Hg; pulse = 68 beats per minute, regular; HGB = 11.5 g/dL.
	1f. Administer liquid supplement as ordered.	1f. Patient may be unable to eat solid food at first.	

18-1 CASE STUDY AND NURSING CARE PLAN—cont'd

Anorexia Nervosa

SHORT-TERM GOAL	INTERVENTION	RATIONALE	EVALUATION
	1g. Observe patient during meals to prevent hiding or throwing away of food and for at least 1 hour after meals and snacks to prevent purging.	1g,1h. The compelling force of the illness is such that these behaviors are difficult to stop. A power struggle between staff and patient may emerge, in which patient appears to comply but defies the rules (appearing to eat but throwing away food).	**WEEK 7:** Patient weighs 71 lb (almost 60% of ideal body weight); calories are mostly from liquid supplement.
	1h. Encourage patient to try to eat some solid food. Preparation of patient's meals should be guided by likes and dislikes list because patient is unable to make own selections to complete menu.		Patient selects balanced meals, eating more varied solid food: turkey, carrots, lettuce, fruit. Patient's HGB = 12.5 g/dL; normal range of BP and pulse are maintained. Patient continues to increase participation in social aspects of eating.
	1i. Be empathetic with patient's struggle to give up control of her eating and her weight as she is expected to make minimum weight gain on a regular basis. Permit patient to verbalize feelings at these times.	1i. Patient is expected to gain at least 0.5 lb on a specific schedule, usually three times a week (Monday, Wednesday, Friday).	**WEEKS 8-12:** Patient gains an average of 2.5 lb/wk and weighs 82 lb (approx. 68% of ideal body weight). Patient is eating more varied solid food, but most caloric intake is still from liquid supplement.
	1j. Monitor patient's weight gain. A weight gain of 2 to 3 lb/wk is medically acceptable.	1j. Weight gain of more than 5 lb in 1 week may result in pulmonary edema.	Patient maintains normal vital signs and HGB levels.
	1k. Provide teaching regarding healthy eating as the basis of a healthy lifestyle.	1k. Healthy aspects of eating (e.g., increased energy, rather than gaining weight) are reinforced.	Patient maintains social interaction during mealtimes and snacks.
	1l. Use a cognitive-behavioral approach to address patient's expressed fears regarding weight gain. Identify and examine dysfunctional thoughts; identify and examine values and beliefs that sustain these thoughts	1l. Confronting irrational thoughts and beliefs is crucial to changing eating behaviors.	**WEEKS 13-16:** Patient has reached medically stable weight at the end of 16th week—92 lb (75% of ideal body weight). Patient continues to eat more solid food with relatively less liquid supplement.
	1m. As patient approaches her target weight, there should be encouragement to make her own choices for menu selection.	1m. Patient can assume more control of her meals, which is empowering for the patient with anorexia.	Patient is not able to participate in planned exercise program until patient reaches 85% of ideal body weight.
	1n. Emphasize social nature of eating. Encourage conversation that does not have the theme of food during mealtimes.	1n. Eating as a social activity, shared with others and with participation in conversation, serves as both a distraction from obsessive preoccupations and a pleasurable event.	
	1o. Focus on the patient's strengths, including her good work in normalizing her weight and eating habits	1o. Patient who is beginning to normalize weight and eating behaviors has achieved a major accomplishment, of which she should be proud. Noneating activities are explored as a source of gratification.	
	1p. Provide for a planned exercise program when patient reaches target weight.	1p. Patient experiences a strong drive to exercise; this measure accommodates this drive by planning a reasonable amount.	
	1q. Encourage patient to apply all the knowledge, skills, and gains made from the various individual, family, and group therapy sessions.	1q. Patient has been receiving intensive therapy and education, which have provided tools and techniques that are useful in maintaining healthy behaviors.	

Evaluation

By the end of the 16th week, Cynthia has achieved a stable weight of 92 lb. This weight is approaching congruency with Cynthia's height, frame, and age. Her vital signs and hemoglobin levels are consistently demonstrated as normal. She is participating in therapy and consistently communicating satisfaction with her body appearance.

Patients may also need monitoring on bathroom trips after seeing visitors and after any hospital pass to ensure they have not had access to and ingested any laxatives or diuretics. Often, patient privileges are linked to weight gain and treatment-plan adherence. The vignette on page 349 demonstrates monitoring the bathroom as a therapeutic intervention.

Advanced Practice Interventions

Anorexia nervosa is a chronic illness that waxes and wanes. The 1-year relapse rate approaches 50%, and long-term studies show that up to 40% of patients continue to meet some criteria for anorexia nervosa after 4 years (Helverskov et al., 2010). Recovery is evaluated as a stage in the process rather than a fixed event. Factors that influence the stage of recovery include percentage of ideal body weight that has been achieved, the extent to which self-worth is defined by shape and weight, and the amount of disruption existing in the patient's personal life.

The patient will require long-term treatment that might include periodic brief hospital stays, outpatient psychotherapy, and pharmacological interventions. The combination of individual, group, couples, and family therapy (especially for the younger patient) provides the patient with the greatest chance for a successful outcome.

Psychotherapy

The advanced practice nurse provides individual, group, or family therapy in a variety of settings. The goals of treatment are weight restoration with normalization of eating habits and initiation of the treatment of psychological, interpersonal, and social issues that personally affect each individual patient.

Outpatient partial hospitalization programs designed to treat eating disorders are structured to achieve outcomes comparable to those of inpatient eating-disorders units. The advanced practice nurse, along with other therapists, might contract with patients with anorexia regarding the terms of treatment. For example, outpatient treatment can continue only if the patient maintains a contracted weight. If weight falls below the goal, other treatment arrangements must be made until the patient returns to the goal weight.

This highly structured approach to treating patients whose weight is below 75% of ideal body weight is necessary, even for therapists who approach treatment from a more emotional or cognitive model of therapy. Assisting the patient with a daily meal plan, reviewing a journal of meals and dietary intake maintained by the patient, and providing for weekly weighing (ideally two to three times a week) are essential if the patient is to reach a medically stable weight.

Families frequently report feeling powerless in the face of behavior that is mystifying. For instance, patients are often unable to experience compliments as supportive and therefore are unable to internalize the support. They often seek attention from others but feel shamed when they receive it. Patients express that they want their families to care for and about them but are unable to recognize expressions of care. When others do respond with love and support, patients do not perceive this as positive. The following vignette demonstrates this phenomenon.

VIGNETTE

Mrs. Demi's daughter, Lila, has gained 40 pounds. Together they attend a family support group where the group leader asks how she regards her daughter now that she has been in treatment. Mrs. Demi replies, "She looks healthy." Her daughter responds with an angry, sullen look. She ultimately verbalizes that she interprets comments about her "healthy" appearance as "You look fat." The group leader points out that it is interesting that Lila equates "healthy" with "fat."

Often, family members and significant others seek ways to communicate clearly with the patient with anorexia but find that they are frequently misunderstood and that overtures of concern are misinterpreted. Consequently, families experience the tension of saying or doing the wrong thing and then feeling responsible if a setback occurs. Advanced practice psychiatric mental health nurses have an important role in assisting families and significant others to develop strategies for improved communication and search for ways to be comfortably supportive to the patient.

EVALUATION

The process of evaluation is built into the outcomes specified by *NOC* (Moorhead et al., 2013). Evaluation is ongoing, and short-term indicators are revised as necessary to achieve the treatment outcomes established. The indicators provide a daily guide for evaluating success and must be continually reevaluated for their appropriateness. Case Study and Nursing Care Plan 18-1 presents a patient with anorexia nervosa.

BULIMIA NERVOSA

APPLICATION OF THE NURSING PROCESS

ASSESSMENT

General Assessment

Initially, patients with bulimia nervosa do not appear to be physically or emotionally ill. They are often at or close to ideal body weight; however, as the assessment continues and the nurse makes further observations, the physical and emotional problems of the patient become apparent. On inspection, the patient demonstrates enlargement of the parotid glands, with dental erosion and caries if the patient has been inducing vomiting. Box 18-5 identifies a number of medical complications that can occur and the laboratory findings that may result in individuals with bulimia nervosa. The disclosed history may reveal great difficulties with both impulsivity and compulsivity. Family relationships are frequently chaotic and reflect a lack of nurturing. Patients' lives reflect instability and troublesome interpersonal relationships as well.

Box 18-6 lists several thoughts and behaviors associated with bulimia nervosa, and Table 18-3 identifies possible signs and symptoms found on assessment and their causes.

BOX 18-5 MEDICAL COMPLICATIONS OF BULIMIA NERVOSA

- Sinus bradycardia
- Orthostatic changes in pulse or blood pressure
- Cardiac arrhythmias
- Cardiac arrest from electrolyte disturbances or Ipecac intoxication
- Cardiac murmur; mitral valve prolapse
- Electrolyte imbalances
- Elevated serum bicarbonate levels (although can be low, which indicates a metabolic acidosis)
- Hypochloremia
- Hypokalemia
- Dehydration, which results in volume depletion, leading to stimulation of aldosterone production, which in turn stimulates further potassium excretion from kidneys; thus, there can be both an indirect renal loss of potassium and a direct loss through self-induced vomiting
- Severe attrition and erosion of teeth, producing irritating sensitivity and exposing the pulp of the teeth
- Loss of dental arch
- Diminished chewing ability
- Parotid gland enlargement associated with elevated serum amylase levels
- Esophageal tears caused by self-induced vomiting
- Severe abdominal pain indicative of gastric dilation
- Russell's sign (callus on knuckles from self-induced vomiting)

Data from Halmi, K. A. (2011). Eating disorders: Anorexia nervosa, bulimia nervosa, and obesity. In R. E. Hales, S. C. Yudofsky, & G. O. Gabbard (Eds.), *Essentials of psychiatry* (3rd ed., pp. 440–441). Washington, DC: American Psychiatric Publishing.

VIGNETTE

During the initial assessment, the nurse wonders if Brittany is actually in need of hospitalization on the eating-disorders unit. The nurse is struck by how well the patient appears, seeming healthy, well-dressed, and articulate. As Brittany continues to relate her history, she tells of restricting her intake all day until early evening, when she buys her food and begins to binge as she is shopping. She arrives home and immediately induces vomiting. For the remainder of the evening and into the early morning hours, she "zones out" while watching television and binge eating. Periodically, she goes to the bathroom to vomit. She does this about 15 times during the evening. The nurse admitting Brittany to the unit reminds her of the goals of the hospitalization, including interrupting the binge-purge cycle and normalizing eating. The nurse further explains to Brittany that she has the support of the eating-disorder treatment team and the milieu of the unit to assist her toward recovery.

Self-Assessment

In working with someone with bulimia, be aware that the patient is sensitive to the perceptions of others regarding this illness and may feel significant shame and totally out of control. In building a therapeutic alliance, try to empathize with the patient's feelings of low self-esteem, unworthiness, and

BOX 18-6 THOUGHTS AND BEHAVIORS ASSOCIATED WITH BULIMIA NERVOSA

- Binge eating behaviors
- Often self-induced vomiting (or laxative or diuretic use) after bingeing
- History of anorexia nervosa in one fourth to one third of individuals
- Depressive signs and symptoms
- Problems with:
  Interpersonal relationships
  Self-concept
  Impulsive behaviors
- Increased levels of anxiety and compulsivity
- Possible chemical dependency
- Possible impulsive stealing

TABLE 18-3 POSSIBLE SIGNS AND SYMPTOMS OF BULIMIA NERVOSA

CLINICAL PRESENTATION	CAUSE
Normal to slightly low weight	Excessive caloric intake with purging, excessive exercising
Dental caries, tooth erosion	Vomiting (HCl reflux over enamel)
Parotid swelling	Increased serum amylase levels
Gastric dilation, rupture	Binge eating
Calluses, scars on hand (Russell's sign)	Self-induced vomiting
Peripheral edema	Rebound fluid, especially if diuretic used
Muscle weakening	Electrolyte imbalance
Abnormal laboratory values (electrolyte imbalance, hypokalemia, hyponatremia)	Purging: vomiting, laxative and/or diuretic use
Cardiovascular abnormalities (cardiomyopathy, electrocardiographic changes)	Electrolyte imbalance—**can lead to death**
Cardiac failure (cardiomyopathy)	Ipecac intoxication

ASSESSMENT GUIDELINES

Bulimia Nervosa

1. Medical stabilization is the first priority. Problems resulting from purging are disruptions in electrolyte and fluid balance and cardiac function; therefore, a thorough medical examination is vital.
2. Medical evaluation usually includes a thorough physical examination, as well as pertinent laboratory testing, including:
   - Electrolyte levels
   - Glucose level
   - Thyroid function tests
   - Complete blood count
   - ECG
3. Psychiatric evaluation is advised because treatment of psychiatric comorbidity is important to outcome.

dysphoria. If you believe the patient is not being honest (e.g., active bingeing or purging goes unreported) or is being manipulative, acknowledge such obstacles and the frustration they provoke and construct alternative ways to view the patient's thinking and behavior. An accepting, nonjudgmental approach, along with a comprehensive understanding of the subjective experience of the patient with bulimia, will help to build trust.

DIAGNOSIS

The assessment of the patient with bulimia nervosa yields nursing diagnoses that result from the disordered eating and weight-control behaviors. Problems resulting from purging are a first priority because electrolyte and fluid balance and cardiac function are affected. Common nursing diagnoses include *decreased cardiac output, disturbed body image, ineffective coping, powerlessness, chronic low self-esteem,* and *social isolation.*

OUTCOMES IDENTIFICATION

Outcome criteria are linked to the diagnoses listed above. Table 18-4 provides an overview of signs and symptoms, nursing diagnoses, and associated outcomes for individuals with bulimia nervosa.

PLANNING

The criteria for inpatient admission of a patient with bulimia nervosa are included in the criteria for inpatient admission of a patient with an eating disorder presented in Box 18-2. Like the patient with anorexia nervosa, the patient with bulimia may be treated for life-threatening complications such as gastric rupture (rare), electrolyte imbalance, and cardiac dysrhythmias in an acute care unit of a hospital. If the patient is admitted to a general inpatient psychiatric unit because of acute suicidal risk, only the acute psychiatric manifestations are addressed short term. Planning will also include appropriate referrals for continuing outpatient treatment.

VIGNETTE

Iris weighs 85% of her ideal body weight. She has a history of diuretic abuse, and she becomes edematous when she stops their use and enters treatment. The nurse informs Iris that the edema is related to the use of diuretics (and thus is transient) and that it will resolve after Iris begins to eat normally and discontinues the diuretics. Iris cannot tolerate the weight gain and the accompanying edema that occurs when she stops taking diuretics. She restarts the diuretics, perpetuating the cycle of fluid retention and the risk of kidney damage. The nurse empathizes with Iris's inability to tolerate the feelings of anxiety and dread she experiences because of her markedly swollen extremities.

IMPLEMENTATION

Acute Care

A patient who is medically compromised as a result of bulimia nervosa is referred to an inpatient eating-disorder unit for comprehensive treatment of the illness. The cognitive-behavioral model of treatment is highly effective and frequently serves as the cornerstone of the therapeutic approach. Inpatient units designed to treat eating disorders are especially structured to interrupt the cycle of binge eating and purging and to normalize eating habits. Therapy is begun to examine the underlying conflicts and body dissatisfaction that sustain the illness. Evaluation for treatment of comorbid disorders, such as major depression and substance abuse, is also undertaken. In most cases of substance dependence, the treatment of the eating disorder must occur after the substance dependence is treated.

Pharmacological Interventions

Antidepressant medication together with cognitive-behavioral psychotherapy has been shown to bring about improvement

TABLE 18-4 SIGNS AND SYMPTOMS, NURSING DIAGNOSES, AND OUTCOMES FOR BULIMIA NERVOSA

SIGNS AND SYMPTOMS	NURSING DIAGNOSES	OUTCOMES
Electrolyte imbalances, esophageal tears, cardiac problems, excessive vomiting, self-destructive behaviors	*Decreased cardiac output* *Risk for injury (electrolyte imbalance)*	Cardiac pump supports systemic perfusion pressure; electrolytes are in balance
Obsession with body, denial of problems, dissatisfied with appearance	*Disturbed body image*	Congruence between body reality, body ideal, and body presentation; satisfaction with body appearance
Obsessed with food, substance abuse, impulsive responses to problems; inappropriate use of laxatives, diuretics, enemas, fasting, inadequate problem solving	*Ineffective coping*	Demonstrates effective coping, reports decrease in stress, uses personal support system, uses effective coping strategies, reports increase in psychological comfort
Loss of control with the binge-purge cycle, feelings of shame and guilt, views self as unable to deal with events, excessive seeking of reassurance	*Chronic low self-esteem* *Powerlessness*	Verbalizes a positive level of confidence, makes informed life decisions, expresses independence with decision-making processes
Absence of supportive significant other(s), hides eating behaviors from others, reports feeling alone	*Social isolation*	Willing to call on others for assistance, develops a confidant relationship, feels a sense of belonging

From Herdman, T. H. (Ed.), (2012). *Nursing diagnoses—Definitions and classification 2012-2014.* Copyright © 2012, 1994-2012 by NANDA International. Used by arrangement with John Wiley & Sons Limited; Moorhead, S., Johnson, M., Maas, M. L., & Swanson, E. (2013). *Nursing outcomes classification (NOC)* (5th ed.). St. Louis, MO: Mosby.

in bulimic symptoms. Limited research suggests that the SSRIs and tricyclic antidepressants helped reduce binge eating and vomiting over short terms. Fluoxetine (Prozac) treatment may help prevent relapse. Bupropion (Wellbutrin) may be effective, but due to an increased risk for seizures, it is contraindicated in patients who purge (Treasure et al., 2010)

Counseling

Compared with the patient with anorexia, the patient with bulimia nervosa often more readily establishes a therapeutic alliance with the nurse because the eating-disordered behaviors are seen as a problem. The therapeutic alliance allows the nurse, along with other members of the multidisciplinary team, to provide counseling that gives useful feedback regarding the patient's distorted beliefs.

Health Teaching and Health Promotion

Health teaching focuses on not only the eating disorder but also meal planning, use of relaxation techniques, maintenance of a healthy diet and exercise, coping skills, the physical and emotional effects of bingeing and purging, and the impact of cognitive distortions. This preparation lays the foundation for the second phase of treatment, in which there are carefully planned challenges to the patient's newly developed skills. For instance, the patient is expected to have an unsupervised meal at home and share the feelings this event provoked with others in a group therapy setting.

Once a patient reaches therapeutic goals, it is recommended that patients seek long-term care to solidify those goals and address the attitudes, perceptions, and psychodynamic issues that maintain the eating disorder and attend the illness.

Teamwork and Safety

The highly structured milieu of an inpatient eating-disorder unit has as its primary goals the interruption of the binge-purge cycle and the prevention of disordered eating behaviors. Observation during and after meals (to prevent purging), normalization of eating patterns, and maintenance of appropriate exercise are integral elements of such a unit. The multidisciplinary team uses a comprehensive treatment approach to address the emotional and behavioral problems that arise when the patient is no longer binge eating or purging. Like the interruption of other obsessive-compulsive behaviors, preventing the binge-purge pattern allows underlying anxiety to come to the surface and be examined.

Advanced Practice Interventions

Psychotherapy

Cognitive-behavioreal therapy is the most effective treatment for bulimia nervosa. Restructuring faulty perceptions and helping individuals develop accepting attitudes toward themselves and their bodies is a primary focus of therapy. When patients do not indulge in bulimic behaviors, issues of self-worth and interpersonal functioning become more prominent.

EVALUATION

Evaluation of treatment effectiveness is ongoing and built into the *NOC* categories. Outcomes are revised as necessary to reach the desired outcomes. Case Study and Nursing Care Plan 18-2 presents a patient with bulimia nervosa.

VIGNETTE

Becky, a 23-year-old patient with a 6-year history of bulimia nervosa, struggles with issues of self-esteem. She expresses much guilt about "letting her father down" in the past by drinking alcohol excessively and binge eating and purging. She is determined that this time she is not going to fail at treatment. After her initial success in stopping the disordered behaviors, she says defiantly, "I'm doing this for *me*." Becky usually experiences her behavior as either pleasing or disappointing to others, but she begins to realize that her feeling of self-worth is very much dependent on how others see her and that she needs to develop a better sense of herself.

BINGE EATING DISORDER

APPLICATION OF THE NURSING PROCESS

ASSESSMENT

Although obesity puts these patients at risk for diabetes, hypertension, and heart disease, hospitalization to treat the binge eating itself is not indicated. Because the stomach must accommodate larger than normal volumes during a binge, there are also gastrointestinal problems associated with this dilation. These patients have significant difficulties with heartburn, dysphagia, bloating, and abdominal pain, as well as diarrhea, urgency, constipation, and a feeling of anal blockage (Cremonini et al., 2009). In addition to reducing binge eating, the nurse will need to help the patient manage the gastric symptoms associated with the disordered eating.

General Assessment

To some extent, all people with obesity have periods when their eating feels out of their control, and to the nurse, the amount of food consumed during meals may look larger than "normal." This presents a major challenge to the accurate discrimination between people who are obese due to metabolic or lifestyle causes and those who have an obsessive bingeing pattern of eating. A careful history of the quantity of food consumed in discrete bingeing episodes and how often they occur is essential to the nursing care plan.

Self-Assessment

It is common for people to believe that obesity is a major personality flaw in people who fail to control their eating and exercise habits. Culturally, obesity is still the subject of jokes and discrimination. In addition, nurses have realistic concerns for their own personal safety when attempting to lift, move, or assist obese patients in the hospital setting (Poon, 2009). It is important that the nurse be aware of possible negative reactions to obese patients. Attitudes among health care providers have changed over time, with more understanding of the etiological factors for obesity, but for many nurses, their personal reactions are still influenced by disgust or displeasure (Creel, 2011).

18-2 CASE STUDY AND NURSING CARE PLAN

Bulimia Nervosa

Sally is a 30-year-old college graduate who reports that she is an aspiring actress. She is being admitted to a partial hospitalization program designed for patients with eating disorders. Sally has bulimia nervosa.

Self-Assessment

Matthew, a seasoned nurse in the area of eating disorders, is assigned to care for Sally. Matthew enjoys working with patients with bulimia because he believes he can help patients move toward health. When he first encounters Sally, he experiences an immediate negative response that surprises him. He speaks to his supervisor about these feelings and raises the question of whether or not he is the appropriate nurse to care for Sally. As he and the supervisor discuss his feelings, Matthew is able to recognize that Sally reminds him of a girlfriend he had many years earlier. The relationship ended badly. Matthew experiences an emotional release with this realization and believes that he will be able to separate his earlier negative experience from his work with Sally.

Assessment

Objective Data

- Height: 65 inches (5 feet 5 inches)
- Weight: 127 lb—95% of ideal body weight
- Blood pressure: 120/80 mm Hg sitting; 90/60 mm Hg standing
- Pulse: 70 beats/min sitting; 96 beats/min standing
- Potassium level of 2.7 mmol/L (normal range, 3.3 to 5.5 mmol/L)
- ECG: abnormal—consistent with hypokalemia
- Erosion of enamel, enlarged parotid glands, consistent with a history of binge eating/purging.

Subjective Data

- "I can't stand to be fat."
- "I'm ashamed that I can't control my bingeing and vomiting—I know it's not good."

Diagnosis

1. *Risk for injury* related to low potassium and other physical changes secondary to binge eating and purging
2. *Powerlessness* related to inability to control bingeing and vomiting cycles

Outcomes Identification

Sally will demonstrate ability to regulate eating patterns, resulting in consistently normal electrolyte balance.

Planning

Sally is admitted to a partial hospitalization program designed for patients with eating disorders. She attends the program 3 or 4 days a week and participates in individual and group therapy. She will continue to work as a "temp" for a publishing house.

Implementation

Sally's care plan is personalized as follows:

SHORT-TERM GOAL	INTERVENTION	RATIONALE	EVALUATION
1. Patient will identify signs and symptoms of low potassium (K^+) level, and K^+ level will remain within normal limits throughout hospitalization.	1a. Educate patient regarding the ill effects of self-induced vomiting, low K^+ level, dental erosion.	1a. Health teaching is crucial to treatment. The patient needs to be reminded of the benefits of normalization of eating behavior.	**WEEK 1:** Patient begins to select balanced meals. Patient demonstrates knowledge of untoward effects of vomiting and K^+ deficiency. Patient begins to demonstrate understanding of repetitive nature of binge-purge cycle.
	1b. Educate patient about binge-purge cycle and its self-perpetuating nature.	1b, 1c. The compulsive nature of the binge-purge cycle is maintained by the sequence of intake restriction, hunger, bingeing, purging accompanied by feelings of guilt, and then repetition of the cycle over and over.	
	1c. Teach patient that fasting sets one up to binge eat.		
	1d. Explore ideas about trigger foods.	1d. Patient needs to understand beliefs about trigger foods to challenge irrational thoughts.	**WEEK 2:** Patient begins to challenge irrational thoughts and beliefs. Patient continues to plan nutritionally balanced meals, including dinner at home. Patient begins to sample "forbidden foods" and discuss thoughts and attitudes about same.
	1e. Challenge irrational thoughts and beliefs about "forbidden" foods.	1e. Challenge forces patient to examine own thinking and beliefs.	**WEEK 3:** Patient discusses triggers to binge and resultant behavior. Patient continues to challenge irrational thoughts and beliefs in individual and group sessions. Patient plans meals, including "forbidden foods."
	1f. Teach patient to plan and eat regularly scheduled, balanced meals.	1f. This teaching helps to ensure success in maintaining abstinence from binge-purge activity.	**WEEK 4:** Patient reports no binge-purge behaviors at day program or outside. Patient demonstrates understanding of repetitive nature of binge-purge cycle. Patient continues to challenge irrational thoughts and beliefs.

Evaluation

At the end of 4 weeks, Sally reports no binge-purge cycles, and her potassium level remains consistently within normal limits. She is beginning to plan meals and challenge irrational thoughts and beliefs.

ASSESSMENT GUIDELINES

Binge Eating Disorder

Determine whether:

1. A thorough physical examination with appropriate blood work has been done.
2. Other medical conditions have been identified.
3. Comorbid psychiatric diagnoses are present.
4. A careful history of bingeing triggers, foods, and frequency has been collected.
5. The patient's self-esteem is overly influenced by his or her physical appearance because this overvaluation tends to indicate a more difficult recovery (Grilo, 2012).

DIAGNOSIS

Imbalanced nutrition: more than body requirements is usually the most appropriate initial nursing diagnosis for individuals with binge eating disorder. Other nursing diagnoses are similar to bulimia nervosa and include *disturbed body image, ineffective coping, anxiety, chronic low self-esteem, powerlessness,* and *social isolation.*

OUTCOMES IDENTIFICATION

To evaluate the effectiveness of treatment, outcome criteria are established to measure treatment results. Patients are included in their development. Table 18-5 provides a summary of signs and symptoms, nursing diagnoses, and general outcomes for binge eating disorder.

PLANNING

Planning the care of these patients includes the usual diet and exercise elements for all weight loss programs. One major difference in binge eating is the complications that arise due to the larger than normal volume of food consumed during a binge. These episodes of abnormal eating cause gastrointestinal problems associated with the periodic dilation of the stomach. These patients have significant difficulties with heartburn, dysphagia, bloating, and abdominal pain as well as diarrhea, urgency, constipation, and a feeling of anal blockage (Cremonini et al., 2009). The nurse will need to help these patients manage dysregulation of the entire gastrointestinal tract.

IMPLEMENTATION

Acute Care

Although obesity puts these patients at risk for diabetes, hypertension, and heart disease, hospitalization to treat the binge eating itself is not indicated. Treatment is usually provided in an outpatient setting.

Psychosocial Interventions

Cognitive behavioral therapy and interpersonal psychotherapy are proven to be effective treatments to reduce the number and severity of binge eating (Wilson et al., 2010); however, without behavioral weight loss programs, the patients may merely stop gaining weight. Variations of cognitive behavioral therapy and dialectical behavior therapy are being developed to address the specific needs of patients with binge eating disorder.

TABLE 18-5 SIGNS AND SYMPTOMS, NURSING DIAGNOSES, AND OUTCOMES FOR BINGE EATING DISORDER

SIGNS AND SYMPTOMS	NURSING DIAGNOSES	OUTCOMES
Dysfunctional eating pattern, eating in response to internal cues, sedentary lifestyle, weight significantly over ideal for height and frame, intake exceeds metabolic need	*Imbalanced nutrition: More than body requirements*	Nutrient intake meets metabolic needs
Embarrassment due to weight gain, fear of negative reactions by others, attempts to hide weight gain, body dissatisfaction	*Disturbed body image*	Congruence between body reality, body ideal, and body presentation; satisfaction with body appearance
Eats as a coping method, absence of other more effective coping methods, eats even when full	*Ineffective coping*	Demonstrates effective coping, reports decrease in stress, uses personal support system, uses effective coping strategies, reports increase in psychological comfort
Feelings of discomfort or dread, feelings of inadequacy, focused on self, increased wariness, irritability, heart pounding, increased blood pressure and pulse	*Anxiety*	Verbalizes a positive level of confidence; makes informed life decisions, expresses independence with decision-making processes
Loss of control of eating, feelings of shame and guilt, views self as unable to deal with events	*Chronic low self-esteem* *Powerlessness*	Verbalizes a positive level of confidence; makes informed life decisions, expresses independence with decision-making processes
Absence of supportive significant other(s), eats normally in the presence of others, hides eating behaviors, reports feeling alone	*Social isolation*	Willing to call on others for assistance, develops a confidant relationship, feels a sense of belonging

From Herdman, T. H. (Ed.), (2012). *Nursing diagnoses—Definitions and classification 2012-2014.* Copyright © 2012, 1994-2012 by NANDA International. Used by arrangement with John Wiley & Sons Limited; Moorhead, S., Johnson, M., Maas, M. L., & Swanson, E. (2013). *Nursing outcomes classification (NOC)* (5th ed.). St. Louis, MO: Mosby.

18-3 CASE STUDY AND NURSING CARE PLAN

Binge Eating Disorder

Angela is a 25-year-old schoolteacher who gives a history of overeating since the age of 10 years. She seeks treatment at a community mental health center because she has recently felt more depressed.

Self-Assessment

The nurse assigned to Angela is Bernice. Bernice is new to the community mental health center, and her experience as a psychiatric nurse is primarily with the seriously mentally ill. She has never worked with a patient with an eating disorder. During Bernice's initial contact with Angela, she feels revulsion with regard to Angela's weight. Bernice speaks to her nurse supervisor about this feeling because she is unable to identify where this feeling comes from and is not sure she can control it. The supervisor recognizes that Bernice's feelings will interfere with creating a therapeutic alliance with Angela and decides to reassign Bernice and provide her with additional support and education regarding the care of the patient with an eating disorder.

Assessment

Objective Data

- Height: 61 inches (5 feet 1 inch)
- Weight: 200 lb—180% of ideal weight
- Uncontrollable eating pattern
- Sad facial expression
- Minimal success with participation in Weight Watchers and Overeaters Anonymous programs

Subjective Data

- "I'll eat anything in sight."
- "I wish I wouldn't wake up in the morning."
- "I once showed promise, and look at me now."
- "I don't take laxatives or diuretics, and I don't vomit."
- "I am not suicidal."

Diagnosis

Imbalanced nutrition: more than body requirements related to compulsive overeating, including episodes of bingeing

Outcomes Identification

Patient will normalize eating pattern and achieve a specific target weight according to a predetermined plan.

Implementation

Angela's care plan is personalized as follows:

SHORT-TERM GOAL	INTERVENTION	RATIONALE	EVALUATION
1. Patient will demonstrate at least two coping strategies that result in adhering to a structured meal schedule.	1a. Clinical nurse specialist can use many techniques of cognitive-behavioral therapy in addressing the issues of overweight and disordered eating. Patient should begin a journal. 1b. Teach the patient to structure and plan ahead for times and places where she will have her meals and snacks for the day.	1a. Cognitive-behavioral techniques can be useful in addressing automatic behaviors. Recording what, when, and where one eats begins to identify patterns that can be modified. 1b. Organization and structure can allow for a different choice.	**WEEK 1:** Patient selects a meal plan with structured times and places; begins journal and maintains it consistently. Patient begins to relate feelings about eating. **WEEK 2:** Patient is able to adhere to structured meal schedule approximately 25% of the time. Patient expresses the struggle and feelings of tension around implementing structured meal schedule; some modifications are made to allow the patient to be more successful. Patient shares contents of journal, which she consistently maintains. Patient reports weight is unchanged; patient was unable to change pattern of exercise.
	1c. Teach patient not to abstain from eating for longer periods of time than planned to avoid rebound binge eating. 1d. Review the nutritional content of dietary intake to ensure consumption of a balanced diet.	1c, 1d. Extended periods of abstinence, restrictive dietary intake, or very-low-calorie diet can result in rebound overeating.	**WEEK 3:** Patient is adhering to schedule 50% of the time. Patient shares journal entries and relates thoughts and feelings concerning eating. Patient reports 0.5-lb weight loss. Patient is beginning to walk for a half hour as part of her daily routine.
	1e. Review journal with patient to identify areas for improvement in adhering to the treatment plan. 1f. Explore with patient the thoughts and feelings she is experiencing about this new regimen. 1g. Identify thoughts, beliefs, and underlying assumptions that reinforce disordered eating patterns. 1h. Establish a once-a-week schedule of weighing.	1e. The journal is an important tool in modifying eating behaviors. 1f, 1g. Nurse must be empathetic and supportive of patient's experience, which is one of struggle accompanied by feelings of tension. 1h. From day to day, there may be minimal or no weight reduction, which can lead to discouragement.	**WEEK 4:** Patient continues to adhere to structured schedule approximately 75% of the time. Patient walks regularly, experiencing a better sense of well-being. Patient thinks she is up to the challenge of continuing the plan to normalize her eating pattern and increase her energy expenditure. Patient's weight is 196 lb (– 4 lb); she acknowledges that progress has and will continue to be slow.

Evaluation

At the end of 4 weeks, Angela's weight is 196 lb. She adheres to a structured meal plan 75% of the time and has increased her exercise by incorporating daily walks into her routine.

Psychobiological Interventions

Pharmacological Interventions

Because of their efficacy with bulimia, the use of SSRIs at or near the high end of the dosage range has been studied to treat binge eating disorder and seems to help in the short term; however, patients regained significant weight after discontinuance of medication. Other medications that are under investigation include the tricyclic antidepressants, antiepileptic agents, and appetite suppressants (Treasure et al., 2010).

The history of "diet pills" has been marked by problems and product withdrawals such as Fen-phen (fenfluramine), a drug that was withdrawn after serious side effects related to heart valves. The first weight-loss drugs in more than a decade were approved in 2012 (Food and Drug Administration [FDA], 2012a, 2012b). While both of the drugs are associated with risks, the advisory panels decided that the risks of untreated obesity were greater. They are approved for persons with body mass index (BMI) of 30 or more or for adults with a BMI of 27 or more who have at least one health condition such as hypertension, high cholesterol, or type 2 diabetes.

Belviq (pronounced bel-veek) (lorcaserin) is designed to make individuals feel full after eating smaller meals by activating a serotonin 2c receptor in the brain and blocking appetite signals. It should be used in combination with exercise and a reduced-calorie diet. Patients who used this drug in clinical trials lost an average of 5% of body weight. The FDA warns that the drug should be stopped if a patient does not experience 5% weight loss after 12 weeks of use. Additionally, while safe at prescribed doses, higher doses affect different serotonin receptors that will create a high response, thereby making this a Schedule IV drug. Pregnant or nursing women should not take this drug. Side effects include headache, dizziness, fatigue, nausea, dry mouth, and constipation, and additional side effects in diabetic patients are low blood sugar (hypoglycemia), headache, back pain, cough, and fatigue.

Qsymia (pronounced kyoo-sim-EE-uh) is made up of two different drugs. One half of Qsymia is the antiseizure medication topiramate; it produces feelings of fullness, reduced taste sensation, and quicker calorie burning. The other half is phentermine, the safer part of Fen-phen, an appetite suppressant that works by neural norepinephrine release that influences blood concentration of the appetite-regulating hormone leptin. Qsymia is a Schedule IV controlled substance due to the amphetamine-like effects of phentermine. Women who take this drug must also use birth control since it is associated with birth defects. Contraindications include glaucoma, monoamine inhibitor use, and hyperthyroidism. The most common side effects of Qsymia are tingling of hands and feet (paresthesia), dizziness, altered taste sensation, insomnia, constipation, and dry mouth.

Surgical Interventions

Bariatric surgery is a controversial option for the treatment of obesity. While all persons who are obese do not suffer from binge eating disorder, the addition of this disorder into the equation has been thought to reduce the effectiveness of bariatric surgery. Malone and Alger-Mayer (2012) investigated the relationship of the severity of binge eating behavior *before* bariatric surgery and binge eating behavior, depression scores, and quality of life *after* surgery. After 12 months, patients who had the most severe binge eating behaviors demonstrated the most improvement.

Health Teaching and Health Promotion

Patients struggling with binge eating disorder have been using food to regulate their mood and will need to learn new coping strategies for the challenges in their lives. Education centered on healthy eating and exercise will need to be reinforced within a caring nurse-patient relationship. At first, the focus of change will be the binge eating itself. Once abstinence has been established, the focus may change to slow and steady weight loss to improve the person's overall health.

Teamwork and Safety

As stated previously, unless patients have a medical complication requiring hospitalization, they are not generally seen in psychiatric settings for this disorder. If the patient can identify emotional or physical triggers to bingeing episodes, the nurse can help with strategies to avoid or alter these triggers. In addition, these patients are emotionally vulnerable and need guidance to seek out people to support them such as self-help groups or supportive group therapies.

Advanced Practice Interventions

Psychotherapy

Cognitive-behavioral therapy, behavior therapy, dialectical behavior therapy, and interpersonal therapy have all been associated with binge frequency reduction rates of 67% or more and significant abstinence rates during active treatment (APA, 2006). Many advanced practice nurses are qualified to provide these therapies. Case Study and Nursing Care Plan 18-3 presents a patient with binge eating disorder.

EVALUATION

Box 18-7 presents relevant *Nursing Interventions Classification (NIC)* interventions for the management of eating disorders (Bulechek et al., 2013).

FEEDING AND ELIMINATION DISORDERS

We have all witnessed children with picky eating habits; children with feeding disorders take this problem to an extreme. One major difference between picky children and children with feeding disorders is that children with feeding disorders are so extremely selective that they will not eat outside of their home environment. The three feeding disorders usually seen in infancy and childhood include **pica, rumination** disorder, and avoidant/restrictive food intake disorder. Box 18-8 identifies the diagnostic criteria for these disorders.

Up to 40% of all toddlers will experience mealtime difficulties that resolve spontaneously with or without caregiver support and education. About 5% to 20% of children without other disorders could be diagnosed with feeding disorders.

BOX 18-7 *NIC* INTERVENTIONS FOR EATING DISORDERS MANAGEMENT

Definition: Prevention and treatment of severe diet restriction and overexercising or bingeing and purging of food and fluids.

Teamwork
- Collaborate with other members of health care team to develop treatment plan; involve patient and/or significant others as appropriate.
- Confer with team and patient to set a target weight if patient is not within a recommended weight range for age and body frame.
- Confer with dietitian to determine daily caloric intake necessary to attain and/or maintain target weight. Encourage patient to discuss food preferences with dietitian.
- Confer with the health care team on a routine basis about patient's progress.

Monitoring
- Monitor physiological parameters (vital signs, electrolyte levels) as needed.
- Weigh on a routine basis (e.g., at same time of day and after voiding).
- Monitor daily caloric intake and intake and output of fluids, as appropriate.
- Restrict food availability to scheduled, pre-served meals and snacks.
- Encourage self-monitoring of daily food intake and weight gain/maintenance as appropriate.
- Observe patient during and after meals/snacks to ensure that adequate intake is achieved and maintained.
- Accompany patient to bathroom during designated observation times following meals/snacks.
- Limit time spent in bathroom during periods when not under direct supervision.
- Limit physical activity as needed to promote weight gain.

Support
- Use behavioral contracting with patient to elicit desired weight gain or maintenance behaviors.
- Use behavior modification techniques to promote behaviors that contribute to weight gain and limit weight-loss behaviors, as appropriate.
- Provide reinforcement for weight gain and behaviors that promote weight gain.
- Provide support (e.g., relaxation therapy, desensitization exercises, opportunities to talk about feelings) as patient integrates new eating behaviors, changing body image, and lifestyle changes.
- Encourage patient use of daily logs to record feelings and circumstances surrounding urge to purge, vomit, or overexercise.
- Assist patient (and significant others, as appropriate) to examine and resolve personal issues that may contribute to the eating disorder.
- Assist patient to develop a self-esteem that is compatible with a healthy body weight.

Promote Increasing Independence
- Allow opportunity to make limited choices about eating and exercise as weight gain progresses in desirable manner.
- Initiate maintenance phase of treatment when patient has achieved target weight and has consistently shown desired eating behaviors for designated period of time.
- Place responsibility for choices about eating and physical activity with patient, as appropriate.
- Institute a treatment program and follow-up care (medical, counseling) for home management.

From Bulechek, G. M., Butcher, H. K., Dochterman, J. M., & Wagner, C. (2013). *Nursing interventions classification (NIC)* (6th ed). St. Louis, MO: Mosby.

BOX 18-8 CHARACTERISTICS OF FEEDING PROBLEMS

PICA	RUMINATION	AVOIDANT/RESTRICTIVE
• Eating nonfood items after maturing past toddlerhood • Not culturally sanctioned • Not part of any other mental illness	• Regurgitation with rechewing, reswallowing or spitting • No GI or medical reason • Not part of other mental illness or eating disorder	• Avoiding or restricting foods starting in childhood • Significantly low BMI • Dependent on enteral feeding or experiencing nutritional deficiencies • No distortion of body image • Not medically explained or part of any other mental illness

Prematurity, failure to thrive, autism, and genetic syndromes result in ranges of 40-80% with feeding disorders (Nationwide Childrens, n.d.). In fact, up to 89% of children with the autism spectrum disorders have strong preferences for certain foods and disrupt mealtimes with food refusal. There are no unifying etiologies for food refusal, and the primary treatment modality is some form of behavioral modification (Sharp et al., 2010). Families caring for a child with a feeding disorder often need support and education in specific behavioral techniques, but family therapy is not usually needed.

Elimination disorders are fairly common and refer to problems related to urinating or defecating at an age or situation where such behavior would be unusual. **Enuresis** is the voiding of urine during the day (diurnal) or at night (nocturnal). **Encopresis** refers to unsuccessful bowel control. Box 18-9 provides characteristics of elimination disorders.

BOX 18-9 CHARACTERISTICS OF ELIMINATION PROBLEMS

ENURESIS	ENCOPRESIS
• Behavioral disorder in children who are developmentally older than age 5 • Involuntary or intentional voiding of urine into clothing or bed • Occurs twice a week for more than 3 months. • Subtypes: Nocturnal, diurnal, or nocturnal and diurnal.	• Behavioral disorder in children who are developmentally older than age 4 • Involuntary or intentional inappropriate passing of feces • Occurs once a month for more than 3 months • Subtypes: With constipation and overflow incontinence or without constipation and overflow incontinence.

From National Institute of Diabetes and Digestive and Kidney Diseases. (2012) *Urinary incontinence in children*. Retrieved from http://kidney.niddk.nih.gov/kudiseases/pubs/uichildren; Har, A. F., & Croffie, J. M. (2010). Encopresis. *Pediatrics in Review, 31*(9) 368–374. Retrieved from http://pedsinreview.aappublications.org/content/31/9/368.extract.

Before any child is given the diagnosis of an elimination disorder, all possible medical explanations for the pattern must be ruled out. If a neurological condition or a medication side effect is responsible, that cause must be resolved before any behavioral intervention is considered. The elimination disorders are also more common in the developmentally disabled pediatric population, and treatments must be suited to the special needs of these children. Nurses can help the caretakers in these families through psychoeducation (Hardy, 2009).

These disorders often cause the child to feel shame, and it is important to teach all caregivers, including schoolteachers, to avoid any punitive measures such as forcing the child to clean soiled clothing. Encopresis often causes unpleasant odors that may require some milieu management to prevent the child from becoming socially isolated. There is little research into effective treatments for the elimination disorders. Generally, the child is assisted in enhancing self-care that includes managing dietary and toileting activities that normalize elimination patterns.

KEY POINTS TO REMEMBER

- A number of theoretical models help explain the origins of eating disorders.
- Neurobiological theories focus on neurotransmitters in the brain that regulate mood and hunger.
- Psychological theories explore issues of control in anorexia and affective instability and poor impulse control in bulimia.
- Genetic theories postulate the existence of vulnerabilities that may predispose people toward eating disorders.
- Sociocultural models look at our present societal ideal of being thin.
- Men with eating disorders share many of the characteristics of women with eating disorders.
- Anorexia nervosa is a potentially life-threatening eating disorder that includes severe underweight; low blood pressure, pulse, and temperature; dehydration; and low serum potassium level and dysrhythmias.
- Anorexia may be treated in an inpatient treatment setting in which milieu therapy, psychotherapy (cognitive), development of self-care skills, and psychobiological interventions can be implemented.
- Long-term treatment is provided on an outpatient basis and aims to help patients maintain healthy weight. It includes treatment modalities such as individual therapy, family therapy, group therapy, psychopharmacology, and nutrition counseling.
- Patients with bulimia nervosa are typically within the normal weight range, but some may be slightly below or above ideal body weight.
- Assessment of the bulimic patient may show enlargement of the parotid glands and dental erosion and caries if the patient has induced vomiting.
- Acute care may be necessary when life-threatening complications such as gastric rupture (rare), electrolyte imbalance, and cardiac dysrhythmias are present.
- The goal of interventions is to interrupt the binge-purge cycle. Psychotherapy and self-care skill training are included in the treatment plan.
- Long-term treatment focuses on therapy aimed at addressing any coexisting depression, substance abuse, and/or personality disorders that are causing the patient distress and interfering with the quality of life. Self-worth and interpersonal functioning eventually become issues that are useful for the patient to target.
- Effective treatment for obese patients with binge eating disorder includes binge abstinence, improvement of depressive symptoms, and achievement of an appropriate weight for the individual.
- Patients with binge-eating disorder often have upper and lower GI problems that bring them to medical professionals for management.
- Feeding disorders have multiple etiologies and are often associated with developmental delays of childhood.
- The primary treatment for feeding disorders involves behavioral interventions to increase food consumption and reduce delaying behaviors.
- The elimination disorders are associated with client shame that is often reinforced by caregivers who do not understand the disorder.

CRITICAL THINKING

1. Logan, a 19-year-old male model, has experienced a rapid decrease in weight over the last 4 months after his agent told him he would have to lose some weight or lose a coveted account. Logan is 6 feet 2 inches tall and weighs 132 pounds, down from his usual 176 pounds. He is brought to the emergency department with a pulse of 40 beats per minute and severe arrhythmias. His laboratory workup reveals severe hypokalemia. He has become extremely depressed, saying, "I'm too fat. . . . I don't want anything to eat. . . . If I gain weight, my life will be ruined. There is nothing to live for if I can't model." Logan's parents are startled and confused, and his best friend is worried and feels powerless to help Logan. "I tell Logan he needs to eat or he will die. . . . I tell him he is a skeleton, but he refuses to listen to me. I don't know what to do."
   a. Which physical and psychiatric criteria suggest that Logan should be immediately hospitalized?
   b. What are some of the questions you would eventually ask Logan when evaluating his biopsychosocial functioning?

c. What are your feelings toward someone with anorexia? Can you make a distinction between your thoughts and feelings toward women with anorexia and toward men with anorexia?
d. What are some things you could do for Logan's parents and friend in terms of offering them information, support, and referrals? Identify specific referrals.
e. Explain the kinds of interventions or restrictions that may be used while Logan is hospitalized (e.g., weighing, observation after eating or visits, exercise, therapy, self-care).
f. How would you describe partial hospitalization programs or psychiatric home care programs when asked if Logan will have to be hospitalized for an extended period?
g. Identify at least five criteria that, if met, would indicate that Logan was improving.

2. You and Heather have been close friends since nursing school and are now working on the same surgical unit. Heather told you that in the past she has made several suicide attempts. Today, you come upon her bingeing off the unit, and she looks embarrassed and uncomfortable when she sees you. Several times you notice that she spends time in the bathroom, and you hear sounds of retching. In response to your concern, she admits that she has been binge-purging for several years but that now she is getting out of control and feels profoundly depressed.
   a. Although Heather does not show any physical signs of bulimia nervosa, what would you look for when assessing an individual with bulimia?
   b. What kinds of emergencies could result from bingeing and purging?
   c. What would be the most useful type of psychotherapy for Heather initially, and what issues would need to be addressed?
   d. What kinds of new skills does a person with bulimia need to learn to lessen the compulsion to binge and purge?
   e. What would be some signs that Heather is recovering?

CHAPTER REVIEW

1. While on an inpatient unit, you are caring for newly admitted Alyssa, a 16-year-old diagnosed with anorexia nervosa. Number the following nursing interventions in order of priority:
   a. ___ Initiate a therapeutic relationship.
   b. ___ Promote caloric consumption.
   c. ___ Assess for suicidal ideation
   d. ___ Review accomplishments made during treatment.
   e. ___ Explore feelings of underlying anxiety and low self-esteem.
2. Brittany is caring for a patient with bulimia. She recognizes which of the following nursing interventions as being most appropriate?
   a. Monitor the patient on bathroom trips after eating.
   b. Allow the patient extensive private time with family members.
   c. Provide meals whenever the patient requests them.
   d. Encourage the patient to select foods that she likes.
3. The nurse is admitting a patient who weighs 100 pounds, is 66 inches tall, and is below ideal body weight. The patient's blood pressure is 130/80 mm Hg, pulse is 72 beats per minute, potassium is 2.5 mmol/L, and ECG is abnormal. Her teeth enamel is eroded, her hands are shaking, and her parotid gland is enlarged. The patient states, "I am really nervous about coming to this unit." What is the priority nursing diagnosis?
   a. Powerlessness
   b. Risk for injury
   c. Imbalanced nutrition: Less than body requirements
   d. Anxiety
4. The nurse is planning care for a patient with a binge eating disorder. What outcomes are appropriate? *Select all that apply.*
   a. The patient will identify stressors that lead to binge eating.
   b. The patient will identify four alternate coping skills.
   c. The patient will increase dietary intake.
   d. The patient will experience satisfaction in eating alone.
5. Which of the following are true regarding feeding disorders in children? *Select all that apply.*
   a. Feeding disorders usually reflect poor parenting.
   b. Feeding disorders are often manifested in children with developmental delays.
   c. Feeding disorders are most often treated with a punishment system.
   d. In many cases, toddler mealtime difficulties spontaneously resolve with no intervention.
   e. Behavior modification has been found to be effective in treating feeding disorders.

Answers to Chapter Review

1. a = 1, b = 3, c = 2, d = 5, e = 4; 2. a; 3. c; 4. a, b; 5. b, d, e.

evolve WEBSITE

Visit the Evolve website for a posttest on the content in this chapter: http://evolve.elsevier.com/Varcarolis

Post-Test interactive review

REFERENCES

American Psychiatric Association (APA). (2006). *Practice guideline for the treatment of patients with eating disorders* (3rd ed.). Washington, DC: Author.

American Psychiatric Association (APA). (2013). *DSM-5 table of contents.* Retrieved from http://www.psychiatry.org/dsm5.

Bienvenu, O. J., Davydow, D. S., & Kendler, K. S. (2011). Psychiatric 'diseases' versus behavioral disorders and degree of genetic influence. *Psychological Medicine, 41*(1), 33–40.

Breuner, C. C. (2010). Complementary, holistic, and integrative medicine: Eating disorders. *Pediatrics in Review, 31*(10), e75–82. doi:10.1542/pir.31-10-e75.

Campbell, I. C., Mill, J., Uher, R., & Schmidt, U. (2011). Eating disorders, gene-environment interactions and epigenetics. *Neuroscience and Biobehavioral Reviews, 35*(3), 784–793.

Caparrotta, L., & Ghaffari, K. (2006). A historical overview of the psychodynamic contributions to the understanding of eating disorders. *Psychoanalytic Psychotherapy, 20*(3), 175–196.

Cremonini, F., Camilleri, M., Clark, M. M., Beebe, T. J., Locke, G. R., Zinsmeister, A. R., et al. (2009). Associations among binge eating behavior patterns and gastrointestinal symptoms: A population-based study. *International Journal of Obesity, 33*(3), 342–353.

Custers, K., & Van, D. B. (2009). Viewership of pro-anorexia websites in seventh, ninth and eleventh graders. *European Eating Disorders Review: The Journal of the Eating Disorders Association, 17*(3), 214–219.

Eisenberg, M. E., & Neumark-Sztainer, D. (2010). Friends' dieting and disordered eating behaviors among adolescents five years later: Findings from project EAT. *Journal of Adolescent Health, 47*(1), 67–73. doi:10.1016/j.jadohealth.2009.12.030.

Ferguson, C., Christopher J., Munoz, M. E., Contreras, S., & Velasquez, K. (2011). Mirror, mirror on the wall: Peer competition, television influences, and body image dissatisfaction. *Journal of Social & Clinical Psychology, 30*(5), 458–483. doi:10.1521/jscp.2011.30.5.458.

Food and Drug Administration. (2012a). *FDA approves Belviq to treat some overweight or obese adults*. Retrieved from http://www.fda.gov/NewsEvents/Newsroom/PressAnnouncements/ucm309993.htm.

Food and Drug Administration. (2012b). *FDA approves weight management drug Qsymia*. Retrieved from http://www.fda.gov/NewsEvents/Newsroom/PressAnnouncements/ucm312468.htm.

Halmi, K. A. (2011). Eating disorders: Anorexia nervosa, bulimia nervosa, and obesity. In R. E. Hales, S. C. Yudofsky, G. O. Gabbard, R. E. Hales, S. C. Yudofsky, & G. O. Gabbard (Eds.), *Essentials of psychiatry* (3rd ed.) (pp. 429–453). Arlington, VA: American Psychiatric Publishing.

Hardy, L. T. (2009). Encopresis: A guide for psychiatric nurses. *Archives of Psychiatric Nursing, 23*(5), 351–358. doi:10.1016/j.apnu.2008.09.002.

Helverskov, J., Clausen, L., Mors, O., Frydenberg, M., Thomsen, P., & Rokkedal, K. (2010). Trans-diagnostic outcome of eating disorders: A 30-month follow-up study of 629 patients. *European Eating Disorders Review, 18*(6), 453–463. doi:10.1002/erv.1025.

Herdman, T. H. (Ed.), (2012). *NANDA international nursing diagnoses: Definitions and classification, 2012-2014*. Oxford, UK: Wiley Blackwell.

Hudson, J. I., Hiripi, E., Pope, H. G., Jr., & Kessler, R. C. (2007). The prevalence and correlates of eating disorders in the national comorbidity survey replication. *Biological Psychiatry, 61*(3), 348–358.

Kaye, W. H., Fudge, J. L., & Paulus, M. (2009). New insights into symptoms and neurocircuit function of anorexia nervosa. *Nature Reviews Neuroscience, 10*(8), 573–584. doi:10.1038/nrn2682.

Kaye, W. H., & Strober, M. A. (2009). Neurobiology of eating disorders. In A. F. Schatzberg, C. B. Nemeroff, A. F. Schatzberg, & C. B. Nemeroff (Eds.), *The American Psychiatric Publishing textbook of psychopharmacology* (4th ed.) (pp. 1022–1043). Arlington, VA: American Psychiatric Publishing.

Kohn, M. R., Madden, S., & Clarke, S. D. (2011). Refeeding in anorexia nervosa: Increased safety and efficiency through understanding the pathophysiology of protein calorie malnutrition. *Current Opinion in Pediatrics, 23*(4), 390–394.

Kong, S., & Bernstein, K. (2009). Childhood trauma as a predictor of eating psychopathology and its mediating variables in patients with eating disorders. *Journal of Clinical Nursing, 18*(13), 1897–1907. doi:10.1111/j.1365-2702.2008.02740.x.

Le Grange, D., Lock, J., Loeb, K., & Nicholls, D. (2010). Academy for eating disorders position paper: The role of the family in eating disorders. *The International Journal of Eating Disorders, 43*(1), 1–5.

Malone, M., & Alger-Mayer, S. (2012). Binge status and quality of life after gastric bypass surgery: A one-year study. *Obesity research, 12*(3), 473–481. doi:10.1038/oby.2004.5.

Moorhead, S., Johnson, M., Maas, M. L., & Swanson, E. (Eds.). (2013). *Nursing outcomes classification (NOC)* (5th ed.). St. Louis, MO: Mosby.

Nationwide Children's Hospital. (n.d.). *Feeding disorders*. Retrieved from http://www.nationwidechildrens.org/feeding-disorders-1.

Ogden, C. L., Carroll, M. D., Kit, B. K., & Flegal, K. M. (2012). *Prevalence of obesity in the United States 2009-2010*. Retrieved from http://www.cdc.gov/nchs/data/databriefs/db82.pdf.

Sansone, R. A., & Sansone, L. A. (2011). Personality pathology and its influence on eating disorders. *Innovations in Clinical Neuroscience, 8*(3), 14–18.

Sharp, W., Jaquess, D. L., Morton, J. F., & Herzinger, C. V. (2010). Pediatric feeding disorders: A quantitative synthesis of treatment outcomes. *Clinical Child and Family Psychology Review, 13*(4), 348–365.

Swanson, S. A., Crow, S. J., Le Grange, D., Swendsen, J., & Merikangas, K. R. (2011). Prevalence and correlates of eating disorders in adolescents: Results from the national comorbidity survey replication adolescent supplement. *Archives of General Psychiatry, 68*(7), 714–723.

Sysko, R., Roberto, C. A., Barnes, R. D., Grilo, C. M., Attia, E., & Walsh, B. T. (2012). Test-retest reliability of the proposed DSM-5 eating disorder diagnostic criteria. *Psychiatry Research, 196*(2–3), 302–308.

Treasure, J., Claudino, A. M., & Zucker, N. (2010). Eating disorders. *Lancet, 375*(9714), 583–593. doi:10.1016/S0140-6736(09)61748-7.

Walsh, B. T., & Sysko, R. (2009). Broad categories for the diagnosis of eating disorders (BCD-ED): An alternative system for classification. *International Journal of Eating Disorders, 42*, 754–764.

Wilson, G. T., Wilfley, D. E., Agras, W. S., & Bryson, M. A. (2010). Psychological treatments of binge eating disorder. *Archives of General Psychiatry, 67*(1), 94-101.

Wright, K. M., & Hacking, S. (2011). An angel on my shoulder: A study of relationships between women with anorexia and healthcare professionals. *Journal of Psychiatric and Mental Health Nursing, 19*(2), 107–115.

Viladrich, A., Yeh, M., Bruning, N., & Weiss, R. (2009). 'Do real women have curves?' Paradoxical body images among Latinas in New York City. *Journal of Immigrant and Minority Health, 11*(1), 20–28. doi:10.1007/s10903-008-9176-9.

CHAPTER

19

Sleep-Wake Disorders

Margaret Trussler

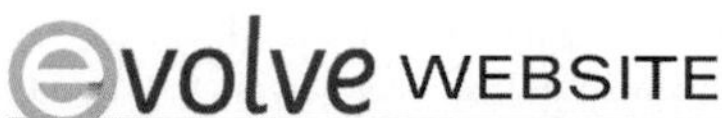

Visit the Evolve website for a pretest on the content in this chapter: *http://evolve.elsevier.com/Varcarolis*

Pre-Test interactive review

OBJECTIVES

1. Discuss the impact of inadequate sleep on overall physical and mental health.
2. Describe the social and economic impact of sleep disturbance and chronic sleep deprivation.
3. Recognize the risks to personal and community safety imposed by sleep disturbance and chronic sleep deprivation.
4. Describe normal sleep physiology and explain the variations in normal sleep.
5. Identify the major categories and medical diagnoses for sleep disorders.
6. Identify the predisposing, precipitating, and perpetuating factors for patients with insomnia.
7. Apply the nursing process in caring for individuals with sleep disorders.
8. Describe the use of two assessment tools in the evaluation of patients experiencing sleep disturbance.
9. Formulate three nursing diagnoses for patients experiencing a sleep disturbance.
10. Develop a teaching plan for a patient with insomnia disorder, incorporating principles of sleep restriction, stimulus control, and cognitive-behavioral therapy.
11. Develop a care plan for the patient experiencing sleep disturbance incorporating basic sleep hygiene principles.

KEY TERMS AND CONCEPTS

basal sleep requirement
circadian drive
excessive sleepiness
hypersomnolence
sleep architecture
sleep continuity
sleep deprivation
sleep drive
sleep efficiency
sleep fragmentation
sleep hygiene
sleep latency
sleep restriction
stimulus control

Sleep and sleep disorders are receiving increased attention in the medical, nursing, research, and social science literature. Obtaining sufficient quality sleep is now recognized as a key determinant of health and well-being (Grandner, 2012). *Healthy People 2020* added sleep health to the list of current health topics, making sleep a national health priority.

The National Center on Sleep Disorder Research (NCSDR) was established in 1996 to facilitate research, training, health information dissemination, and other activities with respect to the basic understanding of sleep and sleep disorders. Under the guidance of the NCSDR, and other organizations such as the National Sleep Foundation (NSF) and the American Academy of Sleep Medicine (AASM), there has been exponential growth in the scientific understanding of sleep over the last 16 years. Despite the increased recognition of the importance of sleep, investment in sleep-related research, and tremendous growth

HEALTH POLICY

Healthy People 2020 and Sleep

Healthy People 2020 added sleep health to the national health agenda with the goal of "increasing public knowledge of how adequate sleep and treatment of sleep disorders improve health, productivity, wellness, quality of life, and safety on roads and in the workplace." Four goals were identified:

1. Increase the proportion of persons with symptoms of obstructive sleep apnea who seek medical evaluation.
2. Reduce the rate of vehicular crashes per 100 million miles traveled that are due to drowsy driving.
3. Increase the proportion of students in grades 9 through 12 who get sufficient sleep.
4. Increase the proportion of adults who get sufficient sleep.

Nurses can be instrumental in advancing the sleep goals of *Healthy People 2020* through increased clinical awareness of the importance of sleep, advocating for policy change that brings the problems of inadequate sleep and its consequences into sharp focus, and developing programs that directly serve to advance the Healthy People goals. *Healthy People 2020* offers a simple guide to implementing the Healthy People goals using the MAP-IT (**M**obilize, **A**ssess, **P**lan, **I**mplement, **T**rack) framework. Consider adopting one of the sleep goals to implement a policy change in your community using this framework. For more information and ideas on how to get started see the *Healthy People 2020* website, http://www.healthypeople.gov/2020/default.aspx, and click on *Implementing Healthy People* (USDHHS, 2012).

in our understanding of sleep physiology and pathology, application of the findings has continued to be slow.

SLEEP

Sleep has become an expendable commodity. In a fast-paced society, sleep is often forfeited, and people subject themselves to schedules that disrupt normal sleep physiology. People frequently cut back on sleep to meet other social and vocational demands with compensated work time, time in academic activities, and travel time to and from work and school being the most potent determinant of total sleep time; the more time devoted to work-related activities, the less time spent sleeping (Knutson et al., 2010).

The NSF (2012a) recommends that the average adult get 7 to 9 hours of sleep each night, yet annual surveys conducted by the NSF between 2002 and 2012 have consistently demonstrated that the average adult gets less than 7 hours of sleep most nights of the week (NSF, 2012b). While currently there seems to be some debate as to whether secular sleep trends have decreased over the last century (Bin et al., 2012), it does seem that the portion of short sleepers (i.e., individuals who sleep 6 hours or less per night) has increased over the last several decades among full-time workers, a period when the prevalence of chronic disease (such as diabetes, cardiovascular disease, and obesity) that may be linked to sleep has also significantly increased (Knutson et al., 2010).

The 2011 NSF *Sleep in America Poll* indicates that 63% of Americans do not believe that they are meeting their sleep needs during the work week; 7% of those between the ages of 13 and 18 and 15% of adults between the ages of 19 and 64 say they sleep less than 6 hours on weeknights due to work- or school-related activities.

Consequence of Sleep Loss

The major consequence of acute or chronic sleep curtailment is **excessive sleepiness**. Excessive sleepiness is a subjective report of difficulty staying awake that is serious enough to impact social and vocational functioning and increase the risk for accident or injury. While self-imposed sleep restriction is a common cause of excessive sleepiness, disruption of the normal sleep cycle (as seen in shift work), underlying sleep disorders, medications, alcohol and substance use, and many medical and psychiatric disorders are important causes of excessive sleepiness.

We need to only look to our own experiences with acute or total sleep loss to recognize its consequences. After a poor night's sleep, we feel tired, lethargic, and out of synch. The effects of chronic sleep deprivation may be less obvious but may have a greater overall impact on health and well-being. A discrepancy between hours of sleep obtained and hours of sleep required for optimal functioning is responsible for a state of **sleep deprivation**, which has widespread implications for quality of life, health, and safety. Since there can be considerable individual variability in total sleep need, the term sleep deprivation applies only to impaired functioning due to sleep loss.

Many of the neurocognitive symptoms of chronic sleep deprivation can mimic psychiatric symptoms, highlighting the importance of a comprehensive sleep evaluation for patients with mental health disorders. In a recent multiethnic, representative sample of U.S. adults, insufficient sleep/rest was shown to be positively associated with poor self-rated health (Geiger et al., 2012). Adults who sleep less than 6 hours per night are more likely to report fair to poor general health, mood disturbance, increase in pain syndromes/perception, impaired cognitive function and memory disturbance, and reduction in measures of overall quality of life (Grandner et al., 2010).

Short and long sleep duration (sleeping less than 6 hours per night or greater than 8 hours per night) is associated with up to a twofold increased risk of obesity, diabetes, hypertension, cardiovascular disease, stroke, depression, substance abuse, and all-cause mortality in multiple studies (NCSDR, 2011). Less than 6 hours of sleep per night is associated with impaired glucose tolerance, elevated cortisol levels, and alterations in sympathetic nervous system activity. Sleep deprivation may be linked to obesity since it is associated with dysregulation of leptin (a hormone that regulates satiety or feelings of fullness) and ghrelin (a hormone that regulates hunger). Less than 6 hours of sleep per night may also increase pro-inflammatory markers such as C-reactive protein, tumor necrosis factor, and interleukin (Luyster et al, 2012). All these problems are common pathways to the development of cardiovascular disease and diabetes. Mechanisms linking long sleep time with vascular and metabolic morbidities are unknown but may be related to cofounders such as depression, inactivity, low socioeconomic status, and overall poor general health (Luyster et al., 2012).

Sleep loss diminishes safety and results in the loss of lives and property. Sleep deprivation can produce psychomotor impairments equivalent to those induced by alcohol consumption at or above the legal limit. Daytime wakefulness in excess of 17 to 19 hours can produce psychomotor deficits equivalent to blood alcohol concentrations (BACs) between 0.05% and 0.1% (the legal limit in most states is 0.08%) (Williamson & Feyer, 2007; Insurance Institute for Highway Safety, 2012).

Acute or chronic sleep deprivation can result in episodes of microsleep lasting from a second up to 10 seconds when a tired person is trying to stay awake. Many of us have experienced this when sitting in a class or in a meeting; this can lead to lower capabilities and efficiency of task performance and increased risk for errors (Orzel-Gryglewska, 2010). Some of the most devastating environmental and human tragedies of our time can be linked to human error due to sleep loss and fatigue. The grounding of the Exxon Valdez, the nuclear meltdown at Three Mile Island, and the explosion of the Union Carbide chemical plant in India are prime examples. Sleepiness with driving has become a national epidemic. The 2011 NSF *Sleep in America Poll* indicates that an alarming 52% of respondents admit to driving while sleepy. An incredible statistic cites one third of Americans report falling asleep while driving once or twice a month (CDC, 2010).

Although researchers have tried to quantify the financial burden associated with sleep disruption, there is relatively little comprehensive data available on the economic burden of sleep-wake disorders; however, considering the prevalence, impact on overall health and quality of life, and the indirect costs associated with property loss and damage, the economic burden is likely in the billions of dollars (Skaer & Sclar, 2010). For example, a recent study estimated that chronic insomnia results in nearly $63.2 billion dollars in direct and indirect expenses annually (Kessler et al., 2011).

Formal training in sleep or sleep disorders within medical and nursing education is limited, and the number of trained clinicians and scientists continues to be insufficient (Institute of Medicine [IOM], 2006). Awareness among health care providers regarding the prevalence and burden of sleep disruption and the problem of inadequate sleep is underappreciated, and providers do not routinely screen for sleep disturbance or inquire about overall sleep quality (Sorscher, 2008). Consequently, sleep disturbances may not be recognized, diagnosed, managed, and treated.

In this chapter, we briefly review the components of normal sleep, sleep regulation, and functions of sleep; give an overview of the most common sleep disturbances encountered in the clinical environment, with a focus on their relationship to psychiatric illness; and discuss the nurse's role in the assessment and management of a patient presenting with sleep disturbance.

Normal Sleep Cycle

Sleep is a dynamic neurological process that involves complex interaction between the central nervous system and the environment. Behaviorally, sleep is associated with low or absent motor activity, a reduced response to environmental stimuli, and closed eyes. Neurophysiologically, sleep is categorized according to specific brain wave patterns, eye movements, and general muscle tone. Sleep is measured electrophysiologically through electroencephalogram (EEG) and consists of two distinct physiological states: non-rapid eye movement (NREM) sleep and rapid eye movement (REM) sleep.

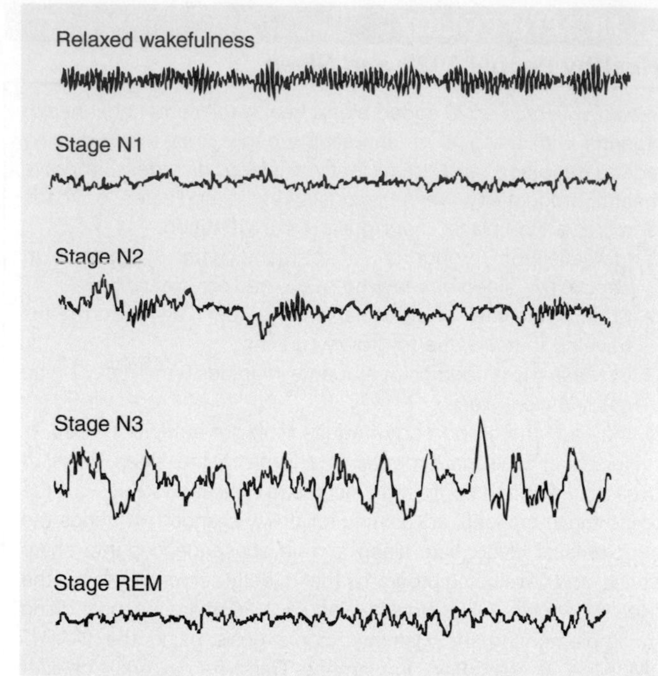

FIG 19-1 Stages of sleep. (Reprinted with permission of Sleep HealthCenters, Boston, MA.)

NREM sleep is divided into three stages (N1, N2, N3) according to criteria by the AASM (2005) and is characterized by progressive or deeper sleep. Stage 1 (N1) is a brief transition between wakefulness and sleep and comprises between 2% to 5% of total sleep time. The time it takes to fall to sleep is referred to as sleep latency. During stage 1 sleep, body temperature declines and muscles relax. Slow, rolling eye movements are common. People lose awareness of their environment but are generally easily aroused. Stage 2 (N2) sleep occupies 45% to 55% of total sleep time; heart rate and respiratory rate decline. Arousal from stage 2 sleep requires more stimuli than stage 1.

Stage 3 (N3) is known as *slow wave sleep* or *delta sleep*. Slow wave sleep is relatively short and constitutes only about 13% to 23% of total sleep time. It is characterized by further reduction in heart rate, respiratory rate, blood pressure, and response to external stimuli. The three stages of NREM sleep make up 75% to 80% of total sleep time. Stage 3 sleep is considered to be "restorative sleep," as it is a time of reduced sympathetic activity.

REM sleep comprises 20% to 25% of total sleep time and is characterized by reduction and absence of skeletal muscle tone (muscle atonia), bursts of rapid eye movement, myoclonic twitches of the facial and limb muscles, reports of dreaming, and autonomic nervous system variability. The atonia in REM sleep is thought to be a protective mechanism to prevent the acting out of nightmares and dreams (Carskadon & Dement, 2011). Figure 19-1 shows the EEG patterns characteristic of these sleep stages.

In the adult, sleep normally begins with NREM sleep. Continuous EEG recordings of sleep demonstrate an alternating cycle between NREM and REM sleep. There are typically four to six cycles of NREM and REM sleep occurring over 90- to 120-minute intervals across the sleep period. There is also a distinct organization to sleep, with NREM predominating during the first half of the sleep period and REM sleep predominating during the second half. The shortest REM period occurs 60-90 minutes after sleep onset and lasts only for several minutes. The longest REM period occurs at the end of the sleep period and can last up to an hour. This is the reason why many people remember dreaming upon awakening in the morning (Carskadon & Dement, 2011).

The structural organization of NREM and REM sleep is known as sleep architecture and is often displayed graphically as a *hypnogram.* Figure 19-2 is a hypnogram depicting the normal progression of the stages of sleep in an adult. The visual depiction of sleep is helpful in identifying sleep continuity (i.e., the distribution of sleep and wakefulness across the sleep period), as well as changes in sleep that may occur as a result of aging, illness, or certain medications. Disruption of sleep stages as indicated by excessive amounts of stage 1 sleep, multiple brief arousals, and frequent shifts in sleep staging is known as sleep fragmentation. Figure 19-3 is a hypnogram of a patient with a complaint of insomnia, indicating multiple brief arousals.

The function of alternations between NREM and REM sleep is not yet understood, but irregular cycling, absent sleep stages, and sleep fragmentation are associated with many psychiatric disorders, sleep disorders, and medication effects. For example, in patients with depression, the latency to REM sleep is frequently reduced, as is the percentage of slow wave sleep. Patients with narcolepsy frequently enter sleep through REM sleep rather than

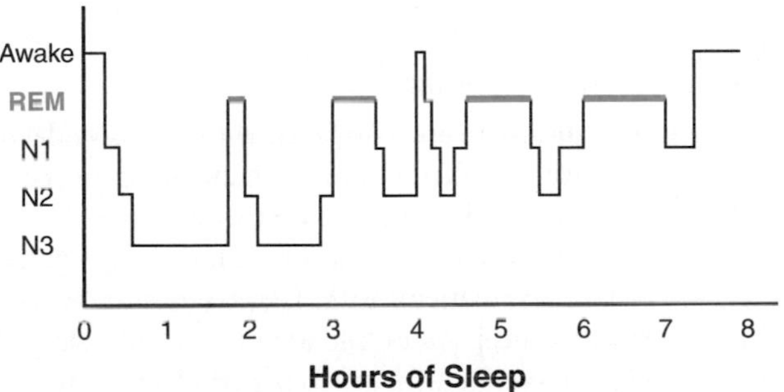

FIG 19-2 Hypnogram depicting the progression of the sleep stages of an adult. (From David N. Neubauer, MD, Johns Hopkins Sleep Disorders Center, Baltimore, MD *[American Family Physician, 59*(9):2551-2558, May 1, 1999].)

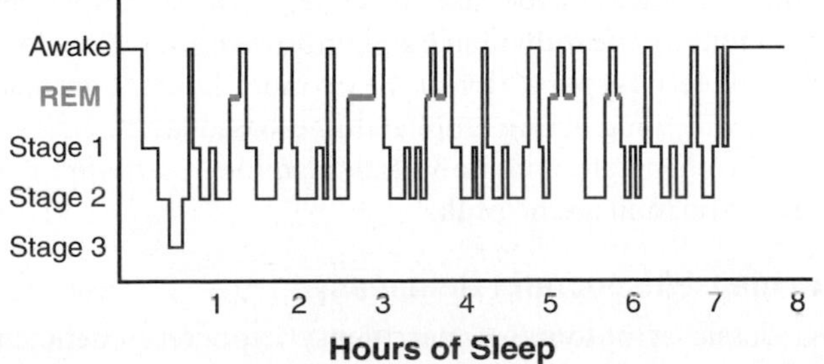

FIG 19-3 Hypnogram depicting multiple awakenings and sleep fragmentation. (From David N. Neubauer, MD, Johns Hopkins Sleep Disorders Center, Baltimore, MD *[American Family Physician, 59*(9):2551-2558, May 1, 1999].)

NREM sleep. Benzodiazepines tend to suppress slow wave sleep whereas serotonergic drugs suppress REM sleep.

Sleep Patterns

Sleep architecture changes over the lifespan. The percentage in each stage of sleep, as well as the overall sleep efficiency, or ratio of sleep duration to time spent in bed, varies according to age. For example, infants sleep 16 to 18 hours a day, enter sleep through REM (not NREM) sleep, and spend up to 50% of sleep time in REM sleep. The percentage of REM sleep decreases to 20% to 25% by age 3 and stays relatively constant throughout old age. The amount of slow wave sleep is maximal in young children and declines with age to almost none, particularly in men. This results in a tendency for middle-of-the-night awakenings and reduced sleep efficiency with age (Bliwise, 2011).

Regulation of Sleep

Although the regulation of sleep and wakefulness is not completely understood, it is believed to be a complex interaction between two processes, one that promotes sleep—known as the homeostatic process, or sleep drive—and one that promotes wakefulness, known as the circadian process, or circadian drive. The homeostatic process, is dependent on the number of hours a person is awake. The longer the period of wakefulness, the stronger the sleeps drive. During sleep, the sleep drive gradually dissipates.

Circadian drives are near-24-hour cycles of behavior and physiology generated and influenced by endogenous and exogenous factors and are wake-promoting. The exogenous factors are various clues from the environment known as *zeitgebers* (time-givers) that help set our internal clock to a 24-hour cycle. The strongest external cue for wakefulness is light whereas darkness is the cue for sleep. Other environmental cues include the timing of social events, such as meals, work, or exercise (Czeisler et al., 2011).

A *master biological clock* is located in the suprachiasmatic nucleus (SCN) of the hypothalamus. This clock regulates not only sleep but also a host of other biological and physiological functions within the body. Information about the lighting conditions of the external environment is relayed to the SCN from the retina. The SCN also receives information from the thalamus and the midbrain. These two pathways transmit photic and nonphotic information to the circadian clock through an expansive network. In addition to regulating sleep/wake cycles, they also exert control over endocrine regulation, body temperature, metabolism, autonomic regulation, psychomotor and cognitive performance, attention, memory, and emotion (Czeisler et al., 2011).

In addition to the circadian and homeostatic processes, several neurotransmitter systems are responsible for sleep and wakefulness. The neurotransmitters responsible for wakefulness are dopamine, norepinephrine, serotonin, acetylcholine, histamine, glutamate, and hypocretin; sleep-promoting neurotransmitters include adenosine, gamma-aminobutyric acid (GABA), and galanin (Carney et al., 2011). Any medication that crosses the blood-brain barrier may have effects on sleep and wakefulness through modulation of these neurotransmitters.

It is important to appreciate the neurotransmitters involved in sleep and wakefulness; many of the medications used in psychiatry manipulate these neurotransmitter systems. For example, amphetamines—which promote wakefulness—increase the release of dopamine and norepinephrine. Caffeine (methylxanthine)—which promotes alertness—functions by blocking adenosine. Patients newly started on selective serotonin reuptake inhibitors (SSRIs) frequently report difficulty sleeping when beginning treatment with one of these agents.

Functions of Sleep

Despite remarkable advances in the understanding of sleep disorders and the biological and physiological process of sleep, very little is known about the true function of sleep. Most of the information regarding the function of sleep comes to us from animal models of sleep deprivation and human models of partial sleep deprivation. Based on these models, several theories are proposed and include brain tissue restoration, body restoration (NREM sleep), energy conservation, memory reinforcement and consolidation (REM sleep), regulation of immune function, metabolism and regulation of certain hormones, and thermoregulation (Bonnet, 2011).

Sleep Requirements

Sleep architecture and efficiency may change over time, but there is little change in the amount of sleep required once we reach adulthood. Sleep requirement varies considerably from individual to individual and to some degree is probably genetically mediated. While most adults require 7 to 8 hours of sleep for optimal functioning, there is a small percentage of individuals defined as *long sleepers* (requiring 10 or more hours per night) and *short sleepers* (requiring less than 5 hours per night). The amount of sleep required is the amount necessary to feel fully awake and able to sustain normal levels of performance during the periods of wakefulness and is known as the **basal sleep requirement**.

For many people, there is a misconception regarding sleep need and a tendency to allow circumstances to dictate the amount of sleep obtained. The most accurate way to determine sleep requirements is to establish a routine bedtime and allow oneself to sleep undisturbed without an alarm for several days. This is usually best accomplished during an extended period of leisure time, such as during a vacation. The average of several nights' sleep undisturbed is a good estimate of the basal sleep requirement.

SLEEP DISORDERS

Sleep testing is often indicated for patients complaining of sleep disturbance or excessive sleepiness that impairs social and vocational functioning. There are four common diagnostic procedures used in the evaluation of sleep disorders: polysomnography (PSG), the multiple sleep latency test (MSLT), the maintenance of wakefulness test (MWT), and actigraphy.

Polysomnography is the most common sleep test and is used to diagnose and evaluate patients with sleep-related breathing disorders and nocturnal seizure disorders (Kushida et al., 2005). The **MSLT** is a daytime nap test used to objectively measure sleepiness in a sleep-conducive setting. Polysomnography and MSLT performed on the day following polysomnography evaluation are routinely indicated in patients suspected of having narcolepsy. **MWT** evaluates a patient's ability to remain awake in a situation conducive to sleep and is used to document adequate alertness in individuals with careers for which sleepiness would pose a risk to public safety (Littner et al., 2005). **Actigraphy** involves using a wristwatch-type device that records body movement over a period of time and is helpful in evaluating sleep patterns and sleep duration. It is used in patients with circadian rhythm disorders and insomnia (Morgenthaler et al., 2007).

CLINICAL PICTURE

In this chapter you will review the major categories of sleep disorders. Insomnia disorders are the most common sleep disorders and will be described along with the application of the nursing process. The American Psychiatric Association (2013) identifies the following disorders:

- Hypersomnolence disorders
- Narcolepsy/hypocretin deficiency
- Breathing-related sleep disorders
- Circadian rhythm disorders
- Disorders of arousal
- Nightmare disorder
- Rapid eye movement sleep behavior disorder
- Restless leg syndrome
- Substance-induced sleep disorders
- Insomnia

Hypersomnolence Disorders

Hypersomnolence disorders are associated with excessive daytime sleepiness and have a prevalence of more than 15% in the general population (Ohayon et al., 2012). Hypersomnolence disorders are chronic (3 months or more) and begin in young adulthood (Ali et al., 2009). The patient with hypersomnolence reports recurrent periods of sleep or unintended lapses into sleep, frequent napping, a prolonged main sleep period of greater than 9 hours, non-refreshing non-restorative sleep regardless of amount of time slept, and difficulty with full alertness during the wake period. Excessive sleepiness significantly impairs social and vocational functioning by impacting the person's ability to participate in and enjoy relationships and function in the workplace. Cognitive impairment is common as is an increased risk for accident or injury associated with the sleepiness.

Treatment for hypersomnolence disorders focuses on maintaining a regular sleep-wake schedule with an ample sleep opportunity. Some individuals will improve if they allow for an extended sleep opportunity of 10 or more hours. Pharmacotherapy with long-acting amphetamine-based stimulants such as methylphenidate and non-amphetamine-based stimulants such as modafinil are helpful.

Narcolepsy/Hypocretin Deficiency

The classic symptoms of narcolepsy/hypocretin deficiency include irresistible attacks of refreshing sleep, cataplexy, hypnagogic hallucinations, and sleep paralysis. Cataplexy is defined as brief episodes of bilateral loss of muscle tone with maintained consciousness. This usually happens along with a strong emotion such as anger, frustration, or laughter. Symptoms may last for up to several minutes, and recovery is generally immediate and complete. Hypnagogic hallucinations may be auditory, visual, and tactile and occur at sleep onset. Sleep paralysis is an inability to move or speak during the transition from sleep to wakefulness. Hynagogic hallucinations and sleep paralysis are quite frightening and may be misdiagnosed as psychiatric symptoms, frequently delaying the identification and treatment of the patient with narcolepsy/hypocretin deficiency.

Additional symptoms of narcolepsy/hypocretin deficiency include disturbed nighttime sleep with multiple middle-of-the-night awakenings and automatic behaviors characterized by memory lapses. Narcolepsy/hypocretin deficiency is distinguished from primary hypersomnia or other hypersomnia disorders in that patients with narcolepsy/hypocretin deficiency generally feel refreshed upon awakening but within 2 or 3 hours begin to feel sleepy again. Individuals with other hypersomnia disorders generally do not feel rested or refreshed regardless of the amount of sleep obtained. Hypocretin measurements in cerebrospinal fluid provide an objective basis for diagnosis (Gever, 2012). Treatment is through lifestyle modifications and long-acting stimulant medication.

Breathing-Related Sleep Disorders

The most common disorder of breathing and sleeping is obstructive sleep apnea hypopnea syndrome (OSAHA), which is characterized by repeated episodes of upper airway collapse and obstruction that result in sleep fragmentation. Patients maintain respiratory effort against an obstructed airway. Essentially, patients with obstructive sleep apnea are not able to sleep and breathe at the same time. Typical symptoms include loud, disruptive snoring, witnessed apnea episodes, and excessive daytime sleepiness. Obesity is an important risk factor for obstructive sleep apnea. Diagnosis is determined by clinical evaluation and polysomnography. Treatment is with continuous positive airway pressure (CPAP) therapy.

Additional breathing-related sleep disorders include central sleep apnea and sleep-related hypoventilation. Central sleep apnea is the cessation of respiration during sleep without associated ventilatory effort and is caused by instability of the respiratory control system. Central sleep apnea is seen in older individuals, those with advanced cardiac or pulmonary disease, or those with neurological disorders. Sleep-related hypoventilation is associated with sustained oxygen desaturation during sleep in the absence of apnea or respiratory events and is seen in individuals with morbid obesity, lung parenchymal disease, or pulmonary vascular pathology.

Circadian Rhythm Sleep Disorder

Circadian rhythm sleep disorders occur when there is a misalignment between the timing of the individual's normal circadian rhythm and external factors that affect the timing or duration of sleep. Diagnosis is determined by clinical evaluation, sleep diaries, and actigraphy. Treatment is with aggressive lifestyle management strategies aimed at adapting to or modifying the required sleep schedule. Examples include delayed sleep phase type, advanced sleep phase type, irregular sleep-wake type, free-running type, jet lag type, and shift work type.

VIGNETTE

Sarah had been living with treatment-resistant schizophrenia for many years. Despite multiple medication trials she was frequently hospitalized. Last year she was started on clozapine and within a few months had a dramatic reduction in her psychotic symptoms.

Despite careful monitoring of her dietary intake and weight by her group home staff, Sarah began to experience weight gain while taking the clozapine. Staff also began to notice a change in her sleeping patterns. She complained of frequently waking in the night and having a morning headache and sore throat. When she returned home from work in the afternoon it was not unusual for her to have a nap for 60 minutes or longer.

While home on a family visit, her mother noted loud snoring and discussed this with the psychiatrist. A polysomnography was performed, which demonstrated a severe degree of obstructive sleep apnea, most likely related to her recent weight gain. Continuous positive airway pressure (CPAP) therapy was initiated, and she was able to return to her baseline level of functioning.

Disorders of Arousal

Unusual or undesirable behaviors of sleep that occur during sleep-wake transitions or during certain stages of sleep are known as disorders of arousal.

Sleepwalking, or somnambulism, consists of a sequence of complex behaviors that begin in the first third of the night during NREM sleep and usually progress (without full consciousness or later memory) to leaving the bed and walking about. The individual may dress, go to the bathroom, leave the house, and, in some extreme cases, drive a car. Because of the possibility of accident or injury, a sleep specialist should always evaluate somnambulism. Polysomnography is sometimes indicated to rule out the possibility of an underlying disorder of sleep fragmentation. Treatment consists of instructing the patient and family regarding safety measures, such as alarms or locks on windows and doors and gating stairways. Attention to sleep hygiene, limiting alcohol prior to bed, obtaining adequate amounts of sleep, and stress reduction are helpful. Benzodiazepines are frequently prescribed when the risk for accident or injury is likely.

Confusional arousals consist of mental confusion or confused behavior during or following arousal from slow wave sleep but also upon attempted awakening from sleep in the morning. Patients may sometimes state that they are not sure they are awake or asleep. Sleepwalking is sometimes difficult to distinguish from confusional arousals because the sleepwalker may frequently seem disoriented. As with sleepwalking, treatment is focused on lifestyle management, safety measures, and gentle reassurance of the confused individual during an episode.

Nightmare Disorder

Nightmare disorder is characterized by long, frightening dreams from which people awaken scared. The nightmares almost always occur during rapid eye movement (REM) sleep and usually after a long REM period late in the night. For some people, this is a lifetime condition; for others, nightmares occur at times of stress and illness. Diagnosis is determined by clinical evaluation. Polysomnography is sometimes necessary to rule out the possibility of an underlying disorder of sleep fragmentation such as obstructive sleep apnea. Nightmare disorder is distinguished from *night terrors* in that night terrors generally occur during the first third of the sleep episode arising out of slow wave sleep, and there is no recollection of dream content. Treatment for nightmare disorder and night terrors is dependent on the frequency and severity of the symptoms as well as the underlying cause. Treatment with hypnotic therapy is sometimes indicated. Many patients do well with lifestyle modification measures, attention to sleep hygiene, and stress reduction.

Rapid Eye Movement (REM) Sleep Behavior Disorder

REM sleep behavior disorder (RSBD) is characterized by absence of muscle atonia during sleep. Patients with this disorder display elaborate motor activity associated with dream mentation (activity). These patients are actually acting out their dreams. RSBD is most frequently seen in elderly men but can be seen as the heralding symptom of neurological pathology such as Parkinson's disease. Serotonergic medications (such as SSRIs or SNRIs) can induce or exacerbate episodes. Diagnosis is determined by clinical evaluation and polysomnography with video recording. Treatment focuses on patient and sleep partner safety. Placing the mattress on the floor is sometimes necessary to prevent injury as a result of falling out of bed. The use of intermediate-acting benzodiazepine can be helpful, especially in cases of severe disruption to the sleep partner and concerns about safety.

VIGNETTE

A primary care provider refers an 80-year-old man with Parkinson's disease to a sleep clinic. The patient's wife became concerned when on several occasions she awoke to find him shouting and thrashing in the bed. It appeared that he was acting out his dreams. The patient reported no memory of these events and had no particular sleep complaint. During one of these episodes, he knocked over the bedside lamp and struck her. When he was awoken, he reported that he was dreaming there was an intruder in the house and he was attempting to save her. A polysomnography examination demonstrated an absence of the muscle atonia normally seen in REM sleep, confirming a diagnosis of REM sleep behavior disorder. He was treated with a low dose of a benzodiazepine and given instructions regarding personal and sleep partner safety.

Restless Leg Syndrome

Restless leg syndrome (RLS) sensory and movement disorder characterized by an unpleasant, uncomfortable sensation in the legs (occasionally the arms and trunk are affected) accompanied by an urge to move. Symptoms begin or worsen during periods of inactivity and are relieved or reduced by physical activity such as walking, stretching, or flexing. Symptoms are worse in the evening and at bedtime and can have a significant impact on the individual's ability to fall asleep and stay asleep. Symptoms may be induced or exacerbated by selective serotonin reuptake inhibitors or selective norepinephrine reuptake inhibitors.

The cause of RLS is unknown, but evidence suggests that it may be related to dysfunction of the brain's basal ganglia circuits that use the neurotransmitter dopamine. There is likely to be a strong genetic component, especially when seen in individuals under 40 years old (National Institute of Neurologic Disorders and Stroke, 2012). Diagnosis is determined by clinical evaluation. Many patients with RLS also have periodic limb movements of sleep that are observed during polysomnography. Treatment is through lifestyle modification and pharmacotherapy. Several classes of medications (narcotics, benzodiazepines, anticonvulsants) have proven effective in the management of RLS, but dopamine agonists such as pramipexole and ropinirole continue to be the mainstay of treatment.

VIGNETTE

Kathy is a 32-year-old woman who was referred by her primary care provider for a psychiatric evaluation for complaints of anxiety and restlessness. She reported feeling fine during the day, but in the evening, she felt nervous and anxious. The symptoms always started at the same time. As soon as she would settle down for the evening to watch some television, she would begin to have a restless sensation in her legs that would make her jump up and pace up and down. She described the sensation as having "soda pop fizzing through my veins." Sometimes she would go out for a walk at night even if it was very late in order to "calm down." These episodes began to occur almost nightly, and as a result, she was having difficulty getting a good night's sleep. She began to dread the approach of nightfall. A full clinical evaluation suggested the diagnosis of restless leg syndrome (RLS), and a course of the dopamine agonist pramipexole was initiated in the evening, with dramatic improvement in her symptoms and total resolution of her sleep complaint.

Substance-Induced Sleep Disorder

A substance-induced sleep disorder can result from the use or recent discontinuance of a substance or medication. While it is quite obvious that many prescriptions and over-the-counter medications may affect sleep, there is less appreciation for the effects of commonly used substances on sleep. Alcohol, nicotine, and caffeine all have an impact on sleep quantity and quality. **Alcohol**—despite its great soporific effects—decreases deep sleep (stage 3) and REM sleep and is responsible for middle-of-the-night awakenings with difficulty returning to sleep. **Nicotine** is a central nervous system stimulant, increasing heart rate, blood pressure, and respiratory rate. As nicotine levels decline through the night, patients wake in response to mild withdrawal symptoms. **Caffeine** blocks the neurotransmitter adenosine, promoting wakefulness. It increases sleep latency, reduces slow wave sleep, and acts as a diuretic, causing middle-of-the-night awakening for urination.

Insomnia Disorder

Patients with insomnia disorder report dissatisfaction with sleep quality and report difficulty with sleep initiation, sleep maintenance, early awakening with difficulty returning to sleep, or nonrefreshing nonrestorative sleep. It is not unusual for a patient to have a combination of complaints. For insomnia disorder to be diagnosed, symptoms must be present at least three times per week for a period of at least 3 months despite adequate sleep opportunity. Key to the diagnosis is a report of some type of daytime consequence associated with the sleep disturbance, such as impaired social or vocational functioning, decreased concentration or memory impairment, somatic complaints, or mood disturbance. Insomnia is best understood as a state of constant hyperarousal that involves biological, psychological, and social factors. As a result of this hyperarousal, patients with insomnia are not generally sleepy but rather complain of generalized fatigue and report somatic symptoms.

In addition to a thorough medical, psychiatric, and substance use history, it is helpful to use Spielman's **3P model of insomnia** to comprehensively assess the causes of insomnia, suggest appropriate interventions, and provide rationales for treatment (Spielman & Glovinsky, 2004). This model suggests that there are three factors that contribute to the insomnia complaint: **predisposing, precipitating,** and **perpetuating** factors (Figure 19-4).

Predisposing factors are individual factors that create a vulnerability to insomnia. These may include a prior history of poor-quality sleep, history of depression and anxiety, or a state of hyperarousal. Patients at risk to develop insomnia may describe themselves as light sleepers and night owls. **Precipitating** factors are external events that trigger insomnia. Personal and vocational difficulties, medical and psychiatric disorders, grief, and changes in role or identity (as seen with retirement) are examples. **Perpetuating** factors are sleep practices and attributes that maintain the sleep complaint, such as excessive caffeine or alcohol use, spending excessive amounts of time in bed or napping, and worry about the consequences of insomnia (Spielman & Glovinsky, 2004).

EPIDEMIOLOGY

Sleep-related problems are highly prevalent and occur across all age groups, cultures, and genders. An estimated 50 to 70 million Americans suffer from a chronic disorder of sleep and wakefulness (IOM, 2006). Obstructive sleep apnea hypopnea syndrome (OSAHS), a disorder of breathing and sleeping, affects 3% to 7% of middle-aged men and 2% to 5% of middle-aged women (Lurie, 2011). OSAHS has been associated with a higher prevalence of psychiatric comorbid conditions, making screening for apnea vital in this population (Sharafkhaneh et al., 2005).

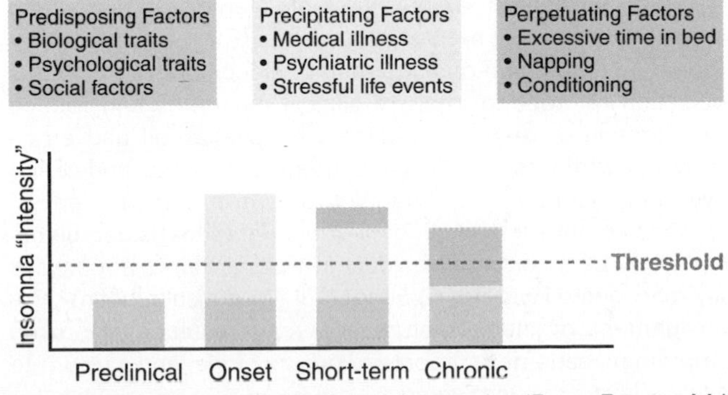

FIG 19-4 Spielman's 3P Model of Insomnia. (From Erman, M.K. [2007]. *Primary Psychiatry, 14*[7].)

CONSIDERING CULTURE

The Role of Sleep in U.S. Culture

Jennifer is a busy 21-year-old college senior. She is working on a degree in social work and has a part-time job working about 20 hours per week as a bartender. She is fully connected, with a smartphone, laptop computer, and television. Despite a long and active day, at night before bed, she surfs the Internet for several hours and sleeps with the television on. She keeps her cell phone on at night and is sometime awoken when she receives email or a text message.

The 2011 NSF *Sleep in America Poll* indicated that 90% of respondents aged 19 to 64 reported using some type of technology (laptop/computer, cell phone, television, electronic music device, video game, reader) in their bedrooms in the hour before going to sleep; individuals under the age of 30 are more likely to do so. Is it possible that our growing cultural attachment to technology is impacting sleep quality by reducing time spent in sleeping and causing sleep fragmentation? The results of the 2011 NSF poll and several recent studies seem to indicate it does.

Results from the 2011 NSF poll indicate that individuals who used their cell phone and/or laptop or computer in the hour before bed were *less* likely to report getting a good night's sleep, *more* likely to be categorized as "sleepy" on the Epworth Sleepiness Scale, and *more* likely to drive drowsy. A study conducted by Brunborg et al. (2010) indicated that respondents who used a computer or cell phone "often," as compared to "rarely," in the bedroom prior to bed reported less total sleep time, more variability in their sleep schedule consistent with a delayed phase, and poorer sleep quality.

Communication technology and media are an important part of American culture but may threaten healthy sleep. Media use, particularly of the computer and cell phone, seem to pose particular threats. The use of these devices at bedtime and during the night, coupled with the brightness of the light that they project onto the retina, are believed to trigger changes in sleep patterns, decrease total sleep time, cause sleep fragmentation, and reduce overall sleep quality (Mesquita & Reimao, 2010).

Many Americans prefer more waking hours and fill these hours with technology that they believe keeps them connected to the world at large. Nurses are in key positions to provide anticipatory guidance regarding the impact technology has on sleep quality and to make recommendations to keep it out of the bedroom and limit its use in the hour before bedtime. Recommend to all patients to engage in a relaxed, quiet activity such as reading, meditating, praying, or crossword puzzles prior to bed. Encourage them to turn off the television, computer, and cell phone.

National Sleep Foundation (2011). *2011 National Sleep in America Poll: Communication technology in the bedroom.* Retrieved from http://www.sleepfoundation.org/sites/default/files/sleepinamericapoll/SIAP_2011_Summary_of_Findings.pdf; Brunborg, G., Mentzoni, R., Molde, H., Myrseth, H., Skouveroe, K., Bjorvatin, B. & Pallesen, S. (2010). The relationship between media use in the bedroom, sleep habits, and symptoms of insomnia. *Journal of Sleep Research, 20(4)*, 569–75; Mesquita, G., & Reimao, R. (2010). Quality of sleep among university students: Effects of nighttime computer and television use. *Arquivos de Neuropsiquiatria, 68*(5), 720–725.

Shift work disorder, a misalignment of the normal sleep/wake pattern to accommodate vocational demands, affects up to 32% of night workers and 26% of rotating workers (Sack et al., 2007). According to the Bureau of Labor Statistics (2012), over 15% of Americans do some type of shift work, thereby increasing their risk for shift work disorder. Analysis from the National Comorbidity Survey Replication Study indicated that between 16% and 25% of Americans report one or more insomnia symptoms over a 12-month period; sleep disturbance was highly correlated with anxiety symptoms, mood disturbance, impulse-control disorders, substance abuse, and role impairment (Roth et al., 2006).

COMORBIDITY

Multiple studies suggest that sleeping less than 6 hours per night may have a significant impact on cardiovascular, endocrine, immune, and neurological function. Short sleep duration has been associated with obesity, cardiovascular disease and hypertension, impaired glucose tolerance and diabetes, and mood disturbance (Cappuccio et al., 2010). Many sleep disorders increase the risk for the development of certain medical conditions. For example, obstructive sleep apnea has been associated with hypertension, diabetes, cardiovascular disease, and stroke (Tracova et al., 2008). Individuals with neurological disease, such as Alzheimer's and Parkinson's disease, frequently experience sleep disturbance that worsens with the progression of the illness. Sleep disturbance is a major factor contributing to nursing-home placement in patients with dementia.

Most psychiatric disorders are associated with sleep disturbance. Insomnia is the most frequent complaint, but reports of hypersomnia are also common. About 85% of patients with a major mood disorder will report some type of a sleep disturbance over the course of the illness. In addition, there is evidence to demonstrate that sleep disruption itself may be a precipitating factor in triggering mood and other psychiatric disorders and increases the risk to relapse, making the identification and management of sleep disturbance in patients with affective disorders critical (Roth et al., 2006). Of special concern is that depressed patients who experience a sleep disturbance demonstrate greater degrees of suicidal ideation (Chellappa & Araujo, 2007).

Sleep disturbance is common in patients with alcoholism, and insomnia occurs in 36% to 72% of patients in early recovery and persists for months or even years. Sleep disturbance increases the risk for relapse to alcohol abuse. Targeting sleep disturbance during recovery may support continued abstinence (Arnedt et al., 2007).

EVIDENCE-BASED PRACTICE

Sleep and Psychiatric Illness

Kaufmann, C., Spira, A., Rae, D., West, J., & Mojtabai, R. (2011). Sleep problems, psychiatric hospitalization, and emergency department use among psychiatric patients with Medicaid. *Psychiatric Services, 62*(9), 1101-1105.

Problem

Sleep disturbance is commonly associated with most psychiatric disorders and may contribute significantly to the symptom burden associated with an illness. The prevalence and implications of sleep problems for patients with serious mental illness are not fully understood.

Purpose

The authors of this study examined the prevalence and severity of sleep problems in a large sample of psychiatric patients who were enrolled in the Medicaid program with a focus on the association of sleep problems with psychiatric hospitalization and use of psychiatric emergency room services.

Methods

The sample consisted of 1560 Medicaid patients of a randomly selected group of psychiatrists who were identified via the American Medical Association's Physician Masterfile. Those psychiatrists who participated in the study were asked to complete a questionnaire concerning two recently treated Medicaid patients. Psychiatrists were asked to provide information regarding the patient's diagnosis, medical comorbidities, medications, current severity of psychiatric symptoms, and reports of sleep disturbance. The patients' health service utilization was measured by a series of items, including psychiatric hospitalization and utilization of emergency department.

Key Findings

- Almost 84% had a least one comorbid medical condition, an important finding in light of the fact that 56% of the sample were under 36 years of age. The presence of a comorbid medical condition was associated with greater severity of sleep disturbance.
- Overall, 78% of patients were rated by their psychiatrist as having sleep problems, with 13% rated as severe sleep disturbance.
- More severe sleep problems were found among patients with mood and substance-use disorders compared to patients without these disorders and among those patients with more than one psychiatric diagnosis.
- Patients with sleep problems had greater odds of psychiatric hospitalization and emergency room use compared to those with no sleep problems.

Implications for Nursing Practice

This study highlights the prevalence of sleep disruption among patients with serious mental illness. It calls for better assessment, monitoring, and management of sleep complaints in this population in order to improve clinical outcomes and reduce the utilization of resources such as hospitalization and emergency departments. In the past, treatment of the underlying psychiatric disorder was thought to result in improvement of the sleep complaint. This study demonstrates that sleep disturbance may be a common residual symptom that is not always fully managed or addressed adequately in clinical practice. Co-management of sleep disturbance may result in improved symptom management, improved quality of life, and a return to baseline levels of functioning.

APPLICATION OF THE NURSING PROCESS

Regardless of the clinical environment or the presenting complaint, all patients can benefit from an evaluation of their sleep. Assessment of the patient's sleep allows the nurse to identify short- and long-term health risks associated with sleep disorders and sleep deprivation, provide health teaching and counseling regarding sleep needs, and improve clinical outcomes in patients experiencing a sleep disturbance.

ASSESSMENT

General Assessment

Sleep Patterns

Patients frequently do not report sleep difficulties or discuss their sleep-related concerns with care providers. People tend to minimize or adapt to the consequences of sleep disturbance. Furthermore, there is a lack of appreciation about the impact sleep disturbance and sleep deprivation have on overall functioning and health. Many patients do not complain of sleep disturbance directly but rather complain of associated symptoms such as fatigue, decreased concentration, mood disturbance, or physical ailments.

When assessing who has a sleep complaint, it is important to recognize the 24-hour nature of the sleep disturbance. Sleep disturbance is not confined to the 7 or 8 hours devoted to sleep. Sleep diaries (see Figure 19-5) are helpful in identifying sleep patterns and behaviors that may be contributing to the sleep complaint. Assigning the patient the homework of completing a sleep diary for 2 weeks will help guide the assessment and direct the plan of care. The following questions and comments provide direction for the assessment:

- When did you begin having trouble with sleep? Have you had trouble with sleep in the past?
- Describe your prebedtime routine. What are the activities you customarily engage in before sleep?
- Describe your sleeping environment. Are there things in your sleep environment that are hampering your sleep (such as noise, light, temperature, or overall comfort)?
- Do you use your bedroom for things other than sleep or sexual activity (such as working, eating, or watching television)?
- What time do you go to bed? How long does it take to fall asleep?
- Once asleep, does middle-of-the-night awakening disturb you? If so, what wakes you up? Are you able to return to sleep?
- If you are unable to sleep, what do you do?
- What time do you wake up? What time do you get out of bed?
- How much time do you actually think you sleep?
- Do you sleep longer on weekends or days off?
- Do you nap? If so, for how long? Do you feel refreshed after napping?
- Can you identify any stress or problem that may have initially contributed to your sleep difficulties?
- Tell me about your daily habits, your diet, exercise, and medications.
- What changes, if any, have you made to improve your sleep? What were the results?

Identifying Sleep-Wake Disorders

It is helpful to think about sleep-wake disorders according to the predominant symptoms of insomnia, hypersomnia, arousal disorders, and circadian rhythm disorders. Box 19-1 provides pertinent screening questions for each diagnosis. An affirmative answer to any of these questions demands further investigation and evaluation.

Functioning and Safety

As previously described, sleep disturbance can result in increased risk for accident and injury and impose serious limitations on quality of life. Several screening tools are available to assist the clinician in evaluating sleep quality and the safety risk associated with excessive sleepiness. The Pittsburgh Sleep Quality Index (PSQI) is a subjective measure of sleep quality.

BOX 19-1 SLEEP DISORDERS SCREENING QUESTIONS

Insomnia

- Do you have difficulty with falling asleep, staying asleep, or early-morning awakenings?
- Do you feel refreshed and restored in the morning?
- Have you noticed any problems with your energy, mood, concentration, or work quality as a result of your sleep problem?

Hypersomnia

- Obstructive sleep apnea hyponea syndrome: Have you ever been told that you snore or that it looks as if you stop breathing in your sleep?
- Restless leg syndrome: Do you have an unpleasant or uncomfortable sensation in your legs (or arms) that prevents you from sleeping or wakes you up from sleep and makes you want to move?
- Narcolepsy: Do you have episodes of sleepiness you cannot control? Have you experienced episodes where you were unable to move as you were about to fall asleep or wake up (sleep paralysis)? Unexplained muscle weakness following a strong emotion (cataplexy)? Have you ever seen or heard something that you knew was not real as you were falling asleep or waking up from sleep (hypnogogic hallucination)?
- Primary hypersomnia: Do you ever feel unrested even after an extended sleep period?

Arousal

- Have you ever been told that you have done anything unusual in your sleep, such as walking or talking? (Somnambulism/somniloquy)?
- Have you ever been told that you act out your dreams? (REM sleep behavior disorder)
- Have you been troubled by nightmares or disturbing dreams?

Circadian Rhythm

- Is your desired sleep schedule in conflict with your social and vocational goals?
- What is your preferred sleep schedule?

A global sum of 5 or greater indicates poor quality and patterns of sleep (Buysse et al., 1989). The PSQI is available online at: http://consultgerirn.org/uploads/File/trythis/try_this_6_1.pdf.

The Epworth Sleepiness Scale (ESS) is a validated psychometric tool used to measure subjective reports of sleepiness and has been validated by objective measures using the MSLT and is shown at http://epworthsleepinessscale.com/1997-version-ess/. Scores of less than 10 are considered normal, 10 to 15 is moderately sleepy, and greater than 15 is excessively sleepy (Johns, 1991). In addition to these screening tools, the following questions provide direction for further assessment:

- Have you had an accident or injury as a result of sleepiness?
- Are you sleepy when you drive a car? What do you do if you are sleepy while driving?
- What kind of work do you do? Do you operate heavy equipment or machinery? How many hours a week do you work? How long is your commute?
- How does your sleep disturbance affect your work performance?
- Do you avoid social obligations as a result of your sleep problems?
- Do you feel as if your sleep disturbance is affecting your physical health? How so?

Self-Assessment

Nurses are especially vulnerable to the effects of sleep deprivation and sleep disruption. Rotating shifts and night work result in circadian rhythm disruption that can cause problems with insomnia and excessive sleepiness. Long shifts and working overtime may lead to a decrease in total available sleep time. Inadequate sleep time and sleep quality have been shown to impair performance and judgment, both of which may affect patient safety and quality of care. In addition, nurses who work rotating or night shifts may pose an increased risk for accident or injury to themselves and the community as a result of excessive sleepiness while driving.

Nurses need to be able to recognize the effects of chronic partial sleep deprivation on their performance and functioning and take measures to assure that they are well rested and able to provide safe and competent care. Self-evaluation for a possible sleep disorder and ability to cope with the rigors of shift work is warranted. Consultation with a sleep professional is indicated if there is significant disruption to sleep, physical and mental health, job performance, job satisfaction, and social functioning. Attention to issues of sleep hygiene, limiting overtime, limiting shift work to 8 hours, and obtaining 7 to 8 hours of sleep within a 24-hour period are essential for personal, patient, and community safety.

DIAGNOSIS

There are four specific North American Nursing Diagnosis Association International nursing diagnoses for sleep disturbance (Herdman, 2012):

1. *Insomnia:* A disruption in amount and quality of sleep that impairs function
2. *Sleep deprivation:* Prolonged periods of time without sleep.
3. *Disturbed sleep pattern:* Changes in sleep routines that cause impairment in social or vocational functioning
4. *Readiness for enhanced sleep:* A pattern of natural, periodic suspension of consciousness that provides adequate rest, sustains a desired lifestyle, and can be strengthened.

OUTCOMES IDENTIFICATION

The *Nursing Outcomes Classification (NOC)* (Moorhead et al., 2013) identifies several appropriate outcomes for the patient experiencing sleep disruption, including *Sleep, Rest, Risk control,* and *Personal well-being.* Table 19-1 provides signs and symptoms, nursing diagnoses, and short-term indicators and long-term indicators for these categories.

PLANNING

The majority of patients with sleep disorders are treated in the community. The exceptions are cases in which the patient has a primary psychiatric disorder or a medical condition that requires hospitalization. Because longstanding sleep problems are associated with a host of occupational, social, interpersonal, psychiatric, and medical conditions, the treatment is multifaceted and frequently requires a team approach under the leadership of a sleep disorder specialist. The role of the nurse is generally to conduct a full assessment, provide support to the patient and family while the appropriate interventions are determined, and teach the patient and family strategies that may improve sleep.

TABLE 19-1 SIGNS AND SYMPTOMS, DIAGNOSES, AND OUTCOMES FOR SLEEP DISORDERS

SIGNS AND SYMPTOMS	NURSING DIAGNOSES	OUTCOMES
Absenteeism, changes in affect and energy; reports changes in mood, quality of life, concentration, and sleep; reports lack of energy, sleep disturbances, early wakening	*Insomnia*	Successful sleep induction, appropriate hours of sleep, consistent sleep pattern, minimal awakening
Acute confusion, agitation, anxiety, apathy, fatigue, poor concentration, irritability, lethargy, malaise, perceptual disorders, slowed reaction	*Sleep deprivation*	Balance between work and sleep, minimal awakening, feeling restored after sleep, sleeping between 7 and 9 hours on average
Changes in normal sleep pattern, decreased ability to function, dissatisfaction with sleep, awakening, no difficulty falling asleep, not feeling well rested	*Disturbed sleep pattern*	Minimal awakening, feeling restored after sleep

From Herdman, T. H. (Ed.), (2012). *Nursing diagnoses—Definitions and classification 2012-2014.* Copyright © 2012, 1994-2012 by NANDA International. Used by arrangement with John Wiley & Sons Limited; Moorhead, S., Johnson, M., Maas, M. L., & Swanson, E. (2013). *Nursing outcomes classification (NOC)* (5th ed.). St. Louis, MO: Mosby.

IMPLEMENTATION

Counseling

The nurse's counseling role begins with the assessment of the sleep disorder. The nurse's questions and responses provide support to the patient and family as well as assurance that the sleep problems are amenable to treatment. For many patients, the distress caused by chronic sleep difficulties results in hopelessness. Through the nurse's counseling approach, this hopelessness is identified and countered with encouragement, positive suggestions, and the belief that the patient will be able to manage sleep difficulties.

Health Teaching and Health Promotion

The nurse's role in health teaching cannot be overemphasized. Most individuals do not think about their sleep. This means that they also do not recognize the importance of a sleep routine or consider factors that influence good sleep. In addition, there are many myths regarding what constitutes "good sleep" and what factors contribute to sleep quality (Box 19-2). The nurse may also be involved in teaching relaxation techniques such as meditation, guided imagery, progressive muscle relaxation, or controlled breathing exercises. Use of these techniques has been linked to sustained benefits for patients with primary insomnia.

Modifying poor sleep habits and establishing a regular sleep/wake schedule can be accomplished using sleep diaries (Figure 19-5). A period of 2 weeks is helpful in establishing overall sleep patterns and determining overall sleep efficiency

BOX 19-2 SLEEP HYGIENE

- Maintain a regular sleep/wake schedule.
- Develop a presleep routine that signals the end of the day.
- Reserve the bedroom for sleep and a place for intimacy.
- Create an environment that is conducive to sleep (taking into consideration light, temperature, and clothing).
- Avoid clock watching.
- Limit caffeinated beverages to 1 or 2 a day and none in the evening.
- Avoid heavy meals before bedtime.
- Use alcohol cautiously and avoid use for several hours before bed.
- Avoid daytime napping.
- Exercise daily but not right before bed.

From Epstein, L. (2007). *The Harvard Medical School guide to a good night's sleep.* New York, NY: McGraw-Hill.

Two-week sleep diary

INSTRUCTIONS:
1 Write the date, day of the week, and type of day: Work, School, Day off, or Vacation.
2 Put the letter "C" in the box when you have coffee, cola or tea. Put "M" when you take any medicine. Put "A" when you drink alcohol. Put "E" when you exercise.
3 Put a line (I) to show when you go to bed. Shade in the box that shows when you think you fell asleep.
4 Shade in all the boxes that show when you are asleep at night or when you take a nap during the day.
5 Leave boxes unshaded to show when you wake up at night and when you are awake during the day.

SAMPLE ENTRY BELOW: On a Monday when I worked, I jogged on my lunch break at 1 PM, had a glass of wine with dinner at 6 PM, fell asleep watching TV from 7 to 8 PM, went to bed at 10:30 PM, fell asleep around midnight, woke up and couldn't get back to sleep at about 4 AM, went back to sleep from 5 to 7 AM, and had coffee and medicine at 7:00 in the morning.

Today's Date	Day of the week	Type of Day Work, School, Off, Vacation	Noon	1 PM	2	3	4	5	6 PM	7	8	9	10	11 PM	Midnight	1 AM	2	3	4	5	6 AM	7	8	9	10	11	
sample	Mon.	Work		E					A				I									C M					
																											Week 1
																											Week 2

FIG 19-5 Two-week sleep diary. (Modified from the American Academy of Sleep Medicine. Retrieved from http.www.sleepeducation.com/pdf/sleepdiary.pdf.)

([time in bed divided by total sleep time] × 100). After reviewing sleep diaries, patients are sometimes surprised to discover that their sleep problems are not as bad as previously believed.

Sleep restriction, or limiting the total sleep time, creates a temporary, mild state of sleep deprivation and strengthens the sleep homeostatic drive. This helps to decrease sleep latency and improves sleep continuity and quality. If, for example, a patient's sleep diary indicates that he or she is in bed for 8 hours but sleeping only 6 hours, sleep is restricted to 6 hours, and the bedtime and wake time are adjusted accordingly. The sleep time should not be reduced below 5 hours, regardless of sleep efficiency, and patients should be cautioned about the dangers of sleepiness with driving while undergoing a trial of sleep restriction. Once sleep efficiency is improved, total sleep time is gradually increased by 10- to 20-minute increments.

Pharmacological Interventions

Many patients use medication to address their sleep problems. Nurses frequently provide education about the benefits of a particular drug, the side effects, untoward effects, and the fact that medications are usually prescribed for no more than 2 weeks, because tolerance and withdrawal may result. In many settings, the nurse also monitors the effectiveness of the medication. See Table 19-2 for the pharmacological treatment of insomnia.

Generally, long-term hypnotic use is discouraged because nonpharmacological treatments have shown superior efficacy in reducing insomnia. Many antidepressants, anticonvulsants, antihistamines, and second-generation antipsychotics are also used off-label (without specific approval from the FDA) for their sedative properties in the treatment of insomnia disorder.

Advanced Practice Interventions

Although psychotherapy offers little value in the treatment of primary insomnia, there is a component of primary insomnia that involves a conditioned response. The initial episode of insomnia is frequently associated with a stressful event or crisis that produces anxiety. This anxiety becomes associated with worry about not being able to get to sleep and leads to preoccupation with getting enough sleep. The more the patient tries to sleep, the more elusive sleep becomes and the greater the patient's experienced anxiety.

Successful treatment of insomnia involves an integration of the basic principles of sleep hygiene (conditions and practices that promote continuous and effective sleep), behavioral therapies, and, in some instances, the use of hypnotic medication. Hypnotic medication is always used with caution, and over-the-counter sleeping aids have limited effectiveness. Melatonin, a naturally occurring hormone, is a popular over-the-counter

TABLE 19-2 DRUG TREATMENT OF PATIENTS WITH INSOMNIA

GENERIC (BRAND) NAME	ONSET OF ACTION (MINUTES)	DURATION OF ACTION	FDA-APPROVED FOR INSOMNIA	HABIT FORMING
Benzodiazepines				
Estazolam (Pro-Som)	15–60	Intermediate	Yes	Yes, all drugs in this class are Schedule IV
Flurazepam (Dalmane)	30–60	Long	Yes	
Quazepam (Doral)	20–45	Long	Yes	
Temazepam (Restoril)	45–60	Intermediate	Yes	
Triazolam (Halcion)	15–30	Short	Yes	
Benzodiazepine-Like Drugs				
Eszopiclone (Lunesta)	60	Intermediate	Yes	Yes, all drugs in this class are Schedule IV
Zaleplon (Sonata)	15–30	Ultra Short	Yes	
Zolpidem (Ambien)	30	Short	Yes	
Melatonin Receptor Agonists				
Ramelteon (Rozerem)	30	Short	Yes	No
Antidepressants				
Trazodone (Desyrel)	60–120	Long	No	No
Silenor (Doxepin)	30	Long	Yes	No
Antihistamines (Generally Discouraged Due to Cholinergic Side Effects)				
Diphenhydramine (Nytol, Sominex)	60–180	Long	No	Tolerance to hypnotic effects develops in 1-2 weeks
Doxylamine (Unisom)	60–120	Long	No	

From Lehne, R. A. (2010). *Pharmacology for nursing care* (7th ed.). Philadelphia, PA: Saunders; Weilburg, J. B., Stakes, J. W., & Roth, T. (2010). Sleep disorders. In T. A. Stern, G. L. Fricchione, N. H. Cassem, M. S. Jellinek, & J. F. Rosenbaum (Eds.), *Massachusetts General Hospital handbook of general hospital psychiatry* (6th ed., pp. 289–302). Philadelphia, PA: Saunders.

product. To date, there is little data to support its use in the management of insomnia disorder, but new research into prolonged release (PR) forms of melatonin are demonstrating some promise.

Cognitive-behavioral therapy for insomnia (CBT-I) includes educational, behavioral, and cognitive components; it targets factors that perpetuate insomnia over time (Morin, 2004). The first objectives are to provide education regarding sleep and sleep needs and to help the patient to set realistic expectations regarding sleep. Patients should be asked what they believe constitutes healthy sleep and have any misconceptions clarified. Eliciting information about the total number of hours spent sleeping typically has little value. Many patients are stuck on a set number of sleep hours rather than on the quality of sleep obtained. Focusing on the number of hours slept rather than the quality of sleep and daytime functioning increases the insomnia experience.

Stimulus control is a behavioral intervention that involves some interventions previously discussed with sleep hygiene. Adherence to five basic principles that decrease the negative associations between the bed and bedroom and strengthen the stimulus for sleep is essential. Patients should be instructed to:

1. Go to bed only when sleepy.
2. Use the bed or bedroom only for sleep and intimacy (no television, reading, or other activities in the bedroom).
3. Get out of bed if unable to sleep and engage in a quiet-time activity such as reading or crossword puzzles (no television, work, or computer).
4. Maintain a regular sleep/wake schedule, with getting up at the same time each day being the most important factor.
5. Avoid daytime napping (if napping is necessary to avoid accident or injury, it should be limited to 20 to 30 minutes maximum, and a timer should be set).

Other objectives of CBT-I are aimed at identifying and correcting maladaptive attitudes and beliefs about sleep that perpetuate insomnia. For example, patients frequently amplify the consequences of their insomnia and attribute most daytime experiences to their sleep complaint. They may rationalize maladaptive coping behaviors such as excessive time in bed to "catch up" on lost sleep and may exhibit unrealistic expectations about sleep. The nurse offers alternative interpretations regarding the sleep complaint to assist the patient to think about his or her insomnia in a different way, empowering the patient to be in control of his or her sleep (Morin, 2004). Because CBT-I approaches are not immediately effective and may take several weeks of practice before improvement is seen, success is dependent on both a high degree of motivation in patients and a commitment on the part of the practitioner.

EVALUATION

Evaluation is based on whether or not the patient experiences improved sleep quality as evidenced by decreased sleep latency, fewer nighttime awakenings, a shorter time to get back to sleep after awakening, and improvement in daytime symptoms of sleepiness. This evaluation is accomplished through patient report and patient maintenance of a sleep diary. Just as important as objective changes in the patient's sleep pattern is the patient's perception that there has been an improvement. Objectively, the improvement may be quite modest, but the patient may perceive that he or she is no longer *controlled by* sleep (or the lack of it) but exerting *control over* sleep through lifestyle changes and a better sleep routine.

KEY POINTS

- Sleep disturbance has major implications for overall health, quality of life, and personal and community safety.
- Research into the physiology of normal sleep, as well as sleep disorders, is expanding.
- Most patients with a mood disorder will report sleep disturbance; recognition and treatment of sleep disturbance in patients with psychiatric disorders improves clinical outcomes.
- Regardless of the clinical environment or the presenting complaint, all patients can benefit from an evaluation of their sleep needs.
- Primary insomnia can be effectively treated with nonpharmacological interventions such as CBT-I, sleep restriction, stimulus control, and attention to issues of sleep hygiene. Long-term pharmacological management is generally not indicated.

CRITICAL THINKING EXERCISES

1. Anthony is a 46-year-old who complains of waking frequently at night. Consequently, he is tired all day and knows that he has not been functioning as well as he should. Whenever he can manage it, he goes out to his car at lunchtime to take a 60-minute nap, because he has fallen asleep at his desk and been given a disciplinary warning. He is drinking 2 to 3 cups of coffee in the afternoon so that he does not feel sleepy while driving home.
   a. What questions would you ask to determine if Anthony might have a sleep disorder?
   b. What recommendations will you make to improve his sleep hygiene?
   c. What instructions and education should you give this patient regarding personal and community safety?
2. Your patient, Vivian, has been using temazepam (Restoril) for several years to treat insomnia. She has been reading that long-term use of hypnotics is not healthy or productive and wants to quit taking them; however, she is focused on needing nine hours of sleep each night and is extremely worried about what will happen when she discontinues the temazepam.
   a. What instructions would you provide to Vivian regarding stimulus control, sleep restriction, and cognitive restructuring of her sleep complaint?
   b. Identify alternative pharmacological therapies.

3. Mrs. Levine is a 72-year-old woman with a history of major depression. She takes fluoxetine (Prozac) 10 mg every day and has experienced significant relief from depression. While reviewing her medications, she tells you she is using a variety of over-the-counter (OTC) sleep aids because she has been having some difficulty sleeping recently. These OTC products include diphenhydramine, melatonin, valerian, and something that her neighbor gave her to try.
   a. In light of the patient's age and history of depression, what are your concerns?
   b. What further assessment is required?
   c. What specific question would you need to ask concerning her use of Prozac?
   d. What instructions and education will you provide?

CHAPTER REVIEW

1. Madelyn, a 29-year-old patient recently diagnosed with depression, comes to the mental health clinic complaining of continued difficulty sleeping. One week ago, she was started on a selective serotonin reuptake inhibitor (SRRI), fluoxetine, for her depressive symptoms. When educating Madelyn, your response is guided by the knowledge that:
   a. SSRIs such as fluoxetine more commonly cause hypersomnolence as opposed to difficulty sleeping.
   b. The sleep problem is caused by the depression and is unrelated to the medication.
   c. The neurotransmitters involved in sleep and wakefulness are the same neurotransmitters targeted by many psychiatric medications and the problem may be temporary.
   d. The medication should be discontinued because sleep is the most important element to her recovery.
2. A patient states that he only needs 6 hours of sleep per night to feel rested. How should the nurse interpret this statement?
   a. The patient is not sleeping enough.
   b. The patient is sleeping too much.
   c. The patient is not getting enough REM sleep.
   d. The patient is sleeping according to his own body's needs.
3. Ed, a registered nurse, is planning care for a patient with primary insomnia. What is an appropriate outcome?
   a. The patient will sleep 12 hours nightly.
   b. The patient will go to sleep and wake up at consistent times.
   c. The patient will take one nap daily to restore energy.
   d. The patient will drink a warm cup of tea before bedtime.
4. You are providing teaching for a patient who has been taking a hypnotic medication to sleep. What education is appropriate?
   a. "You can use this medication for as long as you would like."
   b. "It would be better to take an over-the-counter medication instead."
   c. "Melatonin has been shown to be just as effective as hypnotic medications."
   d. "Be certain to follow up with your care provider regularly while you take this medication."
5. Which patient behavior would alert the nurse to a circadian rhythm sleep disorder?
   a. Excessive sleepiness for at least 1 month, accompanied by prolonged sleep episodes
   b. Multiple episodes of brief daytime sleeping followed by disturbed nighttime sleep
   c. Persistent patterns of sleep disruption after traveling for business
   d. Repeated episodes of upper airway collapse and obstruction that results in sleep fragmentation.

Answers to Chapter Review
1. c; 2. d; 3. b; 4. d; 5. c.

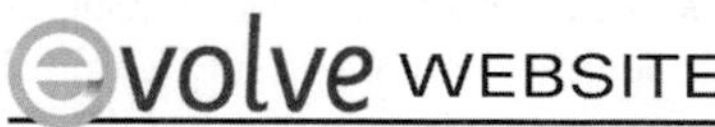

Visit the Evolve website for a posttest on the content in this chapter: http://evolve.elsevier.com/Varcarolis

Post-Test interactive review

REFERENCES

Ali, M., Auger, R. R., Slocumb, N. L., & Morgenthaler, T. I. (2009). Idiopathic hypersomnia: Clinical features and response to treatment. *Journal of Clinical Sleep Medicine, 5*, 562–568.

American Academy of Sleep Medicine (AASM). (2005). *The international classification of sleep disorders (ICSD)* (2nd ed.). Westchester, IL: American Academy of Sleep Medicine.

American Psychiatric Association (APA). (2013). *DSM-5 table of contents.* Retrieved from http://www.psychiatry.org/dsm5.

Arnedt, J. T., Conroy, D. A., & Bower, K. J. (2007). Treatment options for sleep disturbance during alcohol recovery. *Journal of Addictive Diseases, 26*(4), 41–54.

Bin, Y., Marshall, N., & Glozier, N. (2012). Secular trends in adult sleep duration: A systematic review. *Sleep Medicine Review, 16*(3), 223–230. doi:10.1016/j.smrv.2011.07.003.

Bliwise, D. (2011). Normal aging. In M. Kryger, T. Roth, & W. Dement (Eds.), *Principles and practice of sleep medicine* (5th ed.). Philadelphia, PA: Saunders.

Bonnet, M. (2011). Acute sleep deprivation. In M. Kryger, T. Roth, & W. Dement (Eds.), *Principles and practice of sleep medicine* (4th ed.). Philadelphia, PA: Saunders.

Bureau of Labor Statistics. (2012). *Work schedules.* Retrieved from http://www.bls.gov/cps/lfcharacteristics.htm.

Buysse, D. J., Reynolds, C.F., III, Monk, T. H., Berman, S. R., & Kupfer, D. J. (1989). The Pittsburgh Sleep Quality Index: A new instrument for psychiatric practice and research. *Psychiatry Research, 28*(2), 193–213.

Cappuccio, E., Miller, M., & Lockley, S. (2010). *Sleep, health, and society: From aetiology to public health.* Oxford, UK; New York, NY: Oxford University Press. doi:10.1093/acprof:oso/9780199566594.001.0001.

Carney, R., Berry, R., & Geyer, J. (2011). *Clinical sleep disorders* (2nd ed.). Philadelphia, PA: Lippincott, Williams & Wilkins.

Carskadon, M., & Dement, W. (2011). Normal human sleep: An overview. In M. H. Kryger, T. Roth, & W. C. Dement (Eds.), *Principles and practice of sleep medicine* (5th ed.). Philadelphia, PA: Saunders.

Centers for Disease Control (CDC). (2010). Youth risk behavior surveillance—United States, 2009. *Morbidity and Mortality Weekly Report, 59*(SS 5), 1–142.

Chellappa, S. L., & Araujo, J. F. (2007). Sleep disorders and suicidal ideation in patients with depressive disorder. *Psychiatry Research, 153*(2), 131–136.

Czeisler, C., Buxton, O., & Khalsa, S. (2011). The human circadian system and sleep-wake regulation. In M. Kryger, T. Roth, & W. Dement (Eds.), *Principles and practice of sleep medicine* (5th ed.). Philadelphia, PA: Saunders.

Geiger, S. D., Sabanayagam, C., & Shankar, A. (2012). The relationship between insufficient sleep and self-rated health in a nationally representative sample. *Journal of Environmental and Public Health, 2012*, 518263. doi:10.1155/2012/518263.

Geyer, J. (2012). DSM-5: What's in, what's out. *MedPage Today*. Retrieved from http://www.medpagetoday.com/MeetingCoverage/APA/32619.

Grandner, M. A., Patel, N. P., Gehrman, P. R., Perlis, M. L., & Pack, A. I. (2010). Problems associated with short sleep: Bridging the gap between laboratory and epidemiological studies. *Sleep Medicine Reviews, 14*(4), 239–247. doi:10.1016/j.smrv.2009.08.001.

Grandner, M. A. (2012). Sleep duration across the lifespan: Implications for health. *Sleep Medicine Reviews, 16*(3), 199–201. doi:10.1016/j.smrv.201202001.

Herdman, T.H. (Ed.), (2012). *NANDA international nursing diagnoses: Definitions and classification, 2012–2014.* Oxford, UK: Wiley-Blackwell.

Institute of Medicine. (2006). *Sleep disorders and sleep deprivation: An unmet public health problem.*Washington, DC: The National Academies Press.

Insurance Institute for Highway Safety. (2012). *DUI/DWI laws*. Retrieved from http://www.iihs.org/laws/dui.aspx.

Johns, M. W. (1991). A new method for measuring daytime sleepiness: The Epworth Sleepiness Scale. *Sleep, 14*, 540–545.

Kessler, R. C., Berglund, P.A., Coulouvrat, C., Hajak, G., Roth, T., Shahly, V., et al. (2011). Insomnia and performance of U.S. workers: Results from the American insomnia survey. *Sleep, 34*(9), 1161–1171.

Knutson, K., Van Cauter, E., Rathouz, P., DeLeire, T., & Lauderdale, D. (2010). Trends in the prevalence of short sleepers in the USA: 1975–2006. *Sleep, 33*(1), 1085–1095.

Kushida, C., Littner, M., Morgenthaler, T., Alessi, C., Bailey, D., Coleman, J., et al. (2005). Practice parameters for the indications for polysomnography and related procedures. *Sleep, 28*, 499–521.

Littner, M. R., Kushida, C., Wise, M., Davila, D. G., Morgenthaler, T., Lee-Chiong, T., et al. (2005). Practice parameters for clinical use of the multiple sleep latency test and maintenance of wakefulness test. *Sleep, 28*(1), 113–121.

Lurie, A. (2011). Obstructive sleep apnea in adults: Epidemiology, clinical presentation, and treatment options. *Advances in Cardiology, 46*, 1–42.

Luyster, F. S., Strollo, P. J., Zee, P. C., & Walsh, J. K. (2012). Sleep: A health imperative. *Sleep, 35*(6), 727–734.

Moorhead, S., Johnson, M., Maas, M. L., & Swanson, E. (2013). *Nursing outcomes classification (NOC)* (5th ed.). St. Louis, MO: Mosby.

Morgenthaler, T., Alessi, C., Friedman, L., Owens, J., Kapur, V., Boehlecke, B., et al. (2007). Practice parameters for the use of actigraphy in the assessment of sleep and sleep disorders: An update for 2007. *Sleep, 30*, 519–529.

Morin, C. (2004). Cognitive-behavioral approaches to the treatment of insomnia. *Journal of Clinical Psychiatry, 65*(Suppl. 16), 33–40.

National Center on Sleep Disorder Research. (2011). *National Institute of Health: Sleep disorders research plan*. Retrieved from http://www.nhlbi.nih.gov/health/prof/sleep/201101011NationalSleepDisordersResearchPlanDHHSPublication11-7820.pdf.

National Highway Traffic and Safety Administration. (2008). *Drowsy driving and automobile crashes: NCSDR and NHTSA expert panel on driver fatigue and sleepiness*. Retrieved from http://www.nhtsa.dot.gov/people/injury/drowsy_driving1/drowsy.html.

National Institute of Neurologic Disorders and Stroke. (2012). *Restless leg syndrome fact sheet*. Retrieved from http://www.ninds.nih.gov/disorders/restless_legs/detail_restless_legs.htm.

National Sleep Foundation. (2011). *Sleep in America poll: Summary of findings*. Retrieved from http://www.sleepfoundation.org/sites/default/files/sleepinamericapoll/SIAP_2011_Summary_of_Findings.pdf.

National Sleep Foundation. (2012a). *How much sleep do we really need?* Retrieved from http://www.sleepfoundation.org/article/how-sleep-works/how-much-sleep-do-we-really-need.

National Sleep Foundation. (2012b). *Sleep in America™ poll results*. Retrieved from http://www.sleepfoundation.org/secondary-links/media-center.

Ohayon, M. M., Dauvilliers, Y., & Reynolds, C. F. (2012). Operational definitions and algorithms for excessive sleepiness in the general population: Implications for DSM-5 nosology. *Archives of General Psychiatry, 69*, 71–79.

Orzel-Gryglewska, J. (2010). Consequences of sleep deprivation. *International Journal of Occupational Medicine and Environmental Health, 23*(1), 95–114.

Roth, T., Jaeger, S., Jin, R., Kalsekar, A., Stang, P., & Kessler, R. (2006). Sleep problems, comorbid medical disorders and role functioning in the National Comorbidity Survey Replication. *Biological Psychiatry, 60*(12), 1364–1371.

Sack, R., Auckley, D., Auger, R., Carskadon, M., Wright, K., & Vitiello, M. (2007). Circadian rhythms sleep disorders: Part I, basic principles, shift work and jet lag disorders. *Sleep, 30*(11), 1460–1524.

Sharafkhaneh, A., Giray, N., Richardson, P., Young, T., & Hirshkowitz, M. (2005). Association of psychiatric disorders and sleep apnea in a large cohort. *Sleep, 28*(11), 1405–1411.

Skaer, T. L., & Sclar, D. A. (2010). Economic implications of sleep disorders. *Pharmacoeconomics, 28*(11), 1015–1023.

Sorscher, A. (2008). How is your sleep: A neglected topic for health care screening. *Journal of the American Board of Family Medicine, 21*(2), 141–148.

Spielman, A., & Glovinsky, P. (2004). A conceptual framework of insomnia for primary care providers: Predisposing, precipitating, and perpetuating factors. *Sleep Medicine Alert, 9*(1), 1–6.

Tracova, R., Dorkova, Z., Molcanyiova, A., Radikova, Z., Klimes, I., & Tkac, I. (2008). Cardiovascular risk and insulin resistance in patients with obstructive sleep apnea. *Medical Science Monitor, 14*(9), CR438CR444.

U.S. Department of Health and Human Services (USDHHS). (2012). *Healthy People 2020*. Retrieved from http://www.healthypeople.gov/2020/default.aspx.

Williamson, A. M., & Feyer, A. M. (2007). Moderate sleep deprivation produces impairments in cognitive and motor performance equivalent to legally prescribed levels of alcohol intoxication. *Occupational and Environmental Medicine, 57*, 649–655.

CHAPTER

20

Sexual Dysfunctions, Gender Dysphoria, and Paraphilias

Margaret Jordan Halter

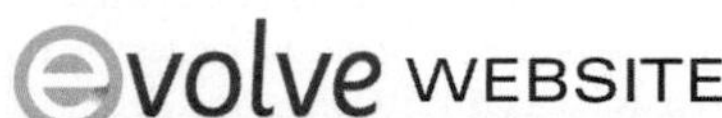

Visit the Evolve website for a pretest on the content in this chapter: http://evolve.elsevier.com/Varcarolis

Pre-Test interactive review

OBJECTIVES

1. Describe the four phases of the sexual response cycle.
2. Describe clinical manifestations of each major sexual dysfunction/disorder.
3. Consider the impact of medical problems and medications on normal sexual functioning.
4. Describe biological, psychological, and environmental factors related to sexual dysfunction.
5. Apply the nursing process to caring for individuals with sexual dysfunction.
6. Examine the importance of nurses being knowledgeable about and comfortable discussing topics pertaining to sexuality.
7. Describe treatments available for sexual dysfunction.
8. Identify the problem of gender dysphoria in children and adults
9. Identify sexual preoccupations considered to be sexual disorders.
10. Discuss personal values and biases regarding sexuality and sexual behaviors.
11. Develop a plan of care for individuals diagnosed with sexual disorders.

KEY TERMS AND CONCEPTS

delayed ejaculation
erectile disorder
exhibitionism
female orgasmic disorder
female sexual interest/arousal disorder
fetishism
frotteurism
gender dysphoria
gender identity
genito-pelvic pain/penetration disorder
male hypoactive sexual desire disorder
paraphilic disorder
pedophilia
premature ejaculation
sex reassignment surgery
sexual disorders
sexual dysfunction
voyeurism

Practicing professional nursing requires us to engage in matter-of-fact discussions with patients regarding topics generally considered to be extremely private and personal. We perform head-to-toe assessments in which we inquire about everything from headaches and sore throats to difficulties urinating and problems with constipation. The realities of providing physical care necessitate becoming comfortable with a number of skills that concern privacy and modesty—performing breast examinations, initiating urinary catheters, and inserting rectal medications to name a few.

Despite a sort of learned fearlessness when it comes to addressing other intimate issues, the topic of sexuality is often a source of discomfort for not only nurses but also other health care providers. Although most recognize that addressing sexuality is part of holistic care, many do not routinely include the topic when doing assessments (Mick, 2007). Nursing curricula typically have a deficiency in training nurses in the fundamentals of sexuality and nursing care. Patients want to know how, for example, medications or treatments will affect their relationships and ability to have satisfying sex lives. Nurses can normalize such issues and foster opportunities to address feelings and fears.

Our views regarding sexuality are based on our individual beliefs about ourselves as women and men, mothers and fathers, and generative individuals who create and give to society in multiple ways. Multiple factors, including societal attitudes and traditions, parental views, cultural practices, spiritual and religious teaching, socioeconomic status, and education affect our sexual beliefs and behaviors and also our attitudes toward the sexual behaviors of others, including our patients.

Health promotion and disease prevention are key responsibilities for nurses. All nurses must assess a patient's sexuality and be prepared to educate, dispel myths, assist with values clarification, refer to appropriate care providers when indicated, and share resources. These actions alleviate or decrease patient illness and suffering and reduce health care costs through prevention. As a nursing student, you are introduced to complex aspects of sexual behavior that should help facilitate thoughtful discussion of the topic, make you aware of your personal belief systems, and help you consider the broader perspective of sexual issues as they exist in contemporary society.

This chapter addresses two general categories of concern related to sexuality. The first half of the chapter examines the normal sexual response cycle, clinical disorders related to the disruption or malfunction of this cycle, and guidelines for nursing care. The second half focuses on problems related to sexual focus and preoccupation. These problems may be sources of discomfort and distress to the person experiencing them (e.g., gender dysphoria) and may be a source of pain and trauma for others whose rights are violated (e.g., pedophilia).

CONSIDERING CULTURE

Female Genital Mutilation and Sexual Functioning

Female genital mutilation is the surgical altering of female sexual organs for nonmedical reasons. The World Health Organization (2008) condemns this practice, as does the United Nations. An estimated 100 million to 140 million females currently are living with the consequences of this surgery, which occurs between birth and 15 years of age. It is performed to decrease libido (ensuring chastity and fidelity to spouses), prevent premarital sex, uphold a cultural tradition, or make the girl more feminine and beautiful by removing parts that are considered "male."

The actual practice varies and may include partial or total removal of the clitoris, the clitoral hood, and labia minora; cutting or fusing of the labia; and narrowing the vaginal opening. The surgery results in severe pain, infection, recurrent urinary tract infections, cysts, infertility, and childbirth complications and may deny women the ability to experience sexual pleasure.

The procedure occurs mainly in Africa, the Middle East, and Asia and is increasingly being protested and restricted by law. Clinicians in the United States are encountering females who have undergone this procedure. Developing a trusting relationship with patients who have been subjected to this custom includes understanding the types of mutilation, as well as the culture in which it occurs.

While research does not demonstrate a difference in desire or pain, there are is an overall decrease in satisfaction between individuals with female genital mutilation and unmutilated women. Additionally, surgically altered women had problems with arousal, lubrication, and orgasm.

Alsibiani, S. A., & Rouzi, A. A. (2010). Sexual function in women with female genital mutilation. *Fertility and Sterility, 93*(3), 722–724; World Health Organization. (2008). *Female genital mutilation.* Retrieved from http://www.who.int/mediacentre/factsheets/fs241/en/.

SEXUALITY

Phases of the Sexual Response Cycle

Before looking more closely at the dysfunctions of sexual functioning, we will first review normal sexual functioning. According to the early experts in sexuality and sexual functioning, Masters and Johnson (1966), there are four distinct phases:

- Phase 1: Desire
- Phase 2: Excitement
- Phase 3: Orgasm
- Phase 4: Resolution

Desire

Many factors may affect interest in sexual activity, including age, physical and emotional health, availability of a sexual partner, and the context of an individual's life. In fact, for a number of individuals, the lack of sexual desire is not a source of distress either to the person or to his or her partner; in such a situation, decreased or absent sexual desire is not viewed as an illness. Furthermore, desire is not a necessary component of sexual functioning.

According to Levine, there are three components to desire: drive, motive, and values (Levine, 2010). He refers to *drive* as the biologically motivated interest based in the cerebral cortex, the limbic, and the endocrine system that prompts a focus on sexually appealing aspects of another, physiological response, and plotting for connection. *Motive* is less physiological and more psychological and is based on choices, aspirations, and motives for interpersonal connection. This is the area that clinicians often target for intervention. *Values* impact sexuality by imparting certain familial, religious, and cultural beliefs and guidelines for our responses and behaviors. It is a significant part of our programming beginning in adolescence; as adults, values are fairly enduring, but they may shift depending on other motivations.

Invariably, there is a difference in sex drive within a relationship, and negotiations are almost always present (Levine, 2010). Low sexual desire may be a source of frustration, both for the one experiencing it and also for partners. It is sometimes associated with psychiatric or medical conditions. Conversely, excessive sexual desire becomes a problem when it creates difficulties for the individual's partner or when such excessive desire drives the person to demand sexual compliance from or to force it upon unwilling partners.

Testosterone (normally present in the circulation of both males and females but in a much higher level in males) appears to be essential to sexual desire in both men and women. Estrogen does not seem to have a direct effect on sexual desire in women. A secondary effect, however, may be present in the requirement of estrogen for the maintenance of normal vaginal elasticity and lubrication.

Excitement

The excitement phase of the normal human sexual response cycle is that period of time during which sexual tension continues to increase from the preceding level of sexual desire. Traditionally, penile erection and vaginal lubrication have been used as indicators of the presence of sexual excitement. If erection or lubrication does not occur in what, for that individual, is a sexually stimulating and appropriate situation, then there has been an inhibition of sexual excitement, regardless of the causative factors.

Orgasm

The orgasm phase of the human sexual response cycle is attained only at high levels of sexual tension in both women and men. Sexual tension (also described as sexual arousal) is produced by a combination of mental activity—including thoughts, fantasies, and dreams—and erotic stimulation of erogenous areas, which may be more or less specific for each individual. Most men require some penile stimulation and most women some clitoral stimulation, either directly or indirectly, to produce the high levels of sexual tension necessary for orgasm to occur.

Some women who have experienced one orgasm may have repeated orgasms during the continuation of the same sexual activity. The occurrence of multiple orgasms depends on the maintenance of high levels of sexual tension through continued stimulation. On the other hand, once men ejaculate as a part of orgasm, they go through a refractory period. This is the time required to produce another ejaculate, which varies primarily with age. In a young man this refractory period is measured in minutes whereas in an older man it may last several hours.

Resolution

During the resolution phase, sexual tension developed in prior phases subsides to baseline levels, provided sexual stimulation has ceased. The physiological changes that occurred during the earlier phases of the response cycle now tend to dissipate. This is a period of psychological vulnerability and can either be experienced as a period of pleasurable "afterglow" or described as being "uncomfortably emotionally exposed." With the restoration of normal physiological pulse, respiratory rate, and blood pressure, individuals frequently experience markedly increased perspiration.

SEXUAL DYSFUNCTION

Sexual dysfunction is an extremely common problem that involves the disturbance in the desire, excitement, or orgasm phases of the sexual response cycle or pain during sexual intercourse. It may prevent or reduce a person's ability to enjoy sex and can be classified according to the phase of the sexual response cycle in which it occurs. In evaluating a patient with a sexual dysfunction, a physical assessment—including laboratory studies—is performed before exploring psychological factors, such as emotional issues, life situation, and experiences. Sexual dysfunctions can be the result of physiological problems, interpersonal conflicts, or a combination of both. Stress of any kind can adversely affect sexual function.

CLINICAL PICTURE

Seven major classes of sexual dysfunction include male hypoactive sexual desire disorder, female sexual interest/arousal disorder, erectile disorder, female orgasmic disorder, delayed ejaculation, premature ejaculation, and genito-pelvic pain/penetration disorder. In addition, there are substance/medication-induced **sexual disorders** and sexual dysfunction that is not classified (American Psychiatric Association, 2013).

It is important to note that some individuals do not have a desire for sexual relations, termed asexuality, and some persons believe that this may be a distinct form of sexual orientation. Asexuality is differentiated from celibacy. Whereas celibacy is a conscious choice to abstain from sex even though the desire is there, asexuality is having no sexual attraction (Brotto, Knudson et al., 2010). Proponents of formalizing this as a sexual orientation maintain that if heterosexuality is attraction to the opposite sex and homosexuality is the attraction to the same sex, then there should be another category that legitimizes the preference for no sexual attraction. Asexual people may have an interest in cuddling and physical contact but no interest in sex, and asexuals may be married and negotiate for sex or simply do without.

Sexual Desire Disorders

The male version of low interest in sex is characterized by a deficiency or absence of sexual fantasies or desire for sexual activity and is called **male hypoactive sexual desire disorder.** It is only considered a disorder if it bothers the person. This problem is determined based on factors such as age and concepts within the culture of the individual where the norm may be to have reduced sexual desire or the reverse. This lack of sexual desire in men can be a lifelong or long-standing problem or may be more acute in nature. The latter, the acquired version, may be situational (the man is not interested in sexual relations with his partner but continues to have interest in another person, others, and/or in masturbation) or generalized (the man has no interest in sexual activity with someone else or solitarily).

The source of this disorder may be physiological, psychological, or a combination of both. Hormonal imbalance, particularly testosterone deficiency, may be an issue. Depression is often implicated in a lack of desire for sexual intimacy in men.

The female version of low sexual desire uses the word "interest" rather than desire and also includes the term "arousal." Brotto (2010) recommended that the two terms be combined in this disorder since it is extremely difficult to separate one from the other. This combination places the disorder across both the "desire" category and also the "excitement" category (below). Female sexual interest/arousal disorder is characterized by emotional distress caused by absent or reduced interest in sexual fantasies, sexual activity, pleasure, and arousal. Some women experience these symptoms their whole lives while others may gradually become less interested in sexual activities.

Reasons for the disorder may be clear, such as having an abusive mate, while in other cases it is a baffling problem to both the woman and her partner. Researchers believe that it is caused by a combination of neurobiological, hormonal, and psychosocial factors (Clayton, 2010). Dopamine, progesterone, estrogen, and testosterone exert an excitatory role while serotonin, prolactin, and opioids inhibit sexual desire. Female sexual interest/arousal disorder is fairly common and is thought to occur in 1 in 10 women (Clayton, 2010).

Sexual Excitement Disorders

Erectile disorder (also called *erectile dysfunction* and *impotence*) refers to failure to obtain and maintain an erection sufficient for sexual activity or decreased erectile turgidity on 75% of sexual occasions and lasting for at least 6 months (Segraves, 2010). This problem may be a rare, lifelong condition in which a man has never been able to obtain an erection sufficient for intercourse. It may also be an acquired condition in which a man has previously been able to have sexual intercourse but has lost the ability.

Orgasm Disorders

Female Orgasmic Disorder

Study of the female orgasm is more complicated than the male orgasm, which results in a noticeable ejaculation. Additionally, there is no reproduction associated with the female analog. Comparing female and male responses to orgasm, men are more focused on performance while women tend to be focused on the subjective quality of having sex (Graham, 2009). Some women are uncertain if orgasm has even occurred. Up to 22% of women experience an orgasmic disorder while only 6% report this problem as distressing.

Female orgasmic disorder is sometimes referred to as *inhibited female orgasm* or *anorgasmia* and is defined as the recurrent or persistent inhibition of female orgasm, as manifested by the recurrent delay in, or absence of, orgasm after a normal sexual excitement phase (achieved by masturbation or coitus). For the recognition of a clinically significant problem, it must happen for at least 6 months and must occur during three fourths of sexual encounters (Graham, 2009).

It may be a lifelong disorder (never having achieved orgasm) or acquired (having had at least one orgasm and then having difficulties). Most cases are lifelong rather than acquired, and once a woman learns how to achieve orgasm it is unusual to lose this capacity (Graham, 2009). Acquired anorgasmia in women tends to be associated with painful intercourse during or after menopause. The prevalence of either type of this disorder is estimated at 30% (Sadock & Sadock, 2008). Psychological factors (including fears of pregnancy, rejection, or loss of control), hostility toward or from men, and cultural/societal restrictions may be causative. There is some evidence to suggest that female orgasmic disorder may be inherited.

Delayed Ejaculation

In delayed ejaculation, formerly referred to as *male orgasmic disorder, inhibited orgasm,* or *retarded ejaculation,* a man achieves ejaculation during coitus only with great difficulty. A man with a *lifelong delayed ejaculation* has never been able to ejaculate during coitus; this uncommon condition may result from a rigid background in which sex is believed to be a sin.

Acquired delayed ejaculation develops after previously normal functioning and is fairly common. Interpersonal problems may be the cause. Physical conditions, substance abuse, and prescribed medication may also cause this problem and should be assessed.

Premature Ejaculation

In premature ejaculation, a man persistently or recurrently achieves orgasm and ejaculation before he wishes to. Diagnosis is made when a man regularly ejaculates before or immediately after the penis enters the vagina. Considerations as to age, newness of the relationship, and how often the man has intercourse should be assessed. About 35% to 40% of men who are treated for sexual disorders complain of premature ejaculation. Physical factors may be involved; some men may be more tactilely sensitive and respond more intensely to stimulation. Psychological factors include fear about performance and stressful relationships where the man feels hurried. There is no disorder in women that corresponds to premature ejaculation.

Genito-Pelvic Pain/Penetration Disorder

The group of disorders previously diagnosed in the psychiatric community included a problem called dyspareunia, which referred to pelvic and/or vaginal pain during or after intercourse. It also included vaginismus, which referred to an involuntary constriction response of the muscles that close the vagina. Researchers believe that the distinction between the two disorders is too blurry and decided to combine them into a single disorder (Svoboda, 2010). Genito-pelvic pain/penetration disorder interferes with penile insertion and intercourse and may even be elicited during a normal gynecological examination with a speculum. Individuals experiencing these problems become fearful that pain and spasms will occur during the next encounter (Binik, 2010). This fear compounds the problem by increasing anxiety and muscle tension.

VIGNETTE

Jessica, a computer programmer, had recently had a baby and was looking forward to renewing her love life with her husband. She said, "My husband would barely begin penetration, and the pain would be awful. The whole area just clenched up." She continued, "I had never had any problems before, and I didn't think I would because I'd had a caesarean, so I didn't think that anything would change. 'Good grief, that hurts,' I thought. 'What is wrong with me?' We were both terribly upset."

Other Sexual Dysfunctions and Problems

Sexual dysfunction due to a general medical condition includes sexual desire disorders, orgasm disorders, and sexual pain disorders, but the cause of each is related to a medical condition, such as cardiovascular, neurological, or endocrine disease.

The diagnosis *substance-induced sexual dysfunction* is used when evidence of substance intoxication or withdrawal is apparent from the history, physical examination, or laboratory findings. Distressing sexual dysfunction occurs within a month of significant substance intoxication or withdrawal. Specified substances include alcohol, amphetamines or related substances, cocaine, opioids, sedatives, hypnotics, antianxiety agents, and other known and unknown substances. Abused recreational substances can have a variety of effects on sexual functioning. In small doses, many substances enhance sexual performance. With continued use, sexual difficulties become the norm.

Sexual dysfunction not elsewhere classified is a category that covers sexual dysfunctions that cannot be classified under one of the other categories. Typically, this is because their presentation is not quite strong enough to meet the criteria for a disorder or because there is not enough information to make a diagnosis.

Box 20-1 provides a discussion regarding the influence of pharmacological treatment for me and psychiatric diagnoses for sexual dysfunction in women.

EPIDEMIOLOGY

Overall, sexual dysfunctions are more common in women than men (Shafer, 2010). There is reasonable descriptive data that indicates that nearly half of adult women (40% to 45%) and about a third of adult men (20% to 30%) have at least one sexual dysfunction (Lewis et al., 2010). The prevalence of male orgasmic disorder has been reported at 5% (Sadock & Sadock, 2008). Acquired erectile disorder is the most common sexual disorder in men and may affect approximately one third of all adult men at some time (Heidelbaugh, 2010). In young men, the disorder is uncommon, and the cause is usually psychological. There are estimates that between 12% to 20% of women experience ongoing genital pain during intercourse (Brotto, 2012).

BOX 20-1 SEXUAL DYSFUNCTION IN WOMEN: THE VIAGRA EFFECT

Experts in psychiatric disorders are expressing concern that women may be overdiagnosed with disorders in sexual function based on criteria in the latest edition of the *Diagnostic and Statistical Manual* (APA, 2013). Normal variation in sexual interest, along with variability within the life cycle, should be taken into consideration when these diagnoses are made (Frances, 2013).

A safeguard in the criteria for female sexual interest/arousal disorder stipulates that emotional distress is necessary. However, the advent of pharmacological innovations such as Viagra that improve sexual performance in men should be factored into this emotional distress. Expectations on the part of men as treated partners, researchers, and pharmaceutical leaders set the social stage for the overdiagnosis of female sexual dysfunction in women. Only a generation ago, both partners in a couple were aging and experiencing a reduction in sexual interest/appetite; now, pharmacological innovations may have created a mismatch between treated men and untreated women.

COMORBIDITY

Sexual functioning may be adversely affected any time there is a disturbance in an individual's ability to develop and maintain stable relationships. This is especially true for patients with schizophrenia, who show difficulty coping with stress, a decrease in reality-based orientation to the world, and defense mechanisms that lead to withdrawn behavior. Sexual dysfunction is often associated with depression and personality disorders (Becker & Stinson, 2008). A history of sexual trauma is also frequently associated with sexual dysfunction.

Obesity and a sedentary lifestyle contribute to sexual dysfunction from both a psychological and a physiological perspective. Psychologically, an obese person may feel undesirable or may have a partner who is no longer attracted. Physiologically, inactivity results in less vitality overall, including sexual ability and responsiveness.

ETIOLOGY

Biological Factors

Aging appears to be a factor in the prevalence of all sexual dysfunction for both men and women. In addition, a variety of physical conditions are related to sexual dysfunction and are presented in Table 20-1.

Psychological Factors

Pioneers in the study of human sexuality include Helen Singer Kaplan (1929-1995). According to Kaplan (1974), sexual dysfunctions are the result of a combination of factors, including the following:

- Misinformation or ignorance regarding sexual and social interaction
- Unconscious guilt and anxiety regarding sex
- Anxiety related to performance, especially with erectile and orgasmic dysfunction
- Poor communication between partners about feelings and what they desire sexually

Additional factors have been identified to explain sexual dysfunction. Unacknowledged or unidentified sexual orientation may lead to poor performance with the opposite sex, or the presence of one sexual problem may lead to another. For example, difficulty maintaining an erection may lead to hypoactive sexual desire (Becker & Stinson, 2008). Education seems to have a buffering effect, and people who have more education have fewer sexual problems and are less anxious about issues pertaining to sex (Shafer, 2010).

TABLE 20-1 MEDICAL CONDITIONS AND SURGICAL PROCEDURES THAT CAUSE SEXUAL DYSFUNCTION

SYSTEM/STATE	ORGANIC DISORDERS	SEXUAL IMPAIRMENT
Endocrine	Hypothyroidism, adrenal dysfunction, hypogonadism, diabetes mellitus	Low libido, impotence, decreased vaginal lubrication, early impotence
Vascular	Hypertension, atherosclerosis, stroke, venous insufficiency, sickle cell disorder	Impotence, but ejaculation and libido intact
Neurological	Spinal cord damage, diabetic neuropathy, herniated disk, alcoholic neuropathy, multiple sclerosis, temporal lobe epilepsy	Sexual disorder—early signs: low or high libido, impotence, impaired orgasm
Genital	*Male*—Priapism, Peyronie's disease, urethritis, prostatitis, hydrocele	Low libido, impotence
	Female—Imperforate hymen, vaginitis, pelvic inflammatory disease, endometriosis	Vaginismus, dyspareunia, low libido, decreased arousal
Systemic	Renal, pulmonary, hepatic, advanced malignancies, infections	Low libido, impotence, decreased arousal
Psychiatric	Depression	Low libido, erectile dysfunction
	Bipolar disorder (manic phase)	Increased libido
	Generalized anxiety disorder, panic disorder, posttraumatic stress disorder (PTSD), obsessive-compulsive disorder (OCD)	Low libido, erectile dysfunction, reduced vaginal lubrication, anorgasmia, "anti-fantasies" focusing on partner's negative qualities (OCD only)
	Schizophrenia	Low desire, bizarre sexual fantasies
	Personality disorders (passive-aggressive, obsessive-compulsive, histrionic)	Low libido, erectile dysfunction, premature ejaculation, anorgasmia
Surgical-postoperative	*Male*—Prostatectomy, abdominal-perineal bowel resection	Impotence, no loss of libido, ejaculatory impairment
	Female—Episiotomy, vaginal prolapse repair, oophorectomy	Dyspareunia, vaginismus, decreased lubrication
	Male and female—Leg amputation, colostomy, ileostomy	Mechanical difficulties in sex, low self-image, fear of odor

Data from Shafer, L. C. (2010). Sexual disorders and sexual dysfunction. In T. A. Stern, G. L. Fricchione, N. H. Cassem, M. S. Jellinek, & J. F. Rosenbaum (Eds.), *Massachusetts General Hospital handbook of general hospital psychiatry* (6th ed., pp. 323-335). Philadelphia, PA: Saunders.

APPLICATION OF THE NURSING PROCESS

ASSESSMENT

General Assessment

Sexual assessment includes both subjective and objective data. Many psychiatric hospitals use a nursing history tool that is biologically oriented but typically has few questions on sexual functioning. Health history questions pertaining to the reproductive system may be limited to menstrual history, parity, history of sexually transmitted diseases, method of contraception, and questions regarding safe sex practices. There may be a few vague questions about sexual functioning or sexual concerns.

While the topic of sex may be uncomfortable to some readers and future nurses, many in our society wonder if we are trying to make everyone fit into a certain mold with our approaches, specifically when interviewing patients about such personal issues. We tend to ask basic questions related to sexual interest and performance, yet one of the most basic questions relates to the congruence of a person's actual sexual life to one that they would like to have. For example, maybe the problem is not in functioning but in fit of the relationship. Perhaps the question to be asked is if there is a type of behavior, a type of partner, or social context that interests the patient more than his or her current situation (Levine, 2010). Perhaps we are asking a homosexual man about arousal and interest in his female partner when the relationship is mismatched in regard to sexual orientation. Also, when approaching non-heterosexual youth about sexual practices, they may be hesitant to truthfully respond, particularly if they have been ostracized or harmed for their sexual choices in the past.

Patients may cue the nurse into the presence of sexual concerns without explicitly verbalizing them. Box 20-2 presents a discussion of these cues.

The nurse may ask the patient if there is concern in the area of sexual functioning. Generally, it is more comfortable for the patient if the nurse firsts asks questions in a general manner and then proceeds to the patient's experience. For example, the nurse might say, "Some people who are prescribed this medication find it difficult to achieve an erection. Have you had this problem?" This allows the patient to feel that he is not alone in what he is experiencing.

Table 20-2 provides facilitative statements for the interviewer conducting a sexual assessment.

The sexual history includes the patient's perception of physiological functioning and behavioral, emotional, and spiritual aspects of sexuality. It also includes cultural and religious beliefs with regard to sexual behavior and sexual knowledge base. During the assessment, both the nurse and the patient are free to ask questions and clarify information. It is reasonable to defer lengthy sexual health assessment when acute psychiatric symptoms preclude a calm, thoughtful discussion. As symptoms subside and rapport is developed, the assessment may be resumed. With experience, the nurse is able to identify those patients who are at greater risk for difficulties in sexual functioning. This includes patients with a history of certain medical problems or surgical procedures (see Table 20-1) and patients taking some drugs (Table 20-3).

Self-Assessment

Discomfort in assessing sexual history may be due to personal embarrassment, concerns about embarrassing the patient, poor training, inexperience, inadequate time, or beliefs that sexual history is not important. Indeed, you may experience discomfort exploring sexual issues with patients, fearing that this discussion will be personally embarrassing as well as embarrassing to the patient. You may fear that you will not know what questions to ask or why the questions should be asked.

Concerns related to age and gender differences are understandable. If the patient is approximately your age and of the opposite sex, you might worry that talking about sexuality may not be appropriate or whether the patient might conclude that you are a little too interested. Discussing issues related to sexuality with people who are your parents' or grandparents' age may also create a level of discomfort, especially if you grew up in a home where such topics were avoided and you had to rely on your friends for your personal information (or misinformation) about sex.

Remembering your position as a professional and addressing the topics in a tone and manner appropriate of a professional will increase your comfort, along with the patient's. Also, letting the patient know *why* you are asking such personal questions increases openness and cooperation. For example, "People who are depressed sometimes find that it affects their sexual desire. Since you have been depressed, have you noticed a change in your interest in sex?" Sometimes a more subtle approach that shifts the focus away from the patient is helpful. "Since you have been depressed, has your husband felt as if you are less interested in him?"

Perhaps the most helpful consideration is recognizing that assessing sexuality is part of holistic nursing care. Your role and responsibility is in assisting the patient in dealing with responses to illness and/or the treatment of the illness. Understanding your patient's concerns, acknowledging the patient's discomfort, and providing useful feedback will enhance your professional abilities to care for your patient and perhaps even improve self-understanding.

BOX 20-2 PATIENT CUES THAT MAY INDICATE CONCERNS ABOUT SEXUALITY

Nonverbal Behaviors

- Showing discomfort by blushing, looking away, making tight fists, fidgeting, crying
- Openly engaging in overt sexual behaviors (e.g., touching own body parts, masturbating, exposing genitals, placing nurse's hand on genitals, making sexually suggestive sounds)

Verbal Behaviors

- Telling sexually explicit jokes
- Making sexual comments about the nurse
- Asking inappropriate questions about the nurse's sexual activity
- Discussing sexual exploits
- Expressing concern about relationship with partner:
  - "I don't feel the same about my partner."
  - "My partner doesn't feel the same about me."
  - "We're not as close."
  - "Our relationship has changed."
  - "My personal life has changed."
- Expressing concern that sexuality has been diminished (e.g., feeling less of a man, less of a woman):
  - "I've lost my manhood."
  - "I'm not as desirable as I once was."
- Expressing concern over lack of sexual desire:
  - "I'm not interested in sex anymore."
  - "My desire has changed."
  - "I'm not the man/woman I used to be."
  - "We don't click anymore."
- Expressing concern over sexual performance:
  - "I've lost my power."
  - "What will happen to my ability to perform?"
  - "I can't perform like I used to."
- Expressing concern about one's love life:
  - "My love life has changed."
  - "The spark is gone."
- Expressing concern over the sexual impact of drugs, surgery, or some other medical treatment:
  - "Will this drug interfere with my sex life?"
  - "Will I still be able to perform sexually after surgery?"

ASSESSMENT GUIDELINES

Sexual Dysfunction

1. A sexual assessment should be conducted in a setting that allows privacy and eliminates distractions.
2. Although note taking may be necessary for the beginner, it can be distracting to the patient and interrupt the flow of the interview. When note taking is necessary, it should be unobtrusive and kept to a minimum.
3. The interviewer should be aware of personal biases and attitudes that could block open discussion of sexual issues.
4. Good eye contact, relaxed posture, and friendly facial expressions facilitate the patient's comfort and communicate openness and receptivity on the part of the nurse.

TABLE 20-2 FACILITATIVE STATEMENTS FOR THE INTERVIEWER CONDUCTING A SEXUAL ASSESSMENT

PURPOSE	FACILITATIVE STATEMENT
To provide a rationale for a question	"As a nurse, I'm concerned about all aspects of your health. Many individuals have concern about sexual matters, especially when they are sick or having other health problems."
To give statements of generality or normality	"Most people are hesitant to discuss. . . ." "Many people worry about feeling. . . ." "Many people have concerns about. . . ."
To identify sexual dysfunction	"Most people have difficulties sometime during their sexual relationships. What have yours been?"
To obtain information	"The degree to which unmarried persons have sexual outlets varies considerably. Some have sexual partners. Some relieve sexual tension through masturbation. Others need no outlet at all. What has been your pattern?"
To identify sexual myths	"While growing up, most of us have heard some sexual myths or half-truths that continue to puzzle us. Are there any that come to mind?"
To determine whether homosexuality is a source of conflict	"What is your attitude toward your homosexual orientation?"
To identify an older person's concerns about sexual function	"Many people, as they get older, believe or worry that this signals the end of their sex life. Much misinformation continues this myth. What is your understanding about sexuality during the later years? How has the passage of time affected your sexuality (sex life)?"
To obtain and give information (miscellaneous areas)	"Frequently people have questions about. . . ." "What questions do you have about. . . ." "What would you like to know about. . . ."
To close the history	"Is there anything further in the area of sexuality that you would like to bring up now?"

Adapted from Green, R. (1975). *Human sexuality: A health practitioner's text.* Baltimore, MD: Williams & Wilkins.

TABLE 20-3 DRUGS THAT CAN CAUSE SEXUAL DYSFUNCTION

CATEGORY	DRUG	SEXUAL SIDE EFFECTS
Cardiovascular drugs	Methyldopa	Low libido, impotence, anorgasmia
	Thiazides	Low libido, impotence, decreased lubrication
	Clonidine	Impotence, anorgasmiaLow libido
	Propranolol	Low libido
	Digoxin	Gynecomastia, low libido, impotence
	Clofibrate	Low libido, impotence
Gastrointestinal drugs	Cimetidine	Low libido, impotence
	Methantheline bromide	Impotence
Hormones	Estrogen	Low libido in men
	Progesterone	Low libido, impotence
Sedatives	Alcohol	Higher doses cause sexual problems
	Barbiturates	Impotence
Antianxiety drugs	Alprazolam	Low libido, delayed ejaculation
	Diazepam	
Antipsychotics	Thioridazine	Retarded or retrograde ejaculation
	Haloperidol	Low libido, impotence, anorgasmia
	Risperidone	Impotence
Antidepressants	MAOIs (Phenelzine)	Impotence, retarded ejaculation, anorgasmia
	Tricyclics (imipramine)	Low libido, impotence, retarded ejaculation
	SSRIs (fluoxetine, sertraline)	Low libido, impotence, retarded ejaculation Priapism, retarded or retrograde ejaculation
	Atypical (trazodone)	Low libido, impotence, retarded ejaculation Priapism, retarded or retrograde ejaculation
Antimanic drugs	Lithium	Low libido, impotence

MAOIs, Monoamine oxidase inhibitors; *SSRIs*, selective serotonin reuptake inhibitors.
Data from Shafer, L. C. (2010). Sexual disorders and sexual dysfunction. In T. A. Stern, G. L. Fricchione, N. H. Cassem, M. S. Jellinek, & J. F. Rosenbaum (Eds.), *Massachusetts General Hospital handbook of general hospital psychiatry* (6th ed., pp. 323-335). Philadelphia, PA: Saunders.

DIAGNOSIS

A comprehensive sexual assessment can reveal areas of sexual concern and dysfunction for the patient. These data are analyzed to determine the appropriate nursing diagnoses. Priority nursing diagnoses, their definitions, and possible etiology follow (Herdman, 2012):

Sexual dysfunction is the state in which an individual experiences a change in sexual function during the sexual response phases of desire, excitation, and/or orgasm. The change is viewed as unsatisfying, unrewarding, or inadequate and may be related to the following:

- Altered body function from medication
- Biopsychosocial alteration of sexuality
- Psychosocial abuse from significant other

Ineffective sexuality pattern is indicated by expressions of concern regarding one's own sexuality. It may be related to the following:

- Lack of significant other
- Conflicts with sexual orientation
- Impaired relationship with significant other
- Knowledge deficit about alternative responses to illness

OUTCOMES IDENTIFICATION

The diagnosis of *sexual dysfunction* may be paired with *NOC* (Moorhead et al., 2013) outcomes listed under the category of sexual functioning. Each is ranked on a 5-point scale where 1 is "never demonstrated" and 5 is "consistently demonstrated." Examples of outcomes include:

- Attains sexual arousal
- Uses hormone replacement therapy as needed
- Expresses ability to be intimate

The diagnosis of *ineffective sexuality pattern* is linked by NOC with the outcome category sexual identity. Useful indicators (ranked the same way as the previous entry) include:

- Exhibits clear sense of sexual orientation
- Reports healthy intimate relationships
- Uses precautions to minimize risks associated with sexual activity

Table 20-4 provides signs and symptoms, nursing diagnoses, and outcomes for sexual disorders.

PLANNING

Planning nursing care for the patient with a sexual dysfunction may occur as part of care for a coexisting disorder. Nurses prepared at the basic level may encounter such patients when they are being treated for a variety of conditions in any setting.

IMPLEMENTATION

An understanding of sexual function and dysfunction is essential for nurses who work in psychiatry as well as most any specialty area in nursing, including oncology, cardiology, and neurology. All nurses need to be able to facilitate a discussion about sexuality with the patient. To be a facilitator, the nurse must be nonjudgmental, have basic knowledge of sexual functioning, and have the ability to conduct a basic sexual assessment. Once the assessment is completed, the nurse needs to know when and to whom to refer the patient with a sexual complaint. Depending on the nature of the problem, the patient may need a referral to a professional such as a marital counselor, psychiatrist, gynecologist, urologist, clinical nurse specialist, or pastoral counselor.

Box 20-3 provides sample interventions from *Nursing Interventions Classification (NIC)* (Bulechek et al., 2013) for *Sexual Counseling.*

Pharmacological Interventions

Treatments for sexual dysfunction increasingly are becoming the target of pharmaceutical industries. Despite the fact that women with sexual dysfunction greatly outnumber men, all of the available pharmacological treatment for sexual dysfunction is aimed at men. There are no treatments approved by the U.S. Food and Drug Administration (FDA) for female sexual disorders. Table 20-5 summarizes treatments for sexual dysfunction.

Pharmacological treatments are available for lifelong premature ejaculation. These treatments include antidepressants in the selective serotonin reuptake inhibitors category or topical anesthetics (Rowland et al., 2010). Conversely, pharmacotherapy may *cause* erectile dysfunction, and medications may need

TABLE 20-4 SIGNS AND SYMPTOMS, DIAGNOSES, AND OUTCOMES FOR SEXUAL DYSFUNCTION

SIGNS AND SYMPTOMS	NURSING DIAGNOSES	OUTCOMES
Alteration in achieving perceived sex role, alteration in relationship with significant other, changes in sexual activities and/or behaviors	*Ineffective sexuality pattern*	Attains sexual arousal, sustains arousal through orgasm, adapts sexual techniques as needed, expresses ability to be intimate, communicates comfortably with partner
Perceived alteration in sexual excitement and/or desire, limitations imposed by disease or therapy, inability to achieve desired satisfaction, verbalization of a problem	*Sexual dysfunction*	Discusses the side effect profile of various antidepressants on sexual functioning, expresses ability to be intimate

From Herdman, T. H. (Ed.), (2012). *Nursing diagnoses—Definitions and classification 2012-2014.* Copyright © 2012, 1994-2012 by NANDA International. Used by arrangement with John Wiley & Sons Limited; Moorhead, S., Johnson, M., Maas, M. L., & Swanson, E. (2013). *Nursing outcomes classification (NOC)* (5th ed.). St. Louis, MO: Mosby.

EVIDENCE-BASED PRACTICE

Testosterone for Postmenopausal Women with Low Libido

Somboonporn, W., Bell, R. J., & Davis, S. R. (2010). Testosterone for peri- and postmenopausal women. *Cochrane Menstrual Disorders and Subfertility Group.* doi: 10.1002/14651858.CD004509.pub2. Retrieved from http://onlinelibrary.wiley.com/doi/10.1002/14651858.CD004509.pub2/abstract.

Problem

Nearly one third of women in the United States may experience lack of sexual interest, and about one fourth cannot achieve orgasm. Postmenopausal women in particular may be distressed by a loss of sexual interest. When taken along with estrogen and progesterone, testosterone has been demonstrated to increase sexual interest in postmenopausal women; however, many women are (understandably) reluctant to take estrogen and/or progesterone due to the increased risk of breast cancer, heart attacks, and strokes.

Purpose of Study

The purpose of this study was to gather information from many strong studies to determine if testosterone, a hormone that is actually more prevalent in the bloodstreams of premenopausal women than estrogen, improves sexual well-being in postmenopausal women. Researchers wondered if adding testosterone therapy to conventional postmenopausal hormone therapy (HT) was effective and safe.

Methods

A total of 4768 participants was included in this review of 35 studies. The typical length of studies was 6 months and the researchers believed that the trials were long enough and had good randomization among participants – i.e., participants were randomly placed into the experimental group or the control group and did not know which group they were in.

Key Findings

- Adding testosterone to hormone therapy improves sexual function in postmenopausal women.
- Combined hormone therapy with testosterone therapy increases unwanted hair growth and acne and also reduces the good high-density lipoprotein cholesterol.
- Doses and routes of administration may impact the degree of these adverse events.
- The addition of testosterone did not increase the number of women who stopped HT therapy.

Implications for Nursing Practice

One of the most basic drives in life is sexuality and intimate expression. While males have benefited by effective pharmacological treatments, there has been little progress made in improving sexual functioning in women. Nurses are in a trusted position to provide recommendations for women who wish to improve sexual functioning. Testosterone may be helpful in improving sexual responsiveness and intimate connection.

BOX 20-3 *NIC* INTERVENTIONS FOR SEXUAL COUNSELING

Definition: Use of an interactive helping process focusing on the need to make adjustments in sexual practice or to enhance coping with a sexual event or disorder.

Activities:*

- Establish a therapeutic relationship based on trust and respect.
- Provide privacy and ensure confidentiality.
- Discuss the effect of the illness or health situation on sexuality.
- Discuss the effect of medications on sexuality, as appropriate.
- Avoid displaying aversion to an altered body part.
- Provide factual information about sexual myths and misinformation that patients may verbalize.
- Provide reassurance that current and new sexual practices are healthy, as appropriate.
- Include the spouse/sexual partner in the counseling as much as possible, as appropriate.
- Refer patient to a sex therapist, as appropriate.

*Partial list.

Data from Bulechek, G. M., Butcher, H. K., Dochterman, J. M., & Wagner, C. (Eds.). (2013). *Nursing interventions classification (NIC)* (6th ed.). St. Louis, MO: Mosby.

to be evaluated for change or dose reduction. Delayed ejaculation may have a biological cause and/or psychogenic etiology. Several strategies for combatting antidepressant-induced sexual dysfunction include the following:

- Waiting to see whether sexual side effects decrease over the course of several weeks.
- Planning for sexual activity prior to taking the antidepressant if the dosing is once a day.
- Switching antidepressants to one with a more favorable side effect profile such as mirtazepine (Remeron), buproprion (Wellbutrin), or vilazodone (Viibrid).

Health Teaching and Health Promotion

Nurses should help patients weigh the pros and cons of any type of pharmacotherapy. Many drugs cause sexual side effects, and notably psychotropic medications used for psychiatric disorders are common offenders. Nurses tend to ignore or minimize the sexual side effects associated with these medications, perhaps in an attempt to promote adherence. The best approach is to help patients to evaluate for themselves the benefits versus the risks of pharmacotherapy empowers patients to choose the best course of action and increases their ability to be informed consumers of mental health services (Higgins, 2007).

TABLE 20-5 PHARMACOLOGICAL, PSYCHOSOCIAL, AND OTHER TREATMENTS FOR SEXUAL DYSFUNCTION

SEXUAL DISORDER	PHARMACOLOGICAL TREATMENT	PSYCHOSOCIAL APPROACHES	OTHER
Male hypoactive sexual desire disorder	Testosterone therapy for males with low levels of this hormone	Individual therapy Couples therapy	
Female sexual interest/ arousal disorder	Testosterone patch for menopausal females Alprostadil cream (Femprox) Tibolone Lubrication (K-Y Jelly)	Sensate focus exercises Individual therapy Couples therapy	EROS-CTD clitoral suction device* Lubrication (e.g., K-Y Jelly)
Male erectile disorder	Sildenafil citrate (Viagra)* Tadalafil (Cialis)* Vardenafil (Levitra)* Avanafil (Stendra)* Alprostadil (MUSE)* penile self-injection and intraurethral suppository Testosterone (for hypogonadism) Yohimbine (Yocon)* Phentolamine (Vasomax)	Sensate focus exercises Group therapy Hypnotherapy Systematic desensitization Psychodynamic therapy Couples therapy	Vacuum pump Penile prostheses
Female orgasmic disorder	Sildenafil (Viagra)	Masturbation training Couples therapy Kegel vaginal exercises	
Male orgasmic disorder	Sildenafil (Viagra)	Masturbatory training Systematic desensitization	
Premature ejaculation	(None with FDA approval) SSRIs to delay or retard ejaculation Topical anesthetics	Start-stop technique Squeeze technique Increased sexual frequency	

*FDA approved.

Data from Shafer, L. C. (2010). Sexual disorders and sexual function. In T. A. Stern, G. L. Fricchione, N. H. Cassem, M. S. Jellinek, & J. F. Rosenbaum (Eds.), *Massachusetts General Hospital handbook of general hospital psychiatry* (6th ed., pp. 323-335). Philadelphia, PA: Saunders; U.S. Food and Drug Administration. (2012). *FDA approves Stendra for erectile dysfunction.* Retrieved from http://www.fda.gov/NewsEvents/Newsroom/PressAnnouncements/ucm302140.htm; Clinicaltrials.gov. (2013). *Safety and efficacy of LibiGel® for treatment of hypoactive sexual desire disorder in postmenopausal women.* Retrieved from http://clinicaltrials.gov/ct2/show/NCT00612742.

Advanced Practice Interventions

Advanced practice nurses (nurse practitioners and clinical nurse specialists) can be qualified to treat sexual dysfunction through advanced training and certification. General therapies include psychoanalytic therapy, couples therapy, group therapy, and hypnotherapy. Some specific therapies available for sexual dysfunction include the following:

- **Sensate focus:** A therapeutic treatment in which patients progress from general touching and cuddling without intercourse to more intimate forms of expression
- **Behavioral therapy:** Useful for men with premature ejaculation when psychogenic or relationship factors are present and is often best combined with medication in an integrated treatment program.
- **Systematic desensitization:** Involves combining relaxation exercises with sexually anxiety- producing stimuli
- **Masturbation training:** Especially helpful in women who have never had an orgasm. This approach helps women learn about their bodies and their responses in order to understand their sexual responsiveness.

VIGNETTE

Maria is a 67-year-old woman, widowed many years, who has recently been approached by a 75-year-old widower with a marriage proposal. Maria is concerned about the sexual implications of a marriage so late in life. She confides in her nurse practitioner, "I really haven't even thought about sex for so many years. I know Joe is just an old goat. He's always after me to take my clothes off." After discussing the possibility of a physiological cause for her lack of interest in sex, Maria's nurse practitioner gives her small doses of testosterone. Within a remarkably short time, Maria stops talking about Joe as "an old goat" and begins talking again about "how great life can be if you have the right partner."

EVALUATION

Evaluation of expected outcomes relates to the level of control and personal satisfaction achieved. Acceptance of sexual dysfunction (e.g., impotence) as being part—but not necessarily the defining characteristic—of sexual behavior can result in greater satisfaction. The degree to which negative attitudes about sex are no longer problematic is also important.

GENDER DYSPHORIA

CLINICAL PICTURE

When we inquire about the birth of an infant, we want to know if it is a boy or a girl; we are asking about the sex of the child (i.e., whether its chromosomes are XX or XY). However, gender identity, the sense of maleness or femaleness, is not usually established until a child is about 3 years old (Becker & Johnson, 2008).

Usually people are comfortable with the fact that they are male or female. Unfortunately, biological assignment does not necessarily determine whether individuals think of themselves as male or female. When biological sex differs from gender identity, the individual may suffer from gender dysphoria, or feelings of unease about their incongruent maleness or femaleness. A man might describe himself as "a woman trapped in a man's body."

It should be noted that gender dysphoria is no longer considered a psychiatric disorder. Until quite recently, this problem was known as gender identity disorder, and all transgender people could be considered mentally ill based on the disorder's criteria (Beredjick, 2012).

Symptoms in children include expressions of desire to be the opposite sex; some children insist that they *are* the opposite sex and ask their families to call them by another name (Grohol, 2011). Boys may wish to wear feminine clothing, play with girls' toys, and choose girls as playmates; girls gravitate toward typically male clothing, play with toys usually associated with boys, and are most comfortable with boys for friends. Fantasy and make-believe are often the vehicle for the expression of their desire to be the opposite sex. Only a small percentage of children who display gender dysphoria characteristics will continue to show these characteristics into adolescence or adulthood.

Teenagers and adults may verbalize a desire to be the other sex and to be treated as such. Dressing up and passing for the opposite sex is common. Adolescents may dread the appearance of secondary sexual characteristics and (along with adults) may seek hormones or surgery to alter their masculinity or femininity. These individuals do not usually consider themselves to be homosexual. The biological female that falls in love with a woman believes she is actually a man who loves that woman.

EPIDEMIOLOGY

This condition is extremely uncommon and affects three to four times as many males as females (Becker & Johnson, 2008). The numbers of people who seek gender reassignment have increased dramatically over the past decade, yet this group is thought to represent the extreme endpoint of persons who actually have gender dysphoric disorder, and no direct studies have been conducted.

COMORBIDITY

Most adolescents with gender dysphoria do not have comorbid conditions (deVries et al., 2011). Anxiety disorders are most common in this population (21%), followed by mood disorders (12.4%) and disruptive disorders (11.4%). Autism spectrum disorder has also been associated with gender dysphoria. Substance abuse and self-destructive behavior are also common parallels found in persons suffering from gender dysphoria.

ETIOLOGY

Biological Factors

While biological factors are not thought to *cause* this problem, they are believed to influence its development (Becker & Johnson, 2008). Hormones may play a role since decreased levels of testosterone in males and increased levels in women are associated with gender dysphoria.

In Klinefelter's syndrome, a condition identified through genetic analysis, the patient has at least one extra X chromosome; the karyotype is XXY instead of the normal XY genetic coding for the male. These patients frequently have immature genitalia, and gender dysphoria is a possibility.

Psychosocial Factors

Learning theorists suggest the absence of same-sex role models may contribute to gender dysphoria. In this scenario, caregivers provide either covert or overt approval for cross-gender identification and behaviors. Psychoanalytic theorists have posited that male children who are deprived of their mothers seek to internally meld or become one with their mothers. This melding prevents them from developing fully as a separate entity. Clinical studies indicate that boys who have gender dysphorias have overly close relationships with their mothers and are disconnected with their fathers.

NURSING CARE FOR GENDER DYSPHORIC DISORDERS

Individuals dealing with gender dysphoric disorders may feel profound social and internal guilt and shame related to their sexual proclivities. "I am disgusted by how hairy my body is," and "I have never wanted to be macho; I have always been sensitive and caring." A nursing diagnosis that goes along with this problem includes disturbed personal identity related to incongruence between expressed (beliefs) and assigned (inborn) gender. Outcomes include seeking social support, using healthy coping behaviors to resolve sexual identity issues, and acknowledging and accepting sexual identity.

Advanced Interventions

Psychotherapy

Long-term psychotherapy is recommended to address gender dysphoria and comorbid conditions (Shafer, 2010). In rare cases, psychotherapy results in the reversal of this dysphoria (Becker & Johnson, 2008).

Pharmacological

In some cases, individuals with gender dysphoria may choose to take hormones to alter their chemistry toward their preferred gender. A female who would like to become a male takes testosterone; this results in more muscle, facial hair, clitoral enlargement, amenorrhea, and increased sex drive. A male becoming a female takes estrogen; this results in decreased size of penis and testicles, less muscle, more fat on the hips, less facial and body hair, and slight increase in breast size.

Surgery

Patients with gender dysphoria tend to resist psychotherapy except, perhaps, as a means to reach the goal of sex reassignment surgery. When gender dysphoria is severe and intractable, this may be an option. If the patient is considered appropriate for sex reassignment, psychotherapy is usually initiated to prepare the patient for the cross-gender role. The patient is then instructed to live in the cross-gender role before surgery is performed—including going to work or attending school—to help the individual determine whether he or she can interact successfully with members of society in the cross-gender mode.

Legal and social arrangements are made: The name is changed on various documents, and new employment is obtained if it is necessary to leave a former job because of discrimination. Relationship issues, such as what to tell parents, children, and former spouses, must be resolved. Males are instructed to have electrolysis and to practice female behaviors. Females are instructed to cut their hair, bind or conceal their breasts, and similarly take on the identity of a man.

After 1 or 2 years, if these measures have been successful and the patient still wishes reassignment, hormone treatment is begun; males take estrogen, and females take androgen. After another 1 to 2 years of hormone therapy, the patient may be considered for surgical reassignment if it is still desired. In men, surgery may include removal of the penis (penectomy) and testes (orchiectomy) and the addition of a vagina (vaginoplasty). In females, surgical procedures may include the removal of the breasts (mastectomy), optional removal of the uterus (hysterectomy) and ovaries (oophorectomy), and the construction of a penis (phalloplasty) in females. Efforts to create an artificial penis have met with mixed results. While surgical reassignment is disturbing to many people, studies show that after sex reassignment 80% of individuals with gender dysphoria reported significant improvement (Murad et al., 2009).

Psychotherapy is indicated after surgery to help the patient adjust to the surgical changes and discuss sexual functioning and satisfaction (Becker & Johnson, 2008). Box 20-4 describes a case of sexual reassignment gone wrong.

BOX 20-4 NATURE OR NURTURE? A CASE OF SEX REASSIGNMENT GONE WRONG

Accidents in early infancy may result in sexual reassignment. One such fascinating case is that of David Reimer, a Canadian-born identical twin male whose penis was destroyed as the result of a botched circumcision. With the advice of health care professionals, the child underwent surgical reassignment and later received hormonal therapy in puberty to induce the development of breasts and secondary female sex characteristics.

While the family psychologist proclaimed the reassignment from male to female a success and concluded that gender identity was primarily based on socialization, David never felt comfortable. He rejected his female designation of Brenda, and began living his life as a male at age 14. Shortly after he learned of his biological sex, he had the reassignment surgically reversed, married a woman, and became stepfather to her three children.

However, David always felt uncomfortable and ultimately committed suicide. His case bolstered support for the biological influence of prenatal and early-life exposure to male hormones on gender identity. David Reimer's life is chronicled in the book *As Nature Made Him*, which raises questions about gender reassignment and the modification of an unconsenting minor's genitals.

From Colapinto, J. (2006). *As nature made him: The boy who was raised as a girl.* New York, NY: Harper Collins.

PARAPHILIC DISORDERS

People do not consciously decide what arouses them sexually. Rather, during the maturation process they discover the nature of their own sexual orientation and interests. Individuals differ from one another in terms of the types of partners they find to be erotically appealing and the types of behaviors they find to be erotically stimulating. They also differ in the intensity of the sexual drive, in the degree of difficulty they experience in trying to resist sexual urges, and in their attitudes about whether or not such urges should be resisted.

Sexual disorders include many forms of paraphilic disorders. These terms refer to acts or sexual stimuli that are outside of what society considers normal, but are required for some individuals to experience desire, arousal, and orgasm (Sadock & Sadock, 2008). Criteria for being diagnosed with this category of disorders include whether the symptoms occur for at least 6 months. A disorder is characterized by discomfort in the individual or persistent risk or danger to themselves or others.

EXHIBITIONISTIC DISORDER

Exhibitionistic disorder involves illegal activity with the intentional display of the genitals in a public place. Almost 100% of cases of exhibitionism involve a man exposing himself to a woman or to women. This may occur as a man walks around exposed in a busy shopping mall or exposes himself on a doorstep after ringing the doorbell. Excitement results from the anticipation of the act, and the individual masturbates during or after exposing himself. The exhibitionist becomes aroused by observers' responses of shock and even disgust, and some fantasize that the person will also be aroused by the experience and actually want to be with them sexually.

On the other hand, some people with exhibitionistic disorder may experience deep shame and judge themselves by the same standard that society does and consider themselves perverts. They may cover their actions and live in intense fear that they will be recognized and shame themselves and their families.

Although these behaviors are illegal, it seems to be done more for shock value than as a precursor to sexual assault or rape. Actual contact is rarely sought. Since few people are arrested for this behavior after age 40, we can speculate that it resolves with age (Shafer, 2010).

FETISHISTIC DISORDER

Fetishistic disorder is characterized by a sexual focus on objects—such as shoes, gloves, pantyhose, and stockings—that are intimately associated with the human body. The particular fetish is linked to someone involved with the individual during childhood and thus is invested with a quality associated with this loved, needed, or even traumatizing person (Sadock & Sadock, 2008). Preferred items are shoes, leather or latex items, and women's underclothing. This interest may replace sexual partners or may include a component of the fetish within a consenting relationship. Fetishes may become all- consuming and destructive. They occur in more men than women.

FROTTEURISTIC DISORDER

Rubbing or touching a nonconsenting person characterizes **frotteuristic disorder.** In fact, the word frotteurism originates from the French word *frotter,* which means to "rub or scrape." The disorder is usually seen in men and typically occurs in busy public places, particularly in subways and buses, where the individual can escape after touching his victim (Becker & Johnson, 2008). People with this disorder often have no close relationships, and this sort of aggressive contact is their only means of sexual gratification (Sadock & Sadock, 2008).

PEDOPHILIC DISORDER

Pedophilic disorder is, unfortunately, the most common paraphilic disorder. It involves a predominant or exclusive sexual interest toward prepubescent children (generally 13 years or younger). Sexual fantasies can lead some individuals to seek physical contact with these sexually immature children. A subtype of this disorder refers to pubescents between ages 11 and 14. Termed hebephilia, this attraction is unacceptable in most cultures and represents a profound violation of the boundaries of the child. Critics of pathologizing this attraction to pubescent young people by calling it a mental disorder say that adults have always had sexual interest in this age group and that it is a legal issue and not a mental disorder (Frances, 2011).

Because pedophilia is illegal, its exact incidence is unknown. For the definition of pedophilia to be met, the perpetrator must be at least 16 years of age and at least 5 years older than the victim (Sadock & Sadock, 2008). The nature of the child molestation ranges from undressing and looking at the child, to genital fondling or oral sex, to penetration, and even torture.

Although most people believe that girls are more frequently molested, there is actually a nearly equal percentage of abuse in boys. Considering homosexual men represent about 5% of the population, you would expect that the rate of sexual abuse in boys would be 5%. Unfortunately, this population appears to be overrepresented, and pedophiles who abuse boys tend to be homosexual adults with unresolved maturational and identity issues (Langfeldt, 2010). Pedophiles who are attracted to females tend to prefer 8- to 10-year-old children whereas those who are attracted to males prefer older children and teens.

HEALTH POLICY

Registered Nurse Advocacy: Eliminating Statutes of Limitations for Reporting Childhood Sexual Abuse

Christine Johnson is a retired nurse whose son was molested by a Catholic priest. While her son's case was tried in time to prosecute the offender, many others are not so lucky. Due to fear and shame many young people suffer in silence. If they eventually summon up the courage that is bolstered by adulthood, it is often too late.

In Hawaii a victim has 2 years from his 18th birthday to come forward. Senate Bill 217 would limit this statute of limitations and open up lawsuits aimed at negligent churches, community organizations, and businesses. The politicians put the bill to a vote and unanimously supported it. Unfortunately, the governor put the bill on his potential veto list.

The governor's concern is that people's due-process rights might be threatened and that it opens the state to unknown legal liability. The Hawaiian Catholic Conference is also opposed to the bill. They note that decades-old allegations are difficult to defend against. Memories fade, witnesses disappear, and the alleged perpetrators are often deceased. He asked for a compromise of expanding the statute of limitations to 8 years from the 18th birthday rather than 2.

Johnson rejects this compromise and wants molesters to know that they are not safe, no matter how much time has passed. As a matter of fact, the bill was her idea based on successful legislation that was passed in Delaware. Johnson contacted her senator, who subsequently introduced the bill. It had the necessary sponsorship of the eight other women in the senate.

DePledge, D. (2012). Veto looms over pedophilia bill. *Honolulu Star Advertiser*. Retrieved from http://www.staradvertiser.com/news/20110711__Veto_looms_over_pedophilia_bill.html?id=.25335948.

SEXUAL SADISM DISORDER AND SEXUAL MASOCHISM DISORDER

Sexual sadism is a term derived from the Marquis de Sade (1740-1814), a well-known French writer who was obsessed with sexual violence. This disorder involves the achievement of sexual satisfaction from the physical or psychological suffering (including humiliation) of the victim. The sadist inflicts pain and suffering on (usually) nonconsenting persons. Most persons with this disorder are male, and the onset usually occurs prior to age 18 (Sadock & Sadock, 2008).

Consenting partners for sadists may be sexual masochists. **Sexual masochism** involves the achievement of sexual satisfaction by being humiliated, beaten, bound, or otherwise made to suffer. Sexual masochistic practices are more common among men than among women (Sadock & Sadock, 2008). In either case, participants tend to know this is a "game," and actual humiliation or pain is avoided.

TRANSVESTIC DISORDER

In **transvestic disorder**, sexual satisfaction is achieved by dressing in the clothing of the opposite gender. This behavior is related to **fetishism** but often goes beyond the use of one particular object. Generally, this behavior develops early in life and is associated with someone with whom the person is closely associated, whether in a loving relationship or through abuse. Unlike gender dysphoria, there are no sexual orientation issues, and people with transvestic disorder do not desire a sex change. Transvestites are usually heterosexual; many cross-dress only in specific sexual situations, and they often receive the cooperation and support of their partners. This paraphilia is more common in men than in women. Over time some men, as well as some women, with transvestic disorder desire to dress and live permanently as the opposite sex.

VOYEURISTIC DISORDER

Voyeurism is another illegal activity that begins in adolescence or early adulthood. It is characterized by seeking sexual arousal through viewing, usually secretly, other people in intimate situations (e.g., naked, in the process of disrobing, or engaging in sexual activity). In the language of the layperson, this behavior is called being a "peeping Tom." The disorder often begins in adolescence and may become a chronic condition and the only type of sexual activity for the person. Voyeurism may be driven by anger and a need to retaliate. Typically, people who engage in voyeurism also engage in other compulsive sexual behavior and are frequently addicted to pornography and going to strip clubs.

Like an exhibitionist, a person who engages in voyeurism may also be consumed by dissonance. The drive to engage in this activity does not make sense, considering the lengths to which the voyeur goes and the risks taken. "Why am I throwing away 2 or 3 hours staring through these binoculars on the off chance that I will see somebody naked when I can rent a movie, buy a magazine, or even find a real relationship? I must be such a loser." As with all obsessions and compulsions, the shame and anxiety is temporarily relieved by engaging in the very activity that brings it about.

PARAPHILIC DISORDER NOT OTHERWISE SPECIFIED

Other paraphilic disorders include various problems that do not meet the criteria for the other categories. Included in this grouping are:

- **Telephone scatalogia disorder:** Obscene phone calling to an unsuspecting person or sending obscene messages or video images by email
- **Necrophilic disorder:** Obsession with having a sexual encounter with a cadaver
- **Zoophilic disorder:** Incorporation of animals into sexual activity
- **Coprophilic disorder:** Fixation on feces in sexual encounters
- **Klismaphilic disorder:** Sexual activity that incorporates enemas
- **Urophilic disorder:** Sexual activity that involves urinating on one's partner or being urinated on
- **Hypoxyphilia:** Desire to achieve an altered state of consciousness secondary to hypoxia while experiencing orgasm; a drug such as nitrous oxide may be used to produce hypoxia

Many of the people involved in nonstandard sexual practices find no need for therapy because their sexual activities are carried out with a consenting adult partner, and they are neither illegal nor physically or emotionally harmful to either partner. If, however, the person is experiencing relationship difficulties, wishes to change the sexual behaviors, becomes involved in illegal activity, or is physically or emotionally harming others or being harmed, therapy is indicated.

EPIDEMIOLOGY

Although the paraphilic disorders are uncommon, the repetitive and consuming nature of the disorders make the occurrence highly frequent (Sadock & Sadock, 2008). Most people with paraphilic disorders are Caucasian males, and in about 50% of these individuals, the onset of the paraphilic arousal is before age 18 years. The behaviors associated with the disorder tend to peak in the decade between 15 and 25 years of age and then become virtually nonexistent by age 50. Patients with paraphilic disorders often have more than one paraphilia, which can occur simultaneously or at different points in their lives.

COMORBIDITY

Attention deficit hyperactivity disorder (ADHD) in childhood, substance abuse, phobic disorders, and major depression/dysthymia are strongly associated with paraphilic disorders (Shafer, 2010). A significant number of pedophiles have previous or current involvement in voyeurism, exhibitionism, or rape (Sadock & Sadock, 2008). Men with paraphilic disorders may have concurrent sexual arousal disorders related to ambivalence created by an altered sexual focus toward the object of their desire (Ahlers et al., 2009). Researchers believe that substance abuse is strongly associated with sex offenses. In one study (Kraanen & Emmelkamp, 2011), nearly 50% of sex offenders misused alcohol, 20% had a history of drug abuse, and 25% were intoxicated at the time of their offense.

ETIOLOGY

Biological Factors

A variety of theories attempt to identify what predisposes an individual to the development of paraphilic disorders, but these theories are far from conclusive since they have focused primarily on violent offenders. Some people with paraphilic disorders have temporal lobe diseases (Becker & Stinson, 2008). Sexual problems can result from head trauma. Patients who have experienced head trauma with damage to the frontal lobe of the brain may display symptoms of promiscuity, poor judgment, inability to recognize triggers that set off sexual desires, and poor impulse control. Inappropriate sexual arousal has been linked to abnormal levels of androgens.

Psychosocial Factors

Psychoanalytic theories also suggest that castration anxiety results in a safer substitution of a symbolic object for the mother, which results in fetishism and transvestism. The need for a safe substitute may result in extreme behaviors such as pedophilia, exhibitionism, and voyeurism (Shafer, 2010). Learning theorists explain paraphilic disorders in terms of timing and reinforcement. During vulnerable periods, especially puberty, sexual exploration is common; if it is pleasurable and there are no negative consequences, the activity becomes reinforced and is repeated. For example, if an adolescent boy experiments sexually with a 7-year-old boy, does not get caught, and continues to fantasize, he may develop arousal to young boys.

Cognitive theorists identify paraphilic disorders as being based on cognitive distortions. Errors in thought make it seem acceptable for deviant and destructive sexual behaviors to occur. For example, belief that there is agreement on the part of a child makes it okay in the individual's mind to have relations with her; or watching others engage in sexual relations is okay "as long as no one gets hurt." Perhaps the perpetrator of exhibitionistic behavior believes that young girls may get as excited as he does when he exposes himself.

APPLICATION OF THE NURSING PROCESS

ASSESSMENT

General Assessment

Patients with paraphilic disorders rarely are hospitalized as a direct result of their condition. However, people with paraphilic disorders may be overrepresented in psychiatric care settings, owing to the frequency of comorbid psychiatric conditions that are undoubtedly exacerbated by the sexual disorder. Nurses who work in forensic settings such as prisons and jails may care for inmates who are imprisoned due to consequences of paraphilic disorders (e.g., sexual impulse disorders). Depression with suicidal ideation and substance abuse are common comorbid conditions and should be assessed using principles outlined in Chapters 22 and 25.

During a thorough assessment for any psychiatric disorder (or medical condition as well), you may discover symptoms of one of the paraphilic disorders. For example, you may ask a patient about his family, and he may remark that he and his wife "aren't getting along so great lately." As you explore this area of concern further, he reveals, "My wife wants to do the same old boring things . . . you know . . . sexually, all the time." As the assessment continues, you may learn that he is focused on sadistic sorts of activities, is obsessed with pornography, and no longer becomes aroused by his wife.

Self-Assessment

It is reasonable for students to read descriptions of sexual disorders and respond with disgust to objectionable behaviors. It is also common to respond with frustration, anger, and hostility to people with disorders such as sexual masochism and pedophilia. A major issue in trying to understand human behavior is where to draw the line between considering a person to be a victim of life experiences and biological makeup and considering him or her (by virtue of having subjective consciousness) to be an active agent capable of transcending previous determinants.

Providing care for someone who has abused others may be nearly impossible for certain individuals. We may have known someone who was the victim of a voyeur or a pedophile, or we may personally have been victimized. Exploring paraphilic disorders, even in an academic context, may evoke significant distress. At this point, talking with a faculty member, a primary care provider, or someone at a mental health clinic can be helpful and important and may even result in better personal understanding and coping.

ASSESSMENT GUIDELINES

Paraphilic Disorders

1. Assess the potential for self-harm, because patients with paraphilic disorders may become despondent and be more of a suicide risk.
2. The main focus of the assessment should be on the presenting problem (e.g., depression with suicidal ideation).
3. Elicit the patient's perception of the impact of the sexual disorder upon the current illness.

DIAGNOSIS

Nursing diagnoses for individuals with paraphilic disorder include *risk for suicide, other-directed violence, ineffective impulse control,* and *ineffective sexuality pattern.* Other diagnoses should be considered, depending upon the comorbid psychiatric condition that has precipitated the admission.

OUTCOMES IDENTIFICATION

NOC (Moorhead et al., 2013) identifies a number of outcomes for patients with either ineffective sexuality patterns or risk for other-directed violence. Included are *sexual identity* and *impulse self-control.* Table 20-6 provides signs and symptoms, nursing diagnoses, and outcomes for paraphilias.

PLANNING

The setting and presenting problem influence the planning of nursing care for the patient with a paraphilic disorder. The basic-level nurse may encounter such a patient during treatment for a comorbid condition, especially when the patient is admitted to the hospital for suicidal thoughts and behavior. Sometimes psychiatric care and treatment are mandated, such as when a voyeur or exhibitionist gets caught.

The care plan will focus on safety and crisis intervention. The patient may also be treated for comorbid depression or

TABLE 20-6 SIGNS AND SYMPTOMS, DIAGNOSES, AND OUTCOMES FOR SEXUAL DISORDERS

SIGNS AND SYMPTOMS	NURSING DIAGNOSES	OUTCOMES
History of exposing self to others, deep remorse and shame over behavior, wants to control the fantasies, urges, and resultant behaviors	*Ineffective impulse control*	Identifies feelings that lead to impulsive actions, consequences of actions, and alternatives; practices self-restraint of impulsive behaviors.
Lacks interest for his spouse,feels an increasing attraction to prepubescent girls, history of arrests	*Risk for other-directed violence (sexual)*	Identifies triggers for maladaptive sexual fantasies and describes techniques to control these fantasies; practices self-restraint of sexual urges and behaviors.
Shame when dressing like a woman, fears loss of community respect,wife found a suicide note, increasingly unable to control sexual impulses	*Risk for suicide*	Expresses a determination to live and a sense of control; identifies strategies to manage his urges, refrains from self-destructive urges
Alteration in relationship with significant other, reports difficulties with sexual activities, values conflict	*Ineffective sexuality pattern*	Seeks social support, reports healthy sexual functioning, sets personal sexual boundaries

From Herdman, T. H. (Ed.), (2012). *Nursing diagnoses—Definitions and classification 2012-2014.* Copyright © 2012, 1994-2012 by NANDA International. Used by arrangement with John Wiley & Sons Limited; Moorhead, S., Johnson, M., Maas, M. L., & Swanson, E. (2013). *Nursing outcomes classification (NOC)* (5th ed.). St. Louis, MO: Mosby.

anxiety disorders in the community setting. Planning will address the major complaint along with the sexual disorder.

IMPLEMENTATION

Interventions are aimed at offering a nonjudgmental emotional presence while exploring identity issues, self-esteem, and anxiety and encouraging an optimal level of functioning. Patients with a potential for violating the boundaries of others may require closer observation and firm limit setting. Box 20-5 lists examples of basic-level *NIC* interventions for paraphilic disorders.

Health Teaching and Health Promotion

Education is typically geared toward reducing symptoms from the presenting problem, typically depression and anxiety. Patients with paraphilic disorders can be taught to journal their feelings and to begin to identify triggers for pathological behavior.

Teamwork and Safety

When the patient who has a paraphilic disorder is in a crisis that requires hospitalization, providing a safe environment is fundamental. All patients on a psychiatric inpatient unit should be informed on admission about unit rules regarding personal contact between patients and between patients and staff. Limit setting is done consistently when it is needed, and staff work together as a team to this end.

Individuals with paraphilic disorders tend to isolate themselves. The unit environment may be a challenge. Sharing meals with others may result in discomfort, and the patient might wonder what other people know about him or her. A particular challenge may be interacting in formal group settings and the expectation of participation. But the group setting may actually provide patients with the greatest opportunity for

BOX 20-5 *NIC* INTERVENTIONS FOR PARAPHILIC DISORDERS

Behavior Management: Sexual

Definition: Delineation and prevention of socially unacceptable sexual behaviors

Activities:*

- Discuss consequences of unacceptable behavior.
- Discuss the negative impact that behavior has on others.
- Encourage expression of feelings about past crises.
- Provide opportunities for caregivers to process their feelings about the patient.

Self-Esteem Enhancement

Definition: Assisting a patient to increase his/her personal judgment of self-worth

Activities:*

- Encourage patient to identify strengths.
- Assist in setting realistic goals to achieve higher self-esteem.
- Assist patient to accept dependence on others, as appropriate.
- Explore previous achievements of success.
- Encourage patient to accept new challenges.

Social Skills Behavior Modification

Definition: Assisting the patient to develop or improve interpersonal social skills

Activities:*

- Assist in identifying problems resulting from social skill deficits.
- Encourage verbalization of feelings regarding social interaction.
- Identify a specific skill to improve.
- Identify steps to reach skill and role-play the steps.

* Partial list.

Data from Bulechek, G. M., Butcher, H. K., & Dochterman, J. M. (Eds.). (2013). *Nursing interventions classification (NIC)* (6th ed.). St. Louis, MO: Mosby.

growth, in that they can experience others as humans with feelings, perhaps learning how much anguish and pain personal violations have caused them. The group milieu can mean having others present who empathize with one's background and current distress.

Pharmacological Interventions

While there is no single treatment for paraphilic disorders, two classes of pharmacological agents, antiandrogens and serotonergic antidepressants, are prescribed during treatment. Medication is not used independently as a treatment without other interventions. Drugs that reduce levels of testosterone may be used to treat sex offenders. The drugs that are frequently used are progestin derivatives, including medroxyprogesterone acetate (MPA) (an analog of progesterone) and cyproterone acetate (CPA) (an inhibitor of testosterone). Both of these drugs act to decrease libido and break the individual's pattern of compulsive deviant sexual behavior. They work best in patients with paraphilic disorders and a high sexual drive, such as pedophiles and exhibitionists, and less well in those with a low sexual drive or an antisocial personality (Becker & Johnson, 2008).

Current research is focusing on the use of SSRIs in the treatment of sexual disorders. Fluoxetine (Prozac) has been used successfully to treat patients with exhibitionism, voyeurism, and pedophilia and persons who have committed rape. These drugs may work to improve mood, reduce impulsivity, decrease sexual obsessions, and cause sexual dysfunction (Rothschild, 2000). In addition to fluoxetine, other drugs, such as clomipramine (Anafranil) and fluvoxamine (Luvox), have been used in the treatment of sexual obsessions, addictions, and paraphilic disorders. The role of the nurse in pharmacotherapy is to educate patients regarding the specific drug prescribed and to monitor the drug's effectiveness and watch for untoward side effects (Becker & Johnson, 2008).

Advanced Practice Interventions

Psychotherapy

The usual treatment plan for working with patients with paraphilic disorders is cognitive-behavioral therapy. An attempt is made to help the person learn a new sexual response pattern that will eliminate the need for the activity that is causing the problem. Techniques range from positive reinforcement for appropriate object choices to aversion techniques, in which mild electrical shocks may be applied for inappropriate choices. Other treatment modalities include psychodynamic techniques designed to help the patient understand the origin of the paraphilia.

Advanced practice nurses may seek specialized training to enable them to work effectively with patients with gender dysphorias and paraphilic disorders. This preparation allows the nurse to practice sex therapy and conduct sex research. The American Association of Sex Educators, Counselors, and Therapists (AASECT) provides credentialing based on academic preparation, clinical supervision, experience, and skills. Credentialing is a method by which consumers of mental health care services can be assured of the professional competency of the therapist treating them.

EVALUATION

Essential evaluative criteria for paraphilic disorders include maintaining the safety of others and self, reducing and/or eliminating behaviors that result in discomfort and shame, and improving interpersonal relationships. Despite progress, people with sexual impulse disorders, especially those that generate victims, may be required to continue treatment, which has been demonstrated to reduce recidivism (relapse into the offending behavior) (Becker & Johnson, 2008).

KEY POINTS TO REMEMBER

- Sexual dysfunction is an extremely common problem that involves a disturbance in the desire, excitement, or orgasm phases of the sexual response cycle or pain during sexual intercourse.
- There are seven different types of sexual dysfunction.
- Sexual problems are considered to be socially atypical, have the potential to disrupt meaningful relationships, and may result in insult or even significant injury to other people.
- Health care workers are often uncomfortable asking questions related to sexuality. Providing professional and holistic care requires that nurses include this vital area of assessment.
- Certain medical and surgical conditions and some drugs result in a variety of sexual dysfunctions, including low libido, impotence, erectile dysfunction, anorgasmia, and priapism.
- There are distinctions between biological sex and gender identity. Gender dysphoria is a strong and persistent cross-gender identification that is accompanied by anxiety, discomfort, and unhappiness.
- *Paraphilia* is a term used to identify repetitive or preferred sexual fantasies or behaviors that involve preference for use of a nonhuman object, repetitive sexual activity with humans involving real or simulated suffering or humiliation, and repetitive sexual activity with nonconsenting partners.
- Paraphilic disorders include exhibitionistic disorder, fetishistic disorder, frotteuristic disorder, pedophilic disorder, sexual masochism disorder, sexual sadism disorder, transvestic disorder, voyeuristic disorder, and paraphilic disorders not otherwise specified.
- In addition to conducting a sexual assessment, nurses are involved in milieu and behavioral therapy, counseling, education, and medication management.
- Nursing interventions for paraphilic disorders involve administration of medications (e.g., medroxyprogesterone [Depo-Provera] and SSRIs) and therapy.
- Advanced practice nurses may specialize in the area of sexual counseling, treatment, and therapy.

CRITICAL THINKING

1. As a nurse on an adolescent psychiatric mental health nursing unit, you often encounter teenagers who are misinformed about growth and development as well as sexuality. What information would you include in a series of teaching sessions that would help these adolescents acquire a greater understanding of the developmental changes they are going through?
2. In order to understand your own beliefs, answer these questions:
   a. Are you comfortable with your own sexuality? With that of others?
   b. Are you judgmental?
   c. Could you be helpful to someone who has a sexual disorder?
   d. What factors have influenced your beliefs and values regarding sexuality?
   e. What do you think is the impact of sexually explicit television, music videos, and movies on your sexual attitudes, values, and beliefs?
3. During a one-to-one session, Mrs. Chase, a patient who was admitted to your inpatient unit with depression and anxiety confides concern about her 17-year-old son, Alex. She becomes tearful and says, "I don't know what I've done wrong. Alex was arrested for exposing himself to a girl at school. I'm worried that he may begin doing even worse things."
   a. Provide Mrs. Chase with information regarding Alex's condition and his probable prognosis.
   b. What sort of feelings in yourself about Alex would you need to be aware of in order to be the most helpful to Mrs. Chase?

CHAPTER REVIEW

1. A 27-year-old patient states that since her marriage ended 2 years ago, she has found herself lacking interest and motivation in sexual activity. Which response is most likely to be therapeutic?
   a. "What is your moral perspective regarding sexual activity outside of marriage?"
   b. "Tell me more about your life since your marriage ended."
   c. "Often physical illness causes decreased desire in women."
   d. "This is a common problem, especially considering all the stress you have been through."
2. A young, newly married man with schizophrenia presents in the emergency department with a complaint of "demons sticking needles in my penis." Which initial response by the triage nurse would be appropriate?
   a. Arrange for the patient to be evaluated by the doctor or advanced practice registered nurse on duty because the patient may be expressing real pain in a delusional manner.
   b. Request an order for labs to rule out a sexually transmitted disease, given that the patient has recently begun sexual relations with his new wife and may have been exposed.
   c. Complete the triage process, and refer the patient for a mental health evaluation, since he appears to be psychotic and possibly having a relapse.
   d. Make the patient feel safe by telling him that it is not possible for demons to be in the emergency room.
3. A young male patient tells you that somehow he feels that he should not be a man and that inside he is a woman. This is likely an example of:
   a. Fetishistic disorder.
   b. Frotteuristic disorder.
   c. Gender dysphoria.
   d. Transvestic disorder.
4. Luisa is the nurse assigned to work with Juan, a male on a step-down unit. He is in counseling as part of the process of seeking sexual reassignment surgery and has female clothing in his hospital locker. Luisa is nervous about working with someone like Juan and spends only the briefest amounts of time responding to his needs. What is/are the best description(s) of what is occurring here? *Select all that apply.*
   a. As long as Juan's minimal care needs are addressed, Luisa is within her rights to respond this way.
   b. Luisa is failing to maintain professional objectivity because of her values and beliefs about this particular patient's decisions and behavior.
   c. Luisa is experiencing a common negative response to a situation about which she has limited knowledge and that she does not understand.
   d. Luisa may be having difficulty looking beyond Juan's gender issues and as a result is failing to see or respond to him simply as a person.
   e. Luisa is avoiding Juan because she is afraid that she cannot mask the disapproval she feels.
5. You are interviewing Matthew, a 39-year-old patient with major depression. You wish to ask Matthew about any sexual dysfunction that may be arising as the result of depression. Which way of opening up the subject may increase the patient's comfort in discussing this with you?
   a. "This is embarrassing for both of us, but I need to ask you about sexual problems."
   b. "I have to ask you about sexual issues, but since I am a professional, you shouldn't feel hesitant to discuss sexual issues with me."
   c. "Many people who have depression also experience sexual problems. Are there any problems you want to talk about?"
   d. "I am going to ask you about sexual problems, but you can be reassured everything we talk about is confidential, and I won't judge you."

Answers to Chapter Review

1. b; 2. a; 3. c; 4. b, c, d, e. 5. c.

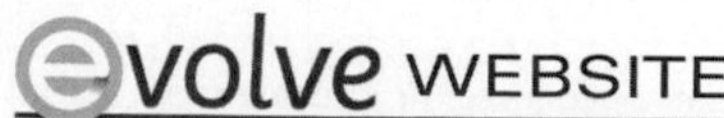

WEBSITE

Visit the Evolve website for a posttest on the content in this chapter: http://evolve.elsevier.com/Varcarolis

Post-Test interactive review

REFERENCES

Ahlers, C. J., Schaefer, G. A., Mundt, I. A., Roll, S., Englert, H., Willich, S.N., et al. (2009). How unusual are the contents of paraphilias? Paraphilia-associated sexual arousal patterns in a community based sample of men. *The Journal of Sexual Medicine, 8*(5), 1362–1370. doi:10.1111/j.1743–6109.2009.01597.x.

American Psychiatric Association (APA). (2013). *DSM-5 table of contents.* Retrieved from http://www.psychiatry.org/dsm5.

Becker, J. V., & Johnson, B. R. (2008). Gender identity disorders and paraphilias. In R. E. Hales, S. C. Yudofsky, & G. O. Gabbard (Eds.), *Textbook of psychiatry* (pp. 729–753). Washington, DC: American Psychiatric Publishing.

Becker, J. V., & Stinson, J. D. (2008). Human sexuality and sexual dysfunctions. In R. E. Hales, S. C. Yudofsky, & G. O. Gabbard (Eds.), *Textbook of psychiatry* (pp. 711–728). Washington, DC: American Psychiatric Publishing.

Beredjick, C. (2012). DSM-V to rename gender identity disorder 'gender dysphoria.' *Advocate.com.* Retrieved from http://www.advocate.com/politics/transgender/2012/07/23/dsm-replaces-gender-identity-disorder-gender-dysphoria.

Binik, Y. M. (2010). The DSM diagnostic criteria for vaginismus. *Archives of Sexual Behavior, 39*(2), 278–91.

Brotto, L. (2012). *Sexual pain disorders.* Retrieved from http://www.obgyn.ubc.ca/SexualHealth/sexual_dysfunctions/pain_disorders.php.

Brotto, L. (2010). The DSM diagnostic criteria for hypoactive sexual disorder in women. *Archives of Sexual Behavior, 39*(2), 221–239. doi:10.1007/s10508-009-9543–1.

Brotto, L., Knudson, G., Inskip, J., Rhodes, K., & Erskine, Y. (2010). Asexuality: A mixed-methods approach. *Archives of Sexual Behavior, 39*(3), 599–618. doi:10.1007/s10508-008-9434-x.

Bulechek, G. M., Butcher, H. K., Dochterman, J. M., & Wagner, C. (2013). *Nursing interventions classification (NIC)* (6th ed.). St. Louis, MO: Mosby.

Clayton, A. H. (2010). The pathophysiology of hypoactive sexual desire disorder in women. *International Journal of Gynecology & Obstetrics, 110(1)*, 7–11.

deVries, A. L. C., Doreleijers, T. A. H., Steensma, T. D., & Cohen-Kettenis, P. T. (2011). Psychiatric comorbidity in gender dysphoric adolescents. *Journal of Child and Adolescent Psychology and Psychiatry, 52*(11), 1195–1202. doi:10.1111/j.1469–7610.2011.02426.x.

Frances, A. (2013). *Essentials of psychiatric diagnosis.* New York, NY: Guilford Press.

Frances, A. (2011). Hebephilia is a crime, not a mental disorder. *Psychiatric Times.* Retrieved from http://www.psychiatrictimes.com/blog/frances/content/article/10168/2006997.

Graham, C. A. (2009). The DSM diagnostic criteria for female orgasmic disorder. *Archives of Sexual Behavior.* Retrieved from http://www.dsm5.org/Documents/Sex%20and%20GID%20Lit%20Reviews/SD/GRAHAM.FOD.DSM.pdf DOI 10.1007/s10508-009-9542-2.

Grohol, J. M. (2011). Gender identity disorder symptoms: Gender dysphoria. *PsychCentral.* Retrieved from http://psychcentral.com/disorders/sx40.htm.

Heidelbaugh, J. J. (2010). Management of erectile dysfunction. *American Family Physician, 81*(3). Retrieved from http://www.mdconsult.com/das/article/body/345935934-227/jorg=journal&source=&sp=22886168&sid=0/N/734254/1.html?issn=0002-838X&issue_id=24414#h1060053601.

Herdman, T. H. (2012). (Ed.). *NANDA international nursing diagnoses: Definitions and classification, 2012-2014.* Oxford, UK: Wiley-Blackwell.

Higgins, A. (2007). Impact of psychotropic medication on sexuality: Literature review. *British Journal of Nursing, 16*, 545–550.

Kaplan, H. S. (1974). *The new sex therapy: Active treatment of sexual dysfunctions.* New York, NY: Brunner/Mazel.

Kraanen, F. L., & Emmelkamp, P. M. G. (2011). Substance misuse and substance use in sex offenders: A review. *Clinical Psychology Review, 31*(3), 478–489.

Langfeldt, T. (2010). Is "pedophilia" a useful or a confusing concept? An empirical study on sexual abuse of children, sexual orientation and typology: Implications for therapy. *Sexual Offender Treatment, 5*(1). Retrieved from http://www.sexual-offender-treatment.org/2-2010_04.98.html.

Levine, H. B. (2010). What patients mean by love, intimacy, and sexual desire. In H. B. Levine, C.B. Risen, & S. E. Althof (Eds.), *Handbook of clinical sexuality for mental health professionals* (pp. 41–56). New York, NY: Taylor and Francis.

Lewis, R. W., Fugl-Meyer, K. S., Corona, G., Hayes, R. D., Laumann, E. O., Moreira, E. D. Segraves, T. (2010). Definitions/epidemiology/risk factors for sexual dysfunction. *The Journal of Sexual Dysfunction, 7*(4 Pt 2), 1598–1607. doi:10.1111/j.1743–6109.2010.01778.x.

Masters, W. H., & Johnson, V. E. (1966). *Human sexual response.* Boston, MA: Little, Brown.

Mick, J. M. (2007). Sexuality assessment: 10 strategies for improvement. *Clinical Journal of Oncology Nursing, 11*, 671–675.

Moorhead, S., Johnson, M., Maas, M. L., & Swanson, E. (2013). *Nursing outcomes classification (NOC)* (5th ed.). St. Louis, MO: Mosby.

Murad, M. H., Elamin, M. B., Garcia, M. Z., Mullan, R. J., Murad, A, Erwin, P. J., & Montori, V. M. (2009). Hormonal therapy and sex reassignment: A systematic review and meta-analysis of quality of life and psychosocial outcomes. *Clinical Endocrinology, 72*(2), 214–231. doi:10.1111/j.1365–2265.2009.03625.x.

Rothschild, A. J. (2000). Sexual side effects of antidepressants. *Journal of Clinical Psychiatry, 61*, 28–36.

Rowland, D., McMahon, C. G., Abdo, C., Chen, J., Jannini, E., Wladinger, M. D., et al. (2010). Disorders of orgasm and ejaculation in men. *The Journal of Sexual Medicine, 7*(4), 1668–1686. doi:10.1111/j.1743–6109.2010.01782.x.

Sadock, B. J., & Sadock, V. A. (2008). *Kaplan & Sadock's concise textbook of clinical psychiatry* (3rd ed.). Philadelphia, PA: Lippincott, Williams & Wilkins.

Segraves, R. T. (2010). Considerations for diagnostic criteria for erectile dysfunction in *DSM-V. The Journal of Sexual Medicine, 7*(2 Pt 1), 654–60.

Shafer, L. C. (2010). Sexual disorders and sexual dysfunction. In T. A. Stern, G. L. Fricchione, N. H. Cassem, M. S. Jellinek, & J. F. Rosenbaum (Eds.), *Massachusetts General Hospital handbook of general hospital psychiatry* (6th ed., pp. 323–335). Philadelphia, PA: Saunders.

Svoboda, E. (2010). The female sex-pain mystery. *The Daily Beast.* Retrieved from http://www.thedailybeast.com/articles/2010/03/27/the-female-sex-pain-mystery.html.

CHAPTER

21

Impulse Control Disorders

*Margaret Jordan Halter**

evolve WEBSITE

Visit the Evolve website for a pretest on the content in this chapter: http://evolve.elsevier.com/Varcarolis

Pre-Test interactive review

OBJECTIVES

1. Describe clinical manifestations of oppositional defiant disorder, intermittent explosive disorder, and conduct disorder.
2. Discuss etiology and comorbidities of the impulse control disorders.
3. Describe biological, psychological, and environmental factors related to the development of impulse control disorders.
4. Compare your feelings about working with someone with an impulse control disorder with someone in your class.
5. Formulate three nursing diagnoses for impulse control disorders, identifying patient outcomes and interventions for each.
6. Identify evidence-based treatments for oppositional defiant, intermittent explosive, and conduct disorders.

KEY TERMS AND CONCEPTS

cognitive-behavioral therapy (CBT)
conduct disorder
dialectical behavioral therapy (DBT)
expressed emotion
intermittent explosive disorder
kleptomania
oppositional defiant disorder
pyromania

The development of a psychiatric illness can be devastating to a person and his or her family. Disorders such as autism and schizophrenia can alter the entire direction of a person's life and also the family's, yet those disorders are generally understood as psychiatric problems, and it is usually evident to others that there is a psychiatric basis to the disorders. However, people with impulse control disorders seem like children whose parents cannot control them or adults who simply do not choose to control their behavior. They are impulsive and exhibit aggressive behaviors and emotions. Problems relating to others in socially acceptable ways result in a lack of healthy relationships, leaving the individual isolated and the family devastated. The behaviors related to these disorders can have severe criminal consequences as well as long-lasting negative personal impact.

Recognizing and treating a person with one of the disorders described in this chapter while he or she is young can prevent further problems and avoid interactions with the criminal justice system; unfortunately, stigma and misconceptions around mental illness may cause individuals and their families to attempt to conceal the conditions or can limit help seeking and professional care, preventing timely intervention.

The disorders presented in this chapter were previously grouped with other disorders usually first diagnosed in infancy, childhood, or adolescence. While the problems presented here have their origins early in life, they may not be diagnosed until the person is an adult. According to the American Psychiatric

*The author would like to acknowledge the contributions of Barbara-Ann Bybel.

Association (2013), major disorders considered under this umbrella include the following:

- Oppositional defiant disorder
- Intermittent explosive disorder
- Conduct disorder

CLINICAL PICTURE

Oppositional Defiant Disorder

Primarily a childhood disorder, **oppositional defiant disorder** is a repeated and persistent pattern of having an angry and irritable mood in conjunction with demonstrating defiant and vindictive behavior. Angry mood can manifest as losing one's temper or becoming easily annoyed by others ("Get away from me! She's bothering me!"). Defiant behavior can be demonstrated through arguing with adults and refusing to comply with adults' requests or rules, as in "NO! I won't do it, and you can't make me!"

Vindictiveness is defined as spiteful, malicious behavior and a particularly chilling aspect of this disorder. This quality increases the chances that revenge will be sought in response to real or imagined slights. Vindictive acts are disturbingly regular for at least 6 months.

The person with this disorder also shows a pattern of deliberately annoying people and blaming others for his or her mistakes or misbehavior. This child may frequently be heard to say "He made me do it!" or "It's not my fault!". Certain aspects of the disorder are seen more in boys than girls. For example, boys are more likely to annoy and blame others, and girls argue more. Additionally, clinicians may view and judge an individual's display of behavior differently depending on their gender. For example, it may be more socially appropriate in many cultures for a boy to express aggression then a girl (de Ancos & Ascaso, 2011).

A child with oppositional defiant disorder is not just a difficult or defiant child. This disorder impairs the child's entire life and makes it extremely difficult for him or her to attend school, to have friends, or be a functioning member of the family. The behaviors may be confined to only one setting or in more severe cases present in multiple settings, such as both at home and in school. Research demonstrates that children with oppositional defiant disorder show a preference for large reward and pay little attention to increasing penalties (Luman et al., 2010).

Left untreated, some children outgrow this disorder; however, most do not and continue to experience social difficulties, conflicts with authority figures, and academic problems that impact their whole lives (Gale, 2011). Oppositional defiant disorder is often predictive of emotional disorders in young adulthood (Rowe et al., 2010).

CONSIDERING CULTURE

Variation of Oppositional Defiant Disorder and Conduct Disorder across Cultures

Various cultures may tolerate conduct disorder and oppositional defiant disorders differently. Prevalence rates can be affected by cultural factors related to the degree to which conduct disorders and oppositional defiant disorder symptoms are considered dysfunctional and/or are differentially tolerated in various cultures and across age groups.

Chinese and Tai cultures suppress external syndromes such as aggression, anger, and strong emotions or overt behaviors. Parents in these cultures may have less tolerance for such externalizing behaviors. When Asian countries are compared to other areas of the world, it is not surprising that there are lower rates of externalizing syndromes in the Asian countries as compared to several Western countries

There is a need to evaluate the validity of conduct disorder or oppositional defiant disorder symptoms across different cultures using several important external and clinical criteria. These criteria include response to pharmacological or evidence-based psychosocial treatment, developmental course, genetic aggregation in families, environmental risk factors (e.g., ineffective parenting) and biological/neuropsychological correlates.

Canino, G., Polanczyk, G., Bauermeister, J. J., Rohde, L. A., & Frick, P. J. (2011). Does the prevalence of CD and ODD vary across cultures? *Social Psychiatry and Psychiatric Epidemiology, 45*(7), 695–704.

Intermittent Explosive Disorder

Intermittent explosive disorder is a pattern of behavioral outbursts in adults 18 years and older characterized by an inability to control aggressive impulses. The aggression can be verbal or physical and targeted toward other persons, animals, property, or even themselves. It was originally termed *monomanie instinctive,* referring to how these impulsive acts seem almost instinctive.

Anything can trigger the inappropriate aggression reaction to the situation. An example may be a person punching his fist through a pane of glass after not being able to locate his favorite video game. He may destroy his room, break furniture, or damage costly property. As the rage continues, he may attack anyone who intervenes and often causes injury. The explosive anger may occur during a competitive sport, such as lashing out at opposing baseball fans when his team loses. The behavior needs to show a repetitive pattern and interference with normal functioning, such as a person being unable to stay employed because they scream and curse at their boss when given any negative feedback (Tamam et al., 2011).

The pattern goes from being upset to being remorseful. The first stage is tension and arousal based on some environmental stimuli, such as someone driving too slowly in the passing lane on the expressway. This is followed by explosive behavior and aggression. A response to the slow driver may be hitting the gas and dangerously passing the person on the shoulder of the road. Immediately thereafter the person experiences a sense of relief and release, taking satisfaction by looking at the offender in the rearview mirror and delivering a negative hand signal. Delayed consequences include feelings of remorse, regret, and embarrassment over the aggressive behavior. After the event, reality may set in. "Wow, I just risked my life to pass an 80-year-old man to get to a party that will go on for hours. I have to stop doing this."

This disorder can impede on a person's functioning by leading to problems with interpersonal relationships and occupational difficulties and can lead to criminal problems as well. Additionally, significant problems with physical health, such as hypertension and diabetes, have been linked to this disease (McCloskey et al., 2010). Being in a heightened state of stress and agitation for a prolonged period of time may be the correlation.

Conduct Disorder

Conduct disorder is a persistent pattern of behavior in which the rights of others are violated and societal norms or rules are disregarded. The behavior is usually abnormally aggressive and can frequently lead to destruction of property or physical injury. Persons with this disorder initiate physical fights and bully others, and they may steal or use a weapon to intimidate or hurt others. Coercion into activity against the will of others, including sexual activity, is characteristic of this disorder. These behaviors are enduring patterns and continue over a period of 6 months and beyond.

It is one of the most frequently diagnosed disorders of childhood and adolescence. The people affected by this disorder may have a normal intelligence, but they tend to skip class or disrupt school so much that they fall behind and may be expelled or drop out. Complications associated with conduct disorder include academic failure, school suspensions and dropouts, juvenile delinquency, drug and alcohol abuse and dependency, and juvenile court involvement (Harvard Medical School, 2011). People with conduct disorder crave excitement and do not worry as much about consequences as others do.

Though the literature tends to focus on children and adolescents with conduct disorder, it is quite a problem in adults as well. In adults, conduct disorder has similar characteristics of aggression, destruction of property, stealing, deceitfulness, and criminal behavior. Adults, like younger persons, have family problems based on self-interest and lack of engagement. Rule breaking takes such forms as parole violation, disregard for general laws such as speed limits, and employment problems such as frequent lateness or absence with unacceptable or unbelievable excuses.

There are two subtypes of conduct disorder—child-onset and adolescent-onset—both of which can occur in mild, moderate, or severe forms. Predisposing factors are ADHD, oppositional child behaviors, parental rejection, inconsistent parenting with harsh discipline, early institutional living, chaotic home life, large family size, absent or alcoholic father, antisocial and drug-dependent family members, and association with delinquent peers.

Childhood-onset conduct disorder occurs prior to age 10 years and is found mainly in males who are physically aggressive, have poor peer relationships, show little concern for others, and lack feelings of guilt or remorse. These children frequently misperceive others' intentions as hostile and believe their aggressive responses are justified. Violent children also often display antisocial reasoning, such as "he deserved it," when rationalizing aggressive behaviors (Farrell et al., 2008). Children with childhood-onset conduct disorder attempt to project a strong image, but they actually have a low self-esteem. Limited frustration tolerance, irritability, and temper outbursts are hallmarks of this disorder. Individuals with childhood-onset conduct disorder are more likely to have problems that persist through adolescence, and without intensive treatment they may later develop antisocial personality disorder as adults.

In **adolescent-onset conduct disorder**, no symptoms are present prior to age 10. Affected adolescents tend to act out misconduct with their peer group (e.g., early onset of sexual behavior, substance abuse, risk-taking behaviors). Males are more likely to fight, steal, vandalize, and have school discipline problems whereas girls tend to lie, be truant, run away, abuse substances, and engage in prostitution. The male-to-female ratio is not as high as for the childhood-onset type, indicating more girls become aggressive during this period of development.

There is a subset of people with conduct disorder who are also referred to as being callous and unemotional. Callousness is characterized by a lack of empathy, such as disregarding and being unconcerned about the feelings of others, having a lack of remorse or guilt except when facing punishment, and being unconcerned about meeting school and family obligations; unemotional traits include a shallow, unexpressive, and superficial affect (Stellwagen & Kerig, 2010). Callousness may be a predictor of future antisocial personality disorder in adults (Burke et al., 2010).

Two problems are related to impulse control disorders and are worthy of mention in this chapter. They are pyromania and kleptomania. **Pyromania** is described as repeated deliberate fire setting. The person experiences tension or becomes excited before setting a fire and shows a fascination with or unusual interest in fire and its contexts such as matches. The person also experiences pleasure or relief when setting a fire, witnessing a fire, or participating in the aftermath of a fire. The fire setting is done solely to satisfy this relief pleasure and not for other reasons, such as to conceal a crime. Like many mental illnesses, this disorder can stem from a form of maladaptive coping a person learned early in life in relation to having unmet needs and poorer social skills (Lyons et al., 2010).

Kleptomania is a repeated failure to resist urges to steal objects not needed for personal use or monetary value. For example, a person may take books even though they cannot read or baby outfits they consider cute even though they have no children and have plenty of money to buy them. The person experiences a buildup of tension before taking the object, and this is followed by relief or pleasure following the theft. Some research has explored whether this disorder is more closely linked to others of addictive behavior, such as substance abuse disorder, since the person is acting to satisfy a compulsion (Talih, 2011).

See Table 21-1 for a summary of the characteristics of impulse control disorders.

EPIDEMIOLOGY

Prevalence

Oppositional defiant disorder is reported to have rates varying between 2% to 16%, depending on the population sampled and the method of measurement. Kessler and colleagues (2012) report the 12-month prevalence at 8.3% among adolescents. Intermittent explosive disorder may affect an alarming number of people—up to 16 million Americans, or about 7% of all adults—in their lifetimes (National Institute of Mental Health, 2006).

TABLE 21-1 **CHARACTERISTICS OF IMPULSE CONTROL DISORDERS**

DISORDER	AGE OF ONSET	LIFETIME PREVALENCE	GENDER	CLINICAL FEATURES	NOTES
Oppositional defiant disorder	Childhood/ Adolescence	12.6%	More males	Anger, disregard for authority, temper tantrums, vengefulness, few friends. Despite behavior, recognizes that others have rights and that there are rules	May become conduct disorder in later years.
Intermittent explosive disorder	14 years of age (diagnosed at age 18); frequently onset is abrupt	7.3%	More males	Impulsive and unwarranted emotional outbursts, violence, destruction of property	Early treatment may prevent worsening pathology
Conduct disorder	Childhood onset (<10 years): worse prognosis. Adolescent onset (no symptoms prior to age 10)	6.8%	Childhood onset: more males Adolescent onset: equal	Unimpulsive violation of the rights of others, aggression to people and animals, destruction of property, deceitfulness, rules violation	More criminal involvement May be a precursor to antisocial personality disorder

Connor, D. F., Ford, J. D., Albert, D. B., & Doerfler, L. A. (2007). Conduct disorder subtype and comorbidity. *Annals of Clinical Psychiatry, 19*(3), 161–168; Kessler, R. C., Coccaro, E. F., Fava, M., Jaeger, S., Jin, R., & Walters, E. (2006). The prevalence and correlates of DSM-IV intermittent explosive disorder in the National Comorbidity Survey Replication. *Archives of General Psychiatry, 63*(6), 669–78; Merikangas, K. R., He, J., Burstein, M., Swanson, S. A., Avenevoli, S., Cui, L., et al. (2010). Lifetime prevalence of mental disorders in U.S. adolescents: Results from the National Comorbidity Survey Replication—Adolescent supplement. *Journal of the American Academy of Adolescent Psychiatry, 49*(10), 980–989.

Conduct disorder prevalence has been on the rise and may be higher in urban settings as compared to rural areas. Rates vary widely from 1% to over 10% based on the population sampled. As previously stated, conduct disorder is one of the most frequently diagnosed disorder in children and adolescents and has an estimated rate of 5.4% in both inpatient and outpatient mental health facilities (Kessler et al., 2012).

Gender Differences

In regard to oppositional defiant disorder, the disorder is more prevalent in males than females prior to puberty, but the rates equal out after puberty. Symptoms are similar in both sexes, but again males tend to have more confrontational behaviors and also more persistent symptoms.

In general, violent behavior is more common in males than in females. This explains why both intermittent explosive disorder and conduct disorder are more common in males. Males also tend to display more confrontational and aggressive behaviors, such as fighting, while females with conduct disorder tend to show less confrontational behaviors, such as lying.

COMORBIDITY

Oppositional defiant disorder is related to a variety of other problems, including attention deficit hyperactivity disorder, anxiety, depression, suicide, bipolar disorder, and substance abuse (Fitzgibbons, 2011). There has long been a theory that disorders within this category are interrelated. Research supports a progression from childhood-onset oppositional defiant disorder to conduct disorder. Some experts even believe that oppositional defiant disorder is a mild form of conduct disorder. A subset of people in this group may progress to antisocial personality disorder (Burke, Waldman, & Lahey, 2010).

Intermittent explosive disorder tends to be associated with mood disorders, anxiety disorders, eating disorders, substance-use disorders and other impulse control disorders.

Conduct disorders are often comorbid with attention deficit hyperactivity disorder, substance use disorders, and learning disabilities. Children with bipolar disorder may often be confused with conduct disorder and may result in delayed detection and treatment (Kovacs & Pollock, 2009).

Kleptomania may be associated with other impulse control disorders and impulse control-related problems such as impulsive buying. It is also associated with mood disorders such as major depression, anxiety disorders, eating disorders (particularly bulimia nervosa), and personality disorders. Individuals who may or may not have pyromania but who do impulsively set fires often have a history of alcohol dependence or abuse. Juvenile fire setting is usually associated with conduct disorder or attention deficit hyperactivity disorder.

ETIOLOGY

Biological Factors

Genetic

Oppositional defiant disorder tends to occur at a young age and may be related to genetics. Many individuals diagnosed with this disorder have a family history of other mental illness. It may be that genetics produces a vulnerability or predisposition to developing oppositional defiant disorder; likewise, intermittent explosive disorder genetics appears to run in families (Coccaro, 2010). Conduct disorders are more common in children and adolescents whose parents were similarly afflicted (Mental Health America, 2012).

Neurobiological

Research demonstrates that gray matter is less dense in the left prefrontal cortex in young patients with oppositional defiant disorder (Fahim et al., 2012). This area is associated with impulse control and self-regulation. The young patients also had an increase in gray matter in the left temporal area. This area is associated with impulsivity, aggression, and antisocial personality. In boys, the structural abnormalities in brains are more pronounced—gray matter density in the orbitofrontal cortex and white matter density in the superior frontal area are reduced.

People with intermittent explosive disorder may have differences in serotonin regulation in the brain. Also, higher levels of the hormone testosterone have been associated with intermittent explosive disorder.

Adolescents with conduct disorder have been found to have significantly reduced gray matter bilaterally in the anterior insulate cortex and the left amygdala (Sterzer et al., 2007). The insulate cortex is believed to be involved in emotion and empathy, and the amygdala also helps to process emotional reactions. Researchers believe that this reduction may be related to aggressive behavior and have found a positive correlation between this deficit and empathy scores. That is, the less gray matter in these regions of the brain, the less likely adolescents are to feel remorse for their actions or victims. Fairchild and colleagues (2011) found that regardless of age of onset gray matter reductions crucial in brain regions for processing emotional stimuli contribute to this disorder.

Psychological Factors

Children with conduct disorders tend to utilize more immature styles of coping and problem solving. People with conduct disorders may be compensating and covering for low self-esteem, which is common with this disorder. They may respond impulsively to situations that remind them either consciously or unconsciously of trauma that they experienced in their childhoods. People who are brought up in chaotic and negligent conditions develop poor emotional responses that are more primitive and id-based, and less ego- and superego-driven. A history of not having their own needs met results in an individual who has a less well-developed sense of empathy.

Intermittent explosive outbursts may be a way of protecting the ego by creating interpersonal distance from others. Vulnerable feelings are compensated for by displays of aggression.

Environmental Factors

During childhood, the main context is the family. While these disorders seem to run in families, they may reflect behavior that is learned from generation to generation rather than be the result of genetics. Parents model behavior and provide the child with a view of the world. To a much greater degree than adults, children are dependent on others, especially their families. If parents are abusive, rejecting, or overly controlling, the child may suffer detrimental effects at the developmental point(s) at which the trauma occurs. Other stressors can include major disruptions such as placement in foster care, severe marital discord, or a separation of parents.

External factors in the environment can either support or put stress on children and adolescents and shape their development. Supportive families that help children with behavioral problems do better, and children without supportive families may have a harder time, but bad parenting does not necessarily cause behavioral problems. A supportive family and environment can help to improve a child's future outcome, however.

Oppositional defiant disorder and conduct disorder are associated with family distress, inadequate parenting, and problems with attachment. Conflict in the marriage is viewed as more important than whether or not the parents separate. Children from larger and impoverished families are also at risk for these disorders (Ursano et al., 2011). Relatively low intelligence, independent of social class, is also associated with conduct disorder.

Intermittent explosive disorder is also associated with conflict and violence in the family of origin. Being exposed to this violence at an early age makes it likely that the behavior will be repeated as the children mature. It is common for these families to have had a history of addiction and substance abuse.

APPLICATION OF THE NURSING PROCESS

ASSESSMENT

General Assessment

Some individuals may be in the health care system based on severe symptoms of an impulse control disorder in order to stabilize them. Patients with these disorders may also be in the health care system based on comorbid disorders such as attention deficit hyperactivity disorder, anxiety, depression, or substance abuse. Careful assessment is important to separate and understand the problems. Especially with children, interviewing the parents along with the child and then separately will enrich the assessment.

Suicide Risk

To determine the cause of the distress and the risk of violence, the nurse must listen carefully to any person expressing the wish to hurt self or others. The number one predictor of suicidal risk is a past suicide attempt. Impulsivity and aggression in this population make the possibility of suicide attempts more likely. Areas to explore when assessing suicidal risk include the following:

- Past suicidal thoughts, threats, or attempts
- Existence of a plan, lethality of the plan, and accessibility of the methods for carrying out the plan
- Feelings of hopelessness, changes in level of energy
- Circumstances, state of mind, and motivation
- Viewpoints about suicide and death (e.g., Has a family member or friend attempted suicide?)
- Depression and other moods or feelings (e.g., anger, guilt, rejection)
- History of impulsivity, poor judgment, or decreased decision making
- Drug or alcohol use

- Prescribed medications and any recent adherence issues
- An assessment of protective factors and coping skills

For the younger person with oppositional defiant disorder or conduct disorder, a distorted concept of death and immature ego functions complicate an assessment of the lethality of a suicide plan. For instance, a child who is highly suicidal may believe a few aspirin will cause death. The incorrect judgment about the lethality does not diminish the seriousness of the intent. Some teens may make a pact to kill themselves or become upset after a friend has committed suicide or died accidentally. Early intervention is essential, and parents need to understand that suicidal thoughts or self-threatening behavior (e.g., cutting, reckless driving, binge drinking) must be taken seriously and evaluated by mental health professionals as an emergency.

Assessment Tools

There are a variety of tools that you can examine to increase your understanding of the important facets of the disorders. Also, they can help you to share information with colleagues and families of patients.

Oppositional defiant and conduct disorder in young people can be examined more carefully with the questions in Figure 21-1. They are subsets of an ADHD scale created by Wolraich (1998). For both scales individually, scores of 2 to 3 are considered to be indicative of a problem

Oppositional Defiant Disorder	Never	Occasionally	Often	Very Often
1. Argues with adults	0	1	2	3
2. Loses temper	0	1	2	3
3. Actively disobeys or refuses to follow an adult's request or rules	0	1	2	3
4. Bothers people on purpose	0	1	2	3
5. Blames others for his or her mistakes or misbehaviors	0	1	2	3
6. Is touchy or easily annoyed by others	0	1	2	3
7. Is angry or bitter	0	1	2	3
8. Is hateful and wants to get even	0	1	2	3

Conduct Disorder	Never	Occasionally	Often	Very Often
1. Bullies, threatens, or scares others	0	1	2	3
2. Starts physical fights	0	1	2	3
3. Lies to get out of trouble or to avoid jobs	0	1	2	3
4. Skips school without permission	0	1	2	3
5. Is physically unkind to people	0	1	2	3
6. Has stolen things that have value	0	1	2	3
7. Destroys others' property on purpose	0	1	2	3
8. Has used a weapon that can cause serious harm (bat, knife, brick, gun)	0	1	2	3
9. Is physically mean to animals	0	1	2	3
10. Has set fire on purpose to do damage	0	1	2	3
11. Has broken into someone else's home, business, or car	0	1	2	3
12. Has stayed out at night without permission	0	1	2	3
13. Has run away from home overnight	0	1	2	3
14. Has forced someone into sexual activity	0	1	2	3

FIG 21-1 Screening for disruptive behaviors: Vanderbilt AD/HD Diagnostic Teacher Rating Scale. (From Wolraich, M. L., Feurer, I. D., Hannah, J. N., Baumgaertel, A., & Pinnock, T. Y. [1998]. Obtaining systematic teacher reports of disruptive behavior disorders utilizing DSM-IV. *Journal of Abnormal Child Psychology, 26*[2], 141–152.)

ASSESSMENT GUIDELINES

Oppositional Defiant Disorder

1. Identify issues that result in power struggles and triggers for outbursts—when they begin and how they are handled.
2. Assess the child's or adolescent's view of his/her behavior and its impact on others (e.g., at home, school, and with peers). Explore feelings of empathy and remorse.
3. Explore how the child or adolescent can exercise control and take responsibility, problem solve for situations that occur, and plan to handle things differently in the future. Assess barriers and motivation to change and potential rewards to engage patient.

Intermittent Explosive Disorder

a. Assess the history, frequency, and triggers for violent outbursts.
b. Identify times in which the patient was able to maintain control despite being in a situation in which the patient might normally lose control of emotions.
c. Explore actual and potential sources of support at home and socially.
d. Assess for substance use (past and present).

Conduct Disorder

1. Assess the seriousness, types, and initiation of disruptive behavior and how it has been managed.
2. Assess anxiety, aggression and anger levels, motivation, and the ability to control impulses.
3. Assess moral development, problem solving, belief system, and spirituality for the ability to understand the impact of hurtful behavior on others, to empathize with others, and to feel remorse.
4. Assess the ability to form a therapeutic relationship and engage in honest and committed therapeutic work leading to observable behavioral change (e.g., signing a behavioral contract, drug testing, and living according to "home rules").
5. Assess for substance use (past and present).

Self-Assessment

People with impulse-control disorders have behaviors that are considered to be objectionable by most people. Concerns for personal emotional and physical safety may be real or exaggerated depending on the nature of the patient's behavior. These concerns should be addressed, and steps should be taken to provide for the safest environment for care.

Negative attitudes may be directed at the patient because the caretaker feels the disorder is controllable and that the patient is choosing not to get better. Our ethical and professional responsibility to provide equal care to all people extends to this population. An empathetic view of people with these disorders is necessary, particularly when considering their environments of origin and a history of constant negative responses from others.

DIAGNOSIS

Children, adolescents, and adults with oppositional defiant disorder, intermittent explosive disorder, and conduct disorder display disruptive behaviors that are impulsive, angry/aggressive, and often dangerous. They are in conflict with others, are noncompliant, do not follow age-appropriate social norms, and have inappropriate ways of meeting their needs. Nursing diagnoses are focused on protection of others and self from impulsive and premeditated acts, improving coping skills, and addressing the family.

OUTCOMES IDENTIFICATION

Outcomes for impulse control disorders relate specifically to reversing the diagnosis that has been identified. Whenever possible, outcomes should be patient-centered and agreed upon by both the nurse and the patient or his/her designee.

Signs and symptoms, nursing diagnoses, and associated outcomes for people with impulse control disorders are paired in Table 21-2.

TABLE 21-2 SIGNS AND SYMPTOMS, NURSING DIAGNOSES, AND OUTCOMES FOR IMPULSE-CONTROL DISORDERS

SIGNS AND SYMPTOMS	NURSING DIAGNOSES	OUTCOMES
History of suicide attempts, aggression and impulsivity, conflictual interpersonal relationships; states, "If I have to stay here, I'm going to kill myself."	*Risk for suicide*	Expresses feelings, verbalizes suicidal ideas, refrains from suicide attempts, plans for the future
Body posture rigid, clenches fists and jaw, paces, invades the personal space of others, history of cruelty to animals, fire setting, and frequent fights, history of childhood abuse and witnessed family violence; states, "That wimp of a roommate better stay out of my way."	*Risk for other-directed violence*	Identifies harmful impulsive behaviors, controls impulses, refrains from aggressive acts, identifies social support
Hostile laughter, projects responsibility for behavior onto others, grandiosity, difficulty establishing relationships	*Defensive coping related to impulse-control problems*	Identifies ineffective and effective coping, identifies and uses support system, uses new coping strategies
Rejection of child or hostility toward the child; unsafe home environment, abusive and/or neglectful; disturbed relationship between parent/caregiver and the child	*Impaired parenting*	Parent/caregiver participates in the therapeutic program, learns appropriate parenting skills

From Herdman, T. H. (Ed.), (2012). *Nursing diagnoses—Definitions and classification 2012-2014*. Copyright © 2012, 1994-2012 by NANDA International. Used by arrangement with John Wiley & Sons Limited; Moorhead, S., Johnson, M., Maas, M. L., & Swanson, E. (2013). *Nursing outcomes classification (NOC)* (5th ed.). St. Louis, MO: Mosby.

IMPLEMENTATION

Psychosocial Interventions

Interventions for severe oppositional defiant, intermittent explosive, and conduct disorders focus on correcting the faulty personality (ego and superego) development, which includes firmly entrenched patterns, such as blaming others and denial of responsibility for personal actions. Children, adolescents, and adults with these disorders also must generate more mature and adaptive coping mechanisms and prosocial goals, a process that is gradual and cannot be accomplished during short-term treatment.

General interventions include the following:

1. Promote a climate of safety for the patient and for others.
2. Establish a rapport with the patient.
3. Set limits and expectations.
4. Consistently follow through with consequences of rule-breaking
5. Provide structure and boundaries.
6. Provide activities and opportunities for achievement of goals to promote a sense of purpose.

Oppositional youth are generally treated on an outpatient basis, using individual, group, and family therapy, with much of the focus on parenting issues. In conduct disorder, inpatient hospitalization for crisis intervention, evaluation, and treatment planning, as well as transfer to therapeutic foster care, group homes, or long-term residential treatment, is often needed.

Unfortunately, studies indicate that many children and adolescents may be simply placed in group homes and in some residential programs and do not maintain improvements following discharge; however, intensive programs such as multisystemic therapy, therapeutic foster care, and use of multidisciplinary, community-based treatment teams for children with serious emotional and behavioral disturbances have been found to improve outcome and reduce offenses over the long term. These types of programs are more promising in improving positive adjustment, decreasing negative behaviors, and improving family stability.

Box 21-1 provides a summary of techniques to manage disruptive behaviors.

Pharmacological Interventions

Pharmacotherapy is generally not indicated for oppositional defiant disorder; however, comorbid conditions that increase defiant symptoms such as attention deficit hyperactivity disorder should be managed.

Medications for intermittent explosive disorder might include the selective serotonin reuptake inhibitor fluoxetine (Prozac), mood stabilizers such as lithium, or some of the anticonvulsant agents (Ploskin, 2012). The use of these medications is considered "off-label" since patients may not have the symptoms for which the drugs are prescribed; however, they may still help reduce the outbursts.

Antipsychotics such as clozapine (Clozaril) and haloperidol (Haldol) may also exert a calming effect on the outbursts associated with intermittent explosive disorder. Antianxiety medications should be avoided since they may reduce inhibitions

EVIDENCE-BASED PRACTICE

Predicting Future Conduct Disorders for Early Intervention

Conduct Problems Prevention Research Group. (2011). The effects of the fast track preventive intervention on the development of conduct disorder across childhood. *Child Development, 82*(1), 331–345.

Problem

Conduct disorder in children and adolescents can often result in antisocial problems further in life, characterized by criminal and violent behavior resulting in devastating personal and financial outcomes. Efforts have been made to develop early screening and prevention programs in hopes of identifying those at risk and intervening, but research is needed to test for efficacy.

Purpose of Study

The purpose of the study was to (1) determine if a screening procedure could accurately predict future disorders, and (2) evaluate if a program called Fast Track could prevent the development of a psychiatric disorder during the implementation period and postintervention, for up to 2 years after completion.

Methods

Kindergarten participants were drawn from three urban sites and one rural site. The predominantly male, African American, and socioeconomically disadvantaged participants were randomly assigned to either a control group or an intervention group. For 10 years, the intervention group was provided with interventions consisting of parent behavior management skills, child social cognitive skills, home visitation, mentoring, and classroom instruction.

Key Findings

- The highest risk kindergarten group demonstrated an 82% probability of ultimate diagnosis.
- Random assignment to the intervention group was found to prevent impulse control disorders over 12 years (including the 2-year period after intervention ended) among the highest risk group.
- The intervention resulted in cumulative benefits across the multiple years of implementation.

Implications of Nursing Practice

Early identification and intervention can reduce future development of lifelong psychiatric illnesses. Nurses have the potential to screen young children and identify those high at risk. In addition to referring them for interventions such as Fast Track to a social worker or guidance counselor through the school system, nurses can apply elements of these treatments into their own nursing care plans. Offering education around parenting skills and social skills for the child are examples of effective interventions for this population.

BOX 21-1 TECHNIQUES FOR MANAGING DISRUPTIVE BEHAVIORS

Behavioral contract: A patient-centered verbal or written agreement between the patient and nurse or other parties (e.g., family, treatment team, teacher) about behaviors, expectations, and needs. The contract is periodically evaluated and reviewed and typically coupled with rewards and other contingencies, positive and negative.

Counseling: Verbal interactions teach, coach, or maintain adaptive behavior and provide positive reinforcement. It is most effective for motivated patients and those with well-developed communication and self-reflective skills.

Modeling: A method of learning behaviors or skills by observation and imitation that can be used in a wide variety of situations. It is enhanced when the modeler is perceived to be similar (e.g., age, interests) and attending to the task is required.

Role playing: A counseling technique in which the nurse, the patient, or a group of patients acts out a specified script or role to enhance their understanding of that role, learn and practice new behaviors or skills, and practice specific situations. It requires well-developed expressive and receptive language skills.

Planned ignoring: When the staff determines behaviors not to be safe and only attention seeking, they may be ignored. Additional interventions may be used in conjunction (e.g., positive reinforcement for on-task actions).

Physical distance and touch control: While touching and closeness may have a positive effect on many patients, patients with oppositional defiant, intermittent explosive, and conduct disorders may need increased personal space and feel threatened by touch.

Redirection: A technique used following an undesirable or inappropriate behavior to engage or re-engage an individual in an appropriate activity. It may involve the use of verbal directives (e.g., setting firm limits), gestures, or physical prompts.

Positive feedback: Emotional support and positive feedback are good for anyone, but they are particularly helpful for individuals who rarely receive such attention.

Clarification as intervention: Sometimes misunderstandings are the source of frustration and potential loss of control. Helping the patient to understand the environment and what is happening can reduce feelings of vulnerability and the urge to strike out.

Restructuring: Changing an activity in a way that will decrease the stimulation or frustration (e.g., shorten the 1:1 session or change to a physical activity). This requires flexibility and planning to have an alternative in mind in case the activity is not going well.

Limit setting: Involves giving direction, stating an expectation, or telling the patient what is required. This should be done firmly, calmly, without judgment or anger, preferably in advance of any problem behavior occurring, and consistently when in a treatment setting among multiple staff.

Simple restitution: Refers to a procedure in which an individual is required or expected to correct the adverse environmental or relational effects of his or her misbehavior by restoring the environment to its prior state, making a plan to correct his or her actions with the nurse, and implementing the plan (e.g., apologizing to the persons harmed, fixing the chairs that are upturned). Simple restitution is not punitive in nature, and there are typically additional activities involved (e.g., counseling).

Physical restraint: For young persons, therapeutic holding may be used to protect the child from impulses to act out and hurt self or others. For stronger adolescents and adults, seclusion and restraint may be necessary.

and self-control further in much the same way as alcohol does. Beta blocking medications may also help to calm individuals with intermittent explosive disorder by slowing the heart rate and reducing blood pressure.

Medications for conduct disorder are directed at problematic behaviors such as aggression, impulsivity, hyperactivity, and mood symptoms (Ursano et al., 2011). These medications include second-generation antipsychotics such as risperidone (Risperdal), olanzapine (Zyprexa), quetiapine (Seroquel), and ziprasidone (Geodon), as well as the third-generation antipsychotic aripiprazole (Abilify). As with oppositional defiant disorder, comorbid conditions aggravate and exacerbate this disorder, and their treatment often improves conduct disorder symptoms.

A variety of medications are used to control aggression. They include tricyclic antidepressants, antianxiety medications, mood stabilizers, and antipsychotics (Strain et al., 2011). Refer to Chapter 27 for further discussion of managing aggression.

Health Teaching and Health Promotion

When the patient is a child or adolescent, families are actively engaged and given support in using parenting skills to provide nurturance and set consistent limits. They are taught techniques for behavior modification, monitoring medication for effects, collaborating with teachers to foster academic success, and setting up a home environment that is consistent, structured, and nurturing to promote achievement of normal developmental milestones. If families are abusive, drug dependent, or highly disorganized, the child may require out-of-home placement. The following nursing interventions are helpful when working with parents and caregivers:

- Explore the impact of the child's behaviors on family life and of the other members' behavior on the child.
- Assist the immediate and extended family to access available and supportive individuals and systems.
- Discuss how to make home a safe environment, especially in regard to weapons and drugs; attempt to talk separately to members whenever possible.
- Discuss realistic behavioral goals and how to set them; problem solve potential problems.
- Teach behavior modification techniques. Role-play them with the parents in different problem situations that might arise with their child.
- Give support and encouragement as parents learn to apply new techniques.
- Provide education about medications.
- Refer parents or caregivers to a local self-help group.
- Advocate with the educational system if special-education services are needed.

Advanced Practice Interventions

There are a variety of psychosocial interventions aimed at the pathology associated with impulse control disorders. The overall goals are to (1) help patients maintain control of their thoughts and behaviors, and (2) assist families to function more adaptively.

Cognitive-Behavioral Therapy (CBT)

Cognitive-behavioral therapy (CBT) is an evidence-based treatment approach that can be used for children, adolescents, and adults. It is a talk therapy that focuses on a patient's feelings, thoughts, and behaviors. It is based on the idea that if we change our thoughts to be more realistic and positive, we can change the way we experience life. Cognitive therapy teaches patients to recognize the onset of the impulse to explode or act aggressively, to identify circumstances or triggers that are associated with the onset, and to develop methods to prevent the maladaptive behaviors from occurring.

Psychodynamic Psychotherapy

One of the older treatment approaches, psychodynamic psychotherapy, continues to have relevance. Its focus is on underlying feelings and motivations and explores conscious and unconscious thought processes. In working with impulse-control problems, the therapist may help the patient to uncover underlying feelings and reasons behind rage or anger. This may help patients to develop better ways to think about and control their behavior.

Dialectical Behavioral Therapy (DBT)

A specific kind of cognitive-behavioral treatment that has a focus on impulse control is dialectical behavioral therapy (DBT). Skills taught include mindfulness, emotional regulation, distress tolerance, and personal effectiveness (Cooper & Parsons, 2010). Shelton and colleagues (2011) found a DBT-Corrections Modified version of this therapy to be effective in reducing physical aggression in incarcerated adolescents.

Parent-Child Interaction Therapy (PCIT)

One evidence-based approach is **parent-child interaction therapy (PCIT).** Therapists such as advanced practice nurses sit behind one-way mirrors and coach parents through an ear audio device while they interact with their children. The advanced practice nurse or other advanced practice provider (e.g., psychiatrist, psychologist, counselor, or therapist) can suggest strategies that reinforce positive behavior in the child or adolescent. The goal is to improve parenting strategies and thereby reduce problematic behavior.

Parent Management Training (PMT)

Parent management training (PMT) has a 65% success rate in significantly improving behavioral problems in children diagnosed with oppositional defiant disorder and conduct disorder (Kazdin, 2005). This evidence-based treatment is for children aged 2 to 14 with mild to severe behavioral problems. Parents of children with oppositional defiant disorder and conduct disorder tend to engage in patterns of negative interactions, ineffective harsh punishments, emotionally charged commands and comments, and poor modeling of appropriate behaviors. This treatment targets the parents rather than the child and focuses attention on reinforcement of positive and prosocial behavior, and on brief, negative consequences of bad behavior.

Multisystemic Therapy (MST)

Of all the treatment approaches presented in this list, multisystemic therapy (MST) is the most extensive. This evidence-based approach is an intensive family and community-based program that takes into consideration all of the environments of violent juvenile offenders. Therapists work with caregivers, are on call 24 hours a day, 7 days a week and go to where the child is. Hanging out with friends is replaced with healthy activities such as sports or recreational activities. MST can improve family functioning, school performance, and peer relationships and can build meaningful social supports (Henggeler et al., 2009).

Teamwork and Safety

Part of teamwork and the promotion of safety is the monitoring of dynamics between staff and patients. Safety is compromised when a power struggle exists between staff and patients. The term expressed emotion refers to the qualitative amount of emotion displayed, usually in the context of family interactions. In the context of the treatment environment, high expressed emotion is a major cause of aggressive responses from patients with impulse-control disorders. Violence increases when persons act in an authoritarian or confrontational way or engage in power struggles. Body language such as standing too close and tone of voice can indicate aggression on the part of staff. Arbitrary or poorly explained denial of privileges can trigger violent retaliation. High expressed emotion includes criticisms, resentment, or annoyance about patient behavior.

Alternatively, staff that use low expressed emotion use calm communication that reduces confrontation and decreases the need for seclusion and restraint and decreases relapse in the patient (Heebner, 2007). The best way to communicate with a potentially hostile patient includes the following techniques:

- Using nonthreatening body posture and a flat, neutral tone of voice (never an angry tone of voice) when correcting behavior
- Using matter-of-fact, easy-to-understand words
- Avoiding personal terms (such as "I" or "you") when setting a limit
- Consistently setting limits

Seclusion and Restraint

Seclusion and restraint may be necessary as a last resort when working with patients with impulse-control disorders. The use of time-out or a quiet area may be helpful in reducing the stimuli of the environment. Please refer to Chapter 6 for more information related to seclusion and restraint.

EVALUATION

Patients with impulse-control disorders exhibit an inability to self-regulate. Care is aimed at providing external boundaries and a safe environment. Ideally, patients on in patient units demonstrate increased levels of self-regulation and ability to interact appropriately with others. In outpatient and community settings patients will progress incrementally from aggressive and impulsive behavior and move on to considering the rights of others and behaviors that are in control.

KEY POINTS TO REMEMBER

- Impulse control disorders include oppositional defiant disorder, intermittent explosive disorder, and conduct disorder. These are disorders of impulse that are seen in mental health care settings and in the criminal justice system.
- Chaotic and punitive environments are strongly correlated with the development of these disorders.
- Impulsivity and aggression in this population make the possibility of suicide attempts and other-directed violence more likely. Continual assessment of suicidal risk and other-directed violence is an essential component of care.
- Nurses are often attracted to health care in order to help people who want and need their assistance. Patients with impulse-control disorders may create a level of discomfort since they resist help and seem to be self-defeating and unkind. Remembering the tragic etiology of these disorders may help increase empathy and therapeutic responses.
- Nursing diagnoses are going to be focused on protection of others and self from impulsive and premeditated acts, improvement of coping skills, and development of an increased self-esteem.
- The three most important interventions with this population promote a climate of safety for the patient and for others, establish rapport with the patient, and set limits and expectations.
- Pharmacological treatments are generally aimed at co-occurring conditions such as attention deficit hyperactivity disorder. Some medications such as second-generation antipsychotics will target aggressive symptoms that accompany each of these disorders.
- A variety of advanced practice interventions should be considered for this population. Most of them are evidence-based and effective.
- An important concept when working with impulse control disorders is expressed emotion. In order to create a positive atmosphere of teamwork and safety, expressed emotion on the part of caregivers should be low to prevent emotional and behavioral reactivity.

CRITICAL THINKING

1. Jacob is a 14-year-old adolescent who has been diagnosed with conduct disorder.
   a. Explain to one of your classmates his probable behaviors in terms of (1) aggression toward others, (2) destruction of property, (3) deceitfulness, and (4) violation of rules.
   b. What are the outcomes for this disorder?
   c. List at least seven ways you could support Jacob's parents. What are some community referrals you could give them in your own locale?
2. Mallory is a 17-year-old female being admitted to the adolescent psychiatric unit after several weeks of impulsive behaviors such as extensive cutting and running away from home.
   a. Put the following areas of assessment in order of priority and provide rationale for your choices:
      1. Suicide risk
      2. Current coping skills
      3. Skin integrity/risk for infection
      4. Childhood development
      5. Current family relationships
   b. Identify at least three appropriate nursing diagnoses for Mallory based on the information above.
   c. Name three nursing interventions to support the nursing diagnosis of ineffective coping.

CHAPTER REVIEW

1. Joshua, a 17-year-old outpatient, has been diagnosed with intermittent explosive disorder. As you care for Joshua, you anticipate that the psychiatric care provider may prescribe which of the following?
   a. A benzodiazepine
   b. An anticonvulsant
   c. A psychostimulant
   d. An anticholinesterase inhibitor
2. You are caring for Gabby, a 12-year-old patient diagnosed with oppositional defiant disorder. Gabby's mother asks you what type of medication is usually prescribed for this diagnosis. Your answer is based on the knowledge that:
   a. Treatment of this disorder does not usually involve any specific medication but focuses on adaptive coping mechanisms.
   b. Interventions for this disorder usually include treatment with mood stabilizers or "off-label" uses of other classifications of medications.
   c. A care plan may include medication, but the patient will outgrow the behavioral problems without any specific treatment.
   d. Psychiatric medications have not been proven to work in the child and adolescent population.
3. Blake is a 15-year-old patient admitted for emergency observation after stealing a car and being pulled over by the police for reckless driving. He also has a history of pyromania. Which of the following is the priority assessment?
   a. Illegal behaviors in the past six months
   b. Assessment of childhood development and family interactions
   c. Suicide risk
   d. Feelings of remorse
4. ________________ disorder is one of the most frequently diagnosed disorders in children and adolescents and is a problem in the adult population as well, with adults experiencing the same type of symptoms. It is characterized by disregard of the rights of others and disdain for societal rules.
5. When working on an in patient adolescent mental health unit, staff may be able to maintain safety and a calm environment when they interact with patients using:
   a. High expressed emotion— "You must stop that immediately!"— using a stern tone.
   b. Strict rule adherence—"There are no snacks after 10 pm. No exceptions!"—using a authoritarian tone.
   c. Suppressed emotion—"Hey, let's just talk about something else that doesn't upset you!"—using a light, friendly tone.
   d. Low expressed emotion—"Please go to your room for quiet time now"—using a neutral, calm tone.

Answers to Chapter Review
1. b; 2. a; 3. c; 4. Conduct; 5. d.

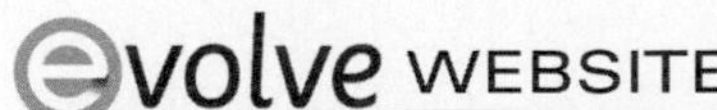

Visit the Evolve website for a posttest on the content in this chapter: http://evolve.elsevier.com/Varcarolis

Post-Test interactive review

REFERENCES

American Psychiatric Association (APA). (2013). *DSM-5 table of contents.* Retrieved from http://www.psychiatry.org/dsm5.

Bulechek, G. M., Butcher, H. K., Dochterman, J. M., & Wagner, C. (2013). *Nursing interventions classification (NIC)* (6th ed.). St. Louis, MO: Mosby.

Burke, J. D., Waldman, I., & Lahey, B. B. (2010). Predictive validity of childhood oppositional defiant disorder and conduct disorder: Implications for the DSM-V. *Journal of Abnormal Psychology, 119*(4), 739–751. doi:10.1037/a0019708.

Coccaro, E. F. (2010). A family history study of intermittent explosive disorder. *Journal of Psychiatric Research, 44*(15), 1101–1105.

Cooper, B., & Parsons, J. (2010). Dialectical behaviour therapy: A social work intervention? Aotearoa New Zealand Social Work Review, *21/22*(4/1), 83–93.

de Ancos, E. T., & Ascaso, L. E. (2011). Sex differences in oppositional defiant disorder. *Psicothema, 23*(4), 666–671.

Fahim, C., Fiori, M., Evans, A. C., & Perusse, D. (2012). The relationship between social defiance, vindictiveness, anger, and brain morphology in eight-year-old boys and girls. *Social Development, 21*(3), 592–609.

Fairchild, G., Passamonti, L., Hurford, G., Hagan, C. C., von dem Hagen, E. A. H., van Goozen, S. H. M., et al. (2011). Brain structure abnormalities in early-onset and adolescent-onset conduct disorder. *American Journal of Psychiatry, 168*, 624–633.

Farrell, A. D., Erwin, E. H., Bettencourt, A., Mays, S., Vulin-Reynolds, M., Sullivan, T., et al. (2008). Individual factors influencing effective nonviolent behavior and fighting in peer situations: A qualitative study with urban African American adolescents. *Journal of Clinical Child & Adolescent Psychology, 37*(2), 397–411.

Fitzgibbons, R. E. (2011). *The angry, defiant (ODD) child.* Retrieved from http://www.maritalhealing.com/conflicts/angrychild.php.

Gale, B. M. (2011). Oppositional defiant disorder. In C. Draper & W. T. O'Donohue (Eds.), Stepped care and e-health (pp. 181–202). New York, NY: Springer.

Harvard Medical School. (2011). Options for managing conduct disorder: Treatment works best when it involves and empowers parents. The Harvard Mental Health Letter, *27*(9), 1–3.

Heebner, E. R. (2007). Expressed emotion and the inpatient psychiatric facility—Expressed emotion and the inpatient psychiatric facility with low functioning psychiatric patients. *International Journal of Psychiatric Nursing Research, 13*(1), 1554–1560.

Henggeler, S. W., Cunningham, P. B., Schoenwald, S. K., Borduin, C. M., & Rowland, M. D. (2009). *Multisystemic therapy for antisocial behavior in children and adolescents.* New York, NY: Guilford Press.

Kazdin, A. E. (2005). *Parent management training: Treatment for oppositional, aggressive, and antisocial behavior in children and adolescents.* New York, NY: Oxford University.

Kessler, R. C., Avenevoli, S., Costello, E. J., Georgiades, K., Green, J. G., Gruber, M. J., et al. (2012). Prevalence, persistence, and sociodemographic correlates of DSM-IV disorders in the national comorbidity survey replication adolescent supplement. *Archives of General Psychiatry, 69*(4), 372–380.

Kovacs, M., & Pollock, M. (2009). *Bipolar disorder and comorbid conduct disorder in childhood and adolescence.* Retrieved from http://www.thebalancedmind.org/learn/library/bipolar-disorder-and-comorbid-conduct-disorder-in-childhood-and-adolescence.

Luman, M., Sergeant, J. A., Knol, D. L., & Ooserlaan, J. (2009). Impaired decision making in oppositional defiant disorder related to altered psychophysiological responses to reinforcement. *Biological Psychiatry, 68*(4), 337–344.

Lyons, J., McClelland, G., & Jordan, N. (2010). Fire setting behavior in a child welfare system: Prevalence, characteristics and co-occurring needs. *Journal of Child & Family Studies, 19*(6), 720–727.

McCloskey, M. S., Kleabir, K., Berman, M. E., Chen, E. Y., & Coccaro, E. F. (2010). Unhealthy aggression: Intermittent explosive disorder and adverse physical health outcomes. *Health Psychology, 29*(3), 324–332.

Mental Health America. (2012). *What is conduct disorder*? Retrieved from http://www.nmha.org/go/conduct-disorder.

National Institute of Mental Health. (2006). Intermittent explosive disorder affects up to 16 million Americans. Retrieved from http://www.nimh.nih.gov/science-news/2006/intermittent-explosive-disorder-affects-up-to-16-million-americans.shtml.

Ploskin, D. (2012). Treatment for intermittent explosive disorder. *Psych Central.* Retrieved from http://psychcentral.com/lib/2007/treatment-for-intermittent-explosive-disorder/.

Rowe, R., Costello, E. J., Angold, A., Copeland, W. E., & Maughan, B. (2010). *Journal of Abnormal Psychology, 119*(4), 726–738. doi:10.1037/a0020798.

Sadock, B. J., & Sadock, V. A. (2008). *Kaplan & Sadock's concise textbook of clinical psychiatry* (3rd ed.). Philadelphia, PA: Lippincott Williams & Wilkins.

Shelton, D., Kesten, K., Zhang, W., & Trestman, R. (2011). Impact of a dialectic behavior therapy-corrections modified upon behaviorally challenged incarcerated male adolescents. *Journal of Child and Adolescent Psychiatric Nursing, 24*(2), 105–113. doi:10.1111/j.1744-6171.2011.00275.x.

Stellwagen, K., & Kerig, P. (2010). Relating callous-unemotional traits to physically restrictive treatment measures among child psychiatric inpatients. *Journal of Child & Family Studies, 19*(5), 588–595.

Sterzer, P., Stadler, C., Poustka, F., & Kleinschmidt, A. (2007). A structural neural deficit in adolescents with conduct disorders and its association with lack of empathy. *NeuroImage, 37*, 335–345.

Strain, J. J., Klipstein, K. G., & Newcorn, J. H. (2011). Adjustment disorders. In R. E. Hales, S. C. Yudofsky, & G. O. Gabbard (Eds.), *Essentials of psychiatry* (3rd ed.). Washington, DC: American Psychiatric Publishing.

Talih, F. R. (2011). Kleptomania and potential exacerbating factors: A review and case report. *Innovations in Clinical Neuroscience, 8*(10), 35–39.

Tamam, L., Eroglu, M. Z., & Paltaci, O. (2011). Intermittent explosive disorder. *Current Approaches in Psychiatry, 3*(3), 387–425.

Ursano, A. M., Kartheiser, P. H., & Barnhill, L. J. (2011). Disorders usually first diagnosed in infancy, childhood, or adolescence. In R. E. Hales, S. C. Yudofsky, & G. O. Gabbard (Eds.), *Essentials of psychiatry* (3rd ed.). Washington, DC: American Psychiatric Publishing.

Wolraich, M. L., Feurer, I. D., Hannah, J. N., Baumgaertel, A., & Pinnock, T. Y. (1998). Obtaining systematic teacher reports of disruptive behavior disorders utilizing DSM-IV. *Journal of Abnormal Child Psychology, 26*(2), 141–152.

CHAPTER

22

Substance-Related and Addictive Disorders

Carolyn Baird and Margaret Jordan Halter

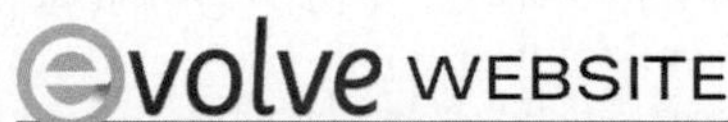

Visit the Evolve website for a pretest on the content in this chapter: http://evolve.elsevier.com/Varcarolis

Pre-Test interactive review

OBJECTIVES

1. Describe the terms substance use, intoxication, tolerance, and withdrawal.
2. Define addiction as a chronic disease.
3. Describe the neurobiological process that occurs in the brain and neurotransmitters involved with substance use.
4. Identify potential co-occurring medical and psychological disorders.
5. Name the common classification of substances used.
6. Identify patterns of substance use
7. Apply the nursing process to caring for an individual who is using substances.

KEY TERMS AND CONCEPTS

addiction
codependence
co-occurring disorders
intoxication
patient-centered care
recovery-oriented systems of care (ROSC)
Screening, Brief Intervention, Referral to Treatment (SBIRT)
substance use disorder
tolerance
transtheoretical model of care
withdrawal

Substance disorders are not disorders of choice. They are complex diseases of the brain represented by craving, seeking, and using regardless of consequences (National Institute on Drug Abuse [NIDA], 2010a). Continuous substance use results in actual changes in the brain structure and function of an area of the brain referred to as the reward or pleasure center. This area of the brain within the limbic system is also the part of the brain that is affected by other mental health disorders such as depression, schizophrenia, or anxiety. More than half the individuals with a substance use disorder can be expected to have some other co-occurring mental health disorder and vice versa, leading researchers to suspect that there is an underlying genetic vulnerability (McCauley, 2009).

Historically, these disorders have been treated in separate systems of care. Individuals received treatment for mental health problems in the mental health system and treatment for substance disorders in chemical dependency units or facilities. If both mental health and substance use disorders were present, the treatment might occur concurrently in different settings or as back-to-back treatment in one system followed by the other.

That care fragmentation began to change in 2001, when the Institute of Medicine (IOM) published a report on the status of the nation's health care. *Crossing the Quality Chasm: A New Health System for the 21st Century* included recommendations for addressing the rising number of individuals with substance and addictive disorders with or without co-occurring mental health disorders. The IOM referred to the United States' delivery of care as being uncoordinated and overly complex, resulting in patients' being handed off from one set of providers to the next. This fragmented care causes errors and slows the process down, wastes resources, and leaves tremendous voids in care.

These concerns are being addressed through a number of federal initiatives. These initiatives include integration of mental health and substance use treatment systems, cross training of health care professionals, and integrated screening and early intervention programs for identifying individuals with substance and addiction problems regardless of where they present for care.

It is important for all nurses regardless of their practice area to develop an understanding of the disease of addiction. Nursing curricula should include the content and practice the skills necessary for addiction screening, early detection, and referral to appropriate treatment. Without an accurate assessment for substance use and other mental health disorders, individuals will be unable to receive comprehensive treatment planning and quality care (Baird, 2011).

CLINICAL PICTURE

A **substance use disorder** is a pathological use of a substance that leads to a disorder of use, intoxication, and, often, withdrawal if the substance is taken away. Substance use disorders encompass a broad range of products that human beings take into their bodies through various means (e.g., swallowing, inhaling, injecting). They range from fairly innocuous and innocent-seeming substances such as coffee to absolutely illegal, mind-altering drugs such as LSD. No matter the substance, use disorders share many commonalities, intoxication characteristics, and withdrawal attributes. The American Psychiatric Association (APA) (2013) identifies the following substance-related and addictive disorders:

- Alcohol
- Caffeine
- Cannabis
- Hallucinogen
- Inhalant
- Opioid
- Sedative, hypnotic, anxiolytic
- Stimulant
- Tobacco
- Other substances

While substances are generally associated as the source of addiction problems, behaviors, too, are gradually being recognized as addictive. Internet gaming, the use of social media, shopping, and sexual activity are also considered to be addictive. Behavioral addictions are also referred to as process addictions. The first behavioral addiction, gambling, was officially declared a disorder in 2013 (APA). Gambling and other compulsive actions activate dopamine and glutamate in the reward or pleasure neural pathways of the brain's limbic system the same as substances do (Potenza, 2008). The activities are reinforced through the dopamine glutamate cycle and may become dysfunctional for the individual, resulting in many of the same problematic behaviors and functional issues as the ingested substances.

See Table 22-1 for information on the commonly abused drugs.

Concepts That Are Central to Substance Use Disorders

A term that people commonly use to describe substance use disorders is **addiction**. The most current definition of addiction states that it is a "primary, chronic disease of brain reward, motivation, memory, and related circuitry" (American Society of Addiction Medicine, 2011, para. 1). It is a disease of dysregulation in the hedonic (pleasure seeking) or reward pathway of the brain (Koob, 2009). Characteristic manifestations

TABLE 22-1 COMMONLY ABUSED DRUGS

CATEGORY AND NAME	*COMMERCIAL* AND STREET NAMES	DEA SCHEDULE*/ ADMINISTRATION	*ACUTE EFFECTS*/HEALTH RISKS
Tobacco			
Nicotine	Found in cigarettes, cigars, bidis, and smokeless tobacco (snuff, spit tobacco, chew)	Smoked, snorted, chewed	*Increased blood pressure and heart rate* Chronic lung disease; cardiovascular disease; stroke; cancers of the mouth, pharynx, larynx, esophagus, stomach, pancreas, cervix, kidney, bladder, and acute myeloid leukemia; adverse pregnancy outcomes; addiction
Alcohol			
Alcohol	Found in liquor, beer, and wine	Swallowed	*Low doses: Euphoria, mild stimulation, relaxation, lowered inhibitions* *High doses: Drowsiness, slurred speech, nausea, emotional volatility, loss of coordination, visual distortions, impaired memory, sexual dysfunction, loss of consciousness* Increased risk of injuries, violence, fetal damage; depression; neurologic deficits, hypertension; live and heart disease; addiction fatal overdose

Continued

TABLE 22-1 COMMONLY ABUSED DRUGS—cont'd

CATEGORY AND NAME	*COMMERCIAL* AND STREET NAMES	DEA SCHEDULE*/ ADMINISTRATION	*ACUTE EFFECTS*/HEALTH RISKS
Cannabinoids			
Marijuana	Blunt, dope, ganja, grass, herb, joint, bud, Mary Jane, pot, reefer, green, trees, smoke, sinsimella, skunk, weed	I/Smoked, swallowed	*Euphoria; relaxation; slowed reaction time; distorted sensory perception; impaired balance and coordination; increased heart rate and appetite; impaired learning, memory; anxiety; panic attacks; psychosis/cough*
Hashish	Boom, gangster, hash, hash oil, hemp	I/Smoked, swallowed	Frequent respiratory infections; possible mental health decline; addiction
Opioids			
Heroin	*Diacetylmorphine*: smack, horse, brown sugar, dope, H., junk, skag, skunk, white horse, China white; cheese	I/Injected, smoked, snorted	*Euphoria; drowsiness; impaired coordination; dizziness; confusion; nausea; sedation; feeling of heaviness in the body; slowed or arrested breathing*
Opium	*Laudanum, paregoric*: big O, black stuff, block, gum, hop	II, III, V/Swallowed, smoked	Constipation; endocarditis; hepatitis; HIV; addiction; fatal overdose
Stimulants			
Cocaine	*Cocaine hydrochloride:* blow, bump, C, candy, Charlie, coke, crack, flake, rock, snow, toot	II/Snorted, smoked, injected	*Increased heart rate, blood pressure, body temperature, metabolism; feelings of exhilaration; increased energy, mental*
Amphetamine	*Biphetamine, Dexedrine:* bennies, black beauties, crosses, hearts, LA turnaround, speed, truck drivers, uppers	II/Swallowed, snorted, smoked, injected	*alertness; tremors; reduced appetite; irritability; anxiety; panic; paranoia; violent behavior; psychosis* Weight loss; insomnia; cardiac or cardiovascular complications; stroke; seizures, addiction
Methamphetamine	*Desoxyn*: meth, ice, crank, chalk, crystal, fire, glass, go fast, speed	II/Swallowed, snorted, smoked, injected	For cocaine: nasal damage from snorting For methamphetamine: severe dental problems
Club Drugs			
MDMA (methylenedioxy-methamphet-amine)	Ecstasy, Adam, clarity, Eve, lover's speed, peace, uppers	I/Swallowed, snorted, injected	*Mild hallucinogenic effects; increased tactile sensitivity, empathic feelings; lowered inhibition; anxiety; chills; sweating; teeth clenching; muscle cramping* Sleep disturbances; depression; impaired memory; hyperthermia; addiction
Flunitrazepam	*Rohypnol:* forget-me pill, Mexican Valium, R2, roach, Roche, roofies, roofinol, rope, rophies	IV/Swallowed, snorted	*Sedation; muscle relaxation; confusion; memory loss; dizziness; impaired coordination* Addiction
GHB	*Gamma-hydroxybutyrate:* G, Georgia home boy, grievous bodily harm, liquid ecstasy, soap, scoop, goop, liquid X	I/Swallowed	*Drowsiness; nausea; headache; disorientation; loss of coordination; memory loss* Unconsciousness; seizures; coma
Dissociative Drugs			
Ketamine	*Ketalar SV:* cat Valium, K, Special K, vitamin K	III/Injected, snorted, smoked	*Feelings of being separate from one's body and environment; impaired motor function; analgesia; impaired memory; delirium; respiratory depression and arrest; death* Anxiety; tremors, numbness; memory loss; nausea
PCP and analogs	*Phencyclidine:* angel dust, boat, hog, love boat, peace pill	I/II/Swallowed, smoked, injected	*Feelings of being separate from one's body and environment; impaired motor function; analgesia; psychosis; aggression; violence; slurred speech; loss of coordination; hallucinations* Anxiety; tremors; numbness; memory loss; nausea

TABLE 22-1 COMMONLY ABUSED DRUGS—cont'd

CATEGORY AND NAME	*COMMERCIAL* AND STREET NAMES	DEA SCHEDULE*/ ADMINISTRATION	*ACUTE EFFECTS*/HEALTH RISKS
Salvia divinorum	Salvia, Shepherdess's Herb, Maria Pastora, magic mint, Sally-D	Chewed, swallowed, smoked	*Feelings of being separate from one's body and environment; impaired motor function* Anxiety; tremors; numbness; memory loss; nausea
Dextromethorphan (DXM)	Found in some cough and cold medications: Robotripping, Robo, Triple C	Swallowed	*Feelings of being separate from one's body and environment; impaired motor function; euphoria; slurred speech; confusion; dizziness; distorted visual perceptions* Anxiety; tremors; numbness; memory loss; nausea
Hallucinogens			
LSD	*Lysergic acid diethylamide*: acid, blotter, cubes, microdot, yellow sunshine, blue heaven	I/Swallowed, absorbed through mouth tissues	*Altered states of perception and feeling; hallucinations; nausea; increased body temperature, heart rate, blood pressure; loss of appetite; sweating; sleeplessness; numbness; dizziness; weakness; tremors; impulsive behavior; rapid shifts in emotion* Flashbacks, Hallucinogen Persisting Perception Disorder
Mescaline	Buttons, cactus, mesc, peyote	I/Swallowed, smoked	*Altered states of perception and feeling; hallucinations; nausea; increased body temperature, heart rate, blood pressure; loss of appetite; sweating; sleeplessness; numbness; dizziness; weakness; tremors; impulsive behavior; rapid shifts in emotion*
Psilocybin	Magic mushrooms, purple passion, shrooms, little smoke	I/Swallowed	*Altered states of perception and feeling; hallucinations; nausea; nervousness; paranoia; panic*
Other Compounds			
Anabolic steroids	*Anadrol, Oxandrin, Durabolin, Depo Testosterone, Equipoise:* roids, juice, gym candy, pumpers	III/Injected, swallowed, applied to skin	*No intoxication effects* Hypertension; blood clotting and cholesterol changes; liver cysts; hostility and aggression; acne; in adolescents – premature stoppage of growth; in males – prostate cancer, reduced sperm production, shrunken testicles, breast enlargement; in females – menstrual irregularities, development of beard and other masculine characteristics
Inhalants	*Solvents (paint thinners, gasoline, glues); gases (butane, propane, aerosol propellants, nitrous oxide); nitrites (isoamyl, isobutyl, cyclohexyl):* laughing gas, poppers, snappers, whippets	Inhaled through nose or mouth	*Varies by chemical – stimulation; loss of inhibition; headache; nausea or vomiting; slurred speech; loss of motor coordination; wheezing* Cramps, muscle weakness; depression; memory impairment; damage to cardiovascular and nervous systems; unconsciousness; sudden death

*Drug Enforcement Agency Schedule I and II drugs have a high potential for abuse. They require greater storage security and have a quota on manufacturing, among other restrictions. Schedule I drugs are available for research only and have no approved medical use; Schedule II drugs are available only by prescription and require a form for ordering. Schedule III and IV drugs are available by prescription, may have five refills in six months, and may be ordered orally. Some Schedule V drugs are available over the counter.

National Institute on Drug Abuse. (2011). *Commonly abused drug chart.* Retrieved from http://www.drugabuse.gov/drugs-abuse/commonly-abused-drugs/commonly-abused-drugs-chart.

usually include loss of behavioral control with craving and inability to abstain, loss of emotional regulation, and loss of the ability to identify problematic behaviors and relationships.

When people are in the process of using a substance to excess they are said be experiencing **intoxication**. Intoxication may manifest itself in a variety of ways depending on the physiological response of the body to the substance that is being abused. Substances may be classified according to their mechanism of action as sedative hypnotics, stimulants, depressants, and hallucinogens. They are often casually referred to as uppers, downers, and all arounders (Palladini, 2011). Individuals who are using substances are considered to be "under the influence," intoxicated, or high. Terminology may vary depending on the substance and the population who is using. Alcohol causes intoxication, but cocaine makes you high. Stimulants cause hyperreactivity, and depressants dampen responses.

There are varying degrees of severity for substance use, and a variety of factors play into how severity is viewed. For example, in some cultures and religions alcohol use is not accepted, and any use would be considered aberrant; in other cultures, alcohol use is a regular part of everyday life, and the amount of consumption would be alarming to people outside the culture.

People with addictions experience tolerance to the effects of the substances. Tolerance is needing increasing amounts of a substance to receive the desired result or finding that using the same amount over time results in a much-diminished effect. Nursing students should know that some prescribed medications might have the same effect, such as some antianxiety medications, analgesics, and beta-blockers. Even antidepressants may result in tolerance (Fava & Offidani, 2011). This type of tolerance is not considered diagnostic when the individual is under medical supervision.

Withdrawal is a set of physiological symptoms that begin to occur as the concentration of the chemical decreases in an individual's bloodstream. It is specific to the substance ingested, and each substance has its own characteristic syndrome. The same substance, or one with a similar action, may be taken to avoid or relieve withdrawal symptoms. Although alcohol is the drug with the greatest potential for and most serious symptoms of withdrawal, the rising numbers of individuals abusing prescription drugs has increased the concern for assessing for withdrawal complications (Office of National Drug Control Policy, 2011). Behavioral addictions such as gambling seldom have clearly identifiable intoxication or withdrawal symptoms, and tolerance is not an issue. Patterns of behavior and consequences are assessed to identify problematic behavior.

EPIDEMIOLOGY

The National Survey on Drug Use and Health is conducted annually on a randomly chosen segment of the population reflecting individuals 12 and older who reside in the United States. It is the primary source for national drug use statistics and trending. According to the 2010 survey, 22.6 million Americans used illicit substances, including the nonmedical use of prescription psychotherapeutics, in the month prior to the survey (Substance Abuse Mental Health Services Administration [SAMHSA], 2011).

While slightly more than half (50.8% or 130.6 million) of the nation's population admits to drinking alcohol, almost a quarter (23.1%) reports binge drinking (five drinks on one occasion on one day in the last month) and about 7% report heavy drinking (five drinks on one occasion on at least five days in the last month). In 2010, 3 million individuals used illicit drugs for the first time, and nearly 5 million individuals tried alcohol; most (82%) of them were younger than 21 years of age (SAMHSA, 2011). Overall, more than 22 million individuals, or nearly 9% of the population of the United States, are estimated to have substance use disorders.

These numbers remained steady overall from 2002 to 2010. In 2010, marijuana had the highest percentage of misuse, followed by cocaine. Marijuana use has remained steady, with almost half of adolescents surveyed reporting that they have easy access to the drug. Cocaine use has been on the decline. It is the rise of prescription drug misuse that has prompted the greatest concern. Over half of individuals using prescription drugs nonmedically got them from a friend or relative for free, more than 10% percent paid a relative or friend for them, and another 9% percent stole them from a friend or relative (SAMHSA, 2011). More than 75% of these persons stated that their friend or relative had gotten them from just one doctor.

Additional statistics are available for all substances abused according to demographics such as gender, race, age, geographic location, education, employment status, driving record, and incarceration status. According to statistics from the 2010 National Survey on Drug Use and Health, the younger the age of first use of drugs or alcohol, the greater the likelihood of misuse as an adult. Adults in their 20s have a higher rate of substance use and addiction than any other age group, and males are twice as likely as females to be

HEALTH POLICY

Bath Salts

Bath salts are a fairly new group of drugs; the salts are sold as tablets, capsules, or powder in sealed envelopes. They are purchased in such places as convenience stores, head shops, and on the Internet. These so-called bath salts are stimulants similar to cocaine, methamphetamine, methylenedioxymethamphetamine (MDMA, Ecstasy), and lysergic acid diethylamide (LSD).

Users of these drugs experience euphoria, elevated mood, and a pleasurable "rush"; however, tachycardia, hypertension, peripheral constriction, chest pain, hallucinations, paranoia, erratic behavior, inattention, lack of memory of substance use, and psychosis are also possible responses to the drugs. Health care workers, including nurses, have been faced with caring for hostile, belligerent, and paranoid patients high on bath salts.

On October 21, 2011, the U.S. Drug Enforcement Administration (DEA) exercised an emergency authority to name three key ingredients in bath salts—MDPV, mephedrone, and methylone—as Schedule I, thereby making them illegal to possess or sell in the United States. Drug sellers have gotten around the law by chemically tweaking the drug just enough to make them fall outside the bounds of the legislation while retaining their psychoactive properties.

In July 2012, President Barack Obama signed a bill that established a federal ban on bath salts, synthetic marijuana, the compounds from which these drugs are produced, and any versions that might be made in the future. This ban includes interstate and online sales and is a part of the Food and Drug Administration (FDA) Safety and Innovation Act (2012).

Data from U.S. Drug Enforcement Administration. (2011). *Chemicals used in "bath salts" now under federal control and regulation.* Retrieved from http://www.justice.gov/dea/pubs/pressrel/pr102111.html; FDA. (2012). *Food and Drug Administration safety and innovation act.* Retrieved from http://www.fda.gov/RegulatoryInformation/Legislation/FederalFoodDrugandCosmeticActFDCAct/SignificantAmendmentstotheFDCAct/FDASIA/ucm20027187.htm.

represented. Around 16% of Alaska Natives and American Indians have substance use disorders as compared with other racial and ethnic groups who are fairly equal at 8% to 9%. Individuals who have higher education levels, are employed, and live in a non-metropolitan county are less likely to misuse substances.

COMORBIDITY

Comorbidity refers to two or more disorders occurring in the same person at the same time with the potential for interaction and exacerbation of symptoms. It may be two or more psychiatric disorders, two or more medical disorders, or a combination of medical and psychiatric disorders (NIDA, 2011b). Although surveys have shown that individuals with substance use disorders have more than a 50% chance of having other mental health disorders of mood and vice versa, it cannot be said that one disorder caused the other, and it is difficult to determine which is primary. It is important that all disorders be identified and treated with a comprehensive approach.

Psychiatric Comorbidity

The high prevalence of psychiatric comorbidity is supported by statistics collected since 1980 using multiple national population surveys. Individuals with mood and anxiety disorders, antisocial behaviors, or histories of conduct or oppositional disorders as adolescents are more than twice as likely to have a substance use disorder (NIDA, 2010b). Three common representations of comorbidity have been identified:

1. The physiological response to certain drugs of abuse presents a cluster of symptoms similar to the symptoms of other mental health disorders (e.g., psychosis, and schizophrenia).
2. Subclinical symptoms from one mental health disorder may result in medication of those symptoms with a psychoactive drug (social anxiety and alcohol or marijuana).
3. Psychiatric illnesses and substance use disorders have common risk factors.

These shared risk factors are genetic vulnerabilities, underlying brain defects in common areas and pathways of the brain, and environmental factors, including exposure to stress or trauma during early developmental stages. Estimates suggest that 40% to 60% of an individual's risk is in genetic vulnerabilities. For this reason, research on substance use and co-occurring disorders has been focusing on trying to identify any genes that may be implicated (NIDA, 2010b). Genes may act individually or in complex interactions of multiple genes to determine an individual's level of susceptibility to risk-taking behavior, response to stress, or metabolism of substances. Research has also identified that the brain circuitry associated with the neurotransmitter dopamine is implicated in addictive disorders, depression, schizophrenia, and other mental health disorders. It has been proposed that deficits or dysfunction in this circuitry may predispose individuals to develop one or multiple psychiatric disorders.

The human brain undergoes dramatic growth from age 5 to 20 and most particularly in adolescence (NIDA, 2010b). Any insult (stress or trauma) during this time may alter the brain circuitry and cause long-term changes in the abilities of decision making, learning and memory, reward, and affect and behavioral control. Early drug use or mental health disorders, such as attention deficit hyperactivity disorder, conduct disorder, posttraumatic stress disorder, or schizophrenia, could be risk factors for all co-occurring disorders but at this time are not considered fully predictive. More research is indicated to determine the role of genetic vulnerabilities and the influence of environmental and psychosocial factors (NIDA, 2010b).

CONSIDERING CULTURE

A Culture of Alcohol and Substance Use

The Monitoring the Future (MTF) survey has been collecting statistics since the mid-1970s on the use of, and attitudes toward, alcohol, tobacco, and other drugs by eighth, tenth, and twelfth grade students. The rate of illicit substance use has been rising and may be related to adolescents' perceptions of risk. It has been suggested that media attention on medical marijuana, the attitude that Ecstasy is a safe drug (10% drop in twelfth graders who believed it was risky to use), and easy availability and nonregulation of synthetic marijuana are responsible for this perception change.

Other illicit drugs (methamphetamine, heroin, and hallucinogens) are increasing or holding steady. Nonmedical use of prescription and over-the-counter drugs, especially opiates such as Vicodin and the stimulant Adderall, is also a problem. Without a change in how the use of substances is viewed and a change in the attitudes voiced in the media, adolescents' perceptions about the risks associated with their behavior will remain unchanged, and their potential for current and future use of alcohol, tobacco, and other drugs will remain the same.

National Institute on Drug Abuse [NIDA]. (2012). *Drug facts: High school and youth trends.* Retrieved from http://www.drugabuse.gov/sites/default/files/drugfactshsyt.pdf.

Medical Comorbidity

According to the 2001-2003 National Comorbidity Survey Replication (NCS-R), 58% of all adults have some type of medical condition while 29% of these adults also have a comorbid psychiatric disorder. At the same time, 68% of adults with a psychiatric disorder have at least one medical disorder. These numbers suggest that 17% (34 million) of the adult population have psychiatric and medical comorbidities (Druss & Walker, 2011).

The more common co-occurring medical conditions are hepatitis C, diabetes, cardiovascular disease, HIV, and pulmonary disorders (NIDA, 2010b). The high comorbidity appears to be the result of shared risk factors, high symptom burden, physiological response to licit and illicit drugs, and complications from the route of administration of substances (Druss & Walker, 2011).

ETIOLOGY

Addiction is a primary and chronic disease that is related to reward, memory, motivation, and circuitry (American Society for Addiction Medicine, 2011). It is characterized by an individual's compulsive seeking of drugs and use despite the amazingly harmful consequences (NIDA, 2009). The parts of the brain most affected by drug use are the brain stem, the limbic system, and the frontal cortex. The reward pathways for motivation and memory are located in the limbic system and are influenced by neurobiological as well as psychological and sociocultural factors (Koob, 2009).

Neurobiological Factors

The human brain is composed of billions of nerve cells called neurons. Each cell has its own receptors and manufactures corresponding neurotransmitters and transporters to convey impulses or messages from cell to cell. In the center of the brain just above the brain stem is the most primitive part. This area is comprised of a number of structures that make up the limbic system and are responsible for survival through a reward system of pleasure and memory coupled with motivational reinforcement or salience (Wright, 2011).

The structures most identified with the reward system or pleasure center are the nucleus accumbens and the ventral tegmental area. The neural pathways between these areas are activated by the neurotransmitter dopamine. Normal activities such as eating, nurturing, and sexual activity are associated with pleasant feelings and cue the amygdala and hippocampus for memories of the experiences. The frontal cortex is stimulated, releasing glutamate and closing the circuit (Koob, 2009).

Psychoactive substances and certain behaviors can hijack this reward pathway circuit, releasing as much as 10 times the amount of dopamine as usual. Over time, the release of dopamine becomes more important than the reward of pleasure, and the increased saliency of the addictive process cancels the inhibitory function of the frontal cortex, leading to craving (McCauley, 2009; Wright, 2011). The brain responds to this imbalance by resetting the pleasure threshold, producing transporter chemicals, and decreasing or down regulating the number of receptors attempting to reach homeostasis. This is the mechanism that is responsible for drug tolerance.

Positron emission tomography (PET) scanning and magnetic resonance imaging (MRI) have made it possible to understand the underlying neurobiology of the brain through imaging studies (Wright, 2011). The brain's response to various psychoactive drugs has been studied, and it has been possible to identify the involved areas of the brain by following the processes as they are activated. The results from these imaging studies also support the theory that other forms of psychopathology share the neurobiology of the same areas of the brain.

Psychological Factors

Shared psychodynamics such as chronic stress and trauma have been identified in the histories of individuals with both substance use and mood disorders. Individuals who experienced abuse or neglect during childhood report more depression and suicidality. Chronic stressors such as poverty, the time and financial obligations of caring for children, and harmful relationships can lead to depression. Domestic violence, combat experience, and exposure to other forms of trauma may lead to posttraumatic stress disorder, major depression, generalized anxiety disorder, and substance use disorders (Druss & Walker, 2011). Many times, there are multiple addictive behaviors that seem to support a shared vulnerability or antecedent.

Sociocultural Factors

Many chronic stressors have their roots in socioeconomic factors. Poverty raises the risk of an unfavorable living environment, lack of parental supervision, poor educational resources, and impaired support systems (Druss & Walker, 2011). A cycle of negative environmental events often begins within disadvantaged neighborhoods, increasing stress and anxiety along with lacking or negative social ties, which contributes to depression. Coping mechanisms may include drugs and acting out behaviors leading to destructive consequences and interaction with the legal system.

APPLICATION OF THE NURSING PROCESS

SCREENING

Screening is essential in order to intervene early and provide treatment for people with substance use disorders and for those at risk of developing these disorders. In one study, about 460,000 individuals were screened for substance use in select medical settings in six different states. A surprisingly high portion of patients screened—23%—was positive for a current or potential substance use problem (Madras et al., 2009). The Screening, Brief Intervention, and Referral to Treatment (SBIRT) (SAMHSA, 2012) is a public health response to this problem. It consists of three major components:

- **Screening:** A nurse or other health care professional in any health care setting assesses a patient for substance use problems using standardized screening tools.
- **Brief Intervention:** A nurse or other health care professional discusses the risks of substance use behaviors with the patient and provides feedback and advice.
- **Referral to Treatment:** A nurse or other health care professional suggests a referral for brief therapy or treatment for patients who screen positively.

People with substance abuse problems often also have psychiatric disorders. These comorbid conditions also need to be treated. Integrated mental health and substance use screenings are valuable in any care setting.

A variety of screening tools are available to assist health care practitioners in gaining important information on which to base plans of care. Simply asking about patterns of use, type of substance, and amounts used is helpful in establishing a baseline. No in-depth knowledge of addiction is necessary for this type of screening. Table 22-2 provides guidelines for assessing excessive amounts of alcohol use. Formalized alcohol screening is as simple as using the Alcohol Use Disorders Identification Test (AUDIT) developed for the World Health Organization (Babor et al., 2006) (Table 22-3). This tool can be administered by a clinician or through self-report. Scores of 8 or more in men and 7 or more in women indicate problematic alcohol use.

The Center for Substance Abuse Treatment and the Center for Substance Abuse Prevention divisions of the Substance Abuse Mental Health Services Administration (SAMHSA) offer

TABLE 22-2 ALCOHOL AMOUNTS THAT INDICATE RISKY/HAZARDOUS DRINKING BASED ON POPULATION

POPULATION	MEN	WOMEN	PREGNANT	ADOLESCENT	ELDERLY
Day/occasion	4	3	0	0	3
Week	14	7	0	0	7

One drink = 12 ounces of beer, 5 ounces of wine, or 1.5 ounces of 80-proof distilled spirits.
Data from U.S. Department of Agriculture and U.S. Department of Health and Human Services. (2010). *Dietary guidelines for Americans, 2010* (7th ed.). Washington, DC: US Government Printing Office.

TABLE 22-3 THE ALCOHOL USE DISORDERS IDENTIFICATION TEST (AUDIT): SELF-REPORT VERSION

Patient: Because alcohol use can affect your health and can interfere with certain medications and treatments, it is important that we ask some questions about your use of alcohol. Your answers will remain confidential so please be honest.
Mark the frequency that best describes your answer to each question.

QUESTIONS	0	1	2	3	4	Score
1. How often do you have a drink containing alcohol?	Never	Monthly or less	2-4 times a month	2-3 times a week	4 or more times a week	
2. How many drinks containing alcohol do you have on a typical day when you are drinking?	1 or 2	3 or 4	5 or 6	7 to 9	10 or more	
3. How often do you have six or more drinks on one occasion?	Never	Less than monthly	Monthly	Weekly	Daily or almost daily	
4. How often during the last year have you found that you were not able to stop drinking once you had started?	Never	Less than monthly	Monthly	Weekly	Daily or almost daily	
5. How often during the last year have you failed to do what was normally expected of you because of drinking?	Never	Less than monthly	Monthly	Weekly	Daily or almost daily	
6. How often during the last year have you needed a first drink in the morning to get yourself going after a heavy drinking session?	Never	Less than monthly	Monthly	Weekly	Daily or almost daily	
7. How often during the last year have you had a feeling of guilt or remorse after drinking?	Never	Less than monthly	Monthly	Weekly	Daily or almost daily	
8. How often during the last year have you been unable to remember what happened the night before because of your drinking?	Never	Less than monthly	Monthly	Weekly	Daily or almost daily	
9. Have you or someone else been injured because of your drinking?	No		Yes, but not in the last year		Yes, during the last year	
10. Has a relative, friend, doctor, or other health care worker been concerned about your drinking or suggested you cut down?	No		Yes, but not in the last year		Yes, during the last year	
					Total	______

Babor, T. F., Higgins-Biddle, J. C., Saunders, J. B., & Monteiro, M. (2001). *The alcohol use disorders identification test* (2nd ed.) (Box 10, p. 31, Appendix B). Geneva, Switzerland: World Health Organization Press. Retrieved from http://whqlibdoc.who.int/hq/2001/who_msd_msb_01.6a.pdf.

links to additional screening tools and resources, such as the informative SAMHSA Treatment Improvement Protocol (TIP) series.

During the screening process, instructions need to be clear and followed carefully. Nonjudgmental attitudes help with objectivity regardless of what the individual reveals. Several trends are important, such as the appearance of progression or loss of control and whether or not tolerance or withdrawal is present. Once the screening process identifies a potential problem, a more complete assessment is warranted

ASSESSMENT

A substance use assessment is part of a more comprehensive assessment that evaluates the individual holistically and ideally involves an addictions professional with specialized knowledge and skills in order to make a diagnosis. Addictions professionals may be nurses certified in addictions or another addictions-certified health care provider. The assessment will include a clinical examination of background, pattern of substance use, and any mental health symptoms. Special note should be made of any history of trauma, a family history of substance use or mental health problems and any disabilities, as well as the individual's strengths and level of willingness to change. As a result of this assessment, the individual may be identified as having a substance-related disorder.

See Tables 22-4 through 22-7 for some of the signs and symptoms of intoxication and withdrawal and some of the more common screening tools for identification of withdrawal.

Family Assessment

Understanding the process of addiction from a family perspective requires careful attention to the family. Living with an individual who abuses alcohol or other substances is a source of stress and requires family system adjustments. Codependence is a cluster of behaviors originally identified through research involving the families of alcoholic patients. People who are codependent often exhibit over responsible behavior—doing for others what others could just as well do for themselves. They have a constellation of maladaptive thoughts, feelings, behaviors, and attitudes that effectively prevent them from living full and satisfying lives. Symptomatic of codependence is valuing oneself by what one does, what one looks like, and what one has, rather than by who one is.

People who are codependent often define their self-worth in terms of caring for others to the exclusion of their own needs. Nurses are at risk for codependency since the very nature of the profession can lead to viewing oneself exclusively as a provider of care. A study conducted by Baldwin and colleagues (2006) surveyed 2646 Midwestern nursing and allied health professions students and found that 48% had a parent, sibling, or grandparent who was affected by addiction. These results suggest that nurses are at higher risk for relationship difficulties related to codependence and having grown up in environments that may have been dysfunctional due to one or more family members being addicted.

Self-Assessment

Substance-related disorders are often thought to be self-inflicted. You should carefully assess personal thoughts, opinions, and feelings as the first step to remaining objective and establishing a therapeutic relationship with a person with a substance use disorder. Most of us have been impacted in some way—either casually or profoundly—by someone whose life has been torn apart by substance use. Recognizing and dealing with our responses is essential to the provision of patient-centered care that is protected from bias or countertransference.

You may be aware that registered nurses themselves might have personal substance use problems. Approximately 1 in 10, or 10% to 15% of all nurses, may suffer from current alcohol or drug addiction or may be in recovery from addiction (Thomas & Siela, 2011). Although the risk for nurses is not higher than the risk for the general public, problems are unique because the work environment provides nurses with greater access to drugs. Kenward (2008) reports that only a third of the nurses who misuse drugs are sanctioned each year.

For those nurses who become aware that they are engaging in risk-taking behaviors or that one of their colleagues may be experiencing difficulties, there are now non punitive alternatives to discipline programs in the form of **peer assistance**. Diversion legislation allows addicted nurses to attend a treatment or recovery program, have their progress monitored, meet specific criteria to return to work, and be spared revocation or suspension of their licenses if they follow the recommendations of their programs. These alternatives to disciplinary programs are available in 41 states, the Virgin Islands, and the District of Columbia (National Council of State Boards of Nursing, 2011).

TABLE 22-4 SIGNS AND SYMPTOMS OF ALCOHOL INTOXICATION

BLOOD ALCOHOL LEVEL	SIGNS AND SYMPTOMS*
20–100 mg percent	Mood and behavioral changes Reduced coordination Impairment of ability to drive a car or operate machinery
101–200 mg percent	Reduced coordination of most activities Speech impairment Trouble walking General impairment of thinking and judgment
201–300 mg percent	Marked impairment of thinking, memory, and coordination Marked reduction in level of alertness Memory blackouts Nausea and vomiting
301–400 mg percent	Worsening of above symptoms with reduction of body temperature and blood pressure Excessive sleepiness Amnesia
401–800 mg percent	Difficulty waking the patient (coma) Serious decreases in pulse, temperature, blood pressure, and rate of breathing Urinary and bowel incontinence Death

*Chronic users of alcohol may show less effect at any given blood alcohol level.
From Substance Abuse and Mental Health Services Administration. (2006). *TIP 45 detoxification and substance abuse treatment* (DHHS Publication No. SMA 06-4224). Washington, DC: U.S. Government Printing Office.

TABLE 22-5 SIGNS AND SYMPTOMS OF ALCOHOL WITHDRAWAL

Uncomplicated or Mild to Moderate Alcohol Withdrawal
Restlessness
Irritability
Anorexia (lack of appetite)
Tremor (shakiness)
Insomnia
Impaired cognitive functions
Mild perceptual changes

Severe Alcohol Withdrawal
Obvious trembling of the hands and arms
Sweating
Elevation of pulse (above 100) and blood pressure (greater than 140/90)
Nausea (sometimes with vomiting)
Hypersensitivity to noises (which seem louder than usual) and light (which appears brighter than usual)
Brief periods of hearing and seeing things that are not present (auditory and visual hallucinations) also may occur
Fever greater than 101° F also may be seen (care should be taken to determine whether the fever is the result of infection)

Most Extreme Forms of Severe Alcohol Withdrawal
Grand mal seizures

Medical Complications of Alcohol Withdrawal
Infections
Hypoglycemia
Gastrointestinal (GI) bleeding
Undetected trauma
Hepatic failure
Cardiomyopathy with ineffective pumping
Pancreatitis
Encephalopathy (generalized impaired brain functioning).

From Substance Abuse and Mental Health Services Administration. (2006). *TIP 45 detoxification and substance abuse treatment* (DHHS Publication No. SMA 06-4224). Washington, DC: U.S. Government Printing Office.

TABLE 22-6 SIGNS AND SYMPTOMS OF OPIOID INTOXICATION AND WITHDRAWAL

OPIOID INTOXICATION	OPIOID WITHDRAWAL
Bradycardia (slow pulse)	Tachycardia (fast pulse)
Hypotension (low blood pressure)	Hypertension (high blood pressure)
Hypothermia (low body temperature)	Hyperthermia (high body temperature)
Sedation	Insomnia
Meiosis (pinpoint pupils)	Mydriasis (enlarged pupils)
Hypokinesis (slowed movement)	Hyperreflexia (abnormally heightened reflexes)
Slurred speech	Diaphoresis (sweating)
Head nodding	Piloerection (gooseflesh)
Euphoria	Increased respiratory rate
Analgesia (pain-killing effects)	Lacrimation (tearing), yawning
Calmness	Rhinorrhea (runny nose)
	Muscle spasms
	Abdominal cramps, nausea, vomiting, diarrhea
	Bone and muscle pain
	Anxiety

From Substance Abuse and Mental Health Services Administration. (2006). *TIP 45 detoxification and substance abuse treatment* (DHHS Publication No. SMA 06-4224). Washington, DC: U.S. Government Printing Office.

TABLE 22-7 SIGNS AND SYMPTOMS OF STIMULANT INTOXICATION AND WITHDRAWAL

STIMULANT INTOXICATION	STIMULANT WITHDRAWAL
Short Term	Depression
Increased energy	Hypersomnia (or insomnia)
Decreased appetite	Fatigue
Mental alertness	Anxiety
Increased heart rate/pressure	Irritability
Dilated pupils	Poor concentration
Long Term	Psychomotor retardation
Irregular heartbeat	Increased appetite
Chest pains	Paranoia
Increased risk of heart attack	Drug craving
Panic attacks	
Depression	
Delusions/hallucinations	
"Cocaine bugs" (skin sensation)	

From Substance Abuse and Mental Health Services Administration. (2006). *TIP 45 detoxification and substance abuse treatment* (DHHS Publication No. SMA 06-4224). Washington, DC: U.S. Government Printing Office.

EVIDENCE-BASED PRACTICE

Adolescent Performance-Enhancing Substance Use

Thorlton, J. R., McElmurry, B., Park, C., & Hughes, T. (2012). Adolescent performance enhancing substance use: regional differences across the US. *Journal of Addictions Nursing, 23*(2), 97–111.

Problem

The use of performance-enhancing substances (PES) has supported the growth of a multibillion dollar industry. Harmful PES are widely available in retail stores, over the Internet, and within schools. Over 1.1 million adolescents have purchased these substances. Side effects of these drugs include psychological and neuropsychiatric symptoms such as violent behavior, changes in mood, suicidal ideation, and premature death.

Purpose of Study

While the dangers of PES use are clearly recognized, not much is known about variations in risk factors. The purpose of this study was to better understand predictors of PES use.

Methods

The authors analyzed data from the National Youth Risk Behavior Survey that had been collected in 2007. More than 14,000 adolescents participated in this study.

Key Findings

- Adolescents who reported sad or hopeless feelings and had serious suicidal ideation were more likely to use PES.
- Involvement with other substances such as drugs, alcohol, and tobacco was associated with PES use.
- Males tend to use performance-enhancing PES and females are more likely to use body composition-altering PES.
- The southern portion of the United States has the highest PES use.

Implications for Nursing Practice

Nurses should be aware that wide varieties of PES are readily available and may have synergistic interactions with similar substances, prescription medications, nicotine, and caffeine. Prevention, screening, and intervention programs that address risk factors may decrease use, cut morbidity and mortality rates, and halt the progression into adult use.

DIAGNOSIS

Once the comprehensive substance use assessment has been completed in a thorough, objective manner, all the data are analyzed and potential or actual problems and needs are identified. Clinical decision-making skills will be used to determine which of the identified problems require a priority intervention. Special attention should be given to an individual's readiness to change. Individuals who are not even contemplating doing something differently may need a counseling intervention rather than referral to treatment.

OUTCOMES IDENTIFICATION

The goals for treatment planning arise from the preferred outcome for each problem. One result of the pursuit for quality in health care is the availability of formal lists of identified outcomes for each type of diagnosis—nursing, substance use, mental health, or co-occurring—that might be given to an individual. Substance use disorder outcome measures may include immediate stabilization for individuals experiencing withdrawal, abstinence if individuals are actively using, motivation for treatment and engagement in early abstinence, and pursuit of a recovery lifestyle for post discharge. Table 22-8 identifies signs and symptoms commonly experienced with substance-related and addictive disorders, offers potential nursing diagnoses, and suggests outcomes.

PLANNING

Planning is focused on identifying the problem, setting a goal, and then determining the interventions that will accomplish the goal. This treatment plan will be developed based on the assessment and diagnoses. For treatment to be successful, a patient-centered approach includes the patient's goals. The plan will take into account acute safety needs, severity and range of symptoms, motivation or readiness to change, skills and strengths, availability of a support system, and the individual's cultural needs (Center for Substance Abuse Treatment, 2006).

Current treatment therapy is changing from an acute illness approach to that of a chronic illness approach, with treatment occurring within recovery-oriented systems of care (ROSC). These are networks composed of formal and informal services that have been organized to support individuals and their families for long-term recovery in the face of substance use and addictive disorders. These systems are part of how a community, state, or nation is organized and not part of a treatment agency (White et al., 2009). Addressing substance use disorders and addiction as a chronic illness promotes the need for comprehensive, ongoing, holistic approaches and continuity of care.

The Care Continuum for Substance Abuse

Continuity of care occurs along a continuum starting with detoxification, rehabilitation, halfway houses, partial programs, intensive outpatient, and outpatient settings. Mutual support groups such as Alcoholics Anonymous (AA) are strongly encouraged throughout the treatment process.

Detoxification

Detoxification (also known as *detox*) is warranted when the individual quits using a psychoactive substance that is known to cause withdrawal or when the individual is already in withdrawal. This is a medically managed inpatient program with 24-hour medical coverage while the patient's body clears itself of drugs. This process is accompanied by uncomfortable and even fatal side effects caused by withdrawal. Detoxification is also available as a medically monitored program with 24-hour professional supervision based on the severity of symptomatology and the presence of comorbid conditions (NIDA, 2010c).

Rehabilitation

Residential rehabilitation programs are available as medically managed and medically monitored inpatient programs. The medically

TABLE 22-8 **SIGNS AND SYMPTOMS, NURSING DIAGNOSES, AND OUTCOMES FOR SUBSTANCE-RELATED AND ADDICTIVE DISORDERS**

SIGNS AND SYMPTOMS	NURSING DIAGNOSES	OUTCOMES
Impulsiveness, loss of relationships and occupation due to focus on substances or gambling, legal problems, social isolation	*Risk for suicide*	Expresses feelings, verbalizes suicidal ideas, refrains from suicide attempts, plans for the future
Impairment from substances, overdose, withdrawal from substances, hallucinations, elevated temperature, pulse, respirations, agitation	*Risk for injury*	Remains free from injury
Reports not feeling well rested, decreased ability to function, reports awakening multiple times	*Disturbed sleep pattern*	Minimal awakening, feels restored after sleep
Substitutes substances for healthy foods, lack of appetite, aversion to food	*Nutrition: less than body requirements*	Maintains a nutrient intake to meet metabolic needs
Increased appetite from cannabis use, dysfunctional eating pattern, weight 20% over ideal for height and frame, excessive intake in relation to metabolic need	*Nutrition: more than body requirements*	Maintains a nutrient intake to meet metabolic needs
Substance use, inadequate environmental hygiene, inadequate personal hygiene, lack of health-seeking behavior, inability to take responsibility for meeting basic health practices, lack of interest in improving health behaviors	*Self-neglect* *Ineffective health maintenance*	Obtains stable health status, adheres to medication and treatment regimen
Focuses on substance use or gambling, decreased use of social support, destructive behavior toward self and others, difficulty organizing information, inadequate problem-solving, poor concentration, reports inability to cope	*Ineffective coping*	Modifies lifestyle as needed to maintain sobriety, maintains abstinence from substances, engages in satisfying relationships
Does not perceive danger of substance use or gambling, minimizes symptoms, refuses healthcare attention, unable to admit impact of disease on life pattern	*Ineffective denial*	Accepts responsibility for behavior, maintains abstinence from substances
Substance use or gambling, lack of initiative, passivity, social isolation, reports seeing no alternatives or personal control, anger, sees no meaning in life	*Hopelessness* *Spiritual distress*	Expresses feelings of self-worth, verbalizes sense of personal identity, expresses meaning in life, sets goals, believes that actions impact outcomes
Substance use	*Risk for impaired liver function*	Abstains from substance use
Substance use edema, loss of appetite, fatigue, shortness of breath, decreased concentration, cough, decreased urine output, palpitations, irregular or rapid pulse	*Decreased cardiac output*	Abstains from substance use, cardiac pump supports systemic perfusion pressure
Agitation, blaming, broken promises, chaos, denial of problems, enabling maintenance of substance use pattern, immaturity, inability to accept help or express feelings, loneliness, lying, manipulation, rationalization, refused to get help social isolation, worthlessness, deterioration of family relationships	*Dysfunctional family processes*	Family members attain cohesion and emotional bonding

From Herdman, T. H. (Ed.). *Nursing diagnoses—Definitions and classification 2012–2014.* Copyright © 2012, 1994-2012 by NANDA International. Used by arrangement with John Wiley & Sons Limited; Moorhead, S., Johnson, M., Maas, M. L., & Swanson, E. (2013). *Nursing outcomes classification (NOC)* (5th ed.). St. Louis, MO: Mosby.

managed programs usually employ 24-hour medical staff and provide intensive and specialized care for those individuals with either biomedical or psychiatric comorbid conditions. Medically monitored programs are also available for individuals with less complex conditions. They offer professionally directed evaluation and treatment in short-term settings for those with acute distress and moderate impairment and long-term settings for those with chronic distress or severe impairment. Short-term rehabilitation aids in the recovery of lost skills and function, while long-term rehabilitation helps to improve functioning that never developed and may have led to addictions (Mee-Lee, 2005).

Halfway Houses

Halfway houses offer residential treatment in a substance-free communal or family environment that provides opportunities for independent growth. Individuals come to continue the work that was begun in other treatment programs, usually that of a long-term or short-term residential rehab. Focus is on extending the period of sobriety, getting case management assistance in addressing educational, economic and social needs, and integrating new life skills into a solid, modeled recovery program. Most residents will live there but work outside (Mee-Lee, 2005).

Other Housing

Opportunities for community reintegration are also available in supportive housing units that are not part of treatment. Three-quarter-way houses, therapeutic communities, and housing programs offer drug-free living environments, peer support, and classes to assist or remediate skills needed for daily living. Residents usually attend some type of outpatient substance use treatment to continue in their recovery program.

Partial Hospitalization

This is an intensive form of outpatient programming for those individuals who do not need 24-hour residential programming but who benefit from a combination of multidisciplinary treatment on at least 3 days a week for at least 10 hours per week of planned programming. This combination of psychotherapy and educational groups does not require the individual to have previous treatment experience. Participants may live in some type of supportive housing program or at an independent home. Medication management is available but it is not usually medically monitored or managed (Mee-Lee, 2005).

Intensive Outpatient

An alternative to partial hospitalization is an intensive outpatient program (IOP). This is a nonresidential program, highly structured with scheduled treatment groups and at least one individual session regularly. Medication oversight is usually available, but it will not be monitored or managed by a healthcare professional. Participants will attend at least 3 days a week for between 5 and 10 hours per week (Mee-Lee, 2005).

Outpatient Treatment

The least-intensive form of substance use treatment is outpatient. Treatment may be a mix of individual sessions and educational or psychotherapy groups as determined by the individuals' needs and their treatment goals. It is structured, drug-free, and non-residential. Programming consists of not more than 5 contact hours a week. Web-based interventions are also available for self-paced, anonymous collective participation in treatment efforts (Finfgeld-Connett, & Madsen, 2008).

Treatment is determined by the severity of the symptoms. One useful approach to evaluating readiness for treatment is the transtheoretical stages of change theory (transtheoretical model of care). Individuals may be at stage one, *precontemplation*, and need assistance in admitting there is a problem. If they have acknowledged the problem, *contemplation*, they may still not be ready to commit to addressing it. The goal of treatment would be to assist in the development of awareness and a commitment. *Preparation,* or getting ready, and *action,* or changing, take place in early treatment phases. The *maintenance* stage is the ongoing commitment to a recovery program. Without continuing action the individual will likely return to previous behavior, *relapse.*

Alcoholics Anonymous

Alcoholics Anonymous (AA) was founded in 1930 and is the oldest and best known of the 12-step fellowships. Anyone with the desire to quit drinking or using substances is welcome to attend meetings (Urshel, 2009). Individuals learn how to be sober through the support of other members and the 12 steps. In most suburban and urban areas, meetings can be found every day and around the clock; they are even available online and are structured for confidentiality and anonymity. Family members and other support are often welcome.

The 12-step model has been adopted worldwide. Specific groups may focus on specific addictions and include specific populations. The size of meetings ranges from small (around 15) to large (more than 50). There are also meetings to address the special needs of family and significant others, such as Al-Anon for friends and family members of alcohol abusers, Alateen for teenage relatives of alcohol abusers, and Nar-Anon for family and friends of drug abusers. Gamblers Anonymous is for individuals with significant gambling problems.

IMPLEMENTATION

Basic nursing interventions are useful in providing a supportive environment for managing substance use disorders. Promoting safety and sleep are essential first-line interventions. Also, nutritional status may be severely compromised due to choosing substances over sustenance; a gradual introduction of healthy food supports body systems and neurological functioning.

Support and encouragement for self-care (hygiene) will help improve self-esteem in individuals who may have long neglected themselves. The development of a therapeutic relationship sets the stage for exploring harmful thoughts, anxiety, hopelessness, and spiritual distress. An understanding of current coping skills along with identification of new skills, provides tools to test in a safe setting. Assistance in goal setting helps a patient to see beyond the current situation and instills hope and direction.

Once the level of intensity and the treatment plan have been established, it is time to begin treatment. Implementation should be undertaken by a substance abuse professional with the necessary knowledge, skills, and attitudes to be competent in providing evidence-based treatment (Center for Substance Abuse Treatment, 2006). These competencies can be applied across a wide variety of disciplines, including nursing. Nurses learn many of the skills as part of their basic education, and a thorough understanding of addiction is necessary. Any nurse interested in skills beyond basic-level assessment and referral to treatment may be interested in focusing on this area of nursing and becoming recognized for advanced expertise. The International Nurses Society on Addictions provides specialty certification through their certification branch, the Addictions Nursing Certification Board (ANCB). Certification is available for both the generalist, as a certified addictions registered nurse (CARN), and the advanced practice nurse, as a (CARN-AP).

Advanced Practice Interventions

The following interventions, brief interventions and counseling, are considered advanced practice. However, they provide a framework of understanding treatment goals and principles that may be understood and used by nurse generalists.

BOX 22-1 THE 5 A's FOR ALCOHOL MISUSE INTERVENTION

Assess alcohol consumption with a brief screening tool
Advise clearly and specifically about effects of alcohol consumption
Agree on goals for reducing use or abstinence
Assist in developing motivation, self-help skills, and supports
Arrange follow up, repeat counseling, or specialty referral

U.S. Preventive Services Task Force. (n.d.). *Evidence-based methods for evaluating behavioral counseling interventions.* Retrieved from http://www.uspreventiveservicestaskforce.org/3rduspstf/behavior/behsum2.htm.

Brief Interventions

The substance abuse professional may choose to start with a brief intervention as a means of providing education, engaging the individual in treatment, or encouraging behavior change as harm reduction. Miller and Sanchez (1994) coined the acronym FRAMES to reflect the six components they believed were necessary for an effective brief intervention (as cited in SAMHSA, 1999). These components include giving **F**eedback about personal risk, encouraging personal **R**esponsibility, and providing **A**dvice to change and a **M**enu of treatment or self-help options using an **E**mpathic communication style. The expected result is **S**elf-efficacy or empowerment.

The Five A's (Box 22-1) encourage harm reduction and movement from the precontemplation or contemplation phases of change toward those of preparation and action. The 5 A's can be adapted to other substance and process misuse situations.

Counseling

Throughout the assessment and treatment planning process, the counselor or therapist has been establishing a therapeutic alliance. Together the counselor and patient will begin to implement the treatment plan. Substance use and addiction treatment professionals use a number of treatment modalities. Those most often employed are cognitive behavioral therapy, motivational interviewing, and mindfulness and meditation (Angres & Bettinardi-Angres, 2008). Cognitive behavioral therapy assists the individual to explore thinking patterns so that core belief systems and any irrational core beliefs can be identified. This allows dysfunctional thought processes to be examined and addressed.

Motivational interviewing is based on the transtheoretical or stages of change theory. It helps the counselor to understand where the individual is in the process, permits matching the stage of change and stage of treatment, and assists in the process of therapy. Motivation can be enhanced and denial broken. Mindfulness and meditation help individuals to be present to the process of living and to reconnect to the community. These practices help to establish activities that enable a sustainable recovery lifestyle.

Relapse Prevention

To maintain long-term sobriety, individuals must prepare for and anticipate the possibility of relapse. This includes identifying potential triggers to substance use, learning skills to regain abstinence in the event of use, and adopting healthy coping, identity, and stress management skills to address triggers before they threaten sobriety. Advances in technology have expanded options for maintaining long-term sobriety, such as the use of applications for smart phones that offer a way to monitor behavioral patterns for precursors to relapse trends. Social media tools such as Facebook and Twitter offer other forms of supportive networking.

One of the biggest downfalls of the utilization of social media is the lack of confidentiality. Mental health and substance use treatment are areas covered by state and federal laws of confidentiality that are even stricter than the Health Information Portability and Accountability Act (HIPAA) of 1996. The Electronic Code of Federal Regulations (2012) spells out confidentiality restrictions, security of records, and penalties for violations. It is important for the nurse or counselor to be knowledgeable about all laws governing privacy and confidentiality and to guard the protected health information of the patient regardless of what the patient chooses to reveal publicly.

Psychobiological Interventions

Pharmacological

Current research into pharmacotherapy approaches has resulted in the availability of medications to treat the disease itself not just the symptoms of use, misuse, and withdrawal. Researchers are also studying genetic markers and potential vaccinations against the particular drugs of abuse. In addition to adding to the body of knowledge, this research will provide alternative options for treatment. See Table 22-9 for some of the common medications and their therapeutic uses.

Health Teaching and Health Promotion

If genetic vulnerability accounts for 40% to 60% of an individual's risk, prevention may be the best answer to the increasing problem of substance use and addiction (NIDA, 2010). Health teaching is a part of the school curriculum, and schools may offer classes on understanding addiction as a brain disorder, its risk factors, and ways to prevent or limit exposure to psychoactive substances. Promoting classes for developing healthy coping and stress management skills and activities for increasing self-confidence and self-efficacy would also lower the risks for use of psychoactive substances.

Social activities that increase supportive relationships reduce the impact of stressful life events and provide a venue for community activities that provide health education and promotion. Special attention should be given to understanding the particular impact of trauma as a risk factor. Physical, sexual, or emotional abuse at any age, physical trauma from accidents, natural disasters, or acts of violence or war can all be predisposing factors for the use of psychoactive substances or processes.

EVALUATION

Evaluation occurs on several levels, assessing the effectiveness of the treatment plan, using objective data to check whether nursing actions addressed the patient's symptoms, and measuring the changes in the patient's behaviors for progress toward meeting

22-1 CASE STUDY AND NURSING CARE PLAN

Alcohol Use Disorder

Mr. Stewart, aged 49 years, and his wife arrive in the emergency department one evening, fearful that he has had a stroke. His right hand is limp, and he is unable to hyperextend his right wrist. Sensation to the fingertips in his right hand is impaired.

Mr. Stewart looks much older than his stated age; in fact, he looks about 65. His complexion is ruddy and flushed. History taking is difficult. Mr. Stewart answers only what is asked of him, volunteering no additional information. He states that he took a nap that afternoon and that when he awakened, he noticed the problems with his right arm.

Ms. Winkler, the admitting nurse, begins the assessment. Mr. Stewart reveals that he has been unemployed for 4 years because the company he worked for went bankrupt. He has been unable to find a new job but has a job interview in 10 days. His wife is now working full time, so the family finances are okay. They have two grown children who no longer live at home. As he relates this, momentarily his lips start to tremble and his eyes fill with tears.

He denies any significant medical illness except for high blood pressure, just diagnosed last year. His father has a history of depression, and his mother is a recovering alcoholic. Ms. Winkler shares with him the fact that depression and alcoholism run in families. She asks Mr. Stewart (1) whether he knows this and (2) whether it concerns him with regard to his own drinking. He says that he knows and that he does not want to think about it.

Ms. Winkler speaks separately with Mr. Stewart's wife and asks if there is anything she would like to add. Mrs. Stewart's shoulders slump; she sighs and says, "I have spent the entire day talking to a counselor at the local treatment center to see if I can get him in. He won't admit that he has a problem." Mrs. Stewart recounts a 6-year history of steadily increasing alcohol use. She says that she could not admit to herself that her husband was an excessive drinker. "He tried to hide it, but gradually I knew. I could tell from little changes that he was intoxicated. I couldn't believe it was happening because he had been through the same thing with his mother. I thought I knew him. Actually, I guess I did when he was working. Being unemployed and unable to find a job has really devastated him. And now he's going to job interviews intoxicated."

She describes her feelings, which are like an emotional roller coaster—elated and hopeful when he seems to be doing okay; dejected and desperate when he loses control. Mrs. Stewart hates going to work for fear of what her husband might do while she is gone. She says she is terrified that one day he will get into a car wreck and kill himself because he often drives when intoxicated. He tells her not to worry because the life insurance policy is paid up.

Meanwhile, the physician in the emergency department has examined Mr. Stewart. The diagnosis is radial nerve palsy. Mr. Stewart most likely passed out while lying on his arm. Because Mr. Stewart was intoxicated, he did not feel the signals (numbness and tingling) that his nerves sent out to warn him to move. He was in this position for so long that the resultant cutoff of circulation was sufficient to cause some temporary nerve damage.

Mr. Stewart's BAL is 0.31 mg%. This is three times the legal limit for intoxication in many states (0.1 mg%). Even though he has a BAL of 0.31 mg%, Mr. Stewart is alert and oriented, not slurring his speech or giving any other outward signs of intoxication. The difference between Mr. Stewart's BAL and his behavior indicates the development of tolerance, a symptom of physical addiction.

Self-Assessment

Ms. Winkler has seen many patients with the disease of alcoholism make radical changes in their lives, and she has learned to view alcoholism as a treatable disease. She is aware also that it is the patient who makes the changes, and she no longer feels responsible when a patient is not ready to make that change.

Assessment

Ms. Winkler organizes her data into objective and subjective components.

Objective Data

- Driving when intoxicated
- Covert references to death
- Nerve damage from passing out while lying on arm
- Increased alcohol use since becoming unemployed
- Ability to find employment impaired by alcohol use
- Disruption in marital relationship because of alcohol use
- Inability to see effects of his drinking
- Family history of alcoholism and depression
- BAL three times the legal limit of intoxication; has developed tolerance

Subjective Data

- Denies he has an alcohol problem
- Denies he has depression

Diagnosis

From the data, the nurse formulates the following nursing diagnoses:

1. *Risk for suicide*

Supporting Data

- Dangerous behavior: driving when drinking
- Full payment of life insurance policy

2. *Ineffective coping* related to alcohol use

Supporting Data

- Increased alcohol use during stressful period of unemployment
- Impairment in capacity to obtain employment caused by alcohol use
- Disruption in marital relationship because of alcohol use
- Inability to see effect of his drinking on his life functioning

Outcomes Identification

Long-term outcomes:

The patient will refrain from attempting suicide.

The patient will report increase in psychological comfort.

Planning

The initial plan is to allow Mr. Stewart to sober up in the emergency department before discussing goals. After he is sober, the nurse establishes realistic outcomes with him.

Implementation

Mr. Stewart's plan of care is personalized as follows:

Nursing diagnosis: *Risk for suicide* as evidenced by dangerous behavior and full payment of life insurance policy

Outcome criteria: Patient will consistently demonstrate suicide self-restraint.

SHORT-TERM GOAL	INTERVENTION	RATIONALE	EVALUATION
1. Patient will seek treatment for depression.	1a. Determine presence and degree of suicidal risk. 1b. Refer patient to mental health care provider for evaluation and treatment.	1a. Risk of suicide is increased in substance-using patients. 1b. Addressing both substance use and mental health treatment needs improves outcomes.	**GOAL MET** After 3 weeks, patient attends appointment at local clinic and has started taking an antidepressant.

22-1 CASE STUDY AND NURSING CARE PLAN—cont'd

Alcohol Use Disorder

Nursing diagnosis: *Ineffective coping* related to alcohol use, as evidenced by increased alcohol use and impairment in life functioning
Outcome criteria: Patient will demonstrate mild to no change in health status and social functioning due to substance addiction.

SHORT-TERM GOAL	INTERVENTION	RATIONALE	EVALUATION
1. Patient will consistently acknowledge personal consequences associated with alcohol misuse.	1a. Identify with patient those factors (genetics, stress) that contribute to chemical addiction. 1b. Assist patient to identify negative effects of chemical dependency.	1a. Emphasis on alcoholism as a disease can lower guilt and increase self-esteem. 1b. Begins to decrease denial and increase problem solving.	**GOAL MET** Patient admits that he cannot find a new job when he is intoxicated.
2. Patient will commit to alcohol-use control strategies.	2a. Determine history of alcohol use. 2b. Identify support groups in community for long-term substance use treatment (for wife also).	2a. Identifies high-risk situations. 2b. Alcohol addiction requires long-term treatment; AA is effective.	**GOAL MET** After 3 weeks, patient states that he attends AA every day. He is learning about his triggers and new coping skills. His wife attends Al-Anon.

Evaluation
See individual outcomes and evaluation in the care plan.

TABLE 22-9 COMMON MEDICATIONS USED FOR TREATMENT OF SUBSTANCE USE DISORDERS

GENERIC (BRAND NAME)	INDICATION	USES	IMPLICATIONS FOR THE THERAPEUTIC PROCESS
Disulfiram (Antabuse)	Alcohol	Maintenance	Ingesting alcohol while taking this medication produces a toxic reaction that causes intense nausea and vomiting, headache, sweating, flushed skin, respiratory difficulties, and confusion. Must be taken consistently for aversion to alcohol to be consistent.
Carbamazepine (Atretol, Tegretol)	Alcohol	Withdrawal	May cause dizziness or drowsiness. Effect is dependent on therapeutic level. Patient will need to take consistently and be tapered off to prevent seizures during detox.
Acamprosate calcium (Campral)	Alcohol	Relapse-prevention agent; rebalance of neurotransmitters	Side effects, although minimal, include diarrhea, nausea, itching, and intestinal gas.
Chlordiazepoxide (Librium)	Alcohol	Increase seizure threshold; reduce withdrawal agitation	Produces sedation. Withdrawal may result in seizures
Phenobarbital (Phenobarbital)	Alcohol	Withdrawal	Produces sedation. Vital signs should be checked frequently during withdrawal
Quetiapine fumarate (Seroquel)	Alcohol	Detoxification with reduced craving	A drop in blood pressure may result when changing position from sitting to standing. May experience dry mouth and restlessness.
Diazepam (Valium)	Alcohol	Withdrawal	Alert patient to potential sedation. Educate about the signs and symptoms of withdrawal, including warnings of seizure activity.
Naltrexone (Vivitrol, injectable, ReVia, Depade, oral)	Alcohol Opiates	Withdrawal; relapse prevention; decreasing cravings	Nausea usually goes away after first month; headache, sedation, and pain at the injection site with each injection
Clonidine (Catapres)	Opiates Presence of hypertension	Heroin withdrawal	Symptoms of opioid withdrawal include tachycardia, fever, runny nose, diarrhea, sweating, nausea, vomiting, irritability, stomach cramps, shivering, unusually large pupils, weakness, difficulty sleeping, and gooseflesh. Take each dose as given.
Levo-alpha-acetylmethadol (LAAM)	Opiates	Withdrawal and maintenance	Contraindicated if pregnant or expecting to get pregnant, if side effects were experienced in the past, or if liver damage is present. Induction takes longer than with methadone.

Continued

TABLE 22-9 COMMON MEDICATIONS USED FOR TREATMENT OF SUBSTANCE USE DISORDERS—cont'd

GENERIC (BRAND NAME)	INDICATION	USES	IMPLICATIONS FOR THE THERAPEUTIC PROCESS
Methadone hydrochloride (Methadone)	Opiates	Detoxification maintenance	An effective but controversial drug. Induction period is required. Safe during pregnancy. Initially and with higher doses sedation is possible.
Buprenorphine (Subutex, oral Buprenex, injectable Suboxone)	Opiates	Detoxification; maintenance	Used for active withdrawal. Levels are adjusted over several days. Typically used for 9-12 months and then tapered.
Naltrexone hydrochloride (Trexan)	Heroin Opiates Pathological gambling	Detoxification; maintenance; reduction of impulsive and compulsive behaviors	Patients should not change dose or use opiates. May experience drowsiness, dizziness, or blurred vision. Nausea or vomiting may require small, frequent meals and frequent mouth care. Contraindicated in pregnancy or while breast-feeding.
Varenicline (Chantix)	Nicotine	Reduction of craving and withdrawal	Patients should stop taking medication and call health care provider immediately if agitation, hostility, depressed mood, changes in behavior or thinking, or suicidal ideation or suicidal behavior develops. It is possible to have vivid, unusual, or strange dreams. Not indicated during pregnancy.
Rimonabant (Zimulti)	Nicotine Obesity	Maintenance of body weight Smoking cessation	May have serious side effects if taken long term. Reports have included depression, suicidal tendencies, nausea, anxiety and nervousness, frequent unpredictable mood swings, tendency to become irritated at most things, and difficulty in sleeping. Any changes should be reported to healthcare provider.
Bupropion (Zyban) Includes patches, gums, lozenges, nasal sprays, and inhalers	Nicotine	Withdrawal from smoking	Take with food to minimize GI discomfort. Agitation and insomnia are possible. Monitor anxiety. Don't take a bedtime dose or double up if doses missed.

From Baird, C., Pancari, J.V., Lutz, P. J., & Baird, T. (2009). Addiction disorders. In J. C. Urbanic, & C. J. Groh (Eds.), *Women's mental health: A clinical guide for primary care providers* (pp. 125–179). Philadelphia, PA: Lippincott, Williams & Wilkins.

stated goals. Problematic behaviors, patterns of expression, or perceptions may improve or only undergo change in small increments, requiring alterations in the action steps or even the goals of the treatment plan to meet the patient's needs. During the treatment experience, ongoing evaluation of the process must be conducted to ensure that any transference or countertransference is managed and that the goals and outcomes of treatment remain patient-centered. Evaluation will also make it possible to make sure that the patient acquires the necessary skills and competencies for continued reflection and maintenance of the new lifestyle identification.

It is important to remember that addiction is a "primary, chronic disease of brain reward, motivation, memory, and related circuitry" (American Society for Addictions Medicine, 2011) and results in the alteration of the neurobiology of the brain. The first 3 to 6 months may be the most difficult as the brain's circuitry and neurochemistry become adjusted. Although substance use and relapse can occur at any time, many individuals repeat these first months of abstinence before attaining long-term sobriety. Research supports that the longer individuals are in treatment, the longer they will remain abstinent.

Men and women differ in the ways in which they are affected by substance use disorders and have different barriers to and supports to treatment and recovery (Baird, 2008). This requires ongoing evaluation to ensure that gender-specific issues and supports are addressed throughout the treatment continuum, thus supporting the process and increasing the likelihood of long-term sobriety.

KEY POINTS TO REMEMBER

- Substance use and addictive disorders occur on a continuum, with dependency developing over a period of time.
- The cause of substance use is a combination of genetic, biological, and environmental factors.
- Assessment of patients with substance use needs to be comprehensive, aimed at identifying common medical and psychiatric comorbidities.
- Patients with a co-occurring diagnosis have more severe symptoms, experience more crises, and require longer treatment for successful outcomes.
- Substance use affects the family system of the patient and may lead to codependent behavior in family members.

- Relapse is an expected complication of substance use, and treatment includes a significant focus on teaching relapse prevention.
- Successful treatments include an integrated approach, self-help groups, psychotherapy, therapeutic communities, and psychopharmacotherapy.
- Nurses need to be aware of their own feelings about substance use so that they can provide empathy and hope to patients.
- Nurses themselves are at higher risk for substance use disorders and should be vigilant for signs of impairment in colleagues to assure patient safety and referral to treatment for the chemically dependent nurse.

CRITICAL THINKING

1. Write a paragraph describing your possible reactions to a drug-dependent patient to whom you are assigned.
   a. Would your response be different depending on the substance (e.g., alcohol versus heroin or marijuana versus cocaine)? Give reasons for your answers.
   b. Would your response be different if the substance-dependent person were a professional colleague? How?
2. Rosetta Seymour is a 15-year-old teenager who has started using heroin nasally.
   a. Briefly discuss the trend in heroin use among teenagers.
   b. When Ms. Seymour asks you why she needs to take more and more to get "high," how would you explain to her the concept of tolerance?
   c. If she had just taken heroin, what would you find on assessment of physical and behavioral-psychological signs and symptoms?
   d. If she came into the emergency department with an overdose of heroin, what would be the emergency care? What might be effective long-term care?
3. Tony Garmond is a 45-year-old mechanic. He has a 20-year history of heavy drinking, and he says he wants to quit but needs help.
   a. Role play with a classmate an initial assessment. Identify the kinds of information you would need to have in order to plan holistic care.
   b. Mr. Garmond tried stopping by himself but is in the emergency department in alcohol withdrawal. What are the dangers for Mr. Garmond? What are the likely medical interventions?
   c. What are some possible treatment alternatives for Mr. Garmond when he is safely detoxified? How would you explain to him the usefulness and function of AA? What are some additional treatment options that might be useful to Mr. Garmond? What community referrals for Mr. Garmond are available in your area?

CHAPTER REVIEW

1. When intervening with a patient who is intoxicated from alcohol, it is useful to first:
   a. Let the patient sober up.
   b. Decide immediately on care goals.
   c. Ask what drugs other than alcohol the patient has recently used.
   d. Gain adherence by sharing your personal drinking habits with the patient.
2. You are caring for Mick, a 32-year-old patient with chemical addiction who will soon be preparing for discharge. A principle of counseling interventions that should be observed when caring for a patient with chemical addiction is to:
   a. Praise the patient for compliant behavior.
   b. Communicate that relapses are always possible.
   c. Confirm that the patient's recovery is considered complete after discharge.
   d. Encourage Mick to resume his former friendships to regain a sense of normalcy.
3. As you evaluate a patient's progress, which treatment outcome would indicate a poor general prognosis for long-term recovery from substance abuse?
   a. Patient demonstrates improved self-esteem.
   b. Patient demonstrates enhanced coping abilities.
   c. Patient demonstrates improved relationships with others.
   d. Patient demonstrates positive expectations for ongoing drug use.
4. You are caring for Leah, a 26-year-old patient who has been abusing CNS stimulants. Which statement provides a basis for planning care for a patient who abuses CNS stimulants?
   a. Symptoms of intoxication include dilation of the pupils, dryness of the oronasal cavity, and excessive motor activity.
   b. Medical management focuses on removing the drugs from the body.
   c. Withdrawal is simple and rarely complicated.
   d. Postwithdrawal symptoms include fatigue and depression.
5. The provision of optimal care for patients withdrawing from substances of abuse is facilitated by the nurse's understanding that severe morbidity and mortality are often associated with withdrawal from:
   a. Alcohol and CNS depressants.
   b. CNS stimulants and hallucinogens.
   c. Narcotic antagonists and caffeine.
   d. Opiates and inhalants.

Answers to Chapter Review
1. c; 2. b; 3. d; 4. d; 5. a.

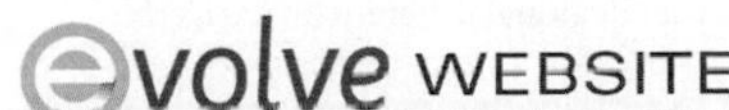

WEBSITE

Visit the Evolve website for a posttest on the content in this chapter: http://evolve.elsevier.com/Varcarolis

Post-Test interactive review

REFERENCES

American Psychiatric Association. (2013). *DSM-5*. Retrieved from http://www.psychiatry.org/practice/dsm/dsm5.

American Society of Addictions Medicine. (2011). *Public policy statement: Definition of addiction*. Retrieved from http://www.asam.org/for-the-public/definition-of-addiction.

Angres, D. H., & Bettinadi-Angres, K. (2008). The disease of addiction: Origins, treatment and recovery. *Disease A Month, 54*, 696–721.

Baird, C. (2008). Treating women with children: What does the evidence say? *Journal of Addictions Nursing, 19*(3), 83–85.

Baird, C. (2009). Spotting alcohol and substance abuse: How to start a screening program for primary care patients. *American Nurse Today, 4*(7), 29–31.

Baird, C. (2011). Addiction care. In J. J. Fitzpatrick & M. W. Kazer (Eds.), *Encyclopedia of nursing research* (pp. 8–11). New York, NY: Springer.

Baird, C., Pancari, J. V., Lutz, P. J., & Baird, T. (2009). Addiction disorders. In J. C. Urbanic & C. J. Groh (Eds.), *Women's mental health: A clinical guide for primary care providers* (pp. 125–179). Philadelphia, PA: Lippincott, Williams & Wilkins.

Center for Substance Abuse Treatment. (2006). *Addiction counseling competencies: The knowledge, skills, and attitudes of professional practice*. Technical Assistance Publication (TAP) Series 21. DHHS Publication No. (SMA) 06-4171. Rockville, MD: Substance Abuse and Mental Health Services Administration.

National Council of State Boards of Nursing. (2011). *Substance use disorder in nursing: A resource manual and guidelines for alternative and disciplinary monitoring programs*. Retrieved from https://www.ncsbn.org/SUDN_11.pdf.

Druss, B. G., & Walker, E. R. (2011). Mental disorders and medical comorbidity. *The Synthesis Project, Research Synthesis Report No. 21*. Retrieved from http://www.rwjf.org/files/research/021011.policysyn thesis.mentalhealth.report.pdf.

Fava, G. A., & Offidani, E. (2011). The mechanism of tolerance in antidepressant action. *Progress in Neuropsychopharmacology and Biological Psychiatry, 35*(7), 1593–602.

Finfgeld-Connett, D., & Madsen, W. (2008). Web-based treatment of alcohol problems among rural women: Results of a randomized pilot investigation. *Journal of Psychosocial Nursing, 46*, 46–53.

Institute of Medicine, & the National Research Council. (2001). *Crossing the quality chasm: A new health system for the 21st century*. Washington, DC: The National Academies Press.

Institute of Medicine [IOM], Committee on Crossing the Quality Chasm: Adaptation to Mental Health and Addictive Disorders. (2006). *Improving the quality of health care for mental and substance-use conditions: Quality chasm series*. Washington, DC: National Academies Press.

Institute of Medicine [IOM]. (2010). *The future of nursing: Leading change, advancing health*. Retrieved from http://thefutureofnursing.org/IOM-Report

Kenward, K. (2008). Discipline of nurses: A review of disciplinary data 1996–2006. *Journal of Nursing Administration, 10*(3), 81–84.

Koob, G. F. (2006). The neurobiology of addiction: A neuroadaptational view relevant for diagnosis. *Addiction, 101*(Suppl. 1), 23–30.

Madras, B. K., Compton, W. M., Avula, D., Stegbauer, T., Stein, J. B., & Clark, H. W. (2009). Screening, brief interventions, referral to treatment (SBIRT) for illicit drug and alcohol use at multiple healthcare sites: Comparison at intake and six months. *Drug and Alcohol Dependence, 99*(1–3), 280–295.

McCauley, K. (2009). *Pleasures unwoven* [documentary]. Salt Lake City, UT: the Institute for Addiction Study.

Mee-Lee, D. (2005). *Overview of the ASAM Patient Placement Criteria, second edition revised (ASAM PPC-2R)* [Slides]. Washington, DC: SAMHSA's Co-occurring Center for Excellence (COCE). Retrieved from http://www.samhsa.gov/co-occurring/topics/screening-and-assessment/ASAMP atientPlacementCriteriaOverview5-05.pdf.

Moorhead, S., Johnson, M., Maas, M., & Swanson, E. (2013). *Nursing outcomes classification (NOC)* (5th ed.). St. Louis, MO: Mosby.

National Institute on Drug Abuse (NIDA). (2012). *Drug facts: High school and youth trends*. Retrieved from http://www.drugabuse.gov/sites/default/files/drugfactshsyt.pdf.

National Institute on Drug Abuse (NIDA). (2011a). *Co-morbidity: Addiction and other mental disorders*. Retrieved from http://www.drugabuse.gov/publications/drugfacts/comorbidity-addiction-other-mental-disorders.

National Institute on Drug Abuse (NIDA). (2011b). *Understanding drug abuse and addiction*. Retrieved from http://www.drugabuse.gov/publications/drugfacts/understanding-drug-abuse-addiction.

National Institute on Drug Abuse (NIDA). (2010a). *Drugs, brains, and behavior: The science of addiction* [NIH Publication No. 10-5605]. Retrieved from http://www.drugabuse.gov/publications/science-addiction.

National Institute on Drug Abuse (NIDA). (2010b). *Co-morbidity: Addiction and other mental illnesses* [NIH Publication No. 10-5771]. Retrieved from http://www.drugabuse.gov/publications/research-reports/comorbidity-addiction-other-mental-illnesses.

National Institute on Drug Abuse (NIDA). (2010c). *Principles of drug addiction treatment: A research-based guide* (3rd ed.). Retrieved from http://www.drugabuse.gov/publications/principles-drug-addiction-treatment.

National Institute on Drug Abuse (NIDA). (2009). *The neurobiology of drug addiction: Section II: the reward pathway and addiction*. Retrieved from http://www.drugabuse.gov/publications/teaching-packets/neurobiology-drug-addiction.

National Quality Forum. (2007). *National voluntary consensus standards for the treatment of substance use conditions: Evidence-based treatment practices: a consensus report*. Princeton, NJ: the Robert Wood Johnson Foundation.

Office of National Drug Control Policy. (2011). *A response to the epidemic of prescription drug abuse*. Retrieved from http://www.whitehouse.gov/ondcp/prescription-drug-abuse.

Palladini, M. (2011). *Drugs of abuse: From doctors to dealers, users and healers*. Beaver, PA: Three Suns.

Pennsylvania Drug and Alcohol Coalition. (2010). *Recovery-oriented system of care: A recovery community perspective*. Retrieved from http://www.facesandvoicesofrecovery.org/pdf/White/rosc_community_perspective_2010.pdf.

Potenza, M. N. (2008). The neurobiology of pathological gambling and drug addiction: An overview and new findings. *Philosophical Transactions of the Royal Society of Behavioral Sciences*, 363(1507), 3181–3189.

Substance Abuse and Mental Health Services Administration (SAMHSA). (2012). *Screening, brief intervention, and referral to treatment (SBIRT)*. Retrieved from http://www.samhsa.gov/prevention/SBIRT/index.aspx.

Substance Abuse and Mental Health Services Administration (SAMHSA). (2011). *Results from the 2010 National Survey on Drug Use and Health* [SMA Publication Number11-4658]. Retrieved from http://store.samhsa.gov/product/Results-from-the-2010-National-Survey-on-Drug-Use-and-Health-NSDUH-/SMA11-4658.

Substance Abuse Mental Health Services Administration (SAMHSA). (2006). *Detoxification and substance abuse treatment* [SMA Publication Number: 06-4131]. http://www.ncbi.nlm.nih.gov/books/NBK64115/.

Substance Abuse and Mental Health Services Administration (SAMHSA). (2005). *Substance abuse treatment for persons with co-occurring disorder* [SMA Publication Number: 05-3922]. Retrieved from http://www.ncbi.nlm.nih.gov/books/NBK64197/.

Substance Abuse and Mental Health Services Administration (SAMHSA). (1999). *Brief interventions and brief therapies for substance abuse* [SMA Publication Number: 99-3353]. Retrieved from http://www.ncbi.nlm.nih.gov/books/NBK64947/.

Thomas, C. M., & Siela, D. (2011). The impaired nurse: Would you know what to do if you suspected substance abuse? *American Nurse Today*, 6(8). Retrieved from http://www.americannursetoday.com/article.aspx?id=8114&fid=8078.

Thorlton, J. R., McElmurry, B., Park, C., & Hughes, T. (2012). Adolescent performance enhancing substance use: Regional differences across the US. *Journal of Addictions Nursing, 23*(2), 97–111.

White, W. L., Evans, A. C., Albright, L., & Flaherty, M. (2009). Recovery management and recovery oriented systems of care: Scientific rationale and promising practices. *Counselor: The Magazine for Addiction Professionals, 10*(1), 24–32.

CHAPTER 23

Neurocognitive Disorders

Jane Stein-Parbury

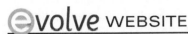

Visit the Evolve website for a pretest on the content in this chapter: http://evolve.elsevier.com/Varcarolis

Pre-Test interactive review

OBJECTIVES

1. Compare and contrast the clinical picture of delirium with that of dementia.
2. Discuss three critical needs of a person with delirium, stated in terms of nursing diagnoses.
3. Identify three outcomes for patients with delirium.
4. Summarize the essential nursing interventions for a patient with delirium.
5. Recognize the signs and symptoms occurring in the stages of Alzheimer's disease.
6. Give an example of the following symptoms assessed during the progression of Alzheimer's disease: (a) amnesia, (b) apraxia, (c) agnosia, and (d) aphasia.
7. Formulate three nursing diagnoses suitable for a patient with Alzheimer's disease and define two outcomes for each.
8. Formulate a teaching plan for a caregiver of a patient with Alzheimer's disease, including interventions for (a) communication, (b) health maintenance, and (c) safe environment.
9. Compose a list of appropriate referrals in the community—including a support group, hotline for information, and respite services—for persons with dementia and their caregivers.

KEY TERMS AND CONCEPTS

agnosia
agraphia
Alzheimer's disease (AD)
aphasia
apraxia
attention
confabulation
delirium
dementia
hallucinations
hypermetamorphosis
hyperorality
hypervigilance
illusions
long-term memory
major neurocognitive disorder
mild neurocognitive disorder
perseveration
short-term memory
social cognition
sundowning

The clarity and purpose of an individual's personal journey through life depend on the ability to reflect on its meaning. Cognition represents a fundamental human feature that distinguishes living from existing. This mental capacity has a distinctive, personalized impact on the individual's physical, psychological, social, and spiritual conduct of life. For example, the ability to remember the connections between related actions and how to initiate them depends on cognitive processing. Moreover, this cognitive processing has a direct relationship to activities of daily living.

Although primarily an intellectual and perceptual process, cognition is closely integrated with an individual's emotional and spiritual values. When human beings can no longer understand facts or connect the appropriate feelings to events, they have trouble responding to the complexity of life's challenges. Profound disturbances in cognitive processing cloud or destroy the meaning of the journey. Caring for people with **neurocognitive disorders** requires a compassionate understanding of the patient and family. Nursing interventions are focused on physical safety, protection of personal dignity, preservation of functional status, and promotion of well-being for cognitively impaired patients.

Cognitive functioning involves a variety of domains. The most obvious is attention, the ability to focus on environmental cues without distraction and to select and register information so that immediate recall (short-term memory) is possible. Other cognitive domains include an ability to do the following: plan and problem solve (executive function); learn and retain information in long-term memory; use language; visually perceive the environment; and "read" social situations in relation to how others might be feeling and determine what is appropriate for the environmental context (social cognition).

The three main neurocognitive syndromes are **delirium**, mild neurocognitive disorders, and major cognitive disorders (American Psychiatric Association, 2013). All of these disorders are caused by physiological changes in brain function, structure, or chemistry, and all involve cognitive deficits that are a decline in the person's previous functioning. The first syndrome is delirium, which is short-term and reversible; the remaining two syndromes, major and mild neurocognitive disorders, encompass what are commonly referred to as **dementia**,which is progressive and irreversible.

DELIRIUM

CLINICAL PICTURE

Delirium is an acute cognitive disturbance and often-reversible condition that is common in hospitalized patients, especially older patients. It is characterized as a syndrome, that is, a constellation of symptoms, rather than a disease state per se. The cardinal symptoms of delirium are an alteration in level of consciousness, which manifests as altered awareness and an inability to direct, focus, sustain, and shift attention; an abrupt onset with clinical features that fluctuate (including periods of lucidity); and disorganized thinking and poor executive functioning. Other characteristics include disorientation (often to time and place and rarely to first person), anxiety, agitation (motor restlessness), poor memory (recall), delusional thinking, and hallucinations, usually visual. Patients experience delirium as a sudden change in reality with a sense that they are dreaming while awake. They experience dramatic scenes that engender strong feelings of fear, panic, and anger (Duppils & Wikblad, 2007).

Delirium is considered a medical emergency that requires immediate attention to prevent irreversible and serious damage (Caplan et al., 2008). Delirium is associated with increased morbidity and mortality (Inouye et al., 2001) and can have lasting long-term consequences (Quinlan & Rudolph, 2011). While delirium is usually short term, there are long-term consequences that are currently better defined through large-scale epidemiological studies (Rudolph & Marcantonio, 2011). In patients with preexisting cognitive impairment (for example, dementia), there is an acceleration of cognitive decline. While there are reports of long-term cognitive impairment (in the absence of preexisting cognitive impairment) and functional decline following delirium, results of studies have been inconsistent. There is an association with depression post delirium, and evidence indicates that younger patients who have been delirious while hospitalized may develop posttraumatic stress disorder-like symptoms (Jones et al., 2001; Jones et al., 2007).

EPIDEMIOLOGY

Delirium is the most common complication of hospitalization in older patients (Rice et al., 2011). The reported incidence of delirium in hospitalized patients ranges from 3% to 56% (Michaud et al., 2007), from 11% to 42% in medically ill older patients (Cerejeira & Mukactova-Ludinska, 2011), and from 4% to 65% in postoperative patients, depending on the type of surgery (Rudolph & Marcantonio, 2011). The high degree of variability in the reported incidence of delirium is most likely due to its underrecognition by both nurses and doctors who work in acute-care settings/hospitals.

COMORBIDITY AND ETIOLOGY

Delirium is always due to underlying physiological causes that are usually multifactorial in nature. There are underlying factors that predispose a patient to developing delirium, and there are immediate factors that precipitate the syndrome.

Predisposing factors for delirium include age, lower education level, sensory impairment, decreased functional status, comorbid medical conditions, malnutrition, and depression (Flagg et al., 2010). Postoperative conditions, systemic disorders, withdrawal of drugs and substances such as alcohol and sedatives, toxicity secondary to drugs or other substances, and impaired respiratory functioning (Tasman & Mohr, 2011).

While the key to offsetting the consequences of delirium is prompt recognition and investigations into possible causes, there is research evidence that the syndrome is poorly recognized and understood by both nurses and doctors (Rice et al., 2011; Flagg et al., 2010). Early recognition and diagnosis is challenging for clinicians due to lack of knowledge about cognitive impairment and its clinical assessment, failure to interpret the signs and symptoms, and nurses' overreliance on disorientation as the only sign of cognitive impairment (Flagg et al., 2010).

At present the best evidence for the prevention and management of delirium in hospitalized patients is having clinical protocols for minimizing the risk factors and for the early detection of delirium (Cerejeira & Mukactova-Ludinska, 2011). The best approach is collaboration between health care providers, with nurses being in the most likely position to first observe the signs and symptoms of delirium (Milisen et al., 2005). In addition, proactive consultation with geriatric specialists has been shown to reduce delirium in hospitalized patients (Siddiqi et al., 2007).

APPLICATION OF THE NURSING PROCESS

ASSESSMENT

Early recognition is the key to offsetting the potential consequences, as the condition if often reversible. While symptoms of delirium must be managed, the goal of treatment is to determine the underlying cause and rectify this when possible (Rudolph & Marcantonio, 2011). This means that clinicians who suspect delirium and note its symptoms should undertake a thorough examination, including mental and neurological status examinations as well as a physical examination. Blood tests should be undertaken along with a urinalysis. In addition, the patient's medication regimen should be examined. A failure to quickly detect and treat delirium is associated with significant increase in morbidity and mortality (Rice et al., 2011).

Overall Assessment

According to Wei and colleagues (2008), there are four cardinal features of delirium:

1. Acute onset and fluctuating course
2. Reduced ability to direct, focus, shift, and sustain attention
3. Disorganized thinking
4. Disturbance of consciousness

Suspect the presence of delirium when a patient abruptly develops a disturbance in consciousness that manifests as reduced clarity of awareness of the environment. The ability to focus, sustain, or shift attention is impaired. Questions must be repeated because the individual's attention wanders, and the person might easily get off track and need to be refocused. Conversation is made more difficult because the person may be easily distracted by irrelevant stimuli. The person may have difficulty with orientation—first to time, then to place, and last to person. For example, a man with delirium may think that the year is 1972, that the hospital is home, and that the nurse is his wife. Orientation to person is usually intact to the extent that the person is aware of the self's identity.

Fluctuating levels of consciousness are unpredictable. Disorientation and confusion are usually markedly worse at night and during the early morning. In fact, some patients may be confused or delirious only at night and may remain lucid during the day.

As nurses, our frequent interaction with hospitalized patients places us in a prime position to detect delirium. Nursing assessment includes observation of (1) cognitive and perceptual disturbances, (2) physical needs, and (3) moods and physical behaviors.

Cognitive and Perceptual Disturbances

It may be difficult to engage patients experiencing delirium in conversation because they are easily distracted, display marked attention deficits, and exhibit memory impairment. In mild delirium, memory deficits are noted only on careful questioning. In more severe delirium, memory problems usually take the form of obvious difficulty in processing and remembering recent events. For example, the person might ask when a son is coming to visit even though the son left only an hour earlier.

Perceptual disturbances are also common. Perception is the processing of information about one's internal and external environment. Various misinterpretations of reality may take the form of illusions or hallucinations.

Illusions are errors in perception of sensory stimuli. A person may mistake folds in the bedclothes for white rats or the cord of

EVIDENCE-BASED PRACTICE

Detecting Delirium in Older Adults

Rice, K., Bennett, M., Gomez, M., Theall, K. P., Knight, M., & Foreman, M. D. (2011). Nurses' recognition of delirium in the hospitalized older adult. *Clinical Nurse Specialist*, Nov/Dec, 299–311.

Problem

Delirium is the most frequent complication of hospitalization in older adults and is costly in relation to fiscal resources; more importantly, delirium is also associated with mortality and morbidity. Timely recognition is essential to offset these negative outcomes. Delirium is often misdiagnosed or not recognized by hospital staff. Nurses are in a prime position to detect delirium.

Purpose of Study

The purpose was to measure staff nurses' recognition of delirium in older hospitalized patients by comparing their delirium ratings with those of expert diagnosticians, using the Confusion Assessment Method (CAM).

Methods

Older patients who were hospitalized in medical-surgical units and were judged to be "at risk of delirium" (n=170) were assessed for delirium at least every other day until discharge. Both staff nurses and experts conducted the assessments using the CAM. The staff nurses' ratings were compared with the experts' ratings to ascertain the level of agreement.

Key Findings

The experts detected delirium in 7% of the patients. The staff nurses failed to recognize delirium 75% of the time, and there was poor agreement between experts and staff nurses for all observations. Predictors of staff nurses' poor recognition of delirium included older age, length of stay, presence of dementia, and hypoactive (quiet) delirium.

Implications for Nursing Practice

Nurses who work with patients at high risk of developing delirium should engage in ongoing education about its detection and management, and regular systems should be put into place to identify those patients most at risk of developing delirium. It is especially important that nurses do not assess older patients who become confused as having dementia. Equally important is that some patients who become delirious will be "quietly confused."

a window blind for a snake. The stimulus is a real object in the environment; however, it is misinterpreted and often becomes the object of the patient's projected fear. Illusions, unlike delusions or hallucinations, can be explained and clarified for the individual.

Hallucinations are false sensory stimuli (refer to Chapter 12). Visual hallucinations are common in delirium, and tactile hallucinations may also be present. For example, individuals experiencing delirium may become terrified when they "see" giant spiders crawling over the bedclothes or "feel" bugs crawling on or under their bodies. Auditory hallucinations occur more often in other psychiatric disorders such as schizophrenia.

The individual with delirium generally is aware that something is very wrong. Statements like "My thoughts are all jumbled" may signal cognitive problems. When perceptual disturbances are present, the emotional response is often one of fear and anxiety, which may be manifested by psychomotor agitation.

Physical Needs

A person with delirium becomes disoriented and may try to "go home." Alternatively, a person may think that he or she *is* home and jump out of a window in an attempt to get away from "invaders." Wandering, pulling out intravenous lines and Foley catheters, and falling out of bed are common dangers that require nursing vigilance.

An individual experiencing delirium has difficulty processing stimuli in the environment, and confusion magnifies the inability to recognize reality. The physical environment should be made as simple and clear as possible. Objects such as clocks and calendars can maximize orientation to time. Eyeglasses, hearing aids, and adequate lighting without glare can maximize the person's ability to interpret more accurately what is going on in the environment. The nurse should interact with the patient whenever the patient is awake. Short periods of social interaction help reduce anxiety and misperceptions.

Self-care deficits, injury, or hyperactivity or hypoactivity may lead to skin breakdown and possible infection. Often this is compounded by poor nutrition, forced bed rest, and possible incontinence. These areas require nursing assessment and intervention.

Autonomic signs, such as tachycardia, sweating, flushed face, dilated pupils, and elevated blood pressure, are often present in delirium. These changes must be monitored and documented carefully and may require immediate medical attention.

Changes in the sleep/wake cycle usually are noted, and in some cases, a complete reversal of the night/day, sleep/wake cycle can occur. The patient's level of consciousness may range from lethargy to stupor or from semi-coma to hypervigilance. In **hypervigilance,** patients are extraordinarily alert, and their eyes constantly scan the room; they may have difficulty falling asleep or may be actively disoriented and agitated throughout the night.

Medications should always be suspected as a potential cause of delirium (Sadock & Sadock, 2008). To recognize drug reactions or anticipate potential interactions before delirium actually occurs, it is important to assess all medications (prescription *and* over-the-counter) the patient is taking.

Moods and Physical Behaviors

The individual's moods and physical behaviors may change dramatically within a short period. A person with delirium may display motor restlessness (agitation), or he or she may be "quietly delirious" and appear calm and settled. When there is agitation, delirium is considered hyperactive; when there is no agitation, delirium is considered hypoactive. Moods may swing back and forth among fear, anger, anxiety, euphoria, depression, and apathy. A person may strike out from fear or anger or may cry, call for help, curse, moan, and tear off clothing one minute and become apathetic or laugh uncontrollably the next. In short, behavior and emotions are erratic and fluctuating. Lack of concentration and disorientation complicate interventions. The following vignette illustrates the fear and confusion a patient may experience when admitted to an intensive care unit (ICU).

VIGNETTE

Peter Wright, age 43, survived numerous life-threatening complications following open-heart surgery to replace his mitral valve. He spent 3 weeks in an ICU. The night before he was to be transferred to a general medical unit he heard a nurse saying, "I need to get a gas." Another nurse answered in a loud voice, "Can you get a large needle for the injection?"

Peter began to get frightened and thought the nurses were going to gas and sedate him. He became suspicious about his bed being moved and thought he was being transported to another country to have his organs removed and donated for transplantation. His fear mounted when he realized that his wife, who had been at his bedside the entire ICU stay, was not there. He wanted her to know that he was being taken away. His incoherent attempts to summon his wife to his bedside confirmed what he suspected: the very people who had saved his life were now out to get him.

Peter began to diligently watch the clock on the wall, recording every movement of the nurses to try to ascertain a pattern to their behavior in order to escape his captors. When he was sure nobody was looking, he climbed over the bedrails and attempted to leave the unit. The nurses responded by calling security personnel to escort him back to bed. Once he was safely in bed, the nurses applied mechanical restraints and then sedated him.

Peter's confusion abated the next day. He was transferred from the ICU to the medical unit. He could recall the details of his confused state. While he realized how distorted his thinking had been during the episode, the anxiety and fear he experienced remained with him for months after discharge from the hospital.

What are some more helpful interventions the nurses could have used? What could the nurses have done differently? What would you have done? For example, the nurses could have told Peter why they were moving his bed, and they could have recognized his need to have his wife return to his bedside. They could have noted signs of his fear and anxiety.

Self-Assessment

Because the behaviors exhibited by the patient with delirium can be directly attributed to temporary medical conditions, intense personal reactions in staff are less likely to arise. In fact, intense, conflicting emotions are less likely to occur in nurses working with a patient with delirium than in nurses working with a patient with dementia, which is discussed later in this chapter. Nonetheless, it can be frustrating to interact with these patients, especially given the fluctuating nature of the clinical picture.

ASSESSMENT GUIDELINES

Delirium

1. Assess for acute onset and fluctuating levels of awareness, which are key in delirium.
2. Assess the person's ability to attend to the immediate environment, including responses to nursing care.
3. Establish the person's normal level of consciousness and cognition by interviewing family or other caregivers.
4. Assess for past cognitive impairment—especially an existing dementia diagnosis—and other risk factors.
5. Identify disturbances in physiological status, especially infection, hypoxia, and pain.
6. Identify any physiological abnormalities documented in the patient's record.
7. Assess vital signs, level of consciousness, and neurological signs.
8. Assess potential for injury, especially in relation to potential for falls and wandering.
9. Maintain comfort measures, especially in relation to pain, cold, or positioning.
10. Monitor situational factors that worsen or improve symptoms.
11. Assess for availability of immediate medical interventions to help prevent irreversible brain damage.
12. Remain nonjudgmental. Confer with other staff readily when questions arise.

DIAGNOSIS

Safety needs to play a substantial role in nursing care. Patients with delirium often perceive the environment in a distorted way, and objects are often misperceived (illusions and/or hallucinations). People and objects may be misinterpreted as threatening or harmful, and patients often act on these misinterpretations. For example, if feeling threatened or thinking that common medical equipment is harmful, the patient may pull off an oxygen mask, pull out an intravenous or nasogastric tube, or try to flee. In such a case, the person demonstrates a *Risk for injury* as evidenced by sensory deficits or perceptual deficits.

Hallucinations, distractibility, illusions, disorientation, agitation, restlessness, and/or misperception are major aspects of the clinical picture. When some of these symptoms are present, *Acute confusion* related to delirium is an appropriate nursing diagnosis.

If fever and dehydration are present, fluid and electrolyte balance will need to be managed. If the underlying cause of the patient's delirium results in fever, decreased skin turgor, decreased urinary output or fluid intake, and dry skin or mucous membranes, then the nursing diagnosis of *Risk for deficient fluid volume* is appropriate. Fluid volume deficit may be related to fever, electrolyte imbalance, reduced intake, or infection.

Because disruption in the sleep/wake cycle may be present, the patient may be less responsive during the day and may become disruptively wakeful during the night. Restful sleep is not achieved, day or night; therefore, *Disturbed sleep pattern* or *Sleep deprivation* related to impaired cerebral oxygenation or disruption in consciousness is a likely nursing diagnosis.

Sustaining communication with a delirious patient is difficult. *Impaired verbal communication* related to cerebral hypoxia or decreased cerebral blood flow, as evidenced by confusion or clouding of consciousness, may be diagnosed.

Fear is one of the most common of all nursing diagnoses and may be related to illusions, delusions, or hallucinations, as evidenced by verbal and nonverbal expressions of fearfulness. Other nursing concerns include *Self-care deficits* and *Impaired social interaction.*

OUTCOMES IDENTIFICATION

The overall outcome is that the delirious patient will return to the premorbid level of functioning. Although the patient can demonstrate a wide variety of needs, *Risk for injury* is always present. Appropriate outcomes include the following:

- Patient will remain safe and free from injury while in the hospital.
- During periods of lucidity, patient will be oriented to time, place, and person with the aid of nursing interventions, such as the provision of clocks, calendars, maps, and other types of orienting information.
- Patient will remain free from falls and injury while confused, with the aid of nursing safety measures.

IMPLEMENTATION

The priorities of treatment are to keep the patient safe while attempting to identify the cause. If the underlying disorder is corrected, complete recovery is possible. If, however, the underlying disorder is not corrected and persists, irreversible neuronal damage can occur. Nursing concerns therefore center on the following:

- Preventing physical harm due to confusion, aggression, or electrolyte and fluid imbalance
- Performing a comprehensive nursing assessment to aid in identifying the cause
- Assisting with proper health management to eradicate the underlying cause
- Using supportive measures to relieve distress

The *Nursing Interventions Classification (NIC)* (Bulechek et al., 2013) can be used as a guide to develop interventions for a patient with delirium (Box 23-1). Medical management of delirium involves treating the underlying organic causes. If the underlying cause of delirium is not treated, permanent brain damage may ensue. Judicious use of antipsychotic or antianxiety agents may also be useful in controlling behavioral symptoms.

BOX 23-1 *NIC* INTERVENTIONS FOR DELIRIUM MANAGEMENT

Definition: Provision of a safe and therapeutic environment for the patient who is experiencing an acute confusional state

- Initiate therapies to reduce or eliminate factors causing delirium.
- Monitor neurological status on an ongoing basis.
- Administer prn (as needed) medications for anxiety or agitation.
- Assist with needs related to nutrition, elimination, hydration, and personal hygiene.
- Use physical restraints, as needed.
- Provide unconditional positive regard.
- Acknowledge patient's fears and feelings.
- Provide optimistic but realistic reassurance.
- Provide patient with information about what is happening and what can be expected
- Limit need for decision making, if frustrating or confusing to patient.
- Accept patient's perceptions or interpretation of reality and respond to the theme or feeling tone
- Avoid frustrating patient by quizzing with orientation questions that cannot be answered.
- Inform patient of person, place, and time, as needed.
- Approach patient slowly and from the front and address patient by name.
- Communicate with simple, direct, descriptive statements.
- Encourage visitation by significant others, as appropriate.
- Maintain a well-lit, hazard-free environment.
- Place identification bracelet on patient.
- Provide a consistent physical environment, daily routine, and caregivers.
- Use environmental cues (e.g., signs, pictures, clocks, calendars, and color coding of environment) to stimulate memory, reorient, and promote appropriate behavior.
- Provide a low-stimulation environment for patient in whom disorientation is increased by overstimulation.
- Encourage use of aids that increase sensory input (e.g., eyeglasses, hearing aids, and dentures).

From Bulechek, G. M., Butcher, H. K., Dochterman, J. M., & Wagner, C. (2013). *Nursing interventions classification (NIC)* (6th ed.). St. Louis, MO: Elsevier.

A patient in acute delirium should never be left alone. Because most hospitals and health facilities are unable to provide one-to-one supervision of the patient, family members can be encouraged to stay with the patient.

EVALUATION

Long-term outcome criteria for a person experiencing delirium include the following:

- Patient will remain safe.
- Patient will be oriented to time, place, and person by discharge.
- Underlying cause will be treated and ameliorated.

DEMENTIA

Dementia is a broad term used to describe progressive deterioration of cognitive functioning and global impairment of intellect with no change in consciousness. It is not a specific disease per se, but rather a collection of symptoms that are due to an underlying brain disorder. These disorders are characterized by cognitive impairments that signal a decline from previous functioning. When mild, the impairments do not interfere with instrumental activities of daily living although the person may need to make extra efforts. While such impairments may be progressive, most people with a mild cognitive impairment will not progress to dementia (Mitchell & Shiri-Feshki, 2009). When progressive, these disorders interfere with daily functioning and independence. While often characterized by memory deficits, dementia affects other areas of cognitive functioning, for example, problem solving (executive functioning) and complex attention.

CLINICAL PICTURE

Dementia is the general term used to describe a variety of progressive conditions that develop when brain cells die or no longer function; **Alzheimer's disease (AD)** is the most common type of dementia, accounting for 60% to 80% of all dementias (Alzheimer's Association, 2012). It is a devastating disease that not only affects the person who has it but also places an enormous burden on the families and caregivers of those affected. Nurses practicing in most any setting will care for patients with AD and must be prepared to respond.

It is important to distinguish between normal forgetfulness and the memory deficit of AD and other dementias. Severe memory loss is *not* a normal part of growing older. Slight forgetfulness is a common phenomenon of the aging process (age-associated memory loss) but not memory loss that interferes with one's activities of daily living. Table 23-1 outlines memory changes in normal aging and memory changes seen in dementia.

TABLE 23-1 MEMORY DEFICIT: NORMAL AGING VERSUS DEMENTIA

TYPICAL AGE-RELATED CHANGES	SIGNS OF ALZHEIMER'S
Making a bad decision once in a while	Poor judgment and decision making
Missing a monthly payment	Inability to manage a budget
Forgetting which day it is and remembering later	Losing track of the date or the season
Sometimes forgetting which word to use	Difficulty having a conversation
Losing things from time to time	Misplacing things and being unable to retrace steps to find them

From Alzheimer's Association. (2013). 10 early signs and symptoms of Alzheimer's disease. Retrieved from http://www.alz.org/alzheimers_disease_10_signs_of_alzheimers.asp.

Many people who live to a very old age never experience significant memory loss or any other symptom of dementia. Most of us know of people in their 80s and 90s who lead active lives with the intellect intact. The slow, mild cognitive changes associated with aging should not impede social or occupational functioning.

Although dementia often begins with a worsening of ability to remember new information, it is marked by progressive deterioration in cognitive functioning and the ability to solve problems and learn new skills and by a decline in the ability to perform activities of daily living. A person's declining intellect often leads to emotional changes such as anxiety, mood lability, and depression, as well as neurological changes that produce hallucinations and delusions.

There are several types of dementia. Dementia is associated with AD, frontotemporal lobar degeneration, Lewy bodies, vascular issues, traumatic brain injury, substances, HIV infection, Prion disease, Parkinson's disease, and Huntington's disease (APA, 2013). Regardless of the cause, dementia is classified as either a mild or a major neurocognitive disorder. Minor neurocognitive disorders are characterized by symptoms that place individuals in a zone between normal cognition and noticeably significant cognitive deterioration. The rationale for the introduction of a mild category is that identifying early-presenting symptoms may aid in earlier interventions at a stage when some disease-modifying therapies may be most neuroprotective (Sperling et al., 2011). Major neurocognitive disorders are characterized by substantial cognitive decline that results in curtailed independence and functioning among affected individuals.

EPIDEMIOLOGY

AD, the most common type of dementia, attacks indiscriminately, striking men and women, people of various ethnicities, rich and poor, and individuals with varying degrees of intelligence. Although the disease can occur at a younger age (early onset), most of those with the disease are 65 years of age or older (late onset). It is estimated that 5.4 million Americans have AD (Alzheimer's Association, 2012). Globally, it is estimated that 24.3 million people have dementia, and the number of people will double every 20 years to 81.1 million by 2040 (Ferri et al., 2005).

It is estimated that one in eight people aged ≥ 65 years has AD and that 45% of the people ≥ 85 years has AD. Of the people with AD:

- 4% are younger than 65 years old.
- 6% are between 65 and 74 years old.
- 44% are between 75 and 84 years old.
- 46% are 85 years old or older. (Alzheimer's Association, 2012)

ETIOLOGY

Although the cause of AD is unknown, most experts agree that, like other chronic and progressive conditions, it is a result of multiple factors that include genetics, lifestyle, and environmental. While many causes are hypothesized, the greatest risk factor is advanced age (Alzheimer's Association, 2012; Lehne, 2013).

Biological Factors

Neuronal Degeneration

In the brains of people with AD there are signs of neuronal degeneration that begins in the hippocampus, the part of the brain responsible for recent memory, and then spreads into the cerebral cortex, the part of the brain responsible for problem solving and higher-order cognitive functioning (Lehne, 2013). There are two processes that contribute to cell death. The first is the accumulation of the protein β-amyloid outside the neurons, which interferes with synapses; the second is an accumulation of the protein tau inside the neurons, which forms tangles that block the flow of nutrients. More research is needed into these mechanisms as some people who have these brain changes do not go on to develop AD (Alzheimer's Association, 2012).

Genetic

There are three known genetic mutations that guarantee that a person will develop AD, although these account for less than 1% of all cases. These mutations lead to the devastating early-onset form of AD, which occurs before the age of 65 and as young as 30 years (Alzheimer's Association, 2012).

A susceptibility gene has been identified for late-onset AD as well. It is a gene that makes the protein apolipoprotein E, APOE ε4, which helps carry cholesterol and is also implicated in cardiovascular disease (Alzheimer's Association, 2012).

Individuals who have or have had family members with AD are understandably concerned about their own risk for developing the disorder. For those who may carry the early-onset gene, genetic counseling, available through the Alzheimer's Disease Research Center, is recommended. Commercial testing is available for one of the three genes that can confirm the disease or predict its onset, but this testing raises significant ethical concerns (Wright et al., 2008). APOE ε4 testing is also available but has limited predictive value.

Risk Factors in Alzheimer's Disease

Cardiovascular Disease

The health of the brain is closely linked to overall heart health, and there is evidence that people with cardiovascular disease are at greater risk of AD. Likewise, lifestyle factors associated with cardiovascular disease, such as inactivity, high cholesterol, diabetes and obesity, are considered risk factors for AD (Alzheimer's Association, 2012).

Social Engagement and Diet

There is some evidence that brain health is affected by modifiable factors, such as remaining mentally and socially active and consuming a health diet, but the research is limited by few studies and low number of participants (Alzheimer's Association, 2012).

Head Injury and Traumatic Brain Injury

Brain injury and trauma are associated with a greater risk of developing AD and other dementias. People who suffer repeated head trauma, such as boxers and football players, may be at greater risk. There is a suggestion that individuals who suffer brain injury and carry the gene APOE ε4 are at greater risk (Alzheimer's Association, 2012).

APPLICATION OF THE NURSING PROCESS

ASSESSMENT

General Assessment

Alzheimer's disease is commonly characterized by progressive deterioration of cognitive functioning. Initial deterioration may be so subtle and insidious that others may not notice. In the early stages of the disease, the affected person may be able to compensate for loss of memory. Some people may have superior social graces and charm that give them the ability to hide severe deficits in memory, even from experienced health care professionals. This hiding is actually an unconscious protective defense against the terrifying reality of losing one's place in the world. Family members may also unconsciously deny that anything is wrong as a defense against the painful awareness that a loved one is deteriorating. As time goes on, symptoms become more obvious, and other defense mechanisms become evident, including (1) denial, (2) confabulation, (3) perseveration, and (4) avoidance of questions.

Confabulation is the creation of stories or answers in place of actual memories to maintain self-esteem. For example, the nurse addresses a patient who has remained in a hospital bed all weekend:

Nurse: Good morning, Ms. Jones. How was your weekend?

Patient: Wonderful. I discussed politics with the president, and he took me out to dinner.

or

Patient: I spent the weekend with my daughter and her family.

Confabulation is not the same as lying. When people are lying, they are aware of making up an answer; confabulation is an unconscious attempt to maintain self-esteem.

Perseveration (the repetition of phrases or behavior) is eventually seen and is often intensified under stress. The avoidance of answering questions is another mechanism by which the person is able to maintain self-esteem unconsciously in the face of severe memory deficits.

Symptoms observed in AD include the following:

- **Memory impairment:** Initially the person has difficulty remembering recent events. Gradually, deterioration progresses to include both recent and remote memory.
- **Disturbances in executive functioning** (planning, organizing, abstract thinking): The degeneration of neurons in the brain results in the wasting away of the brain's working components. These cells contain memories, receive sights and sounds, cause hormones to secrete, produce emotions, and command muscles into motion.
- Aphasia (loss of language ability): Initially the person has difficulty finding the correct word, then is reduced to a few words, and finally is reduced to babbling or mutism.
- Apraxia (loss of purposeful movement in the absence of motor or sensory impairment): The person is unable to perform once-familiar and purposeful tasks. For example, in apraxia of dressing, the person is unable to put clothes on properly (may put arms in trousers or put a jacket on upside down).
- Agnosia (loss of sensory ability to recognize objects): For example, a person may lose the ability to recognize familiar sounds (auditory agnosia), such as the ring of the telephone. Loss of this ability extends to the inability to recognize familiar objects (visual or tactile agnosia), such as a glass, magazine, pencil, or toothbrush.

Diagnostic Tests

A wide range of problems may be mistaken for dementia or AD. Depression in the older adult is the disorder frequently confused with dementia. In fact, many persons diagnosed with Alzheimer's dementia also meet the diagnostic criteria for a depressive disorder. In addition, dementia and depression or dementia and delirium *can* coexist. It is important that nurses and other health care professionals be able to assess some of the important differences among depression, dementia, and delirium. Table 23-2 outlines important differences among these three phenomena.

When symptoms of dementia are present, a comprehensive assessment must be completed in order to rule out conditions that mimic dementia but are treatable. Making a diagnosis of Alzheimer's disease includes ruling out all other pathophysiological conditions through the history and through physical and laboratory tests, many of which are identified in Box 23-2.

Brain imaging with CT, positron emission tomography (PET), and other developing scanning technologies have diagnostic capabilities because they reveal brain atrophy and rule out other conditions such as neoplasms. The use of mental status questionnaires, such as the Mini-Mental State Examination and various other tests to identify deterioration in mental status and brain damage, is an important part of the assessment.

In addition to performing a complete physical and neurological examination, it is important to obtain a complete medical and psychiatric history, description of recent symptoms, review of medications used, and nutritional evaluation. The observations and history provided by family members are invaluable to the assessment process.

Progression of Alzheimer's Disease

Alzheimer's disease is classified according to the stage of the degenerative process. The number of stages defined ranges from three to seven, depending on the source. Table 23-3 outlines the seven stages as identified and described by the Alzheimer's Association. These stages can be used as a guide to understand the progressive deterioration seen in those diagnosed with AD.

Recently, the Alzheimer's Association and the National Institute on Aging (Alzheimer's Association, 2012) have proposed new staging of the illness. The recommendations are that AD be identified in three stages: preclinical AD, mild cognitive impairment (MCI) due to AD, and dementia due to AD. The first stage occurs prior to any symptoms and is identified through AD biomarkers, such as β-amyloid and tau; at present, further scientific evidence about biomarkers is needed before use in clinical setting.

TABLE 23-2 COMPARISON OF DELIRIUM, DEMENTIA, AND DEPRESSION

	DELIRIUM	DEMENTIA	DEPRESSION
Onset	Sudden, over hours to days	Slowly, over months	May have been gradual, with exacerbation during crisis or stress
Cause or contributing factors	Hypoglycemia, fever, dehydration, hypotension; infection, other conditions that disrupt body's homeostasis; adverse drug reaction; head injury; change in environment (e.g., hospitalization); pain; emotional stress	Alzheimer's disease, vascular disease, human immunodeficiency virus infection, neurological disease, chronic alcoholism, head trauma	Lifelong history, losses, loneliness, crises, declining health, medical conditions
Cognition	Impaired memory, judgment, calculations, attention span; can fluctuate through the day	Impaired memory, judgment, calculations, attention span, abstract thinking; agnosia	Difficulty concentrating, forgetfulness, inattention
Level of consciousness	Altered	Not altered	Not altered
Activity level	Can be increased or reduced; restlessness, behaviors may worsen in evening (sundowning); sleep/wake cycle may be reversed	Not altered; behaviors may worsen in evening (sundowning)	Usually decreased; lethargy, fatigue, lack of motivation; may sleep poorly and awaken in early morning
Emotional state	Rapid swings; can be fearful, anxious, suspicious, aggressive, have hallucinations and/or delusions	Flat; agitation	Extreme sadness, apathy, irritability, anxiety, paranoid ideation
Speech and language	Rapid, inappropriate, incoherent, rambling	Incoherent, slow (sometimes due to effort to find the right word), inappropriate, rambling, repetitious	Slow, flat, low
Prognosis	Reversible with proper and timely treatment	Not reversible; progressive	Reversible with proper and timely treatment

BOX 23-2 BASIC MEDICAL WORKUP FOR DEMENTIA

- Chest and skull radiographic studies
- Electroencephalography
- Electrocardiography
- Urinalysis
- Sequential multiple analyzer 12-test serum profile
- Thyroid function tests
- Folate level
- Venereal Disease Research Laboratories (VDRL), human immunodeficiency virus tests
- Serum creatinine assay
- Electrolyte assessment
- Vitamin B_{12} level
- Liver function tests
- Vision and hearing evaluation
- Neuroimaging (when diagnostic issues are not clear)

The proposed second and third stages correspond to the *DSM-5* criteria for Mild and Major Neurocognitive Disorders as the major differentiation is based on how much the disease is disrupting functional daily living. In relation to the seven stages outlined in Table 23-3, Stage 1 relates to the preclinical stage, stages 3-4 to MCI (Mild ND), and stages 5-7 are consistent with dementia due to AD (Major ND).

Mild Cognitive Impairment Due to Alzheimer's Disease

The loss of intellectual ability is insidious. The person with mild AD loses energy, drive, and initiative and has difficulty learning new things. Because personality and social behavior remain intact, others tend to minimize and underestimate the loss of the individual's abilities. The individual may still continue to work, but the extent of the dementia becomes evident in new or demanding situations. Depression may occur early in the disease but usually lessens as the disease progresses.

As AD progresses the person is often unable to identify familiar objects or people, even a spouse **(agnosia).** The person needs repeated instructions and directions to perform the simplest tasks **(apraxia):** "Here is the face cloth; pick up the soap. Now, put water on the face cloth, and rub the face cloth with soap." Often the individual cannot remember where the toilet is and becomes incontinent. Total care is necessary at this point, and the burden on the family can be emotionally, financially, and physically devastating. The world is very frightening to the person with AD because nothing makes sense any longer. Agitation, violence, paranoia, and delusions are commonly seen. Another problem that is frightening to family members and caregivers is wandering behavior.

TABLE 23-3 **STAGES OF ALZHEIMER'S DISEASE**

STAGE	HALLMARKS
Stage 1 No impairment	No memory problems
Stage 2 Very mild cognitive decline (may be age-related or due to dementia)	Aware of memory lapses Forgetting familiar words or the location of everyday objects. No symptoms of dementia can be detected during a medical examination or by friends, family, or co-workers.
Stage 3 Mild cognitive decline (early-stage Alzheimer's can be diagnosed in some, but not all, individuals with these symptoms)	Others begin to notice difficulties. Noticeable problems coming up with the right word or name Trouble remembering names when introduced to new people Noticeable difficulty performing tasks in social or work settings Forgetting material that one has just read Losing or misplacing a valuable object Increasing trouble with planning or organizing
Stage 4 Moderate cognitive decline (mild or early-stage Alzheimer's disease)	Forgetfulness of recent events Impaired ability to perform challenging mental arithmetic Difficulty performing complex tasks, such as planning dinner for guests, paying bills, or managing finances Becoming moody or withdrawn, especially in socially or mentally challenging situations
Stage 5 Moderately severe cognitive decline (moderate or midstage Alzheimer's disease)	Gaps in memory and thinking are noticeable, and individuals begin to need help with day-to-day activities. At this stage, individuals may: Be unable to recall their own addresses or telephone numbers or the high schools or colleges from which they graduated Become confused about where they are or what day it is Have trouble with less challenging mental arithmetic Need help choosing proper clothing for the season or the occasion Still remember significant details about themselves and their families Still require no assistance with eating or using the toilet
Stage 6 Severe cognitive decline (moderately severe or midstage Alzheimer's disease)	Personality changes may take place, and sufferers may need extensive help with daily activities. At this stage, individuals may: Lose awareness of recent experiences as well as of their surroundings Remember their own names but have difficulty with their personal histories Distinguish familiar and unfamiliar faces but have trouble remembering the name of a spouse or caregiver Need help dressing properly and may, without supervision, make mistakes such as putting pajamas over daytime clothes or shoes on the wrong feet Experience major changes in sleep patterns (sleeping during the day, becoming restless at night) Need help handling details of toileting Have increasingly frequent trouble controlling their bladder or bowels Experience major behavioral changes, including suspiciousness and delusions or compulsive, repetitive behavior Tend to wander or become lost
Stage 7 Very severe cognitive decline (severe or late-stage Alzheimer's disease)	In the final stage of this disease, individuals lose the ability to respond to their environment, to carry on a conversation, and, eventually, to control movement. They may still say words or phrases. At this stage, individuals need help with much of their daily personal care, including eating and using the toilet. They may also lose the ability to smile, sit without support, and hold their heads up. Reflexes become abnormal. Muscles grow rigid. Swallowing is impaired.

Adapted from Alzheimer's Association. (2013). *Seven stages of Alzheimer's*. Retrieved from http://www.alz.org/alzheimers_disease_stages_of_alzheimers.asp.

VIGNETTE

Mrs. White, 78 years old, a retired teacher, has always enjoyed an active life and good health, other than an overactive thyroid, which has been successfully treated and controlled. Remarkably, her only hospitalizations were for the births of her two children, now grown and married. She is a vibrant person who takes enormous pride in her appearance and in her beautifully clean home. She is beginning to forget things that she previously has taken for granted, but jokes about her failing memory as "senior moments."

During a recent visit, her daughter found Mrs. White quite distressed while in the kitchen. Mrs. White was attempting to make dinner for family guests and planned on her famous specialty, lasagna. The ingredients were strewn all over the kitchen, and Mrs. White was frantically searching for a recipe. Her daughter was quite taken aback as neither of them had ever used a written recipe. Her daughter managed to settle Mrs. White and helped with step-by-step instructions in the construction of the lasagna. Quietly, she was quite worried about her mother's failing memory, fearing that it was more than usual aging. Her daughter tried to broach the subject with her dad, a loving and loyal companion to Mrs. White. When she shared her concerns, his reply was simply, "I don't know what you are talking about." Clearly, he was not able to admit what was becoming obvious to others.

The situation reached a crisis point when her daughter discovered that Mrs. White was no longer taking her thyroid medications as she was confused between them and a calcium-sparing medication. As Mrs. White had taken medication for her thyroid for 30 years and yet she could not remember, this signaled a progression in her condition.

It was painful, but her husband too began to realize that Mrs. White was not functioning. Her once-clean house was in a state of disarray and dirty; she no longer could coordinate her clothing and often wore the same outfit for a number of days as she became overwhelmed by having to make a clothing choice; often, her clothes were dirty, and her makeup was applied in a haphazard manner.

Late in AD, the following symptoms may occur: **agraphia** (inability to read or write), **hyperorality** (the need to taste, chew, and put everything in one's mouth), blunting of emotions, visual agnosia (loss of ability to recognize familiar objects), and **hypermetamorphosis** (manifested by touching of everything in sight).

VIGNETTE

Mrs. White no longer was able to participate in or enjoy previous activities such as reading the newspaper and watching the morning television shows. She would stare at both the paper and television, attempting to understand but unable to retain any information. She was often restless during the day, going from one random activity to another, often rearranging her favorite knickknacks in her curio cupboard. She would attempt to wash clothes but forget to put laundry detergent in the machine. She would empty half-filled drinking glasses into the gas range top in her kitchen. If these mistakes were pointed out, she would become defensive and angry, stating, "I have always done it this way."

Eating became difficult as she did not seem to recognize food on her plate, and she was unable to use a knife and fork to cut her food. Sometimes, she would pick up a spoon and ask what it was. Her weight began to decrease.

While Mrs. White always slept well throughout her adult life, she began to wander around in the middle of the night, often waking her husband to ask questions. She would go to the kitchen and empty the cupboards for no apparent reason. She would enter her wardrobe and rearrange her clothing, often leaving articles of clothing lying on the floor.

When she set kitchen paper towels on fire by leaving them on the gas range and then lighting it, her family and husband realized that she could no longer function safely at home. Her husband was unable to leave her alone, even for short periods of time, as she would be become extremely distressed, almost to the point of panic. She and her husband moved into an assisted-living facility.

Self-Assessment

Working with cognitively impaired people in any setting should make us aware of the tremendous responsibility placed on caregivers. The behavioral problems these patients may display can cause tremendous stress for professionals and family caregivers alike. Caring for people who are unable to communicate and have lost the ability to relate and respond to others is extremely difficult, especially for nursing students or nurses who do not understand dementia or AD.

Nurses working in facilities for residents who are cognitively impaired (e.g., nursing homes and extended-care facilities) need special education and skills. Education must include information about the process of the disease and effective interventions, as well as knowledge regarding antipsychotic drugs. Support and educational opportunities should be readily available, not just to nurses but also to nurse aides, who are often directly responsible for administering basic care.

Because stress is a common occurrence when working with persons with cognitive impairments, nurses need to be proactive in minimizing its effects, which can be facilitated by:

- Having a realistic understanding of the disease so that expectations for the person are realistic.
- Establishing realistic outcomes for the person and recognizing when they are achieved. These outcomes may be as minor as *patient feeds self with spoon*, yet remember that even the smallest achievement can be a significant accomplishment for the impaired individual.
- Maintaining good self-care. As nurses, we need to protect ourselves from the negative effects of stress by obtaining adequate sleep and rest, eating a nutritious diet, exercising, engaging in relaxing activities, and addressing our own emotional and spiritual needs.

ASSESSMENT GUIDELINES

Dementia

1. Evaluate the person's current level of cognitive and daily functioning.
2. Identify any threats to the person's safety and security and arrange their reduction.
3. Evaluate the safety of the person's home environment (e.g., with regard to wandering, eating inedible objects, falling, engaging in provocative behaviors toward others).
4. Review the medications (including herbs, complementary agents) the patient is currently taking.
5. Interview family to gain a complete picture of the person's background and personality.
6. Explore how well the family is prepared for and informed about the progress of the person's dementia, depending on cause (if known).
7. Discuss with the family members how they are coping with the patient and their main issues at this time.
8. Review the resources available to the family. Ask family members to describe the help they receive from other family members, friends, and community resources. Determine if caregivers are aware of community support groups and resources.
9. Identify the needs of the family for teaching and guidance (e.g., how to manage catastrophic reactions, lability of mood, aggressive behaviors, and nocturnal delirium and increased confusion and agitation at night [**sundowning**]).

DIAGNOSIS

Caring for a person with dementia requires a great deal of patience, creativity, and maturity. The needs of such a person can be enormous for nursing staff and for families who care for their loved ones in the home. As the disease progresses, so do the needs of the person and the demands on the caregivers, staff, and family.

One of the most important areas of concern identified by both staff and families is the patient's safety. Many people with AD wander and may be lost for hours or days. Wandering, along with behaviors such as rummaging, may be perceived as purposeful to the person with AD. Wandering may result from changes in the physical environment, fear caused by hallucinations or delusions, or lack of exercise.

Injuries from falls and accidents can occur during any stage as confusion and disorientation progress. The potential for burns exists if the person is a smoker or is unattended when using the stove. Prescription drugs can be taken incorrectly, or bottles of noxious fluids can be mistakenly ingested, which results in a medical crisis; therefore, *Risk for injury* is always present.

As the person's ability to recognize or name objects is decreased, *Impaired verbal communication* becomes a problem. As memory diminishes and disorientation increases, *Impaired environmental interpretation syndrome, Impaired memory,* and *Confusion* occur.

Additional family issues may emerge. Perhaps some of the most crucial aspects of the patient's care are support, education, and referrals for the family. The family loses an integral part of its unit. Family members lose the love, the function, the support, the companionship, and the warmth that this person once provided. *Caregiver role strain* is always present, and planning with the family and offering community support is an integral part of appropriate care. *Anticipatory grieving* is also an important phenomenon to assess and may be an important target for intervention. Helping the family grieve can make the task ahead somewhat clearer and at times less painful. Review Table 23-4 for examples of the types of everyday problems faced by people with dementia as these provide potential nursing diagnoses for confused patients.

OUTCOMES IDENTIFICATION

Families who have a member with dementia are faced with an exhaustive list of issues that need to be addressed. Table 23-4 provides a checklist that may help nurses and families identify areas for intervention. Self-care needs, impaired environmental interpretation, chronic confusion, ineffective individual coping, and caregiver role strain are just a few of the areas nurses and other health care members will need to target. Table 23-5 identifies signs and symptoms commonly experienced with dementia or delirium, offers potential nursing diagnoses, and suggests outcomes.

PLANNING

Planning care for a person with dementia is geared toward the person's immediate needs. The Functional Dementia Scale (Figure 23-1) can be used by nurses and families to plan strategies for addressing immediate needs and to track progression of the dementia.

Identifying level of functioning and assessing caregivers' needs help focus planning and identify appropriate community resources. Does the person or family need the following?

- Transportation services
- Supervision and care when primary caregiver is out of the home
- Referrals to day care centers
- Information on support groups within the community
- Meals on Wheels
- Information on respite and residential services
- Telephone numbers for help lines
- Home health services

IMPLEMENTATION

The attitude of unconditional positive regard is the nurse's single most effective tool in caring for people with dementia. It induces patients to cooperate with care, reduces catastrophic outbreaks, and increases family members' satisfaction with care. Box 23-3 lists *NIC* interventions related to the management of dementia, and Table 23-6 provides special guidelines for nurses, family members, and other caregivers to use in communicating with a cognitively impaired person.

TABLE 23-4 PROBLEMS THAT MAY AFFECT PEOPLE WITH DEMENTIA AND THEIR FAMILIES

PROBLEM	EXAMPLES
Memory impairment	Forgets appointments, visits, etc. Forgets to change clothes, wash, go to the toilet Forgets to eat, take medications Loses things
Disorientation	Time: mixes night and day, mixes days of appointments, wears summer clothes in winter, forgets age Place: loses way around house Person: has difficulty recognizing visitors, family, spouse
Need for physical help	Dressing Washing, bathing Toileting Eating Performing housework Maintaining mobility
Risks in the home	Falls Fire from cigarettes, cooking, heating Flooding Admission of strangers to home Wandering out
Risks outside the home	Competence, judgment, and risks at work Driving, road sense Getting lost
Apathy	Little conversation Lack of interest Poor self-care
Poor communication	Dysphasia
Repetitiveness	Repetition of questions or stories Repetition of actions
Uncontrolled emotion	Distress Anger or aggression Demands for attention
Uncontrolled behavior	Restlessness day or night Vulgar table or toilet habits Undressing Sexual disinhibition Shoplifting
Incontinence	Urine Feces Urination or defecation in the wrong place
Emotional reactions	Depression Anxiety Frustration and anger Embarrassment and withdrawal
Other reactions	Suspiciousness Hoarding and hiding
Mistaken beliefs	Still at work Parents or spouse still alive Hallucinations
Decision making	Indecisive Easily influenced Refuses help Makes unwise decisions
Burden on family	Disruption of social life Distress, guilt, rejection Family discord

TABLE 23-5 SIGNS AND SYMPTOMS, DIAGNOSES, AND OUTCOMES FOR THE CONFUSED PATIENT

SYMPTOMS	NURSING DIAGNOSES	OUTCOMES
Wanders, has unsteady gait, acts out fear from hallucinations or illusions, forgets things (leaves stove on, doors open), falls	*Risk for injury*	Remains safe in hospital or at home
Awake and disoriented during the night *(sundowning),* frightened at night	*Disturbed sleep pattern* *Fear* *Acute confusion*	Sleep pattern is regular, balances rest and activity
Unable to take care of basic needs, incontinence, imbalanced nutrition, insufficient fluid intake,	*Self-care deficit (bathing/hygiene, dressing, feeding, toileting)* *Ineffective coping* *Functional urinary incontinence* *Imbalanced nutrition: less than body requirements* *Risk for deficient fluid volume*	Self-care needs are met with optimal participation by the patient
Sees frightening things that are not there *(hallucinations),* mistakes everyday objects for something sinister and frightening *(illusions),* may become paranoid and think that others are doing things to confuse him or her *(delusions)*	*Anxiety* *Impaired environmental interpretation syndrome*	Anxiety is reduced to a mild-moderate level, acknowledges the reality of an object or sound after it is pointed out
Does not recognize familiar people or places, has difficulty with short- and/or long-term memory, forgetful, confused	*Acute/chronic confusion*	Reports feeling safe, responds well to orientation interventions

Continued

TABLE 23-5 SIGNS AND SYMPTOMS, DIAGNOSES, AND OUTCOMES FOR THE CONFUSED PATIENT—cont'd

SYMPTOMS	NURSING DIAGNOSES	OUTCOMES
Has difficulty with communication, cannot find words, has difficulty in recognizing objects and/or people, incoherent	*Impaired verbal communication* *Impaired social interaction*	Communicates needs, connects with other patients, visitors, and staff at an optimal level with a variety of verbal and nonverbal methods.
Devastated over losing place in life as known (during lucid moments), fearful and overwhelmed by what is happening	*Spiritual distress* *Hopelessness* *Situational low self-esteem* *Grieving*	Expresses feelings, demonstrates a decreased preoccupation with loss
Family and loved ones overburdened and overwhelmed, unable to care for patient's needs	*Disabled family coping* *Interrupted family processes* *Impaired home maintenance* *Caregiver role strain*	Family members: express feelings in a supportive environment, have access to counseling and support groups, participate in care, utilize respite care

Herdman, T. H. (Ed.). *Nursing diagnoses—Definitions and classification 2012–2014.* Copyright © 2012, 1994-2012 by NANDA International. Used by arrangement with John Wiley & Sons Limited; Moorhead, S., Johnson, M., Maas, M. L., & Swanson, E. (2013). *Nursing outcomes classification (NOC)* (5th ed.). St. Louis, MO: Mosby.

FUNCTIONAL DEMENTIA SCALE

Circle one rating for each item:
1. None or little of the time
2. Some of the time
3. Good part of the time
4. Most or all of the time

Client: ______________________
Observer: ______________________
Position or relation to patient: ______________
Facility: ______________________
Date: ______________________

1	2	3	4	1. Has difficulty in completing simple tasks on own (e.g., dressing, bathing, doing arithmetic).
1	2	3	4	2. Spends time either sitting or in apparently purposeless activity.
1	2	3	4	3. Wanders at night or needs to be restrained to prevent wandering.
1	2	3	4	4. Hears things that are not there.
1	2	3	4	5. Requires supervision or assistance in eating.
1	2	3	4	6. Loses things.
1	2	3	4	7. Appearance is disorderly if left to own devices.
1	2	3	4	8. Moans.
1	2	3	4	9. Cannot control bowel function.
1	2	3	4	10. Threatens to harm others.
1	2	3	4	11. Cannot control bladder function.
1	2	3	4	12. Needs to be watched so doesn't injure self (e.g., by careless smoking, leaving the stove on, falling).
1	2	3	4	13. Destructive of materials around him/her (e.g., breaks furniture, throws food trays, tears up magazines).
1	2	3	4	14. Shouts or yells.
1	2	3	4	15. Accuses others of doing bodily harm or stealing his or her possessions — when you are sure the accusations are not true.
1	2	3	4	16. Is unaware of limitations imposed by illness.
1	2	3	4	17. Becomes confused and does not know where he or she is.
1	2	3	4	18. Has trouble remembering.
1	2	3	4	19. Has sudden changes of mood (e.g., gets upset, angered, or cries easily).
1	2	3	4	20. If left alone, wanders aimlessly during the day or needs to be restrained to prevent wandering.

FIG 23-1 Functional Dementia Scale. (From Moore, J. T., Bobula, J. A., Short, T. B., & Mischel, M. [1983]. A functional dementia scale. *Journal of Family Practice, 16,* 498, Fig 17-2.)

BOX 23-3 *NIC* INTERVENTIONS FOR DEMENTIA MANAGEMENT

Definition: Provision of a modified environment for the patient who is experiencing a chronic confusional state

- Include family members in planning, providing, and evaluating care, to the extent desired.
- Determine and monitor cognitive deficit(s), using standardized assessment tool.
- Identify usual patterns of behavior for such activities as sleep, medication use, elimination, food intake, and self-care.
- Provide rest periods to prevent fatigue and reduce stress.
- Monitor nutrition and weight.
- Place identification bracelet on patient.
- Address patient by name when initiating interaction, and speak slowly.
- Give one simple direction at a time in a respectful tone of voice.
- Avoid frustrating patient by quizzing with orientation questions that cannot be answered.
- Use distraction, rather than confrontation, to manage behavior.
- Provide consistent caregivers, physical environment, and daily routine.
- Provide a low-stimulation environment with adequate lighting.
- Identify and remove potential dangers in environment for patient.
- Provide cues—such as current events, seasons, location, and names—to assist orientation.
- Seat patient at small table in groups of three to five for meals, as appropriate.
- Provide finger foods to maintain nutrition for patient who will not sit and eat.
- Select television or radio programs based on cognitive processing abilities and interests.
- Select one-to-one and group activities geared to patient's cognitive abilities and interests.
- Limit number of choices patient has to make so as not to cause anxiety.
- Place patient's name in large block letters in room and on clothing, as needed.
- Use symbols, rather than written signs, to assist patient in locating room, bathroom, or other area.

From Bulechek, G. M., Butcher, H. K., Dochterman, J. M., & Wagner, C. (2013). *Nursing interventions classification (NIC)* (6th ed.). St. Louis, MO: Mosby.

TABLE 23-6 GUIDELINES FOR COMMUNICATION WITH PEOPLE WITH DEMENTIA

INTERVENTION	RATIONALE
Always identify yourself and call the person by name at each meeting.	The person's short-term memory is impaired—requires frequent orientation to time and environment.
Speak slowly.	The person needs time to process information.
Use short, simple words and phrases.	The person may not be able to understand complex statements or abstract ideas.
Maintain face-to-face eye contact.	Verbal and nonverbal clues are maximized.
Be near the person when talking, one or two arm-lengths away.	This distance can help the person focus on speaker as well as maintain personal space.
Focus on one piece of information at a time.	Attention span of the person is poor, and the person is easily distracted—helps the person focus. Too much data can be overwhelming and can increase anxiety.
Talk with the person about familiar and meaningful things.	Self-expression is promoted, and reality is reinforced.
Encourage reminiscing about happy times in life.	Remembering accomplishments and shared joys helps distract the person from deficit and gives meaning to existence.
When the person is delusional, acknowledge the person's feelings and reinforce reality. Do not argue or refute delusions.	Acknowledging feelings helps the person feel understood. Pointing out realities may help the person focus on realities. Arguing can enhance adherence to false beliefs.
If the person gets into an argument with another person, stop the argument and temporarily separate those involved. After a short while (5 minutes), explain to each person matter-of-factly why you had to intervene.	Escalation to physical acting out is prevented. The person's right to know is respected. Explaining in an adult manner helps maintain self-esteem.
When the person becomes verbally aggressive, acknowledge the person's feelings and shift the topic to more familiar ground (e.g., "I know this is upsetting for you because you always cared for others. Tell me about your children.")	Confusion and disorientation easily increase anxiety. Acknowledging feelings makes the person feel more understood and less alone. Topics the person has mastery over can remind him or her of areas of competent functioning and can increase self-esteem.
Have the person wear prescription eyeglasses or hearing aid.	Environmental awareness, orientation, and comprehension are increased, which in turn increases awareness of personal needs and the presence of others.
Keep the person's room well lit.	Environmental clues are maximized.
Have clocks, calendars, and personal items (e.g., family pictures or Bible) in clear view of the person while he or she is in bed.	These objects assist in maintaining personal identity.
Reinforce the person's pictures, nonverbal gestures, Xs on calendars, and other methods used to anchor the person in reality.	When aphasia starts to hinder communication, alternate methods of communication need to be instituted.

From Bulechek, G. M., Butcher, H. K., Dochterman, J. M., & Wagner, C. (2013). *Nursing interventions classification (NIC)* (6th ed.). St. Louis, MO: Mosby.

Person-Centered Care Approach

The conventional construction of dementia, based on a biological model and focusing on deficits, has been that the person is eventually "lost" to the disease (Davis, 2004). When viewed in this way, people with dementia can be isolated into a "social death" by being treated "as if" they are already dead (Tappen, Williams, Fishman, & Touhy, 1999). In fact, the social aspects of a person's life are the first to be threatened by dementia as other people change the way they respond to the person (Buron, 2008).

These views are currently being challenged with a model of care that focuses on the preservation of the personhood of people with dementia and attends to their psychosocial world as possible triggers for observed behaviors. For example, when treated as if "they are no longer there," people with dementia can become withdrawn or agitated. Thus, their behavior is a result of the way they are being treated, rather than symptoms of a disease.

Called *person-centered care* (PCC) (Kitwood, 1997), this model is based on an ethical stance that personhood in dementia remains and should be honored. It is especially relevant to nursing care because it is based on an appreciation that people exist in a social, relational world. More importantly, forming positive and enriching interpersonal relationships with people who have dementia can offset the disabling effects of the disease (Brooker, 2007; Davis, 2004; Dewing, 2008). For example, if verbalization becomes difficult for the person with dementia through the loss of language and difficultly with word retrieval, nurses may view their communication as confused and meaningless. When interpreted in this manner, attempts to establish social connection diminish, thus further isolating the person with dementia and denying a basic human need for belonging (Acton, Yauk, Hopkins, & Mayhew, 2007).

PCC is being used and tested throughout the world (Edvardsson, Winblad, & Sandman, 2008). A recent randomized trial demonstrated that this approach reduced agitation in people with dementia who were being treated in residential aged care settings (Chenoweth et al., 2009).

Health Teaching and Health Promotion

Educating families who have a cognitively impaired member is one of the most important health-teaching duties nurses encounter. Families who are caring for a member in the home need to know about strategies for communicating and for structuring self-care activities (Table 23-7).

Most importantly, families need to know where to get help. Help includes professional counseling and education regarding the process and progression of the disease. Families especially need to know about and be referred to community-based groups that can help shoulder this tremendous burden (e.g., day care centers, senior citizen groups, organizations providing home visits and respite care, and family support groups). A list with definitions of some of the types of services available in the person's community, as well as the names and telephone numbers of the providers of these services, should be given to the family.

Referral to Community Supports

The Alzheimer's Association is a national umbrella agency that provides various forms of assistance to persons with the disease and their families. Additional resources that might be available in some communities are found in Table 23-8.

EVIDENCE-BASED PRACTICE

Addressing Unmet Needs in Older Adults

Chenoweth, L., King, M., Jeon, Y., Brodaty, H., Stein-Parbury, J., Norman, R., Haas, M., & Luscombe, G. (2009). Caring for Aged Dementia Care Resident Study (CADRES) of person-centred care, dementia-care mapping, and usual care in dementia: a cluster-randomised trial. *Lancet Neurology, 8*, 317–325.

Problem

Caring for people with dementia can be challenging for nursing staff, especially when people with dementia demonstrate behaviors such as agitation, sleep disturbance, pacing, crying, and calling out. Such behaviors are not always a result of the dementia but can signal distress from unmet needs (Algase, et al., 1996). More importantly, the way that nurses respond to such behavior can influence the well-being of people with dementia, for better or worse.

Purpose of Study

The purpose of this study was to test the effectiveness of person-centered care (PCC) and dementia care mapping (a method of implementing PCC) compared to usual care in residential care settings for people with dementia.

Methods

A cluster-randomized trial was used to compare the implementation of PCC, dementia care mapping, and usual care based on outcomes for residents (n=289) in 15 residential care settings. A host of measures was used, including resident well-being, and were taken at baseline, at 4 months after intervention, and again at 4-month follow-up.

Key Findings

There was significant reduction in agitation (as measured by the Cohen-Mansfield Agitation Inventory) in both the dementia care mapping and the PCC interventions sites when compared to the usual care sites. In addition, an economic analysis revealed that PCC was costeffective.

Implications for Nursing Practice

When caring for people with dementia, nurses must attend to how they are approaching and treating the person. Interpreting behavior not as a biological sign of an illness but rather as a sign of unmet needs can improve well-being for people with dementia. Nurses must realize that their care approach has considerable impact on the person with dementia, and that agitation is not necessarily a sign of dementia per se but a result of the psychosocial environment.

TABLE 23-7 **PATIENT AND FAMILY TEACHING: GUIDELINES FOR SELF-CARE IN DEMENTIA**

INTERVENTION	RATIONALE
Dressing and Bathing	
Always have the person perform all tasks within his or her present capacity.	Maintains the person's self-esteem and uses muscle groups; impedes staff burnout; minimizes further regression.
Always have the person wear own clothes, even if in the hospital.	Helps maintain the person's identity and dignity.
Use clothing with elastic and substitute fastening tape (Velcro) for buttons and zippers.	Minimizes the person's confusion and eases independence of functioning.
Label clothing items with the person's name and name of item.	Helps identify the person if he or she wanders and gives the person additional clues when aphasia or agnosia occurs.
Give step-by-step instructions whenever necessary (e.g., "Take this blouse. Put in one arm . . . now the other arm. Pull it together in front. Now . . . .")	The person can focus on small pieces of information more easily; allows the person to perform at optimal level.
Make sure that water in faucets is not too hot.	Judgment is lacking in the person; the person is unaware of many safety hazards.
If the person is resistant to performing self-care, come back later and ask again.	Moods may be labile, and the person may forget but often complies after short interval.
Nutrition	
Monitor food and fluid intake.	The person may have anorexia or be too confused to eat.
Offer finger food that the person can take away from the dinner table.	Increases input throughout the day; the person may eat only small amounts at meals.
Weigh the person regularly (once a week).	Monitors fluid and nutritional status.
During periods of hyperorality, watch that the person does not eat nonfood items (e.g., ceramic fruit or food-shaped soaps).	The person puts everything into mouth; may be unable to differentiate inedible objects made in the shape and color of food.
Bowel and Bladder Function	
Begin bowel and bladder program early; start with bladder control.	Establishing same time of day for bowel movements and toileting—in early morning, after meals and snacks, and before bedtime—can help prevent incontinence.
Evaluate use of disposable diapers.	Prevents embarrassment.
Label bathroom door, as well as doors to other rooms.	Additional environmental clues can maximize independent toileting.
Sleep	
Because the person may awaken, be frightened, or cry out at night, keep area well lighted.	Reinforces orientation, minimizes possible illusions.
Maintain a calm atmosphere during the day.	Encourages a calming night's sleep.
Order nonbarbiturates (e.g., chloral hydrate) if necessary.	Barbiturates can have a paradoxical reaction, causing agitation.
If medications are indicated, consider neuroleptics with sedative properties, which may be the most helpful (e.g., haloperidol [Haldol]).	Helps clear thinking and sedates.
Avoid the use of restraints.	Can cause the person to become more terrified and fight against restraints until exhausted to a dangerous degree.

Although many families manage the care of their loved one until death, other families eventually find that they can no longer deal with the labile and aggressive behavior, incontinence, wandering, unsafe habits, or disruptive nocturnal activity. Family members need to know where and how to place their loved one for care if this becomes necessary. Families need information, support, and legal and financial guidance at this time. When the nurse is unable to provide the relevant information, proper referrals by the social worker are needed. Information regarding advance directives, durable power of attorney, guardianship, and conservatorship should be included in the communication with the family. Useful guidelines for families in structuring a safe environment and planning appropriate activities are found in Table 23-9.

Pharmacological Interventions

Table 23-10 presents drugs used in the United States to treat AD.

Cognitive Impairment

There is currently no cure for Alzheimer's disease; however, there are five AD drugs approved by the U.S. Food and Drug Administration (FDA) that are considered to be "disease

CONSIDERING CULTURE

The Influence of Culture on Caregiving in Dementia

It has long been recognized that caregivers suffer a great deal of burden in relation to caring for a person with dementia. They are prone to emotional distress, depression, and decreased quality of life as they cope with caregiving. It also has been recognized that the experience of stress and coping varies among cultural groups. Research studies on caregiving in dementia frequently use race/ethnicity as a control variable and therefore fail to capture the role of cultural values in the caregiving process.

A systematic review of the studies that investigated caregiving in dementia among Chinese Americans revealed two major themes. The first is that Chinese Americans hold cultural beliefs about dementia that differ from Western culture. Rather than view dementia as a "disease," Chinese Americans depicted dementia as "fate" or "wrongdoing." In addition, they perceived the memory loss associated with dementia, especially in the early stages, as part of normal aging. As the disease progresses, dementia is viewed as a mental illness with associated stigma and "loss of face," resulting in feelings of humiliation. The second theme identified in the review was the importance of "filial piety" and family harmony, which emphasizes an honor and devotion to parents, with an accompanying obligation to sacrifice individual needs and wants in order to be of benefit to parents.

The beliefs and values of Chinese Americans in their caregiving role place enormous stress on coping resources. They are more likely to just "grin and bear" the burden of caregiving; in fact, they may not perceive their caregiving role as burdensome. They are less likely to seek help from others than other cultural groups.

This review highlights the importance of cultural awareness and understanding when addressing the needs of family caregivers in dementia.

Sun, F., Ong, R., & Burnette, D. (2012). The influence of ethnicity and culture on dementia caregiving: a review of empirical studies on Chinese Americans. *American Journal of Alzheimer's Disease & Other Dementias*, 27(1), 13–32.

TABLE 23-8 TYPES OF SERVICES THAT MAY BE AVAILABLE TO PEOPLE WITH DEMENTIA

TYPE OF SERVICE	SERVICES PROVIDED
Family/caregiver Some people may live by themselves in the community; active case management is vital.	Caregivers have a right to: Easy access to services Respite care Full involvement in decision making Assessment of the needs of both the caregiver and the person with dementia Information and referral Case management: coordination of community resources and follow-up
Community services	Adult day care: provides activities, socialization, supervision Physician services Protective services: prevent, eliminate, and/or remedy effects of abuse or neglect Recreational services Transportation Mental health services Legal services
Home care	Meals on Wheels Home health aide services Homemaker services Hospice services Occupational therapy Paid companion or sitter services Physical therapy Skilled nursing Personal care services: assistance in basic self-care activities Social work services Telephone reassurance: regular telephone calls to individuals who are isolated and homebound* Personal emergency response systems: telephone-based systems to alert others that a person who is alone is in need of emergency assistance*

*Vital for those living alone.

modifying" and may slow the progression of the illness (Lehne, 2013). Since a deficiency of acetylcholine has been linked to AD, medications aimed at preventing its breakdown (cholinesterase inhibitors) have been developed, including tacrine hydrochloride, donepezil, rivastigmine, and galantamine. Memantine (Namenda) normalizes levels of glutamate, a neurotransmitter that may contribute to neurodegeneration (Lehne, 2013). Refer to Chapter 3 for a more-detailed discussion of drugs used to treat AD.

Although these medications are used widely and have been shown to have statistically significant effects when compared to placebos, it seems that they produce only a clinically marginal effect on cognition, behavior, or quality of life (Raina et al., 2008); nonetheless, they do delay the cognitive progression of dementia and assist with some of the behavioral symptoms.

Tacrine (Cognex) was the first cholinesterase inhibitor to be approved by the FDA for the treatment of mild to moderate

TABLE 23-9 PATIENT AND FAMILY TEACHING: GUIDELINES FOR CARE AT HOME

INTERVENTION	RATIONALE
Safe Environment	
Gradually restrict use of the car.	As judgment becomes impaired, the person may be dangerous to self and others.
Remove throw rugs and other objects in person's path.	Minimizes tripping and falling.
Minimize sensory stimulation.	Decreases sensory overload, which can increase anxiety and confusion.
If the person becomes verbally upset, listen briefly, give support, then change the topic.	Goal is to prevent escalation of anger. When attention span is short, the person can be distracted to more productive topics and activities.
Label all rooms and drawers. Label often-used objects (e.g., hairbrushes and toothbrushes).	May keep the person from wandering into other persons' rooms. Increases environmental clues to familiar objects.
Install safety bars in bathroom.	Prevents falls.
Supervise the person when he or she smokes.	Danger of burns is always present.
If the person has history of seizures, keep padded tongue blades at beside. Educate family on how to deal with seizures.	Seizure activity is common in advanced Alzheimer's disease.
Wandering	
If the person wanders during the night, put mattress on the floor.	Prevents falls when the person is confused.
Have the person wear medical alert bracelet that cannot be removed (with name, address, and telephone number). Provide police department with recent pictures.	The person can easily be identified by police, neighbors, or hospital personnel.
Alert local police and neighbors about wanderer.	May reduce time necessary to return the person to home or hospital.
If the person is in hospital, have him or her wear brightly colored vest with name, unit, and phone number printed on back.	Makes the person easily identifiable.
Put complex locks on door.	Reduces opportunity to wander.
Place locks at top of door.	In moderate and late Alzheimer's-type dementia, ability to look up and reach upward is lost.
Encourage physical activity during the day.	Physical activity may decrease wandering at night.
Explore the feasibility of installing sensor devices.	Provides warning if the person wanders.
Useful Activities	
Provide picture magazines and children's books when the person's reading ability diminishes.	Allows continuation of usual activities that the person can still enjoy; provides focus.
Provide simple activities that allow exercise of large muscles.	Exercise groups, dance groups, and walking provide socialization, as well as increased circulation and maintenance of muscle tone.
Encourage group activities that are familiar and simple to perform.	Activities such as group singing, dancing, reminiscing, and working with clay and paint all help to increase socialization and minimize feelings of alienation.

symptoms of AD. It improves functioning and slows the progress of the disease, particularly in the areas of cognition and memory, in about 20% to 50% of patients. Unfortunately, tacrine is associated with a high frequency of side effects, including elevated liver transaminase levels, gastrointestinal effects, and liver toxicity (Healy, 2005). As a result, it is no longer actively marketed for use with dementia (Wright et al., 2008).

Donepezil (Aricept), approved by the FDA in 1996, inhibits acetylcholine breakdown. It also appears to slow down deterioration in cognitive functions but without the potentially serious liver toxicity attributed to tacrine. This is the drug of choice for AD because of its once-per-day dosing and fewer side effects (Lehne, 2013). In studies of donepezil, some individuals with AD did experience diarrhea and nausea while taking the drug.

Rivastigmine (Exelon), a brain-selective acetylcholinesterase inhibitor, was approved in 2000. The most common side effects are nausea, vomiting, loss of appetite, and weight loss. In most cases, these side effects are temporary (Lehne, 2013). Rivastigmine should always be taken with food to reduce gastrointestinal side effects.

TABLE 23-10 DRUG TREATMENT FOR ALZHEIMER'S DISEASE

GENERIC (TRADE)	ACTION	INDICATIONS	SIDE EFFECTS	WARNINGS
Cholinesterase Inhibitors				
Tacrine* (Cognex) Donepezil* (Aricept) Rivastigmine* (Exelon) Galantamine* (Razadyne)	Prevent the breakdown of acetylcholamine and thereby increase its availability at cholinergic synapses	Modestly improves cognition, behavior, function. Slows disease progression.	Nausea, vomiting, diarrhea, insomnia, fatigue, muscle cramps, incontinence, bradycardia, and syncope	Tacrine no longer used extensively, owing to hepatotoxicity. Donepezil is better tolerated; dosage is only once a day and is preferred. Rivastigmine available as a once-daily patch.
***N*-methyl-d-aspartate (NMDA) Antagonist**				
Memantine* (Namenda, Namenda XR)	Normalizes levels of glutamate, which in excessive quantities contributes to neurodegeneration	Treatment of moderate to severe Alzheimer's disease; no evidence that it modifies underlying disease	Dizziness, agitation, headache, constipation, and confusion	Clearance is reduced with renal impairment. Use cautiously with moderate renal impairment. Do not use with severe renal impairment.
Antidepressants—Selective Serotonin Reuptake Inhibitors				
Citalopram (Celexa) Escitalopram (Lexapro) Fluoxetine (Prozac) Paroxetine (Paxil) Sertraline (Zoloft)	Blocks the reuptake of serotonin, thereby making more available and improving mood	Useful with depression, irritability, sleep disturbances, and anxiety	Agitation, insomnia, headache, nausea and vomiting, sexual dysfunction, and hyponatremia	Discontinuation syndrome—dizziness, insomnia, nervousness, irritability, nausea, and agitation—may occur with abrupt withdrawal (depending on half-life). Taper slowly.
Antianxiety Agents				
Lorazepam (Ativan) Oxazepam (Serax)	Facilitates the action of the inhibitory neurotransmitter GABA	Anxiety, restlessness, verbally disruptive behavior, and resistance	Drowsiness, dizziness, headaches. Restlessness, insomnia, and increased anxiety possible	Use cautiously due to risk for further memory impairment, sedation, and falls.
Antipsychotics				
Aripiprazole (Abilify) Olanzapine (Zyprexa) Quetiapine (Seroquel) Risperidone (Risperdal) Ziprasidone (Geodon)	Blockade of serotonin and dopamine receptors	**Used with extreme caution** for paranoid thinking, hallucinations, and agitation; questionable efficacy in clinical trials	Many; refer to Chapters 3 and 12. Weight gain, increased serum glucose, and hyperlipidemia.	Lower dose used in the elderly. Nighttime dose is preferred. FDA Alert for increased risk of CVA and death in dementia patients issued in 2005.
Anticonvulsants				
Carbamazepine (Tegretol) Divalproex (Depakote)	Reduces the excitability of neurotransmission	Agitated and aggressive behavior and emotional lability	Ataxia, sedation, confusion, and (rarely) bone marrow suppression	Monitor the complete blood count and liver-associated enzymes.

*Approved by the U.S. Food and Drug Administration for treatment of Alzheimer's disease.

Data from Bourgeois, J. A., Seaman, J. S., & Servis, M. E. (2008). Delirium, dementia, and amnestic and other cognitive disorders. In R. E. Hales, S. C. Yudofsky, & G. O. Gabbard (Eds.), *Textbook of psychiatry.* Arlington, VA: American Psychiatric Association; Lehne, R. A. (2013). *Pharmacology for nursing care* (8th ed.). St. Louis, MO: Elsevier; Wright, C. I., Trinh, N., Blacker, D., & Falk, W. E. (2008). Dementia. In T. A. Stern, J. F. Rosenbaum, M. Fava, J. Biederman, & S. L. Rauch (Eds.), *Massachusetts General Hospital comprehensive clinical psychiatry* (pp. 231–246). St. Louis, MO: Mosby.

Galantamine (Razadyne [formerly known as *Reminyl*]) is a reversible cholinesterase inhibitor approved for use in the United States in 2001 (Lehne, 2013). Galantamine also works to increase the concentration of acetylcholine by blocking the action of acetylcholinesterase, the enzyme that breaks down acetylcholine. Galantamine is prescribed in the first and second stages of AD.

All of the cholinesterase inhibitors have the potential to cause nausea, diarrhea, and vomiting. In addition, they should be used with caution when patients are taking nonsteroidal antiinflammatory drugs (NSAIDs).

Memantine (Namenda) (approved for treatment of Alzheimer's disease in 2003) is the first drug to target symptoms during the moderate to severe stages of the disorder, but it is not approved by the FDA for mild symptoms. This drug works by regulating the activity of glutamate, a chemical involved in learning and memory (Lehne, 2013).

Behavioral Symptoms

Other medications are often useful in managing the behavioral symptoms of individuals with dementia, but these need to be used with extreme caution. The rule of thumb for elderly people is "start low and go slow." In addition, because people with dementia are at high risk of developing delirium, adding medications should always be done with caution.

Some of the troubling behaviors exhibited by people with dementia, with which their caregivers must cope, are (1) psychotic symptoms (hallucinations, paranoia), (2) severe mood swings (depression is very common), (3) anxiety (agitation), and (4) verbal or physical aggression (combativeness).

In June 2008, the FDA warned that the use of antipsychotics, both conventional and atypical, is no longer indicated for dementia-related psychosis because they are associated with increased risk of death (USFDA, 2008).

Of clinical relevance to nurses is the evidence that suggests that personalized nursing care, in which the idiosyncratic needs of the person are recognized and met, is as effective as nonpharmacological treatment for the behavioral problems associated with dementia (Ayalon et al., 2006). With this evidence in mind, nurses should try to decipher patients' needs as expressed in their behavior; people with dementia do not always communicate their needs verbally (see Evidence-Based Practice box on page 446).

Integrative Therapy

A number of herbal or all-natural drugs are under investigation; however, currently there is not enough scientific evidence concerning their effectiveness or harmfulness. Keep in mind that the designation *all-natural* or *herbal* does not mean that a substance is safe. Some alternative treatments being investigated include *Ginkgo biloba*. According to Kidd (2008), omega-3 fatty acids, other antioxidant nutrients, and vitamins—especially folate, B_6, B_{12}, C, and E—may also be helpful in the treatment of AD.

EVALUATION

The outcome criteria for people with cognitive impairments need to be measurable, within the capabilities of the individual person, and evaluated frequently. As the person's condition continues to deteriorate, outcomes must be altered to reflect the person's diminished functioning. Frequent evaluation and reformulation of outcome criteria and short-term indicators also help reduce staff and family frustration and minimize the patient's anxiety by ensuring that tasks are not more complicated than the person can accomplish.

The overall outcomes for treatment are to promote the person's optimal level of functioning and to delay further regression whenever possible. Working closely with family members and providing them with the names of available resources and support sources may help increase the quality of life for both the family and the patient with AD (Case Study and Nursing Care Plan 23-1).

23-1 CASE STUDY AND NURSING CARE PLAN

Cognitive Impairment

During the past 4 years, Mr. Ludwig has demonstrated rapidly progressive memory impairment, disorientation, and deterioration in his ability to function, related to Alzheimer's disease. He is a 67-year-old man who retired at age 62 to spend some of his remaining "youth" with his wife and to travel, garden, visit family, and finally to get to do the things they always wanted to do. At age 63, he was diagnosed with Alzheimer's disease.

Mr. Ludwig has been taken care of at home by his wife and his daughter, Kelly. Kelly is divorced and has returned home with her two young daughters.

The family members find themselves close to physical and mental exhaustion. Mr. Ludwig is becoming increasingly incontinent when he cannot find the bathroom. He wanders away from home, despite close supervision. The police and neighbors bring him back home an average of four times a week. Once, he was lost for 5 days after he somehow boarded a bus for Pittsburgh, 1000 miles from home. He was robbed and beaten before being found by the police and returned home.

He frequently wanders into his granddaughters' rooms at night while they are sleeping and tries to get into bed with them. Too young to understand that their grandfather is lonely and confused, they fear that he is going to hurt them. Four times in the past 2 weeks, he has fallen while getting out of bed at night, thinking he is in a sleeping bag, camping out in the mountains. After a conflicted and painful 2 months, the family places him in a care facility for persons with Alzheimer's disease.

Mrs. Ludwig tells the admitting nurse, Mr. Jackson, that her husband wanders almost all the time. He has difficulty finding the right words for things (aphasia) and becomes frustrated and angry when that happens. Sometimes he does not seem to recognize the family (agnosia). Once, he thought that Kelly was a thief breaking into the house and attacked her with a broom handle. Telling this story causes Kelly to break down into heavy sobs: "What's happened to my father? He was so kind and gentle. Oh, God . . . I've lost my father."

Mrs. Ludwig tells Mr. Jackson that her husband can sometimes participate in dressing himself; at other times, he needs total assistance. At this point, Mrs. Ludwig begins to cry uncontrollably, saying, "I can't bear to part with him . . . but I can't do it anymore. I feel as if I've betrayed him."

Mr. Jackson then focuses his attention on Mrs. Ludwig and her experience. He states, "This is a difficult decision for you. "Mr. Jackson suggests that Mrs. Ludwig talk to other families who have a cognitively impaired member. "It might help you to know that you are not alone, and having contact with others to share your grief can be healing." One of the groups he suggests is the Alzheimer's Association, a well-known self-help group.

Self-Assessment

Mr. Jackson has worked on his particular unit for 4 years. It is a unit especially designed for cognitively impaired individuals, which makes nursing care easier than on a regular unit. He applied for this position shortly after his own father died of complications secondary to Alzheimer's disease. Mr. Jackson refers to the process of living and dying with this disease as horrifying; his goal is to help others go through this with caring, dignity, and the highest level of functioning possible.

Caring for Mr. Ludwig and his family is becoming especially personal. Mr. Jackson is struck by the similarity between this family's situation and his own. Mr. Ludwig is about the same age his father had been, looks similar to him, and has many of his mannerisms. Mrs. Ludwig and her daughter Kelly seem to be responding in much the same way his family did. He finds that he is having stronger than usual transference feelings with this family and even became teary when Mrs. Ludwig did.

The evening after he met the Ludwigs, Mr. Jackson went home utterly exhausted and continued to think about them and his own father. He shared these feelings with his wife, and the two of them spent some time talking about his father and all they had been through together, good and bad. In the end, Mr. Jackson sat back, breathed a long, deep sigh of relief, and thanked his wife for being there for him. He told his wife that he supposed he will never really get over the death of his father, but he is getting better every day.

When Mr. Jackson returned to work, he nearly walked right into Mr. Ludwig, who was standing at the doorway wearing two shirts, a pair of pajama bottoms, and a baseball cap. "Are you the man who's taking me to pick up my car?" he asks. Mr. Jackson smiles and says, "It looks like you have quite a day planned. Let's start with a cup of coffee," and redirects him to the day hall.

Assessment

Objective Data

- Patient wanders away from home about four times a week.
- Was lost for 5 days and was robbed and beaten.
- Often incontinent when he cannot find the bathroom.
- Has difficulty finding words.
- Has difficulty identifying members of the family at times.
- Has difficulty dressing himself at times.
- Falls out of bed at night.
- Has memory impairment.
- Is disoriented much of the time.
- Gets into bed with granddaughters at night when wandering.
- Family undergoing intense feelings of loss and guilt.

Subjective Data

- "I can't bear to part with him."
- "I feel as if I've betrayed him."
- "I've lost my father."

Diagnosis

1. *Risk for injury*

Supporting Data

- Wanders away from home about four times a week.
- Wanders despite supervision.
- Falls out of bed at night.
- Gets into other people's beds.
- Wanders at night.

2. *Functional urinary incontinence* related to disturbed cognition, as evidenced by inability to find the toilet

Supporting Data

- Incontinent when he cannot find the bathroom

3. Dressing/grooming *self-care deficit* (self-dressing deficits) related to impaired cognitive functioning, as evidenced by impaired ability to put on and take off clothing

Supporting Data

- Sometimes is able to dress with help of wife.
- At other times is too confused to dress self at all.

23-1 CASE STUDY AND NURSING CARE PLAN—cont'd

Cognitive Impairment

4. *Anticipatory grieving* related to loss and deterioration of family member

Supporting Data

- "I can't bear to part with him."
- "I feel as if I've betrayed him."
- "I've lost my father."
- Family undergoing intense feelings of loss and guilt.

Outcomes Identification

Although Mr. Ludwig has many unmet needs that require nursing interventions, Mr. Jackson decides to focus on the four initial nursing diagnoses. As other problems arise, they will be addressed.

NURSING DIAGNOSIS	LONG-TERM GOALS	SHORT-TERM GOALS
1. *Risk for injury* as evidenced by wandering	1. Resident will remain safe in nursing home.	1a. Throughout nursing home stay, resident will not fall out of bed. 1b. Throughout nursing home stay, resident will wander only in protected area. 1c. Resident will be returned within 2 hours if he succeeds in escaping from the unit.
2. *Functional urinary incontinence* related to disturbed cognition, as evidenced by inability to find the toilet	2. Resident will experience less incontinence (fewer episodes) by fourth week of hospitalization.	2a. By the end of 4 weeks, resident will participate in toilet training. 2b. By the end of 4 weeks, resident will find the toilet most of the time.
3. *Self-care deficit* (self-dressing) related to impaired cognitive functioning, as evidenced by impaired ability to put on and take off clothes	3. Resident will participate in dressing himself 80% of the time.	3a. By the end of 4 weeks, resident will follow step-by-step instructions for dressing most of the time. 3b. By the end of 4 weeks, resident will dress in own clothes with aid of fastening tape.
4. *Anticipatory grieving* related to loss and deterioration of family member	4. In 3 months' time, all family members will state that they feel they have more support and are able to talk about their grieving.	4a. After 3 months, family members will state that they have opportunity to express "unacceptable" feelings in supportive environment. 4b. After 3 months, family members will state that they have found support from others who have a family member with Alzheimer's disease.

Planning

Mr Jackson plans care to ensure Mr. Ludwig's safety, provide for the maintenance of his hygiene needs and incontinence, and assist Mrs. Ludwig as she deals with her husband's deterioration.

Implementation

Using the concepts of *NIC*, Mr. Jackson's plan of care (Nursing diagnosis: *Risk for injury* as evidenced by wandering) was personalized as follows:

SHORT-TERM OUTCOME	INTERVENTION	RATIONALE	EVALUATION
1. Throughout nursing home stay, resident will not fall out of bed.	1a. Spend time with resident on admission. 1b. Label resident's room in big, colorful letters. 1c. Remove mattress from bed and place on floor. 1d. Keep room well lit at all times. 1e. Show resident clock and calendar in room. 1f. Keep window shade up.	1a. Lowers anxiety, provides orientation to time and place. Resident's confusion is increased by change. 1b. Offers clues in new surroundings. 1c. Prevents falling out of bed. 1d. Provides important environmental clues; helps lower possibility of illusions. 1e. Fosters orientation to time. 1f. Allows day-night variations.	**GOAL MET** Mattress on floor prevents falls out of bed.
2. Throughout nursing home stay, resident will wander only in protected area.	2a. At night, take resident to large, protected, well-lit room. 2b. Alert physician to check resident for cardiac decompensation. 2c. Offer snacks when resident is awake (e.g., milk, decaffeinated tea, sandwich). 2d. Allow soft music on radio. 2e. Spend short, frequent intervals with resident. 2f. Take resident to bathroom after snacks. 2g. During day, offer activities that include use of large muscle groups.	2a. Resident is able to wander safely in protected environment. 2b. Addresses possible underlying cause of nocturnal wakefulness and wandering. 2c. Helps replace fluid and caloric expenditure. 2d. Helps induce relaxation. 2e. Decreases resident's feelings of isolation and increases orientation. 2f. Helps prevent incontinence. 2g. For some residents helps decrease wandering.	**GOAL MET** Resident continues to wander at night; with supervision, keeps out of other residents' rooms most of the time. By fourth week, resident starts to nap on couch in large room after snacks during the night.

Continued

23-1 CASE STUDY AND NURSING CARE PLAN—cont'd

Cognitive Impairment

SHORT-TERM OUTCOME	INTERVENTION	RATIONALE	EVALUATION
3. Resident will be returned within 2 hours if he succeeds in escaping from the unit.	3a. Order MedicAlert bracelet for resident (with name, unit, hospital, and phone number). 3b. Place brightly colored vest on resident with name, unit, and phone number taped on back. 3c. Check resident's whereabouts periodically during the day and especially at night.	3a. If resident gets out of hospital, he can be identified. 3b. If resident wanders in hospital, he can be identified and returned. 3c. Helps monitor resident's activities.	**GOAL MET** By fourth week, resident wanders off unit only once; is found in lobby and returned by security guard within 45 minutes.

Evaluation

Although Mr. Ludwig continues to display wandering behaviors, his wandering is contained to safe areas of the unit except for one instance when he wanders to the lobby. He is stopped by security and safely returned to the unit within 45 minutes. He has not fallen out of bed. Nursing interventions, such as placing his mattress on the floor and ensuring adequate lighting, increase his safety while at the same time acknowledging that he continues to exhibit wandering behaviors.

KEY POINTS TO REMEMBER

- *Neurocognitive disorder* is a term that refers to disorders resulting from changes in the brain and marked by disturbances in orientation, memory, intellect, judgment, and affect.
- Delirium and dementia are discussed in this chapter because they are the neurocognitive disorders most frequently seen by health care workers.
- Delirium is marked by acute onset, disturbance in consciousness, and symptoms of disorientation and confusion that fluctuate by the minute, hour, or time of day.
- Delirium is always secondary to an underlying condition; therefore, it is temporary, transient, and may last from hours to days once the underlying cause is treated. If the cause is not treated, permanent damage to neurons can result.
- Dementia usually has a more insidious onset than delirium. Global deterioration of cognitive functioning (e.g., memory, judgment, ability to think abstractly, and orientation) is often progressive and irreversible, depending on the underlying cause.
- Dementia may be primary (e.g., Alzheimer's disease [AD], vascular dementia, Pick's disease, Lewy body disease). In this case, the disease is irreversible.
- All types of dementia are diagnosed as either mild (modest cognitive decline) or major (substantial cognitive decline).
- Alzheimer's disease accounts for up to 70% of all cases of dementia, and vascular dementia accounts for about 20%.
- There are various theories regarding the cause of AD, but none is definitive.
- Signs and symptoms change according to the four stages of AD: stage 1 (mild), stage 2 (moderate), stage 3 (moderate to severe), and stage 4 (late).
- The behavioral manifestations of AD include confabulation, perseveration, aphasia, apraxia, agnosia, and hyperorality.
- No known cause or cure exists for AD, although a number of drugs that increase the brain's supply of acetylcholine (a nerve-communication chemical) are helpful in slowing the progress of the disease.
- People with AD have many unmet needs and present numerous management challenges to both their families and health care workers.
- Specific nursing interventions for cognitively impaired individuals can increase communication, safety, and self-care and are described in the chapter. The need for family teaching and support is strong.

CRITICAL THINKING

1. Mrs. Kendel is an 82-year-old woman who has Alzheimer's disease. She lives with her husband, who has been trying to care for her in their home. Mrs. Kendel is having trouble dressing. She has put her blouse on backwards and sometimes puts her bra on over her blouse. She often forgets where things are. She makes an effort to cook but has recently attempted to "put out" the electric burners of the stove with pitchers of water. Once in a while, she cannot find the bathroom in time, often mistaking it for a closet. At times, she cries because she is aware that she is losing her sense of her place in the world. She and her husband have always been close, loving companions, and he wants to keep her at home as long as possible.
   a. Assist Mr. Kendel by writing out a list of suggestions that he can try at home that might help facilitate (a) communication, (b) activities of daily living, and (c) maintenance of a safe home environment.
   b. Identify at least three interventions that are appropriate to this situation for each of the areas cited above.
   c. Identify resources available for maintaining Mrs. Kendel in her home for as long as possible. Provide the name of a self-help group that you would urge Mr. Kendel to join.
2. Share with your class or clinical group the name and function of at least three community agencies in your area that could be an appropriate referral for a family with a member with dementia. (For one, you can contact the Alzheimer's Association to find a local chapter; www.alz.org.)

CHAPTER REVIEW

1. Evelyn, a 73-year-old woman with pneumonia becomes agitated after being admitted to the intensive care unit through the emergency department. Her vital signs are erratic, and her thinking seems disorganized. During her first 24 hours in ICU, the patient varies from somnolent to agitated and from laughing to angry shouting. Her daughter reports that the patient "was never like this at home." What is the most likely explanation for the situation?
   - **a.** Pneumonia has worsened the patient's early-stage dementia.
   - **b.** The patient is experiencing delirium secondary to the pneumonia.
   - **c.** The patient is sundowning due to the decreased stimulation of the intensive care unit.
   - **d.** The patient does not want to be in the hospital and is angry that staff will not let her leave.
2. Intervention(s) appropriate for Evelyn and other hospitalized patients experiencing delirium include which of the following? *Select all that apply.*
   - **a.** Immediately placing the patient in restraints if she begins to hallucinate or act irrationally or unsafely
   - **b.** Ensuring that a clock and a sign indicating the day and date are displayed where the patient can see them easily
   - **c.** Being prepared for possible hostile responses to efforts to take vital signs or provide direct physical care
   - **d.** Preventing sensory deprivation by placing the patient near the nurses' station and leaving the television and multiple lights turned on 24 hours per day
   - **e.** Speaking with the patient frequently for short periods for reassurance, assisting the patient in remaining oriented, and ensuring the patient's safety
   - **f.** Anticipating that the patient may try to leave if agitated and providing for continuous direct observation to prevent wandering
3. Mrs. Smith dies at the age of 82. In the 2 months following her death, her husband, aged 84 and in good health, has begun to pay less attention to his hygiene and seems less alert to his surroundings. He complains of difficulty concentrating and sleeping and reports that he lacks energy. His family sometimes has to remind and encourage him to shower, take his medications, and eat, all of which he then does. Which response is most appropriate?
   - **a.** Reorient Mr. Smith by pointing out the day and date each time you have occasion to interact with him.
   - **b.** Meet with family and support persons to help them accept, anticipate, and prepare for the progression of his stage II dementia.
   - **c.** Avoid touch and proximity; these are likely to be uncomfortable for Mr. Smith and may provoke aggression when he is disoriented.
   - **d.** Arrange for an appointment with a therapist for evaluation and treatment of suspected depression.
4. You are preparing Genevieve, an 86-year-old patient diagnosed with Alzheimer's disease, for discharge and giving discharge education to Genevieve's family, who will be caring for her. Which of the following intervention(s) would be beneficial to teach Genevieve's family? *Select all that apply.*
   - **a.** Recommend switching to hospital-type gowns to facilitate bathing, dressing, and other physical care of the patient.
   - **b.** Discourage wandering by installing complex locks or locks placed at the tops of doors where the patient cannot readily reach them.
   - **c.** For situations in which the patient becomes upset, teach loved ones to listen briefly, provide support, and then change the topic.
   - **d.** Recognize that the patient can no longer successfully interact with others; provide a darkened, quiet room for her to spend her time.
   - **e.** Encourage caregivers to care for themselves, as well as the patient, via use of support resources such as adult day care or respite care.
   - **f.** If the patient is prone to wandering away, encourage family to notify police and neighbors of the patient's condition, wandering behavior, and description.
5. Which statement about dementia is accurate?
   - **a.** The majority of people over age 85 are affected by dementia.
   - **b.** Disorientation is the dominant and most disruptive symptom of dementia.
   - **c.** People with early dementia do not tend to be distressed by symptoms.
   - **d.** Hypertension, diminished activity levels, and head injury increase the risk of dementia.

Answers to Chapter Review

1. b; 2. b, c, e, f; 3. d; 4. a, b, c, e, f; 5. d.

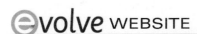

Visit the Evolve website for a posttest on the content in this chapter: http://evolve.elsevier.com/Varcarolis

Post-Test interactive review

REFERENCES

Acton, G .J., Yauk, S., Hopkins, B. A., & Mayhew, P. A. (2007). Increasing social communication in persons with dementia. *Research and Theory for Nursing Practice, 21*(1), 32–44.

Algase, D., Beck, C., Kolanowski, A., Whal, A., Berent, S. K., & Richards, K. (1996). Need-driven compromised behavior: An alternative view of disruptive behavior. *American Journal of Alzheimer's Disease, 11*(6), 10–19.

Alzheimer's Association. (2007). *FDA-approved treatments for Alzheimer's.* Retrieved from http://alz.org.national/documents/topicsheet_treatments.pdf.

Alzheimer's Association. (2012). Alzheimer's disease facts and figures. *Alzheimer's and Dementia, 8,* 131–168.

American Psychiatric Association. (2013). *Diagnostic and statistical manual of mental disorders (DSM 5)* (5th ed.). Washington, DC: Author.

Ayalon, L., Gunn, A. M., Feliciano, L., & Areân, P. A. (2006). Effectiveness of nonpharmacological interventions for the management of neuropsychiatric symptoms in patients with dementia. *Archives of Internal Medicine, 166,* 2182–2188.

Brooker, D. (2007). Person-centred dementia care: Making services better. In M. Downs (Series Ed.), *Bradford dementia group good practice guides*. London, UK: Jessica Kingsley Publishers.

Bulechek, G. M., Butcher, H. K., Dochterman, J. M., & Wagner, C. (2013). *Nursing interventions classification (NIC)* (6th ed.). St. Louis, MO: Mosby.

Buron, B. (2008). Levels of personhood: A model for dementia care. *Geriatric Nursing, 29*(5), 324–332.

Caplan, J. P., Cassem, N. H., Murray, G. B., Park, J. M., & Stern, T. A. (2008). Delirium. In T.A. Stern, J. F. Rosenbaum, M. Fava, J. Biederman, & S. L. Rauch (Eds.), *Massachusetts General Hospital comprehensive clinical psychiatry* (pp. 217–229). St. Louis, MO: Mosby.

Cerejeira, J., & Mukactova-Ludinska, E. B. (2011). A clinical update on delirium: From early recognition to effective management. *Nursing Research and Practice, 2011*. doi:10.1155/2011/875196.

Chenoweth, L., King, M., Jeon, Y., Brodaty, H., Stein-Parbury, J., Norman, R., et al. (2009). Caring for Aged Dementia Care Resident Study (CADRES) of person-centred care, dementia-care mapping, and usual care in dementia: A cluster-randomised trial. *Lancet Neurology, 8*, 317–325.

Davis, D. H. J. (2004). Dementia: Sociological and philosophical constructions. *Social Science and Medicine, 58*, 369–378.

Dewing, J. (2008). Personhood and dementia: Revisiting Tom Kitwood's ideas. *International Journal of Older People Nursing, 3*, 3–13.

Duppils, G. S., & Wikblad, K. (2007). Patients' experiences of being delirious. *Journal of Clinical Nursing, 16*, 810–818.

Edvardsson, D., Winblad, B., & Sandman, P. (2008). Person-centred care of people with severe Alzheimer's disease: Current status and ways forward. *Lancet Neurology*, 7, 362–67.

Ferri, C. P., Prince, M., Brayne, C., Brodaty, H., Fratiglioni, L., Ganguli, M., et al. (2005). Global prevalence of dementia: A Delphi consensus study. *The Lancet, 366*(9503), 2112–2117.

Flagg, B., Cox, L., McDowell, S., Mwose, J. M., & Buelow, J. M. (2010). Nursing identification of delirium. *Clinical Nurse Specialist, 24*(5), 260–266.

Healy, D. (2005). *Psychiatric drugs explained* (4th ed.). Edinburgh, UK: Churchill Livingstone.

Herdman, T. H. (Ed.), (2012). *NANDA international nursing diagnoses: Definitions and classification 2012–2014*. Oxford, UK: Wiley-Blackwell.

Holmes, C., Boche, D., Wilkinson, D., Yadegarfar, G., Hopkins, V., Bayer, A., et al. (2008). Long-term effects of A beta(42) immunisation in Alzheimer's disease: Follow-up of a randomized, placebo-controlled phase I trial. *The Lancet, 372*(9634), 216–223.

Holtzman, D. M., (2008). Moving towards a vaccine. *Nature, 454*, 418–420.

Jones, C., Bäckman, C., Capuzzo, M., Flaatten, H., Rylander, C., & Griffiths, R. D. (2007). *Intensive Care Medicine, 33*, 978–985.

Jones, C., Griffiths, R. D., Humphris, G., & Skirrow, P. M. (2001). Memory, delusions, and the development of acute posttraumatic stress disorder-related symptoms after intensive care. *Critical Care Medicine, 29*, 573–580.

Kidd, P. M. (2008). Alzheimer's disease, amnestic mild cognitive impairment, and age-associated memory impairment: Current understanding and progress toward integrative prevention. *Alternative Medicine Review, 13*(2), 85–115.

Kitwood, T. (1997). *Dementia reconsidered: The person comes first*. Buckingham, UK: Open University Press.

Lehne, R. A. (2013). *Pharmacology for nursing care* (8th ed.). St. Louis, MO: Elsevier.

Michaud, L., Büla, C., Berney, A., Camus, V., Voellinger, R., Stiefel, F., & Burnand, B. (2007). Delirium: Guidelines for general hospitals. *Journal of Psychosomatic Research, 62*, 371–383.

Milisen, K., Lemiengre, J., Braes, T., & Foreman, M. D. (2005). Multicomponent intervention strategies for managing delirium in hospitalized older people: Systematic review. *Journal of Advanced Nursing, 52*(1), 79–90.

Mitchell, A. J., & Shiri-Feshki, M. (2009). Rate of progression of mild cognitive impairment to dementia—meta-analysis of 41 robust inception cohort studies. *Acta Psychiatrica Scandinavica, 119*(4), 252–265.

Moorhead, S., Johnson, M., Maas, M., & Swanson, E. (2013). *Nursing outcomes classification (NOC)* (5th ed.). St. Louis, MO: Mosby.

Quinlan, N., & Rudolph, J. L. (2011). Postoperative delirium and functional decline after noncardiac surgery. *Journal of the American Geriatric Society, 59*(S2), S301–S304.

Raina, P., Santaguida, P., Ismaila, A., Patterson, C., Cowan, D., Levine, M., et al. (2008). Effectiveness of cholinesterase inhibitors and memantine for treating dementia: Evidence review for a clinical practice guideline. *Annals of Internal Medicine, 148*(5), 379–397.

Rice, K. L., Bennett, M., Gomez, M., Theall, K. P., Knight, M., & Foreman, M. D. (2011). Nurses' recognition of delirium in the hospitalized older adult. *Clinical Nurse Specialist, 2011*, 299–311.

Rudolph, J. L., & Marcantonio, E. R. (2011). Postoperative delirium: Acute change with long-term implications. *Anesthesia & Analgesia, 112*(5), 1202–1211.

Sadock, B. J., & Sadock, A. (2008). *Kaplan and Sadock's concise textbook of clinical psychiatry* (3rd ed.). Philadelphia, PA: Lippincott Williams & Wilkins.

Shankar, G., Li, S., Mehta, T., Garcia-Munoz, A., Shepardson, N., Smith, I., et al. (2008). Amyloid-protein dimers isolated directly from Alzheimer's brains impair synaptic plasticity and memory. *Nature Medicine, 14*, 837–842.

Siddiqi, N., Stockdale, R., Britton, A. M., & Holmes, J. (2007). Interventions for preventing delirium in hospitalized patients. *Cochrane Database of Systematic Reviews 2007*, (Issue 2), Art. No.: CD005563. doi:10.1002/14651858.CD005563.pub2.

Sperling, R. A., Aisen, P. S., Beckett, L. A., Bennett, D. A., Craft, S., Fagan, A. M., et al. (2011). Toward defining the preclinical stages of Alzheimer's disease: Recommendations from the National Institute on Aging. *Alzheimer's Dementia, 7*(3), 280–292. doi:10.1016/j.jalz.2011.03.003.

Tappen, R. M., Williams, C., Fishman, S., & Touhy, T. (1999). Persistence of self in advanced Alzheimer's disease. *Image: The Journal of Nursing Scholarship, 31*(2), 121–125.

Tasman, A., & Mohr, W. K. (2011). *Fundamentals of psychiatry*. Oxford, UK: Wiley-Blackwell.

U.S. Food and Drug Administration [USFDA]. (2008). *Information for healthcare professionals: Antipsychotics; FDA ALERT [6/16/2008]*. Retrieved from http://www.fda.gov/CDER/drug/InfoSheets/HCP/antipsychotics_conventional.htm

Wei, L. A., Fearing, M. A., Sternberg, E. J., & Inouye, S. K. (2008). The confusion assessment method: A systematic review of current usage. *Journal of the American Geriatrics Society, 56*, 823–830.

Wright, C. I., Trinh, N., Blacker, D., & Falk, W. E. (2008). Dementia. In T. A. Stern, J. F. Rosenbaum, M. Fava, J. Biederman, & S. L. Rauch (Eds.), *Massachusetts General Hospital comprehensive clinical psychiatry* (pp. 231–246). St: Louis, MO: Mosby.

CHAPTER

24

Personality Disorders

Claudia A. Cihlar

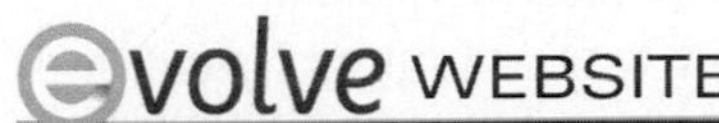

Visit the Evolve website for a pretest on the content in this chapter: http://evolve.elsevier.com/Varcarolis

Pre-Test interactive review

OBJECTIVES

1. Identify characteristics of each of the 10 personality disorders.
2. Analyze the interaction of biological determinants and psychosocial stress factors in the etiology of personality disorders.
3. Describe the emotional and clinical needs of nurses and other staff when working with patients who meet criteria for personality disorders.
4. Formulate a nursing diagnosis for each of the personality disorders.
5. Discuss two nursing outcomes for patients with antisocial and borderline personality disorder.
6. Plan basic interventions for a patient with impulsive, aggressive, or manipulative behaviors.
7. Identify the role of the advanced practice nurse when working with patients with personality disorders.

KEY TERMS AND CONCEPTS

antisocial personality disorder
avoidant personality disorder
borderline personality disorder
dependent personality disorder
diathesis-stress model
dialectical behavior therapy (DBT)
emotional dysregulation
emotional lability
histrionic personality disorder
narcissistic personality disorder
obsessive-compulsive personality disorder
paranoid personality disorder
personality
personality disorder
schizoid personality disorder
schizotypal personality disorder
separation-individuation
splitting

We may often meet someone and think, "She's quite a strange person" or "What an unusual character he is." When we make evaluations such as these about other people, we are reacting to their personalities. Personality comes from the Latin word *persona,* which means mask, and it may refer to what other people see.

Western scholars such as Hippocrates suggested that personality and general health problems were the results of an imbalance of essential bodily fluids. These fluids, or "humors," were phlegm (mucous), blood, and bile. The scientist Galen proposed that these humors produced personality profiles of *phlegmatic* (calm and unemotional), *sanguine* (lighthearted and unemotional), *melancholic* (creative and depressive), and *choleric* (energetic and passionate) (Kagan, 2005).

In the 19th century, Sigmund Freud proposed a construct of personality that created a paradigm shift from a biological imbalance to a psychological perspective for both healthy and disordered personality. Freud's hypothesis that personality emerged from childhood experiences rather than one's chemistry gave birth to the psychoanalytic movement.

Personality can be described operationally in terms of functioning. We know that personality can be protective for a person in times of difficulty but may also be a liability if one's personality results in ongoing relationship problems or leads to emotional distress on a regular basis (Clarkin & Huprich, 2011). **Personality** determines the quality of experiences among people and serves as a guide for one-to-one interaction and in social groups. Based on this description, we can tell when a personality is unhealthy, that is, "when it interferes with, or complicates, social and interpersonal function" (Blais et al., 2008, p. 527). In contemporary society there is a consensus that personality disorders exist on a continuum of severity and likely represent more extreme variations in normal personality development.

CLINICAL PICTURE

Personality disorders are among the most challenging and complex group of disorders to treat. Individuals who meet criteria for these disorders display significant challenges in self-identity or self-direction, and they have problems with empathy or intimacy within their relationships.

People with these disorders have difficulty recognizing or owning that their difficulties are problems of their personality. They may truly believe the problems originate outside of themselves. Still others may be unaware that their behavior is unusual, and they may not experience any distress (Skodol & Gunderson, 2008).

Judgments about an individual's personality functioning must take into account the person's ethnic, cultural, and social background. Patients who differ from the majority culture or the culture of the clinician may be at risk for overdiagnosis of a personality disorder; therefore, it is important to obtain additional information from others knowledgeable of the particular cultural or ethnic norms before determining the presence of a personality disorder.

According to the American Psychiatric Association (2013), there are 10 personality disorders (Box 24-1; also see Table 24-1). Eight of these disorders will be described in terms of prevalence, characteristic pathological responses, and etiology. A vignette is also provided to illustrate each of these disorders. Afterwards, two common and challenging personality disorders, antisocial and borderline, will be described in more depth along with an application of the nursing process.

BOX 24-1 PERSONALITY DISORDERS

- Paranoid personality disorder
- Schizoid personality disorder
- Schizotypal personality disorder
- Histrionic personality disorder
- Narcissistic personality disorder
- Avoidant personality disorder
- Dependent personality disorder
- Obsessive-compulsive personality disorder
- Antisocial personality disorder
- Borderline personality disorder

Paranoid Personality Disorder

Paranoid personality disorder occurs at a prevalence rate of about 1.7% in community samples (Torgersen, 2009). This disorder is characterized by a longstanding distrust and suspiciousness of others based on the belief (unsupported by evidence) that others want to exploit, harm, or deceive the person. These individuals are hypervigilant, anticipate hostility, and may provoke hostile responses by initiating a "counterattack." They demonstrate jealousy, controlling behaviors, and unwillingness to forgive. Paranoid persons are difficult to interview because they are reluctant to share information about themselves. Underneath the guarded surface, they are actually quite anxious about being harmed.

Paranoid personality disorder may be found in people who grew up in households where they were the objects of excessive rage and humiliation, which resulted in feelings of inadequacy (Skodol & Gunderson, 2008). Projection is the dominant defense mechanism; they blame others for their shortcomings.

People with this disorder tend to reject treatment. Antianxiety agents may be accepted as a method to improve relaxation. Agitation and delusions may be treated with antipsychotic medication.

VIGNETTE

Mrs. Alonzo is a 54-year-old unemployed female who comes to a mental health clinic complaining of depression and pain. She walks stiffly and uses two old, broken canes. She provides elaborate details about "nerve pain" all over her body resulting from an accident 5 years earlier. She states that multiple doctors refused to help her because of instructions from her insurance company. She believes that her health maintenance organization has circulated her medical record to all health care providers in the region to prevent her from being treated. She refuses to give any social history and is reluctant to share her telephone number. When the nurse indicates that the psychiatrist will not prescribe pain medications, she smiles bitterly and says, "So they already got to you."

Schizoid Personality Disorder

Schizoid personality disorder is fairly uncommon and is estimated to occur in around 0.9% of the population (Torgersen, 2009). People with schizoid personality disorder exhibit a poor ability to function in their lives. Relationships are particularly affected due to the prominent feature of emotional detachment. People with this disorder do not seek out or enjoy close relationships and are viewed as loners. Neither approval nor rejection from others seems to have much effect. Friendships, dating, and sexual experiences are rare. Employment may be jeopardized if interpersonal interaction is necessary; individuals with this disorder may be able to function well in a solitary occupation such as a security guard on the night shift. Feelings of being an observer rather than a participant in life are common. Depersonalization, or feelings of detachment from oneself and the world, may be present.

From a psychological perspective, people with this disorder are often raised in a cold and neglectful atmosphere in which they may conclude that relationships are unsatisfying and unnecessary. Genetically, this disorder may be based on a predisposition to shyness. Schizoid personality disorder can be a precursor to schizophrenia or delusional disorder, and there is

TABLE 24-1 PREVALENCE OF PERSONALITY DISORDERS BY TOTAL POPULATION, GENDER, AND COMMON COMORBIDITIES

PERSONALITY DISORDER	TOTAL POPULATION	GENDER	COMORBIDITY
Avoidant	1.7%	Equal in men and women	Mood disorders Anxiety disorders
Antisocial	1.1%	More men	Anxiety disorders Depressive disorders Substance use disorders Somatization disorders
Borderline	1.6%	More women	Mood disorders Substance use disorders Eating disorders Posttraumatic stress disorders Attention deficit hyperactivity disorder
Dependent	0.7%	More women	Mood disorders Anxiety disorders Adjustment disorders
Histrionic	1.5%	More women	Major depressive disorder Somatization disorder Conversion disorder
Narcissistic	<1%	More women	Depressive disorders Substance use disorders Anorexia nervosa
Paranoid	1.7%	More men	Major depressive disorder Agoraphobia Obsessive-compulsive disorders Substance abuse disorders
Obsessive-compulsive	2.1%	More men	Anxiety disorders Mood disorders Eating disorders
Schizoid	0.9%	More men	Major depressive disorder
Schizotypal	<1%	More men	Major depressive disorder

Data from Torgersen, S. (2009). Prevalence, sociodemographics, and functional impairment. In J. M. Oldham, A. E. Skodol, & D. S. Bender (Eds.), *Essentials of personality disorders* (pp. 83–102). Washington, DC: American Psychiatric Publishing.

increased prevalence of the disorder in families with a history of schizophrenia or schizotypal personality disorder.

Antidepressants such as bupropion (Wellbutrin) may help to increase pleasure in life. Second-generation antipsychotics, such as risperidone (Risperdal) or olanzapine (Zyprexa) are used to improve flattened emotions. Psychotherapy can help to improve sensitivity to others' social cues; group therapy provides experience in practicing interactions and feedback from others.

VIGNETTE

Mr. Gray is a 30-year-old single male who is a graduate student in mathematics at a large state university. He lives alone and has never been married. He works as an assistant in a math classroom in which the professor teaches the course via television. He wears thick eyeglasses, and his clothing is inconspicuous. He rarely smiles and seldom looks directly at the students, even when answering questions. He does get somewhat animated when he writes lengthy solutions to math problems on the blackboard. He is content with his low-paying job and has never been in psychiatric treatment.

Schizotypal Personality Disorder

Schizotypal personality disorder is more common in men than women and occurs at a rate of less than 1% in the general population (Torgersen, 2009). Despite its low prevalence, schizotypal personality disorder is so unusual and debilitating that it is one of the most studied personality disorders (Hummelen et al., 2011). In the *Diagnostic and Statistical Manual of Mental Illness*, 5th edition (DSM-5) (APA, 2013), it is identified as a both a personality disorder and the first of the schizophrenia spectrum disorders, which are, in general, listed from least to most severe. Chapter 12 discusses the schizophrenia spectrum disorders in greater detail.

Like schizoid personality disorder, persons with schizotypal personality disorder have severe social and interpersonal deficits. They experience extreme anxiety in social situations and contributions to conversations tend to ramble with lengthy, unclear, overly detailed, and abstract content. An additional feature of this disorder is paranoia; individuals with schizotypal personality disorder are overly suspicious and anxious. They tend to misinterpret the motivations of others as being out to get them and blame others for their social isolation. Odd beliefs (e.g., being overly superstitious) or magical thinking (e.g., thinking of themselves as psychic) are also common.

Psychotic symptoms seen in persons with schizophrenia, such as hallucinations and delusions, might also exist with schizotypal personality disorder, but to a lesser degree and only briefly (Skodol et al., 2011). A major difference between this disorder and schizophrenia is that people with schizotypal personality disorder can be made aware of their misinterpretations of reality. Schizophrenia results in a far stronger grip on delusions.

Although schizotypal personality disorder is generally diagnosed in adulthood, signs of the disorder tend to be present in childhood and adolescence. Prominent characteristics include being an underperformer in school and difficulty in connecting with peers. Characteristic communication eccentricities combined with unusual beliefs tend to make the child or adolescent a target for teasing and bullying.

As a schizophrenia spectrum disorder, schizotypal personality disorder is genetically linked. There is a higher incidence of schizophrenia-related disorders in family members of people with schizotypal personality disorder. There is growing evidence to support that persons with schizotypal personality disorder have structural abnormalities of the brain such as ventricular enlargement, reductions in the volume of their striatal structures, and altered dopamine transmission mechanisms (Skodol et al., 2011).

While there is no specific medication for schizotypal personality disorder, associated conditions may be treated. Persons with schizotypal personality disorders seem to benefit from low-dose antipsychotic agents for psychotic-like symptoms and day-to-day functioning (Ripoll et al., 2011). Depression and anxiety may be treated with antidepressants and antianxiety agents.

VIGNETTE

Raymond is a 55-year-old single male who lives with his mother. He is the youngest of seven children raised in a farming community. Three of his siblings are deaf, and Raymond also has some hearing loss. Raymond started therapy with Jenny, an advanced practice registered nurse in psychiatric mental health, after he suffered a career-ending injury from which he is completely disabled. Jenny and Raymond have been working together for several years on quality-of-life issues and depression. Raymond is frequently distressed by his unwavering belief that everyone in his hometown greets him with sexual gestures and believes he is gay. This fixation extends to truck drivers who come through the town; he thinks that they talk about his sexuality on their CB radios. These beliefs create great distress and anxiety for him. He occasionally yells at people or gestures back. Jenny has been helping Raymond to understand how his perceptions may be faulty and how his hearing loss may contribute to his perceptual difficulties and anxiety. Raymond and Jenny have invited his mother into the discussion so she can support him at home.

Histrionic Personality Disorder

Histrionic personality disorder is thought to occur at a rate of about 1.5 % in community samples (Torgersen, 2009). Persons with histrionic traits do not generally experience a reduction in quality of life. Studies focusing on heritability traits suggest there may be common risk factors for impulsivity, reduced levels of agreeableness and introversion (Skodol et al., 2001). This disorder is characterized by emotional attention-seeking behaviors, including self-centeredness, low frustration tolerance, and excessive emotionality. The person with histrionic personality disorder is often impulsive and melodramatic and may act flirtatiously or provocatively. Relationships do not last, because the partner often feels smothered or reacts to the insensitivity of the histrionic person. The individual with histrionic personality disorder does not have insight into his or her role in breaking up relationships and may seek treatment for depression or another comorbid condition. In the treatment setting, the person demands "the best of everything" and can be very critical.

Histrionic personality disorder has been explained from a psychodynamic perspective as beginning at 3 to 5 years of age with an overly intense attachment to the opposite-sex parent, which results in fear of retaliation by the same-sex parent. Inborn character traits such as emotional expressiveness and egocentricity have also been identified as predisposing an individual to this disorder.

In general, people with this disorder do not think they need psychiatric help. They may go into treatment for associated problems such as depression that may be precipitated by losses, such as loss of a relationship. Psychotherapy is the treatment of choice for this disorder. Medications such as antidepressants and antianxiety agents may be helpful in treating associated symptoms.

VIGNETTE

Ms. Lombard is a 35-year-old, twice-divorced female admitted to an inpatient unit after an overdose of asthma medications and antibiotics. She took all of her pills after her primary care doctor refused to order a sleeping pill for her. On the first night, she is withdrawn and tearful in her room. But the next morning, she is neatly groomed, even wearing makeup, and socializes with everyone. She denies thoughts of self-harm. Over the next 2 days, Ms. Lombard monopolizes the community meetings by talking about how unappreciated she is by her family and physician. She seeks special attention from an evening-shift male RN, asking if he can stay late after his shift to sit with her. When he refuses, she demands to be placed back on one-to-one precautions because she suddenly feels suicidal again.

Narcissistic Personality Disorder

Narcissistic personality disorder is thought to be one of the least frequently occurring personality disorders. In the community it exists at less than 1%, but it is seen in clinical populations more frequently (Torgersen, 2009). Narcissistic personality disorder is also associated less than other personality disorders with impairment in individual functioning and the quality of one's life.

These persons come across as arrogant with an inflated view of their self-importance. The individual with this disorder has a need for constant admiration, along with a lack of empathy for others, a factor that strains most relationships over time.

A sense of personal entitlement paired with a lack of social empathy may result in the exploitation of other people.

Underneath the surface of arrogance, persons with narcissistic personality disorder feel intense shame and have a fear of abandonment. In keeping with these descriptions, the main pathological personality trait of narcissism is antagonism, represented by the grandiosity and attention-seeking behaviors of these individuals. As a result, narcissistic individuals may seek help for depression or may seek to be validated by therapists and/or loved ones for their emotional pain of not being appreciated enough by others for their efforts or special qualities.

Narcissistic personality disorder may be the result of childhood neglect and criticism. The child does not learn that other people can be the source of comfort and support. As adults, they hide feelings of emptiness with an exterior of invulnerability and self-sufficiency. Little is known about inborn traits or heritability for this disorder.

There is no medication indicated for this disorder. Treatment includes individual cognitive-behavioral therapy, family therapy, and group therapy,

VIGNETTE

Dr. Abigail McLaughlin is a 40-year-old female attending psychiatrist at a university outpatient center. She is twice divorced and has no children. Her grooming and makeup are impeccable, and she likes to chat about her expensive shopping habits. She is quite intelligent and is the only doctor on the staff trained in psychoanalysis. In clinical team meetings, she often discusses this fact, repeatedly telling others that psychoanalysis is the best treatment for mental illness. She frequently makes derogatory remarks to psychiatric residents if they suggest alternative treatment approaches for new cases. She is usually late to staff meetings, and when she is not speaking, she yawns and shifts noisily in her seat. She has a reputation for exhibiting angry outbursts at therapists in the hallway for minor mistakes, such as a scheduling error for a patient. She underwent 7 years of psychoanalysis but does not consider it to have been therapy—it "was only for training purposes."

Avoidant Personality Disorder

Avoidant personality disorder is fairly common and is believed to occur in about 1.7% of the U.S. population (Torgersen, 2009). The main pathological personality traits are low self-esteem that is associated with functioning in social situations, feelings of inferiority compared to peers, and a reluctance to engage in unfamiliar activities involving new people.

Avoidant personality disorder has been linked with parental and peer rejection and criticism. A biological predisposition to anxiety and physiological arousal in social situations has also been suggested. Genetically, this disorder may be part of a continuum of disorders related to social anxiety disorder; studies have found a shared association between persons who have avoidant personality disorder and persons with social anxiety disorder (Skodol et al., 2011). A timid temperament in infancy and childhood may also be associated with this disorder.

CONSIDERING CULTURE

Ageism, Culture of Aging, and Personality Disorders in Older Adults

Ageism, or the discrimination of persons based upon their age, is ubiquitous in our Western culture with its emphasis on youth. This bias even permeates health care settings that are designed to serve the needs of older adults. Stereotypes regarding older adults interfere with accurate assessment of older adults. The presence of personality disorders further complicates the provision of their care.

In addition, aging brings with it natural changes in social relationships, most notably more social isolation and loss. Since personality disorders profoundly affect the ability to function effectively in relationship with others, there is a greater likelihood that issues will become exacerbated and affect their care in later life.

While the traditional belief is that personality disorders "age out," new research indicates that these problems continue throughout the lifespan. Nurses are more successful in addressing the needs of older adults with personality disorders when they examine their biases about aging and personality disorders. A flexible approach supporting a "goodness of fit" style that recognizes strength-based values of the client, the family members, and the system of care involved with them may be followed.

Magoteaux, A. L., & Bonnivier, J. F. (2009). Distinguishing between personality disorders, stereotypes, and eccentricities in older adults. *Journal of Psychosocial Nursing, 47*(7), 19–24.

Persons with avoidant personality disorders seem to respond positively to antidepressant medications such as selective serotonin reuptake inhibitors like citalopram and selective norepinephrine reuptake inhibitors such as venlafaxine (Ripoll et al., 2011). Individual and group therapy is useful in processing anxiety-provoking symptoms and in planning methods to approach and handle anxiety-provoking situations.

VIGNETTE

Ms. Lowell is a 35-year-old single female who works for a computer repair company. As a child, she had few friends and never participated in extracurricular activities. She lives alone in her own apartment and has never had an adult intimate relationship. On the job, she rarely talks to co-workers and prefers to work alone. If she has any questions, she asks the supervisor and carefully follows directions. Although she has 7 years of experience and a good work record, she refuses the offer of a promotion because it would require her to interact with customers.

Dependent Personality Disorder

The prevalence rate of dependent personality disorder is about 0.7 % in community samples and has been found to be associated with moderate to low problems in functioning (Skodol et al., 2011). However, there are discrepant studies that suggest this disorder may be more common.

Persons with dependent personality disorder have a high need to be taken care of, which can lead to patterns of submissiveness with fears of separation and abandonment by others. This may create problems for sufferers by leaving them more vulnerable to exploitation by others because of their passive and submissive nature. Feelings of insecurity about their self agency may interfere with attempts at becoming more independent in their life roles.

Persons with dependent personality disorder are thought to have early and profound learning experiences during childhood in which disordered attachment and dependency on the caretaker develop. Dependent personality disorder may be the result of chronic physical illness or punishment of independent behavior in childhood. Childhood trauma has been suggested as a stress factor associated with the development of personality disorders in general and, as such, has also been found to be linked to neuroendocrine changes, both cortisol and adrenocorticotropin-releasing hormone (Birgenheir & Pepper, 2011). The inherited trait of submissiveness may also be a factor, which has been found to be 45% heritable.

There are no specific medications indicated for this disorder, but symptoms of depression and anxiety may be treated with the appropriate medications. Psychotherapy is the treatment of choice for this disorder. The goal is for the person to be more independent and to form meaningful relationships. The therapeutic relationship can provide a testing ground for increased assertiveness. Cognitive behavioral therapy can help in the development of new perspectives and attitudes about other people.

VIGNETTE

Ashley is a 32-year-old, married, former engineer, and she is mother to two young children, ages 3 years and 11 months. Her therapist, an advanced practice registered nurse, recommended that she come for brief treatment of depression and anxiety at the partial hospitalization program. Ashley's depression and anxiety have been more severe since she stopped working. She feels inadequate and overwhelmed by her responsibilities, so her mother moved in with the young family at her daughter's request. Ashley bonded quickly with her case manager and psychiatrist, both older women. She frequently asks them for reassurance that she is doing the "right thing" by coming to treatment. She seeks them out frequently for extra individual sessions. During her group therapies over the course of treatment, Ashley begins to realize that excessive dependence on her mother contributes to longstanding feelings of ineffectiveness, helplessness, and invalidation of her own parenting skills.

Obsessive-Compulsive Personality Disorder

Obsessive-compulsive personality disorder is the most prevalent personality disorder in the general community and in clinical populations; its prevalence rate is estimated at 2.1% (Torgersen, 2009). Along with borderline personality disorder, this disorder is associated with the highest burden of medical costs, and obsessive-compulsive personality disorder affects workplace productivity losses (Skodol et al., 2011).

The main pathological personality traits are rigidity and inflexible standards of self and others along with persistence to goals long after it is necessary, even if it is self-defeating or relationship-defeating. Persons with obsessive-compulsive personality disorder feel genuine affection for friends and family but do not have insight about their own difficult behavior. Internally, they are fearful of imminent catastrophe. They rehearse over and over how they will respond in social situations. These individuals do not have full-blown obsessions or compulsions but may seek treatment for anxiety or mood disorders. This disorder has been associated with increased relapse rates of depression and an increase in suicidal risks in persons with co-occurring depression.

Obsessive-compulsive personality disorder is associated with excessive parental criticism, control, and shame. The child in this atmosphere responds to this negativity by trying to control his environment through perfectionism and orderliness. Heritable traits such as compulsivity, oppositionality, lack of emotional expressiveness, and perfectionism have all been implicated in this disorder.

Selective serotonin reuptake inhibitors such as fluoxetine (Prozac) are Food and Drug Administration (FDA) approved for the treatment of the more severe version of this disorder, obsessive-compulsive disorder. Drugs such as Prozac may help reduce the obsessions, anxiety, and depression associated with this disorder. Psychotherapy may provide additional support. Group therapy and self-help groups have been found to be especially helpful in sharing and learning from others.

VIGNETTE

Mr. Wright is a 45-year-old single male postal worker in a small town. He lives alone and has never married. He is well groomed and wears a clean, neatly ironed uniform every day. He carefully follows all policies and procedures and is quite resistant whenever there is any update or change. He frequently challenges the supervisor about policy details and has been referred to the regional personnel office countless times for resolution of these conflicts. In staff meetings, he gives excessive circumstantial details and writes extra material on the back of any required report form. When dealing with the public, he sometimes gets into arguments with customers about postal rules or the schedule. The other staff do not consider him to be a team player because he seldom volunteers to help others. Even if he is asked to help someone, he is quick to criticize his peer's performance. Although he has worked in the same office for 10 years, he has never advanced beyond the front-line position. He is fairly content with his work and has never been in psychiatric treatment.

EPIDEMIOLOGY AND COMORBIDITY

While studies vary in their estimates of prevalence depending upon methodologies, personality disorders affect about 6% of the global population (Huang et al., 2009). In the U.S. population the overall prevalence rate of personality disorders among community samples is higher—around 10% (Sansone & Sansone, 2011).

Culture has a definite influence on the rate of diagnosing personality disorders. For example, Australian and North American studies reflect higher prevalence rates (Samuels, 2011). Differences may reflect personality and behavior as being viewed as deviant rather than normative in a particular culture and study methods. It is generally agreed that there are insufficient studies to address the role that ethnicity and race have on the prevalence of personality disorders (McGilloway et al., 2010).

Personality disorders frequently co-occur with disorders of mood and eating, anxiety, and substance abuse. Personality disorders often amplify **emotional dysregulation**, a term that describes poorly modulated mood characterized by mood swings. Individuals with emotion regulation problems have ongoing difficulty managing painful emotions in ways that are healthy and effective.

Other studies confirm that personality disorders are more common among persons who are homeless or incarcerated. Recent studies have also suggested that personality disorders affecting older adults are more common than originally thought and frequently become evident when accompanied by major depression or anxiety (Magoteaux & Bonnivier, 2009).

ETIOLOGY

Personality disorders are the result of complex biological and psychosocial phenomena that are influenced by multifaceted variables involving genetics, neurobiology, chemistry, and environmental factors. An overview of the possible causes of personality disorders is provided.

Biological Factors

Genetic

Genetics are thought to influence the development of personality disorders (Skodol & Gunderson, 2008). Recently, studies have led to a consensus that personality disorders represent extreme variations of normal personality traits in four areas: anxious-dependency traits, psychopathy-antisocial, social withdrawal, and compulsivity (Svrakic et al., 2008). These findings support a genetic or inherited trait transmission in families.

Neurobiological

The chemical neurotransmitter theory proposes that certain neurotransmitters, including neurohormones, may regulate and influence temperament. Research in brain imaging has also revealed some differences in the size and function of specific structures of the brain in persons with some personality disorders (Coccaro & Siever, 2005).

Psychological Factors

Several psychological theories may help to explain the development of personality disorders. Learning theory emphasizes that the child developed maladaptive responses based on modeling or reinforcement by important people in the child's life. Cognitive theories emphasize the role of beliefs and assumptions in creating emotional and behavioral responses that influence one's experiences within the family environment.

Psychoanalytic theory focuses on the use of primitive defense mechanisms by individuals with personality disorders. Defense mechanisms such as repression, suppression, regression, undoing, and splitting have been identified as dominant (Kernberg, 1985). The role of psychoanalytic theory, while historically relevant and interesting, is not confirmable through evidence-based research methods.

Environmental Factors

Behavioral genetics research has shown that about half of the variance accounting for personality traits emerges from the environment (Paris, 2005). These findings suggest that while the family environment is influential on development, there are other environmental factors besides family upbringing that shape an individual's personality. One need only think about the individual differences among siblings raised together to illustrate this point.

Childhood neglect or trauma has been established as a risk factor for personality disorders (Samuels, 2011). This association has been linked to possible biological mechanisms involving corticotropin-releasing hormone in response to early life stress and emotional reactivity (Lee et al., 2011).

Diathesis-Stress Model

The **diathesis-stress model** is a general theory that explains psychopathology using a systems approach. This theory helps us understand how personality disorders emerge from the multifaceted factors of biology and environment (Paris, 2005). *Diathesis* refers to genetic and biological vulnerabilities and includes personality traits and temperament. *Temperament* is our tendency to respond to challenges in predictable ways. Descriptors of temperament may be "laid back," referring to a calm temperament, or "uptight," as an example of an anxious temperament. These characteristics remain stable throughout a person's life.

In this model, *stress* refers to immediate influences on personality, such as the physical, social, psychological, and emotional environment. Stress also includes what happened in the past, such as growing up in one's family with exposure to unique experiences and patterns of interaction. Under conditions of stress, the diathesis-stress model proposes that personality development becomes maladaptive for some people, resulting in the emergence of a personality disorder (Paris, 2005).

There is a two-way directionality among stressors and diatheses. Genetic and biological traits are believed to influence the way an individual responds to the environment, while at the same time, the environment is thought to influence the expression of inherited traits. Many studies have suggested a strong correlation between trauma, neglect, and other dysfunctional family or social patterns of interaction on the development of personality disorders among individuals with certain personality traits and temperament.

Table 24-2 provides an overview of nursing and other therapies for the treatment of all the personality disorders discussed above. Two additional personality disorders, antisocial

TABLE 24-2 **NURSING AND THERAPY GUIDELINES FOR PERSONALITY DISORDERS**

PERSONALITY DISORDER	CHARACTERISTICS	NURSING GUIDELINES	SUGGESTED THERAPIES
Antisocial	Can seem normal Exhibits no anxiety or depression Manipulative Exploitive of others Aggressive Seductive Callous toward others	1. Try to prevent or reduce untoward effects of manipulation (flattery, seductiveness, instilling of guilt): Set clear and realistic limits on specific behavior. Ensure that limits are adhered to by all staff. Carefully document signs of manipulation or aggression. Document behaviors (give times, dates, circumstances). Provide clear boundaries and consequences. 2. Be aware that antisocial patients can instill guilt when they are not getting what they want. Guard against being manipulated through feelings of guilt. 3. Substance abuse is best handled through a well-organized treatment program before counseling and other forms of therapy are started.	1. More responsive to psychotherapy when hospitalized than when jailed 2. Pharmacotherapy for anxiety, rage, and depression 3. Careful use of addictive agents (e.g., benzodiazepines) 4. Ritalin may help ADHD 5. Anticonvulsants may help impulsive behavior
Avoidant	Excessively anxious in social situations Hypersensitive to negative evaluation Desire social interaction	1. A friendly, accepting, reassuring approach is the best way to treat patients. 2. Being pushed into social situations can cause extreme and severe anxiety.	1. Psychotherapy focuses on trust 2. Group therapy 3. Assertiveness training 4. Antidepressants and antianxiety agents helpful; β-adrenergic receptor antagonists (e.g., atenolol) help reduce autonomic nervous system hyperactivity
Borderline	Shows separation anxiety Manifests ideas of reference Impulsive (suicide, self-mutilation) Engages in splitting (adoring then devaluing persons)	1. Set realistic goals; use clear action words. 2. Be aware of manipulative behaviors (flattery, seductiveness, instilling of guilt). 3. Provide clear and consistent boundaries and limits. 4. Use clear and straightforward communication. 5. When behavioral problems emerge, calmly review the therapeutic goals and boundaries of treatment. 6. Avoid rejecting or rescuing. 7. Assess for suicidal and self-mutilating behaviors, especially during times of stress.	1. Individual psychotherapy 2. Dialectical behavior therapy 3. Group therapy 4. Antipsychotics may control anger and brief psychosis 5. Antidepressants such as SSRIs and MAOIs 6. Benzodiazepines help anxiety
Dependent	Excessively clinging Self-sacrificing, submissive Needy, gets others to care for him or her	1. Identify and help address current stresses. 2. Try to satisfy patient's needs at the same time that limits are set up in such a manner that patient does not feel punished and withdraw. 3. Be aware that strong countertransference often develops in clinicians because of patient's excessive clinging (demands of extra time, nighttime calls, crisis before vacations); therefore, supervision is well advised. 4. Teach and role-model assertiveness.	1. Insight-oriented psychotherapy, behavioral therapy, assertiveness training. 2. Family and group therapy 3. Antianxiety agents and antidepressants used for specific symptoms. Panic attacks can be helped with imipramine.
Histrionic	Seductive Flamboyant Attention seeking Shallow Depressive and suicidal when admiration withdrawn	1. Understand seductive behavior as a response to distress. 2. Keep communication and interactions professional, despite temptation to collude with the patient in a flirtatious and misleading manner. 3. Encourage and model the use of concrete and descriptive rather than vague and impressionistic language. 4. Teach and role-model assertiveness.	1. Group therapy 2. Treatment of comorbid personality disorders 3. Antidepressants as needed

TABLE 24-2 NURSING AND THERAPY GUIDELINES FOR PERSONALITY DISORDERS—cont'd

PERSONALITY DISORDER	CHARACTERISTICS	NURSING GUIDELINES	SUGGESTED THERAPIES
Narcissistic	Exploitive Grandiose Disparaging Filled with rage Very sensitive to rejection, criticism Cannot show empathy Handles aging poorly	1. Remain neutral; avoid engaging in power struggles or becoming defensive in response to the patient's disparaging remarks. 2. Convey unassuming self-confidence.	1. Psychotherapy only works after patient acknowledges narcissism 2. Group therapy may help empathy 3. Lithium may help those with mood swings; antidepressants also used
Obsessive-compulsive	Perfectionistic Has need for control Inflexible, rigid Preoccupied with details Highly critical of self and others	1. Guard against power struggles with patient. Need for control is very high. 2. Intellectualization, rationalization, reaction formation, isolation, and undoing are the most common defense mechanisms.	1. Supportive or insightful psychotherapy 2. Clomipramine and SSRIs for obsessional thinking and depression
Paranoid	Projects blame Suspicious and mistrustful Hostile and violent Shows cognitive and perceptual distortions	1. Avoid being too "nice" or "friendly." 2. Give clear and straightforward explanations of tests and procedures beforehand. 3. Use simple, clear language; avoid ambiguity. 4. Project a neutral but kind affect. 5. Warn about any changes, side effects of medication, and reasons for delay. Such interventions may help allay anxiety and minimize suspiciousness. A written plan may help encourage cooperation.	1. Psychotherapy is treatment of choice; later, cognitive-behavioral techniques 2. Group therapy may help with social skills 3. Antidepressant or antianxiety agents as needed; antipsychotics may be of use, especially if they become acutely psychotic
Schizoid	Reclusive Avoidant Uncooperative	1. Avoid being too "nice" or "friendly." 2. Do not try to increase socialization. 3. Perform thorough diagnostic assessment as needed to identify symptoms or disorders the patient is reluctant to discuss.	1. Supportive psychotherapy 2. Group therapy 3. Antipsychotics, antidepressants, antianxiety agents as needed
Schizotypal	Manifests ideas of reference Shows cognitive and perceptual distortions Socially inept Anxious	1. Respect patient's need for social isolation. 2. Be aware of patient's suspiciousness, and employ appropriate interventions. 3. Perform careful diagnostic assessment as needed to uncover any other medical or psychological symptoms that may need intervention (e.g., suicidal thoughts).	1. Supportive psychotherapy 2. Cognitive and behavioral measures 3. Group therapy may improve social skills 4. Low-dose antipsychotics and antidepressants

Data from Sadock, B. J., & Sadock, V. A. (2008). *Concise textbook of clinical psychiatry* (3rd ed.). Philadelphia, PA: Lippincott Williams & Wilkins.

and borderline, are included in this table for a quick reference, and they are also addressed in more depth in the remainder of the chapter.

ANTISOCIAL PERSONALITY DISORDER

CLINICAL PICTURE

People with **antisocial personality disorder** may be more commonly referred to as sociopaths. This diagnosis is reserved for adults, but symptoms are evident by the midteens. Symptoms tend to peak during the late teenage years and into the mid twenties. By around 40 years of age, the symptoms may abate and improve even without treatment.

The main pathological traits that characterize antisocial personality disorder are antagonistic behaviors, such as being deceitful and manipulative for personal gain or hostile if needs are blocked. The disorder is also characterized by disinhibited behaviors such as high-risk taking, disregard for responsibility, and impulsivity. Criminal misconduct and substance abuse are common in this population.

Persons with this disorder are mostly concerned with gaining personal power or pleasure, and in relationships they focus on their own gratification to an extreme that defies conforming to ethical or community standards consistent with their culture. They have little to no capacity for intimacy and will exploit others if it benefits them in relationships. One of the most disturbing qualities associated with antisocial personality disorder is a profound lack of empathy, also known as callousness. This callousness results in a lack of concern about the feelings of others, the absence of remorse or guilt except when facing punishment, and a disregard for meeting school, family, and other obligations.

These individuals tend to exhibit a shallow, unexpressive, and superficial affect; however, they may also be adept at portraying themselves as concerned and caring if these attributes help them to manipulate and exploit others. A person with antisocial personality disorder may be able to act witty and charming and be good at flattery and manipulating the emotions of others.

EPIDEMIOLOGY

Antisocial personality disorder is the most researched personality disorder, probably due to its marked impact on society in the form of criminal activity. The prevalence of antisocial personality disorder is about 1.1% in community studies (Skodol et al., 2011). While the disorder is much more common in men (3% versus 1%), women may be underdiagnosed due to the traditional close association of this disorder with males.

ETIOLOGY

Biological Factors

Antisocial personality disorder is genetically linked, and twin studies indicate a predisposition to this disorder. Kendler and colleagues (2012) note that the main two dimensions of genetic risk include the trait of aggressive-disregard (violent tendencies without concern for others) and the trait of disinhibition (lack of concern for consequences).

An alteration in serotonin transmission has also been implicated with the aggression and impulsivity that frequently accompany this disorder. Levels of a metabolite of serotonin, 5-hydroxyindoleacetic acid, can be measured in urine and cerebrospinal fluid. It has been found to be lower in individuals with antisocial personality disorder. Lower levels of serotonin along with dopamine hyperfunction may contribute to aggression, disinhibition, and comorbid substance abuse (Seo et al., 2008).

Environmental Factors

It is likely that a genetic predisposition for characteristics of antisocial personality disorder such as a lack of empathy may be set into motion by a childhood environment of inconsistent parenting and discipline, significant abuse, and extreme neglect. Children reflect parental attitudes and behaviors in the absence of more prosocial influences. Virtually all individuals who eventually develop this disorder have a history of impulse control and conduct problems as children and adolescents. Chapter 21 describes impulse control and conduct disorders in greater detail.

Cultural Factors

Assigning a diagnosis of personality disorder cannot be entirely separated from the cultural context of both the individual and the person diagnosing. Cultural bias, including race, ethnicity, ageism, religion, and gender expectations may unintentionally enter into the categorization. Some studies have found a higher prevalence rate of antisocial personality disorder in African Americans and in persons with co-occurring substance dependence (McGilloway et al, 2010).

VIGNETTE

Richard is a 25-year-old divorced cab driver who is referred to the hospital by the court for competency evaluation after an assault charge. He told the arresting officer that he has bipolar disorder. He has a history of substance abuse and multiple arrests for disorderly conduct or assault. During his intake interview, he is polite and even flirtatious with the female registered nurse. He insists that he is not responsible for his behavior because he is manic. The only symptom he describes is irritability. Richard points out that he cannot tolerate any psychotropic medications because of the side effects. He also notes that he has dropped out of three clinics after several visits because "the staff don't understand me."

APPLICATION OF THE NURSING PROCESS

ASSESSMENT

People with antisocial personality disorder do not enter the health care system for treatment of this disorder unless they have been court-ordered to do so. Psychiatric admissions may be initiated for anxiety and depression. Entering treatment may also be a way to avoid or address legal, financial, occupational, or other circumstances. Health care workers also encounter people with this disorder based on the physical consequences of high-risk behaviors, such as acute injury and substance use. Keep in mind that questions asked during the assessment phase may not always result in accurate responses since the patient may become defensive or simply not tell the truth.

Self-Assessment

You may respond to a person with antisocial personality disorder in a variety of ways. Because these individuals have the capacity to be charming, you may want to defend the person as someone who is being unfairly treated and misunderstood. These feelings should be explored with your faculty or other experienced personnel. Conversely, if you are aware that your patient has a history of criminal acts, you may feel disdain or personally threatened. Again, share your concerns with people who are experienced in caring for this population. Awareness and monitoring of one's own stress responses to patient behaviors facilitate more effective and therapeutic intervention, regardless of the specific approach to their care.

ASSESSMENT GUIDELINES

Antisocial Personality Disorder

1. Assess current life stressors.
2. Assess for suicidal, violent, and/or homicidal thoughts.
3. Assess anxiety, aggression, and anger levels.
4. Assess motivation for maintaining control.
5. Assess for substance misuse (past and present).

DIAGNOSIS

This disorder presents a challenge for health care providers, who should consider the potential for disruption in psychiatric and medical-surgical settings. While there is little evidence that it can be successfully treated, diagnoses and nursing care plans should be geared toward maintaining safety and providing structure for this safety. Nursing diagnoses are focused on protection of others and self from impulsive and premeditated acts, and on improving coping skills.

NANDA-I nursing diagnoses (Herdman, 2012) with the most relevance to this disorder include *Risk for other-directed violence, Defensive coping, Impaired social interaction,* and *Ineffective health maintenance.*

OUTCOMES IDENTIFICATION

Pertinent categories of nursing outcomes based on the Nursing Outcomes Classification (NOC) include abusive behavior self-restraint, aggression self-restraint, coping, social interaction, social isolation, health promotion knowledge, and health promoting behavior (Moorhead et al., 2013). Successfully achieving these outcomes when working with this population is extremely difficult, but maintaining safety is the priority. Small, incremental changes and progress will likely be the best outcomes. Table 24-3 lists common signs and symptoms, suggests nursing diagnoses, and identifies potential outcomes associated with antisocial personality disorders.

PLANNING

Distrust, hostility, and a profound inability to connect with others will impair the usual process of developing a therapeutic relationship. In the context of antisocial personality disorder, the role of the nurse will be to provide consistency, support, boundaries, and limits. Providing realistic choices (e.g., selection of a particular group activity) may enhance adherence to treatment.

IMPLEMENTATION

Persons with antisocial personality disorder may be involuntarily admitted to psychiatric units for evaluation. With their freedom thus limited they tend to be angry, manipulative, aggressive, and impulsive. Refer to Boxes 24-2, 24-3, and 24-4 for interventions to address these behaviors based on the *Nursing Interventions Classification (NIC)* (Bulechek et al., 2013).

Teamwork and Safety

The safety of patients and staff is a prime consideration in working with individuals in this population. In order to promote safety, the whole treatment team should follow a solid treatment plan that emphasizes realistic limits on specific behavior, consistency in responses, and consequences for actions. Careful documentation of behaviors will aid in providing effective interventions and in promoting teamwork

Therapeutic communication techniques are still valuable tools for working with individuals with antisocial personality

TABLE 24-3 SIGNS AND SYMPTOMS, NURSING DIAGNOSES, AND OUTCOMES FOR ANTISOCIAL PERSONALITY DISORDER

SIGNS AND SYMPTOMS	NURSING DIAGNOSES	OUTCOMES
Rigid posture, hyperactivity, pacing, history of child abuse, history of violence, violates rights of others, anger and aggression, impulsivity, substance abuse, negative role models	*Risk for other-directed violence*	Patient will not harm others, uses conflict resolution methods, controls impulses, expresses needs in a nondestructive manner, refrains from verbal outbursts, avoids violating others' personal space
Denial of obvious problems and weaknesses, difficulty establishing and maintaining, grandiosity, hostile laughter, lack of follow-through to care, projection of blame and responsibility, rationalization of failures, ridicule of others, superior attitude toward others	*Defensive coping*	Uses effective coping strategies, uses strategies to promote safety, takes responsibility for own actions, uses strategies to avoid violent situations, obtains needed support, self-initiates goal-directed behavior, expresses belief in ability to perform actions
Unstable relationships, lacks empathy, projects hostility, shows behaviors unaccepted by dominant cultural group, grandiose, dysfunctional interactions, unaccepted social behavior	*Impaired social interaction*	Exhibits receptiveness, exhibits sensitivity to others, cooperates with others, interacts with other, exhibits consideration
History of lack of health-seeking behavior, inability to take responsibility for meeting basic health practices, impairment of personal support systems, lack of expressed interest in improving health behaviors	*Ineffective health maintenance*	Performs healthy behaviors, follows healthy diet, balances activity and rest, avoids substance use, obtains assistance from health professionals

From Herdman, T. H. (Ed.), (2012). *Nursing diagnoses—Definitions and classification 2012-2014.* Copyright © 2012, 1994-2012 by NANDA International. Used by arrangement with John Wiley & Sons Limited; Moorhead, S., Johnson, M., Maas, M. L., & Swanson, E. (2013). *Nursing outcomes classification (NOC)* (5th ed.). St. Louis, MO: Mosby.

BOX 24-2 *NIC* INTERVENTIONS FOR MANIPULATIVE BEHAVIOR

Limit Setting

Definition: Establishing the parameters of desirable and acceptable patient behavior

Activities (partial list):

- Discuss concerns about behavior with patient.
- Identify (with patient input when appropriate) undesirable patient behavior.
- Discuss with patient, when appropriate, what is desirable behavior in a given situation or setting.
- Establish consequences (with patient input when appropriate) for occurrence or nonoccurrence of desired behaviors.
- Communicate established behavioral expectations and consequences to patient in language that is easily understood and nonpunitive.
- Refrain from arguing or bargaining with patient about established behavioral expectations and consequences.
- Monitor patient for occurrence or nonoccurrence of desired behaviors.
- Modify behavioral expectations and consequences, as needed, to accommodate reasonable changes in patient's situation.

Data from Bulechek, G. M., Butcher, H. K., Dochterman, J. M., & Wagner, C. (2013). *Nursing interventions classification (NIC)* (6th ed.). St. Louis, MO: Mosby.

BOX 24-3 *NIC* INTERVENTIONS FOR AGGRESSIVE BEHAVIOR

Anger Control Assistance

Definition: Facilitation of the expression of anger in an adaptive, nonviolent manner

Activities (partial list):

- Determine appropriate behavioral expectations for expression of anger, given patient's level of cognitive and physical functioning.
- Limit access to frustrating situations until patient is able to express anger in an adaptive manner.
- Encourage patient to seek assistance from nursing staff during periods of increasing tension.
- Monitor potential for inappropriate aggression, and intervene before its expression.
- Prevent physical harm if anger is directed at self or others (e.g., restraint and removal of potential weapons).
- Provide physical outlets for expression of anger or tension (e.g., sports, modeling clay, journal writing).
- Provide reassurance to patient that nursing staff will intervene to prevent patient from losing control.
- Assist patient in identifying source of anger.
- Identify function that anger, frustration, and rage serve for patient.
- Identify consequences of inappropriate expression of anger.

Data from Bulechek, G. M., Butcher, H. K., Dochterman, J. M., & Wagner, C. (2013). *Nursing interventions classification (NIC)* (6th ed.). St. Louis, MO: Mosby.

BOX 24-4 *NIC* INTERVENTIONS FOR IMPULSIVE BEHAVIOR

Impulse Control Training

Definition: Assisting the patient to mediate impulsive behavior through application of problem-solving strategies to social and interpersonal situations

Activities (partial list):

- Assist patient to identify the problem or situation that requires thoughtful action.
- Assist patient to identify courses of possible action and their costs and benefits.
- Teach patient to cue himself or herself to "stop and think" before acting impulsively.
- Assist patient to evaluate the outcome of the chosen course of action.
- Provide positive reinforcement (e.g., praise and rewards) for successful outcomes.
- Encourage patient to self-reward for successful outcomes.
- Provide opportunities for patient to practice problem solving (role playing) within the therapeutic environment.
- Encourage patient to practice problem solving in social and interpersonal situations outside the therapeutic environment, followed by evaluation of outcome.

Data from Bulechek, G. M., Butcher, H. K., Dochterman, J. M., & Wagner, C. (2013). *Nursing interventions classification (NIC)* (6th ed.). St. Louis, MO: Mosby.

disorder. Simply being heard can defuse an emotionally charged situation. For example, the nurse can listen to a patient's emotional complaints about the staff and the hospital without correcting any errors, simply noting that the patient truly feels hurt. Showing empathy may also decrease aggressive outbursts if the patient feels that staff members are trying to understand feelings of frustration. Table 24-4 depicts a therapeutic nurse-patient interaction after an antisocial patient initiates a fight with a peer in an inpatient unit.

Pharmacological Interventions

In the United States, there are no FDA specifically approved medications for treating antisocial personality disorder (Ripoll et al., 2011). This means that prescribers are using medications "off label" until evidence-based pharmacotherapies are proven to be safe and effective. Persons with antisocial personality disorder respond to mood-stabilizing medications such as lithium to help with aggression and impulsivity. See Chapter 27 for a more detailed discussion on medications that target aggression.

Advanced Practice Interventions

The advanced practice registered nurse treats patients with personality disorders in a variety of inpatient and community settings. New research shows that persons with these disorders do benefit from therapies to address other mental health conditions and their personality disorder. Advanced practice nurses with training in psychotherapy, pharmacology, and the management of complex health challenges are in an excellent position to deliver and coordinate care across the continuum of health systems

TABLE 24-4 **DIALOGUE WITH A PATIENT WITH MANIPULATIVE, AGGRESSIVE, AND IMPULSIVE TRAITS**

DIALOGUE	THERAPEUTIC TOOL/COMMENT
Nurse: Donald, I would like to talk with you about what happened this morning.	Be clear as to purpose of interview.
Donald: OK, shoot.	
Nurse: Tell me what started the incident.	Use open-ended statements. Maintain a nonjudgmental attitude.
Donald: Well, as I told you before, I always had to fight to get what I wanted in life. My father and mother abandoned me emotionally when I was a child.	
Nurse: Yes, but tell me about this morning.	Redirect patient to present problem or situation.
Donald: OK. I disliked Richard from the first. He has it in for me, I just know it. He doesn't get along with anyone here. Just 2 days ago, he almost had a fight.	
Nurse: Donald, what do you mean, Richard has it in for you?	Explore situation.
Donald: When I'm talking to one of the nurses, he stares and makes comments under his breath.	
Nurse: What does he say?	Encourage description.
Donald: How I'm "in" with the nurses. I'm just trying to do what's expected of me here.	
Nurse: You mean that Richard is envious of your relationship with the nurses?	Validate patient's meaning.
Donald: Right. He really doesn't want to be here. He doesn't care about all that therapeutic junk.	
Nurse: You seem to know a lot about how Richard thinks. I wonder how that is.	Assist patient to make association to present situation.
Donald: He reminds me of someone I knew when I was young. His name was Joe. We called him "Bones."	
Nurse: Tell me more about Bones.	Explore situation further.
Donald: We called him Bones because he was skinny. He was into drugs and never ate. He was also called Bones because he was selfish. He never shared anything. He never even had a girl that I knew about.	
Nurse: So Richard reminds you of someone who is selfish and lonely?	Make interpretation of information. Note increasing anxiety.
Donald: That's right. I've had three marriages and girlfriends on the side. No one can take them away from me. (Angrily.) Just let them try!	
Nurse: What makes you so angry now?	Identify feelings and explore threat or anxiety.
Donald: Richard! I know he wants to be like me, but he can't. I'll hurt him if he makes any more comments about me.	
Nurse: Donald, you will not hurt anyone here on the unit.	Set limits on, and expectations of, patient's behavior.
Donald: I'm sorry, I didn't mean that.	
Nurse: It's important that we examine your part in the incident this morning and ways to cope without threats or violence.	Focus on patient's responsibility and suggest alternative methods of coping with situation.
Donald: Listen, I know I've gotten into trouble because I can't control my temper, but that's because I won't get any respect until I can show them I don't fear them.	Patient exhibits rationalization.
Nurse: Who are "they"?	Clarify pronoun.
Donald: People like Richard.	
Nurse: You've told me that fighting was a way of survival as a child, but as an adult, there are other ways of handling situations that make you angry.	Show understanding and suggest other means of coping.
Donald: You're right. I've thought about this. Do you think it would help if you give me some meds to control my anger?	Patient exhibits superficial and concrete thinking—possible manipulation.
Nurse: I wasn't thinking of medications but of a plan for being aware of your anger and talking it out instead of fighting it out.	Clarify meaning toward behavior change. Start to explore alternatives Donald can use when angry instead of fighting.
Donald: I told you before, I *have* to fight.	
Nurse: Have you thought about the consequences of your fighting?	Identify results of impulsive behavior.
Donald: I feel bad afterwards. Sometimes I wish it hadn't happened.	Patient continues to explore.

for these individuals who often require intense and long term treatment.

EVALUATION

Evaluating treatment effectiveness in this patient population is difficult. Nurses may never know the real results of their interventions, particularly in acute-care settings. Even in long-term outpatient treatment, many patients with antisocial personality disorder find the relationship too intimate an experience to remain long enough for successful treatment. However, some motivated patients may be able to learn to change their behavior, especially if positive experiences are repeated.

Each therapeutic experience offers an opportunity for the patient to observe himself or herself interacting with caregivers who consistently try to teach positive coping skills. Perhaps effectiveness can be measured by how successfully the nurse is able to be genuine with the patient, maintain a helpful posture, offer substantial instruction, and still care for himself or herself. Specific short-term outcomes may be accomplished, and overall, the patient can be given the message of hope that quality of life can always be improved.

BORDERLINE PERSONALITY DISORDER

CLINICAL PICTURE

Borderline personality disorder is the most well known and dramatic of the personality disorders. Borderline personality disorder is characterized by severe impairments in functioning. The major features of this disorder are patterns of marked instability in emotional control or regulation, impulsivity, identity or self-image distortions, unstable mood, and unstable interpersonal relationships

One of the primary features of borderline personality disorder is emotional lability, that is, rapidly moving from one emotional extreme to another. Typically, these emotional shifts include responding to situations with emotions that are out of proportion to the circumstances, pathological fear of separation, and intense sensitivity to perceived personal rejection.

Another disruptive trait common in persons with borderline personality disorder is **impulsivity**. Impulsivity is manifested in acting quickly in response to emotions without considering the consequences. This impulsivity results in damaged relationships and even in suicide attempts.

Self-destructive behaviors are prominent in this disorder. Ineffective and often harmful self-soothing habits, such as cutting, promiscuous sexual behavior, and numbing with substances are common and may result in unintentional death. Chronic, suicidal ideation is also a common feature of this disorder and influences the likelihood of accidental deaths. Co-occurring mood, anxiety, or substance disorders complicate the treatment and prognosis of the condition.

Another characteristic of borderline personality disorder is that of antagonism; it is marked by hostility, anger, and irritability in relationships. This area of externalized aggressive behavior has received little research and clinical attention (Sansone & Sansone, 2012). There is evidence that people with this disorder may be physically violent toward intimate partners and nonintimate partners alike, engage in destructive behaviors such as property damage, and, rarely, commit homicide of family members or others.

An unusual feature of this disorder is the use of splitting as a primary defense or coping style. Splitting refers to the inability to view both positive and negative aspects of others as part of a whole. This results in viewing someone as either a wonderful person or a horrible person. This kind of dichotomous thinking and coping behavior is believed to be partly a result of the person's failed experiences with adult personality integration and likely is influenced by exposure to earlier psychological, sexual, or physical trauma. For example, the individual may tend to idealize another person (friend, lover, health care professional) at the start of a new relationship, hoping that this person will meet all of his or her needs. But at the first disappointment or frustration, the individual's status quickly shifts to one of devaluation, and the other person is despised.

Persons with borderline personality disorder seek out treatment for depression, anxiety, suicidal and self-harming behaviors, and other impulsive behaviors, including substance use. The person with borderline personality disorder frequently pursues repeated hospitalizations. While hospitalization may decrease self-destructive risk for patients with borderline personality disorder, it is not regarded as an effective long-term solution.

EPIDEMIOLOGY AND COMORBIDITY

Borderline personality disorder occurs at a rate of about 1.6% in community studies (Skodol et al., 2011). It carries a high mortality rate—nearly 10%—and results in extensive utilization of services from the health care system (Soeteman et al., 2008). The disorder seems to decrease with age. Gunderson (2011) found that over the course of a decade, people with borderline personality disorder experienced high rates of remission and low rates of relapse.

About 85% of people with borderline personality disorder also meet the diagnostic criteria for another mental illness (Lenzenweger et al., 2007). Substance abuse in individuals with borderline personality disorder is extremely common, with some studies suggesting the rate of co-occurrence above 50% (Pennay et al., 2011). Women with this disorder are more likely to have major depression and anxiety disorders (Tadic et al., 2009). Men are more likely to have substance use disorders or antisocial personality disorder.

Nonpsychiatric diagnoses are also associated with borderline personality disorder. They include diabetes, high blood pressure, chronic back pain, fibromyalgia, and arthritis.

ETIOLOGY

Biological Factors

This disorder has been found to run in families and is highly associated with genetic factors such as hypersensitivity, impulsivity, and emotional dysregulation (Gunderson, 2011). Persons with borderline personality disorder may have a hyperresponsive amygdala and impairment in the prefrontal cortex that make them more vulnerable to emotionally charged words, facial expressions, and interpersonal exchanges.

Psychological Factors

Borderline personality disorders have traditionally been thought to develop as a result of early abandonment, which results in an unstable view of self and others. However, this abandonment is made more intense by a biological predisposition.

Margaret Mahler (1895-1985), a Hungarian-born child psychologist who worked with emotionally disturbed children, developed a framework that is useful in considering borderline personality disorder. Mahler and colleagues (1975) believed that psychological problems are a result of the disruption of the normal **separation-individuation** of the child from the mother.

According to Mahler, an infant progresses from complete self-absorption with an inability to separate itself from its mother, to a physically and psychologically differentiated toddler. Mahler emphasized the role of the significant other (traditionally the mother) in providing a secure, psychic base of support that promotes enough confidence for the child to separate. This support is achieved through a balance of holding (emotionally and physically) a child enough for the child to feel safe, while at the same time fostering and encouraging independence and natural exploration.

Problems may arise in this separation-individuation. If a toddler leaves his or her mother on the park bench and wanders off to the sandbox, two things ideally should accompany the action. First, the child should be encouraged to set off into the world with smiles and reassurance: "Go on, honey, it's safe to go away a little." Second, the mother needs to be reliably present when the toddler returns, thereby rewarding his or her efforts. Clearly, parents are not perfect and are sometimes distracted and short-tempered. Mahler notes that raising healthy children does not require that parents never make mistakes and that "good enough parenting" will promote successful separation-individuation.

Stages of this process are as follows:

- **Stage 1 (birth to 1 month): Normal autism.** The infant spends most of its time sleeping.
- **Stage 2 (1-5 months): Symbiosis.** The infant perceives the mother-infant as a single fused entity. Infants gradually distinguish the inner from the outer world.
- **Stage 3 (5-10 months): Differentiation.** The infant recognizes distinctness from mother. Progressive neurological development and increased alertness draw the infant's attention away from self to the outer world.
- **Stage 4 (11-18 months): Practicing.** The ability to walk and explore greatly expands the toddler's sense of separateness.
- **Stage 5 (18-24 months): Rapprochement.** Toddlers move away from their mothers and come back for emotional refueling. Periods of helplessness and dependence alternate with the need for independence.
- **Stage 6 (2-5 years): Object constancy.** When children comprehend that objects (in this case, the object is the mother) are permanent even when they are not in their presence, the individuation process is complete.

Children who later develop borderline personality may have had this process disrupted. The Rapprochement stage is particularly crucial and coincides with the terrible twos that are characterized by darting away and clinging and whining; some experts suggest that this phase is not a desirable time for extended separation between parent and child.

Consider the previous ideal example of the child who wants to play in the sandbox with alterations. If the child wanders off to the sandbox and returns to a caregiver who is emotionally unavailable, perhaps hurt by the attempt at independence, the child feels unsafe to explore. Alternately, if the caregiver has personal issues related to dependency and abandonment, he or she may be threatened by the child's attempts at independence and respond with clinging and halting exploration. The child cannot safely move on to the next stage of development. A fear of abandonment from others, along with a sense of anger, carries over into adulthood.

VIGNETTE

Devon is a 38-year-old married woman with a young son. She works full time as a dietitian at a large medical center. Devon was diagnosed with fibromyalgia two years ago and is in treatment at a pain clinic. Most days, she comes home from work fatigued and goes to bed, leaving her son to play by himself after school or with friends until her husband gets home from work. Devon also has struggled with an eating disorder since she was a teenager. When she feels guilty for ignoring her son's needs, she binges and then purges to relieve her negative emotions. Devon recognizes that it helps only temporarily and adds to her fatigue, but she still feels helpless to stop it. When her son asks her to play with him or take him to an activity, she becomes angry with him and then feels angry with herself. The palliative care nurse at the pain clinic refers Devon to a dialectical behavior therapy group (discussed later in this chapter). There, she will learn skills to deal with her chronic pain and discover alternative self-soothing strategies for her bingeing and purging behaviors.

APPLICATION OF THE NURSING PROCESS

ASSESSMENT

Assessment Tools

The preferred method for determining a diagnosis of borderline personality disorder is the semistructured interview obtained by clinicians. Self-report inventories, such as the well-known Minnesota Multiphasic Personality Inventory (MMPI), are useful because they have built-in validity and reliability scales for the clinician to refer to when interpreting test results.

Areas of assessment that are typically included on questionnaires and rating scales related to borderline personality disorder include the following:

- Feelings of emptiness
- An inclination to engage in risky behaviors such as reckless driving, unsafe sex, substance use, binge eating, gambling, or overspending
- Intense feelings of abandonment that result in paranoia or feeling spaced out
- Idealization of others and becoming close quickly
- A tendency toward anger, sarcasm, and bitterness
- Self mutilation and self-harm
- Suicidal behaviors, gestures, or threat
- Sudden shifts in self-evaluation that result in changing goals, values, and career focus
- Extreme mood shifts that occur in a matter of hours or days
- Intense, unstable romantic relationships

Patient History

Borderline personality disorder usually begins prior to adulthood. Important issues in assessment for borderline personality disorder include a history of suicidal or aggressive ideation or actions, treatment history, and medication (prescribed and illicit) use.

Significant areas about which further details must be obtained include current or past physical, sexual, or emotional abuse and level of current risk of harm from self or others. At times, immediate interventions may be needed to ensure the safety of the patient or others. Information regarding prior use of any medication, including psychopharmacological agents, is important. This information gives evidence of other contacts the patient has made for help and indicates how the health care provider found the patient at that time.

Self-Assessment

Because interpersonal difficulties are central to the problems faced by persons diagnosed with borderline personality disorder, it is understandable that these problems surface in the treatment milieu and within the relationships between patients and caregivers. Anticipating that persons with borderline personality disorder will likely have a disrupted, intense interpersonal experience with caregivers is helpful in monitoring personal stress responses when working with these individuals. Keep in mind that without the necessary skills to be effective in their lives, these dysfunctional behaviors may really represent the person's best effort to cope.

With borderline personality disorder, the therapeutic alliance often follows an initial hesitancy on the part of patient, then an upward curve of idealization by the patient toward the caregiver, followed by a devaluation of the staff member when the patient is disappointed by his or her own unmet expectations of the treatment team. This process is often acted out in the treatment milieu and can interrupt the delivery of care.

For example, a female patient may briefly idealize her male nurse on the inpatient unit, telling staff and patients alike that she is "the luckiest patient because [she has] the best nurse in the hospital." The rest of the team understands that this comment is an exaggeration. After days of constant dramatic praise for the nurse, with subtle insults to the rest of the staff, some members of the team may start to feel inadequate and resentful of the nurse. They begin to make critical remarks about minor events to prove that the nurse is not perfect. A similar scenario can occur if the patient constantly complains about one staff member; some staff are torn between defending and criticizing the targeted staff member.

EVIDENCE-BASED PRACTICE

Family Members' Experiences with Borderline Personality Disorder

Ekdahl, S., Idvall, E., Samuelsson, M., & Perseius, K. I. (2011). A life tiptoeing: Being a significant other to persons with borderline personality disorder. *Archives of Psychiatric Nursing, 25*(6), 369–376.

Problem

Persons with borderline personality disorder characteristically struggle to create effective interpersonal relationships due to challenges with heightened emotional sensitivity, a reduced ability to be empathic to others, and a preoccupation fearing abandonment by others. These issues negatively impact both family and professional provider relationships. This is especially important because the support of family is a major factor in recovery from a psychiatric illness episode or crisis. Research in the area of the family's lived experience with borderline personality disorder is scarce.

Purpose of Study

The purpose of this study was to explore how family members experience living close to a person with borderline personality disorder and how they experience their encounters with health care providers.

Methods

The study was qualitative and used a purposeful sampling method, which means that persons believed to have the best knowledge of the problem were invited to participate. Participants were recruited from a Swedish association of family members with borderline personality disorder. Nineteen participants emerged from a possible population of thirty members. The majority were parents (N=17); one participant was a spouse, and one was an adult child. Data was collected from a questionnaire that related to the patient's health condition, strain in the family, and their encounters with health care. Narrative data were collected through group interviews that focused on living close to someone with borderline personality disorder and their experiences of encountering health and psychiatric care.

Key Findings

Themes that emerged include the following:

- Referred to as "tiptoeing," family members identified the 24-hour-a-day burden of worry and duty, especially in regard to self-harm or suicide attempts, and living in constant crisis.
- Powerlessness was manifested in guilt that included perceived neglect of other family members, strained marital relationships, and a lack of support from others, including health care providers, due to prejudice toward the disorder.
- Feeling left out when the patient was hospitalized but burdened without help once the patient was discharged. They felt like providers viewed them as obstacles in the treatment process. Privacy and confidentiality contributed to secrecy in treatment.
- Care providers did not view the person and family in context. They described nurses as kind and caring, yet they felt betrayed by the inability of these providers to keep their loved one safe.

Implications for Nursing Practice

This study supports findings from other research on family involvement. Specifically, families and patients benefit from more involvement in the treatment process before a patient is discharged home. Nurses and other team members have both an obligation and opportunity to consider the needs of the patient in the context of their family. Family education groups that focus on teaching skills about interpersonal effectiveness with the loved one with the borderline personality disorder and individual family meetings to identify the needs of families around discharge planning are two steps that nurses can be leaders in facilitating.

ASSESSMENT GUIDELINES

Borderline Personality Disorder

1. Assess for suicidal or violent thoughts toward others. If these are present, the patient will need immediate attention.
2. Determine whether the patient has a medical disorder or another psychiatric disorder (especially a substance use disorder) that may be responsible for the symptoms.
3. View the assessment about personality functioning from within the person's ethnic, cultural, and social background.
4. Ascertain whether the patient experienced a recent important loss. Borderline personality disorder is often exacerbated after the loss of significant supporting people or in a disruptive social situation.
5. Evaluate for a change in personality in middle adulthood or later, which signals the need for a thorough medical workup or assessment for unrecognized substance use disorder.

Clinical supervision and additional education are helpful and supportive to staff on the front lines of care. Awareness and monitoring of one's own stress responses to patient behaviors facilitate more effective and therapeutic intervention, regardless of the specific approach to their care.

DIAGNOSIS

Persons with borderline personality disorder are usually admitted to psychiatric treatment programs because of symptoms with comorbid disorders or dangerous behavior. Emotions such as anxiety, rage, and depression, and behaviors such as withdrawal, paranoia, and manipulation are among the most frequent that health care workers must address.

The nursing diagnosis *Self-mutilation* is most often associated with this disorder. It is defined as "deliberate self-injurious behavior causing tissue damage with the intent of causing nonfatal injury to attain relief of tension" (Herdman, 2012, p. 449). Related characteristics include:

- Borderline personality disorder
- Disturbed interpersonal relationships
- Feels threatened with loss of significant relationship
- History of self-directed violence
- Impulsivity
- Irresistible urge to cut self
- Labile behavior
- Mounting tension that is intolerable
- Use of manipulation to obtain nurturing relationship with others

Other nursing diagnoses that are directly relevant to borderline personality disorder are *Risk for suicide, Risk for self-directed violence, Risk for other-directed violence, Social isolation, Impaired social interaction, Disturbed personal identity, and Ineffective coping*

OUTCOMES IDENTIFICATION

Realistic outcomes are established for individuals with borderline personality disorder based on the perspective that personality change occurs with one behavioral solution and one learned skill at a time. This can be expected to take much time and repetition. In the acute-care setting, the focus is on the presenting problem, which may be depression or severe anxiety. Health care providers do not expect resolution of chronic behavior problems during the hospital stay, but rather to be met with appropriate therapeutic feedback and incremental steps toward recovery.

The *Nursing Outcomes Classification (NOC)* provides useful scales for measuring improvement in mutilation self-restraint, suicide self-restraint, aggression self-control, impulse self-control, social interaction skills, abusive behavior self-restraint, social interaction, social isolation, identity, self-awareness, coping, and stress level (Moorhead et al., 2013). Table 24-5 lists common signs and symptoms associated with borderline personality disorder, suggests nursing diagnoses, and identifies potential outcomes.

PLANNING

A therapeutic relationship is essential with patients who have borderline personality disorder because most of them have experienced failed relationships, including therapeutic alliances. Their distrust and hostility can be a setup for failure. When patients blame and attack others, the nurse needs to understand the context of their complaints; that is, these attacks spring from the feeling of being threatened. The more intense their complaints are, the greater their fear of potential harm or loss is. Case Study and Nursing Care Plan 24-1 presents a patient with borderline personality disorder.

IMPLEMENTATION

People with borderline personality disorder are impulsive (e.g., suicidal, self-mutilating), aggressive, manipulative, and even psychotic during periods of stress. Refer to Boxes 24-2, 24-3, and 24-4 for interventions to address these behaviors based on the *Nursing Interventions Classification (NIC)* (Bulechek et al., 2013).

Finding an approach that works with patients in the setting in which they are treated is important. Therapies such as dialectical behavior therapy and mindfulness-based therapies offer staff evidence-based interventions, clinical structure, and formalized support for identifying best practices.

Teamwork and Safety

When individuals with borderline personality disorders are admitted to the hospital, partially hospitalized, or in day treatment settings, team management is a significant part of treatment. The primary goal is management of the patient's affect in a group context. Community meetings, coping skills groups, and socializing groups are all helpful for these patients. They have the opportunity to interact with peers and staff to discuss goals and learn problem-solving skills. Dealing with emotional issues that arise in the milieu requires a calm, united approach by the staff to maintain safety and to enhance self-control.

Common problems resulting from staff splitting can be minimized if the unit leaders hold weekly staff meetings in which staff members are allowed to ventilate their feelings

24-1 CASE STUDY AND NURSING CARE PLAN

Borderline Personality Disorder

Brianna Drake is a 24-year-old single administrative assistant who lives alone. She has been seen in the emergency department several times for superficial suicide attempts. She is admitted because she has cut her wrists, ankles, and vagina with glass and has lost a lot of blood. This event is precipitated by her graduation from a community college.

Upon admission she is sweet, serene, and grateful to all the nurses, calling them "angels of mercy." Within a week, she is angry at half of the nurses and demands a new primary nurse, saying that the one she has (to whom she had grown attached) hates her. She has a history of heavy drinking and has managed to sneak alcohol onto the unit. She has been found in bed with a young male patient. She continually breaks unit rules and then pleads to have this behavior forgiven and forgotten. When angry, she threatens to cut herself again. When asked why she cut herself, Brianna states, "I was tired." She appears restless and tense and frequently asks for antianxiety medication. When asked what she is anxious about, she says, "Uh . . . don't know . . . I feel so empty inside." Brianna frequently paces up and down the halls, looking both angry and bored. Her admitting diagnoses include substance use disorder and borderline personality disorder.

Self-Assessment

Salma, a recent graduate and Brianna's primary nurse, talks to Brianna's therapist twice a week in staff meetings. The therapist impresses upon Salma the difficulty health care workers have in dealing effectively with persons with borderline personality disorders. These patients constantly act out their feelings in self-destructive and maladaptive ways. They usually are not aware of their feelings or what triggered their actions.

The most difficult area for many health care workers is dealing with the intense feelings and reactions these patients can provoke in others. Salma sets a time twice a week for supervision with Brianna's therapist. At the next meeting, common goals and intervention strategies are discussed.

Assessment

Objective Data

- Makes frequent, superficial suicide attempts.
- Requests antianxiety medication frequently.
- Paces up and down the hall much of the day.
- Threatens self-mutilation when anxious.
- Brings alcohol onto the unit after pass.
- Is found in bed with male patient.

Subjective Data

- Initially "loved" her primary nurse, now "hates" her and wants another nurse.
- States she is restless and tense.
- Complains of feeling empty inside.
- Describes self as angry and bored much of the time.

Diagnosis

Salma formulates two initial nursing diagnoses that have the highest priority during this time:

1. *Ineffective coping* related to inadequate psychological resources, as evidenced by self-destructive behaviors

Supporting Data

- After stating that she feels frustrated, patient goes on pass and comes back with alcohol.
- After stating that she is in love with her therapist, patient is found in bed with a male patient.
- After stating that she hates her primary nurse, patient demands a new primary nurse.

2. *Self-mutilation* related to borderline personality disorder, as evidenced by suicidal gestures and poor impulse control

Supporting Data

- Is admitted following self-mutilation
- Threatens self-mutilation when anxious
- Threatens self-mutilation on unit

Outcomes Identification

1. Patient will consistently demonstrate the use of effective coping strategies.
2. Patient will refrain from injuring self.

Planning

The initial plan is to maintain patient safety and to encourage verbalization of feelings and impulses instead of action.

Implementation

Brianna's plan of care is personalized as follows:

Nursing diagnosis: *Ineffective coping* related to inadequate psychological resources, as evidenced by self-destructive behaviors

Outcome criteria: Patient will consistently demonstrate the use of effective coping strategies.

SHORT-TERM GOAL	INTERVENTION	RATIONALE	EVALUATION
Brianna will consistently demonstrate a decrease in stress as evidenced by talking about feelings with staff every day and an absence of acting-out behaviors.	1. Encourage verbalization of feelings, perceptions, and fears. 2. Support the use of appropriate defense mechanisms.	1. Discussing and understanding the dynamics of frustration help reduce the frustration by helping patient take positive action. 2. Discussing and understanding the meaning of defenses help reduce the potential for acting out.	**GOAL MET** Brianna was able to experience problems and deal with them appropriately. Acting out was minimal or absent. *Example:* Patient had an appointment for a job interview. She wanted to stay in bed and avoid the interview, but instead she talked with the nurse about her fear of "growing up" and was able to get up and go to the interview.

24-1 CASE STUDY AND NURSING CARE PLAN—cont'd

Borderline Personality Disorder

Nursing diagnosis: *Self-mutilation* related to borderline personality disorder, as evidenced by suicidal gestures and poor impulse control
Outcome criteria: Patient will refrain from injuring self.

SHORT-TERM GOAL	INTERVENTION	RATIONALE	EVALUATION
Brianna will consistently demonstrate that she will seek help when feeling the urge to injure self as evidenced by the absence of self-injurious behaviors and talking to staff about her troubling feelings on a daily basis.	1. Assist patient to identify situations and/or feelings that may prompt self-harm. 2. Instruct patient in coping strategies. 3. Provide ongoing surveillance of patient and environment.	1. Observing, describing, and analyzing thoughts and feelings reduce the potential for acting them out destructively. 2. Alternative behaviors are offered that can be more satisfying and growth promoting. 3. Times of increased anxiety, frustration, or anger without external controls could increase probability of patient using self-mutilating behaviors.	**GOAL MET** Brianna was able to experience troubling thoughts and feelings without self-mutilation. Stated, "I was mad at my therapist today and decided to cut my arms after the session. Instead, I told her I was angry, and together we figured out why."

Evaluation
See individual outcomes and evaluation in the care plan.

TABLE 24-5 SIGNS AND SYMPTOMS, NURSING DIAGNOSES, AND OUTCOMES FOR BORDERLINE PERSONALITY DISORDER

SIGNS AND SYMPTOMS	NURSING DIAGNOSES	OUTCOMES
Impulsivity, abrading, biting, cuts on body, hitting, ingestion of harmful substances, inhalation of harmful substances, insertion of object into body orifice, picking at wounds, scratches on body, self-inflicted burns	*Self-mutilation*	Patient refrains from intentional self-inflicted injury, maintains self-control without supervision, obtains assistance as needed, uses support groups, follows treatment regimen
History of self-mutilation and suicide attempts, family history of self-destructive behavior, disturbed interpersonal relationships, isolation, impulsivity, manipulation to obtain nurturing relationships	*Risk for self-mutilation* *Risk for suicide* *Risk for self-directed violence*	Patient remains free from harm, maintains healthy connections, upholds suicide contract, maintains control without supervision, uses social support group, plans for the future
Impulsivity, history of other-directed violence, threats	*Risk for other-directed violence*	Expresses needs in a constructive manner, monitors anger, maintains self-control without supervision
Behavior unaccepted by dominant cultural group, hypersensitivity to negative evaluation, unstable relationships, reports feeling rejected, experiences feelings of differences from others, inability to achieve a sense of social engagement, intense and unstable relationships	*Social isolation* *Impaired social interaction*	Exhibits receptiveness and sensitivity to others, cooperates with others, uses assertive behaviors as appropriate, interacts with others
Dependency, excessive emotional responses, attention-seeking, reports feeling emptiness, uncertainty about goals, uncertain boundaries with others	*Disturbed personal identity*	Verbalizes clear sense of personal identity, performs social roles, challenges negative images of self, establishes personal boundaries, maintains awareness of thoughts and feelings
Difficulty in relationships, manipulation, destructive behavior toward others and self, inability to meet role expectations, inadequate problem solving, uses self-mutilation to calm and summon nurturing	*Ineffective coping*	Uses effective coping strategies, expresses emotion, seeks emotional support, uses strategies to promote safety, takes responsibility for own actions, identifies available community resources, obtains needed support, self-initiates goal-directed behavior, expresses belief in ability to perform action

From Herdman, T. H. (Ed.), (2012). *Nursing diagnoses—Definitions and classification 2012-2014.* Copyright © 2012, 1994-2012 by NANDA International. Used by arrangement with John Wiley & Sons Limited; Moorhead, S., Johnson, M., Maas, M. L., & Swanson, E. (2013). *Nursing outcomes classification (NOC)* (5th ed.). St. Louis, MO: Mosby.

about conflicts with patients and each other. Consistency and a team approach helps to ensure productive use of therapeutic time and structure for the patient. Patient-centered approaches allow the patient to be part of the treatment planning.

A final approach that is useful for patients with borderline personality disorder relates to the response to superficial self-destructive behaviors. Acting in accordance with unit policies, the nurse remains neutral and dresses the wound in a matter-of-fact manner. Then the patient is instructed to write down the sequence of events leading up to the injury, as well as the consequences, before staff will discuss the event. This cognitive exercise encourages the patient to think independently about his or her own behavior instead of merely ventilating feelings. It facilitates the discussion with staff about alternative actions.

Pharmacological Interventions

In the United States, there are no medications specifically approved by the FDA for treating personality disorders (Ripoll et al., 2011). This means that prescribers are using the medications "off label" until evidenced-based pharmacotherapies are proven to be safe and effective. Psychotropic medications geared toward maintaining patients' cognitive function, symptom relief, and improved quality of life are available (Ripoll 2012; Ripoll et al., 2011). Persons with borderline personality disorder often respond to anticonvulsant mood-stabilizing medications, low-dose antipsychotics, and omega-3 supplementation for mood and emotion dysregulation symptoms. Naltrexone, an opioid receptor antagonist has been found to reduce self-injuring behaviors.

Advanced Practice Interventions

Advanced practice nurses are likely to interact with staff members regarding the treatment of individuals with borderline personality disorders as part of their practice and clinical supervision responsibilities. The advanced practice registered nurse can assist staff members in engaging these patients in a therapeutic alliance.

Psychotherapy

Advanced practice registered nurses are highly involved and often the clinical leaders in providing individual and group psychotherapy. There are three essential therapies for borderline personality disorder:

1. **Cognitive behavioral therapy (CBT):** CBT can help individuals to identify and change inaccurate core perceptions of themselves and others and problems interacting with others. CBT may result in a reduction of mood and anxiety symptoms and reduce the number of self-harming or suicidal behaviors.
2. **Dialectical behavior therapy (DBT):** DBT is an evidence-based therapy developed by Dr. Marsha Linehan to successfully treat chronically suicidal persons with borderline personality disorder (Linehan, 1993). Data on the use of DBT with individuals experiencing comorbid personality disorders (such as obsessive-compulsive personality disorder) and other psychiatric disorders (such as major depression, generalized anxiety, substance abuse and eating disorders) have been confirmed. DBT combines cognitive and behavioral techniques with *mindfulness*, which emphasizes being aware of thoughts and actively shaping them. The goals of DBT are to increase the patient's ability to manage distress, improve interpersonal effectiveness skills, and enhance the therapist's effectiveness in working with this population. Treatment focuses on behavioral targets, beginning with identification of and interventions for suicidal behaviors and then progressing to a focus on interrupting destructive behaviors (Figure 24-1). Finally, DBT addresses quality-of-life behaviors across a hierarchy of care (Figure 24-2).
3. **Schema-focused therapy:** This therapy combines parts of CBT with other forms of therapy that focus on the ways that people view themselves. This reframing of "schemas" is based on the notion that borderline personality disorder is the result of a dysfunctional self-image, probably brought about by a dysfunctional childhood, and that it affects how people respond to stress, react to their environment, and interact with others (Kellogg & Young, 2006).

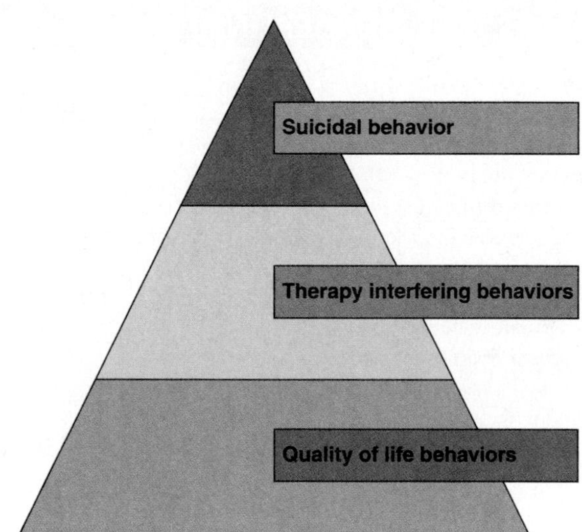

FIG 24-1 Dialectical behavior therapy treatment targets.

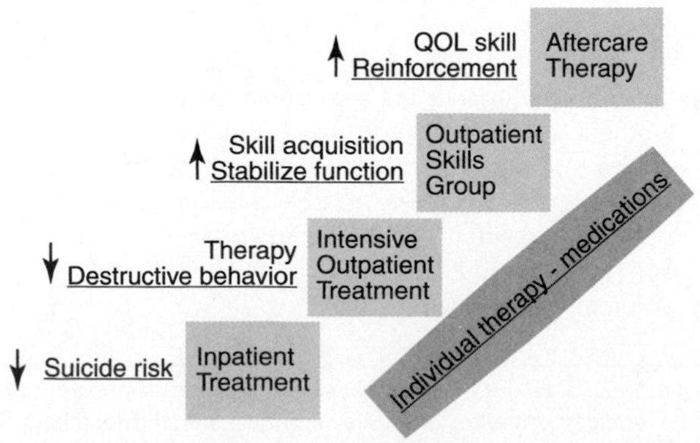

FIG 24-2 Dialectical behavior therapy treatment hierarchy. *QOL*, Quality of life.

EVALUATION

Evaluating treatment effectiveness in this patient population is difficult. Freedom from harm to self and others is a tangible and satisfying positive evaluation. Nurses may never know the real results of their intervention, particularly in acute-care settings. Even in long-term outpatient treatment, patients with borderline personality disorder experience too many disruptions to relationships to remain long enough for successful treatment. As noted earlier, however, some motivated patients may be able to learn to change their behavior, especially if positive experiences are repeated.

Each therapeutic experience offers an opportunity for the patient to observe himself or herself interacting with caregivers who consistently and reliably try to teach positive coping skills. Perhaps effectiveness can be measured by how successfully the nurse is able to be genuine with the patient, maintain a helpful posture, offer substantial instruction, and still care for himself or herself. Specific short-term outcomes may be accomplished, and overall, the patient can be given the message of hope that quality of life can always be improved.

KEY POINTS TO REMEMBER

- All personality disorders share characteristics of inflexibility and difficulties in interpersonal relationships that impair social or occupational functioning.
- Personality disorders are most likely caused by a combination of biological and psychosocial factors.
- Patients with personality disorders often enter psychiatric treatment because of distress from a comorbid mental illness.
- Nurses may experience intense emotional reactions to patients with personality disorders and need to make use of clinical supervision to maintain objectivity.
- Despite the relatively fixed patterns of maladaptive behavior, some patients with personality disorders are able to change their behavior over time as a result of treatment.

CRITICAL THINKING

1. Mr. Beech is undergoing surgery for a broken leg. He is suspicious of the staff and believes that the IV he is receiving for hydration and pre-anesthesia will be used for harmful purposes. He keeps his eyes closed and refuses to answer or look at his family, who describe him as odd. He has schizotypal personality disorder.
   a. Explain how being friendly and outgoing may be threatening to Mr. Beech.
   b. Explain how being matter-of-fact and neutral and sticking to the facts would be effective to Mr. Beech.
   c. What could be done to give Mr. Beech some control over his situation as a hospitalized patient?
   d. How could you best handle his beliefs and lack of interpersonal comfort with caregivers so that both you and he would feel most comfortable?
2. Cherie is brought to the emergency department after slashing her wrist with a razor. She has previously been in the emergency department for drug overdose and has a history of addictions. Cherie can be sarcastic, belittling, and aggressive to those who try to care for her. She has a history of difficulty with interpersonal relationships at her job. When the psychiatric triage nurse comes in to see her, Cherie is initially adoring and compliant, telling him, "You are the best nurse I've ever had, and I truly want to change." But when he refuses to support her request for diazepam (Valium) and meperidine (Demerol) for "pain," she yells at him, "You are a stupid excuse for a nurse. I want to see the doctor immediately." Cherie has borderline personality disorder.
   a. What defense mechanisms is Cherie using?
   b. How could the nurse handle this situation while setting limits and demonstrating concern?

CHAPTER REVIEW

1. Josie, a 27-year-old patient, complains that most of the staff do not like her or care what happens to her, but you are special and she can tell that you are a caring person. She talks with you about being unsure of what she wants to do with her life and her "mixed-up feelings" about relationships. When you tell her that you will be on vacation next week, she becomes very angry. Two hours later, she is found using a curling iron to burn her underarms and explains that it "makes the numbness stop." Given this presentation, which personality disorder would you suspect?
   a. Obsessive-compulsive
   b. Borderline
   c. Antisocial
   d. Schizotypal
2. Which statement about persons with personality disorders is accurate?
   a. They, unlike those with mood or psychotic disorders, are at very low risk of suicide.
   b. They tend not to perceive themselves as having a problem but instead believe their problems are caused by how others behave toward them.
   c. They are believed to be purely psychological disorders, that is, disorders arising from psychological rather than neurological or other physiological abnormalities.
   d. Their symptoms are not as disabling as most other mental disorders; therefore, their care tends to be less challenging and complicated for staff.
3. Lacey, a 19-year-old patient, shows you multiple fresh, serious (but non-life-threatening) self-inflicted cuts on her forearm. Which response would be most therapeutic?
   a. "I'm so sorry you felt so bad that you cut yourself! Let's discuss what led up to this action while I take care of your wounds."
   b. "I will take care of the wounds first, then you will have to be searched for anything else you could injure yourself with."
   c. "I can give you some Band-Aids for you to put on your cuts, but you need to stop this attention-seeking behavior."
   d. "After I care for your wounds, I'd like you to write down what you were thinking and feeling before you cut yourself; then we will discuss it."

4. Alicia, a 31-year-old patient, is flirting with a peer. She is overheard asking him to convince staff to give her privileges to leave the inpatient mental health unit. Later she offers you a backrub in exchange for receiving her 10:00 p.m. Xanax an hour early. Which response(s) to such behaviors would be most therapeutic? *Select all that apply.*
   a. Label the behavior as undesirable, and explore with Alicia more effective ways to meet her needs.
   b. By role-playing, demonstrate other approaches Alicia could use to meet her needs.
   c. Advise the other patients that Alicia is being manipulative and that they should ignore her when she behaves this way.
   d. Bargain with Alicia to determine a reasonable compromise regarding how much of such behavior is acceptable before she crosses the line.
   e. Explain that such behavior is unacceptable, and give Alicia specific examples of consequences that will be enacted if the behavior continues.
   f. Ignore the behavior for the time being so Alicia will find it unrewarding and in turn seek other, and hopefully more adaptive, ways to meet her needs.

5. A patient becomes frustrated and angry when trying to get his MP3 player and headset to function properly and angrily throws it across the room, nearly hitting a peer with it. Which intervention(s) would be the most therapeutic? *Select all that apply.*
   a. Place the patient in seclusion for 1 hour to allow him to de-escalate.
   b. Tell the patient that any further outbursts will result in a loss of privileges.
   c. Offer to help the patient learn how to operate his music player and headset.
   d. Explore with the patient how he was feeling as he worked with the music player.
   e. Point out the consequences of such behavior and note that it cannot be tolerated.
   f. Limit the patient's exposure to frustrating experiences until he attains improved coping skills.
   g. Encourage the patient to recognize signs of mounting tension and seek assistance.

Answers to Chapter Review
1. b; 2. b; 3. d; 4. a, b, e; 5. a, d, e, g.

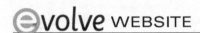
WEBSITE

Visit the Evolve website for a posttest on the content in this chapter: http://evolve.elsevier.com/Varcarolis

Post-Test interactive review

REFERENCES

American Psychiatric Association. (2013). *DSM-5*. Retrieved from http://www.psychiatry.org/practice/dsm/dsm5.

Birgenheir, D. G., & Pepper, C. M. (2011). Negative life experiences and the development of cluster C personality disorders: A cognitive perspective. *Cognitive Behavior Therapy*, *40*(3), 190–205.

Blais, M. A., Smallwood, P., Groves, J. E., & Rivas-Vazquez, R. A. (2008). Personality and personality disorders. In T. A. Stern, J. F. Rosenbaum, M. Fava, J. Biederman, & S. L. Rauch (Eds.), *Massachusetts General Hospital comprehensive clinical psychiatry* (pp. 527–540). St. Louis, MO: Mosby.

Bulechek, G. M., Butcher, H. K., Dochterman, J. M., & Wagner, C. (2013). *Nursing interventions classification (NIC)* (6th ed.). St. Louis, MO: Mosby.

Clark, J. F., & Huprich, S. K. (2011). Do DSM-5 personality disorder proposals meet criteria for clinical utility? *Journal of Personality Disorders*, *25*(2), 192–205.

Coccaro, E. F., & Siever, L. J. (2005). Neurobiology. In J. M. Oldham, A. E. Skodol, & D. S. Bender (Eds.), *Textbook of personality disorders* (pp. 155–169). Washington, DC: American Psychiatric Publishing.

Ekdahl, S., Idvall, E., Samuelsson, M., & Perseius, K. I. (2011). A life tiptoeing: Being a significant other to persons with borderline personality disorder. *Archives of Psychiatric Nursing*, *25*(6), 369–376.

Gunderson, J. G. (2011). Borderline personality disorder. *The New England Journal of Medicine*, *364*, 2037–2042.

Gunderson, J. G., Stout, R. L., McGlashan, T. H., Shea, M. T., Morey, L. C., Grilo, C. M., Zanarini, M. C., et al. (2011). Ten year course of borderline personality disorder: Psychopathology and function from the collaborative longitudinal personality disorders study. *Archives of General Psychiatry*, *68*(8), 827–837.

Hayward, B. A. (2007). Cluster A personality disorders: considering the "odd-eccentric" in psychiatric nursing. *International Journal of Mental Health Nursing*, *16*, 15–21.

Hazlett, E. A., Speiser, L. J., Goodman, M., Roy, M., Carrizal, M., Wynn, J. K., et al. (2007). Exaggerated affect-modulated startle during unpleasant stimuli in borderline personality disorder. *Biological Psychiatry*, *62*(3), 250–255.

Herdman, T. H. (Ed.), (2012). *NANDA international nursing diagnoses: Definitions and classification, 2012–2014*. Oxford, UK: Wiley-Blackwell.

Huang, Y., Kotov, R., de Girolamo, G., Preti, A., Angermeyer, M., Benjet, C., et al. (2009). DSM-IV personality disorders in the WHO World Mental Health Surveys. *British Journal of Psychiatry*, *195*(1), 46–53. doi:10.1192/bjp.bp.108.058552

Hummelen, B., Pedersen, G., & Karterud, S. (2011). Some suggestions for the DSM-5 schizotypal personality disorder construct. *Comprehensive Psychiatry*, *53*(4), 341–349.

Kagan, J. (2005). Personality and temperament. In M. Rosenbluth, S. H. Kennedy, & R. M. Bagby (Eds.), *Depression and personality: Conceptual and clinical challenges* (pp. 3–18). Washington, DC: American Psychiatric Publishing.

Kellogg, S. H., & Young, J. E. (2006). Schema therapy for borderline personality disorder. *Journal of Clinical Psychology*, *62*(4), 445–58.

Kendler, K. S., Aggen, S. H., & Patrick, C. J. (2012). A multivariate twin study of the DSM-IV criteria for antisocial personality disorder. *Biological Psychiatry*, *71*(3), 247–253.

Kernberg, O. (1985). *Internal world and external reality*. London, UK: Aronson.

Lee, R. J., Hempel, J., TenHarmsel, A., Tianmin, L., Mathe, A. A., & Klock, A. (2011). The neuroendocrinology of childhood trauma in personality disorder. *Psychoneuroendocrinology*, *37*(1), 1–9. doi:10.1016/j.psyceuen.2011.05.006.

Lenzenweger, M. F., Lane, M. C., Loranger, A. W., & Kessler, R. C. (2007). DSM-IV personality disorders in the National Comorbidity Survey Replication. *Biological Psychiatry*, *62*(6), 553–564.

Linehan, M. M. (1993). Cognitive behavioral treatment of borderline personality disorder. New York, NY: Guilford.

Magoteaux, A. L., & Bonnivier, J. F. (2009). Distinguishing between personality disorders, stereotypes and eccentricities in older adults. *Journal of Psychosocial Nursing, 47*(7), 19–24.

Mahler, M. S., Pine, F., & Bergman, A. (1975). *The psychological birth of the human infant.* New York, NY: Basic Books.

McGilloway, A., Hall, R. E., Lee, T., & Bhui, K. S. (2010). A systematic review of personality disorder, race, and ethnicity: Prevalence, aetiology and treatment. *BMC Psychiatry, 10*(33), 1–14.

Miller, J. D., Campbell, W. K., & Widiger, T. A. (2010). Narcissistic personality disorder and the DSM-5. *Journal of Abnormal Psychology, 119*(4), 640–649.

Moorhead, S., Johnson, M., Maas, M. L., & Swanson, E. (2013). *Nursing outcomes classification (NOC)* (5th ed.). St. Louis, MO: Mosby.

Paris, J. (2005). A current integrative perspective on personality disorders. In J. M. Oldham, A. E. Skodol, & D. S. Bender (Eds.), *Textbook of personality disorders* (pp. 119–128). Washington, DC: American Psychiatric Publishing.

Pennay, A., Cameron, J., Reichert, T., Strickland, H., Lee, N. K., Hall, K., & Lubman, D. I. (2011). A systematic review of interventions for co-occurring substance use disorder and borderline personality disorder. *Journal of Substance Abuse Treatment, 41*, 363–373.

Ripoll, L. H. (2012). Clinical psychopharmacology of borderline personality disorder. *Current Opinion in Psychiatry, 25*(1), 52–58.

Ripoll, L. H., Triebwasser, J., & Siever, L. (2011). Evidence-based pharmacotherapy for personality disorders. *International Journal of Neuropsychopharmacology,14*, 1257–1288.

Sadock, B. J., & Sadock, V. A. (2008). *Kaplan & Sadock's concise textbook of clinical psychiatry* (3rd ed.). Philadelphia, PA: Lippincott Williams & Wilkins.

Samuels, J. (2011). Personality disorders: Epidemiology and public health issues. *International Review of Psychiatry, 23*(3), 223–233.

Samuel, D. B., Lynam, D. R., Widiger, T. A., & Ball, S. A. (2011). An expert consensus approach to relating the proposed DSM-5 types and traits. *Personality disorders: Theory, research and treatment, 3*(1), 1–16.

Sansone, R. A. & Sansone, L. A. (2012). Borderline personality and externalized aggression. *Innovations in clinical neuroscience, 9*(3), 23–26.

Sansone, R. A. & Sansone, L. A. (2011). Personality disorders: A nation-based perspective on prevalence. *Innovations In Clinical Neuroscience, 8*(4), 13–18.

Seo, D., Patrick, C. J., & Kennealy, P. J. (2008). Role of serotonin and dopamine system interactions in the neurobiology of impulsive aggression and its comorbidity with other clinical disorders. *Aggression and Violent Behavior, 13*(5), 383–395. doi:10.1016/j.avb.2008.06.003.

Skodol, A. E., Bender, D. S., Morey, L. C., Clark, L. A., Oldham, J. M., Alarcon, R. D., et al. (2011). Personality disorder types proposed for DSM-5. *Journal of Personality Disorders, 25*(2), 136–169.

Skodol, A. E., & Gunderson, J. G. (2008). Personality disorders. In R. E. Hales, S. C. Yudofsky, & G. O. Gabbard (Eds.), *Textbook of psychiatry* (5th ed.) (pp. 821–860). Washington, DC: American Psychiatric Publishing.

Soeteman, D. I., Hakkaart-VanRoijen, L., Verheul, R., & Busschbach, J. J. (2008). The economic burden of personality disorders in mental health care. *The Journal of Clinical Psychiatry, 69*(2), 259–265.

Supiano, K. P., & Carroll, A. M. (2009). Personality disorders in older clients and their families: A challenge for geriatric case managers. *Care Management Journals, 10*(4), 146–150.

Svrakic, D. M., Leck-Tosevski, D., & Divac-Jovanovic, M. (2008). DSM axis II: Personality disorders or adaptation disorders? *Current Opinions in Psychiatry, 22*, 11–117.

Tadic, A., Wagner, S., Hoch, J., Baskaya, O., von Cube, R., Skaletz, C., et al. (2009). Gender differences in axis I and axis II comorbidity in patients with borderline personality disorder. *Psychopathology, 42*(4), 257–63.

Torgersen, S. (2009). Prevalence, sociodemographics and functional impairment. In J. M. Oldham, A. E. Skodol, & D. S. Bender (Eds.), *Essentials of personality disorders* (pp. 83–102). Washington, DC: American Psychiatric Publishing.

Widiger, T. A. (2011). A shaky future for personality disorders. *Personality Disorders: Theory, Research and Treatment, 2*(1), 54–67.

Widiger, T. A., & Mullins-Sweatt, S. N. (2010). Clinical utility of a dimensional model of personality disorder. *Professional Psychology: Research and Practice, 41*(6), 488–494.

Widiger, T., & Mullins-Sweatt, S. (2008). Personality disorders. In A. Tassman, J. Kay, J. Lieberman, M. B. First, & M. Maj (Eds.), *Psychiatry* (pp. 1718–1753). London, UK: John Wiley & Sons.

CHAPTER

25

Suicide and Non-Suicidal Self-Injury

Faye J. Grund and M. Selena Yearwood

evolve WEBSITE

Visit the Evolve website for a pretest on the content in this chapter: http://evolve.elsevier.com/Varcarolis

Pre-Test interactive review

OBJECTIVES

1. Describe the profile of suicide in the United States, noting psychosocial and cultural factors that affect risk.
2. Identify three common precipitating events for suicide attempts.
3. Describe risk factors for suicide, including coexisting psychiatric disorders.
4. Name the most frequent coexisting psychiatric disorders.
5. Use the SAD PERSONS scale to assess suicide risk.
6. Describe three expected reactions a nurse may have when beginning work with suicidal patients.
7. Give examples of primary, secondary, and tertiary interventions.
8. Describe basic-level interventions that take place in the hospital or community.
9. Identify key elements of suicide precautions and environmental safety factors in the hospital.
10. Describe the problem of non-suicidal self-injury.

KEY TERMS AND CONCEPTS

completed suicides
copycat suicide
lethality
non-suicidal self-injury
no-suicide contract
parasuicide
postvention
primary intervention
psychological autopsies
SAD PERSONS scale
secondary intervention
suicidal ideation
suicide
suicide attempt
tertiary intervention

Don't grieve for me, for now I'm free,
I'm following the path that God laid for me.
I took his hand when I heard him call,
I turned away, and left it all.
Tasks left undone must stay that way,
I've found true peace at the close of day.
If parting now has left a void,
Then fill it with remembered joy.
Perhaps my time seemed all too brief,
Don't lengthen it now with undue grief.
Lift up your hearts and remember me,
God wants me now, he set me free.

—From a suicide note

Suicide is devastating for those who lose a family member or friend; for those who contemplate suicide, the feelings are powerful and overwhelming. Approximately every 14 minutes, a human life ends as the result of suicide, leading to the loss of approximately 105 American lives daily (Centers for Disease Control and Prevention [CDC], 2012). Pain and hopelessness too frequently culminate in a suicide attempt or completed suicide.

Suicide is largely preventable; yet too often, efforts are only directed toward individuals who are at immediate risk. In the month prior to their deaths, 45% of suicide completers had contact with their primary care provider as compared to 20% who were in contact with mental health providers (Schreiber, Culpepper, & Fife, 2011). It is critical for health care providers to be advocates for this problem and to mobilize the community in reducing and preventing factors that may contribute to suicide. This chapter reviews the facts about suicide, discusses assessment and care of patients who may be suicidal, and addresses the needs of families of these patients. A second, related category of behavior disturbance, non-suicidal self-injury, is addressed in a separate section at the end of the chapter.

CLINICAL PICTURE

Suicide is the intentional act of killing oneself by any means. A history of suicide attempts puts a person at a high probability of actually completing the suicide in the future, particularly in the 24 months following the attempt. Nock and colleagues (2010) note that while these suicide behaviors are most often associated with other psychiatric disorders, especially major depression, suicidal behaviors share similar pathological features and require similar treatment plans no matter what other disorder is present.

Suicidal intent and behaviors are symptoms that are manifested in association with mood disorders and psychotic disorders. Clinical attention is directed to individuals who exhibit these behaviors because of the serious outcomes that may result.

EPIDEMIOLOGY

In the United States, suicide is the tenth-leading cause of death—38,364 people ended their lives by suicide in 2011 (CDC, National Center for Injury Prevention and Control, 2012). Suicide is the fourth-leading cause of death among children ages 10 to 14, the third-leading cause of death among 15- to 24-year-olds, the fourth-leading cause of death among persons ages to 44, and the eighth-leading cause of death among 45- to 64-year-olds (Centers for Disease Control, 2012).

Attempted suicide or suicidal ideation led to 666,000 annual visits to the emergency room, and outcomes may be catastrophic for the individual. Consider the young man with schizophrenia who is so depressed and confused from his illness that he takes an overdose and kneels down in front of his couch to pray for forgiveness as he dies. His father finds him lifeless. The young man lives, but since he was in a kneeling position for so long, the circulation to his legs was compromised. This necessitated their amputation and led to lifelong physical disability.

It is important to consider that the number of suicides may actually be double or triple those reported due to underreporting in general. Purposefully aiming the car at a bridge abutment and crashing may look like an accident; however, many reported accidents, homicides, and deaths ruled as "undetermined" are actually suicides.

In a study on war veterans, the rate of significant depressive symptoms was 31% higher than that of the general population. According to the Department of Defense, completed suicides of military personnel between 2005 and 2009 accounted for more than 1100 deaths, an average of 1 suicide every 36 hours during the 5-year period (Cassels, 2010). More recent statistics reveal that active-duty military personnel complete suicide at the rate of 1 per day, and when veterans are included in the count, the rate is 1 suicide every 80 minutes (Gibbs & Thompson, 2012). Box 25-1 provides some facts about suicide, including data for specific age groups.

Risk Factors

Suicidal ideation is the manifestation of inner pain, hopelessness, and helplessness suffered by individuals. Psychiatric disorders accompany 90% of **completed suicides** (Brendel et al., 2008, National Institute of Mental Health, 2012). The percentage of completed suicides attributable to specific psychiatric disorders is listed in Table 25-1.

It is estimated that two thirds of those who complete suicide are experiencing depression at the time. About 15% of patients who have major depression or bipolar disorder (during the depressed phase) will complete suicide (Brendel et al., 2008). Loss of relationships, financial difficulty, and impulsivity are factors in this population.

Suicide is more than 50 times higher among patients with schizophrenia than in the general population, especially during the first few years of the illness (Limosin et al., 2007). It is the leading cause of early death in this population. About 40% of all patients with schizophrenia attempt suicide at least once; males have a rate of 60%. Up to 10% of these patients die from suicide, usually related to depressive symptoms rather than to command hallucinations or delusions.

Patients with alcohol or substance use disorders also have a higher suicide risk. Years of abuse and comorbidity with depression or antisocial personality disorder are also factors associated with increased risk. Up to 15% of alcohol/substance abusers complete suicide (Sadock & Sadock, 2008). Studies have indicated that 50% of the individuals who end their life by suicide have alcohol in their blood at the time of death. Alcohol, a depressant, tends to dull one's senses, and individuals who are otherwise ambivalent about whether to end their lives may act on suicidal thoughts.

Suicide is usually accompanied by intensely conflicted feelings of pain, hopelessness, guilt, and self-loathing, coupled with the belief that there are no solutions and that that things will not improve. However, the hope of appropriate treatment to relieve patients' suicidal symptoms does exist, and health care providers are important in communicating this hope with patients.

People who survive serious **suicide attempts** often report that it is these feelings that fuel the sense of isolation and despair. They describe an all-consuming psychic pain that shuts out thoughts of the loved ones and heartache they will leave behind. To understand this phenomenon, imagine the pain of your hand on a hot stove burner. At that moment, you are unlikely to think of anything but putting an immediate end to

BOX 25-1 SUICIDE FACTS

General

- Suicide is the tenth-leading cause of death for all ages.
- More than 34,000 suicides occur annually in the U.S. This is the equivalent of 105 suicides per day or 1 suicide every 14 minutes.
- The National Violent Death Reporting System examined toxicology tests of those who committed suicide in 16 states; 33.3% tested positive for alcohol and 21% for opiates or prescription painkillers.

Gender Statistics

- Males take their own lives at nearly four times the rate of females and represent 79.8% of all U.S. suicides.
- During their lifetime, women attempt suicide about two to three times more often than men.
- Suicide is the seventh-leading cause of death for males and the fifteenth-leading cause for females.
- Among males, adults aged 75 years and older have the highest rate of suicide (nearly 36.1 per 100,000 population).
- Among females, those in their 40s and 50s have the highest rate of suicide (8.8 per 100,000 population).
- Firearms are the most commonly used method of suicide among males (approximately 56.7%).
- Poisoning is the most common method of suicide for females (37%).

Racial and Ethnic Statistics

- Among American Indians/Alaska Natives ages 15 to 34 years, suicide is the second-leading cause of death.
- Suicide rates among American Indian/Alaskan Native adolescents and young adults ages 15 to 34 (31 per 100,000) are 2.5 times higher than the national average for that age group (12 per 100,000).
- Of female students in grades 9 to 12, significantly more Hispanic (13.5%) attempt suicide than black non-Hispanics (9%) and white non-Hispanics (8%).

Age Statistics

- In 2011, 16% of U.S. high school students reported that they had seriously considered attempting suicide during the 12 months preceding the survey. About 8% of students reported that they had actually attempted suicide one or more times during the same period.
- Suicide is the third-leading cause of death among 15- to 24-year-olds, accounting for 20% of all deaths annually.
- Suicide is the second-leading cause of death among 25- to 34-year-olds.
- The rate of suicide for adults ages 75 years and older was 16 per 100,000.

Attempted Suicide

- In 2011, nearly 500,000 people were treated in emergency departments for self-inflicted injuries.
- There is 1 suicide for every 25 attempted suicides.

Data from Centers for Disease Control and Prevention. (2012). *Suicide facts at a glance: 2012.* Retrieved from http://www.cdc.gov/violenceprevention/pdf/suicide_dataSheet-2012-a.pdf.

TABLE 25-1 PERCENTAGE OF SUICIDES ATTRIBUTABLE TO PSYCHIATRIC DISORDERS

DISORDERS	PERCENTAGE
Affective illnesses (major depression and bipolar disorder)	50
Drug or alcohol abuse	25
Schizophrenia	10
Personality disorders	5

From Brendel, R. W., Lagomasino, I. T., Perlis, R. H., & Stern, T. A. (2008). The suicidal patient. In T. A. Stern, J. R. Rosenbaum, M. Fava, J. Biederman, & S. L. Rauch (Eds.), *Massachusetts General Hospital comprehensive clinical psychiatry* (pp. 733–745). St. Louis, MO: Mosby.

the pain. Emotional pain often renders the individual void of thought and without enough motivation to leave a suicide note. Only about 33% of individuals who complete suicide leave a note (Haines et al., 2011).

Besides psychiatric disorders, other risk factors for suicide include the following (Sadock & Sadock, 2008):

- **Male gender:** Men commit suicide four times more often than women.
- **Increasing age:** For men, suicide rates peak after the age of 45; for women, rates peak after 55.
- **Race:** White males commit two out of every three suicides in the United States.
- **Religion:** Religiosity is associated with decreased rates of suicide. Protestants and Jews have higher rates of suicide than Roman Catholics.
- **Marriage:** Being married, especially with children in the home, significantly reduces the risk of suicide. Divorced men are more likely than divorced women to kill themselves.
- **Profession:** Professionals are generally considered at higher risk for suicide, particularly if there is a fall in status. Law enforcement personnel, dentists, artists, mechanics, insurance agents, and lawyers are also at higher risk.
- **Physical health:** About half of those who complete suicide have physical illnesses. Loss of mobility, disfigurement, and chronic pain are especially associated with suicide.

Since individuals with suicidal ideation are often ambivalent about death, helping them examine alternative actions to reduce their pain is critical. Extensive data are available about risk factors for suicide, based on epidemiological studies and psychological autopsies (i.e., retrospective reviews of the deceased person's life within several months of death to establish likely diagnoses at the time of death). There is also evidence concerning protective factors (those that tend to reduce risk). Refer to Box 25-2 for a description of significant psychosocial risk and protective factors for suicide.

BOX 25-2 SUICIDE RISK FACTORS AND PROTECTIVE FACTORS

Risk Factors
- Suicidal ideation with intent
- Lethal suicide plan
- History of suicide attempt
- Co-occurring psychiatric illness
- Co-occurring medical illness
- History of childhood abuse
- Family history of suicide
- Recent lack of social support (isolation)
- Unemployment
- Recent stressful life event (e.g., death, other loss)
- Hopelessness
- Panic attacks
- Feeling of shame or humiliation
- Impulsivity
- Aggressiveness
- Loss of cognitive function (e.g., loss of impulse control)
- Access to firearms and other highly lethal means
- Substance abuse (without formal disorder)
- Impending incarceration
- Low frustration tolerance
- Sexual orientation issues

Protective Factors
- Sense of responsibility to family (spouse, children)
- Pregnancy
- Religious beliefs
- Satisfaction with life
- Positive social support
- Access to health care
- Effective coping skills
- Effective problem-solving skills
- Intact reality testing

Data from American Psychiatric Association. (2003). Practice guidelines for the assessment and treatment of patients with suicidal behaviors. *American Journal of Psychiatry, 160*(11 Suppl), 12.

EVIDENCE-BASED PRACTICE

SAFE-T: Benchmarking Suicide Risk and Recommendations for Interventions

Fowler, J. (2012). Suicide risk assessment in clinical practice: Pragmatic guidelines for imperfect assessments. *Psychotherapy, 49*(1), 81–90.

Problem

Conducting assessments for the relative risk of suicide that are both sensitive and accurate is challenging. After suicide attempts, the assessment, management, and treatment of patients who survive is a challenging task for clinicians.

Purpose of Study

The purpose of the study was to evaluate tools for suicide risk assessment that summarize the risk factors, warning signs, and protective factors; benchmark the risk; and suggest targeted interventions when the outcome of the assessment is heightened risk.

Methods

The researcher reviewed the risk and protective factors known from the literature to have the strongest evidence base. The researcher also reviewed recent recommendations in the literature for clinicians to enhance therapeutic alliances with patients and to consider recent situations that contributed to the patient's suicidal ideation.

Key Findings

Risk factors associated with suicide attempts include the following:
- Past suicide attempts remain the strongest consistent predictor of suicide attempts and completed suicide.
- Comorbid psychiatric diagnosis is a greater risk with substance, mood, and personality disorders.
- Single diagnoses of eating disorders and substance abuse disorders have the greatest risk.
- Severity of mental disorder, regardless of the disorder, may be a risk factor.
- Psychological vulnerabilities, including aggressiveness/impulsivity, anxiety, and depressive symptoms, increase the risk.
- Genetic markers; 5-HTT serotonin-gene is a moderate risk factor.
- Demographic factors convey risk, albeit inconsistently. At higher risk are males (who complete more suicides), persons who are unmarried, the elderly, adolescent and young adult age groups, and Caucasian race.
- Diathesis-stress models may confer greater risk where underlying genetic and psychological vulnerabilities may be triggered by environmental stressors.

Warning Signs
- Suicidal ideation/plan
- Stressful life events
- Posthospitalization transition

Protective Factors
- Religious affiliation/beliefs
- Reasons for living, including social and religious/moral reasons
- Marriage except in high-conflict and violent relationships
- Children in the home except in postpartum depression and extreme financial hardships
- Supportive social networks, including religious and school environments and close familial ties
- Therapeutic contacts, particularly for borderline personality disorders
- Psychotropic medications, including lithium prophylaxis for mood disorders and clozapine for psychotic disorders
- Brief, supportive contacts including caring communication and concern

The assessment tool that encompasses both risk and protective factors, provides the clinician with a tool to benchmark risk, and suggests interventions when the outcome is heightened risk is the Suicide Assessment Five-step Evaluation and Triage (SAFE-T). This tool was established based on sponsored research outcomes from the Substance Abuse and Mental Health Services Administration and the recommendations of the American Psychiatric Association Practice Guidelines (2003). Students are encouraged to download a free pocket guide may be downloaded from *http://store.samhsa.gov/product/SMA09-4432*. The tool allows the clinician to benchmark relative risk (high, moderate, low) and to develop a treatment plan, in consultation with the patient, to reduce current risk.

Implications for Nursing Practice

Nurses have an important role in the assessment of suicidal risk in both inpatient and outpatient settings. Assessment of risk factors, warning signs, and protective factors is an ongoing responsibility, as is establishing therapeutic alliances with patients. Nurses are in a unique position to establish therapeutic alliances with patients while communicating care and concern. Use of the SAFE-T risk assessment will provide valuable information for development of a plan of care to keep the patient safe.

ETIOLOGY

Biological Factors

Suicidal behavior is often prevalent among family members. Margaux Hemingway's death in 1996 was the fifth suicide among four generations of writer Ernest Hemingway's (1899-1961) family. Twin and adoption studies suggest the presence of genetic factors in suicide. Suicide rates in twins are higher among monozygotic (identical) twins than among dizygotic (fraternal) twins. Studies found a significantly higher incidence of suicide among biological relatives of adoptees who completed suicide than among the biological relatives of control subjects. With the identification of the human genome, the number of studies examining both protective and risk genetic variants is increasing is number.

Murphy et al. (2011) obtained blood samples for DNA from 159 patients with diagnosed mental disorders (76 suicide attempters and 83 non-attempters). They examined the contribution of individual genetic variants to the prediction of suicide attempters and whether single nucleotide polymorphisms (SNPs) have potential for gene-gene and gene-environmental interactions. The researchers identified four SNPs that were positively associated with suicide attempters when compared to the non-attempter group. Further studies examining the complex relationship of genetic and environmental factors in the suicidal behavior of individuals with mental disorders have promise to provide insight into treatment strategies.

Low serotonin levels are related to depressed mood. Studies have found low levels of serotonin or its metabolites in the cerebrospinal fluid of patients who are suicidal (Brendel et al., 2008). Postmortem exams of individuals who complete suicide also reveal a low level of serotonin in the brainstem or the frontal cortex.

Psychosocial Factors

Sigmund Freud originally theorized that suicide resulted from unacceptable aggression toward another person that is turned inward. Karl Menninger added to Freud's thought by describing three parts of suicidal hostility: the wish to kill, the wish to be killed, and the wish to die (Sadock & Sadock, 2008). Aaron Beck identified a central emotional factor underlying suicide intent: hopelessness. Cognitive styles that contribute to higher risk are rigid all-or-nothing thinking, inability to see different options, and perfectionism (APA, 2003).

Recent theories of suicide have focused on the lethal combination of suicidal fantasies accompanied by loss (love, self-esteem, job, and freedom due to imminent incarceration), rage or guilt, and identification with an individual who completed suicide (copycat suicide). A **copycat suicide** follows a highly publicized suicide of a public figure, an idol, or a peer in the community. Adolescents are at especially high risk, due to their immature prefrontal cortex, the portion of the brain that controls the executive functions involving judgment, frustration tolerance, and impulse control.

Cultural Factors

Cultural factors, including religious beliefs, family values, sexual orientation (see the Considering Culture box), and attitude toward death, have an impact on suicide rates. In 2009, ethnicity was a significant factor in the number of deaths by suicide in the United States. White, non-Hispanics had the highest number of deaths by suicide, about 14 per 100,000. Other groups with high rates of suicide are American Indians and Alaskan Natives, about

CONSIDERING CULTURE

Suicide and Sexual Identity

Suicide among lesbian, gay, and bisexual (LGB) youth is on the rise in the United States. In the 15- to 24-year-old population, suicide is the third-leading cause of death, and LGB youth are more likely to attempt suicide than their heterosexual peers (CDC, National Center for Injury Prevention and Control, 2011). Hatzenbuehler (2012) utilized the Oregon Healthy Teens survey to study youth in the 11th grade between 2006 and 2008. Of the 33,714 students who participated in the study, about 90% identified themselves as heterosexual, about 1% identified themselves as gay or lesbian, about 3% identified themselves as bisexual, about 2% reported they were not sure about their sexual identity, and 4% did not respond. Of those students who reported their sexual identity, nearly 20% of lesbian and gay youth, and 22% of bisexual youth reported having attempted suicide as compared to only 4% of the heterosexual youth.

In all instances, self-identified lesbian or gay and self-identified bisexual youth reported significantly higher percentages of the suicide risk factors than their heterosexual peers. The study also suggests that an environment that is supportive of LGB results in fewer suicide attempts. A supportive environment includes a higher number of same-sex couples, registered Democrats, the presence of gay-straight alliances in schools, and school policies that protect LGB from discrimination and bullying.

From Hatzenbeuhler, M. (2011). The social environment and suicide attempts in lesbian, gay, and bisexual youth. *Pediatrics, 127*, 896–903.

12 per 100,000, and Asian or Pacific Islanders, about 6 per 100,000 (Centers for Disease Control, 2012).

Among African Americans, men complete suicide more often than women, and the peak rate occurs in adolescence and young adulthood. Protective factors for this group as a whole include religion and the role of the extended family, both of which provide a strong social support system. Similarly, among Hispanic Americans, Roman Catholic religion (in which suicide is a sin) and the importance given to the extended family decrease the risk for suicide. There is also the philosophy of *fatalismo*, a belief that divine providence regulates the world; the individual is deemed unable to control adverse events and is more likely to accept misfortune instead of blaming the self.

Among Asian Americans, suicide rates are noted to increase with age. Beliefs that reduce suicide attempts include the adherence to religions that emphasize interdependence between the individual and society (i.e., self-destruction is seen as disrespectful to the group or selfish). The high value given to the reputation of the family, however, may lead to the conclusion that suicide is preferable if it prevents shame to the family. A belief in reincarnation may make death a potentially honorable solution to life problems.

Suicide bombing has grown exponentially in recent years, most recently in the Middle East. While not condoned by Islam, suicide bombers may believe that it is an honor to die in defense of their faith, that real happiness exists beyond this life, and that for martyrs, dying is not real death but an honorable ticket straight to heaven. However, there is debate in the literature regarding the difference between martyrdom and suicide. Further research will bring clarity to how mental health professionals might indeed prevent suicide for those who clearly have personal suicidal intent versus those who choose to conduct suicide bombings for martyrdom's purpose.

Societal Factors

Assisted suicide, as a societal factor, is both a moral and ethical issue. In the United States, Oregon's Death with Dignity Act of 1994 allowed terminally ill patients to legally seek a physician-assisted suicide. The patient must be thoroughly screened by a physician and deemed to be both terminally ill and psychiatrically sound; however, concern has been raised that as many as 25% of the patients in Oregon who were assisted to die actually have clinical depression (Ganzini & Dobscha, 2008).

In 2009, Washington state also approved legislation allowing physicians to prescribe lethal medication. Montana's Supreme Court determined that assisted suicide is a medical treatment (Marker & Hamlon, 2010). The Netherlands allows for this practice in nonterminal cases of "lasting and unbearable" suffering (Appel, 2007). Belgium authorizes physician-assisted suicide for nonterminal cases when suffering is deemed to be "constant and cannot be alleviated." Switzerland, where assisted suicide has been legal since 1918, has the most liberal laws; it allows nonresidents to terminate their lives without a physician involved in the process (Appel, 2007).

The ethical and moral dilemmas in this evolving trend are clear. There are now debates about whether chronic and serious mental illness is no different in the depth and breadth of suffering than chronic and serious physical illness. Until more effective treatment or a cure is found, some individuals who obtain little or no benefit from existing psychiatric treatments may choose to end suffering through suicide. As such, individuals do have the power to end their lives by suicide; however, suicide is an all too often tragic, individual act. Assisted suicide, on the other hand, is not a private act, rather one person facilitating the death of another. The ethical dilemma over assisted suicide will continue as individuals attempt to determine the definition of "terminal illness" as a reason to support assisted suicide (Marker & Hamlon, 2010).

APPLICATION OF THE NURSING PROCESS

The process of suicide risk assessment is comprehensive and based on identifying specific risk and protective factors, taking a psychosocial and health history, and establishing a therapeutic alliance with the patient during the interview. The nurse usually completes this assessment in conjunction with other clinicians since comparison of data from two interviewers is often a significant element of the evaluation.

ASSESSMENT

Verbal and Nonverbal Clues

Individuals considering suicide generally provide some indication of their thoughts, especially to people whom they perceive to be supportive of them. Nurses often fit into this category. There may be overt or covert verbal clues and nonverbal signals. Examples include the following:

Overt Statements

- "I can't take it anymore."
- "Life isn't worth living anymore."
- "I wish I were dead."
- "Everyone would be better off if I died."

Covert Statements

- "It's okay now. Soon everything will be fine."
- "Things will never work out."
- "I won't be a problem much longer."
- "Nothing feels good to me anymore and probably never will."
- "How can I give my body to medical science?"

Most often it is a relief for people contemplating suicide to finally talk to someone about their despair and loneliness. Asking about suicidal thoughts does not "give a person ideas" and is, in fact, a professional responsibility similar to asking about chest pain in cardiac conditions. Talking openly leads to a decrease in isolation and can increase problem-solving alternatives for living. People who contemplate suicide, attempt suicide, and even those who regret the failure of their attempt, are often extremely receptive to talking about their suicide crisis. Specific questions to ask about suicidal ideation include the following (APA, 2003):

- Have you ever felt that life was not worth living?
- Have you been thinking about death recently?
- Did you ever think about suicide?

- Have you ever attempted suicide?
- Do you have a plan for completing suicide?
- If so, what is your plan for suicide?

The following dialogue illustrates how the nurse can make covert messages more open:

Nurse: You haven't eaten or slept well for the past few days, Mary.

Mary: No, I feel pretty low lately.

Nurse: How low are you feeling?

Mary: Oh, I don't know. Nothing seems to matter to me anymore. It's all so meaningless . . . .

Nurse: Tell me about it, Mary. I want to understand how you're feeling. What is meaningless?

Mary: Life . . . the whole thing . . . nothingness. Life is a bad joke.

Nurse: Are you saying you don't think life is worth living?

Mary: Well . . . yes. It's all so hopeless anyway.

Nurse: Are you thinking of killing yourself?

Mary: Oh, I don't know. Well, sometimes I think about it. I probably would never go through with it.

Nurse: Mary, let's talk more about what you're thinking and feeling. This is important. I'll need to share your thoughts with other members of the staff.

The nurse should be alert for nonverbal behavioral clues, including showing a sudden brightening of mood with more energy (especially after recently being prescribed an antidepressant medication), giving away possessions, or organizing financial affairs. Individuals may be at greater risk as their mood lifts and they have enough energy to act on their feelings of ambivalence regarding suicide. The risk of suicide is highest in the first year after a suicide attempt (Simon, 2011).

Evidence-based clinical practice guidelines emphasize the importance of establishing a therapeutic relationship with the patient and asking directly about suicidal feelings (APA, 2003). This is the single most important assessment (and intervention), yet health care professionals report a surprisingly small amount of probing. Possible reasons for this lack of probing include lack of personal comfort, lack of professional confidence, and time constraints. Crisis intervention techniques involve listening for the emotional feeling message underlying the verbal message, especially when the patient presents as angry, hostile, and overwhelmed. The therapeutic alliance established with a patient is a dynamic, changeable interaction that may change between interactions. Thus, it must be constantly assessed and documented. The presence of the therapeutic alliance may be a protective factor, while the absence of a therapeutic alliance may be a risk factor for suicide (Simon, 2011).

Lethality of Suicide Plan

The evaluation of a suicide plan is extremely important in determining the degree of suicidal risk. Three main elements must be considered when evaluating lethality: (1) Is there a specific plan with details? (2) How lethal is the proposed method? (3) Is there access to the planned method? People who have definite plans for the time, place, and means are at high risk.

Based on the lethality of a method, which indicates how quickly a person would die by that mode, a method can be classified as higher or lower risk. Higher-risk methods, also referred to as *hard methods*, include:

- Using a gun
- Jumping off a high place
- Hanging
- Poisoning with carbon monoxide
- Staging a car crash

Examples of lower-risk methods, also referred to as *soft methods*, include:

- Slashing one's wrists
- Inhaling natural gas
- Ingesting pills

When the proposed method is available, the situation is more serious. A man who has access to a high building and states that he will jump from it or a woman who has a gun and says that she will shoot herself is at serious risk for suicide. When people are experiencing psychotic episodes, they are at high risk—regardless of the specificity of details—because impulse control and judgment are grossly impaired. A person suffering psychosis is particularly vulnerable when depressed or having command hallucinations.

Assessment Tools

Many tools have been developed to aid a health care worker in assessing suicidal potential. Patterson, Dohn, Bird, and Patterson (1983) devised an assessment aid with the acronym *SAD PERSONS* to evaluate 10 major risk factors for suicide (Table 25-2). The SAD PERSONS scale is a simple and practical

TABLE 25-2 SAD PERSONS SCALE

S	Sex	1 if male
A	Age	1 if 25 to 44 years or 65+ years
D	Depression	1 if present
P	Previous attempt	1 if present
E	Ethanol use	1 if present
R	Rational thinking loss	1 if psychotic for any reason
S	Social supports lacking	1 if lacking, especially recent loss
O	Organized plan	1 if plan with lethal method
N	No spouse	1 if divorced, widowed, separated, or single male
S	Sickness	1 if severe or chronic

Guidelines for Action

POINTS	CLINICAL ACTION
0-2	Send home with follow-up
3-4	Closely follow up; consider hospitalization
5-6	Strongly consider hospitalization
7-10	Hospitalize or commit

From Patterson, W. M., Dohn, H. H., Bird, J., & Patterson, G. A. (1983). Evaluation of suicidal patients: The SAD PERSONS scale. *Psychosomatics, 24*(4), 343–349.

guide for triaging patients who are potentially suicidal, particularly in an emergency department environment. Ten categories are described in the assessment tool, and the person being evaluated is assigned 1 point for each applicable characteristic. The total point score for the individual correlates with an action scale assisting health care workers in determining whether hospital admission is advisable. If a patient scores in the 3- to 4-point ranges, it is then necessary for a psychiatric/mental health professional to conduct a full mental status examination and interview.

The SAD PERSONS tool does not address whether or not the individual is taking either illicit or prescribed drugs that may have a significant impact on the patient. Although the tool is dated (1983), it remains a quick assessment of risk factors to determine need for further evaluation.

Prescription medications such as antidepressants should be evaluated for their contribution to suicide risk. The U.S. Federal Drug Administration (FDA) (2007) black box warning for all classes of antidepressants includes children and young adults between 18 and 24 years old. It states that careful monitoring should occur during the first few weeks of treatment as well as when the dosage is changed. The use of selective serotonin reuptake inhibitors (SSRIs) in patients with depression related to undiagnosed bipolar disorder may result in mania, which carries an especially high risk for suicide. This type of mania can also be the result of steroid use.

Self-Assessment

Health care professionals working with individuals who are suicidal need collaboration with other clinicians. Fear, grief, anger, puzzlement, and condemnation of suicidal feelings/intent are common. If these intense emotional responses are not acknowledged, countertransference may limit effective intervention. Understanding the patient with suicidal behavior disorder, as well as acknowledging, understanding, and accepting the emotions that arise from working with and caring for these patients, is essential.

ASSESSMENT GUIDELINES

Suicide

1. Assess risk factors, including history of suicide (in family, friends), degree of hopelessness and helplessness, and lethality of plan.
2. Assess protective factors that may be built upon.
3. If there is a history of suicide attempt, assess intent, lethality, and injury.
4. Determine whether the patient's age, medical condition, psychiatric diagnosis, or current medications put the patient at higher risk.
5. A change from sad or depressed to happy and peaceful may be a red flag. Often a decision to commit suicide gives a feeling of relief and calm.
6. If the patient is to be managed on an outpatient basis, also assess social supports and helpfulness of significant others.

DIAGNOSIS

The nursing diagnosis with the highest priority is *Risk for suicide*. Feelings of hopelessness, anger, frustration, abandonment, and rejection are common among people who are suicidal. Nursing diagnoses that address problems related to depressed mood, anxiety, mania, or disturbed thought include *Self-care deficit, Sleep pattern disturbance, Altered nutrition,* and *Anxiety*. See the clinical chapters focusing on depressive disorders, bipolar disorders, and schizophrenia spectrum disorders for more information.

OUTCOMES IDENTIFICATION

Relevant *Nursing Outcomes Classification (NOC)* outcomes include *Suicide Self-Restraint, Coping, Hope, Social Support, Spiritual Health*, and *Self-Esteem* (Moorhead et al., 2013). Table 25-3 describes signs and symptoms, potential nursing diagnoses, and outcomes for suicidal behavior.

PLANNING

The plan of care for the patient who is suicidal is based on risk and protective factors. When there is a comorbid psychiatric disorder, the treatment plan includes appropriate nursing approaches (e.g., care for patients with depression or schizophrenia). The patient's significant others need to be involved because the patient's perception of isolation is a significant cause of hopelessness. Case Study and Nursing Care Plan 25-1 represents the case of a young woman with suicidal ideation treated in an outpatient setting.

IMPLEMENTATION

Nursing interventions for patients with suicidal ideation and suicide attempts take place at three different levels: primary, secondary, and tertiary. Improving *overall* community mental health may reduce the incidence of suicide more effectively than extensive efforts directed at identifying individuals who are imminently suicidal; therefore, more attention focused on primary interventions that involve community-wide participation will lead to improved outcomes.

Primary Intervention

Primary intervention includes activities that provide support, information, and education to prevent suicide (Box 25-3). Primary intervention is practiced in a wide variety of community settings such as schools, homes, churches, clinics, hospitals, and work settings. Elementary school children are screened using evidence-based tools that focus on both risk factors and warning signs (Joe & Bryant, 2007). Some high schools are adopting suicide prevention curricula that involve elements of education, peer support and referral, discussions about risk and prevention factors, and warning signs (Ciffone, 2007, American Association of Suicidology, 2008).

A suicide prevention model where nurses may be educated as gatekeepers as well as be involved in educating the community is the Question, Persuade, Refer (QPR) model (Quinnett, 2007). This model, originally developed in1995, is a simple educational "train the trainer" program that provides ordinary

25-1 CASE STUDY AND NURSING CARE PLAN

A Patient with Suicidal Ideation in the Outpatient Setting

Kaitlin is a 23-year-old single waitress who is brought to the emergency department by ambulance after a suicide attempt. Her live-in boyfriend had narrowly prevented her from fatally shooting herself with a gun kept in their apartment. She has a minor scalp wound and remains under observation for a few hours after treatment. The psychiatric nurse and psychiatrist on call then interview her.

She states that she has been under increasing stress for the past 2 months since entering a management-training program at work. Kaitlin ultimately failed at this venture and lost her job. She expresses a great deal of desperation owing to the accumulation of several bills and the upcoming Christmas holidays. She admits to keeping these feelings to herself and self-medicating her growing fear and anxiety with drugs and alcohol. She states that she feels "like a total loser."

Because Kaitlin continues to state that she wants to kill herself, because of her reluctance to open up and share her feelings with anyone, and because her scoring a 4 on the SAD PERSONS scale, the decision is made to hospitalize her. After careful assessment, Kaitlin is placed on antidepressant therapy and carefully monitored. Additionally, problems relating to her depressive state are assessed and monitored (poor appetite, insomnia, self-care deficit, and anxiety). After 3 days on suicide precautions, she is no longer acutely suicidal and agrees to continue treatment in the outpatient division of the hospital.

Self-Assessment

Mrs. Ruiz is a registered nurse with a bachelor's degree and 5 years' experience. She remembers Kaitlin from the emergency evaluation and expresses reluctance to take the assignment. She seeks out the clinical supervisor to discuss the case. In talking about her feelings, she realizes that she wants to avoid this patient for two reasons. The first is that Kaitlin's impatience, agitation, and anger cause Mrs. Ruiz to feel anxious and inadequate. The second is that Mrs. Ruiz disapproves of Kaitlin's attempt to end her life. "She is so young and has her whole life in front of her. How bad can her problems be? My Catholic faith makes suicide difficult to accept."

Mrs. Ruiz also notes the countertransference involved, in that Kaitlin reminds her of her own daughter. Mrs. Ruiz recognizes her own feelings and can now better focus on Kaitlin's issues. Kaitlin feels angry and helpless after losing her job and facing financial concerns; her isolation seems self-imposed because she pushes people away and keeps her feelings to herself, probably because of low self-esteem. After consultation, Mrs. Ruiz agrees with her supervisor that she can work with Kaitlin.

Assessment

Objective Data

- Reported first suicide attempt in a 23-year-old female
- Self-medicating with alcohol and substances (denies chronic use)
- Isolated without social support systems
- Recent failure at work and subsequent loss of job
- Mounting debt at holiday season
- No history of bipolar disorder or related behaviors

Subjective Data

- "I love my boyfriend, but I don't like to talk about my problems."
- "I have a lot of friends, but they don't really know me; I keep secrets from everyone."
- "I just feel so down and depressed."
- "I'm constantly getting in over my head and screwing up."
- "I don't want my family to find out what a mess I've made of things . . . again."

Diagnosis

1. *Risk for suicide* related to feeling overwhelmed and depressed secondary to loss of job and mounting debt, as evidenced by suicide attempt

Supporting Data

- Suicide attempt with lethal intent
- "I don't want to live and have to face everyone with this mess I've made."
- Mounting debt at the holiday season
- Recent job loss

2. *Impaired social interaction* related to feelings of fear and shame, as evidenced by avoiding disclosure of issues and feelings with family and significant others.

Supporting Data

- "I'm too ashamed to face everyone now."
- "I feel like I'm all alone with my mess. I'm so disgusted and angry!"
- "My job was where my friends were."
- "I can't even tell my boyfriend."

Outcomes Identification

1. Patient will consistently use suicide prevention resources and social support groups within the community (long-term outcome).
2. Patient will develop insight and trust in order to establish supportive social contacts (long-term outcome).

Planning

The initial plan is to establish a working relationship with Kaitlin, involving her in planning her own treatment and identifying alternative actions for suicidal ideation in the future.

Implementation

Kaitlin's plan of care is personalized as follows:

Nursing diagnosis: *Risk for suicide* related to feeling overwhelmed and depressed secondary to loss of job and mounting debt

Outcome criteria: Patient will consistently use suicide prevention resources and social support groups within the community.

25-1 CASE STUDY AND NURSING CARE PLAN—cont'd

A Patient with Suicidal Ideation in the Outpatient Setting

SHORT-TERM GOAL	INTERVENTION	RATIONALE	EVALUATION
1. Kaitlin will immediately seek help when feeling self-destructive.	1a. Assess suicide status.	1a. Ongoing periodic check of suicidal status. Higher rate of suicide for those who have attempted suicide.	**GOAL MET** Kaitlin agrees to talk to the nurse about suicidal feelings. If clinic is closed, she will call the crisis hotline (first session). Kaitlin also agreed to a family session that included her boyfriend, and the gun was removed from her apartment.
	1b. Even if Kaitlin denies suicidal ideas, make a future plan.	1b. Demonstrates concern and offers alternatives if suicidal thoughts return.	
	1c. Monitor efficacy of antidepressant therapy and assess for side effects.	1c. Ongoing periodic. Important to assess for agitation and increase in suicidal feelings and to monitor for lifting of depressive state.	1c. No adverse side effects noted. Noted increase in socialization, improved hygiene, reported improvement in sleep and appetite. Patient states her mood is improving, and she feels more hopeful.
2. Kaitlin will talk about painful feelings by the first week.	2a. Remain neutral in face of anger.	2a. Diminishes power struggles and discourages continuing acting-out behaviors.	**GOAL MET** During the initial sessions, angry communication is constant. By the end of the first week, Kaitlin states, "You really want to know." Kaitlin talks of feeling like a failure as a daughter, girlfriend, and employee.
	2b. Refocus attention back to Kaitlin and the emotions underlying her anger.	2b. Arguments and power struggles keep attention away from important issues.	
	2c. Give frequent opportunities for discussion of feelings through verbal invitation and stated concern.	2c. Aggressive, hostile communications are a cover for painful feelings. When patient can express feelings in words, there is less need to act them out.	
3. Kaitlin will explore other employment opportunities by the end of the second week.	3. Alternative solutions can be problem-solved once feelings and problems are identified.	3. Acceptable alternatives increase a future orientation and decrease hopelessness. Patient can experience feelings of control over situation.	**GOAL MET** By the end of the second week, Kaitlin talks about attending a regional job fair that will be held after the holidays. She has accepted a referral to social services for the purpose of registering for unemployment benefits and debt management.

Nursing diagnosis: *Impaired social interaction* related to feelings of fear and shame, as evidenced by avoiding disclosure of issues and feelings with family and significant others

Outcome criteria: Patient will develop insight and trust in order to establish supportive social contacts.

SHORT-TERM GOAL	INTERVENTION	RATIONALE	EVALUATION
1. Kaitlin will discuss feelings of isolation and loneliness by the end of the third week.	1. Provide opportunities for Kaitlin to honestly express feelings and thoughts regarding her self-imposed isolation.	1. Before change can take place, clarification of personal feelings and thoughts is necessary.	**GOAL MET** By the end of the third week, Kaitlin speaks of feeling alone and demonstrates insight into the dynamics of keeping secrets, yet desperately wanting a real and honest connection to loved ones.
2. Kaitlin will identify three positive aspects of self by the end of the third week.	2a. Validate Kaitlin's strengths.	2a. Both positive and negative feedback aid in more realistic perception of self.	**GOAL MET** By the end of the third week, Kaitlin states that she thinks she is a hard worker, good friend, and a caring daughter and girlfriend.
	2b. Encourage self-evaluation of both positive and negative aspects of Kaitlin's life.	2b. Patient can begin to see herself more clearly, with increase in self-esteem	
3. Kaitlin will state that she enjoys one new, healthy activity with at least one other person by the end of the fourth week.	3a. Review previous activities that Kaitlin enjoyed before she lost her job.	3a. Change focus from negative present to positive aspects of patient's past. Can help increase hope and self-esteem.	**GOAL MET** By the end of the fourth week, Kaitlin states that she started skiing again and is surprised that she and her boyfriend had a good time.
	3b. Have Kaitlin choose an activity she is willing to participate in.	3b. Participating in own problem solving and decision making offers patient a sense of control and an increase in self-esteem.	

Evaluation

See individual outcomes and evaluation within the care plan.

TABLE 25-3 SIGNS AND SYMPTOMS, NURSING DIAGNOSES, AND OUTCOMES FOR A PATIENT WITH SUICIDAL IDEATION

SIGNS AND SYMPTOMS	POTENTIAL NURSING DIAGNOSES	OUTCOMES
Gives overt or covert clues (e.g., "I can't stand the pain"), has a plan (gun), is in high-risk category on assessment (elderly or teenager, isolated, depressed, has had a recent loss), has a psychiatric diagnosis (substance abuse, depression, borderline personality disorder, psychosis)	*Risk for suicide* *Risk for injury* *Risk for self-directed/other-directed violence*	Remains free from injury, expresses will to live, discloses plan for suicide if present, refrains from attempting suicide
Overwhelmed with situational crises, relies heavily on drugs or alcohol, has few supportive systems, shows poor problem-solving skills, has "tunnel vision"; no family available or crisis in the family, poor family communication	*Ineffective coping* *Disabled family coping* *Impaired social interaction*	Identifies coping mechanisms to assist with situational crisis, identifies social support within community.
Lacks hope for the future; believes nothing can change intolerable situation; has intense feelings of isolation, deprivation, and lack of love; has nowhere to turn; has no control over the future; lacks spiritual resources; has no close relationships	*Hopelessness* *Powerlessness* *Social isolation* *Spiritual distress* *Loneliness* *Chronic sorrow*	Expresses willingness to call on others for help, identifies one support system within community.
Believes that he or she is no good, worthless, ineffective, a burden to others, can't do anything right	*Situational low self-esteem* *Chronic low self-esteem*	Describes feelings of self-worth
Does not understand age-related crises; does not know of available resources	*Deficient knowledge*	Patient and family identify developmental crisis as age-related and identify community resources.

From Herdman, T. H. (Ed.) *Nursing diagnoses—Definitions and classification 2012-2014.* Copyright © 2012, 1994-2012 by NANDA International. Used by arrangement with John Wiley & Sons Limited; Moorhead, S., Johnson, M., Maas, M. L., & Swanson, E. (2013). *Nursing outcomes classification (NOC)* (5th ed.). St. Louis, MO: Mosby.

BOX 25-3 GOALS OF THE NATIONAL STRATEGY FOR SUICIDE PREVENTION

- Promote awareness that suicide is a preventable public health problem.
- Develop broad-based support for suicide prevention.
- Develop and implement strategies to reduce the stigma associated with being a consumer of mental health, substance abuse, and suicide-prevention services.
- Develop and implement suicide-prevention programs.
- Promote efforts to reduce access to lethal means and methods of self-harm.
- Implement training for recognition of at-risk behavior and delivery of effective treatment.
- Develop and promote effective clinical and professional practices.
- Improve access to and community linkages with mental health and substance abuse services.
- Improve reporting and portrayals of suicidal behavior, mental illness, and substance abuse in the entertainment and news media.
- Promote and support research on suicide and suicide prevention.
- Improve and expand surveillance systems.

From U.S. Department of Health & Human Services. (2001). *National strategy for suicide prevention: Goals and objectives for action.* Rockville, MD: Author; Office of the Surgeon General. (1999). *The Surgeon General's call to action to prevent suicide.* Washington, DC: Author.

citizens with education about how to recognize a mental health emergency, get individuals at risk the help they need, and provide hope through the process.

An evolving role for nurses that has significant influence on positive primary interventions community-wide is that of the parish nurse. The Behavioral Health and Family Institute Society at Indiana University, Purdue University (2011) recognizes the importance of faith-based communities in prevention of youth suicide. Parish nurses are encouraged to learn suicide prevention strategies and to teach these strategies to parishioners. Evidence suggests that enhanced education for nurses is needed to change attitudes and increase competence and compassion in caring for patients with suicidal behaviors (Patterson et al., 2007).

Secondary Intervention

Secondary intervention is treatment of the actual suicidal crisis. It is practiced in clinics, hospitals, jails, and on telephone hotlines. Involving the entire community, especially in primary and secondary interventions, is essential to reducing the number of suicides. Oftentimes, secondary interventions are the

HEALTH POLICY

Preventing Teen Suicide

A study sponsored by the National Institutes of Health indicated that youth are attempting suicide at increasingly younger ages. Mazza, Catalono, Abbott, and Haggerty (2011) investigated 883 youth, aged 18 or 19, who had previously attempted suicide and found that 40% reported their first suicide attempt was before they entered high school. The earliest reported attempt was third or fourth grade with a peak being in eighth or ninth grade.

After the death of his 22-year-old son by suicide, Senator Gordon Smith introduced a bill that promoted the development of effective strategies and best practices to prevent youth suicide. The Garrett Lee Smith Memorial Act was passed, and President George W. Bush signed the bill into law in 2004.

Senator Jack Reed sponsored legislation in 2011 to increase suicide prevention programs in communities and on college campuses across the country. The Garrett Lee Smith Memorial Act Reauthorization of 2011 (Senate Bill 740) promotes continued development of effective strategies and best practices to prevent youth suicide. Since then, other senators and representatives have championed the reauthorization of the bill to provide much-needed funding to prevent youth suicide.

Reauthorization of the bill is required to continue funding, and challenges related to balancing the federal budget put this bill at risk. Proponents of the bill cite statistics regarding increasing suicide at younger ages in American. The fate of reauthorization bills in each Congressional session is dependent on advocacy efforts by nurses and proponents of suicide prevention.

Mazza, J., Catalono, R., Abbott, R., & Haggerty, K. (2011). An examination of the validity of retrospective measures of suicide attempts in youth, *Journal of Adolescent Health*, *49*, 532–537.

determinants of life or death, and nurses with good crisis intervention skills are in a position to use, role model, and teach these skills to others.

Tertiary Intervention

Tertiary intervention (or **postvention**) refers to interventions with the circle of survivors of a person who has completed suicide (Jordan & McIntosh, 2010). This is done to both reduce the traumatic aftereffects and explore effective means of addressing survivor problems using primary and secondary interventions. Knowledge regarding grief and loss counseling positions nurses to refer, consult, and collaborate in the best interests of friends and family. This is vital since the suicide rate increases for those who experience loss from suicide. Survivors of suicide are in immediate need of supportive avenues for coping with such complicated grief.

General Interventions

The *Nursing Interventions Classification (NIC)* offers the following topics pertinent to the care of the suicidal patient: Suicide Prevention, Hope Instillation, Coping Enhancement, Self-esteem Enhancement, Family Mobilization, and Support System Enhancement (Bulechek et al., 2013).

In the hospital or community setting, the registered nurse utilizes counseling, health teaching, case management, and psychobiological interventions to provide care to patients who have suicidal ideation. During the acute suicidal crisis, suicide precautions are carried out as a specialized form of milieu therapy. It is important to understand that when a patient is admitted to an inpatient psychiatric unit, the nurse must carefully assess and prioritize care. As previously noted, the vast majority (90%) of patients with suicidal behavior disorder have a comorbid psychiatric illness underlying their suicide attempt. Oftentimes, these patients self-medicate with alcohol and/or other drugs to treat their emotional pain; this may lead to reduced rational thought, low frustration tolerance, and impulsivity and may require close monitoring for harm directed at self and also toward others.

Teamwork and Safety

Effective management of patients manifesting suicidal behavior requires an interprofessional collaborative approach to care. This interprofessional collaborative approach maximizes patient safety through timely communication and improved coordination of care leading to best outcomes for patients.

Suicide Precautions

In accordance with unit policies and procedures, patients who are suicidal are observed continuously by nursing staff. Refer to Table 25-4 for a general description of suicide precautions. This intense attention from the nurse provides for safety and allows for constant reassessment of risk. Monitoring flow sheets for suicide precautions is more clinically useful if they include a description of affect as well as behavior. For example, instead of noting "Patient watching television," the nurse will describe the patient's affect (hostile, fearful, calm, etc.) at each observation interval. Flow sheets should also indicate clear accountability for staff starting and ending their periods of observation. In addition to observing the patient, the nurse is responsible for monitoring the environment for safety hazards. Review Box 25-4 for guidelines on how to minimize physical risks in the environment.

Studies show that acute care of patients who are suicidal is usually effective. Suicide risk is highest in the first few days of admission and during times of staff rotation. Assessment of suicidal risk must be an ongoing process; assessment should be performed particularly before a change in level of observation or upon sudden improvement or worsening of symptoms.

Counseling

Counseling skills, including interviewing, crisis care, and problem-solving techniques, are used in both inpatient and outpatient settings. The key element is establishing a therapeutic alliance to encourage the patient to engage in more realistic problem solving. Helpful staff characteristics include warmth, sensitivity, interest, and consistency. After hospitalization, the nurse may see these patients in the clinic, in a partial hospital program, or in home care. One particular aspect of counseling is the use of a **no-suicide contract** (also called a *no-harm contract*). This is a written contract in which the patient agrees not to harm himself or herself but to take an alternative action if feeling suicidal (e.g., talk with staff, call a crisis line). Although no literature is available to verify the effectiveness of these contracts, they are used to form a clinical agreement between

TABLE 25-4 SUICIDE PRECAUTIONS WITH CONSTANT ONE-TO-ONE OBSERVATION

STAFF ASSESSMENT	POSSIBLE PATIENT SYMPTOMS	NURSING RESPONSIBILITIES
Patient with suicidal ideation or delusions of self-mutilation who, according to assessment by unit staff, presents clinical symptoms that suggest a clear intent to follow through with the plan or delusion	1. Patient is currently verbalizing a clear intent to harm self. 2. Patient is unwilling to make a no-suicide contract. 3. Patient shows no insight into existing problems. 4. Patient has poor impulse control. 5. Patient has already attempted suicide in the recent past by a particularly lethal method (e.g., hanging, gun, carbon monoxide poisoning).	1. Conduct one-to-one nursing observation and interaction 24 hours a day (never let patient out of staff's sight). 2. Chart patient's whereabouts and record mood, verbatim statements, and behavior every 15 to 30 minutes per protocol. 3. Ensure that meal trays contain no glass or metal silverware. 4. During observation when patient is sleeping, **hands should always be in view**, not under the bedcovers. 5. Carefully observe patient swallow each dose of medication. 6. The nurse and physician should explain to the patient what they will be doing and why; both document this in the chart.

BOX 25-4 ENVIRONMENTAL GUIDELINES FOR MINIMIZING SUICIDAL BEHAVIOR ON THE PSYCHIATRIC UNIT

- Use plastic eating utensils, and count utensils upon collection.
- Do not assign patient to a private room, and ensure the door remains open at all times.
- Jump-proof and hang-proof the bathrooms by installing breakaway shower rods and recessed shower nozzles.
- Keep electrical cords to a minimal length.
- Install unbreakable glass in windows. Install tamper-proof screens or partitions too small to pass through. Keep all windows locked.
- Lock all utility rooms, kitchens, adjacent stairwells, and offices. All nonclinical staff (e.g., housekeepers, maintenance workers) should receive instructions to keep doors locked.
- Take all potentially harmful gifts (e.g., flowers in glass vases) from visitors before allowing them to see patients. Search all items brought to patients by visitors.
- Go through personal belongings with patient present, and remove all potentially harmful objects (e.g., belts, shoelaces, metal nail files, tweezers, matches, razors, perfume, and shampoo).
- Ensure that visitors do not bring in or leave potentially harmful objects in patient's room (e.g., matches, nail files).
- Search patient for harmful objects (e.g., drugs, sharp objects, cords) if allowed to leave unit on pass.

the patient and the clinician regarding established collaboration to prevent suicide (Simon, 2011).

Health Teaching and Health Promotion

The nurse teaches the patient about psychiatric diagnoses, medications and complementary therapies, and age-related developmental crises. Teaching is also important regarding community resources, coping skills, stress management, and communication skills. When possible, the family or significant others are included to strengthen the patient's support system.

Case Management

Case management is an important aspect of nursing care for the patient with suicidal ideation. The patient's perception of being alone without supports often blinds the person to the real support figures who are present. Reconnecting the patient with family and friends is a major focus, whether in the hospital or the community. Aftercare referrals may include information on the following resources: substance treatment centers, crisis hotlines, support groups for patients or families, and recreational activities to enhance socialization and self-esteem. Encouraging the patient to get reacquainted with a previous spiritual support system may also be beneficial.

Pharmacological Interventions

A significant nursing intervention to assist the patient with suicidal ideation in regaining self-control is the careful administration of medication. Medications prescribed to high-risk patients are monitored carefully. Lethal overdose is nearly impossible with selective serotonin reuptake inhibitors (SSRIs); however, overdose remains a concern with tricyclic antidepressants and monoamine oxidase inhibitors. Mouth checks may be used to be sure that patients are not saving (hoarding) medications in the hospital; in the community, provision of a limited-day supply or family supervision is required.

The American Psychiatric Association (2003) recommends treatment strategies for patients with suicidal ideation. Antidepressants should be ordered for patients who have depressive or anxiety disorders, with an emphasis on administering an adequate dosage and providing appropriate clinical evaluation. The treatment guidelines recommend initial use of an SSRI antidepressant. Close monitoring must occur, especially when medication is initiated and during times of dosage adjustment. Astute nursing care involves careful patient (and family, if appropriate) teaching about the identified benefits and risks of antidepressant therapy.

There is clear evidence that long-term lithium treatment for bipolar disorder and major depression significantly reduces suicide and suicide attempts. Since lithium does frequently cause serious side effects and necessitates periodic blood work to test for therapeutic levels, patient and family education is important to support adherence.

For patients experiencing psychotic or bipolar manic episodes, antipsychotic medication is usually ordered. Second-generation antipsychotics are preferable to first-generation antipsychotics because they have fewer adverse effects. Some studies have shown a reduced suicide rate among patients with schizophrenia receiving clozapine. The use of clozapine must be monitored closely, however, because of the risk of severe side effects (e.g., agranulocytosis, myocarditis, and altered glucose metabolism).

Finally, antianxiety medication may help to treat panic and insomnia. Thus far, no clinical studies have examined the effect of antianxiety treatment on suicide risk, but short-term use of long-acting benzodiazepines may be helpful for management of panic symptoms.

An alternative somatic treatment for acute suicidal risk is electroconvulsive therapy (ECT). Evidence suggests that ECT decreases acute suicidal ideation. This treatment is useful for certain types of patients with depression or psychosis whose behavior is considered life threatening and for whom waiting for medication to take effect is not feasible. It is also safe and effective for pregnant patients, patients with certain medical conditions who cannot tolerate medication, and patients who do not respond to multiple trials of medication. Refer to Chapter 14 for further discussion of ECT.

Postvention for Survivors of Completed Suicide

A discussion of patients with suicidal behavior disorder is incomplete without noting the issues surrounding a completed suicide. Surviving family and friends may experience overwhelming guilt and shame, compounded by the difficulty of discussing the frequently taboo subject of suicide. The usual social supports of neighbors and church are sometimes lacking for these mourners. Adolescent friends who suffer traumatic grief are more likely to report suicidal ideation within 6 years of the suicide (APA, 2003). Family members of individuals who complete suicide develop a 4.5-times greater risk of suicide than those in families in which no suicide occurred. Despite their suffering, only approximately 25% of survivors seek treatment.

One survivor wrote a personal account several years after the suicide of her daughter:

If only I hadn't responded with anger and frustration during our last phone call . . . she was angry with herself and seemed to want to pick a fight with me—which was the pattern. If I could have looked past her angry words and instead tuned into the desperation behind them, maybe I could have gotten her to open up to me. Now I can only look back and consider the many, many times I should have picked up on the severity of her illness and how she struggled with it. Her experience has also caused me to look at my own depression and realize how especially vulnerable I am now. If I have any advice for others based on my experience, it is to get connected, listen, and be a real part of the lives of those you love. That's the only way you'll know when something is just not right and how desperate someone really is. That also applies to friends and family of us survivors. Don't treat us like we're "contagious." And please do talk about our loss. The worst thing possible is to avoid mention of our lost loved one.

Survivors give the following suggestions to health care professionals:

- If being a survivor is the main reason treatment has been sought, remember that the survivor, not the deceased, is the patient. Focus on the patient's thoughts and feelings, and do a thorough assessment as you usually would.
- If you are a friend or relative of a suicide survivor, remember that the most difficult time for these survivors is not so much in the immediate aftermath of the suicide; rather, it is in the weeks, months, and *years* following their loss. Make frequent efforts to reach out to these individuals, especially on the most difficult anniversary dates. Do not be afraid of talking about the deceased person; in fact, speak of them often. While this may seem counterintuitive and uncomfortable for most, survivors of suicide universally want their loved one to be remembered in this way. Talking reduces the hurt, isolation, and stigma.
- If being a survivor comes out as an incidental finding during an assessment, ask open-ended questions and evaluate how much the loss has been resolved.
- Recommend community resources and survivor support groups and show empathy about the loss of someone to suicide. Know about local Survivors of Suicide (SOS) support groups in your area, and refer the survivors and their families as soon as possible following the suicide.

Staff members who have cared for a patient who completed suicide within the treatment facility are similarly traumatized by suicide. Staff may also experience symptoms of posttraumatic stress disorder, with guilt, shock, anger, shame, and decreased self-esteem (APA, 2003). Group support is essential as the treatment team conducts a thorough psychological postmortem assessment. The event is carefully reviewed to identify the potential overlooked clues, faulty judgments, or changes that are needed in agency protocols. Most facilities have a clear policy about communication with families after suicide. Although some lawyers advise having no contact except through them, others recommend designating a spokesperson who can address the feelings of the family without discussing the details of the patient's care. Referrals should be given to family members to assist them in dealing with their grief and to address any emotional problems that develop, especially in adolescents.

As for documentation, staff must ensure that the record is complete and that any late entries are identified. Courts require that the patient be periodically evaluated for suicidal risk, that the treatment plan provide for high-level security, and that staff members follow the individual treatment plan. Despite following institution protocols, treatment plans, and the appropriate standards of practice, suicides do occasionally still happen.

This is especially the case for patients in the community. Human behavior is simply not predictable.

Advanced Practice Interventions

The psychiatric advanced practice nurse (APRN) may treat suicidal patients directly with psychotherapy, psychobiological interventions, clinical supervision for direct care staff, or consultation in nonpsychiatric settings (e.g., health care unit, nursing home, or forensic site). Following hospitalization, the APRN provides aftercare for the patient with coexisting psychiatric disorders, including individual therapy and family therapy.

EVALUATION

Evaluation of a patient with suicidal ideation is ongoing. The nurse must be constantly alert to changes in the patient's mood, thinking, and behavior. The nurse also looks for indications that the patient is communicating thoughts and feelings more readily and that the patient's social network is widening. For example, if the person is able to talk about his or her feelings and engage in problem solving with the nurse, this is a positive sign.

The nurse must remember that *suicidal behavior is the result of interpersonal turmoil*. If an episode of major depression is the main admitting diagnosis and a serious suicidal gesture resulted from this depression, both problems are initially assessed and treated. When the patient is no longer an acute suicide risk, treating the suicidal ideation and depressive disorder becomes the main focus of care. Essentially, the nurse evaluates each short-term goal and establishes new ones as the patient progresses toward the long-term goal of resolving suicidal ideation.

Once stabilized, the patient may qualify for transfer to an intensive outpatient (IOP) treatment program, which involves continuing treatment after discharge, or a partial hospitalization program (PHP) that allows patients to go home in the evening to practice new coping skills. Community-based support groups are also available that are effective and financially affordable for the patient. Nurses should be knowledgeable about, and proactive in, referring patients to these support groups. Due to the increasing numbers of uninsured and underinsured patients, nurses should familiarize themselves regarding reimbursement systems and treatment options available in their communities.

QUALITY IMPROVEMENT

Quality improvement is imperative to ensure the provision of safe care, a primary factor in caring for patients with suicidal behavior. Ongoing research provides evidence-based practices to improve both the quality and safety of care. Suicide prevention and risk assessment are primary focuses for quality improvement.

The Clinical Care and Intervention Task Force to the National Action Alliance for Suicide Prevention identified best practices for suicide care (Covington & Hogan, 2011). Three critical factors for suicide prevention programs were determined, including core values, systems management, and evidence-based clinical care practice. This task force believes that suicide is a "never event" and that suicide may be eliminated by improved access to care and continuous quality improvement.

The quality improvement task force concluded that collaborative care must be established as the standard of care for the detection, treatment, and management of behavioral health problems. To be effective in achieving suicide as a never event, care coordination that is patient-centered and encompasses both inpatient and community-based care is essential.

NON-SUICIDAL SELF-INJURY

Another closely related problem to suicidal behavior is **non-suicidal self-injury**. This problem is manifested by deliberate and direct attempts to cause bodily harm that does not result in death (Nock, 2010). Sometimes referred to as **parasuicide**, this behavior most commonly consists of cutting/carving, burning, scraping/scratching skin, biting, hitting, skin picking, and interfering with wound healing. Half of self-injurers report multiple methods (Klonsky, 2011). For these behaviors to be considered significant, they typically last at least a year and happen repeatedly.

Even when they are not engaged in the behaviors, self-injurers tend to be thinking about self-injury. Self-injurious actions are most often done with the intent to either alleviate psychic pain or to pierce the psychic numbness these individuals describe. Other times, these actions are used to punish themselves, to connect with others, to get attention, to escape a responsibility or to avoid a situation.

Prevalence

The lifetime prevalence of non-suicidal self-injury in adolescents was estimated from 13% to 23% (Jacobson & Gould, 2007). It is a global problem with similar prevalence rates worldwide (Muehlenkamp et al., 2012). Non-suicidal self-injury begins between 10 to 15 years of age, peaking in the late teens. Hospital admission data confirm a decline in the behavior between 25 to 29 years of age (Crosby, Ortega, & Melanson, 2011). Klonsky (2011) estimates that 5.9% of the U.S. population have engaged in non-suicidal self-injury within their lifetime.

Research regarding prevalence by gender is inconclusive. Some studies demonstrate that it is more common among females while other studies find a higher prevalence in males. What does seem to be clear is that self-injury is more visible among females than males (Whitlock et al., 2009).

Comorbidity

In a study of college students, risk factors for non-suicidal self-injury were depression in either parent, non-heterosexual orientation, and depression (Wilcox et al., 2012). Personality disorders, particularly borderline personality disorder, are associated with non-suicidal self-injury in adolescence and adulthood (Nitkowski & Petermann, 2011). Anxiety and substance use disorders are considered to be co-occurring disorders with self-injurious behaviors.

Etiology

Biological Factors

Studies related to the physiological mechanism of action in non-suicidal self-injury are inconclusive; however, researchers continue to investigate the neurobiological mechanisms behind the disorder. Several neurochemical pathways in the brain are proposed to play a role in the development of these behaviors (Bloom & Holly, 2011). Recently, studies have determined that individuals who engage in self-injury have lower levels of cerebrospinal fluid endogenous opiods when compared with individuals who do not engage in the behaviors (Stanley et al., 2010). Although studies are inconclusive, the neurotransmitter group of monoamines including serotonin, dopamine, and norepinephrine may play a role in the mediation of self-injury, and research is ongoing. As practitioners continue to search for an effective treatment, clinical research will seek to find the neurobiological basis of non-suicidal self-injury.

Cultural Factors

Recent studies have investigated the prevalence of non-suicidal self-injury behaviors internationally to determine best practices for treatment and whether culturally different approaches to care are relevant. Similar rates of the behavior are reported among adolescents in the Midwestern states and southern Germany; however, these rates differ significantly from the Netherlands and Belgium. In European countries, German adolescents have the highest rates of the behavior (10.4%) with the lowest rates among Romanian youth (1.9%)(Kaess et al., 2011). The behavior has stabilized among youth over the last 5 years, with no significant increases internationally (Muehlenkamp et al., 2012). With this stabilization in occurrence, researchers will have opportunity to further investigate cultural differences in the behavior and whether these differences lead to different treatment modalities.

Societal Factors

Many people believe that self-injurious behaviors such as cutting are a social phenomenon that is rampant in society. Social media such as YouTube may have a tremendous impact on the culture at-large. In one study researchers found that top 100 videos related to self-injurious behaviors were viewed over 2 million times (Lewis et al., 2011). Viewers tended to rate these videos positively despite the explicit imagery of self-injury, most commonly self-cutting.

Summary of Nursing Implications

Nonacute suicidal or self-destructive thoughts and feelings are generally treated in the outpatient setting. Alternate services available to patients with suicidal ideation include crisis intervention and assertive community treatment (ACT), addiction treatment, social services, and legal assistance. These types of interventions are evidence based and cost effective, as well as individualized and realistic—all essential aspects of the person-centered recovery model (American Psychiatric Nurses Association & International Society of Psychiatric Nurses, 2007).

KEY POINTS TO REMEMBER

- Suicide is a significant public health problem in the United States.
- Specific biological, psychosocial, and cultural factors are known to increase the risk of suicide.
- Most patients with suicidal ideation may be helped by treatment of a coexisting psychiatric disorder.
- Certain health conditions and psychiatric diagnoses are associated with increased risk for suicide.
- Every suicide attempt must be taken seriously, even if the person has a history of multiple attempts.
- The nurse may have a real impact on suicide prevention through primary, secondary, and tertiary interventions.
- Nursing care of the patient who is suicidal is challenging but rewarding; patients' desperate feelings evoke intense reactions in staff, but most people with suicidal behaviors respond to treatment and do not complete suicide.
- If a patient completes suicide, family, friends, and health care workers are traumatized and need support, possibly including referrals for psychiatric treatment.
- A principle of quality improvement is that suicide is a "never event" that should be eliminated by improved access to care, continuous quality improvement, and collaborative care.
- Non-suicidal self-injury is a problem that is becoming increasingly important, especially among young people.

CRITICAL THINKING

1. Locate and review the suicide protocol at your hospital unit or community center. Are there any steps you anticipate having difficulty carrying out? Discuss these difficulties with your peers or clinical group.
2. How would you respond to another staff member who expresses guilt over the completed suicide of a patient on your unit?
3. Identify three common and expected emotional reactions that a nurse might have when initially working with persons who manifest suicidal behavior disorder.
   a. How do you think you might react?
   b. What actions could you take to deal with the event and obtain support?

CHAPTER REVIEW

1. Griffin is a 19-year-old student who volunteers for a depression screening at his college. He identifies himself as gay. Which of the following is true based on current knowledge of the gay, lesbian, and bisexual community and suicide risk?
   a. Griffin's sexual preference has no bearing on suicide risk.
   b. Griffin has a higher suicide risk than his heterosexual peers.
   c. Griffin has a lower suicide risk than his heterosexual peers.
   d. Griffin may experience a threefold risk for a mood disorder in his lifetime because of his sexual preference.

2. You are admitting Joel, a 39-year-old patient with depression. Which assessment statement(s) would be appropriate to ask Joel to assess suicide risk? *Select all that apply.*
   a. Do you ever think about suicide?
   b. Are you thinking of hurting yourself?
   c. Do you sometimes wish you were dead?
   d. Has it ever seemed as if life is not worth living?
   e. If you were to kill yourself, how would you do it?
   f. Does it seem as if others might be better off if you were dead?
3. Which person is at the highest risk for suicide?
   a. A 50-year-old married white male with depression who has a plan to overdose if circumstances at work do not improve.
   b. A 45-year-old married white female who recently lost her parents, suffers from bipolar disorder, and attempted suicide once as a teenager.
   c. A young, single white male who is alcohol dependent, hopeless, impulsive, has just been rejected by his girlfriend, and has ready access to a gun he has hidden.
   d. An older Hispanic male who is Catholic, is living with a debilitating chronic illness, is recently widowed, and states: "I wish that God would take me too."
4. Which intervention(s) maximize the safety of a patient who is actively suicidal on an inpatient mental health unit? *Select all that apply.*
   a. Place the patient on every-15-minute checks.
   b. Place the patient in a room near the nurses' station.
   c. Allow the patient periods of time alone for reflection to promote self-awareness.
   d. Install breakaway curtain rods, coat hooks, and shower rods.
   e. Allow the patient to keep personal objects such as a razor and hair dryer in his room to demonstrate trust.
   f. Assign the patient to a private room to facilitate monitoring.
5. Kara is a 23-year-old patient admitted with depression and suicidal ideation. Which intervention(s) would be therapeutic for Kara? *Select all that apply.*
   a. Focus primarily on developing solutions to the problems that are leading the patient to feel suicidal.
   b. Assess the patient thoroughly, and reassess the patient at regular intervals as levels of risk fluctuate.
   c. Avoid talking about the suicidal ideation as this may increase the patient's risk for suicidal behavior.
   d. Meet regularly with the patient to provide opportunities for the patient to express and explore feelings.
   e. Administer antidepressant medications cautiously and conservatively because of their potential to increase the suicide risk in Kara's age group.
   f. Help the patient to identify positive self-attributes and to question negative self-perceptions that are unrealistic.

Answers to Chapter Review

1. b; 2. a, b, c, d, e, f; 3. c; 4. a, b, d; 5. b, d, e, f.

evolve WEBSITE

Visit the Evolve website for a posttest on the content in this chapter: http://evolve.elsevier.com/Varcarolis

Post-Test interactive review

REFERENCES

American Association of Suicidology. (2008). *School suicide prevention accreditation programs.* Retrieved from http://www.suicidology.org/c/document_library/get_file?folderId=234&name=DLFE-43.pdf.

American Foundation for Suicide Prevention. (2009). *Facts and figures: National statistics.* Retrieved from http://www.afsp.org/index.cfm?fuseaction=home.viewpage&page_id=050fea9f-b064-4092-b1135c3a70de1fda.

American Psychiatric Nurses Association (APNA), & International Society of Psychiatric-Mental Health Nurses (ISPN). (2007). *Psychiatric mental health nursing: Scope and standards of practice.* Silver Spring, MD: American Nurses Association.

American Psychiatric Association. (2003). *American Psychiatric Association practice guideline for the assessment and treatment of suicidal behaviors.* Arlington, VA: American Psychiatric Publishing.

American Psychiatric Association. (2003). Practice guideline for the assessment and treatment of patients with suicidal behaviors. *American Journal of Psychiatry, 160*(11 Suppl.), 1–60.

Appel, J. (2007). A suicide right for the mentally ill? A Swiss case opens a new debate. *Hastings Center Report, 37*(3), 21–23.

Behavioral Health and Family Studies Institute. (2011). *Faith based communities: Suicide prevention recommendations.* Fort Wayne, IN: Indiana University-Purdue University. Retrieved from http://www.indianacares.org/Faith%20based%20Community%20Suicide%20Prevention%20Recommendations.draft1.pdf.

Brendel, R., Lagomasino, I., Perlis, R., & Stern, T. (2008). The suicidal patient. In T. Stern, J. Rosenbaum, M. Fava, J. Biederman & S. Rauch (Eds.), *Massachusetts General Hospital comprehensive clinical psychiatry* (pp. 733–745). St. Louis, MO: Mosby.

Bulechek, G. M., Butcher, H. K., Dochterman, J. M., & Wagner, C. (2013). *Nursing interventions classification (NIC)* (6th ed.). St. Louis, MO: Mosby.

Cassels, C. (2010, August 26). DoD report aims to halt escalating suicide rates in military. *Medscape News.* Retrieved from http://www.medscape.com/viewarticle/727542.

Centers for Disease Control and Prevention. (2012). *Suicide facts at a glance: 2012* Retrieved from http://www.cdc.gov/violenceprevention/pdf/suicide_datasheet_2012-a.pdf.

Centers for Disease Control and Prevention, National Center for Injury Prevention and Control. (2012). *Deaths: Final data for 2010* (NVSR Volume 61, Number 6). Atlanta, GA: Centers for Disease Control and Prevention.

Centers for Disease Control and Prevention, National Center for Injury Prevention and Control. (2011). *Injury statistics query and reporting system.* Retrieved from http://www.cdc.gov/injury/wisqars/index.html

Ciffone, J. (2007). Suicide prevention: An analysis and replication of a curriculum-based high school program. *Social Work, 52*(1), 41–49.

Covington, D., & Hogan, M. (2011). *Suicide care in systems framework.* Retrieved from http://actionallianceforsuicideprevention.org/sites/actionallianceforsuicideprevention.org/files/taskforces/ClinicalCareIntervention-Report.pdf.

Crosby, A., Ortega, L., & Melanson, C. (2011). *Self-directed violence surveillance: Uniform definitions and recommended data elements* (Vol. 1). Atlanta, GA: Centers for Disease Control, National Center for Injury Prevention and Control.

Eisenberg, M., & Resnick, M. (2006). Suicide among gay, lesbian, and bisexual youth: The role of protective factors. *Journal of Adolescent Health, 39*(5), 662–668.

Fowler, J. (2012). Suicide risk assessment in clinical practice: Pragmatic guidelines for imperfect assessments. *Psychotherapy, 491*(1), 81–90. doi:10.1037/a0026148.

Ganzini, L., & Dobscha, K. (2008). Prevalence of depression and anxiety in patients requesting physicians' aid in dying: A cross-sectional survey. *British Medical Journal, 337*, a1682. doi:10.1136/bmj.a1682.

Gibbs, N., & Thompson, M. (2012, July 23). The war on suicide? Time Magazine. Retrieved from http://www.time.com/time/magazine/article/0,9171,2119337,00.html.

Haines, J., Williams, C. L., & Lester, D. (2011). The characteristics of those who do and do not leave suicide notes: Is the method of residuals valid? *Omega, 63*(1), 79–94.

Hatzenbuehler, M. (2011). The social environment and suicide attempts in lesbian, gay, and bisexual youth. *Pediatrics, 127*(5), 896–903. doi:10.1542/peds.2010-3020.

Herdman, T. H. (Ed.), (2012). *NANDA international nursing diagnoses: Definitions and classification, 2012–2014*. Oxford, UK: Wiley Blackwell.

Joe, S., & Bryant, H. (2007). Evidence-based suicide prevention screening in schools. *Children and Schools, 29*(4), 219–227.

Jordan, J. R., & McIntosh, J. L. (2010). *Grief after suicide: Understanding the consequences and caring for the survivors*. New York, NY: Taylor and Francis.

Kaess, M., Parzer, P., Klug, K., Fischer, G., Schonbach, N., Resch, F., & Brunner, R. (2011). Saving and Empowering Young Lives in Europe (SEYLE). Presented at the Deutsche Gesellschaft für Kinder und Jugendpsychiatrie, Psychosomatik und Psychotherapie's 32nd Annual Meeting, Rostock, Germany.

Klonsky, E. D. (2011). Non-suicidal self-injury United States adults: Prevalence, sociodemographics, topography and functions. *Psychological Medicine, 41*(9), 1981–1986.

Lewis, S. P., Heath, N. L, St. Denis, J. M., & Noble, R. (2011). The scope of nonsuicidal self-injury on Youtube. *Pediatrics, 127*(3), 552-557. doi:10.1542/peds.2010-2317.

Limosin, F., Lose, J., Philippe, A., Casadebaig, F., & Rouillon, F. (2007). Ten-year prospective follow-up study of the mortality by suicide in schizophrenic patients. *Schizophrenia Research, 94*(1), 23–28.

Marker, R., & Hamlon, K. (2010). *Euthanasia and assisted suicide: Frequently asked questions*. Retrieved from http://www.patientsrightscouncil.org/site/frequently-asked-questions/.

Mazza, J., Catalono, R., Abbott, R., & Haggerty, K. (2011). An examination of the validity of retrospective measures of suicide attempts in youth. *Journal of Adolescent Health, 49*, 532–537. doi:10.1016/j.jadohealth.2011.04.009.

MedicineNet.com. (2002). *Definition of parasuicide*. Retrieved from http://www.medterms.com/script/main/art.asp?articlekey=21820.

Moorhead, S., Johnson, M., Maas, M. L., & Swanson, E. (2013). *Nursing outcomes classification (NOC)* (5th ed.). St. Louis, MO: Mosby.

Muehlenkamp, J., Claes, L., Havertape, L., & Plener, P. (2012). International prevalence of adolescent non-suicidal self-injury and deliberate self-harm. *Child and Adolescent Psychiatry and Mental Health, 6*(10). doi: 10.1186/1753-2000-6-10. Retrieved from http://www.capmh.com/content/6/1/10.

National Institute of Mental Health. (2012). *Suicide in the United States: Statistics and prevention*. Retrieved from http://www.nimh.nih.gov/health/publications/suicide-in-the-us-statistics-and-prevention/index.shtml#factors.

Nitkowski, D., & Petermann, F. (2011). Non-suicidal self-injury and comorbid mental disorders: A review. *Fortschritte der Neurologie-Psychiatrie, 79*(1), 9–20 (in German).

Nock, M. K. (2010). Self-injury. *Annual Review of Clinical Psychology, 6*, 339–363.

Nock, M., Hwang, I., Sampson, N., & Kessler, R. (2010). Mental disorders, comorbidity and suicidal behavior: Results from the national comorbidity survey replication. *Molecular Psychiatry, 15*(8), 868–876. doi: 10.1038/mp.2009.29.

Patterson, P., Whittington, R., & Boggs, J. (2007). Testing the effectiveness of an educational intervention aimed at changing attitudes to self-harm. *Journal of Psychiatric and Mental Health Nursing, 14*, 100–105.

Patterson, W., Dohn, H., Bird, J., & Patterson, G. (1983). Evaluation of suicidal patients: The SAD PERSONS scale. *Psychosomatics, 24*, 343–349.

Price, N. (2007). Improving emergency care for patients who self harm. *Emergency Nurse, 15*(8), 30–36.

Quinnett, P. (2007). QPR gatekeeper training for suicide prevention: The model, rationale, and theory. Unpublished manuscript. Retrieved from http://www.uwlax.edu/conted/pdf/2012QPRtheoryPaper.pdf.

Sadock, B., & Sadock, V. (2008). *Kaplan and Sadock's concise textbook of clinical psychiatry* (3rd ed.). Philadelphia, PA: Lippincott Williams & Wilkins.

Saewyc, E., Homma, Y., Skay, C., Bearinger, L., Resnick, M., & Reis, E. (2009). Protective factors in the lives of bisexual adolescents in North America. *American Journal of Public Health, 99*(1), 110–117.

Schreiber, J., Culpepper, L. & Fife, A. (2011). *Suicidal ideation and behavior in adults*. Retrieved from http://www.uptodate.com/contents/suicidal-ideation-and-behavior-in-adults.

Simon, R. (2011). Suicide. In R. Hales, S. Yudofsky & G. Gabbard (Eds.), *Essentials of psychiatry* (pp. 699–717). Washington, DC: American Psychiatry Publishing, Inc.

Stanley, B., Sher, L., Wilson, S., Ekman, R., Huang, Y. Y., & Mann, J. J. (2010). Non-suicidal self-injurious behavior, endogenous opiods, and monoamine neurotransmitters. *Journal of Affective Disorders, 124*(1–2), 134–140.

U.S. Department of Health & Human Services. (2001). *National strategy for suicide prevention: Goals and objectives for action* (No. O2NLM:HV 6548.A1 2001). Rockville, MD: Public Health Service.

U.S. Food and Drug Administration. (2007). *Questions and answers on antidepressant use in children, adolescents, and adults: May, 2007*. Retrieved from http://www.fda.gov/Drugs/DrugSafety/InformationbyDrugClass/ucm096321.htm.

Whitlock, J., Muehlenkamp, J., Purington, A., Eckenrode, J., Barreira, J., Baral-Abrahms, G., Knox, K, et al. (2011). Primary and secondary non-suicidal self-injury characteristics in a college population: General trends and gender differences. *Journal of American College Health, 59*(8), 691–698.

Wilcox, H. C., Arria, A. M., Caldeira, K. M., Vincent, K. B., Pinchevsky, G. M., & O'Grady, K. E. (2012). Longitudinal predictors of past-year non-suicidal self-injury and motives among college students. *Psychological Medicine, 42*(4), 717–726.

CHAPTER

26

Crisis and Disaster

Margaret Jordan Halter and Christine Heifner Graor

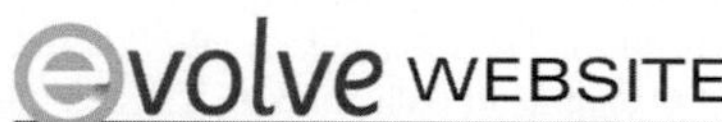

Visit the Evolve website for a pretest on the content in this chapter: http://evolve.elsevier.com/Varcarolis

Pre-Test interactive review

OBJECTIVES

1. Differentiate among three types of crisis and provide an example of each.
2. Delineate six aspects of crisis that have relevance for nurses involved in crisis intervention.
3. Develop a handout describing areas to assess during crisis. Include at least two sample questions for each area.
4. Discuss four common problems in the nurse-patient relationship that are frequently encountered by beginning nurses when starting crisis intervention. Discuss two interventions for each problem.
5. Compare and contrast the differences among primary, secondary, and tertiary intervention, including appropriate intervention strategies.
6. Explain to a classmate four potential crisis situations that patients may experience in hospital settings.
7. Provide concrete examples of interventions to minimize the situations.
8. List at least five resources in the community that could be used as referrals for a patient in crisis.
9. Recognize disaster occurrences and management as global concerns.
10. Differentiate among disaster types.
11. Describe three reasons why professional nurses should have disaster-preparedness training.

KEY TERMS AND CONCEPTS

adventitious crisis
crisis intervention
critical incident stress debriefing (CISD)
disaster
maturational crisis
mitigation
preparedness
primary care
recovery
response
secondary care
situational crisis
tertiary care

The Homeland Security Department raises the terror alert to high and warns American citizens to be watchful for any suspicious behavior. A tornado touches down in a small town, levels an entire neighborhood, and leaves 10 residents dead and many more homeless. A hurricane rips into a coastline, levees fail, 80% of a major city floods, and nearly 2,000 die. A teenage boy armed with automatic weapons enters a crowded movie theater and shoots everyone he can. A young nursing student discovers she is pregnant, and the father of the baby abandons her. What do these situations have in common? Each of these situations could be the precipitant of a crisis—leaving individuals, families, and whole communities struggling to cope with the impact of the event.

Crisis is not defined by the experience itself. Crisis is defined by the struggle for equilibrium and adaptation in its aftermath. Roberts (2005) defines a crisis as a profound disruption of a person's normal psychological homeostasis. Normal coping mechanisms fail to deal with this distress, resulting in an inability to function as usual. The primary cause of crisis is the actual traumatic event, but two other conditions are also involved:

The individual perceives the event as significantly distressing.

The individual is unable to resolve the disruption by previously used coping mechanisms.

Crisis threatens personality organization, but it also presents an opportunity for personal growth and development. Successful crisis resolution results from the development of adaptive coping mechanisms, reflects ego development, and suggests the employment of physiological, psychological, and social resources.

Crises are acute and time-limited, usually lasting 4 to 6 weeks. They are associated with events that are experienced with overwhelming emotions of increased tension, helplessness, and disorganization.

As shown in Figure 26-1 (Aguilera, 1998), the outcome of crisis depends on (a) the realistic perception of the event, (b) adequate situational supports, and (c) adequate coping mechanisms.

- **Perception of the event:** People vary in the way they absorb, process, and use information from the environment. Some people may respond to a minor event as if it were life threatening. Conversely, others may assess a life-threatening event and carefully consider options.
- **Situational supports:** Situational supports include nurses and other health professionals who use crisis intervention to assist those in crisis. Crisis intervention is "a short-term therapeutic process that focuses on the rapid resolution of an immediate crisis or emergency using available personnel, family, and/or environmental resources" (American Psychiatric Nurses Association [APNA], 2007, p. 65).
- **Coping mechanisms:** Coping mechanisms and skills are acquired through a variety of sources, such as cultural responses, the modeling behaviors of others, and life opportunities that broaden experience and promote the adaptive development of new coping responses (Aguilera, 1998). Many factors compromise a person's ability to cope with a crisis event. These may include the number of other stressful life events with which the person is currently coping, other unresolved losses, concurrent psychiatric disorders, concurrent medical problems, excessive fatigue or pain, and the quality and quantity of a person's usual coping skills.

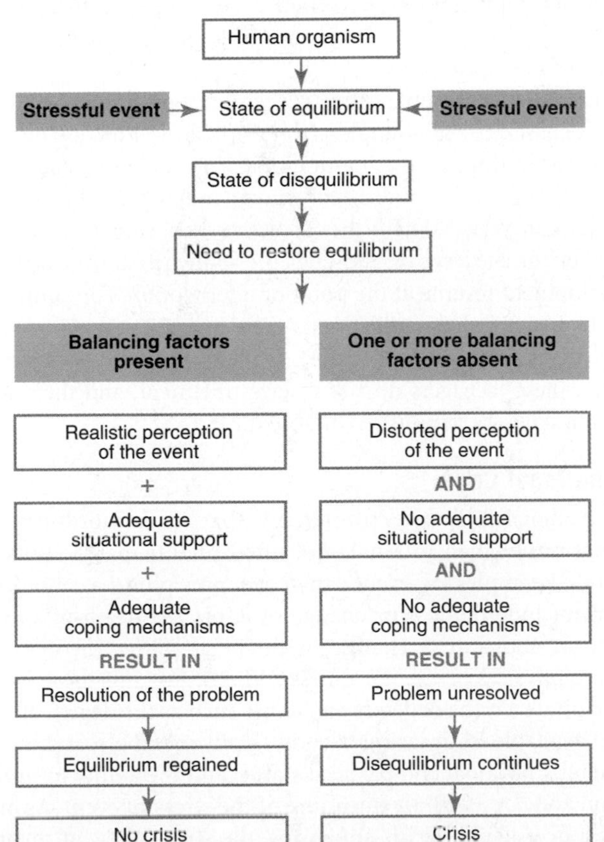

FIG 26-1 Paradigm: The effect of balancing factors in a stressful event. (From Aguilera, D.C. [1998]. *Crisis intervention: Theory and methodology* [8th ed.]. St. Louis, MO: Mosby.)

CRISIS THEORY

An early crisis theorist, Erich Lindemann, conducted a classic study in the 1940s on the grief reactions of close relatives of the 492 victims who died in the Cocoanut Grove nightclub fire in Boston. This tragedy was due, in part, to exits being blocked to prevent customers from leaving without paying and inward swinging exit doors that trapped crowds as they desperately tried to escape; laws requiring outward swinging exit doors were enacted as a result of this fire.

This study formed the foundation of crisis theory and clinical intervention. Lindemann was convinced that even though acute grief is a normal reaction to a distressing situation, preventive interventions could eliminate or decrease potential serious personality disorganization and the devastating psychological consequences of the sustained effects of severe anxiety. He believed that the same interventions that were helpful in bereavement would prove just as helpful in dealing with other types of stressful events; therefore, he proposed a crisis intervention model as a major element of preventive psychiatry in the community.

In the early 1960s, Gerald Caplan (1964) advanced crisis theory and outlined crisis intervention strategies. Since that time, our understanding of crisis and effective intervention has continued to be refined and enhanced by numerous contemporary clinicians and theorists (Behrman & Reid, 2002; Roberts, 2005). The 1961 report of the Joint Commission on Mental Illness and Health addressed the need for community mental health centers throughout the country. This report stimulated the establishment of crisis services, which are now an important part of mental health programs in hospitals and communities.

Donna Aguilera and Janice Mesnick (1970) provided a framework for nurses for crisis assessment and intervention, which has grown in scope and practice. Aguilera continues to set a standard in the practice of crisis assessment and intervention.

Albert R. Roberts's seven-stage model of crisis interventions (Figure 26-2) (Roberts, 2005; Roberts & Ottens, 2005) is a model that is useful in helping individuals who have suffered from an acute situational crisis as well as people who are diagnosed with acute stress disorder.

In an effort to establish consensus on mass trauma intervention principles, Hobfoll and colleagues (2007) identified

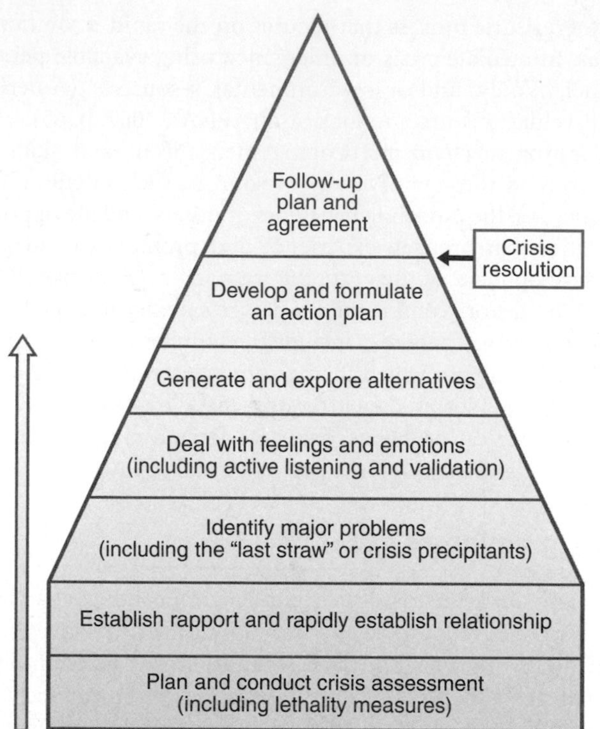

FIG 26-2 Roberts's seven-stage model of crisis intervention. (From Roberts, A. R., & Ottens, A. J. [2005]. The seven-stage crisis intervention model: A road map to goal attainment, problem solving, and crisis resolution. *Brief Treatment and Crisis Intervention, 5,* 329–339.)

five essential, empirically supported elements of mass trauma interventions that promote: (1) a sense of safety, (2) calming, (3) a sense of self-efficacy and collective efficacy, (4) connectedness, and (5) hope.

The effects of disasters such as the 9/11 World Trade Center terrorist attack, the earthquake in Haiti in 2010, and a dozen billion-dollar weather disasters in the United States in 2011 have emphasized the need for crisis assessment and intervention by community and general mental health providers. Regardless of the type of crisis and whether traumatized individuals are victims, families, rescue workers, or observers, those with access to crisis assessment and intervention are more likely to feel safe, supported, and empowered. Individuals are also better able to make sense of their response to the disaster, compared to those without access to supportive care providers (Phoenix, 2007).

Components of crisis assessment are derived from established crisis theory and constitute a sound knowledge base for the application of the nursing process to treatment of a patient in crisis. An understanding of the types of crises and phases of crises lays the groundwork for the application of the nursing process.

TYPES OF CRISIS

There are three basic types of crisis situations: (1) maturational (or developmental) crises, (2) situational crises, and (3) adventitious crises. Identifying which type of crisis the individual is experiencing or has experienced helps in the development of a patient-centered plan of care.

Maturational Crisis

A process of maturation occurs across the life cycle. Erik Erikson (1902-1994) conceptualized the process by identifying eight stages of ego growth and development (see Table 2-2 in Chapter 2). Each stage represents a time when physical, cognitive, instinctual, and sexual changes prompt an internal conflict or crisis, which results in either psychosocial growth or regression. Therefore, each developmental stage represents a **maturational crisis** that is a critical period of increased vulnerability and, at the same time, heightened potential.

When a person arrives at a new stage, formerly used coping styles are no longer effective, and new coping mechanisms have yet to be developed. Thus, for a time the person is without effective defenses. This often leads to increased tension and anxiety, which may manifest as variations in the person's normal behavior. Examples of events that can precipitate a maturational crisis include leaving home during late adolescence, marriage, birth of a child, retirement, and the death of a parent. Successful resolution of these maturational tasks leads to development of basic human qualities.

Erikson believed that the way these crises are resolved at one stage affects the ability to pass through subsequent stages because each crisis provides the starting point for movement toward the next stage. If a person lacks support systems and adequate role models, successful resolution may be difficult or may not occur. Unresolved problems in the past and inadequate coping mechanisms then adversely affect what is learned in each developmental stage. When a person experiences severe difficulty during a maturational crisis, professional intervention may be indicated.

Factors may disrupt individuals' progression through the maturational stages. For example, alcohol and drug addiction disrupts progression through the maturational stages. Unfortunately, this interruption occurs too often among individuals during their adolescent years. When the addictive behavior is controlled (e.g., by the late teens or mid-20s), the young person's growth and development resume at the point of interruption. For example, a young person whose addiction is arrested at 22 years of age may have the psychosocial and problem-solving skills of a 14-year-old. Often these teenagers do not receive treatment, and their adult coping skills are diminished or absent.

Situational Crisis

A **situational crisis** arises from events that are extraordinary, external rather than internal, and often unanticipated (Roberts, 2005). Examples of events that can precipitate a situational crisis include the loss or change of a job, the death of a loved one, an abortion, a change in financial status, divorce, and severe physical or mental illness. Whether or not these events precipitate a crisis depends on factors such as the degree of support available from caring friends, family members, and others; general emotional and physical status; and the ability to understand and cope with the meaning of the stressful event. As in all crises or potential crisis situations, the stressful event involves loss or change that threatens a person's self-concept and self-esteem. To varying degrees, successful resolution of a crisis depends on resolution of the grief associated with the loss.

Adventitious Crisis

An adventitious crisis is not a part of everyday life; it results from events that are unplanned and that may be accidental, caused by nature, or human-made. This type of crisis results from (1) a natural disaster (e.g., flood, fire, earthquake), (2) a national disaster (e.g., acts of terrorism, war, riots, airplane crashes), or (3) a crime of violence (e.g., rape, assault, or murder in the workplace or school; bombing in crowded areas; spousal or child abuse).

Commonly experienced, posttrauma phenomena include acute stress disorder, posttraumatic stress disorder, and depression; therefore, the need for psychological first aid (crisis intervention) and debriefing after any crisis situation for all age groups cannot be overstressed.

It is also possible to experience more than one type of crisis situation simultaneously, and as expected, the presence of more than one crisis further taxes individual coping skills. Consider a 51-year-old woman who may be going through menopause (maturational) when her husband dies suddenly of cancer (situational). Think about the victims of Hurricane Katrina, many of whom were members of vulnerable groups—racially, socially, and financially—and may have been experiencing maturational or situational crises prior to the hurricane. They were then confronted with the devastation of the hurricane and the simultaneous onset of multiple losses. Many of them lost family members and friends, homes and belongings, employment, community supports, and even personal identification.

PHASES OF CRISIS

Through extensive study of individuals experiencing crisis, Caplan (1964) identified behaviors that followed a fairly distinct path. These behaviors were categorized in four distinct phases of crisis.

Phase 1

A person confronted by a conflict or problem that threatens the self-concept responds with increased feelings of anxiety. The increase in anxiety stimulates the use of problem-solving techniques and defense mechanisms in an effort to solve the problem and lower anxiety.

Phase 2

If the usual defensive response fails and the threat persists, anxiety continues to rise and produce feelings of extreme discomfort. Individual functioning becomes disorganized. Trial-and-error attempts at solving the problem and restoring a normal balance begin.

Phase 3

If the trial-and-error attempts fail, anxiety can escalate to severe and panic levels, and the person mobilizes automatic relief behaviors, such as withdrawal and flight. Some form of resolution (e.g., compromising needs or redefining the situation to reach an acceptable solution) may be made in this stage.

Phase 4

If the problem is not solved and new coping skills are ineffective, anxiety can overwhelm the person and lead to serious personality disorganization, depression, confusion, violence against others, or suicidal behavior.

APPLICATION OF THE NURSING PROCESS

Nurses, perhaps more than any other group of health professionals, deal with people who are experiencing disruption in their lives. Because people typically experience increased stress and anxiety in medical, surgical, and psychiatric hospital settings, as well as in community settings, nurses are often positioned and primed to initiate and participate in crisis intervention. Crisis theory defines aspects of crisis that are basic to crisis intervention and relevant for nurses (Box 26-1).

ASSESSMENT

General Assessment

As shown in Figure 26-1, a person's equilibrium may be adversely affected by one or more of the following: (1) an unrealistic perception of the precipitating event, (2) inadequate situational supports, and (3) inadequate coping mechanisms (Aguilera, 1998). It is crucial to assess these factors when a crisis situation is evaluated because data gained from the assessment guide both

BOX 26-1 FOUNDATION FOR CRISIS INTERVENTION

- A crisis is self-limiting and usually resolves within 4 to 6 weeks.
- At the resolution of a crisis, the patient will emerge at one of three different functional levels:
  - A higher level of functioning.
  - The same level of functioning.
  - A lower level of functioning.
- The goal of crisis intervention is to return the patient to at least the pre-crisis level of functioning.
- The form of crisis resolution depends on the patient's actions and others' interventions.
- During a crisis, people are often more receptive than usual to outside intervention. With intervention, the patient can learn different adaptive means of problem solving to correct inadequate solutions.
- The patient in a crisis situation is assumed to be mentally healthy, to have functioned well in the past, and to be presently in a state of disequilibrium.
- Crisis intervention deals only with the patient's present problem and resolution of the immediate crisis (e.g., the "here and now").
- The nurse must be willing to take an active, even directive, role in intervention, which is in direct contrast to conventional therapeutic intervention that stresses a more passive and nondirective role.
- Early intervention probably increases the chances for a good prognosis.
- The patient is encouraged to set realistic goals and plan a focused intervention with the nurse.

the nurse and the patient in setting realistic and meaningful goals and in planning possible solutions to the problem situation.

The nurse's initial task is to promote a sense of safety by assessing the patient's potential for suicide or homicide. If the patient is suicidal, homicidal, or unable to take care of personal needs, hospitalization should be considered (Aguilera, 1998). Sample questions to ask include the following:

- Do you feel you can keep yourself safe?
- Have you thought of killing yourself or someone else? If yes, have you thought of how you would do this?

After establishing that the patient poses no danger to self or others, the nurse assesses three main areas: (1) the patient's perception of the precipitating event, (2) the patient's situational supports, and (3) the patient's personal coping skills.

> **VIGNETTE**
> Madison, a 25-year-old woman, is brought to the emergency department by police after being beaten by her husband. Madison is seen by the medical personnel and then interviewed by the psychiatric mental health nurse working in the emergency department. The nurse calmly introduces herself and tells Madison she would like to spend some time with her. The nurse says, "It looks as if things are pretty overwhelming. Is that how you're feeling?" The nurse makes the observation that things must be very bad if Madison stays with an abusive husband. Madison sits slumped in a chair, her hands in her lap, head hanging down, and tears in her eyes.

Assessing Perception of Precipitating Event

The nurse's task is now to assess the individual or family and the problem. The more clearly the problem can be defined, the more likely effective solutions will be identified. Sample questions that may facilitate assessment include the following:

- Has anything particularly upsetting happened to you within the past few days or weeks?
- What was happening in your life before you started to feel this way?
- What leads you to seek help now?
- Describe how you are feeling right now.
- How does this situation affect your life?
- How do you see this event affecting your future?
- What would need to be done to resolve this situation?

Assessing Situational Supports

Next the nurse determines available resources by assessing the patient's support systems. Family and friends are often involved to aid the patient by offering material or emotional support. If these resources are unavailable, the nurse or counselor acts as a temporary support system while relationships with individuals or groups in the community are established. Sample questions include the following:

- Who do you live with?
- Who can you talk with when you feel overwhelmed?
- Who can you trust?
- Who is available to help you?
- How important is spirituality in your life?

> **VIGNETTE**
> **Nurse:** Madison, tell me what has happened.
> **Madison:** I can't go home . . . . No one cares . . . . No one believes me . . . . I can't go through it again.
> **Nurse:** Tell me what you can't go through again.
> (Madison starts to cry, shaking with sobs. The nurse sits quietly for a while and then speaks.)
> **Nurse:** Tell me what is so terrible. Let's look at it together.
> After a while, Madison tells the nurse that her husband has been beating her regularly, although particularly after a night of drinking. The beatings have become much worse over time, and Madison states, "I'm afraid that eventually I'll end up dead."

- Do you take part in organized religious services?
- Where do you go to school or to other community-based activities?
- During difficult times in the past, whom did you want most to help you?
- Who is the most helpful?

> **VIGNETTE**
> **Nurse:** Madison, who can you go to? Do you have any other family?
> **Madison:** No. My family is in another state. We stay pretty much alone.
> **Nurse:** Do you have anyone you can talk to?
> **Madison:** I really don't have any friends. My husband's jealousy makes it difficult for me to have friends. He doesn't like anyone that I would want as a friend.
> **Nurse:** What about people at your place of worship or co-workers?
> **Madison:** My co-workers are nice, but I can't tell them things like this. They wouldn't believe me anyway.
> The nurse learns that Madison does well at her job. Madison explains that her job helps her forget her problems for a little while. Getting good job reviews also has another reward: it is the only time her husband says anything nice about her.

Assessing Personal Coping Skills

Finally, the nurse assesses the patient's personal coping skills by evaluating the patient's anxiety level and identifying the patient's established patterns of coping. Common coping mechanisms may be overeating, drinking, smoking, withdrawing, seeking out someone to talk to, yelling, fighting, or engaging in other physical activity. Sample questions to ask include the following:

- What do you usually do to feel better?
- Did you try it this time? If so, what was different?
- What helped you through difficult times in the past?
- What do you think might happen now?

> **VIGNETTE**
> **Nurse:** What do you think would help your situation?
> **Madison:** I don't want to be in an abusive marriage. I just don't know where to turn.
> The nurse tells Madison that she wants to work with her to find a solution and that she is concerned for Madison's safety and well-being.

Self-Assessment

Nurses need to constantly monitor and acknowledge personal feelings and thoughts when dealing with a patient in crisis. It is important to recognize your own level of anxiety to prevent the patient from closing off his or her expression of painful feelings to you. Self-awareness of your negative feelings and reactions can prevent unconscious suppression of the patient's personal distress in an effort to manage your own discomfort.

There may be times when, perhaps for personal reasons, you feel you cannot deal effectively with a patient's situation. If this happens, ask another colleague to work with the individual. Consulting a more experienced colleague or mentor or seeking supervision will help you separate the patient's needs from your own and identify how to work through uncomfortable or painful personal issues or bias to better care for those in crisis.

New nurses working in crisis intervention often face common problems that must be dealt with before they can become comfortable and competent in the role of a crisis counselor. Four of the more common problems include the following:

1. The nurse needs to be needed.
2. The nurse sets unrealistic goals for patients.
3. The nurse has difficulty dealing with the issue of suicide.
4. The nurse has difficulty terminating the nurse-patient relationship.

Table 26-1 gives examples, results, appropriate interventions, and desired outcomes of common problems in the nurse-patient

TABLE 26-1 COMMON PROBLEMS IN THE NURSE-PATIENT RELATIONSHIP

EXAMPLE	RESULT	INTERVENTION	OUTCOME
Problem 1: Nurse Needs to Feel Needed			
Nurse: Allows excessive phone calls between sessions. Gives direct advice without sufficient knowledge of patient's situation. Attempts to influence patient's lifestyle on a judgmental basis.	Patient becomes dependent on nurse and relies less on own abilities. Nurse reacts to patient's not getting "cured" by projecting feelings of frustration and anger onto patient.	Nurse: Evaluates personal needs versus patient's needs with an experienced professional. Discourages patient's dependency. Encourages goal setting and problem solving by patient. Takes control only if patient is suicidal or homicidal.	Patient is free to grow and problem-solve own life crises. Nurse's skills and effectiveness grow as comfort with role increases and own goals are clarified.
Problem 2: Nurse Sets Unrealistic Goals for Patients			
Nurse: Expects physically abused woman to leave battering partner. Expects man who abuses alcohol to stop drinking when loss of family or job is imminent.	Nurse feels anxious and responsible when expectations are not met; anxiety resulting from feelings of inadequacy are projected onto the patient in the form of frustration and anger.	Nurse: Examines realistic expectations of self and patient with an experienced professional. Reevaluates patient's level of functioning and works with patient on his level. Encourages setting of goals by patient.	Patient feels less alienated, and a working relationship can ensue. Nurse's ability to assess and problem solve increases as anger and frustration decrease.
Problem 3: Nurse Has Difficulty Dealing with a Suicidal Patient			
Nurse is selectively inattentive by: Denying possible clues. Neglecting to follow up on verbal suicide clues. Changing topic to less threatening subject when self-destructive themes come up.	Patient is robbed of opportunity to share feelings and find alternatives to intolerable situation. Patient remains suicidal. Nurse's crisis intervention ceases to be effective.	Nurse: Assesses own feelings and anxieties with help of an experienced professional. Evaluates all clues or slight suspicions and acts on them (e.g., "Are you thinking of killing yourself?"—if yes, nurse assesses suicide potential and need for hospitalization).	Patient experiences relief in sharing feelings and evaluating alternatives. Suicide potential can be minimized. Nurse becomes more adept at picking up clues and minimizing suicide potential.
Problem 4: Nurse has Difficulty Terminating after Crisis Has Resolved			
Nurse is tempted to work on other problems in patient's life to prolong contact with patient.	Nurse steps into territory of traditional therapy without proper training or experience.	Nurse works with an experienced professional to: Explore own feelings about separations and termination. Reinforce crisis model; crisis intervention is a preventive tool, not psychotherapy. Nurse becomes better able to help patient with his/her feelings when nurse's own feelings are recognized.	Patient is free to go back to his or her life situation or request appropriate referral to work on other issues of importance to patient.

From Wallace, M. A., & Morley, W. E. (1970). Teaching crisis intervention. *American Journal of Nursing, 70*(7), 1484–1487.

relationship faced by beginning nurses. It is crucial that expert supervision be available as an integral part of the crisis-intervention training process.

Even experienced nurses working in disaster situations can become overwhelmed when witnessing catastrophic loss of human life (e.g., acts of terrorism, plane crashes, school shootings) and/or mass destruction of homes and belongings (e.g., floods, fires, tornadoes). In fact, researchers find that mental health care providers may experience psychological distress from working with traumatized populations, a phenomenon of secondary traumatic stress or "vicarious traumatization" (Dunkley & Whelan, 2006). As stressed before, nurses need to constantly monitor personal feelings and thoughts when dealing with patients in crisis (Phoenix, 2007), and disaster nurses need both supportive ties and access to debriefing.

Debriefing is an important step for staff in coming to terms with overwhelmingly violent or otherwise disastrous situations. Such intervention helps staff put the crisis in perspective and begin their own recovery. Debriefing is discussed in detail later in the chapter.

ASSESSMENT GUIDELINES

Crisis

1. Identify whether the patient's response to the crisis warrants psychiatric treatment or hospitalization to minimize decompensating (suicidal behavior, psychotic thinking, violent behavior).
2. Identify whether the patient is able to identify the *precipitating event.*
3. Assess the patient's understanding of his or her present *situational supports.*
4. Identify the patient's usual *coping styles,* and determine what coping mechanisms may help the present situation.
5. Determine whether there are certain religious or cultural beliefs that need to be considered in assessing and intervening in this patient's crisis.
6. Assess whether this situation is one in which the patient needs primary intervention (education, environmental manipulation, or new coping skills), secondary intervention (crisis intervention), or tertiary intervention (rehabilitation).

CONSIDERING CULTURE

Examining a Gun Culture in the United States

On December 12, 2012, Adam Lanza, 24, shot and killed his mother. He then proceeded to an elementary school where he killed 20 children and 6 staff members with semiautomatic weapons at Sandy Hook Elementary School in Newtown, Connecticut. As police arrived on the scene, he shot himself in the head. The news scenes of crying and horrified children being led from the school holding hands have been etched in the memory of many Americans. Pictures of the first-grade victims and their teachers were published in newspapers and shown on television. Seeing these innocent faces was so heartbreaking that many people could not bring themselves to look at them.

As the crisis unfolded, a debate quickly ensued regarding gun control and the issue of a gun culture in the United States. One post on Facebook read, "Before you go blaming assault rifles for this tragedy, folks, he [Lanza] used handguns." Another said, "More people get killed by hammers and clubs than by rifles." A response to this post was, "If Lanza had walked into that school with a hammer, those six staff members could have taken him down."

The United States has a strong gun culture. The Wild West is romanticized for its gun slinging, wars are part of the fabric of our history, and guns are associated with strength and virility. The Second Amendment right from the Constitution is frequently cited as a right to bear arms. A general argument is that if only bad people have guns, then good people cannot defend themselves.

Rights of gun owners are being challenged in unprecedented ways In response to the shooting and ensuing crisis, President Barack Obama called for tighter regulations on assault rifles and magazines (clips) with multiple rounds and stringent background checks for people buying guns. Attention has been directed toward preventing people like Lanza, who was believed to have a psychiatric disorder, from having access to guns. Violent video games where young males act out virtual killings have also been on the radar for outright bans.

How this clash between the two cultures, the gun culture and gun-control culture, will play out is yet to be seen. The murders that took place in Sandy Hook Elementary dramatically energized a nation and will likely be a force for a change in laws that will impact the gun culture in the United States.

DIAGNOSIS

The North American Nursing Diagnosis Association International (NANDA-I) (Herdman, 2012) provides nursing diagnoses that can be considered for patients experiencing anxiety and anxiety disorders. When a person is in crisis, the nursing diagnosis of *Ineffective coping* is often useful. Because anxiety may escalate to moderate or severe levels, the ability to solve problems is usually impaired. Ineffective coping may be evidenced by inability to meet basic needs, inability to meet role expectations, alteration in social participation, use of inappropriate defense mechanisms, or impairment of usual patterns of communication. The "related-to" component will vary with the individual patient.

VIGNETTE

In the preceding vignette, the assessment of Madison's (1) perception of the precipitating event, (2) situational supports, and (3) personal coping skills provides the nurse enough data to formulate two diagnoses and work with Madison in setting goals and planning interventions:

Anxiety (moderate/severe) related to mental and physical abuse, as evidenced by ineffectual problem solving and feelings of impending doom

Compromised family coping related to the constant threat of violence

OUTCOMES IDENTIFICATION

Relevant outcomes from the *Nursing Outcomes Classification (NOC)* (Moorhead et al., 2013) for a person experiencing a crisis include *Coping, Decision Making, Role Performance,* and *Stress Level.* The planning of realistic outcomes is patient-centered and includes the patient and family, which result in outcomes congruent with the patient's cultural and personal values. Without the patient's involvement, the outcome criteria (goals at the end of 4 to 8 weeks) may be irrelevant or unacceptable solutions to that person's crisis. Table 26-2 identifies signs and symptoms commonly experienced in crises, offers potential nursing diagnoses, and suggests outcomes.

PLANNING

Nurses are called upon to plan and intervene through a variety of crisis-intervention modalities, such as disaster nursing, mobile crisis units, group work, health education and crisis prevention, victim outreach programs, and telephone hotlines; therefore, the nurse may be involved in planning and intervention for an individual (e.g., cases of physical abuse), for a group (e.g., students after a classmate's suicide or shooting), or for a community (e.g., disaster nursing after tornadoes, shootings, and airplane crashes). Data from the answers to the following questions guide the nurse in determining immediate actions (Aguilera, 1998):

- How much has this crisis affected the patient's life? Can the patient still go to work? Attend school? Care for family members?
- How is the state of disequilibrium affecting significant people in the patient's life (wife, husband, children, other family members, boss, boyfriend, girlfriend)?

VIGNETTE

The nurse consults a social worker about Madison, and the three meet together. All agree that Madison should not return to her home. Madison and the nurse then establish goals and plan interventions. The goals are as follows:

- Madison will return to her pre-crisis state within 2 weeks.
- With the support of the staff, Madison will find a safe environment.
- With the support of the staff, Madison will have at least two outside supports available within 24 hours.
- Madison will receive continued evaluation and support until the immediate crisis is over (6 to 8 weeks).

TABLE 26-2 SIGNS AND SYMPTOMS, DIAGNOSES, AND OUTCOMES FOR CRISIS INTERVENTION

SIGNS AND SYMPTOMS	NURSING DIAGNOSES	OUTCOMES
Inability to meet basic needs, decreased use of social support, inadequate problem solving, inability to attend to information, isolation	*Ineffective coping* *Risk for compromised resilience*	Modifies lifestyle as needed, uses effective coping strategies, reports decrease in physical symptoms of stress, reports decrease in negative feelings
Denial, exaggerated startle response, flashbacks, horror, hypervigilance, intrusive thoughts and dreams, panic attacks, feeling numb, substance abuse, confusion, incoherence	*Posttrauma syndrome* *Rape-trauma syndrome* *Anxiety (moderate, severe, panic)* *Acute confusion* *Sleep deprivation*	Exhibits nonlabile mood, impulse control; reports adequate sleep, exhibits concentration, tends to ADLs, shows interest in surroundings
Minimizes symptoms, delays seeking care, displays inappropriate affect, makes dismissive comments when speaking of distressing events	*Ineffective denial*	Recognizes reality of health situation, maintains relationships, copes with health situation, makes decisions about health, reports sense of life being worth living
Overwhelmed, depressed, states has nothing in life worthwhile, self-hatred, feelings of being ineffectual, sees limited alternatives, feels strange, perceives a lack of control	*Risk for suicide* *Chronic low self-esteem* *Disturbed personal identity* *Hopelessness* *Powerlessness*	Remains free from harm, expresses feelings of self-worth, verbalizes sense of personal identity, expresses meaning in life, sets goals, believes that actions impact outcomes
Difficulty with interpersonal relationships, isolated, has few or no social supports	*Social isolation* *Impaired social interaction*	Expresses a sense of belonging, effects meaningful relationships
Changes in family relationships and functioning, difficulty performing family caregiver role	*Compromised family coping* *Interrupted family processes* *Caregiver role strain*	Manages family problems, expresses feelings openly among family members, respite for caregiver, sense of control for caregiver

From Herdman, T.H. (Ed.) *Nursing diagnoses—Definitions and classification 2012-2014.* Copyright © 2012, 1994–2012 by NANDA International. Used by arrangement with John Wiley & Sons Limited; Moorhead, S., Johnson, M., Maas, M. L., & Swanson, E. (2013). *Nursing outcomes classification (NOC)* (5th ed.). St Louis, MO: Elsevier.

IMPLEMENTATION

Crisis intervention is a function of the basic-level nurse. The focus is on the present problem only and has two initial goals:

1. **Patient safety.** External controls may be applied for protection of the patient in crisis if the patient is suicidal or homicidal.
2. **Anxiety reduction.** Anxiety-reduction techniques are used so that inner resources can be mobilized.

During the initial interview, the patient in crisis first needs to gain a feeling of safety. Solutions to the crisis may be offered so that the patient is aware of other options. Feelings of support and hope will temporarily diminish anxiety. The nurse needs to play an active role by indicating that help is available. The availability of help is conveyed by the competent use of crisis-intervention skills and genuine interest and support. It is not conveyed by the use of false reassurances and platitudes, such as "everything will be all right." Crisis intervention requires a creative and flexible approach through the use of traditional and nontraditional therapeutic methods. The nurse may act as educator, advisor, and role model, always keeping in mind that it is the patient who solves the problem, not the nurse. The following are important assumptions when working with a patient in crisis:

- The patient is in charge of his or her own life.
- The patient is able to make decisions.
- The crisis counseling relationship is one between partners.

The nurse helps the patient refocus to gain new perspectives on the situation. The nurse supports the patient during the process of finding constructive ways to solve or cope with the problem. It is important for the nurse to be mindful of how difficult it is for the patient to change behavior. Table 26-3 offers guidelines for nursing interventions and corresponding rationales.

VIGNETTE

After talking with the nurse and the social worker, Madison seems open to going to a safe house for battered women. She also agrees to talk to a counselor at a mental health facility. The nurse sets up an appointment at which she, Madison, and the counselor will meet. The nurse will continue to see Madison twice a week.

Counseling

Primary Care

Psychotherapeutic crisis interventions are directed toward three levels of care: (1) primary, (2) secondary, and (3) tertiary. **Primary care** promotes mental health and reduces mental illness to decrease the incidence of crisis. On this level the nurse can:

- Work with a patient to recognize potential problems by evaluating the patient's experience of stressful life events.
- Teach the patient specific coping skills, such as decision making, problem solving, assertiveness skills, meditation, and relaxation skills.
- Assist the patient in evaluating the timing or reduction of life changes to decrease the negative effects of stress as much as possible. This may involve working with a patient to plan environmental changes, make important interpersonal decisions, and rethink changes in occupational roles.

Secondary Care

Secondary care establishes intervention during an acute crisis to *prevent* prolonged anxiety from diminishing personal effectiveness and personality organization. The nurse's primary focus is to ensure the safety of the patient. After safety issues are dealt with, the nurse works with the patient to assess the patient's problem, support systems, and coping styles. Desired goals are

TABLE 26-3 GUIDELINES FOR CRISIS INTERVENTION

INTERVENTION	RATIONALE
Assess for suicidal or homicidal thoughts or plans.	Safety is always the first consideration.
Take initial steps to make patient feel safe and less anxious.	A person who feels safe and less anxious is able to more effectively problem solve solutions with the nurse.
Listen carefully (e.g., make eye contact, give frequent feedback to verify and convey understanding, summarize what patient says).	A person who believes someone is really listening is more likely to believe that someone cares about his or her situation and that help may be available. This offers hope.
Crisis intervention calls for directive and creative approaches. Initially the nurse may make phone calls to arrange babysitters, schedule a visiting nurse, find shelter, or contact a social worker.	A person who is confused, frightened, or overwhelmed may be temporarily unable to perform usual tasks.
Identify needed social supports (with patient's input) and mobilize the priority.	A person's need for shelter, help with care for children or elders, medical workup, emergency medical attention, hospitalization, food, safe housing, and self-help groups is determined.
Identify needed coping skills (problem solving, relaxation, assertiveness, job training, newborn care, self-esteem building.	Increasing coping skills and learning new ones can help with current crisis and help minimize future crises.
Involve patient in identifying realistic, acceptable interventions.	The person's involvement in planning increases his or her sense of control, self-esteem, and adherence to plan.
Plan regular follow-up (e.g., phone calls, clinic visits, home visits) to assess patient's progress.	Plan is evaluated to see what works and what does not.

explored and interventions planned. Secondary care lessens the time a patient is mentally disabled during a crisis. Secondary-level care occurs in hospital units, emergency departments, clinics, or mental health centers, usually during daytime hours.

Tertiary Care

Tertiary care provides support for those who have experienced a severe crisis and are now recovering from a disabling mental state. Social and community facilities that offer tertiary intervention include rehabilitation centers, sheltered workshops, day hospitals, and outpatient clinics. Primary goals are to facilitate optimal levels of functioning and prevent further emotional disruptions. People with severe and persistent mental problems are often extremely susceptible to crisis, and community facilities provide the structured environment that can help prevent problem situations. Box 26-2 lists *Nursing Interventions Classification (NIC)* interventions for responding to a crisis (Bulechek et al., 2013).

Critical Incident Stress Debriefing. Critical incident stress debriefing (CISD) is an example of a tertiary intervention directed toward a group that has experienced a crisis (Everly, Lating, & Mitchell, 2000). CISD consists of a seven-phase group meeting that offers individuals the opportunity to share their thoughts and feelings in a safe and controlled environment. It is used to debrief staff on an inpatient unit following a patient suicide or an incident of violence, to debrief crisis hotline volunteers, to debrief schoolchildren and school personnel after multiple school shootings, and to debrief rescue and health care workers who have responded to a natural disaster or a terrorist attack such as that on the World Trade Center (Hammond & Brooks, 2001).

The phases of CISD are:

- *Introductory phase:* Meeting purpose is explained; an overview of the debriefing process is provided; confidentiality is assured; guidelines are explained; team members are identified; and questions are answered.
- *Fact phase:* Participants discuss the facts of the incident; participants introduce themselves, tell their involvement in the incident, and describe the event from their perspective.
- *Thought phase:* Participants discuss their first thoughts of the incident.
- *Reaction phase:* Participants talk about the worst thing about the incident—what they would like to forget, and what was most painful.
- *Symptom phase:* Participants describe their cognitive, physical, emotional, or behavioral experiences at the incident scene and describe any symptoms they felt following the initial experience.
- *Teaching phase:* The normality of the expressed symptoms is acknowledged and affirmed; anticipatory guidance is offered regarding future symptoms; group is involved in stress-management techniques.
- *Reentry phase:* Participants review material discussed, introduce new topics, ask questions, and discuss how they would like to bring closure to the debriefing. Debriefing team members answer questions, inform, and reassure; provide written material; provide information on referral sources; and summarize the debriefing with encouragement, support, and appreciation.

BOX 26-2 CRISIS INTERVENTION

Definition: Use of short-term counseling to help the patient cope with a crisis and resume a state of functioning comparable to or better than the precrisis state

Activities:

- Provide an atmosphere of support.
- Avoid giving false reassurances.
- Provide a safe haven.
- Determine whether the patient presents a safety risk to self or others.
- Initiate necessary precautions to safeguard the patient or others at risk for physical harm.
- Encourage expression of feelings in a nondestructive manner.
- Assist in identification of the precipitants and dynamics of the crisis.
- Encourage patient to focus on one implication at a time.
- Assist in identification of personal strengths and abilities that can be used in resolving the crisis.
- Assist in identification of past/present coping skills and their effectiveness.
- Assist in development of new coping and problem-solving skills, as needed.
- Assist in identification of available support systems.
- Link the patient and family with community resources, as needed.
- Provide guidance about how to develop and maintain support systems.
- Introduce the patient to persons (or groups) who have successfully undergone the same experience.
- Assist in identification of alternative courses of action to resolve the crisis.
- Assist in evaluation of the possible consequences of the various courses of action.
- Assist the patient to decide on a particular course of action.
- Assist in formulating a time frame for implementation of the chosen course of action.
- Evaluate with the patient whether the crisis has been resolved by the chosen course of action.
- Plan with the patient how adaptive coping skills can be used to deal with crises in the future.

Adapted from Bulechek, G. M., Butcher, H. K., Dochterman, J. M., & Wagner, C. (2013). *Nursing interventions classification (NIC)* (6th ed.). St. Louis, MO: Mosby.

VIGNETTE

The nurse performs secondary crisis intervention and meets with Madison twice weekly for 4 weeks. Madison is motivated to work with the social worker and the nurse to find another place to live. The nurse suggests several times that Madison start to see a counselor in the outpatient clinic after the crisis is over so that she can talk about some of her pain. Madison is ambivalent and is already thinking she will return to her husband.

EVALUATION

NOC includes a built-in measurement for each outcome and for the indicators that support the outcome. Each indicator is measured on a 5-point Likert scale, which helps the nurse evaluate the effectiveness of the crisis intervention. This evaluation is usually performed 4 to 8 weeks after the initial interview although it can be done earlier (e.g., by the end of the visit, the anxiety level will decrease from 1 = severe to 3 = moderate). If the intervention has been successful, the patient's level of anxiety and ability to function should be at pre-crisis levels. Often a patient chooses to follow up on additional areas of concern and is referred to other agencies for more long-term work. Crisis intervention frequently serves to prepare a patient for further treatment.

VIGNETTE

Madison returned to her husband 3 weeks after the battering episode. She has convinced herself that he has changed his behavior, despite the fact that he has not sought any help to control his anger.

After 6 weeks, Madison and the nurse decide that the crisis is over. Madison is aloof and distant. The nurse evaluates Madison as being in a moderate amount of emotional pain, but Madison feels she is doing well. The nurse's assessment indicates that Madison has other serious issues (e.g., low self-esteem, childhood abuse), and the nurse strongly suggests that she could benefit from further counseling. The decision, however, is up to Madison, who says she is satisfied with the way things are and again states that if she has any future problems, she will return to the safe house counselor.

DISASTERS IN THE CONTEXT OF PSYCHIATRIC NURSING

Disaster research reflects global attempts to learn from present and past disaster experiences. Professionals attending informational conferences promoting international dialogue, together with world leaders and burgeoning national and international organizations, are all stakeholders underscoring society's need to collaborate (World Health Organization [WHO], 2010).

There is a growing awareness of interdependencies that exist among all members of the global community. Each successive large-scale earthquake, tsunami, hurricane, flood, or wildfire has ripple effects regardless of where in the world it occurs. Directly or remotely, we experience some element of the far-reaching depletion of human, economic, and natural resources. Consider the declining values of international stocks, illness-ravaged citizens in Haiti, or the devastation of flood victims on the U.S. Gulf Coast.

A decade of 21st century disaster literature supports disaster preparedness by developing resilient communities and assessing disaster risks on a local level. Considering the unique forms of devastation connected with any disaster, reducing risk within local communities is expedient, eventually extending into networking communities then to larger societal and national programs (Federal Emergency Management Agency [FEMA], 2012)

Professional nurses regularly provide strong and dynamic core contributions to the multiple facets of disaster and recovery relief efforts around the world. Professional nurses are experienced care providers and managers of care, adaptable with critical thinking and problem-solving expertise. Also, professional nurses are visibly emerging around the world both as disaster researchers and authors and as pivotal spokespeople in disaster management planning arenas (Powers, 2010).

Increasing demands for contributions by advanced practice psychiatric nurses are also expected in view of persistent research strongly emphasizing a pivotal facet of building resilient communities lies in making systematic, comprehensive mental health services available to people in need worldwide (Herrman, 2012; WHO, 2010).

Climactic events inflicting significant damage to life and property exceeding the resource capabilities of local communities are considered natural disasters (Powers, 2010). Having a clear understanding about the specific characteristics of natural and man-made disasters enhances the usefulness of information in disaster plans. Earthquakes, wildfires, floods, tsunami, tornadoes, droughts, extreme heat and cold periods, and blizzards are some of the more recent global events. Man-made occurrences are direct, identifiable human actions, deliberate or otherwise, and include technological events such as power outages, major industrial accidents, or the unplanned release of nuclear energy. More complex events include war, civil or political strife, or some combination of natural and man-made events.

Each catastrophic event will set in operation a five-phase disaster management continuum including the following:

1. **Preparedness**: The protective plan designed before the event to structure the response, assess risk, and evaluate damage.
2. **Mitigation**: Attempt to limit a disaster's impact on human health and community function.
3. **Response**: Actual implementation of the disaster plan.
4. **Recovery**: Actions focus on stabilizing the community and returning it to its previous status.
5. **Evaluation**: Evaluating the response effort to prepare for the future (FEMA, 2012).

Unexpected occurrences that create needs beyond the capabilities of victims to address without assistance can be expected to result in crisis experiences. Everyone experiences a crisis at some time.

Disaster Management Context

On November 25, 2002, the events of 9/11 prompted the creation of a government cabinet, the Department of Homeland Security (DHS), subsuming FEMA and its charge to coordinate responses to U.S. disasters, particularly in situations where local and state resources were inadequate to the presenting challenges. As a result the DHS has ultimate governmental responsibility for the safety of U.S. citizens and territories while assuring adequate preparedness, response, and recovery protocols are immediately available.

To achieve its objectives the DHS uses civilian first responders, local emergency response professionals who prepare for and respond to natural disasters or terrorist threats or any other large-scale event. In 2004 DHS furthered its agenda and created the National Incident Management System (NIMS) to help first responders from different disciplines and areas to effectively work together when a community exhausted its available resources in addressing a large-scale occurrence.

To understand NIMS operations, incident command system training (ICS) is required. ICS provides a common organizational structure facilitating an immediate response to occurrences by establishing a clear chain of command that supports the coordination of personnel and equipment at the event site. Minimal core competencies for individuals expected to participate in an event have been developed by the DHS and are included in established training programs (FEMA, 2012). The Citizen's Core created by President George W. Bush in 2002 affords American citizens opportunities to participate in emergency preparedness-enhancing efforts to develop greater resiliency at local community levels (Office of the Press Secretary, Citizen Corps Guide Book).

Relative to the following research, FEMA programs provide opportunities to volunteer or otherwise participate at various preparedness, relief, and recovery efforts. The study highlighted in Evidence-Based Practice describes college students' evacuation experience, implementing one university's initial disaster response and recovery plans, respectively.

EVIDENCE-BASED PRACTICE

The Impact of Disaster on the Process of Higher Education

Watson, P. G., Loffredo, V. J., & McKee, J. C. (2011). When a natural disaster occurs: Lessons learned in meeting students' needs. *Journal of Professional Nursing, 27*(6), 362–369.

Problem

Extreme weather conditions are frequently accompanied by catastrophic events and disruption to lives. Students at colleges and universities who are assaulted by such events may be unprepared for these events and experience acute distress.

Purpose of the Study

This study was conducted to understand the experience of students who go through emergency evacuation and then return to their academic studies.

Methods

A Hurricane Needs Survey was administered to students 7 months after an emergency evacuation of a Texas campus during a hurricane. It included 26 structured questions and 3 open-ended questions:

1. What information could have served you better for storm preparation?
2. While you were away from [campus] immediately after the storm, what information could have served you better?
3. What information could have better assisted you in your return to campus after the storm?

513 responses represented 37.2% of the University of Texas Medical Branch student population.

Key Findings

- The majority of the 513 respondents had not seen a health care provider, and they reported functioning at prestorm levels physically and mentally.
- Nearly 25% of the sample reported physical distress and fatigue following the evacuation.
- Almost all of the students reported that the storm had a negative effect on their academic performance.
- International respondents and graduate students reported slightly more difficulties and moderate financial losses.
- Three themes were identified from the open-ended questions: Students want the university to be prepared for weather-related disasters; they want to be connected with the university after the storm; and returning to normalcy after such a disruption is important.

Implications for Nursing Practice

Given the uniqueness of each catastrophic event, nurses benefit from ongoing qualitative inquiries into the lived experiences of disaster victims. As health care leaders, nurses promote physical and mental well-being through health service programs in universities across the country. Nurses are in pivotal positions to influence and strengthen the resiliency of college communities through their participation in disaster research, planning, and preparedness.

26-1 CASE STUDY AND NURSING CARE PLAN

Crisis

Ms. Greg, the psychiatric clinical nurse specialist, is called to the neurological unit. She is told that Mr. Raymond, a 43-year-old man with Guillain-Barré syndrome, is presenting a serious nursing problem, and the staff has requested a consult. The disease has caused severe muscle weakness to the point that Mr. Raymond is essentially paralyzed; however, he is able to breathe on his own.

The nurse manager says that Mr. Raymond is hostile and sexually abusive, and his abusive language, demeaning attitude, and angry outbursts are having an adverse effect on the unit as a whole. The staff nurses state that they feel ineffective and angry and have tried to be patient and understanding; however, nothing seems to get through to him. The situation has affected the morale of the staff and, the nurses believe, the quality of their care.

Mr. Raymond, a American Indian, was employed as a taxicab driver. Six months before his hospital admission, he had given up drinking after years of episodic alcohol abuse. His fiancée visits him every day. He needs a great deal of assistance with every aspect of his activities of daily living. Because of his severe muscle weakness, he has to be turned and positioned every 2 hours and fed through a gastrostomy tube.

Assessment

Ms. Greg gathers data from Mr. Raymond, the nursing staff, and Mr. Raymond's fiancée.

Perception of the Precipitating Event

During the initial interview, Mr. Raymond speaks to Ms. Greg angrily, using profanity and making lewd sexual suggestions. He also expresses anger about needing a nurse to "scratch my head and help me blow my nose." He still cannot figure out how his illness suddenly developed. He says the doctors told him that it was too early to know for sure if he would recover completely but that the prognosis was good.

Support System

Ms. Greg speaks with Mr. Raymond's fiancée. Mr. Raymond's relationships with his fiancée and with his American Indian cultural group are strong. With minimal ties outside their reservation, neither Mr. Raymond nor his fiancée has much knowledge of supportive agencies.

Personal Coping Skills

Mr. Raymond comes from a strongly male-dominated subculture where the man is expected to be a strong leader. His ability to be an independent person with the power to affect the direction of his life is central to his perception of being acceptable as a man.

Mr. Raymond feels powerless, out of control, and enraged. He is handling his anxiety by displacing these feelings onto the environment, namely, the staff and his fiancée. This redirection of anger temporarily lowers his anxiety and distracts him from painful feelings. When he intimidates others, he feels temporarily in control and experiences an illusion of power. He uses displacement to relieve his painful levels of anxiety when he feels threatened.

Mr. Raymond's unconscious use of displacement is maladaptive because the issues causing his distress are not being resolved. His anxiety continues to escalate; furthermore, his behavior leads others to minimize interactions with him, which increases his sense of isolation and helplessness.

Self-Assessment

Ms. Greg meets with the staff twice. The staff discuss feelings of helplessness and lack of control stemming from their feelings of rejection by Mr. Raymond. They talk of their anger about Mr. Raymond's demeaning behavior and frustration about the situation. Ms. Greg points out to the staff that Mr. Raymond's feelings of helplessness, lack of control, and anger at his situation are the same feelings the staff are experiencing. Displacement of his feelings of helplessness and frustration by intimidating the staff gives Mr. Raymond a brief feeling of control. It also distracts him from his own feelings of helplessness.

The nurses become more understanding of the motivation for the behavior Mr. Raymond employs to cope with moderate to severe levels of anxiety. They begin to focus more on the patient, less on personal reactions, and decide on two approaches they can try as a group. First, they will not take Mr. Raymond's behavior personally. Second, Mr. Raymond's displaced feelings will be refocused back to him.

On the basis of her assessment, Ms. Greg identifies three main problem areas of importance and formulates the following nursing diagnoses:

Diagnosis

1. *Ineffective coping* related to inadequate coping methods, as evidenced by inappropriate use of defense mechanisms (displacement)
   - Anger directed toward staff and fiancée
   - Profanity and crude sexual remarks aimed at staff
   - Isolation related to staff withdrawal
   - Continued escalation of anxiety
2. *Powerlessness* related to lack of control over his health care environment, as evidenced by frustration over inability to perform previously uncomplicated tasks
   - Anger over nurses' having to "scratch my head and blow my nose"
   - Minimal awareness of available supports in larger community

Outcomes Identification

Ms. Greg speaks to Mr. Raymond and tells him she would like to spend time with him for 15 minutes every morning to talk about his concerns. She suggests that he might be able to handle his feelings in alternative ways and notes that they can also explore community resources. Mr. Raymond gruffly agrees, saying, "You can visit me if it will make you feel better." They make arrangements to meet each morning at 7:30 AM for 15 minutes.

For each nursing diagnosis, the following outcomes are set:

NURSING DIAGNOSIS	SHORT-TERM GOAL
1. *Ineffective coping* related to inadequate coping methods, as evidenced by inappropriate use of defense mechanisms (displacement)	1. Mr. Raymond will be able to name and discuss at least two feelings about his illness and lack of mobility by the end of the week.
2. *Powerlessness* related to lack of control over health care environment, as evidenced by frustration over inability to perform previously uncomplicated tasks .	2. Mr. Raymond will be able to name two community organizations that can offer him information and support by the end of 2 weeks.

26-1 CASE STUDY AND NURSING CARE PLAN—cont'd

Crisis

Planning

Ms. Greg creates a nursing care plan and shares it with the staff.

Nursing diagnosis: *Ineffective coping* related to inadequate coping methods, as evidenced by inappropriate use of defense mechanisms (displacement)

Supporting Data:

- Anger directed toward staff and fiancée
- Profanity and crude sexual remarks aimed at staff
- Isolation related to staff withdrawal
- Continued escalation of anxiety

Outcome criteria: By discharge, Mr. Raymond will state that he feels more comfortable discussing difficult feelings.

SHORT-TERM GOAL	INTERVENTION	RATIONALE	EVALUATION
1. By the end of the week, Mr. Raymond will be able to name and discuss at least two feelings about his illness and lack of mobility.	1a. Nurse will meet with patient daily for 15 minutes at 7:30 AM.	1a. Night is usually the most frightening for patient; in early morning, feelings are closer to surface.	**GOAL MET** Within 7 days, Mr. Raymond speaks to nurse more openly about feelings.
	1b. When patient lashes out, nurse will remain calm.	1b. Patient perceives that nurse is in control of her feelings. This can reassure patient and increase patient's sense of security.	
	1c. Nurse will consistently redirect and refocus anger from environment back to patient (e.g., "It must be difficult to be in this situation").	1c. Refocusing feelings offers patient opportunity to cope effectively with his anxiety and decreases need to act out.	
	1d. Nurse will come on time each day and stay for allotted time.	1d. Consistency sets stage for trust and reinforces that patient's anger will not drive nurse away.	

Nursing diagnosis: *Powerlessness* related to lack of control over health care environment, as evidenced by frustration over inability to perform previously uncomplicated tasks

Supporting Data

- Anger over nurses' having to "scratch my head and help me blow my nose"
- Minimal awareness of available supports in larger community

Outcome criteria: By discharge, Mr. Raymond will contact at least one community support source.

SHORT-TERM GOAL	INTERVENTION	RATIONALE	EVALUATION
1. By the end of the 2 weeks, Mr. Raymond will name and discuss at least two community organizations that can offer information and support.	1a. Nurse will spend time with patient and fiancée. Role and use of specific agencies will be discussed.	1a. Both patient and fiancée will have opportunity to ask questions with nurse present.	**GOAL MET** By the end of 10 days, Mr. Raymond and his fiancée can name two community resources they are interested in. At the end of 6 weeks, Mr. Raymond has contacted the Guillain-Barré Society.
	1b. Nurse will introduce one agency at a time.	1b. Gradual introduction allows time for information to sink in and minimizes feeling of being pressured or overwhelmed.	
	1c. Nurse will not push patient to contact any of the agencies.	1c. Patient is able to make own decisions once he has appropriate information.	

Implementation

Ms. Greg goes into Mr. Raymond's room at 7:30 AM the following morning and sits by his bedside. At first, Mr. Raymond's comments are hostile.

DIALOGUE	THERAPEUTIC TOOL/COMMENT
Nurse: Mr. Raymond, I'm here as we discussed. I'll be spending 15 minutes with you every morning. We could use this time to talk about some of your concerns.	Nurse offers herself as a resource, gives information, and clarifies her role and patient expectations. Night is Mr. Raymond's most difficult time. In the early morning, he will be the most vulnerable and open for therapeutic intervention and support.
Mr. Raymond: Listen, sweetheart, my only concern is how to get a little sexual relief, get it?	
Nurse: Being hospitalized and partially paralyzed can be overwhelming for anyone. Perhaps you wish you could find some relief from your situation.	Nurse focuses on the process "need for relief," not the sexual content, and encourages discussion of feelings. Sexual issues often challenge new nurses, and discussing their feelings and appropriate interventions with an experienced professional is important for their growth and the quality of the care they give.
Mr. Raymond: What do you know, Ms. Know-it-all? I can't even scratch my nose without getting one of those fools to do it for me . . . and half the time those bitches aren't even around.	

Continued

26-1 CASE STUDY AND NURSING CARE PLAN—cont'd

Crisis

DIALOGUE	THERAPEUTIC TOOL/COMMENT
Nurse: It must be difficult to have to ask people to do everything for you.	Nurse restates what the patient says in terms of his feelings and continues to refocus away from the environment back to the patient.
Mr. Raymond: Yeah . . . . The other night a fly kept landing on my face. I had to shout for 5 minutes before one of those stupid aides came in, just to take the fly out of the room.	
Nurse: Having to rely on others for everything can be a terrifying experience for anyone. It sounds extremely frustrating for you.	Nurse acknowledges that frustration and anger would be a natural response for anyone in this situation. This encourages the patient to talk about these feelings instead of acting them out.
Mr. Raymond: Yeah . . . . It's a bitch . . . like a living hell.	

Ms. Greg continues to spend time with Mr. Raymond. He gradually talks more about his feelings and acts with less hostility toward the staff. As he begins to feel more in control, he becomes less defensive about others' caring for him. After 2 weeks, Ms. Greg decreases her visits to twice a week. Mr. Raymond is beginning to experience gross motor movements but is not walking yet. He still displaces much of his frustration and lack of control onto the environment, but he is better able to acknowledge the reality of his situation. He can also identify and briefly talk about his feelings.

DIALOGUE	THERAPEUTIC TOOL/COMMENT
Nurse: What's happening? Your face looks tense this morning, Mr. Raymond.	Nurse observes the patient's clenched fists, rigid posture, and tense facial expression.
Mr. Raymond: I had to wait 10 minutes for a bedpan last night.	
Nurse: And you're angry about that.	Nurse verbalizes the implied.
Mr. Raymond: Well, there were only two nurses on duty for 30 people, and the aide was on her break . . . . You can't expect them to be everywhere . . . but still	
Nurse: It may be hard to accept that people can't be there all the time for you.	Nurse validates the difficulty of accepting situations one does not like when one is powerless to make changes.
Mr. Raymond: Well . . . that's the way it is in this place.	

Evaluation

After 6 weeks, Mr. Raymond is able to get around with assistance, and his ability to perform his activities of daily living is increasing. Although Mr. Raymond still feels angry and overwhelmed at times, he is able to identify more of his feelings and acts them out less often. He is able to talk to his fiancée about his feelings, and he lashes out at her less. He is looking forward to going home, and his boss is holding his old job.

Mr. Raymond makes arrangements with the Guillain-Barré Society for a meeting, and he is thinking about Alcoholics Anonymous but believes he can handle this problem himself.

Staff feel more comfortable and competent in their relationships with Mr. Raymond. The goals have been met. Mr. Raymond and Ms. Greg agree that the crisis is over and terminate their visits. Mr. Raymond is given the number of the crisis unit and encouraged to call if he has questions or feels the need to talk.

KEY POINTS TO REMEMBER

- Crises can lead to personality disorganization but also offer opportunities for emotional growth.
- There are three types of crisis: maturational, situational, and adventitious.
- Crises are usually resolved within 4 to 6 weeks.
- Crisis intervention therapy is short term, from 1 to 6 weeks, and focuses on the present problem only.
- Resolution of a crisis takes three forms: a patient emerges at a higher level, at the pre-crisis level, or at a lower level of functioning.
- Social support and intervention can promote successful resolution.
- Crisis therapists take an active and directive approach with the patient in crisis.
- The patient is an active participant in setting goals and planning possible solutions.
- Crisis intervention is usually aimed at the mentally healthy patient who generally is functioning well but is temporarily overwhelmed and unable to function.
- The crisis model can be adapted to meet the needs of patients in crisis who have long-term and persistent mental problems.
- The steps in crisis intervention are consistent with the steps of the nursing process.
- Specific qualities in the nurse that can facilitate effective intervention are a caring attitude, flexibility in planning care, an ability to listen, and an active approach.
- The basic goals of crisis intervention are to reduce the individual's anxiety level and to support the effort to return to the patient's precrisis level of functioning.
- Critical incident stress debriefing is a group approach that helps groups of people who have been exposed to a crisis situation.
- Disaster occurrences and management are global concerns that involve nursing.
- Current trends in disaster management are being directed toward preparedness and developing resilient communities.
- Disaster-preparedness training can optimize nursing contributions to disaster planning and management.

CRITICAL THINKING

1. List the three important areas of the crisis assessment once safety concerns have been identified. Give examples of two questions in each area that need to be answered before planning can take place.
2. Barbara, 21 years old and a junior in nursing school, tells her nursing instructor that her father (age 45 years) has just lost his job. Her father has been drinking heavily for years, and Barbara is having difficulty coping. Because of her father's alcoholism and the increased stress in her family, Barbara wants to leave school. Her mother has multiple sclerosis and thinks Barbara should quit school to take care of her.
   a. How many different types of crises are going on in this family? Discuss the crises from the viewpoint of each family member.
   b. If this family came for crisis counseling, what areas would you assess, and what kinds of questions would you ask to evaluate each member's individual needs and the needs of the family as a unit (perception of events, social supports, coping styles)?
   c. Formulate some tentative goals you might set in conjunction with the family.
   d. Identify—by name—appropriate referral agencies in your area that would be helpful if members of this family were willing to expand their use of outside resources and stabilize the situation.
   e. How would you set up follow-up visits for this family? Would you see the family members together, alone, or in a combination during the crisis period (4 to 6 weeks)? How would you decide whether follow-up counseling was indicated?

CHAPTER REVIEW

1. Which statement about crisis theory will provide a basis for nursing intervention?
   a. A crisis is an acute, time-limited phenomenon experienced as an overwhelming emotional reaction to a problem perceived as unsolvable.
   b. A person in crisis has always had adjustment problems and has coped inadequately in his or her usual life situations.
   c. Crisis is precipitated by an event that enhances a person's self-concept and self-esteem.
   d. Nursing intervention in crisis situations rarely has the effect of ameliorating the crisis.
2 Lilly, a single mother of four, comes to the crisis center 24 hours after an apartment fire in which all the family's household goods and clothing were lost. Lilly has no other family in the area. Her efforts to mobilize assistance have been disorganized, and she is still without shelter. She is distraught and confused. You assess the situation as:
   a. A maturational crisis.
   b. A situational crisis.
   c. An adventitious crisis.
   d. An existential crisis.
3. When responding to the patient in question 2, the intervention that takes priority is to:
   a. Reduce anxiety.
   b. Arrange shelter.
   c. Contact out-of-area family.
   d. Hospitalize and place the patient on suicide precautions.
4. Which belief would be least helpful for a nurse working in crisis intervention?
   a. A person in crisis is incapable of making decisions.
   b. The crisis counseling relationship is one between partners.
   c. Crisis counseling helps the patient refocus to gain new perspectives on the situation.
   d. Anxiety-reduction techniques are used so the patient's inner resources can be accessed.
5. The highest-priority goal of crisis intervention is:
   a. Patient safety.
   b. Anxiety reduction.
   c. Identification of situational supports.
   d. Teaching specific coping skills that are lacking.

Answers to Chapter Review
1. a; 2. b; 3. a; 4. a; 5. a.

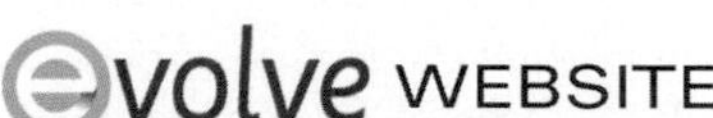

WEBSITE

Visit the Evolve website for a posttest on the content in this chapter: http://evolve.elsevier.com/Varcarolis

Post-Test interactive review

REFERENCES

Aguilera, D. C. (1998). *Crisis intervention: Theory and methodology* (8th ed.). St. Louis, MO: Mosby.

Aguilera, D. C., & Mesnick, J. (1970). *Crisis intervention: Theory and methodology.* St. Louis, MO: Mosby.

American Nurses Association, American Psychiatric-Mental Health Nurses Association, & International Society of Psychiatric-Mental Health Nurses. (2007). *Psychiatric mental health nursing: Scope and standards of practice.* Silver Spring, MD: American Nurses Association.

Blacklock, E. (2012). Intervention following a critical incident: Developing a critical incident stress management team. *Archives of Psychiatric Nursing, 26,* 2–8.

Bulechek, G. M., Butcher, H. K., Dochterman, J. M., & Wagner, C. (2013). *Nursing interventions classification (NIC)* (6th ed.). St. Louis, MO: Mosby.

Caplan, G. (1964). *Symptoms of preventive psychiatry.* New York, NY: Basic Books.

Dunkley, J., & Whelan, T. (2006). Vicarious traumatization: Current status and future directions. *British Journal of Guidance and Counseling, 34*(1), 107–116.

Everly, G. S. Jr., Lating, J. M., & Mitchell, J. T. (2000). Innovations in group crisis intervention: Critical incident stress debriefing (CISD) and critical incident stress management (CISM). In A. R. Roberts (Ed.), *Crisis interventions handbook: Assessment, treatment, and research* (pp. 77–100). New York, NY: Oxford University Press.

Federal Emergency Management Agency (FEMA). (2012). *FEMA: Plan and prepare*. Retrieved from http://www.fema.gov/plan-prepare-mitigate/ and www.fema.gov/preparedness-1.

Hammond, J., & Brooks, J. (2001). The world trade center attack: Helping the helpers: the role of critical incident stress management. *Critical Care, 5*(6), 315–317.

Herdman, T. H. (Ed.), (2012). *NANDA international nursing diagnoses: Definitions and classification, 2012–2014*. Oxford, UK: Wiley-Blackwell.

Herrman, H. (2012). Promoting mental health and resilience after a disaster. *Journal of Experimental and Clinical Medicine, 4*(2), 82–87. doi:10.1016/j.jecm.2012.01.003.

Hobfoll, S., Watson, P., Bell, C., Bryant, R., Brymer, M., Friedman, M. J., . . . Ursano, R.J. (2007). Five essential elements of immediate and mid-trauma mass trauma intervention: Empirical evidence. Psychiatry, 70(4): 283-315.

Joint Commission on Mental Illness and Health. (1961). *Action for mental health: Final report, 1961*. New York, NY: Basic Books.

Moorhead, S., Johnson, M., Maas, M. L., & Swanson, E. (2013). *Nursing outcomes classification (NOC)* (5th ed.) St. Louis, MO: Elsevier.

Phoenix, B. (2007). Psychoeducation for survivors of trauma. *Perspectives of Psychiatric Care, 43*, 123–131.

Powers, R. (2010). Introduction to disaster nursing. In R. Powers, & E. Daily (Eds.), *International disaster nursing* (pp. 1–55). New York, NY: Cambridge University Press.

Roberts, A. R. (2005). *Crisis intervention handbook: Assessment, treatment, and research* (3rd ed.). New York, NY: Oxford.

Roberts, A. R., & Ottens, A. J. (2005). The seven-stage crisis intervention model: A road map to goal attainment, problem solving, and crisis resolution. *Brief Treatment and Crisis Intervention, 5*, 329–339.

Smoyak, S. (2005). Disaster response for mental health professionals: Interview with Thomas H. Bornemann, Ed. D., Director of the Mental Health Program at the Carter Center, Atlanta, Georgia. *Journal of Psychosocial Nursing, 43*(11), 18–21.

Wallace, M. A., & Morley, W. E. (1970). Teaching crisis intervention. *American Journal of Nursing, 70*(7), 1484–1487.

World Health Organization (WHO). (2010). *Mental health and development: A model for practice*. Geneva, CH: WHO Press. Retrieved from www.who.int/mental_health/policy/mhtargeting/en/index.html.

CHAPTER

27

Anger, Aggression, and Violence

Lorann Murphy

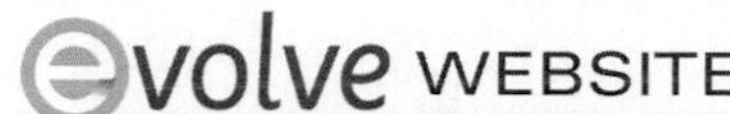

WEBSITE

Visit the Evolve website for a pretest on the content in this chapter: http://evolve.elsevier.com/Varcarolis

Pre-Test interactive review

OBJECTIVES

1. Compare and contrast three theories that explore the determinants for anger, aggression, and violence.
2. Compare and contrast interventions for a patient with healthy coping skills with those for a patient with marginal coping behaviors.
3. Apply at least four principles of de-escalation with a moderately angry patient.
4. Describe two criteria for the use of seclusion or restraint over verbal intervention.
5. Discuss two types of assessment and their value in the nursing process.
6. Role-play with classmates by using understandable but unhelpful responses to anger and aggression in patients; discuss how these responses can affect nursing interventions.

KEY TERMS AND CONCEPTS

aggression
anger
de-escalation techniques
restraint
seclusion
trauma-informed care
validation therapy
violence

Anger, aggression, and violence are the subject of daily news headlines. In the United States, the National Football League recently suspended coaches and players for promoting and using unnecessary aggression against players of other teams (Maske, 2012). Evidence of the scope and prevalence of the problem can been seen in an expanding list of terminology used to describe specific types of aggression. *Road rage* is a dangerous habit rampant in high-stress, industrialized societies and is accompanied by cursing, offensive gestures, and cutting others off while driving. *Air rage* is manifested as objectionable behavior, aggressive utterances, threats, and violence within the confines of an aircraft. *Desk rage* includes lashing out at work. Hospitals, as 24-hour-a-day, high-stress environments, have even earned a term for their own brand of confrontation: *ward rage.*

CLINICAL PICTURE

Anger is an emotional response to frustration of desires, a threat to one's needs (emotional or physical), or a challenge. It is a normal emotion that can even be viewed as positive when it is expressed in a healthy way. It can be used as a motivator or an aid in survival (Kassinove & Tafrate, 2006), but problems begin to occur when anger is expressed through aggression or violence.

Aggression is an action or behavior that results in a verbal or physical attack. Aggression tends to be used synonymously with violence; however, aggression is not always inappropriate and is sometimes necessary for self-protection. On the other hand, **violence** is always an objectionable act that involves intentional use of force that results in, or has the potential to result in, injury to another person.

Coping with a patient's anger is a challenge. Effective nursing intervention becomes more difficult when the anger is directed at the nurse. Nursing interventions for anger and aggression should begin when patients experience increased anxiety. Refer to Chapter 15 for interventions that can be used when anxiety is escalating.

EPIDEMIOLOGY

As a nurse, it is likely that you will deal with violent behavior. In a preliminary report, the Centers for Disease Control and Prevention (CDC)(2012) reported more than 40,000 deaths from suicide and homicide in 2010. The National Hospital Ambulatory Medical Care Survey reported that in 2008 there were 1.8 million emergency room visits for treatment of assault. Violence can occur anywhere in the hospital, but it is most frequent in the following areas (Estryn-Chandler, 2008):

- Psychiatric units
- Emergency departments
- Geriatric units

Refer to Chapter 28 for statistics related to abuse of children, elders, and intimate partners; refer to Chapter 29 for statistics on sexual assault.

COMORBIDITY

Although anger is a universal emotion, not everyone responds to anger with aggression and violence. A great deal of research has been done on aggression and violence in persons with post traumatic stress disorders (PTSD) and substance use disorders (Sirotich, 2008). Anger also coexists with depression, anxiety, psychosis, and personality disorders (Kassinove & Tafrate, 2006).

Anger and hostility have effects on physical well-being; they are risk factors for hypertension and cardiovascular disease, including ischemic heart disease and cerebral vascular attacks (Kassinove & Tafrate, 2006). Suppression of anger has been shown to increase the rate of major cardiac events, and anger has also been shown to increase a person's perception of pain (Denollet et al., 2010; Middendorp et al., 2010).

ETIOLOGY

Biological Factors

Many neurological conditions are associated with anger and aggression. For example, certain brain tumors, Alzheimer's disease, temporal lobe epilepsy, and traumatic injury to certain parts of the brain result in changes to personality that include increased violence. Many patients with brain injury have severe behavior disorders, including aggressiveness, that disrupt their lives.

One area of the brain known to be associated with aggression is the limbic system, which mediates primitive emotion and behaviors necessary for survival. The limbic system contains several structures that appear to have a role in the production of aggression. The area of the brain called the *amygdala* mediates anger experiences, judging events as either aversive or rewarding. In animal studies, stimulation of the amygdala produces rage responses, whereas lesions in the same structure produce docility. The temporal lobe of the brain shares some structures with the limbic system. Memory is thought to be integrated in the temporal lobe; memory of previous insult is important in the cognitive appraisal of threat in the face of new stimuli. This lobe is also the source of complex partial seizures, which may give rise to aggressive behavior (Ito et al., 2007).

The prefrontal cortex also has been identified as playing an important role in aggressive behavior. This was first noted in persons who had lesions or injury that caused aggressive behavior (Siever, 2008). Individuals with antisocial personality disorder have been shown to have less gray matter in their prefrontal cortexes (Narayan et al., 2007). Neurotransmitters play a vital role in anger and aggression. Serotonin, dopamine, norepinephrine, gamma-aminobutyric acid (GABA), glutamate, and acetylcholine all have an impact on anger and aggression (Comai, 2012). Studies have shown a relationship between impulsive aggression and low levels of serotonin (Gross & Sanders, 2008). Dopamine has also been linked to aggressive outbursts in patients with neurological impairment (Ramírez-Bermudez et al., 2010).

Some individuals are biologically more predisposed than others to respond to life events with irritability, easy frustration, and anger. This predisposition may be a function of genetics or of neurological development that occurs in the context of certain infant and childhood environments. Individuals who have a history of aggression have been shown to be more acutely aware of subtle facial cues of anger (Wilkowski et al., 2012). If all the dimensions of anger are centrally mediated, then successful interventions can be designed to target any of its manifestations. This is likely the reason biological, pharmacological, behavioral, and cognitive strategies are all useful in the management of anger and aggression.

Psychological Factors

Freud wrote in *Civilization and Its Discontents* that the conflict between sexual needs and societal norms was the source of mankind's dissatisfaction, aggression, hostility, and ultimately violence. More recently, Menninger (2007) asserted that the struggle for control over our lives is fundamental in every person. If that control is threatened, we experience trauma, and it is from that trauma that anger, aggression, and violence may originate. Interventions should be focused on realizing that the patient may be experiencing trauma and helping the patient feel as though he has some control in his or her life.

Early behaviorists held that emotions, including anger, were learned responses to environmental stimuli (Skinner, 1953). The stimulus is often a perceived threat, and this cognition leads to the emotional and physiological arousal necessary to take action. Although the threat is usually understood as an alert to physical danger, Beck (1976) noted that perceived assault on areas of personal domain, such as values, moral code, and protective rules, can also lead to anger. For example, clinic patients kept waiting for long periods of time without explanation may interpret this as neglect and a lack of respect. Anger may escalate when the initial appraisal is followed by cognitions such as, "They have no right to treat me this way. I am a person too." These additional cognitions lead to escalating behavior that can erupt into violence unless the situation is defused through successful interventions.

In some individuals, the period of escalation can be rapid. In contrast, patients less predisposed to anger might interpret the wait as a sign that the clinic is busy. These patients might be frustrated by the situation, but in the absence of anger, they might access and utilize skills such as asking how much longer the wait is likely to be, finding distractions in the environment, or rescheduling the appointment.

Social learning theorists conducted research that showed that children learn aggression by imitating others and that persons repeat behavior that is rewarded (Bandura, 1973). Thus children who watch television violence or experience violence in the home learn violent ways of resolving problems. Not only is television violence portrayed as an option for resolving conflict, but most of those violent acts are presented as having no negative consequences. Bullying is another less extreme form of violence that is far more prevalent and has significant consequences. *Bullying* is any negative activity, including teasing, kicking, hitting, and spitting, intended to bother or harm someone else.

CONSIDERING CULTURE

The Anger Sundrome

Cho Hyun-Ja, a 42-year-old Korean female, comes to the clinic with complaints of irritability, quick to anger, feelings of emptiness, insomnia, and general feelings of unfairness. She also complains of dry mouth, headaches, and palpitations. You note that she is sighing frequently during the interview. She may be suffering from hwa-byung, an anger syndrome that is found in 4.1% of Koreans, mostly in middle aged or older women. Anger, irritability, cardiovascular symptoms, generalized anxiety, depression, anorexia, insomnia, and frequent sighing are characteristics of this syndrome. The best approach to treating hwa-byung is a holistic approach consisting of stress management education, psychotherapy, psychopharmacology, acupuncture, music, and drama therapy.

Choi, M., & Yeon, H.A. (2011). Identifying and treating the culture-bound syndrome of hwa-byung among older Korean immigrant women: Recommendations for practitioners. *Journal of the American Academy of Nurse Practitioners, 23*(5), 226-232.

APPLICATION OF THE NURSING PROCESS

ASSESSMENT

General Assessment

When patients are experiencing anger, it may manifest as increased demands, irritability, frowning, redness of the face, pacing, twisting of the hands, or clenching and unclenching of the fists. Speech may either be increased in rate and volume or may be slowed, pointed, and quiet. Any change in behavior from what is typical for that patient must be addressed. Box 27-1 identifies signs and symptoms that indicate the risk of escalating anger leading to aggressive behavior.

It is also important to assess the patient's history of aggression or violence. Most of our reactions to stimuli come from our previous experiences; therefore, identifying patients' triggers is essential. Initial and ongoing assessment of the patient can reveal problems before they escalate to anger and aggression. Such assessment also leads directly to the appropriate nursing diagnosis and intervention.

HEALTH POLICY

Workplace Violence Legislation

Assault on inpatient psychiatric units is of worldwide concern. Recently, there has been an increased emphasis on violence toward emergency room nurses. These concerns have resulted in the development of laws and policies regarding violence against hospital workers. In 2008, the American Psychiatric Nurses Association wrote a position statement on workplace violence. Its recommendations included calls for creating a culture of safety, increased intervention and reporting of incidents from nurses, increased education regarding how to deal with aggressive patients, and increased research on workplace violence.

The Emergency Nurses Association recently released the results of a 2-year survey of violence against emergency room nurses. It found that 54.4% of the nurses reported being victims of workplace violence over the past 7 days.

Growing recognition of this problem in many states has resulted in the passage of legislation to protect health care workers. States such as Massachusetts, New York, and Ohio have passed laws that increase penalties for convicted offenders.

American Nurses Association. (2011). *Workplace violence.* Retrieved from http://ana.nursingworld.org/workplaceviolence; American Psychiatric Nurses Association. (2008). *Position statement on workplace violence.* Retrieved from http://www.apna.org/i4a/pages/index.cfm?pageid53786; Emergency Nurses Association (2011). *Emergency Department Violence Surveillance Study.* Retrieved from http://www.ena.org/IENR/Documents/ENAEDVSReportNovember2011.pdf.

Trauma-informed care is an older concept of providing care that has recently been reintroduced. It is based on the notion that disruptive patients often have histories that include violence and victimization (Sansone et al., 2012). These traumatic histories can impede patients' ability to self-soothe, result in negative coping responses, and create a vulnerability

BOX 27-1 PREDICTORS OF VIOLENCE

1. Signs and symptoms that usually *(but not always)* precede violence:
   - Hyperactivity: most important predictor of imminent violence (e.g., pacing, restlessness)
   - Increasing anxiety and tension: clenched jaw or fist, rigid posture, fixed or tense facial expression, mumbling to self (patient may have shortness of breath, sweating, and rapid pulse)
   - Verbal abuse: profanity, argumentativeness
   - Loud voice, change of pitch; or very soft voice, forcing others to strain to hear
   - Intense eye contact or avoidance of eye contact
2. Recent acts of violence, including property violence
3. Stone silence
4. Alcohol or drug intoxication
5. Possession of a weapon or object that may be used as a weapon (e.g., fork, knife, rock)
6. Isolation that is new
7. Milieu characteristics conducive to violence.
   - Overcrowding
   - Staff inexperience
   - Provocative or controlling staff
   - Poor limit setting
   - Arbitrary revocation of privileges

to coercive interventions (such as restraint) by staff. Trauma-informed care focuses on the patient's past experiences of violence or trauma and on the role these experiences currently play in their lives.

Careful assessment can reduce the potential for violence. In a study conducted at New York State Psychiatric Institute, patients filled out a questionnaire that identified things that made them upset, how they responded to being upset, and how they wanted to be treated when they became upset. Examples of how they wanted to be treated included talking with them and allowing them time out alone. Making use of the patients' suggestions resulted in a decreased amount of time in restraints and seclusion and a reduction in the number of fights and assaults on the unit (Hellerstein et al., 2007).

EVIDENCE-BASED PRACTICE

Reducing the Use of Restraints

Vernberg, E. M., Nelson, T. D., Fonagy, P., & Twemlow, S. W. (2011). Victimization, aggression and visits to the school nurse for somatic complaints, illnesses, and physical injuries. *Pediatrics, 27*(5), 842–848.

Problem

Children who have been bullied have an increased risk for anxiety, depression, and psychiatric problems as adults. Children who have been identified as aggressors also are at increased risk for psychiatric problems. Children who are either aggressors or victims of bullying have been shown to display more somatic complaints and physical illnesses than other children. In the past most emphasis has been identifying victims of bullying. We also must be aware of the aggressors and intervene appropriately with them as well.

Purpose of Study

The purpose of the study was to examine how aggressors and victims of bullying are linked to somatic complaints, physical illnesses, and injuries in elementary-aged children.

Methods

This study looked at third- to sixth-grade students from six elementary schools who visited the school nurse during the school year. The researcher collected school nurse logs with types of complaints during the school year. The children also filled out a self-report of victimization.

Key Findings

- Being involved in bullying as an aggressor or victim is associated with an increase in school nurse visits for somatic complaints, physical illnesses, and physical injury.
- Children who are viewed by peers as aggressive are also at risk for an increased amount of school nurse visits.

Implications for Nursing Practice

The school nurse is integral in the identification and intervention of peer victimization in schools. The nurse should be aware that frequent visits might be an indicator of a child's involvement in aggressive episodes either as a victim or as a perpetrator. The nurse's plan of care will focus on early intervention for the victim as well as for the aggressor to assist in promoting mental and physical well-being for each child.

Self-Assessment

Like patients, nurses have their own histories. The nurse's ability to intervene safely depends on self-awareness of strengths, needs, concerns, and vulnerabilities. Without this awareness, nursing interventions are marked by impulsive or emotion-based responses, which may be nontherapeutic. Self-awareness includes knowledge of personal responses to anger and aggression, including choice of words and tone of voice, as well as nonverbal communication via body posture and facial expressions. Awareness of the personal and cultural norms is also essential. In addition, staff must be aware of personal dynamics that may trigger emotions and reactions that are not therapeutic with specific patients. Finally, the nurse must assess situational factors (e.g., fatigue, insufficient staff) that may decrease normal competence in the management of complex patient problems.

Self-assessment promotes calm responses to patient anger and potential aggression. The following further supports these responses:

- Creation of an environment that encourages staff to speak openly about their feelings
- Use of humor
- Development of a professional support system
- Variance of clinical work

ASSESSMENT GUIDELINES

Anger and Aggression

Aggression assessment tools have been developed to assist in predicting violent behavior on inpatient psychiatric units (Oglaff, 2006). These tools can beneficial, but general risk identification includes the following:

1. A history of violence is the single best predictor of future violence.
2. Patients who are delusional, hyperactive, impulsive, or predisposed to irritability are at higher risk for violence.
3. Assess patient risk for violence:
   - Does the patient have a wish or intent to harm?
   - Does the patient have a plan?
   - Does the patient have means available to carry out the plan?
   - Does the patient have demographic risk factors: male gender, age 14 to 24 years, low socioeconomic status, inadequate support system, and prison time?
4. Aggression by patients occurs most often in the context of limit setting by the nurse.
5. Patients with a history of limited coping skills, including lack of assertiveness or use of intimidation, are at higher risk of using violence.
6. Assess self for personal triggers and responses likely to escalate patient violence, including patient characteristics or situations that trigger impatience, irritation, or defensiveness.
7. Assess personal sense of competence when in any situation of potential conflict; consider asking for the assistance of another staff member.

DIAGNOSIS

Patients may have coping skills that are adequate for day-to-day events but may be overwhelmed by the stresses of illness or hospitalization. Other patients may have a pattern of maladaptive coping that is marginally effective and consists of a set of coping strategies that is unhealthy and may increase the possibility of anger and aggression. When the nursing assessment identifies potential for anger or aggression, *Risk for other-directed violence*, *Risk for self-directed violence*, *Ineffective coping* (overwhelmed or maladaptive), *Stress overload*, and *Impaired impulse control* are important nursing diagnoses to consider (Herdman, 2012).

OUTCOMES IDENTIFICATION

When interventions are planned for angry and aggressive patients, having clearly defined outcome criteria is important for identifying the behaviors that staff can encourage if their interventions have been successful. The *Nursing Outcomes Classification (NOC)* outlines specific outcome criteria for use with angry and aggressive patients (Moorhead et al., 2013). Table 27-1 identifies signs and symptoms commonly experienced with anger and aggression, offers potential nursing diagnoses, and suggests outcomes.

PLANNING

Planning interventions necessitates having a sound assessment, including patient history (previous acts of violence, comorbid disorders), present coping skills, and willingness and capacity of the patient to learn alternative and nonviolent ways of handling angry feelings.

Does the patient have:

- Good coping skills but is presently overwhelmed?
- Marginal coping skills and uses anger or violence as a way to cover other feelings and gain a sense of mastery or control?
- A personality disorder or chronic psychotic disorder and is prone to violence?
- Cognitive deficits that predispose to anger in the form of misinterpretation of environmental stimuli?

Does the situation call for:

- Psycho educational approaches to teach the patient new skills for handling anger?
- Immediate intervention to prevent overt violence (de-escalation techniques, restraint/seclusion, and/or medications)?

Does the environment provide:

- Privacy for the patient?
- Enough space for patients, or is there overcrowding?
- A healthy balance between structured time and quiet time?
- Adequate personnel available to safely and effectively deal with a potentially violent situation?

Do the skills of the staff call for:

- Additional education for staff in verbal de-escalation techniques?
- Counseling of staff regarding use of punitive and arbitrary approaches to patients?
- Additional training in restraint techniques?

IMPLEMENTATION

Ideally, intervention begins prior to any sign of escalation. It is important to develop a relationship of trust with the patient by having numerous brief, nonthreatening, nondirective interactions

TABLE 27-1 SIGNS AND SYMPTOMS, NURSING DIAGNOSES, AND OUTCOMES FOR AGGRESSION

SIGNS AND SYMPTOMS	NURSING DIAGNOSES	OUTCOMES
Body language (rigid posture, clenching of fists and jaw, hyperactivity, pacing), history of violence, history of family violence, history of substance abuse, impulsivity	*Risk for other-directed violence* *Impaired impulse control*	Identifies when angry, identifies alternatives to aggression, refrains from verbal outbursts, avoids violating others' personal space, maintains self-control
Impulsivity, suicidal ideation (has plan, ability to carry it out), overt or covert statements regarding killing self, feelings of worthlessness, hopelessness, helplessness	*Risk for self-directed violence* *Risk for suicide*	Expresses feelings, verbalizes suicidal ideas, refrains from suicide attempts, plans for the future.
Difficulty with simple tasks, inability to function at previous level, poor problem solving, poor cognitive functioning, verbalizations of inability to cope	*Ineffective coping*	Identifies ineffective and effective coping, uses support system, uses new coping strategies, engages in personal actions to manage stressors effectively
Demonstrates feelings of anger, impatience; reports feelings of pressure, tension, difficulty in functioning, anger, impatience; experiences negative impact from stress; reports problems with decision making	*Stress overload*	Expresses feelings constructively, reports feelings of calmness and acceptance; physical symptoms of stress are reduced or absent; decision-making is optimal

From Herdman, T. H. (Ed.) *Nursing diagnoses—Definitions and classification 2012–2014*. Copyright © 2012, 1994-2012 by NANDA International. Used by arrangement with John Wiley & Sons Limited; Moorhead, S., Johnson, M., Maas, M. L., & Swanson, E. (2013). *Nursing outcomes classification (NOC)* (5th ed.). St. Louis, MO: Elsevier.

(e.g., talking about the weather, sports, or something of interest to the patient).

In settings in which staff can reasonably expect episodes of patient anger and aggression, regular teaching and practice of verbal and nonverbal interventions are essential. This fosters nurses' increased confidence in their own abilities and those of co-workers.

Psychosocial Interventions

As you try to determine what the patient is feeling, you have already begun to intervene. During this process, you are attempting to hear the patient's feelings and concerns. Frequently, this can be accomplished by telling the patient that you are concerned and want to listen. The patient needs reassurance that others are interested and willing to help. It is essential to acknowledge the patient's needs, regardless of whether the expressed needs are rational or possible to meet. It is important to clearly and simply state your expectations for the patient's behavior: "I expect that you will stay in control."

However, patient behavior may escalate quickly, or the patient may mask early signs of distress. Nurses may be distracted and miss those early signs. Other patients may be acutely ill and not amenable to early nursing interventions. In these situations, the problem with anger may not be resolved before the risk for violence arises. When anger and aggression are the priority problems, de-escalation of anger is the primary nursing intervention. Seclusion, restraint, or pharmacological means of de-escalation may be necessary to ensure the safety of patients and staff.

When you approach the patient, convey that you are calm, controlled, open, nonthreatening, and caring. Maintain a relaxed posture. If you are experiencing fear, you may find that this is quite challenging. Maintaining a calm exterior while your interior is in an upheaval requires considerable self-discipline and will come with experience.

It is important to demonstrate respect for the patient's personal space. Your eyes should be on the same level as the patient's to decrease a sense of intimidation and communicate to the patient that you are speaking as equals. Allow the patient enough personal space so that you are not perceived as intrusive but not so much space that the patient cannot speak in a normal voice. Be sure you have left yourself an escape route if the patient becomes out of control. Always stay about 1 foot farther than the patient can reach with arms or legs.

Patients who are poised for violence need much more space than those who are not. While you are giving the patient space, the patient may be invading your space with verbal abuse and the use of profanity. This may be the only way feelings can be expressed. As uncomfortable as this may be, you cannot take the patient's words personally or respond in kind. It is also important not to end the conversation because of the patient's verbal abusiveness or to forbid the patient from communicating in this way.

When anger is escalating, a patient's ability to process decreases. It is important to speak to the patient slowly and in short sentences, using a low and calm voice. Never yell but continue to model controlled behavior. Use open-ended statements and questions such as "You think people are always unkind to you?" rather than challenging statements such as "What is wrong with you?" Avoid ending statements with "okay?" because it may create ambivalence in the patient and give the erroneous impression that choices exist. It is also important to avoid punitive, threatening, accusatory, or challenging statements to the patient; rather, find out what is behind the angry feelings and behaviors. Honestly verbalize the patient's options, and encourage the individual to assume responsibility for choices made. You may want to give two options, such as, "Do you want to go to your room or to the quiet room for a while?" This approach decreases the sense of powerlessness that often precipitates violence.

It is vital to pay attention to the environment. Choose a quiet place to talk to the patient but one that is visible to staff. This is most beneficial in helping a patient regain control. Staff should know who is working with the patient, keep an eye on the interaction, and be prepared to intervene if the situation escalates. At this point, other patients should be moved away, and the environment around the patient should be free from any object that could be used as a weapon.

Considerations for Staff Safety

There are six basic considerations for ensuring safety:

1. Avoid wearing dangling earrings or necklaces. The patient may become focused on these and grab at them, causing serious injury. Such jewelry should be removed before dealing with an agitated patient.
2. Ensure that there is enough staff for backup. Only one person should talk to the patient, but staff need to maintain an unobtrusive presence in case the situation escalates.
3. Always know the layout of the area. Correct placement of furniture and elimination of obstacles or hazards are important to prevent injury if the patient requires physical interventions.
4. Do not stand directly in front of the patient or in front of the doorway; this position could be interpreted as confrontational. It is better to stand off to the side and encourage the patient to have a seat.
5. If a patient's behavior begins to escalate, provide feedback: "You seem to be very upset." Such an observation allows exploration of the patient's feelings and may lead to de-escalation of the situation.
6. Avoid confrontation with the patient, either through verbal means or through a "show of support" with security guards. Verbal confrontation and discussion of the incident must occur when the patient is calm. A show of force by security guards may serve to escalate the patient's behavior; therefore, security personnel are better kept in the background until they are needed to assist.

Box 27-2 lists some principles underlying de-escalation techniques.

Pharmacological Interventions

When a patient is showing increased signs or symptoms of anxiety or agitation, it is perfectly appropriate to offer the patient a prn (as-needed) medication to alleviate symptoms.

BOX 27-2 DE-ESCALATION TECHNIQUES: PRACTICE PRINCIPLES

- Maintain the patient's self-esteem and dignity.
- Maintain calmness (your own and the patient's).
- Assess the patient and the situation.
- Identify stressors and stress indicators.
- Respond as early as possible.
- Use a calm, clear tone of voice.
- Invest time.
- Remain honest.
- Establish what the patient considers to be his or her need.
- Be goal-oriented.
- Maintain a large personal space.
- Avoid verbal struggles.
- Give several options.
- Make clear the options.
- Utilize a nonaggressive posture.
- Use genuineness and empathy.
- Attempt to be confidently aware.
- Use verbal, nonverbal, and communication skills.
- Be assertive (not aggressive).
- Assess for personal safety.

From Mason, T., & Chandley, M. (1999). *Management of violence and aggression* (p. 73). Philadelphia, PA: Churchill Livingstone.

When used in conjunction with psychosocial interventions and de-escalation techniques, this can prevent an aggressive or violent incident. The nurse's ongoing assessment of behavioral changes will give the patient the opportunity to obtain pharmacological relief from symptoms.

Antianxiety agents and antipsychotics are used in the treatment of acute symptoms of anger and aggression. These agents, their form of delivery, and considerations are listed in Table 27-2. During aggressive or violent incidents, haloperidol has historically been the most widely used antipsychotic, but with the introduction of intramuscular (IM) second-generation antipsychotics, the use of olanzapine and ziprasidone has become more widespread, in part because of the severe side effects of haloperidol. A combination of antipsychotic (haloperidol or perphenazine) and a benzodiazepine (lorazepam) can be given IM. Diphenhydramine or benztropine is added to the injection to reduce extrapyramidal side effects.

It is the nurse's role to assess for appropriateness of prn medications. It is important to remember that patients often feel traumatized by the use of IM injections, so oral medications should always be used if appropriate (Gilburt et al., 2008). The nurse also educates the patient about the medication, the reason it is being given, and the potential side effects of the medication, even if the patient is out of control.

The long-term treatment of anger, aggression, and violence is based on treating the underlying psychiatric disorder. SSRIs, lithium, anticonvulsants, benzodiazepines, second-generation antipsychotics, and beta-blockers are all used successfully for specific patient populations. Anger and aggression related to attention deficit disorder/attention deficit hyperactivity disorder may be reduced through the use of psychostimulants. Table 27-3 gives an overview of the drugs used to treat chronic aggression.

Health Teaching and Health Promotion

One of the most important roles a nurse plays in a patient's recovery is that of role model and educator. You can model appropriate responses and ways to cope with anger, teach patients a variety of methods to appropriately express anger, and educate patients regarding coping mechanisms, de-escalation techniques, and self-soothing skills that can be used to manage behavior. It is also helpful to assist the patient in identifying triggers for angry or aggressive behavior. One method that can be used if the patient is not out of control is a "do over." The patient who responds inappropriately can try again to respond in a more appropriate way while being coached by the nurse.

Interest in using alternative interventions such as forgiveness Osterndorf et al., 2011) and mindfulness (Robins et al., 2012) in healthy individuals has been gaining interest. Nurses may introduce these concepts and educate the patient on how to incorporate them into their lives.

Case Management

A multidisciplinary approach is important for all patients but especially for a patient with behavioral issues. A plan of care must be implemented and carried out by all members of the health care team. A focus on intervention strategies should be discussed during treatment team meetings. The plan for discharge with appropriate follow-up, possibly with an anger-management course, must be put into place. The consistency of intervention among all team members is key to the patient's success.

Teamwork and Safety

A thorough consideration of the environment is important when considering anger and aggression on the unit. It is important to be proactive and not reactive. It is hard to imagine how the stimulation of a psychiatric unit might be experienced by someone whose anxiety is extremely high or who is delusional or confused. If the patient has enough control, sometimes simply taking a timeout in his own room is sufficient. A multisensory room is another form of timeout. It is also known as a *Snoezelen*, named partly from the Dutch word for "dozing." This quiet room is partially lit, has relaxing music available, and comfortable furniture and soft pillows. It promotes feelings of security and safety.

Realize that behavior rarely occurs in a vacuum. The nurse must examine the milieu as a whole and identify the stressors patients have to deal with, especially patients who have an antisocial personality disorder. These individuals have a tendency to create havoc and make it appear that another patient is at fault, either for their own pleasure or for their own purposes (e.g., escaping the unit or getting into the medication room). So even while dealing with an incident, staff must be aware of what could be happening in the surrounding environment.

Use of Restraints or Seclusion

Occasionally, despite numerous interventions, a patient will become violent and require restraint or seclusion. When this happens, it is essential to have an organized approach to the seclusion or restraint. According to the U.S. Department of Health & Human Services, Centers for Medicare and Medicaid

TABLE 27-2 DRUGS USED FOR ACUTE MANAGEMENT OF VIOLENT BEHAVIOR

GENERIC (TRADE)	FORMS	CONSIDERATIONS
Antianxiety Agents (Benzodiazepines)		
Lorazepam (Ativan)	PO, SL, IM, IV	Drug of choice in this class Use with caution with hepatic dysfunction
Alprazolam (Xanax)	PO	Paradoxical (opposite response) with personality disorders and elderly
Diazepam (Valium)	PO, IM, IV	Rapid onset of calming and sedating Long half-life; use with caution in elderly
First-Generation Antipsychotics		
Haloperidol (Haldol)	PO, IM, IV	Favorable side-effect profile. Due to risk of neuroleptic malignant syndrome, keep hydrated, check vital signs, and test for muscle rigidity
Chlorpromazine (Thorazine)	PO, PR, IM	Very sedating Injections can cause pain; watch for hypotension
Second-Generation Antipsychotics		
Risperidone (Risperdal)	PO	Calms while treating underlying condition. Watch for hypotension. Increased risk of stroke in elderly.
Olanzapine (Zyprexa)	PO, IM	Useful in patients unresponsive to haloperidol Calms while treating underlying condition Avoid when using lorazepam Increased risk of stroke in elderly
Ziprasidone (Geodon)	PO, IM	Use cautiously with QT prolongation Less sedating
Aripiprazole (Abilify)	PO, IM	Avoid when using lorazepam
Combinations		
Haloperidol (Haldol), lorazepam (Ativan), and diphenhydramine (Benadryl) or benztropine (Cogentin)	IM	Commonly used in the acute setting Men who are young and athletic are at increased risk of dystonia Consider akathisia if agitation increases
Perphenazine, lorazepam (Ativan), and diphenhydramine (Benadryl) or benztropine (Cogentin)	IM	Consider this combination if patient has difficulty taking haloperidol

Data from Gross, A. F., & Sanders, K. M. (2008). Aggression and violence. In T. S. Stern, J. F. Rosenbaum, M. Fava, J. Biederman, & S. L. Rauch (Eds.), *Massachusetts General Hospital comprehensive clinical psychiatry* (pp. 895–905). St. Louis: Mosby; and Martinez, M., Marangell, L. B., & Martinez, J. M. (2008). Psychopharmacology. In R. E. Hales, S. C. Yudofsky, & G. O. Gabbard (Eds.), *Textbook of psychiatry*. Arlington, VA: American Psychiatric Publishing; Buckley, P., Citrome, L., Nichita, C., & Vitacco, M. (2011). Psychopharmacology of aggression in schizophrenia. *Schizophrenia Bulletin, 37*(5), 930–936; Stahl, S. M. (2008). *Stahl's essential psychopharmacology: Neuroscientific basis and practical applications* (3rd ed.). New York, NY: Cambridge University Press.

Services (2008), **seclusion** refers to "the involuntary confinement of a patient alone in a room, or area from which the patient is physically prevented from leaving" (p. 96). The goal of seclusion is never punitive; rather, *the goal is safety of the patient and others.*

Restraint is defined as "any manual method, physical or mechanical device, material, or equipment that immobilizes or reduces the ability of a patient to move his or her arms, legs, body, or head freely" (p. 90). Seclusion or physical restraint is used only after alternative interventions have been tried, including verbal intervention, behavioral care plan, medication, decrease in sensory stimulation, removal of a particular problematic stimulus, presence of a significant other, frequent observation, or use of a sitter who provides 24-hour, one-on-one observation of the patient. Seclusion or restraint is used only if the patient presents a clear and present danger to self or others.

Prior to an episode of seclusion, a patient must be assessed for contraindications for seclusion: pregnancy, COPD, head or spinal injury, seizure disorder, abuse, history of surgery or fracture, morbid obesity, and sleep apnea. A patient may not be held in seclusion or restraint without an order from a licensed practitioner. Once in restraint, a patient must be directly observed and formally assessed at frequent, regular intervals for level of awareness, level of activity, safety within the restraints, hydration, toileting needs, nutrition, and comfort. The frequency of observation is mandated by licensing and accreditation agencies.

Each team member is trained in the correct use of physical restraining maneuvers as well as the use of physical restraints. The team is organized before approaching the patient so that each team member knows his or her individual responsibility regarding limb securing. Before approaching the patient, the team is prepared with the correct number and size of restraints

TABLE 27-3 **DRUGS USED FOR LONG-TERM MANAGEMENT OF CHRONIC AGGRESSION**

CLASS	POPULATION	CONSIDERATIONS
Selective serotonin reuptake inhibitors (SSRIs)	Antisocial personality, schizophrenia, dementia, brain injury	Reduces irritability, impulsivity, and aggression Stabilizes mood Use cautiously with bipolar disorder
Lithium	Antisocial personality, prison inmates, mental retardation, brain injury	TSH levels measured prior to treatment Due to anti-aggressive properties, blood levels can be lower than those necessary to treat bipolar mania
Anticonvulsants	Prison inmates, antisocial/borderline personality, substance use, attention-deficit disorders, brain injury, schizophrenia	Significantly reduces impulsive aggression Similar doses with bipolar disorder Multiple drug interactions Periodic blood levels Monitor CBC and LFTs
Gabapentin	Anxiety disorder, personality disorders	No interactions with other anticonvulsants
Benzodiazepines	Anxiety disorder	Potential for abuse, dependence, and withdrawal May cause paradoxical aggression
Second-generation antipsychotics	Schizophrenia, psychosis, mania, borderline personality, mental retardation	Clozapine superior to other second-generation drugs Fewer side effects and greater adherence than first-generation antipsychotics Risperidone reduces irritability in autistic disorder
Beta-blockers	Schizophrenia, brain injury, dementia, mental retardation	Propranolol contraindicated with asthma, COPD, and IDDM Sedation side effects may explain anti-aggressive effects
Psychostimulants	ADD/ADHD in children and adults	Potential for addiction and abuse

ADD/ADHD, Attention deficit disorder/attention deficit hyperactivity disorder; *CBC,* complete blood count; *COPD,* chronic obstructive pulmonary disease; *IDDM,* insulin-dependent diabetes mellitus; *LFT,* liver function test; *TSH,* thyroid-stimulating hormone.
Data from Buckley, P., Citrome, L., Nichita, C., & Vitacco, M. (2011). Psychopharmacology of aggression in schizophrenia. *Schizophrenia Bulletin, 37*(5), 930–936; Stahl, S. M. (2008). *Stahl's essential psychopharmacology: Neuroscientific basis and practical applications* (3rd ed.). New York, NY: Cambridge University Press; Comai, S., Tau, M., & Gobbi, G. (2012). The psychopharmacology of aggressive behavior, a translational approach: Part 1 neurobiology. *Journal of Clinical Psychopharmacology, 32*(1), 83–94.

and with medication, if ordered. The patient must be given every opportunity to regain control so that the least restrictive method can be used. If restraints are to be used, the patient is informed at this point of the team's intent and the reason for the actions. The team remains calm and acts as quickly as possible.

Once the patient is restrained, the nurse must get an order for the restraint episode from the appropriate health care provider. The nurse may also get an order for medication and administer it to the patient. The team leader continues to relate to the patient in a calm, steady voice, communicating decisiveness, consistency, and control. A restraint episode is typically not planned, so these may not be an accurate reflection of what happens. Guidelines for the use of mechanical restraints are given in Box 27-3.

While the patient is restrained and in seclusion, close monitoring to determine the patient's ability to reintegrate into unit activities is mandatory. Reintegration should be gradual and geared to the patient's ability to handle increasing amounts of stimulation. If the reintegration proves to be too much for the patient and results in increased agitation, the individual is returned to the room or another quiet area. Patients must be able to follow commands and control behaviors before reintegration can occur.

Generally, a structured reintegration is the best approach. It can begin by reducing four-point restraints to three-point restraints. Once the patient no longer requires the locked seclusion room or restraints and is able to exercise self-control, he or she can return to the unit. After being returned to the unit the patient should be observed carefully to maintain safety. In some cases, the patient may require further seclusion or restraint, and another order must be obtained.

Immediately after the seclusion or restraint episode, the staff must debrief with one another. Staff analysis of the episode of violence, referred to as *critical incident debriefing*, is crucial for a number of reasons. First, a review is necessary to ensure that quality care was provided to the patient. Staff members need to critically examine their response to the patient. Questions to be answered include the following:

- Could we have done anything that would have prevented the violence? If yes, then what could have been done, and why was it not done in this situation?
- Did the team respond as a team? Were team members acting according to the policies and procedures of the unit? If not, why not?
- How do staff members feel about this patient? About this situation? Feelings of fear and anger are discussed and handled. Employee morale, productivity, use of sick leave time, transfer

BOX 27-3 GUIDELINES FOR USE OF MECHANICAL RESTRAINT

Indications for Use
- To protect the patient from self-harm
- To prevent the patient from assaulting others

Legal Requirements
- Multidisciplinary involvement
- Appropriate health care provider's signature according to state law
- Patient advocate or relative notification
- Restraint/seclusion discontinuation as soon as possible
- No use of weapons

Documentation
- Patient's behavior leading to restraint/seclusion
- Least-restrictive measures used prior to restraint
- Interventions used
- Patient response to interventions
- Plan of care for restraint/seclusion use implemented
- Ongoing evaluations by nursing staff and appropriate health care providers

Clinical Assessments
- Patient's mental state at time of restraint
- Physical exam for medical problems possibly causing behavioral changes
- Need for restraints

Observation
- Have staff in constant attendance
- Complete written record every 15 minutes
- Range of movement
- Monitor vital signs
- Observe blood flow in hands/feet
- Observe that restraint is not rubbing
- Provide for nutrition, hydration, and elimination

Release Procedure
- Patient must be able to follow commands and stay in control.
- Termination of restraints
- Debrief with patient

Restraint Tips
- Patient must be able to follow commands and stay in control.
- Physical holding of a patient against his or her will is a restraint.
- Physical holding of a patient for medication administration is a restraint.
- Four side rails up is a restraint except in seizure precautions.
- Keeping a patient in his room by physical intervention is seclusion.
- Tucking sheets in so tightly patient cannot move is a restraint.
- Orders for seclusion/restraint cannot be prn ("as needed").

requests, and absenteeism are all affected by patient violence, especially if a staff member has been injured. Staff members must feel supported by their peers as well as by the organizational policies and procedures established to maintain a safe environment.

- Is there a need for additional staff education regarding how to respond to violent patients?
- How did the actual restraining process go? What could have been done differently? Do not focus only on whether staff members were acting like a team.
- If injury occurred, has it been reported and cared for? It has been shown that there is vast underreporting of violence against health care staff.

When the patient is reintegrated into the unit, discussion with the patient is an important part of the therapeutic process. Going over what has occurred allows the patient to learn from the situation, to identify the stressors that precipitated the out-of-control behavior, and to plan alternative ways of responding to these stressors in the future.

The nurse must provide documentation in situations in which violence was either averted or actually occurred, including the following:

- Assessment of behaviors that occurred as the patient was escalating
- Nursing interventions and the patient's responses
- Evaluation of the interventions used
- Detailed description of the patient's behaviors during the assaultive stage
- All nursing interventions used to defuse the crisis
- Patient's response to those interventions
- Observations of the patient and interventions performed while the patient was in restraints and/or seclusion
- The way the patient was reintegrated into the unit milieu
- Documentation required by the Centers for Medicare and Medicasid Services and The Joint Commission

Box 27-4 lists selected *Nursing Interventions Classifications (NIC)* for *Anger Control Assistance* (Bulechek et al., 2013).

Let's take a closer look at intervening in different settings with patients who are exhibiting anger and have the potential for aggression and violence.

Caring for Patients in General Hospital Settings

Patients with Healthy Coping Who Are Overwhelmed

A patient loses autonomy and control when hospitalized, which can cause a great deal of related distress. When this stress is combined with the uncertainty of illness, a patient may respond in ways that are not usual for him or her. A careful nursing assessment, with history and information from family members, helps evaluate whether a patient's anger is a usual or an unusual way of managing stress. Interventions for patients whose usual coping strategies are healthy involve finding ways to reestablish or substitute similar means of dealing with the hospitalization. This problem solving occurs in collaboration with the patient in interactions that demonstrate the nurse acknowledges the patient's distress, validates it as understandable under the circumstances, and indicates a willingness to search for solutions. Validation includes making an apology to the patient when appropriate, such as when a promised intervention (e.g., changing a dressing by a certain time) has not been delivered, or sympathizing with the patient

BOX 27-4 *NIC* INTERVENTIONS FOR ANGER-CONTROL ASSISTANCE

Definition: Facilitation of the expression of anger in an adaptive, nonviolent manner

Activities (partial list):

- Establish basic trust and rapport with patient.
- Use calm, reassuring approach.
- Determine appropriate behavioral expectations for expression of anger, given patient's level of cognitive and physical functioning.
- Limit access to frustrating situations until patient is able to express anger in an adaptive manner.
- Encourage patient to seek assistance from nursing staff or responsible others during periods of increasing tension.
- Monitor potential for inappropriate aggression and intervene before its expression.
- Prevent physical harm if anger is directed at self or others (e.g., restrain and remove potential weapons).
- Provide reassurance to patient that nursing staff will intervene to prevent patient from losing control.
- Use external controls (e.g., physical or manual restraint, timeouts, and seclusion) as needed to calm patient who is expressing anger in a maladaptive manner.

Adapted from Bulechek, G. M., Butcher, H. K., Dochterman, J. M., & Wagner, C. (2013). *Nursing interventions classification (NIC)* (6th ed.). St. Louis, MO: Mosby.

about the "horrible food" and assisting him or her to make tastier choices on the menu.

Patients who have become angry may be unable to moderate this emotion enough to problem solve with their nurses; others may be unable to communicate the source of their anger. Often, the nurse—knowing the patient and the context of the anger—can make an accurate guess at what feeling is behind the anger. Naming this feeling can lead to a dissipation of the anger, help the patient to feel understood, and lead to a calmer discussion of the distress. Some of the feelings that can precipitate anger are listed in Box 27-5. The following vignette provides an example of nursing interventions that are helpful in dissipating anger in a hospital situation. In this situation, it is most important that the medical nurse take time to sit down with the patient while listening.

BOX 27-5 FEELINGS THAT MAY PRECIPITATE ANGER

- Discounted
- Embarrassed
- Frightened
- Found out
- Guilty
- Humiliated
- Hurt
- Ignored
- Inadequate
- Insecure
- Unheard
- Out of control of the situation
- Rejected
- Threatened
- Tired
- Vulnerable

VIGNETTE

Rachel, a 41-year-old woman with a history of peripheral vascular disease, surgeries for vascular grafts, and repair of graft occlusions, is admitted to the hospital with severe pain in her left foot. Tests reveal that vessels to the foot are occluded. Additional surgery is ruled out, and medication is prescribed. Unfortunately, the medication is ineffective, and the foot begins to necrotize. Physicians discuss amputation with the patient. Rachel refuses the surgery, demands a series of unproven alternative therapies, and is extremely angry with all members of the hospital staff. The treatment team becomes increasingly impatient to schedule surgery before the tissue death worsens and because the patient is beginning to exhibit signs of systemic infection. This impatience aggravates the patient's feelings of being out of control and erodes her belief that she is a competent partner in her treatment.

Intervention. The nurse is aware that before Rachel became disabled by progressive vascular disease, she had been employed for many years as a buyer at a local department store. The nurse knows too that the patient's family lives some distance from the hospital and is unable to visit regularly. Nursing intervention is twofold. First, Rachel's anger and unwillingness to discuss her condition ends when the nurse empathizes with her feelings of fear and being out of control. Once the anger is reduced, the nurse is able to help Rachel negotiate more time for the final decision; this allows her to process anticipatory grieving (including stages of denial, anger, and bargaining). In this interval, the patient's wish to explore alternative therapies is addressed via second and third medical opinions. Rachel is also able to spend more time discussing her concerns with her family.

Patients with Marginal Coping Skills

Patients whose coping skills were marginal before hospitalization need a different set of interventions than those with basically healthy ways of coping. Patients with maladaptive coping are poorly equipped to use alternatives when their initial attempts to cope are unsuccessful or are found to be inappropriate. Such patients frequently manifest anger that moves quickly from anxiety to aggression. For some, anger and intimidation are primary strategies used to obtain their short-term goals of feelings of control or mastery. For others, the anger occurs when limited or primitive attempts at coping are unsuccessful and alternatives are unknown. For these patients, anger and violence are particular risks in inpatient settings.

This is especially true for hospitalized patients with chemical dependence who may be anxious about being cut off from their substance of choice. They may have well-founded concerns that any physical pain will be inadequately addressed. Many patients with marginal coping also have personality styles that externalize blame. That is, they see the source of their discomfort and anxiety as being outside themselves; relief must therefore also come from an outside source (e.g., the nurse, medication).

Interventions begin with attempts to understand and meet the patient's needs. For instance, baseline anxiety can be moderated by the provision of comfort items before they are requested (e.g., decaffeinated coffee, deck of cards). This can build rapport and acts symbolically to reassure. Anxiety can also be minimized by reducing ambiguity. This strategy includes clear and concrete communication. An interaction providing clarity about what the nurse can and cannot do is most usefully ended by offering something within the nurse's power to provide (e.g., leaving the patient with a "yes"). Most hospitals have some sort of withdrawal protocol assuring the patient that he or she will not go through withdrawal without medication. This can be very anxiety relieving if the patient has a chemical dependency problem.

Interventions for anxiety might also include the use of distractions such as magazines, action comics, and video games. Generally, distractions that are colorful and do not require sustained attention work best, although this varies according to the patient's interests and abilities. Finally, patients with a high level of baseline anxiety and limited coping skills are helped when their interactions with the treatment team are predictable. This may include speaking with the physician at a specific time each day and consistency in nursing assignments. Individuals from outside the unit such as a chaplain or a volunteer may help by giving the patient more attention.

Because these patients have limited coping skills, once anxiety is moderated, nursing interventions include teaching alternative behaviors and strategies. For patients who externalize blame, such teaching may best be preceded by a gentle challenge. The challenge serves to engage the patient's interest in teaching that might otherwise be seen as irrelevant. This intervention is also important in that the nurse has (1) avoided a punitive or demeaning response that might have fueled escalation of the patient's anger, (2) taught a number of strategies, and (3) provided the patient with choices and thus with more control.

Often anger may be communicated via long-term verbal abuse. If attempts to teach alternatives have not been successful, three interventions can be used:

1. The first is to leave the room as soon as the abuse begins; the patient can be informed that the nurse will return in a specific amount of time (e.g., 20 minutes) when the situation is calmer. A matter-of-fact, neutral manner is important because fear, indignation, and arguing are gratifying to many verbally abusive patients. Alternatively, if the nurse is in the midst of a procedure and cannot leave immediately, the nurse can break off conversation and eye contact, completing the procedure quickly and matter-of-factly before leaving the room. The nurse avoids chastising, threatening, or responding punitively to the patient.
2. Withdrawal of attention to the abuse is successful only if a second intervention is also used. This step requires attending positively to, and thus reinforcing, non abusive communication by the patient. Interventions can include discussing non–illness related topics, responding to requests, and providing emotional support.
3. Patients who are verbally abusive may respond best to the predictability of routine, such as scheduled contacts with the nurse (e.g., every 30 or 60 minutes). Use of such contacts provides nursing attention that is not contingent on the patient's behavior and therefore does not reinforce the abuse. Of course, the patient's illness or injury may sometimes require nursing visits for assessment or intervention outside the scheduled contact times. These visits can be carried out in a calm, brief, matter-of-fact manner.

Implementing appropriate interventions can be difficult when the nurse is feeling threatened. Remaining matter-of-fact with patients who habitually use anger and intimidation can be difficult; these patients are often skillful at making personal and pointed statements. It is important to remember that patients do not know their nurses personally and thus have no basis on which they can make judgments. Nurses can also vent their own responses elsewhere with other staff or family members (while maintaining confidentiality) or via critical incident debriefing.

VIGNETTE

A 21-year-old man who was in an automobile accident is bedridden with a pelvic fracture. During his first day of admission, he yells at each nurse who walks by his room, using expletives in his demands that the nurse enter the room.

Intervention. The nurse who is assigned to the patient for the evening stops in his doorway after he yells at her and asks in mild disbelief, "Is this working for you? Do nurses really come in here when you yell at them that way?" The patient responds sullenly, justifying his behavior by complaining about his care; however, the nurse's challenge has caught his attention, and she goes on to suggest (i.e., teach) alternative strategies for contacting her and other nurses. The strategies are immediately put into use by the patient.

Caring for Patients in Inpatient Psychiatric Settings

It is important to know that not all psychiatric patients are violence-prone, and aggression appears to be correlated less with certain illnesses than with certain patient characteristics. The two most significant predictors of violence are a history of violence and a history of impulsivity.

Situational factors contribute to patient anger and aggression. For instance, feelings of vulnerability and powerlessness resulting from trying to come to grips with depersonalized hospital routines, intrusive procedures, and restrictions on freedom can lead to anger and possibly aggression. Additional causes of patients' anger include (1) unrealistic expectations that their nurses will be angels of mercy, (2) the feeling that their physical and psychological needs are being ignored, and (3) the feeling that health care providers fail to recognize the uniqueness and wholeness of the patient.

If staff can identify patients who have a potential for violence, early intervention becomes possible. Nurses can work with these patients to recognize early signs of anger and can teach them strategies to manage the anger and prevent aggression.

VIGNETTE

A 19-year-old man has a 2-year history of quadriplegia. He also has a history of drug abuse that began in grade school, an inability to set or work toward long-term goals, and a primary coping style of anger and intimidation. The patient is admitted to an inpatient psychiatric unit because of increasing suicidal ideation. He clearly communicates to staff that his preferred means of coping with anger is to "cuss people out" and run into them with his wheelchair. In the hospital, however, the consequence of wheelchair assaults is that the patient is secluded in his room, which he finds intolerable. The patient asks the staff to help him manage his anger.

Intervention. The nurse assigned to this young man sets aside time to interview him regarding the triggers for his anger. He identifies several issues that "make him angry." These typically relate to feeling unheard and controlled by the staff. Together, the nurse and patient examine alternative ways for him to deal with these situations, such as telling the staff he doesn't feel they are listening to him and letting them know he needs to be involved in planning his care so that he can have an increased sense of control. The patient and nurse role-play a situation in which the patient is told by a staff member that he must attend a group session. Such a situation would usually result in the patient's becoming angry and aggressive, but in the role play he is willing to "try out" alternative communication techniques to communicate his feelings to the staff member and thus to handle his anger. In addition, the patient is willing to enter into a behavioral contract with the nurse stating that he will not curse at staff nor assault anyone with his wheelchair. Instead, he will let the staff know when he is feeling angry and what the triggering issue is so that a nonaggressive resolution can be found.

Response. Because this patient is intelligent and motivated to gain increased personal control, he responds positively to these suggestions. In addition, once it becomes clear that his issues of feeling unheard and out of control underlie most episodes of anger, the patient is able to target these issues for problem solving. He rapidly develops effective and appropriate ways to make himself heard and understood. He also becomes adept at communicating when he feels out of control and at finding ingenious ways of negotiating control on issues that are particularly important to him. The patient's suicidal impulses, which occur when he is frustrated, also diminish.

Caring for Patients with Cognitive Deficits

Patients with cognitive deficits are particularly at risk for acting aggressively. Such deficits may result from delirium, dementias (e.g., Alzheimer's disease, multi-infarct dementia), or brain injury (refer to Chapter 23). Traditional approaches to disorientation and to the agitation it can cause have relied heavily on reality orientation and medication. Reality orientation consists of providing the correct information to the patient about place, date, and current life circumstances. For many patients, this is comforting because it reminds them of pertinent information and helps them feel grounded. For others, reality orientation does not work. Because of their cognitive disorder, they can no longer "enter into our reality"; they become frightened and more agitated and may become aggressive. Orientation aids, such as a calendar and a clock, can provide easy reference and increased autonomy. Such aids must be prominent and easily read by patients with diminished eyesight. Sedating medication may calm agitation, but the risks often outweigh the benefits. Sedation only further clouds a patient's sensorium, which makes disorientation worse and increases the risk of falls and injuries. It is better to examine alternative interventions.

Typically, patients experiencing delirium will be in and out of reality. At times they will appear perfectly fine, and at others they will have a clouded sensorium. They will sometimes fall asleep as you are talking to them. Often, patients with delirium will have visual hallucinations, commonly of children, animals, or bugs. Occasionally they will show periods of paranoia. The best intervention for delirium is to find and treat the medical cause. The next choice is to medicate the symptoms with a low-dose antipsychotic and discontinue it as the delirium clears.

Patients with any clouding of the sensorium have difficulty interpreting environmental stimuli. Another set of interventions involves making the environment as simple, predictable, and comfortable as possible. Simplicity includes decreasing sensory stimuli. In the hospital, this might include placing the patient's bed away from doorways that enter onto the hall and choosing not to turn on the television. Establishing a routine of activities for each day and displaying the day's schedule prominently in the patient's room can provide predictability. The comfort of the patient is enhanced by provision of familiar photographs and objects from home. The availability of a rocking chair can provide a rhythmic source of self-soothing.

Sometimes the patient with a cognitive disorder experiences such severe agitation and aggression that it is referred to as a *catastrophic reaction*. The patient may scream, strike out, or cry because of overwhelming fear. Adopting a calm and unhurried manner is the best approach to take with such a patient. To respond effectively to episodes of agitation, it is crucial to identify the antecedents (i.e., what preceded the episode) and the consequences of such episodes. Once antecedents are understood, interventions are often obvious.

VIGNETTE

An 81-year-old woman with Alzheimer's disease always becomes agitated during her morning care; this comes to be a time dreaded by her caregivers. Careful observation of antecedents to the episodes of agitation reveals a natural course to the morning problems. The patient is initially calm when care begins; however, one staff person gives morning care to the patient and her roommate at the same time, moving between the two. Observation of the process reveals that the patient becomes distracted by cues being given to her roommate and often startles when the caregiver returns to her. As this process continues over several minutes, the patient becomes increasingly distressed and then agitated. The patient's morning agitation ends when a change is made so that the patient's care is provided by one person who remains with her throughout the process.

Patients who misperceive their setting or life situation may be calmed by **validation therapy**. Some disoriented older patients believe that they are young and feel the need to return to important tasks that were a significant part of those earlier years.

For example, a woman may insist that she must go home to take care of her babies. Telling the patient that her babies have grown up and there is no home to return to is not only cruel but nontherapeutic and will result in increased agitation. It is often more helpful to reflect back to the patient the feelings behind her demand and to show understanding and concern for her worry.

Rather than attempting to reorient the patient, the nurse should ask the patient to further describe the setting or situation that is reported to be a problem (e.g., the need to return home). During the conversation, the nurse can comment on what appears to be underlying the patient's distress, thus validating it. In the earlier example, the woman who believes that she needs to return home to care for her children is asked to tell the nurse more about her children. The nurse may note that the patient misses her children and that the current setting gets lonely at times:

Nurse: "Mrs. Green, you miss your children, and this can be a lonely place."

As the nurse shows interest in aspects of the patient's life, the nurse establishes himself or herself as a safe, understanding person. In turn, the patient often becomes calmer and more open to redirection. As patients reminisce in this fashion, they often bring themselves into the present:

Patient: "Of course, they're all grown and doing well on their own now."

Refer to Chapter 23 for a more detailed discussion of interventions for people with cognitive impairments. Refer to Chapter 30 for a more detailed discussion of the use of validation and reminiscent therapeutic modalities for older adults.

EVALUATION

Evaluation of the care plan is essential for patients who are potentially angry and aggressive. A well-considered plan has specific outcome criteria (see Table 27-1). Evaluation provides information about the extent to which the interventions have achieved the outcomes. Revision focuses on all aspects of the nursing process:

- Was the assessment accurate and thorough?
- Were the nursing diagnoses applicable to the assessment data? Did the nursing diagnoses accurately drive nursing interventions?
- Was the plan comprehensive and individualized?

The initial plan may have included assessment of the environmental stimuli that precede a patient's agitation. Once these are identified, the plan provides interventions that are specific to those stimuli; however, the plan can work only if staff members evaluate the effectiveness of the approach by noting the extent to which agitation is decreased. Evaluation may reveal that the patient's agitation has decreased except in specific situations. The plan is then revised to include these situations.

KEY POINTS TO REMEMBER

- Angry emotions and aggressive and violent actions are difficult targets for nursing intervention.
- Nurses benefit from an understanding of how the angry, aggressive, or violent patient should be handled.
- Understanding patient cues to escalating aggression, appropriate goals for intervention for individuals in a variety of situations, and helpful nursing interventions is important for nurses in any setting.
- The expression of anger can lead to increased anger and to negative physiological changes.
- Psychosocial, cognitive, and biological theories provide explanations for anger and aggression.
- It is helpful for providers of care to know what cues should be looked for and what should be assessed when a patient's anger is escalating (verbal cues; nonverbal cues that include facial expression, breathing, body language, and posture).
- A patient's past aggressive behavior is the most important indicator of future aggressive episodes.
- Working with angry and aggressive patients is a challenge for all nurses, and a careful understanding and recognition of one's personal responses to angry or threatening patients can be crucial.
- Many approaches are effective in helping patients de-escalate and maintain control.
- Different interventions are used, depending on the patient's coping abilities, cognitive status, and potential for violence.
- Specific medications such as antipsychotics, mood stabilizers, and antianxiety medications may be useful.
- Restraints may be necessary to ensure the safety of the patient, other patients, and the staff.
- Each unit has a clear protocol for the safe use of restraints and for the humane management of care during the time the patient is restrained as well as clear guidelines for understanding and protecting the patient's legal rights.

CRITICAL THINKING

1. Jennifer admits a 24-year-old man with mania to an inpatient unit. She notes that the patient is irritable, has trouble sitting during the interview, and has a history of assault.
   a. Identify appropriate responses the nurse can make to the patient.
   b. What interventions should be built into the care plan?
   c. Identify at least three long-term outcomes to consider when planning care.
2. What are the two indicators for the use of seclusion and restraint rather than verbal interventions? Give rationales for your answers.
3. Discuss the use of restraint and seclusion with your clinical group or in class. Choose a side and defend it (even if you do not necessarily believe it) regarding the following:
   a. There are always better alternatives to seclusion and restraint.
   b. Seclusion and restraint are underutilized; people who have tried to limit their use have gone too far.
   c. Using chemical restraint with medication is/is not preferable to seclusion and restraint.

CHAPTER REVIEW

1. You are caring for Malcolm, an 83-year-old African American patient with Alzheimer's disease. Malcolm exhibits agitated behavior at times, especially when he feels he is missing work, and he sometimes attempts to leave the unit to "get to the school where I teach." Which of the following interventions is appropriate for de-escalating Malcolm's agitation?
   a. Medicate Malcolm with prn medication at regular intervals to prevent agitation.
   b. Repeatedly explain to Malcolm that he is retired and no longer teaches as the repetition will reinforce the patient's orientation.
   c. Use validation therapy and ask Malcolm about the school and his job.
   d. Reduce stimulation in the environment by having Malcolm sit by himself in his room until the agitation passes.
2. Ian makes the following statements to you while admitting him. Which statement indicates an increased likelihood of violent behavior?
   a. "When I get mad, I want to be left alone."
   b. "Last time I was in here I ended up in seclusion for punching my roommate."
   c. "My old man was meek and mild, and I've always said I'm not going to be like him."
   d. "My girlfriend says I yell way too much, and she's threatened to leave me."
3. You respond to a loud, angry voice coming from the day room, where you find that Alex is pacing and shouting that he isn't "going to take this (expletive) anymore." Which of the following responses is likely to be helpful in de-escalating Alex? *Select all that apply.*
   a. Remain calm, quiet, and in control.
   b. Tell Alex that his actions are unacceptable and that he must go to his room.
   c. Match Alex's volume level so that he is able to hear over his own shouting.
   d. Ask Alex if he can tell you what is upsetting him so you may be able to help.
   e. Stand close to Alex so you can intervene physically if needed to protect others.
   f. Tell Alex that he could be placed in seclusion if he cannot control himself so that the patient is aware of negative consequences.
4. Andie is a patient anxiously waiting her turn to speak with you. As you are very busy, you ask Andie if she can wait a few minutes so that you can finish your task. Unfortunately the task takes longer than anticipated and you are delayed getting back to Andie. On seeing you approach her, Andie accuses you of lying and refuses to speak with you. Which response is most likely to be therapeutic at this time?
   a. "You are angry that I didn't speak with you when I promised I would."
   b. "I'm sorry for being late, but screaming at me is not the best way to handle it."
   c. "You are too angry to talk right now. I'll come back in 20 minutes, and we can try again."
   d. "Why are you angry? I told you that I was busy and would get to you as soon as I could."
5. Which statement about violence and nursing is accurate?
   a. Unless working in psychiatric mental health settings, nurses are unlikely to experience patient violence.
   b. To date, no legislation exists that addresses workplace violence against nurses.
   c. Emergency, psychiatric, and step-down units have the highest rates of violence toward staff.
   d. Violence primarily affects inexperienced or unskilled staff who cannot calm their patients.

Answers to Chapter Review
1. c; 2. b; 3. a, d; 4. a; 5. c.

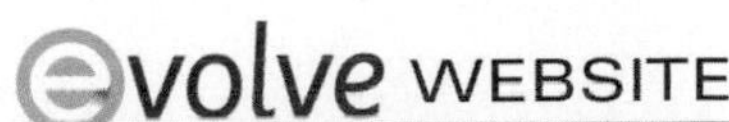
WEBSITE

Visit the Evolve website for a posttest on the content in this chapter: http://evolve.elsevier.com/Varcarolis

Post-Test interactive review

REFERENCES

Bandura, A. (1973). *Aggression: A social learning analysis.* New York, NY: Prentice Hall.

Beck, A. (1976). *Cognitive therapy and the emotional disorders.* New York, NY: International Universities Press.

Bulechek, G. M., Butcher, H. K., Dochterman, J. M., &. Wagner, C. (2013). *Nursing interventions classification (NIC)* (6th ed.). St. Louis, MO: Mosby.

Centers for Disease Control. (2010). Surveillance for violent deaths—national violent death reporting system, 16 states. *Morbidity and Mortality Weekly Report, 59*(SS04), 1–50. Retrieved from http://www.cdc.gov/mmwr/pdf/ss/ss5904.pdf.

Choi, M., & Yeon, H. A. (2011). Identifying and treating the culture-bound syndrome of hwa-byung among older Korean immigrant women: Recommendations for practitioners. *Journal of the American Academy of Nurse Practitioners, 23*(5), 226–232.

Denollet, J., Gidron, Y., Vrints, C. J., & Conraads, V. M. (2010). Anger, suppressed anger, and risk of adverse events in patients with coronary artery disease. *American Journal of Cardiology, 105*(11), 555–1560.

Gilburt, H., Rose, D., & Slade, M. (2008). The importance of relationships in mental health care study of service users' experiences of psychiatric hospital admission in the UK. *BioMed Central Health Services Research,* (92), 1–22.

Gross, A. F., & Sanders, K. M. (2008). Aggression and violence. In T. S. Stern, J. F. Rosenbaum, M. Fava, J. Biederman, & S. L. Rauch (Eds.), *Massachusetts General Hospital comprehensive clinical psychiatry* (pp. 895–905). St. Louis, MO: Mosby.

Hellerstein, D. J., Staub, A. M., & Lequesne, E. (2007). Decreasing the use of restraint and seclusion among psychiatric inpatients. *Journal of Psychiatric Practice, 13*(5), 1–16.

Herdman, T. H. (Ed.), (2012). *NANDA International nursing diagnoses: Definitions and classification, 2012–2014.* Oxford, UK: Wiley Blackwell.

Kassinove, H., & Tafrate, R. F. (2006). Anger related disorders: Basic issues, models, and diagnostic considerations. In E. L. Feindler (Ed.), *Anger-related disorders: A practitioner's guide to comparative treatments* (pp. 1–27). New York, NY: Springer.

Ito, M., Okazaki, M., Takahashi, S., Muramatsu, R., Kato, M., & Onuma, T. (2007). Subacute postictal aggression in patients with epilepsy. *Epilepsy Behavior*, *10*(4), 611–614.

Maske, M. (2012). NFL commissioner Roger Goodell upholds penalties against Saints' coaches, team in bounty scheme. *Washington Post*. Retrieved from http://www.washingtonpost.com/blogs/football-insider/post/nfl-commissioner-roger-goodell-upholds-penalties-against-saints-coaches-team-in-bounty-scheme/2012/04/09/gIQA7gbK6S_blog.html.

Menninger, W. W. (2007). Uncontained rage: A psychoanalytic perspective on violence. *Bulletin of the Menninger Clinic*, *71*(2), 115–131.

Moorhead, S., Johnson, M., Maas, M. L., & Swanson, E. (2013). *Nursing outcomes classification (NOC)* (5th ed.). St. Louis, MO: Elsevier.

Narayan, K. L., Narr, V., Kumari, R. P., Woods, P. M., Thompson, A. W., Toga, T., & Sharma, V. M. (2007). Regional cortical thinning in subjects with violent antisocial personality disorder or schizophrenia. *American Journal of Psychiatry*, *164*, 1418–1427.

Ogloff, J., & Daffern, M. (2006). The dynamic appraisal of situational aggression: An instrument to assess risk for imminent aggression in psychiatric patients. *Behavioral Sciences and the Law*, *24*, 799–813.

Osterndorf, C. L., Enright, R. D., Holter, A. C., & Klatt, J. S. (2011). Treating adult children of alcoholics through forgiveness therapy. *Alcoholism Treatment Quarterly*, *29*(3), 274–292.

Ramirez-Bermudez, J., Perez-Neri, I., Montes, S., Rairez-Abascal, M., Nente, F., Abundes-Corona, A., Soto-Herandez, J. L., & Rios, C. (2010). Imbalance between nitric oxide and dopamine may underlie aggression in acute neurological patients. *Neurochemical Research*, *35*(10), 1659–1665.

Robins, C. J., Keng, S. L., Ekblad, A.G., & Brantley, J. G. (2012). Effects of mindfulness-based stress reduction on emotional experience and expression: A randomized controlled trial. *Journal of Clinical Psychology*, *68*(1), 117–131.

Sansone, R. A., Farukhi, S., & Wiederman, M. W. (2012). History of childhood trauma and disruptive behaviors in the medical setting. *International Journal of Psychiatry in Clinical Practice*, *16*(1), 68–71.

Sirotich, F. (2008). Correlates of crime and violence among persons with mental disorder: An evidence-based review. *Brief Treatment Crisis Interventions*, *8*(2), 171–194.

Skinner, B. (1953). *Science and human behavior*. New York, NY: Macmillan.

U.S. Department of Health and Human Services, Centers for Medicare and Medicaid Services. (2008). *Revised interpretive guidelines for seclusion and restraint*. Retrieved from http://www.cms.hhs.gov/EOG/downloads/EO%.

Van Middendorp, H., Lumley, M. A., Jacobs, J. W. G., Bijlsma, J. W. J., & Geenan, R. (2010). The effects of anger and sadness on pain reports and experimentally induced pain thresholds in women with fibromyalgia. *Arthritis Care and Research*, *62*(10), 1370–1376.

Wilkowski, B. M., & Robinson, M. D. (2012). When aggressive individuals see the world more accurately: The case of perceptual sensitivity to subtle facial expressions of anger. *Personality and Social Psychology Bulletin*, *38*(1), 540–543.

CHAPTER

28

Child, Older Adult, and Intimate Partner Violence

Judi Sateren

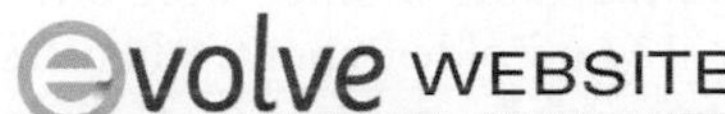

Visit the Evolve website for a pretest on the content in this chapter: http://evolve.elsevier.com/Varcarolis

Pre-Test interactive review

OBJECTIVES

1. Identify the nature and scope of family violence and factors contributing to its occurrence.
2. Identify three indicators of (a) physical abuse, (b) sexual abuse, (c) neglect, and (d) emotional abuse.
3. Describe risk factors for both victimization and perpetration of family violence.
4. Describe four areas to assess when interviewing a person who has experienced abuse.
5. Identify two common emotional responses the nurse might experience when faced with a person subjected to abuse.
6. Formulate four nursing diagnoses for the survivor of abuse, and list supporting data from the assessment.
7. Write out a safety plan for a victim of intimate partner abuse.
8. Discuss the legal and ethical responsibilities of nurses when working with families experiencing violence.
9. Compare and contrast primary, secondary, and tertiary levels of intervention, giving two examples of intervention for each level.
10. Describe at least three possible referrals for an abusive family, including the telephone numbers of appropriate agencies in the community.
11. Discuss three psychotherapeutic modalities useful in working with abusive families.

KEY TERMS AND CONCEPTS

crisis situation
economic abuse
emotional abuse
family violence
neglect
perpetrators
physical abuse
primary prevention
safety plan
secondary prevention
sexual abuse
shelters or safe houses
survivor
tertiary prevention
vulnerable person

There's no place like home. This is a statement familiar to most of us, and home is considered by many to be a source of refuge and peace. Yet for many children, adults, and elders the home is a dangerous place where family members or intimate partners demonstrate complete disregard for the rights of others. Family violence (also called domestic violence) is among the most important public health issues in the United States. Nurses are in a unique position to respond to family violence and are educated to identify, evaluate, and treat both victims and perpetrators of violence.

CLINICAL PICTURE

Types of Abuse

The American Academy of Family Physicians defines **family violence** as the "intentional intimidation, abuse, or neglect of children, adults, or elders by a family member, intimate partner, or caretaker in order to gain power and control over the victim" (2008, para. 1). Legal definitions of family or domestic violence vary from state to state; 46 states have specific definitions in their civil statutes (U.S. Department of Health and Human Services [USDHHS], 2011).

Specific types of abuse have been identified as physical abuse, sexual abuse, emotional abuse, neglect, and economic abuse. **Physical abuse** is the infliction of physical pain or bodily harm (e.g., slapping, punching, hitting, choking, pushing, restraining, biting, throwing, and burning). **Sexual abuse** is any form of sexual contact or exposure without consent, or in circumstances in which the victim is incapable of giving consent. Sexual abuse is also referred to as *sexual assault* or *rape* and is discussed in Chapter 29. **Emotional abuse** is the infliction of mental anguish (e.g., threatening, humiliating, intimidating, and isolating). **Neglect** is the failure to provide for physical, emotional, educational, and medical needs. **Economic abuse** is controlling a person's access to economic resources. Each of these types of abuse will be addressed in more depth in this chapter.

EPIDEMIOLOGY

It is estimated that half of all people in the United States have experienced abuse in their families. While the true prevalence of child, elder, and intimate partner abuse is unknown because of underreporting and variability in reporting methods, instruments, sites, and reporters, it is clear that abuse is a significant problem.

Child Abuse

In 2010 there were 3.3 million referrals for child abuse, 20% of which were substantiated (USDHHS, 2011). The most common form of abuse was neglect (78%), followed by physical abuse (17%), sexual abuse (9%), and emotional abuse (8%). Table 28-1 gives statistics related to abuse rates and fatalities among different ethnicities.

Girls are slightly more likely to be abused, comprising 51% of victims. In general, the younger the child the more vulnerable she or he is to abuse. Tragically, children under the age of 1 account for about 21% of all abuse cases (USDHHS, 2011). Approximately 80% of children who die are younger than 4 years of age, and boys die at a slightly higher rate than girls. The abuse of neglect is the most common cause of death. The prevalence of sexual abuse in children is difficult to determine due to the fact that children are often unable to describe their experience. Relatively uncommon in infants, sexual abuse increases with age. Beginning at puberty, the rate of sexual abuse is about 9% of all abuse cases (USDHHS, 2011).

It is estimated that 80% of perpetrators are the victim's parents (USDHHS, 2011). Mothers abuse more frequently and account for 37% of cases, fathers acting alone account for 19% of abuse cases, both parents as abusers occurs in 18% of cases, and in 7% of the cases the abusers are a parent along with another person.

Intimate Partner Abuse

According to the National Intimate Partner and Sexual Violence Survey (Black et al., 2011), more than 1 in 3 women and 1 in 4 men have experienced physical violence, rape, and/or stalking by an intimate partner at some time in their lives. Females are victimized about 6 times more often than males. In persons aged 12 and older, about 4 females per 1000 persons report abuse while males report abuse at a rate of 0.8 per 1000 persons (U.S. Bureau of Justice Statistics, 2007).

The gender gap of physical violence in intimate partner relationships seems to be narrower. Nearly 1 in 3 women and 1 in 4 men have been slapped, pushed, or shoved by an intimate partner in their lifetimes (Black et al., 2011). Nearly half of married couples have instances of abuse, and evidence suggests that intimate partner violence affects same-sex relationships at about the same rates as heterosexual relationships (Stephenson et al., 2011). One out of 10 homicides is due to spousal murder, and about a third of females who are killed are or were in an intimate relationship with their killer.

Older Adult Abuse

According to the American Psychological Association (APA) (2012), every year about 2 million older adults in the United States are reported to be physically abused, psychologically abused, or neglected. The APA suggests that the number may be far higher and that for every case reported, five go unreported. Further complicating the picture is that the older adult may be caring for himself or herself, which creates the potential for self-neglect. Elder abuse occurs in both institutional and family settings. Family members are reported to be the perpetrators in about 76% of incidents (Acierno et al., 2010).

TABLE 28-1 VICTIMS OF ABUSE AND FATALITIES AMONG DIFFERENT ETHNICITIES: 2010

RACE OR ETHNICITY	% OF TOTAL ABUSE CASES	% OF TOTAL CHILD FATALITIES
African American	21.9%	28.1%
American Indian or Alaska Native	1.1%	0.8%
Children of multiple races	3.5%	4.4 %
Hispanic	21.4%	16.6%
White	44.8%	43.6%
Asian	0.9%	0.9%

Data from the U.S. Department of Health & Human Services. (2011). *Child maltreatment 2010.* Washington, DC: U.S. Government Printing Office.

VIGNETTE

Walter, a 73-year-old man, came to the ambulatory care clinic looking very fatigued and complaining of pain in his left shoulder "since last night." Holding his left arm close to his side, Walter averted his eyes from those of the receptionist, nurse, and doctor. When asked if anything had occurred that might have caused the pain, he answered, "I fell." Asked why he had not sought care the previous night, Walter stated, "I . . . I . . . thought it would go away overnight." Upon further examination and X-ray imaging, it was determined that the patient had sustained a fractured clavicle. Additional direct, supportive questioning elicited the information that the patient had been injured when pushed to the floor by his son.

COMORBIDITY

The occurrence of one type of abuse is a fairly strong predictor of the occurrence of another type. The secondary effects of abuse, such as anxiety, depression, and suicidal ideation, are health care issues that can last a lifetime. Depression and post-traumatic stress disorder (PTSD) are two of the most prevalent disorders resulting from childhood trauma. Family violence is common in the childhood histories of juvenile offenders, runaways, violent criminals, prostitutes, and those who in turn are violent toward others. Exposure to abuse can adversely affect a child's development because the energy needed to successfully accomplish developmental tasks goes instead to coping with abuse (Bensley et al., 2003; Desai et al., 2002).

Abused adolescents exhibit more psychopathological changes, poorer coping and social skills, a higher incidence of dissociative identity disorder, and poorer impulse control than do other adolescents. Women who are victims of prolonged childhood sexual abuse are more likely to develop major psychiatric distress. Box 28-1 identifies some of the long-term effects of family violence.

BOX 28-1 LONG-TERM EFFECTS OF FAMILY VIOLENCE

People involved in family violence are found to have a higher incidence of:

- Depression
- Suicidal feelings
- Self-contempt
- Inability to trust
- Inability to develop intimate relationships in later life

Victims of severe violence are also at higher risk for experiencing recurring symptoms of posttraumatic stress disorder:

- Flashbacks
- Dissociation—out-of-body experiences
- Poor self-esteem
- Compulsive or impulsive behaviors (e.g., substance abuse, excessive spending, gambling, and promiscuity)
- Multiple somatic complaints

Children who witness violence in their homes:

- After the age of 5 or 6 years show an indication of identifying with the aggressor and losing respect for the victim.
- Are at greater risk for developing behavioral and emotional problems throughout their lives.

Some mental and behavioral disorders are associated with violence in childhood:

- Depressive disorders
- Posttraumatic stress disorder
- Somatic complaints, technically not a "disorder"
- Low self-esteem, same as above
- Phobias (agoraphobia, social and specific phobias)
- Antisocial behaviors
- Child or spouse abuse

Adolescents are more likely to have behavioral symptoms such as:

- Failing grades
- Difficulty forming relationships
- Increased incidence of theft, police arrest, and violent behaviors
- Seductive or promiscuous behaviors
- Running away from home

ETIOLOGY

Environmental Factors

Abuse occurs across all segments of society in the United States. Social factors that reinforce violence include the wide acceptance of corporal punishment; increasingly violent movies, video games, websites, and comic books; violent themes in music; and the increase in the total volume of pornography.

The occurrence of abuse requires the following participants and conditions:

1. A perpetrator
2. Someone who by age or situation is vulnerable (children, women, older adults, and mentally ill or physically challenged persons)
3. A crisis situation

Perpetrator

The propensity for violence is rooted in childhood and manifested by a general lack of self-regard, dissatisfaction with life, and inability to assume adult roles. Often the abuser lacked good role models and was deprived of the opportunity to develop problem-solving skills. Witnessing or experiencing family violence, neglect, or abusive parenting (Box 28-2) are contributing factors. **Perpetrators**, those who initiate violence, often consider their own needs to be more important than anyone else's and look toward others to meet their needs.

The term *perpetrator* applies to any member of a household who is violent toward another member (e.g., siblings, same-sex partners, extended family members). Both male and female perpetrators perceive themselves as having poor social skills. They describe their relationships with their partners as being the closest they have ever known, and they typically lack supportive relationships outside the relationship.

Men who abuse believe in male supremacy, being in charge, and being dominant. "Acting out" physically makes them feel more in control, more masculine, and more powerful. Parent-child interactions, peer group experiences, observations of the

BOX 28-2 CHARACTERISTICS OF ABUSIVE PARENTS

- A history of abuse, neglect, or emotional deprivation as a child
- Family authoritarianism: raise children as they were raised by their own parents
- Low self-esteem, feelings of worthlessness, depression
- Poor coping skills
- Social isolation (may be suspicious of others): few or no friends, little or no involvement in social or community activities
- Involvement in a crisis situation: unemployment, divorce, financial difficulties
- Rigid, unrealistic expectations of child's behavior
- Frequent use of harsh punishment
- History of severe mental illness, such as schizophrenia
- Violent temper outbursts
- Looking to child for satisfaction of needs for love, support, and reassurance (often unmet because of parenting deficits in family of origin)
- Projection of blame onto the child for parents' "troubles" (e.g., stepparent may project hostility toward new mate onto a child)
- Lack of effective parenting skills
- Inability to seek help from others
- Perception of the child as bad or evil
- History of drug or alcohol abuse
- Feeling of little or no control over life
- Low tolerance for frustration
- Poor impulse control

partner dyad, and the influence of the media (television, comics, video games, movies) all support the same message: Males can expect to be in a position of power in relationships and may use physical aggression to maintain that position.

Extreme pathological jealousy is characteristic of an abuser. Many refuse to allow their partners to work outside the home; others demand that their partners work in the same place as they do so that they can monitor activities and friendships. Many accompany their partners to and from all activities and forbid them to have personal friends or to participate in recreational activities outside the home. When this is not possible, a perpetrator may restrict mobility by monitoring the odometer and keeping stopwatches. Even after imposing such restrictions, abusers often accuse their partners of infidelity. Many perpetrators maintain their possessiveness by controlling the family finances so tightly that there is barely enough money for daily living.

Cycle of Violence. Walker (1979) describes a pattern of behavior that perpetrators of violence may use to control their partners. While there is little empirical evidence testing Walker's theory, it is commonly cited to describe the dynamics of an abuser's behavior. The **tension-building stage** is characterized by relatively minor incidents, such as pushing, shoving, and verbal abuse. During this time, the victim often ignores or accepts the abuse for fear that more severe abuse will follow. Abusers then rationalize that their abusive behavior is acceptable. As the tension escalates, both participants may try to reduce it. The abuser may try to reduce the tension with the use of alcohol or drugs, and the victim may try to reduce the tension by minimizing the importance of the incidents ("I should have had the house neater . . . dinner ready").

During the **acute battering stage**, the abuser releases the built-up tension by brutal beatings, which can result in serious injuries. After the abuse occurs, the abuser and victim enter a period of calm known as the **honeymoon stage** that is characterized by kindness and loving behaviors. The abuser, at least initially, feels remorseful and apologetic and may bring presents, make promises, and tell the victim how much she or he is loved and needed. The victim usually believes the promises, feels needed and loved, and drops any legal proceedings or plans to leave that may have been initiated during the acute battering stage.

Unfortunately, without intervention, the cycle will repeat itself. Over time, the periods of calmness and safety become briefer, and the periods of anger and fear are more intense. There are intervals of stability, but the violence increases over time. With each repeat of the pattern, the victim's self-esteem becomes more and more eroded. The victim either believes the violence was deserved or accepts the blame for it. This can lead to feelings of depression, hopelessness, immobilization, and self-deprecation. Figure 28-1 illustrates the cycle of violence.

Minority groups, particularly those experiencing poverty and social marginalization, may have the label of perpetrator or abuser applied to them more often than those who are more socioeconomically advantaged (Malley-Morrison & Hines, 2004). It is important to recognize that a wide variety of cultural norms dictate relationships among intimate partners and child-rearing practices. Learning about the cultural backgrounds of patients can prevent mistaking common cultural norms for abuse.

Individuals are more likely to engage in family violence when they use substances. Alcohol and other drugs (illicit or prescribed) tend to weaken inhibitions and lead to a disregard of social rules prohibiting violence. The victim may rationalize the abuse as being caused by alcohol and drugs. "He was drunk and didn't know what he was doing." However, even when drug and alcohol use is reduced or eliminated, family violence still occurs.

Vulnerable Person

The vulnerable person is the family member upon whom abuse is perpetrated. This individual is variously referred to as the *victim, survivor*, or *victim/survivor*. Using the term survivor recognizes the recovery and healing process that follows victimization and does not have the connotation of passivity that *victim* has. In some intimate relationships, violence does not occur until after the legal marriage of couples who have lived together or dated for a long time.

Women. Pregnancy may trigger or increase violence. National estimates of assaults to pregnant women range from 1% to 20%, depending on the definition of assault and the population studied (Saltzman et al., 2003). The partner may resent the added responsibility a baby entails, or he may resent the relationship the baby will have with his mate. Violence also escalates when the woman makes a move toward independence, such as visiting friends without permission, getting a job, or going back to

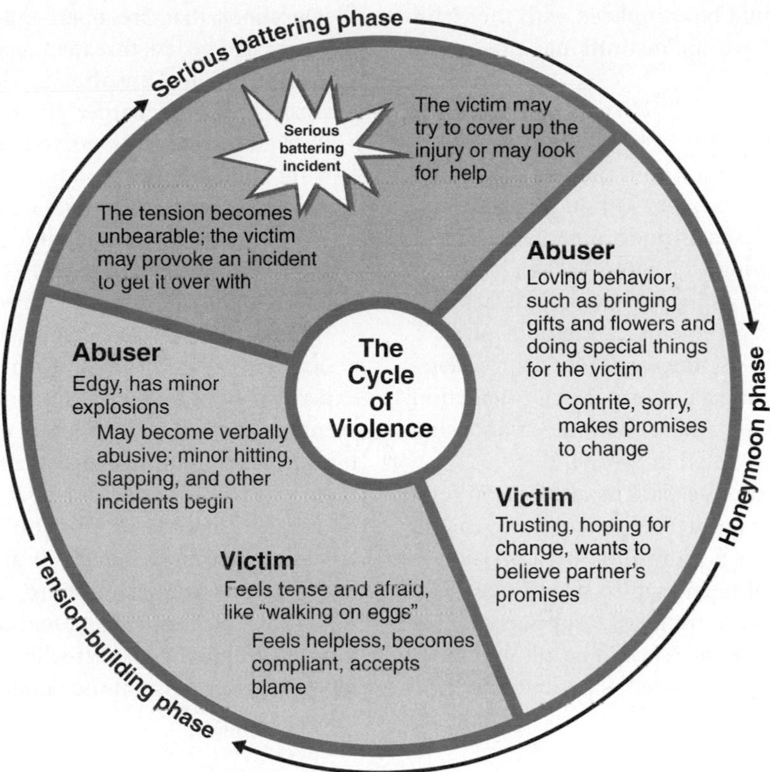

FIG 28-1 The cycle of violence. (Redrawn from YWCA of Annapolis and Anne Arundel County, 1517 Ritchie Highway, Arnold, MD 21012.)

school. Victims are at greatest risk for violence when they threaten to or actually leave the relationship.

Children. Children are most likely to be abused if they are younger than 3 years of age; are perceived as being different because of temperamental traits, congenital abnormalities, or chronic disease; remind the parents of someone they do not like (perhaps an ex-spouse); are different from the parents' fantasy of what the child should be like; or are a product of an unwanted pregnancy. Interference with emotional bonding between parents and child, which can occur because of a premature birth or prolonged illness requiring hospitalization, has also been found to increase the risk for future abuse. Adolescents are abused at least as frequently as younger children; however, such abuse is often overlooked, perhaps because adolescents tend to be viewed as capable of defending themselves.

Older Adults. Older adults may become vulnerable because they are in poor mental or physical health or are disruptive due to disorders such as Alzheimer's disease. The dependency needs of older adults are usually what put them at risk for abuse. The typical victim is female, over 75 years of age, Caucasian, living with a relative, and experiencing a physical and/or mental impairment. Caring for older adults can be stressful in the best of cases, but in families in which violence is a coping strategy, the potential for abuse is great. Other situations in which abuse occurs include the older man cared for by a daughter he abused as a child and who now is abusive toward him, the older woman abused by her husband as part of a longstanding abusive relationship, or the caregiver who becomes angry because of the failing health of a loved one.

Crisis Situation

Anyone may be at risk for abuse in a **crisis situation**—a situation that puts stress on a family with a violent member. A person with effective impulse control, problem-solving skills, and a healthy support system is less likely to resort to violence; however, stressful life events tax coping skills, leaving the perpetrator incapable of dealing with the situation. Social isolation caused by frequent moves or an inability to make friends contributes to ineffective coping during crisis situations.

APPLICATION OF THE NURSING PROCESS

ASSESSMENT

General Assessment

Victims of violence are encountered in every health care setting; therefore, all patients should be screened for possible abuse. Due to the number of victims of violence seen in emergency departments, the Emergency Nurses Association (2006) issued a formal position statement urging nurses in this specialty area to be active in promoting hospital and community teams to treat and protect people from domestic violence, abuse, and neglect.

Symptoms may be vague and can include chronic pain, insomnia, hyperventilation, or gynecological problems. Attention to the interview process and setting are important to facilitate accurate assessment of physical and behavioral indicators of family violence. All assessments should include questions to elicit a history of sexual abuse, family violence, and drug use or abuse. Any assessment should be completed with the victim alone, and it is helpful to have an institutional policy that facilitates screening in private.

Interview Process and Setting

Important and relevant information about the family situation can be gathered by routine assessment conducted with tact, understanding, and a calm, relaxed attitude. A person who feels judged or accused of wrongdoing is likely to become defensive and may not be receptive to changing behavior. It is better to ask about ways of solving disagreements or methods of disciplining children rather than to use the words *abuse* or *violence.* It is also important not to assume a person's sexual orientation; rather, use the term *partner* when asking about the relationship. Key interviewing guidelines are listed in Box 28-3.

When interviewing, sit near the patient and spend some time establishing trust and rapport before focusing on the details of the violent experience. Establishing trust is crucial if the patient is to feel comfortable enough to self-disclose. The interview should be non-threatening and supportive. The person who experienced the violence should be allowed to tell the story without interruption. Reassure the patient that he or she did nothing wrong. Verbal approaches may include the following:

- Tell me about what happened to you.
- Who takes care of you? (for children and dependent older adults)
- What happens when you do something wrong? (for children) *or* How do you and your partner/caregiver resolve disagreements? (for women and dependent older adults)
- What do you do for fun?
- Who helps you with your child(ren)/parent?
- What time do you have for yourself?

Questions that are open-ended and require a descriptive response can be less threatening and elicit more relevant information than questions that are direct or can be answered with *yes* or *no* (refer to Chapter 9):

- What arrangements do you make when you have to leave your child alone?
- How do you discipline your child?
- When your infant cries for a long time, how do you get him/her to stop?
- What about your child's behavior bothers you the most?

When trust has been established, openness and directness about the situation can strengthen the relationship with those experiencing or perpetrating violence. A five-question assessment tool developed by Soeken and colleagues (1998) has been used extensively to assist in the routine identification of intimate partner abuse (Figure 28-2).

Areas to include in an abuse assessment include: (a) violence indicators, (b) levels of anxiety and coping responses, (c) family coping patterns, (d) support systems, (e) suicide potential, (f) homicide potential, and (g) drug and alcohol use. The following vignette illustrates the key points in assessing a woman in crisis at the initial interview, as well as suggested follow-up.

BOX 28-3 INTERVIEW GUIDELINES

Do

- Do conduct the interview in private.
- Do be direct, honest, and professional.
- Do use language the patient understands.
- Do ask the patient to clarify words not understood.
- Do be understanding.
- Do be attentive.
- Do inform the patient if you must make a referral to Children's or Adult Protective Services, and explain the process.
- Do assess safety and help reduce danger (at discharge).

Do Not

- Do *not* try to "prove" abuse by accusations or demands.
- Do *not* display horror, anger, shock, or disapproval of the perpetrator or situation.
- Do *not* place blame or make judgments.
- Do *not* allow the patient to feel "at fault" or "in trouble."
- Do *not* probe or press for answers the patient is not willing to give.
- Do *not* conduct the interview with a group of interviewers.
- Do *not* force a child or anyone else to remove clothing.

VIGNETTE

Darnell Peters is a 42-year-old married woman in a relationship she describes as "bad for a long time. We don't communicate." She is brought to the emergency department by ambulance with swollen eyes, lips, and nose and lacerations to her face. She tells the nurse that her husband had been in bed asleep for hours before she joined him. On getting into bed, she attempted to redistribute the blankets. Suddenly he leaped from the bed, started punching her in the face, and began to throw her against the wall. She called out to her 11-year-old son to call the police. The police arrived, called an ambulance, and took Mr. Peters to jail.

The nurse takes Mrs. Peters to a private examination room for a full assessment. Mrs. Peters states that her relationship with her husband is always stormy. "She states that he constantly puts me down and yells." She states that he started hitting her 5 years earlier when she became pregnant with her second and last child. The beatings have increased in intensity over the past year, and this emergency department visit is the fifth this year. Tonight is the first time she has ever called the police.

Mrs. Peters has visibly lost control. Periods of crying alternate with periods of silence. She appears apathetic and depressed. The nurse remains calm and objective. After Mrs. Peters has finished talking, the nurse explores alternatives designed to help her reduce the danger when she is discharged. "I'm concerned that you will be hurt again if you go home. What options do you have?" Acknowledging the escalating intensity of the violence, Mrs. Peters is able to make arrangements with a shelter to take in her and her two children until after she has secured a restraining order.

The nurse charts the abuse referrals. Keeping careful and complete records helps ensure that Mrs. Peters will receive proper follow-up care and will assist her when and if she pursues legal action.

ABUSE ASSESSMENT SCREEN

1. Within the last year, have you been hit, slapped, kicked, or otherwise physically hurt by someone?

☐ Yes ☐ No

If yes, by whom? ____________________

Total number of times: ____________________

2. Since you've been pregnant, have you been hit, slapped, kicked, or otherwise physically hurt by someone?

☐ Yes ☐ No

If yes, by whom? ____________________

Total number of times: ____________________

Mark the area of injury on the body map below.

3. Within the last year, has anyone forced you to have sexual activities?

☐ Yes ☐ No

If yes, who? ____________________

Total number of times: ____________________

4. Have you ever been emotionally or physically abused by your partner or someone important to you?

☐ Yes ☐ No

If yes, by whom? ____________________

Total number of times: ____________________

5. Are you afraid of your partner or anyone listed above?

☐ Yes ☐ No

Score each incident according to the following scale:

1 = Threats of abuse including use of a weapon
2 = Slapping, pushing; no injuries and/or continuing pain
3 = Punching, kicking, bruises, cuts, and/or continuing pain
4 = Beating up, severe contusions, burns, broken bones
5 = Head injury, internal injury, permanent injury
6 = Use of weapon, wound from weapon

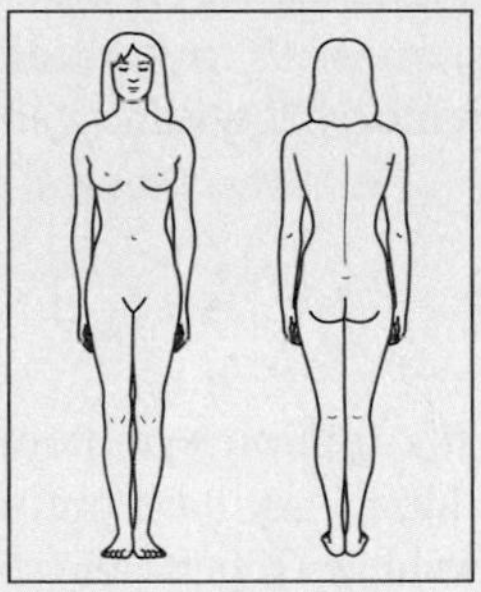

SCORE

____
____
____
____
____
____

FIG 28-2 Abuse assessment screen. (From Soeken, K., McFarlane, J., Parker, B., & Lominack, M. [1998]. The abuse assessment screen: A clinical instrument to measure frequency, severity and perpetrator of abuse against women. In J. Campbell [Ed.], *Empowering survivors of abuse: Health care for battered women and their children* [pp. 575-579]. New Brunswick, NJ: Transaction.)

Types of Abuse

Physical Abuse

A series of minor complaints, such as headaches, back trouble, dizziness, and accidents (especially falls), may be a covert indicator of violence. Overt signs of battering include bruises, scars, burns, and other wounds in various stages of healing, particularly around the head, face, chest, arms, abdomen, back, buttocks, and genitalia. Injuries that should arouse the nurse's suspicion are listed in Box 28-4.

If the explanation does not match the injury seen, or if the patient minimizes the seriousness of the injury, abuse may be suspected. Ask patients directly, but in a nonthreatening

BOX 28-4 COMMON PRESENTING PROBLEMS OF VICTIMS OF ABUSE

Emergency Department
- Bleeding injuries, especially to head and face
- Internal injuries, concussions, perforated eardrum, abdominal injuries, severe bruising, eye injuries, strangulation marks on neck
- Back injuries
- Broken or fractured jaw, arms, pelvis, ribs, clavicle, legs
- Burns from cigarettes, appliances, scalding liquids, acids
- Psychological trauma, anxiety, attacks of hyperventilation, heart palpitations, severe crying spells, suicidal tendencies
- Miscarriage

Ambulatory Care Settings
- Perforated eardrum, twisted or stiff neck and shoulder muscles, headache
- Depression, stress-related conditions (e.g., insomnia, violent nightmares, anxiety, extreme fatigue, eczema, loss of hair)
- Talk of having "problems" with husband or son, describing person as very jealous, impulsive, or an alcohol or drug abuser
- Repeated visits with new complaints
- Bruises of various ages and specific shapes (fingers, belt)

Any Setting
- Signs of stress due to family violence: emotional, behavioral, school, or sleep problems and increase in aggressive behavior
- Injuries in a pregnant woman
- Recurrent visits for injuries attributed to being "accident-prone"

manner, if someone close to them has caused the injury. Observe the nonverbal response, such as hesitation or lack of eye contact, as well as the verbal response. Then ask specific questions such as: "When was the last time it happened? How often does it happen? In what ways are you hurt?" Inconsistent explanations serve as a warning that further investigation is necessary. Vague explanations should alert the nurse to possible abuse. ("She fell from a chair [from a lap, down the stairs]." "He was running away." "The hot water was turned on by mistake.") The key to identification is a high index of suspicion.

Nonspecific bruising in older children is common. Any bruises on an infant younger than 6 months of age should be considered suspicious. **Shaken baby syndrome**, the leading cause of death as a result of physical abuse, usually occurs in children younger than 2 years old. Injuries are a result of the brain moving in the opposite direction as the baby's head. A baby who has been shaken may present with respiratory problems, bulging fontanels, retinal hemorrhages, and central nervous system damage, resulting in seizures, vomiting, and coma.

Sexual Abuse

Sexualized behavior is one of the most common symptoms of sexual abuse in children. Younger children may have precocious sexual knowledge, may draw sexually explicit images, demonstrate sexual aggression, or act out sexual interactions in play, for example, with dolls. Masturbation may be excessive in sexually abused children. In older children, sexual promiscuity is one of the most common symptoms of sexual abuse, and there is a strong connection between sexual abuse and later prostitution in females.

PTSD symptoms, such as nightmares, somatic complaints, and feelings of guilt, are also common in children who are sexually abused. There are a variety of emotional, behavioral, and physical consequences of sexual abuse, with depression being the most commonly reported symptom by adults who were sexually abused as children. Other consequences include anxiety, suicide, aggression, chronic low self-esteem, chronic pain, obesity, substance abuse, self-mutilation, and PTSD.

> **VIGNETTE**
> Ms. Randall, 83 years old, is admitted from an adult foster home for evaluation of deterioration in her mental status. She is confused and disoriented as to time and place and is unable to give a coherent history. Blood and urine are collected for diagnostic evaluation. The laboratory report notes semen in the urine. Adult Protective Services is called to begin an investigation into the adult family home.

Emotional Abuse

Emotional abuse may exist on its own or in conjunction with physical or sexual abuse. Although it is less obvious and more difficult to assess than physical violence, it can be identified through indicators such as low self-esteem, reported feelings of inadequacy, anxiety and withdrawal, learning difficulties, and poor impulse control. Many consider emotional abuse to have the most negative and enduring effects on victims.

Neglect

Neglected children and older adults often appear undernourished, dirty, and poorly clothed. Neglect is also manifested by inadequate medical care, such as lack of immunizations or untreated medical conditions.

Economic Abuse

Economic abuse may take the form of failure to provide for the needs of the victim when adequate funds are available. Bills may be left unpaid by the person in charge of finances, which may result in disconnection of the heat or electricity. Economic abuse may limit the victim's capacity to support himself or herself and forces the victim to depend on the perpetrator for support. This type of abuse may include preventing the victim from pursuing education or finding a job, thereby ensuring dependency.

Level of Anxiety and Coping Responses

Nonverbal responses to the assessment interview can be indicative of the victim's anxiety level. Agitation and anxiety bordering on panic are often present in victims experiencing violence. Because they live in terror, abused individuals remain vigilant, unable to relax or sleep. Signs of the effects of living with chronic stress and severe levels of anxiety may be present (e.g., hypertension, irritability, gastrointestinal disturbances). Hesitation, lack of eye contact, and use of vague statements such as "It's been rough lately" indicate that the situation is difficult to talk about.

Coping mechanisms used by many victims to endure living in violent and terrifying situations often prevent the dissolution of the relationship. These coping mechanisms may take the form of flawed beliefs or myths (Table 28-2). Because of feelings of confusion, shame, despair, and powerlessness, victims may withdraw from interaction with others, increasing their isolation.

> **VIGNETTE**
> The nurse in a walk-in clinic assesses Janet for bilateral corneal abrasions. The nurse becomes suspicious as she notes the patient's vague responses to history questions and her unrelenting checking of the clock, followed by the urgent statement, "I've got to get home." On further questioning, Janet reveals that she is often quite fatigued because of caring for her five children, all under the age of 7. Her husband, who works until 2 AM, expects her to be awake when he comes home from work and have a warm meal ready in the oven. "He hits me if I'm asleep." She had taped her eyes open so that even if she were lying down when he came home she would look awake. "I didn't even think about taking my contacts out."

TABLE 28-2 MYTH VERSUS FACT: FAMILY ABUSE

MYTH	FACT
The victim's behavior often causes violence.	The victim's behavior is *not* the cause of the violence. Violence is the abuser's pattern of behavior, and the victim cannot learn how to control it.
Men have the right to keep their wives and/or children in line.	No person has the right to beat or hurt another person.
Intimate partner abuse is a minor problem.	There is a *real* danger that abusive partners may kill victims.
Battered women are masochistic and like to be beaten. (The abuse cannot be that bad or they would leave.)	Women do not like, ask, or deserve to be abused. Economic considerations are usually the only reason they stay.
Victims of intimate partner abuse could leave if they really wanted to.	There are numerous factors influencing a decision to leave, including fear of injury or death, financial dependence, welfare of children, etc.
Family abuse is most prevalent in poorly educated people from poor, working-class backgrounds.	Abuse occurs in families of all socioeconomic, religious, cultural, and educational backgrounds.
Family matters are private, and families should be allowed to take care of their own problems.	Intervention in family abuse is justified; abuse always escalates in frequency and intensity, can end in death, and is passed on to future generations.
Victims of abuse tacitly accept the abuse by trying to conceal it, by not reporting it, or by failing to seek help.	When attempting to disclose their situation, many victims are met with disbelief. This discourages them from persevering.
Myths victims commonly believe: "I can't live without him/her." "If I hadn't done ____, it wouldn't have happened." "She/he will change." "I stay for the sake of the children." "Jealousy and possessiveness prove his/her love."	These myths are coping mechanisms used to allay panic in a situation of random and brutal violence. They give the illusion of control and rationality.
Alcohol and stress are the major causes of physical and verbal abuse.	This myth offers an explanation of and tolerance for verbal abuse and battering. There are no excuses, and it is not acceptable behavior. Abuse is a learned behavior, not an uncontrollable reaction. People are abusive because they have acquired the belief that violence and aggression are acceptable and effective responses to real or imagined threats.
Violence occurs only between heterosexual partners.	Gay and lesbian partners experience violence for reasons similar to those in heterosexual relationships.
Pregnancy protects a woman from battering.	Battering frequently begins or escalates during pregnancy.

Family Coping Patterns

To effectively assess abuse, the nurse must show a willingness to listen and avoid any judgmental tone. It is important to assess family strengths as well as stressors. Questioning about memories of early family relationships can provide additional information about attitudes in the home and the way they might influence coping. Asking parents about how they were disciplined as children may provide insight into their child-rearing attitudes and practices. Living with and caring for children and older adults can cause frustration, stress, and anger. Unless there are appropriate outlets for stress, abuse can occur. Box 28-5 is a useful guide for assessing the risk of child and/or older adult abuse in the home.

Support Systems

The person experiencing abuse is usually in a dependent position, relying on the perpetrator for basic needs. This dependence, along with the isolation the perpetrator imposes on the person, limits the victim's access to support systems. Children's options are especially limited, as are those of the physically and mentally challenged. Assessing for support should focus on intrapersonal, interpersonal, and community resources (e.g., the school system for school-aged victims).

Suicide Potential

A person experiencing violence may feel desperate to leave yet be trapped in a detrimental relationship, and suicide may seem like the only option. An emotionally abusive person may also use the threat of suicide in an attempt to manipulate the victim. Statements such as "Don't leave me or I'll kill myself" and "I took all my pills . . . I said I would the next time you were late" may cause the victim to submit to the perpetrator's demands.

A suicide attempt may be the presenting symptom in the emergency department. With sensitive questioning conducted in a caring manner, the nurse can elicit the history of violence. Often the means of attempted suicide is overdose with a combination of alcohol and other central nervous system depressants, or sleeping medications that have been prescribed in previous visits to physicians' offices, clinics, or emergency departments.

When the crisis of the immediate suicide attempt has been resolved, careful questioning to determine lethality is in order.

BOX 28-5 FACTORS TO ASSESS DURING A HOME VISIT

For a Child
- Responsiveness to infant's signals
- Caregiver's facial expressions in response to infant
- Playfulness of caregiver with infant
- Nature of physical contact during feeding and other caretaking activities
- Temperament of infant
- Caregiver's history of harsh discipline or abuse as a child
- Parental attitudes:
  - Feelings of inadequacy as a parent
  - Unrealistic expectations of child
  - Fear of "doing something wrong"
  - Attribution of negative qualities to newborn
  - Misdirected anger
  - Continued evidence of isolation, apathy, anger, frustration, projection
  - Adult conflict
- Environmental conditions:
  - Sleeping arrangements
  - Child management
  - Home management
  - Use of supports (formal and informal)
- Need for immediate services for situational (economics, child care), emotional, or educational information:
  - Information about hotlines, baby-sitters, homemakers, parent groups
  - Information about child development
  - Information about child care and home management services

For an Older Adult
- Absence of or lack of access to basic necessities (food, water, medications)
- Unsafe housing
- Lack of or inadequate utilities, ventilation, space
- Poor physical hygiene
- Lack of assistive devices, such as hearing aids, eyeglasses, wheelchair
- Medication mismanagement (outdated prescriptions, unmarked bottles)

For example, if the patient still feels that life is not worth living, has a suicide plan, and has the means to carry it out, admission to an inpatient psychiatric unit must be considered. On the other hand, if the patient is talking about future plans and about staying "for the sake of the children," outpatient referrals are appropriate.

Homicide Potential

Ask whether the patient feels safe going home and if so, whether a safety plan is in place for when the violence recurs. The potential for lethality should always be assessed. Certain factors place a vulnerable person at greater risk for homicide, including the following:

- The presence of a gun in the home
- Alcohol and drug abuse
- History of violence on the part of the perpetrator in other situations
- Extreme jealousy and obsessiveness on the part of the perpetrator regarding the relationship with the victim and attempt to control all the victim's daily activities

Persons victimized by violence should be asked if they have ever felt like killing the perpetrator and if so, whether they have the current desire and means to do so. If the answer is yes, intervention is required.

Drug and Alcohol Use

A person experiencing violence may self-medicate with alcohol or other drugs as a way of escaping an intolerable situation. The drugs are usually central nervous system depressants, such as benzodiazepines, prescribed by physicians for stress-related symptoms (e.g., insomnia, gastrointestinal upsets, anxiety, and difficulty concentrating).

The degree of intoxication can be determined by history, physical examination, and blood alcohol level. If an abused patient is intoxicated on presentation, allow the patient time to sober up before initiating referral. Referral information will not be understood or assimilated if the patient is intoxicated. Assess for a chronic alcohol or drug problem (refer to Chapter 22) and provide appropriate treatment referrals. The patient should not be discharged to the abuser. Treatment choices can include both inpatient and outpatient options.

Maintaining Accurate Records

Because of the possibility of future legal action, it is essential that the health care record contain an accurate and detailed description of the victim's medical history, the psychosocial history of the family, and observations of the family interactions during the interviews. Especially important in documentation of findings from the initial assessment are (1) verbatim statements of who caused the injury and when it occurred; (2) a body map to indicate size, color, shape, areas, and types of injuries, with explanations (see Figure 28-2); and (3) physical evidence of sexual abuse, when possible. Procedures for evidence collection must be followed carefully, or legal action can be thwarted. If the abuse has just occurred, ask the patient to return in a day or two for more photographs; bruises may be more evident at that time. The patient must be assured of the confidentiality of the record and of its power, should legal action be initiated. Even if intervention does not occur at this time, the record is begun; the next provider will be aware of the problem and will be in a better position to offer support.

Self-Assessment

In all areas of psychiatric mental health nursing and counseling, the nurse should be aware of personal emotions and thoughts. Acknowledging feelings that arise in response to those experiencing abuse stimulates an examination of personal views toward abuse and the status of children, women, and older adults. Strong negative feelings can cloud one's judgment and interfere with objective assessment and

TABLE 28-3 COMMON RESPONSES OF HEALTH CARE PROFESSIONALS TO VIOLENCE

RESPONSE	SOURCE
Anger	Anger may be felt toward the person responsible for the abuse, toward those who allowed it to happen, and toward society for condoning its occurrence through attitudes, traditions, and laws.
Embarrassment	The victim is a symbol of something close to home: the stress and strain of family life unleashed as uncontrollable anger.
Confusion	One's view of the family as a haven of safety and privacy is challenged.
Fear	A small percentage of perpetrators are dangerous to others.
Anguish	The nurse may have experienced abuse.
Helplessness	The nurse may want to do more, eliminate the problem, or cure the victim and/or perpetrator.
Discouragement	Discouragement may result if no long-term solution is achieved.
"Blame the victim" mentality	Health care workers can get caught up in "blaming the victim" for behaviors they see as provoking the abuse. There is never an excuse for abuse, and no one has the right to hurt another person. "Blaming the victim" can occur when health care professionals feel overwhelmed. Supervision is a must for therapeutic intervention.

intervention, no matter how much one tries to cover or deny personal bias. Working with those who experience violence may arouse intense and overwhelming feelings. Common responses of health care professionals to violence are listed in Table 28-3.

The nurse who has a personal history of abuse may identify too closely with the victim, and personal issues connected with the abuse may surface, further clouding judgment. Many nurses do not believe they are adequately prepared or have not had enough supervisory experience to intervene in cases of abuse. Supervision needs to be made available to nurses working with victims of abuse.

Multidisciplinary team conferences can be especially helpful in clarifying reactions and neutralizing intense emotions. Information from other nurses, physicians, psychologists, nurses, and social workers can assist in refocusing efforts to work constructively with a family in crisis. Sharing perceptions and feelings with other professionals can help reduce feelings of isolation and discomfort.

ASSESSMENT GUIDELINES

Family Violence

During your assessment and counseling, maintain an interested and empathetic manner. Refrain from displaying horror, anger, shock, or disapproval of the perpetrator or the situation. Assess:

1. Presenting signs and symptoms of victims of abuse
2. Potential problems in vulnerable families; for example, some indicators of vulnerable parents who might benefit from education and instruction in effective coping techniques
3. Physical, sexual, and/or emotional abuse and neglect and economic maltreatment of older adults
4. Family coping patterns
5. Patient's support system
6. Drug or alcohol use
7. Suicidal or homicidal ideas
8. Posttrauma syndrome

DIAGNOSIS

Nursing diagnoses are focused on the underlying causes and symptoms of family violence. While many of the diagnoses are directed toward protecting vulnerable family members, the perpetrator may also be included in plans of care. Safety is the number one concern and is addressed in *Risk for violence* (other-directed or self-directed), *Risk for suicide*, *Pain*, and *Risk for infection*. *Rape-trauma syndrome* is addressed in Chapter 29.

Living in a situation where vulnerable individuals feel unsafe and helpless warrants the nursing diagnoses of *Anxiety*, *Fear*, *Hopelessness*, and *Powerlessness*. Constant negative messages and being treated in a disrespectful manner suggest the diagnoses of *Situational* and *Chronic low self-esteem*. Deficits in managing day-to-day responsibilities are addressed in *Ineffective individual coping*. The family as patient gets focus with diagnoses of *Dysfunctional family process*, *Impaired parenting*, *Disabled family coping*, *Caregiver role strain*, and *Ineffective role performance*.

OUTCOMES IDENTIFICATION

The *Nursing Outcomes Classification (NOC)* (Moorhead et al., 2013) provides an overall outcome where the individual is free from being hurt or exploited, or Abuse Cessation. The following indicators address specific types of abuse:

- Physical abuse has ceased.
- Emotional abuse has ceased.
- Sexual abuse has ceased.
- Financial exploitation has ceased.

Ratings that you may find quite useful in determining the degree to which an outcome has been met are available in *NOC* (pp. 71-76). These scales include Abuse Protection, Abuse Recovery, Abuse Recovery: Emotional; Abuse Recovery: Financial; Abuse Recovery: Physical; and Abuse Recovery: Sexual. An additional outcome addresses the perpetrator with Abusive Behavior Self-Restraint (p. 77). Other outcomes focus

TABLE 28-4 SIGNS AND SYMPTOMS, NURSING DIAGNOSES, AND OUTCOMES FOR FAMILY VIOLENCE

SIGNS AND SYMPTOMS	POTENTIAL NURSING DIAGNOSES	OUTCOMES
History of child abuse, history of violence, substance use, impulsivity, suicidal behavior	*Risk for violence (self- or other-directed)* *Risk for suicide*	Family members remain free of harm
Bruises, cuts, broken bones, lacerations, scars, burns, wounds in various phases of healing, vaginal-anal bruises, sores, discharge, peritoneal pain	*Pain* *Risk for infection*	Timely treatment of injuries, healing of physical injuries, absence of pain, protection from further injuries
Restlessness, scanning, vigilance, uncertainty, isolation, fear, depression, feelings of helplessness, decreased control over environment, abuse	*Anxiety* *Fear* *Hopelessness* *Powerlessness*	Behavioral manifestations of anxiety absent, reports a decrease in anxiety, reports feeling safe, expresses expectations of a positive future, sets goals
Poor eye contact and body posture, lack of respect from significant others, traumatic situation, neglect, feelings of shame and low self-esteem, feelings of worthlessness	*Situational low self-esteem* *Chronic low self-esteem*	Maintains eye contact and erect posture, describes positive level of confidence, expects positive responses from others, describes feelings of success and self-worth
Poor coping skills, hostility, impulsivity, inadequate problem solving, substance abuse	*Ineffective individual coping*	Discusses the abusive behavior, obtains needed treatment, controls impulses, refrains from substance abuse
Family disorganization, conflict, denial of problems, resistance to change, ineffective problem solving, chaotic family environment, abandonment, aggression, neglect, domestic violence	*Dysfunctional family process* *Impaired parenting* *Disabled family coping* *Caregiver role strain* *Ineffective role performance*	Emotional, physical, sexual, and neglectful behaviors have ceased, alternative coping methods for stress are used, mental health and community resources are utilized effectively

From Herdman, T. H. (Ed.) *Nursing diagnoses—Definitions and classification, 2012–2014.* Copyright © 2012, 1994–2012 by NANDA International. Used by arrangement with John Wiley & Sons Limited; Moorhead, S., Johnson, M., Maas, M. L., & Swanson, E. (2013). *Nursing outcomes classification (NOC)* (5th ed.). St. Louis, MO: Mosby.

on addressing the nursing diagnoses described in the previous section.

The identification of desired outcomes should be patient-centered, and therefore developed in conjunction with the survivor and primary support person. These outcomes should be continually reassessed and revised as new information about the survivor's needs emerges.

Table 28-4 identifies signs and symptoms, potential nursing diagnoses, and outcomes for victims of child, intimate partner, and elder abuse, as well as for abusers.

PLANNING

Nurses and other health care workers encounter abuse frequently, not only in health care settings but also in their communities and families. Unfortunately, those outside the family, including nurses, seldom recognize abuse within families. The nurse is often the first point of contact for people experiencing abuse and thus is in an ideal position to contribute to prevention, detection, and effective intervention. The Joint Commission requires staff education in family violence and abuse, as well as the development of standards of care to guide clinical practice (Family Violence Prevention Fund, 2004).

The Nursing Network on Violence Against Women encourages the development of a nursing practice that focuses on health issues relating to the effects of abuse on women's lives. Altering the pattern of violence against women can also affect child abuse because a key predictor of violence toward children is violence toward their mothers. Ultimately, the general tolerance of violence in the United States must be addressed if long-lasting changes are to be made.

Most hospitals and community centers provide protocols for dealing with child, intimate partner, or elder abuse that may or may not meet all the needs of a given patient. Unless it is a case of child abuse in which the child has been removed from the home, most interventions performed after necessary emergency care will take place within the community. Plans should center on the patient's safety first. Whenever it is possible or in the best interests of the patient, plans should be discussed with the patient. Planning should also take into consideration the needs of the abuser(s) (e.g., parents, caretakers, spouse or partner) if he or she is willing to learn alternatives to abuse and violence.

IMPLEMENTATION

Reporting Abuse

Nurses are legally mandated to report suspected or actual cases of child and vulnerable adult abuse. The appropriate agency may be the state or county child welfare agency, law enforcement agency, juvenile court, or county health department. Each state has specific guidelines for reporting, including whether the report can be oral, written, or both, and within what time period the suspected abuse or neglect must be reported (immediately, within 24 hours, or within 48 hours). Every abused person is a crime victim, and assault with a weapon is reportable in most states. All 50 states have marital rape statutes. The following vignette gives an example of a child-abuse case to report.

VIGNETTE

Two nurses who work in a family practice clinic are suspicious of child abuse. Hannah, 12 years old, has recurrent urinary tract infections. Her father, who accompanies her into the bathroom when she is providing urine samples, always brings her to clinic visits. He answers all questions for Hannah, even when they are directed to her. He has recently refused the next diagnostic test to attempt to ascertain the reason for the recurrent infections.

After pressure by the nurses, the physician agrees to ask Hannah some questions in private. The nurses think the physician has discounted the problem, asked superficial questions, and dismissed their concerns; however, the nurses are not successful in their attempt to separate Hannah from her father for a discussion. They decide to report their concerns to Children's Protective Services. They inform the father, who becomes outraged at their accusations and threatens to change doctors. Subsequent investigation confirms the likelihood of sexual abuse, and Hannah is placed in temporary foster care with follow-up counseling. The father refuses treatment and threatens to sue the nurses. Four months later, the father leaves the family.

The case in the preceding vignette illustrates that a reasonable basis for suspecting abuse, not proof, is all that is required to report. Nurses must attempt to maintain both an appropriate level of suspicion and a neutral, objective attitude. One can be too concerned and jump to conclusions (which are what the physician in this case thought the nurses were doing) or not be concerned enough and rationalize an incomplete examination to avoid confrontation (which is what the nurses thought the physician was doing). Given these opposing stances, the case was reported, as required by law and ethical standards, and Children's Protective Services was given the opportunity to investigate.

Competency may be a consideration in a situation of elder abuse. Unless the older adult has been found legally incompetent, he or she has the right to self-determination. Many older abused women are battered women who have grown old. They are not incompetent simply by virtue of their age; therefore, they would not legally be considered vulnerable adults.

Some institutions and health care agencies have developed guidelines for dealing with actual or suspected situations of abuse. These protocols list possible behaviors or conditions of older adults and the most appropriate intervention. Establishing such protocols is highly recommended because it gives support to the nurse's actions.

Quality nursing care for those experiencing abuse must be culturally sensitive. This means the nurse must be aware of the cultural issues that may affect response to violence and to intervention. For example, Cambodian women control their responses to stress and violence through non confrontation and withdrawal, which are designed to restore equilibrium. Culture is important because it is central to how people organize their experience. Even the most acculturated people have a tendency to revert to their cultural past in organizing coping strategies after a stressful event. If there is a language barrier, the nurse should speak slowly and clearly in English, without using jargon, and allow time for the response. If the patient speaks no English, a trained medical interpreter should be provided. A family member should *not* be used as interpreter in order to ensure confidentiality and protect the person from future retaliation.

Counseling

Counseling includes crisis intervention measures. It is important to emphasize that people have a right to live without fear of violence, physical harm, or assault. Telling an abused person that "no one deserves to be hit" can be a powerful statement in and of itself. The role of the nurse is to support the victim, counsel about safety, and facilitate access to other resources as appropriate. By listening, giving support, discussing options, and describing alternative ways of living, the nurse initiates an awareness of other possibilities.

All persons experiencing abuse should be counseled about developing a **safety plan**, a plan for a rapid escape when abuse recurs. Patients should be asked to identify the signs of escalation of violence and to pick a particular sign that will tell them in the future that "now is the time to leave." If children are present, they can all agree on a code word that, when spoken by the parent, means "It is time to go." If the individual plans ahead, it may be possible to leave before the violence occurs. It is important that the plan include a destination and transportation. The nurse should suggest packing the items listed in Box 28-6 ahead of time. The packed bag should be kept in a place where the perpetrator will not find it.

If the abused person chooses to leave, **shelters or safe houses** (for both sexes) are available in many communities. They are open 24 hours a day and can be reached through hotline information numbers, hospital emergency departments, YWCAs, or the local office of the National Organization for Women. The address of the house is usually kept secret to protect abused persons from attack by the perpetrator. Besides

BOX 28-6 PERSONALIZED SAFETY GUIDE

Suggestions for Increasing Safety While in the Relationship

- I will have important phone numbers available to my children and myself.
- I can tell _____ and _____ about the violence and ask them to call the police if they hear suspicious noises coming from my home.
- If I leave my home, I can go to (list four places) ______, ______, ______, or ______.
- I can leave extra money, car keys, clothes, and copies of documents with _______.
- If I leave, I will bring _______ (see checklist below).
- To ensure safety and independence, I will open my own savings account, rehearse my escape route with a support person, and review safety plan on _______ (date).

Suggestions for Increasing Safety When the Relationship Is Over

- I can change the locks; install steel or metal doors, a security system, smoke detectors, and an outside lighting system.
- I will inform ______ and _______ that my partner no longer lives with me and ask them to call the police if he or she is observed near my home or my children.
- I will tell people who take care of my children the names of those who have permission to pick them up. The people who have permission are ______, ______, and ______.
- I can tell ______ at work about my situation and ask ______ to screen my calls.
- I can avoid stores, banks, and _______ that I used when living with my battering partner.
- I can obtain a protective order from _______. I can keep it on or near me at all times, as well as have a copy with _______.
- If I feel down and ready to return to a potentially abusive situation, I can call ______ for support or attend workshops and support groups to gain support and strengthen my relationships with other people.

Important Phone Numbers

- Police ____________
- Hotline ____________
- Friends ____________
- Shelter ____________

Checklist of Items to Take

- Identification
- Birth certificates for me and my children
- Social Security card
- School and medical records
- Money, bank books, credit cards
- Keys to house, car, office
- Driver's license and registration
- Medications
- Change of clothes
- Welfare identification
- Passport(s), green card, work permit
- Divorce papers
- Lease or rental agreement, house deed
- Mortgage payment book, current unpaid bills
- Insurance papers
- Address book
- Pictures, jewelry, items of sentimental value
- Children's favorite toys and/or blankets

offering protection, many of these shelters and safe houses serve important educational and consciousness-raising functions. Patients should be given the number of the nearest available shelter, even if they decide for the present to stay with their partners. Referral phone numbers may be kept for years before the decision to call is made. Having the number and a contact person during that time contributes to thinking about options.

Case Management

Community mental health centers are becoming increasingly involved in the delivery of services to victims and perpetrators of abuse. Nurses working in these settings have the opportunity to coordinate community, medical, criminal justice, and social services to provide comprehensive assistance to families in crisis. Strategies must encompass needs for housing, child care, economic stability, physical and emotional safety, counseling, legal protection, career development or job training, education, ongoing support groups, and health care.

The myriad of agencies and people that those seeking help must reach can be daunting and confusing. A nurse functioning in a case manager role can assist the patient in choosing the best options and coordinating the interventions of several agencies. Box 28-7 lists selected *NIC* interventions for *Abuse protection support* for children, intimate partners, and older adults (Bulechek et al., 2013).

Therapeutic Environment

Interventions are geared toward stabilizing the home situation and maintaining an abuse-free environment. Some mental health agencies have family-based units in which a caseworker or clinician visits the home instead of the family going to the agency. Providing and maintaining a therapeutic environment in the home ideally involves three levels of help for abusive families:

1. Provide the family with economic support, job opportunities, and social services.
2. Arrange social support in the form of a public health nurse, lay home visitor, day care teacher, schoolteacher, social worker, respite worker, or any other potential contact person who has a good relationship with the family.
3. Encourage and provide family therapy.

Promotion of Self-Care Activities

The primary goal of intervention is empowerment. Supporting the patient to act on her or his own behalf can decrease feelings of helplessness and hopelessness. The initial phase of recovery begins when a patient first makes steps to leave the abusive relationship. Giving referral numbers and providing an opportunity

BOX 28-7 INTERVENTIONS FOR ABUSE PROTECTION SUPPORT FOR CHILDREN, INTIMATE PARTNERS, AND OLDER ADULTS

Abuse Protection Support: Children

Definition: Identification of high-risk, dependent child relationships and actions to prevent possible or further infliction of physical, sexual, or emotional harm or neglect of basic necessities of life

Activities:*

- Identify mothers who have a history of late (4 months or later) or no prenatal care.
- Identify parents who have had another child removed from the home or have placed previous children with relatives for extended periods.
- Identify parents with a history of domestic violence or a mother who has a history of numerous "accidental" injuries.
- Determine whether a child demonstrates signs of physical abuse, including numerous injuries in various stages of healing; unexplained bruises and welts; unexplained pattern, immersion, and friction burns; facial, spiral, shaft, or multiple fractures; unexplained facial lacerations and abrasions; human bite marks; intracranial, subdural, intraventricular, and intraocular hemorrhaging; whiplash shaken infant syndrome; and diseases that are resistant to treatment and/or have changing signs and symptoms.
- Encourage admission of child for further observation and investigation as appropriate.
- Monitor parent-child interactions and record observations.
- Report suspected abuse or neglect to proper authorities.

Abuse Protection Support: Intimate Partners

Definition: Identification of high-risk, dependent domestic relationships and action to prevent possible or further infliction of physical, sexual, or emotional harm or exploitation of a domestic partner

Activities:*

- Screen for risk factors associated with domestic abuse (e.g., history of domestic violence, abuse, rejection, excessive criticism, or feelings of being worthless and unloved; difficulty trusting others or feeling disliked by others; feeling that asking for help is an indication of personal incompetence; high physical care needs; intense family care responsibilities; substance abuse; depression; major psychiatric illness; social isolation; poor relationships between domestic partners; multiple marriages; pregnancy; poverty; unemployment; financial dependence; homelessness; infidelity; divorce; or death of a loved one).
- Document evidence of physical or sexual abuse using standardized assessment tools and photographs.
- Listen attentively to individual who begins to talk about own problems.
- Encourage admission to a hospital for further observation and investigation, as appropriate.
- Provide positive affirmation of worth.
- Report any situations in which abuse is suspected in compliance with mandatory reporting laws.

Abuse Protection Support: Older Adults

Definition: Identification of high-risk, dependent elder relationships and actions to prevent possible or further infliction of physical, sexual, or emotional harm; neglect of basic necessities of life; or exploitation

Activities:*

- Identify older patients who perceive themselves to be dependent on caretakers due to impaired health status, functional impairment, limited economic resources, depression, substance abuse, or lack of knowledge of available resources and alternatives for care.
- Identify family caretakers who have a history of being abused or neglected in childhood.
- Monitor patient-caretaker interactions and record observations.
- Report suspected abuse or neglect to proper authorities.

*Partial list.

Adapted from Bulechek, G. M., Butcher, H. K., Dochterman, J. M., & Wagner, C. (2013). *Nursing interventions classification (NIC)* (6th ed.). St. Louis, MO: Mosby.

for the patient to call from your office, or inquiring at the next visit whether the patient was successful in reaching the appropriate agency, demonstrates confidence in the patient's ability to take care of herself or himself.

Specific referrals regarding emergency financial assistance and legal counseling should be made available to each patient. Vocational counseling is another referral that may be appropriate. Patients should be given referrals to parenting resources that enable them to explore alternative approaches to discipline (e.g., no hitting, slapping, or other expressions of violence).

Health Teaching and Health Promotion

In families at risk for abuse, health teaching and health promotion includes meeting with both the individual and the family to help them learn to recognize behaviors and situations that might trigger violence.

Normal developmental and physiological changes should be explained to enable family members to gain a more positive view of the victim and the crisis situation. Gaining a more complete understanding can help family members broaden their insight and thus increase their compassion. They may then begin to anticipate new stress situations and be able to prepare for them before a crisis occurs.

Nurses who work on a maternity unit are often in a position to identify risk factors for abuse between new parents and initiate appropriate interventions, including education about effective parenting and coping techniques. Information about these interventions should be shared with the patient's health care team for appropriate monitoring and follow-up. Parents who are candidates for special attention include the following:

- New parents whose behavior toward the infant is rejecting, hostile, or indifferent.
- Teenage parents who require special help in handling the baby and discussing their expectations of the baby and their support systems.

- Parents with cognitive deficits, for whom careful, explicit, and repeated instructions on caring for the child and recognizing the infant's needs are indicated.
- Parents who grew up watching their mothers being abused. This is a significant risk factor for perpetuation of family violence.

Nurses can also recognize when children are at risk and make referrals to community resources, including emergency child care facilities, emergency telephone numbers, numbers of 24-hour crisis centers or hotlines, and respite programs in which volunteers take the child for an occasional weekend so that parents can get some relief. Community health nurses can make home visits to identify risk factors for abuse in the crucial first few months of life during which the style of parent-child interactions is established. See Box 28-5 for important factors for the community health nurse to assess during a home care visit. Such observations made by nurses in clinic and public health settings are fundamental in case finding and evaluation.

Prevention of Abuse

Primary Prevention

Primary prevention consists of measures taken to prevent the occurrence of abuse. Identifying individuals and families at high risk, providing health teaching, and coordinating supportive services to prevent crises are examples of primary prevention. Specific strategies include (1) reducing stress, (2) reducing the influence of risk factors, (3) increasing social support, (4) increasing coping skills, and (5) increasing self-esteem. Community health nurses are in a unique position to assess family functioning in the home during visits for other medical problems. In addition, the community health nurse and clinic nurse maintain contact with the family over time, which allows for assessment of changes. They are also in an excellent position to connect parents to appropriate resources in the community that can meet their needs. All nurses can work to reduce society's acceptance of violence by working toward social policy change.

Secondary Prevention

Secondary prevention involves early intervention in abusive situations to minimize their disabling or long-term effects. Nurses can establish screening programs for individuals at risk, participate in the medical treatment of injuries resulting from violent episodes, and coordinate community services to provide continuity of care. Stress and depression can be reduced by providing supportive psychotherapy, support groups, pharmacotherapy, and contact information for community resources. Social dysfunction or lack of information can be addressed by counseling and education. Caregiver burden can be reduced by arranging assistance in caring for the family member, housekeeping, or, in cases in which caregiving needs exceed even optimal caregiver capacity, by placing the patient in a more appropriate setting. The following vignette illustrates a successful secondary prevention effort.

VIGNETTE

Gavin, aged 6 years, is brought to the school nurse by his teacher, who said he had complained of an upset stomach. When the nurse examines Gavin, she notices bruises on his arms and abdomen. Gavin appears frightened and hesitant to speak.

Nurse: How did you hurt yourself, Gavin? *(Gavin looks down and starts to cry.)* It's OK if you don't want to talk about it.

Gavin: *(Does not look at the nurse and speaks softly.)* My mom hit me.

Nurse: Tell me what happened before that.

Gavin: Mom was mad because I didn't put my toys away.

Nurse: What does your mom usually do when she gets mad?

Gavin: She yells mostly. Sometimes she hits me.

Nurse: Tell me about the hitting.

Gavin: Mom hits me a lot since my dad left. *(Gavin starts to cry to himself.)*

Gavin appears well-nourished and properly dressed. He is at his approximate developmental age except for some language delay; however, because of the physical evidence and history, the nurse notifies Children's Protective Services, and the family situation is evaluated for possible placement of Gavin in protective custody. The initial evaluation concludes that there is no indication of serious potential harm to the child and that Gavin should return home. The mother, who is initially defensive, starts to cry and states, "I can't cope with being alone, and I don't know where to turn."

Nursing interventions center on caring for Gavin's immediate health needs, finding supports for the mother to help her cope with crises, providing a counseling referral for the mother to learn alternative ways of expressing anger and frustration, and informing the mother of parents' groups.

Tertiary Prevention

Tertiary prevention, which often occurs in mental health settings, involves nurses facilitating the healing and rehabilitative process by counseling individuals and families, providing support for groups of survivors, and assisting survivors of violence to achieve their optimal level of safety, health, and well-being. Legal advocacy programs for survivors of intimate partner violence are an example of tertiary prevention (Chamberlain, 2008). Complementary therapies, such as mindfulness-based stress reduction, can also assist survivors in the healing process.

Advanced Practice Interventions

Psychotherapy is carried out by a nurse who is educated at the master's or doctoral level and is certified in advanced practice psychiatric nursing. Therapy is most effective after crisis intervention, when the situation is less chaotic and tumultuous. A variety of therapeutic modalities are available for treatment of abusive families.

Individual Psychotherapy

The goals of individual therapy for a survivor are empowerment, the ability to recognize and choose productive life options, and the development of a solid sense of self. People who have experienced abuse as a child or have left a violent relationship may choose individual therapy to address symptoms of depression, anxiety, somatization, or PTSD.

Many of the psychological symptoms shown by women who have been abused can be understood as complex survival strategies and responses to violence. Nurses must address the guilt, shame, and stigmatization experienced by survivors of abuse. It is helpful for nurses to understand that the individual's feelings and behaviors may be reflective of the grieving process since he or she has experienced numerous losses as a result of the abusive relationship. Helping the survivor work through the stages of grieving can promote healing.

Individual psychotherapy is often indicated for the perpetrator, particularly when an individual psychopathological process is identified. Therapy for the perpetrator is most effective when it is court mandated because the perpetrator is more likely to complete the course of treatment. Nurses engaged in therapy with perpetrators have a duty to warn potential victims if they conclude that the perpetrator is a danger. Refer to Chapter 6 for a more detailed discussion of the duty to warn and duty to protect.

Family Psychotherapy

Because abuse is a symptom of a family in crisis, each part of the family system needs attention. Also, because change in one member of the family system affects the whole system, support and understanding are needed by all members. Interventions may maximize positive interactions among all family members. Family or marital therapy should take place *only* if the perpetrator has had individual therapy and has demonstrated change as a result and if both parties agree to participate.

Expected outcomes are that the perpetrator will recognize destructive patterns of behavior, learn alternative responses, control impulses, and refrain from abusive behavior. Intermediate goals are that members of the family will openly communicate and learn to listen to one another. Refer to Chapter 34 for a more detailed discussion of family therapy.

Group Psychotherapy

Participation in therapy groups provides assurances that one is not alone and that positive change is possible. Because many survivors of abuse have been isolated over time, they have been deprived of validation and positive feedback from others. Working in a group can help diminish feelings of isolation, strengthen feelings of self-esteem and self-worth, and increase the potential for realistic problem solving in a supportive atmosphere.

The real problem in an abusive relationship is the perpetrator. Groups often use cognitive-behavioral techniques to help the abuser see abusive actions as behavioral patterns that can be changed. In therapy groups, perpetrators are taught to recognize the thoughts preceding an abusive incident, the responses to the thoughts, and how to interrupt negative feelings about their partners. Perpetrators who have never discussed problems with anyone before are encouraged to discuss their thoughts and feelings. Group therapy can help create a community of healing and restoration. Refer to Chapter 33 for a more detailed discussion of group therapy.

EVALUATION

Failures of interventions with abusive families often are due to problems within the social, economic, and political systems in which we live. Nurses can direct their interventions to the social environment and can question, among other things, the acceptance of corporal punishment as a technique for guiding behavior in children, the unequal burden of caregiving responsibilities placed on women, the low priority given to education and preparation for parenthood, and the belief that older adults have little social value.

Evaluation of brief interventions can be based on whether the survivor acknowledges the violence, is willing to accept intervention, and is removed from the abusive situation. Evaluation of long-term interventions should be made on an ongoing basis. Because abuse is a symptom of a family in crisis, a multidisciplinary team that includes a physician, a nurse, a social worker, an attorney, and perhaps a psychiatrist should carry out diagnosis, interventions, and evaluation. Follow-up is crucial in helping decrease the frequency of family abuse.

28-1 CASE STUDY/NURSING CARE PLAN

Family Violence

Mrs. Robb, a recently widowed 84-year-old woman, moved to her son's apartment 3 months ago. She had been living in her third-floor walk-up in the city. Because of her declining health, crime in the neighborhood, and the need to climb three flights of stairs, and with her son John's encouragement, she went to live with him. He and his wife Judy, who have been married for almost 20 years, have five children 6 to 18 years of age, all living in a rather cramped three-bedroom apartment.

A visiting nurse, who monitors her blood pressure and adjusts her medication, is caring for Mrs. Robb. Over a series of visits, the nurse, Ms. Green, notices that Mrs. Robb is looking unkempt, pale, and withdrawn. While taking her blood pressure, Ms. Green observes bruises on Mrs. Robb's arms and neck. When questioned about the bruises, Mrs. Robb appears anxious and nervous. She says that she slipped in the bathroom. Mrs. Robb becomes increasingly apprehensive and stiffens up in her chair when her daughter-in-law Judy comes into the room, asking when the next visit is. The nurse notices that Judy avoids eye contact with Mrs. Robb.

When the injuries are brought to Judy's attention, she responds by becoming angry and agitated, blaming Mrs. Robb for causing so many problems. She will not explain the reason for the change in Mrs. Robb's behavior or the origin of the bruises to the nurse. She merely comments, "I have had to give up my job since my mother-in-law came here. It's been difficult and crowded ever since she moved in. The kids are complaining. We are having trouble making ends meet since I gave up my job, and my husband is no help at all."

Self-Assessment

Ms. Green has worked in a number of situations with violent families, but this is the first time she has encountered elder maltreatment. She discusses her reactions with the other team members. She is especially angry at Judy although she is able to understand the daughter-in-law's frustration. The team concurs with Ms. Green that there seems to be potential for positive change in this family. If abuse does not abate, more drastic measures will need to be taken and legal services contacted.

Assessment

Objective Data

- Physical symptoms of violence (bruises, unkempt appearance, withdrawn attitude)
- Stressful, crowded living conditions
- No eye contact between Mrs. Robb and her daughter-in-law
- Economic hardships leading to stress
- No support for the daughter-in-law from the rest of the family for care of Mrs. Robb

Subjective Data

- Mrs. Robb states she slipped in the bathroom, but physical findings do not support this explanation.
- Judy states, "It's been difficult and crowded ever since she moved in."
- Mrs. Robb exhibits withdrawn and apprehensive behavior.

Diagnosis

On the basis of the data, the nurse formulates the following nursing diagnoses:

1. *Risk for injury* related to increase in family stress, as evidenced by signs of violence

Supporting Data

- Mrs. Robb states she slipped in the bathroom, but physical findings do not support this explanation.
- Physical symptoms of violence (bruises, unkempt appearance, withdrawn attitude)
- Stressful, crowded living conditions

2. *Ineffective coping* related to helplessness, as evidenced by inability to meet role expectations

Supporting Data

- Mrs. Robb appears unkempt, anxious, depressed.
- Mrs. Robb exhibits withdrawn and apprehensive behavior.

3. *Risk for other-directed violence* related to increased stressors within a short period, as evidenced by probable elder abuse and feelings of helplessness verbalized by the primary caregiver

Supporting Data

- Judy states, "It's been difficult and crowded ever since she moved in."
- No eye contact between Judy and Mrs. Robb
- Signs and symptoms of physical abuse on Mrs. Robb
- Judy says, "My husband is no help at all."

4. *Caregiver role strain* related to extreme feelings of being overwhelmed and of helplessness

Supporting Data

- Family not helping with care of mother-in-law; burden of care on Judy
- Economic hardships leading to stress when Judy gave up her job to care for Mrs. Robb

Outcomes Identification

Overall outcome: Abuse cessation: Evidence that the victim is no longer hurt or exploited

Short-term indicators:

- Evidence that physical abuse has ceased
- Evidence that emotional abuse has ceased

Planning

Ms. Green discusses several possible outcomes with members of her team, giving attention to the priority of outcomes and to whether they are realistic in this situation. She also plans to report the elder abuse to Adult Protective Services and to work with Mrs. Robb, Judy, and the rest of the family to improve this situation for everyone.

Implementation

Mrs. Robb's plan of care is personalized as follows:

Nursing diagnosis: *Risk for injury* related to increase in family stress, as evidenced by signs of violence

Outcome criteria: Abuse cessation

28-1 CASE STUDY/NURSING CARE PLAN—cont'd

Family Violence

SHORT-TERM GOAL	INTERVENTION	RATIONALE	EVALUATION
1. On each visit made by the nurse, the patient will state that abuse has decreased, using a scale from 1 to 5 (1 being the least abuse).	1a. Provides maximum protection under the law. Provides data for future use.	1a. Follow state laws and guidelines for reporting elder abuse.	**GOAL MET** Patient states that after family talked to the nurse and planned strategies, physical abuse no longer occurs.
	1b. Assess severity of signs and symptoms of abuse.	1b. Accurate charting (body map, pictures with permission, verbatim statements) helps follow progress and provides legal data.	
	1c. Do a careful home assessment to identify other areas of abuse and neglect.	1c. Check for inadequacy of food, presence of vermin, blocked stairways, medication safety issues, etc. All indicate abuse and neglect. Determine the kinds of problems in the home, and plan intervention. Identify community resources that could help the elder and caregivers.	
	1d. Discuss with patient factors leading to abuse and concern for safety.	1d. Allows family stressors and potential areas for intervention to be identified. Validates that situation is serious and increases patient's knowledge base.	
2. Within 2 weeks, patient will be able to identify at least two supportive services to deal with emergency situations.	2. Discuss with patient supportive services such as hotlines and crisis units to call in case of emergency situations.	2. Maximizes patient's safety through use of support systems.	**GOAL MET** Patient has been talking to two old friends she had stopped talking to because of shame and depression. She has called the hotline once to get information on transportation to the senior center in town.
3. Within 3 weeks, family members will be able to identify difficult issues that increase their stress levels.	3. Discuss with family members their feelings and identify at least four areas that are most difficult for the various family members.	3. Listening to each family member and identifying unmet needs helps both family and nurse identify areas that require changing and appropriate interventions.	**GOAL MET** Family members identify areas such as overwork, lack of free time, lack of privacy, and financial difficulties, all of which increase their stress levels.
4. Within 3 weeks, family will seek out community resources to help with anger management, need for homemaker support, and other needs.	4. Identify potential community supports, skills training, respite places, homemakers, financial aids, etc., that might help meet family's unmet needs.	4. When stressed, individuals solve problems poorly and do not know about or cannot manage to organize outside help. Finances are often a problem.	**GOAL MET** The daughter-in-law is glad to get out of the house for anger management classes, and the son states he will try to take on more responsibility, but he often feels guilty and angry too. Reluctantly, he and his wife agree to try a support group with other caregivers in similar situations.

Evaluation

Eight weeks after Ms. Green's initial visit, Mrs. Robb appears well groomed, friendly, and more spontaneous in her conversation. She comments, "Things are better with my daughter-in-law." No bruises or other signs of physical violence are noticeable. She is considerably more outgoing and has even taken the initiative to contact an old friend. Mrs. Robb has talked openly to her son and daughter-in-law about stress in the family. Mrs. Robb says that she went for a walk when her daughter-in-law Judy appeared tense and returned to find that the tension had lessened. Neither Mrs. Robb nor her family has initiated plans for alternative housing.

KEY POINTS TO REMEMBER

- Abuse can occur in any family and can be predicted with some accuracy by examining the characteristics of perpetrators, vulnerable people, and crisis situations in which violence is likely.
- Abuse can be physical, sexual, emotional, or economic or can be caused by neglect.
- Assessment includes identifying indicators of abuse, levels of anxiety, coping mechanisms, support systems, suicide and homicide potential, and alcohol and drug abuse.

CRITICAL THINKING

1. A colleague who has witnessed a child being abused states, "I don't think it's any of our business what people do in the privacy of their own homes."
   a. What would you be legally required to do?
   b. What are your ethical responsibilities?
2. You successfully convinced your colleagues to assess routinely for abuse, and now they want to know how to do it. How would you go about teaching them to assess for child abuse? Intimate partner abuse? Elder abuse?
3. Your health maintenance organization's routine health screening form for adolescents, adults, and older adults has just been changed to include questions about family abuse. How would you respond to patients who indicate on this form that abuse occurs in their home?
4. Write out a safety plan that could be adopted by individuals who are being abused.
   a. Identify at least four referrals in your community for a victim of family violence.
   b. Identify two referrals in your community for a perpetrator of family violence.

CHAPTER REVIEW

1. An appropriate expected outcome in family therapy regarding the perpetrator of abuse would be:
   a. A decrease in family interaction so that there are fewer opportunities for abuse to occur.
   b. The perpetrator will recognize destructive patterns of behavior and learn alternate responses.
   c. The perpetrator will no longer live with the family but have supervised contact while undergoing intensive inpatient therapy.
   d. A triad of treatment modalities, including medication, counseling, and role-playing opportunities.
2. You are discharging Vanessa, a 30-year-old victim of domestic violence, from the emergency department. She has sustained bruises and abrasions but no serious trauma. She is fearful that Children's Services will take custody of her daughter. Her daughter has not been harmed and is safe with Vanessa's mother. Which intervention on your part is indicated?
   a. Report the assault to the police, because reporting of domestic violence is mandatory.
   b. Probe Vanessa for information to use as evidence in prosecuting the perpetrator.
   c. Advise Vanessa to leave her abusive partner and move in with her mother.
   d. Assist Vanessa to develop a safety plan for rapid escape should abuse happen again.
3. Nathan, a nursing student, is assigned to care for Shawna, who is recovering from injuries received during an episode of domestic violence, the third such assault for which she has received treatment. Nathan left home at age 17 to escape an abusive father. Which statements about Nathan's situation are accurate? *Select all that apply.*
   a. He may be prone to blame the patient for her injuries and abuse.
   b. His personal experiences give him special insight into the needs of this patient.
   c. His experiences are likely to make him more empathetic towards victims.
   d. Caring for victims of abuse will help him cope with his own abuse experiences.
   e. He may experience overwhelming emotions as a result of caring for abuse victims.
   f. He would likely benefit from clinical supervision related to caring for abuse victims.
4. Perpetrators of domestic violence tend to: *Select all that apply.*
   a. Have relatively poor social skills and to have grown up with poor role models.
   b. Believe they, if male, should be dominant and in charge in relationships.
   c. Force their mates to work and expect them to handle the financial decisions.
   d. Be controlling and willing to use force to maintain their power in relationships.
   e. Prevent their mates from having relationships and activities outside the family.
5. You are assessing Lindy, a 25-year-old woman who came to the emergency department with a broken arm. She states she slipped on the ice on the steps outside her home. She has numerous other bruises in different stages of healing. Her boyfriend, with whom she lives, accompanied her to the emergency department and aggressively responds to questions posed to the patient, while the patient remains silent. What is your best response to the boyfriend?
   a. "It sounds as if you care a lot about Lindy. She is lucky to have such support."
   b. "By answering the questions for her, it sounds as if you don't want her to answer. What are you afraid of?"
   c. "I now need to examine Lindy in private. Please wait outside the room. I will come get you when we are finished."
   d. "I am calling security to have you escorted out because you are being obnoxious."

Answers to Chapter Review
1. b; 2. d; 3. b, c, e, f; 4. a, b, d, e; 5. c.

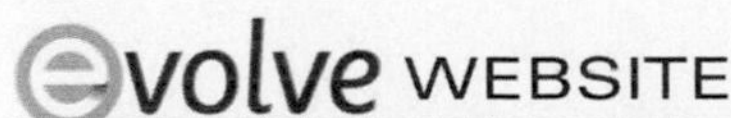

Visit the Evolve website for a posttest on the content in this chapter: http://evolve.elsevier.com/Varcarolis

Post-Test interactive review

REFERENCES

Acierno, R., Hernandez, M. A., Amstadter, A. B., Resnick, H. S., Steve, K., Mizzy, W., & Kilpatrick, D. G. (2010). Prevalence and correlates of emotional, physical, sexual, and financial abuse and potential neglect in the United States: The National Elder Mistreatment Study. *American Journal of Public Health, 100*(2), 292–297.

American Academy of Family Physicians. (2008). *Family and intimate partner violence and abuse.* Retrieved from http://www.aafp.org/online/en/home/policy/policies/f/familyandintimatepartner-violenceandabuse.html

American Psychological Association. (2012). *Elder abuse and neglect: In search of solutions.* Retrieved from http://www.apa.org/pi/aging/resources/guides/elder-abuse.aspx.

Black, M. C., Basile, K. C., Breiding, M. J., Smith, S. G., Walters, M. L., Merrick, M. T., Chen, J., & Stevens, M. R. (2011). *The national intimate partner and sexual violence survey (NISVS): 2010 summary report.* Atlanta, GA: National Center for Injury Prevention and Control, Centers for Disease Control and Prevention.

Bulechek, G. M., Butcher, H. K., Dochterman, J. M., & Wagner, C. (2013). *Nursing interventions classification (NIC)* (6th ed.). St. Louis, MO: Mosby.

Chamberlain, L. (2008). A prevention primer for domestic violence: Terminology, tools, and the public health approach. In P. A. Harrisburg (Ed.), *VAWnet, a project of the National Resource Center on Domestic Violence/Pennsylvania Coalition Against Domestic Violence.* Retrieved from http://www.vawnet.org/applied-research-papers/print-document.php?doc_id=1313.

Emergency Nurses Association. (2006). *Emergency Nurses Association position statements: Domestic violence, maltreatment, and neglect.* Retrieved from http://www.ena.org/SiteCollectionDocuments/Position%20Statements/Violence_-_Intimate_Partner_and_Family_-_ENA_PS.pdf.

Family Violence Prevention Fund. (2004). *Comply with JCAHO Standard PC.3.10 on victims of abuse.* Retrieved from http://www.futureswithoutviolence.org/section/our_work/health/_health_material/_jcaho.

Herdman, T.H. (Ed.), (2012). *NANDA international nursing diagnoses: Definitions and classification, 2012–2014.* Oxford, UK: Wiley Blackwell.

Malley-Morrison, K., & Hines, D. (2004). *Family violence in a cultural perspective: Defining, understanding and combating abuse.* Thousand Oaks, CA: Sage Publications.

Moorhead, S., Johnson, M., Maas, M. L., & Swanson, E. (2013). *Nursing outcomes classification (NOC)* (5th ed.). St. Louis, MO: Mosby.

Stephenson, R., Rentsch, C., Salazar, L., & Sullivan, P. (2011). Dyadic characteristics and intimate partner violence among men who have had sex with men. *Western Journal of Emergency Medicine, 12*(3), 324–332.

Soeken, K., McFarlane, J., Parker, B., & Lominack, M. (1998). The abuse assessment screen: A clinical instrument to measure frequency, severity and perpetrator of abuse against women. In J. Campbell (Ed.), *Empowering survivors of abuse: Health care for battered women and their children* (pp. 575–579). New Brunswick, NJ: Transaction.

U.S. Bureau of Justice Statistics. (2007). *Intimate partner violence in the U.S.: Victim characteristics.* Retrieved from http://www.bjs.gov/content/intimate/victims.cfm.

U.S. Department of Health & Human Services, Administration for Children and Families, Administration on Children, Youth and Families Children's Bureau. (2011). *Child maltreatment 2010.* Retrieved from http://www.acf.hhs.gov/programs/cb/pubs/cm10/index.htm.

Walker, L. E. (1979). *The battered woman* (2nd ed.). New York, NY: Springer.

CHAPTER

29

Sexual Assault

Jodie Flynn and Margaret Jordan Halter

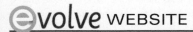

Visit the Evolve website for a pretest on the content in this chapter: http://evolve.elsevier.com/Varcarolis

Pre-Test interactive review

OBJECTIVES

1. Define sexual assault, sexual violence, rape, and attempted rape.
2. Discuss the implications for the underreporting of sexual assault.
3. Describe the profile of the victim and the perpetrator of sexual assault.
4. Distinguish between the acute and long-term phases of the rape-trauma syndrome, and identify some common reactions during each phase.
5. Identify five areas to assess when working with a person who has been sexually assaulted.
6. Analyze personal thoughts and feelings regarding rape and its impact on survivors.
7. Formulate two long-term outcomes and two short-term goals for the nursing diagnosis posttrauma syndrome.
8. Identify six overall guidelines for nursing interventions related to sexual assault.
9. Describe the role of the sexual assault nurse examiner to a colleague.
10. Discuss the long-term psychological effects of sexual assault that might lead a patient to seek psychological care.
11. Identify three outcome criteria that would signify successful interventions for a person who has suffered a sexual assault.

KEY TERMS AND CONCEPTS

acquaintance (or date) rape
attempted rape
rape
rape-trauma syndrome
sexual assault
sexual violence
spousal (or marital) rape

In 2008, a 42-year-old Austrian woman, Elisabeth Fritzl, reported to police that she had been imprisoned in the soundproofed, windowless cellar of her family home since the age of 18. Her own father, Josef Fritzl, lured her there, locked her in, and repeatedly raped her for the next 24 years. This abuse resulted in seven children, one of whom died shortly after birth. Three of the surviving children were taken upstairs to be raised by Fritzl and his wife. He explained to his wife that their daughter, Elisabeth, had run away to join a cult and had left the children on the doorstep. The other three children remained in the cellar with their mother, never seeing the light of day, and were forced to be present for the continual rape of their mother by their father/grandfather. When the moldy, dark conditions caused the eldest daughter, Kersten, 19, to become mortally ill, Elisabeth begged Fritzl to get her treatment. Fritzl relented and took her to a hospital, where Elisabeth would later be taken to visit. It was there that Elisabeth revealed the nature of her daughter's illness and her own abuse, on the condition that she would never have to see her father again.

This story is horrific and demonstrates some of the most contemptible violations that can be perpetrated by one human being on another. In this chapter, we will further explore these violations. **Sexual assault** and **sexual violence** are broad terms that encompass unwanted sexual advances and sexual harassment to stranger rape, marital rape, date rape, and drug-facilitated sexual assault. Incest, human sex trafficking, and female genital mutilation are other examples of sexual assault. Although sexual assault generally involves adult males assaulting adult females, it includes any combination of females, males, adults, and children. Vulnerable individuals such as the disabled and the elderly are often targets. Sexual violence also includes denying emergency contraception or measures to prevent sexually transmitted infections, organized rape during conflict or war, and sexual homicide.

In 2012, U.S. Attorney General Eric Holder announced revisions to the Uniform Crime Report's definition of rape (U.S. Department of Justice, FBI, 2012). **Rape** is defined in the context of nonconsensual activity and involves any penetration of the vagina or anus with any object or body part or the oral penetration by a sex organ of another person. This comprehensive definition will lead to a more uniform statistical reporting of rapes and replaces a decades-old one that did not account for men as victims. **Attempted rape** refers to threats of rape or intention to rape that is unsuccessful.

Because state laws vary in regard to sexual assault, it is important for you to identify how sexual acts are medically and legally defined within your community. Based on your jurisdiction and legal mandates, health care providers may be required to report a sexual assault to law enforcement. Patient identification may be withheld if the individual wishes to remain anonymous; evidence can be stored until the individual decides whether he or she wishes to report the assault. Regardless of whether individuals report the sexual assault to police, states and tribal governments are required to pay for or reimburse for sexual assault exams (109th Congress of the United States, 2005). Failure to comply with this mandate results in loss of funding from the Violence Against Women grant initiatives. This mandate is patient centered and gives control back to individuals who should be the primary decision makers in personal health and legal matters.

The Federal Bureau of Investigation (FBI) (2008) considers rape to be the second-most violent crime in a group of crimes that includes murder, robbery, and aggravated assault. Victims are traumatized, both physically and emotionally, and are often seen in health care settings. Nurses are instrumental in providing holistic care for those who have been sexually assaulted and also in helping to preserve evidence. Preservation of evidence can lead to the prosecution of a crime or the exoneration of a person of interest; therefore, it is essential that nurses be informed adequately about their roles and responsibilities with regard to providing both medical and legal care and ensuring that nursing policies and procedures effectively manage the care of sexual assault patients.

For the remainder of this chapter, victims of sexual assault will be referred to using the female pronoun in recognition of the fact that women are more frequently sexually assaulted; however, the principles discussed apply to anyone. In health care settings, victims of sexual assault are referred to as *patients;* advocacy groups use the term *survivor;* and legal systems use the term *victim.* Within this chapter, individuals will often be referred to as *patients* because those individuals are cared for in health care settings.

EPIDEMIOLOGY

Nearly 1 in 5 women and 1 in 71 men in the United States have been raped at some time in their lives (Black, et al., 2011). According to the National Intimate Partner and Sexual Violence Survey (NISVS) (2011), most female victims will experience their first rape before the age of 25, with 42.2% reporting a rape before the age of 18 years. More than one quarter of male victims experienced their first rape when they were 10 years of age or younger. Each year, women experience about 4.8 million intimate partner-related physical assaults and rapes (Centers for Disease Control, 2011).

Lifetime prevalence of rape is 18% among U.S. adult women, and few rape survivors seek immediate medical attention, even with serious injury (Tjaden & Thomas, 2008). For male victims, more than half (52.4%) reported being raped by an acquaintance and 15.1% by a stranger (Black et al., 2011). A male who is raped is more likely to experience physical trauma and to have been victimized by several assailants. Reports of male-to-male rape occur primarily in locked institutions, such as prisons and maximum-security hospitals. Males experience the same devastation, physical injury, and emotional consequences as females. Although they may cover their responses, they too benefit from care and treatment.

Race and ethnicity are important variables in rape statistics. The NISVS (2011) reports that approximately 22% of black women, nearly 19% of white non-Hispanic women, and about 15% of Hispanic women in the United States have experienced rape at some point in their lives. More than 25% of women who identify themselves as American Indian or as Alaskan Natives and about 33% of women who identified as multiracial non-Hispanic have reported rape victimization.

Precise estimates of sexual violence are impossible since this crime is greatly underreported, but there is reason for optimism. According to the 2011 FBI Uniform Crime Reporting Program, there was a decrease of about 5% for a majority of population groups. A reduction of sexual assault cases is part of an overall trend that may be due to several factors: policies that support longer sentences for perpetrators, mandatory sentences, and trained health care providers who specialize in caring for victims of sexual assault. Women and men today may be willing to report sexual violence, which may be a deterring factor.

Prevention efforts should include a multidisciplinary response in caring for victims of sexual violence. Nurses are often frontline health care providers who are needed to help coordinate these efforts. Men and women need to receive timely, competent care and help navigating both the health care and legal systems. Collective action is needed to help ensure short-term and long-term recovery as well as to prevent future adverse health consequences as a result of sexual victimization.

Sexual Offenders and Relationships with Victims

While we often think of a stranger lurking in the shadows of parking lots as the typical sexual offender, this is not true. The terms **spousal (or marital) rape** and **acquaintance (or date) rape** describe the nature of the relationship between victim and rapist. In recent years, courts have recognized spousal (or marital) rape, in which the perpetrator (nearly always the male) is married to the person raped. In acquaintance (or date) rape, the perpetrator is known to, and presumably trusted by, the person raped. The psychological and emotional outcomes of rape seem to vary depending on the level of intimacy between the victim and the perpetrator. Sexual distress is more common among women who have been sexually assaulted by intimates, and fear and anxiety are more common in those assaulted by strangers. Depression occurs in both groups.

Females know their offenders in almost 70% of all violent crimes committed against them; males know their offenders 45% of the time (Truman & Rand, 2010). Acquaintance (or date) rape has increased in incidence in the United States in recent years, with drugs, often combined with alcohol, being used to commit sexual assault. Date-rape drugs may render a woman incapable of resisting the attack and are purported to facilitate acquaintance rape. Often these drugs are given to the unknowing victim. Once the drugs are ingested, victims lose their ability to ward off attackers, develop amnesia, and become unreliable witnesses. Because the symptoms mimic those of alcohol, victims are not always screened for these drugs. The increase in prevalence and incidence of drug-assisted rape led to the passage of the Drug-Induced Rape Prevention and Punishment Act in 1996. This law allows up to 20 years imprisonment and fines for anyone who intends to commit a violent crime by administering a controlled substance to an unknowing individual (U.S. Department of Justice, 1997). Table 29-1 provides information about date-rape drugs.

CLINICAL PICTURE

Just as there is no typical patient presentation following a sexual assault, psychological presentation will vary from person to

TABLE 29-1 DRUGS ASSOCIATED WITH DATE RAPE

DRUG, ALTERNATE NAMES, AND STATUS IN THE UNITED STATES	FORM, MECHANISM OF ACTION, AND ONSET	EFFECT ON VICTIM	OVERDOSE SYMPTOMS AND TREATMENT
GHB (γ-hydroxy-butyric acid) Also known as *G, Georgia home boy, liquid ecstasy, salty water, and scoop* Legal in the United States for narcolepsy Often made in home labs	Liquid, white powder, or pill with a salty taste Schedule III central nervous system depressant A metabolite of γ-aminobutyric acid Onset within 5-20 minutes; duration is dose related and from 1-12 hours	Produces relaxation, euphoria, and disinhibition Incoordination, confusion, deep sedation, and amnesia Tolerance and dependence exhibited by agitation, tachycardia, insomnia, anxiety, tremors, and sweating	Respiratory depression, seizures, nausea, vomiting, bradycardia, hypothermia, agitation, delirium, unconsciousness, and coma Intubation for severe respiratory distress; atropine for bradycardia, and benzodiazepines for seizure activity. Vomiting should be induced when possible.
Rohypnol (flunitrazepam)* Also known as *forget-me pill, roofies, club drug, roachies, R2, and rophies* Not legal in the United States	Pill that dissolves in liquids Schedule IV potent benzodiazepine; 10 times stronger than diazepam Impact is within 10-30 minutes and lasts 2-12 hours	More potent when combined with alcohol; causes sedation, psychomotor slowing, muscle relaxation, and amnesia Dependence and tolerance may develop	Overdose unlikely Airway protection and gastrointestinal decontamination
Ketamine Also known as *black hole, bump, K, kit kat, purple, and Special K* Legal in the United States for anesthesia	Comes as a liquid or a white powder An anesthetic frequently used in veterinary practice; also a hallucinogenic substance related to PCP (phencyclidine) Onset within 30 seconds intravenously and 20 minutes orally; duration only 30-60 minutes; amnesia effects may last longer	Causes dissociative reaction, with a dreamlike state leading to deep amnesia and analgesia and complete compliance of the victim May become confused, paranoid, delirious, combative, with drooling and hallucinations	Airway maintenance and use of anticholinergics such as atropine and benzodiazepines

*Two other benzodiazepines, clonazepam (Klonopin) and alprazolam (Xanax), are also used.

Data from Lehne, R. A. (2010). *Pharmacology for nursing care* (7th ed.). Philadelphia, PA: Saunders; U.S. Department of Health and Human Services. (2008). *Date rape drugs.* Retrieved from http://www.womenshealth.gov/faq/date-rape-drugs.cfm.

person. Psychological effects include those found in acute stress disorder and posttraumatic stress disorder.

Acute stress disorder is a psychological reaction to a serious trauma, such as witnessing a death, suffering a serious injury, or a sexual violation. Those who suffer from acute stress disorder following sexual assault are at an increased risk for psychological problems as a result of that trauma (Gaffney, 2011).

Sexual assault is deemed a traumatic event that may incite vivid dreams, flashbacks, illusions, recurring images, and marked avoidance of stimuli (e.g., sights, smells, sounds, places) that provides recall of the event. Symptoms usually begin immediately after the sexual assault, persist at least 3 days, and can extend for up to 1 month.

Acute stress can lead to **posttraumatic stress disorder** (PTSD) if symptoms extend beyond 1 month. According to the National Institute of Mental Health (2009), PTSD symptoms can be grouped into three main categories:

1. Reexperiencing: Repeated reliving of the event that interferes with daily activity. This category includes flashbacks, frightening thoughts, recurrent memories or dreams, and physical reactions to situations that remind you of the event.
2. Avoidance: Changing routines to escape similar situations to the trauma. Victims might avoid places, events, or objects that remind them of the experience. Emotions related to avoidance are numbness, guilt, and depression. Some have a decreased ability to feel certain emotions, such as happiness. They also might be unable to remember major parts of the trauma and feel that their future offers fewer possibilities than other people have.
3. Hyperarousal: Difficulty concentrating or falling asleep, being easily startled, feeling tense, and angry outbursts. These can combine to make it difficult for victims to complete normal daily tasks.

Psychological Effects of Sexual Assault

Most people who are raped suffer severe and long-lasting emotional trauma. Long-term psychological effects of sexual assault may include depression, suicide, anxiety, and fear; difficulties with daily functioning; low self-esteem; sexual dysfunction; and somatic complaints. Victims of incest may experience a negative self-image, depression, eating disorders, personality disorders, self-destructive behavior, and substance abuse. A history of sexual abuse in psychiatric patients is associated with a characteristic pattern of symptoms that may include depression, anxiety disorders, chemical dependency, suicide attempts, self-mutilation, compulsive sexual behavior, and psychosis-like symptoms (Read et al., 2007).

Specialized Sexual Assault Services

Facilities may have trained **Sexual Assault Nurse Examiners (SANEs)** or other specially trained clinicians to provide care to patients who have been sexually assaulted. A SANE is a registered nurse who has specialized training in caring for sexual assault patients, has demonstrated competency in conducting medical and legal evaluations, and has the ability to be an expert witness in court. A SANE is a member of the Sexual Assault Response Team (SART), a multidisciplinary team approach to caring for victims of sexual assault. Members include nurses, physicians, attorneys, social service workers, advocates, mental health professionals, forensic lab personnel, and other collaborative agencies that provide services for sexual assault patients. If a SANE or specially trained clinician is not available in your facility, nurses should be prepared to provide both the medical and legal aspects of care.

APPLICATION OF THE NURSING PROCESS

ASSESSMENT

According to the Centers for Disease Control and Prevention (2010), sexual assault represented 8% of all nonfatal violence-related injury visits to emergency departments for females in 2008. According to the U.S. Department of Justice, 32% of sexual assault victims seek help in a hospital emergency department. The attention the patient receives depends on the policy of the health care facility.

The U.S. Department of Justice (2004) publishes *A National Protocol for Sexual Assault Medical/Forensic Examinations* to assist health care facilities in establishing protocols in caring for adult and adolescent sexual assault patients. This protocol has been instrumental in guiding care toward a more comprehensive approach to sexual assault care. According to the protocol, the medical exam should include the following:

1. Information from the patient
2. An examination
3. Documentation of biological and physical findings
4. Collection of evidence
5. Follow-up as needed to document additional evidence

The Emergency Nurses Association (2010) position statement on care of sexual assault and rape victims suggests:

1. An individualized, multidisciplinary, multiagency approach.
2. A physical and social environment conducive to private, empathetic, and unbiased care by health care providers, family members, law enforcement officers, and members of the justice system.
3. A private and safe environment, with personnel limited to examining health care providers during sexual assault care. Translators must be available if needed. With the consent of the patient, a specially trained advocate also may be present.
4. Comprehensive, competent, and sensitive emergency health care.
5. Employment of SANE nurses in the emergency department is highly recommended.
6. Emergency nurses should collaborate to promote and establish ongoing community education focused on preparing the public and emergency nurses to better identify, prevent, care for, and report incidents of sexual assault and rape.
7. Emergency nurses should be involved in research concerning the identification, assessment, and treatment of victims of sexual assault and rape.

Historically, patients who were sexually assaulted and went to health care facilities for medical care and evidence collection had to wait for long periods of time to be evaluated. Often, they were not considered in need of acute care because they lacked visible physical injuries. Now, a patient who is sexually assaulted is considered a priority due to the intense psychological impact and potential hidden physical injury. Collecting legal evidence is also a priority, and delays may result in its destruction or contamination.

The care of sexual assault victims varies from facility to facility. In one Midwestern study, researchers found that virtually all emergency departments provided acute medical care (Patel et al., 2008); however, only two thirds of these agencies offered rape counseling and sexually transmitted infection management. Counseling and emergency contraceptives were provided by 40% of facilities, and HIV management was provided by 30% of the facilities. Just 10% of the emergency departments provided all of these services to victims of sexual assault.

General Assessment

The nurse should talk with the patient, the family or friends who accompany the patient, and the police to gather as much data as possible for assessing the crisis. The nurse then assesses the patient's (1) level of anxiety, (2) coping mechanisms, (3) available support systems, (4) signs and symptoms of emotional trauma, and (5) signs and symptoms of physical trauma. Information obtained from the assessment is then analyzed, and nursing diagnoses are formulated.

Level of Anxiety

Patients experiencing severe-to-panic levels of anxiety will not be able to problem solve or process information. Support, reassurance, and appropriate therapeutic techniques can lower the patient's anxiety and facilitate mutual goal setting and the assimilation of information. Refer to Chapters 10 and 15 for more detailed discussions of the levels of anxiety and therapeutic interventions.

Coping Mechanisms

The same coping skills that have helped the survivor through other difficult problems in her lifetime will be used in adjusting to the rape. In addition, new ways of getting through the difficult times may be developed for both the short- and long-term adjustment. Behavioral responses include crying, withdrawing, smoking, abusing alcohol and drugs, talking about the event, becoming extremely agitated, confused, disoriented, incoherent, and even laughing or joking.

Cognitive coping mechanisms are the thoughts people have that help them deal with high anxiety levels. A positive cognitive response might be "At least I am alive and will get to see my children again." Not-so-positive responses may become generalized as a way to sum up the situation: "It's my fault this happened; my mother warned me about working in such a trashy place" may develop into an ego-damaging refrain. If such thoughts are verbalized, the nurse will know what the patient is thinking. If not, the nurse can ask questions such as "What are you thinking and feeling?" or "What can I do to help you in this difficult situation?" or "What has helped in the past?"

Available Support Systems

The availability, size, and usefulness of a patient's social support system must be assessed. Often partners or family members do not understand the survivor's feelings about the sexual assault, and they may not be the best supports available. Pay careful attention to verbal and nonverbal cues of the patient that may communicate the strength of the social network.

Involve the patient, family, or friends, who accompany the patient, or other health care providers in collaborative holistic data collection. Obtaining information from others is particularly important if the patient is unable to provide details surrounding the sexual assault (i.e., the patient is unconscious, nonverbal, or has a disability). If interpreting services are needed, please contact a certified medical interpreter to assist.

VIGNETTE

Celia, a home care provider, brings Ms. Smith, a 64-year-old woman with a history of schizophrenia, to the emergency department. Celia shared with the triage nurse that Ms. Smith, who is also a paraplegic, has been reclusive for the last few days and behaving strangely. According to Celia, Ms. Smith does not eat, sleeps all day, and repeatedly says that she is pregnant.

The triage nurse asked Ms. Smith, "Can you tell me why you are here?" Ms. Smith began to sob, stared at the floor, began rocking back and forth in her wheelchair, and muttered, "Someone is hurting me, and I am pregnant." A physical assessment reveals bruises on her upper thigh and breasts. The triage nurse has been trained as a sexual assault nurse examiner (SANE) and immediately recognizes that Ms. Smith needs a sexual assault evaluation. She states, "I believe you, and I will help you. You are safe here." Ms. Smith speaks, "Thank you."

Signs and Symptoms of Emotional Trauma

The first challenge for any health care provider is to identify if a forensic patient exists, as in the clinical situation above. A forensic patient is anyone who seeks treatment that interfaces with the law or has the potential to interface with the law. Patients may disclose a history of sexual assault or report a history that is inconsistent with physical findings; others may demonstrate a behavioral change that causes a concern for family, friends, caregivers, or other health care providers. Patients may present to a health care facility after a sexual assault occurs, visit their primary care physician, or contact law enforcement. No matter how or where the initial presentation occurs, sexual assault patients need acute intervention.

Nurses work with sexual assault survivors most frequently in the emergency department soon after a sex crime has occurred. Rape is a psychological emergency and should receive immediate attention. Some emergency departments provide the services of sexual assault nurse examiners (SANEs) or clinicians specially trained to meet the needs of patients who are sexually assaulted. They are trained to assess the extent of psychological and emotional trauma that may not be readily apparent.

A nursing history should be obtained and carefully recorded. When taking a history, the nurse determines only the details of the assault that will be helpful in addressing the immediate physical and psychological needs of the patient. The nurse allows the patient to talk at a comfortable pace; poses questions in nonjudgmental, descriptive terms; and refrains from asking "why" questions. The patient frequently finds that relating the events of the rape is traumatic and embarrassing.

If suicidal thoughts are expressed, ask direct questions, such as "Are you thinking of harming yourself?" or "Have you ever tried to kill yourself before or after this attack occurred?" If the answer is yes, the nurse conducts a thorough suicide assessment (plan, means to carry it out), as described in Chapter 25.

Signs and Symptoms of Physical Trauma

It is essential that nurses provide psychological support while collecting and preserving legal evidence. The nurse should be conscientious of the patient's reactions during the physical exam and advise her to report any signs of pain or discomfort immediately.

During the examination, the nurse will inspect and palpate for any signs of injury. Recent injuries may not show visible bruising; therefore, failure to palpate the skin can prevent evidence collection and further documentation of an injured site. The most characteristic physical signs of sexual assault are injuries to the face, head, neck, and extremities. Any physical injuries should be carefully documented (i.e., size, color, description, and location of injury should be noted), both in narrative and pictorial form using preprinted body maps, hand-drawn copies, or photographs. If an injury is present, ask the patient if she knows how that injury occurred.

The nurse will collect and preserve legal evidence, such as a blood standard, hair samples, oral swabs, nail swabs or scrapings, and anal, genital, or penile swabs. Facilities may have standardized Sexual Assault Evidence Collection Kits (SAECKs) that provide direction in how to collection and preserve evidence. This can be helpful to nurses and other clinicians who do not have specialized training in evidence collection and preservation.

The nurse takes a gynecological history, including the date of the last menstrual period and the likelihood of current pregnancy, and assesses for a history of sexually transmitted infections. A detailed genital examination, with speculum insertion, is needed to observe for signs of injury for the female patient. If the patient has never undergone a genital examination, the steps of the examination will need to be explained. The nurse plays a crucial role in giving support and minimizing the trauma of the examination because the patient may experience it as another violation of her body. Recognizing this, the nurse can explain the examination procedure in a way that will be reassuring and supportive. Providing details of this procedure helps prevent revictimization. Allowing the patient to participate in all decisions affecting care helps her regain a sense of control.

Best Practice Guidelines. The examination involves five steps:

1. Head-to-toe physical assessment, observing for signs of injury
2. Detailed genital examination, observing for signs of injury
3. Evidence collection and preservation
4. Documentation of physical findings (both written and photo documentation)
5. Treatment, discharge planning, and follow-up care

The patient has the right to decline parts of the legal or medical examination. Informed consent must be provided and consent forms signed before photographs are taken, a physical examination occurs, and any other procedures that might be needed to collect evidence and provide treatment. A shower and change of clothing should be made available to the patient as soon as possible after the examination and collection of evidence.

Providing prophylactic treatment for sexually transmitted diseases—according to guidelines of the Centers for Disease Control and Prevention (2010)—is common practice. Historically, sexual assault patients are noncompliant with follow-up visits after a sexual assault (Ackerman et al., 2006). Sexually transmitted diseases, including HIV and hepatitis exposure, are often a concern of patients who are sexually assaulted. This concern should always be addressed and the patient given information needed to evaluate the likelihood of risk and follow-up care. With this information, the person and her sexual partner(s) can make educated choices about testing and safer sex practices until further testing can be done.

About 5% of women who are raped become pregnant as a result (Rape, Abuse & Incest National Network, 2008). Pregnancy prevention is offered in the emergency department once pregnancy tests establish that the patient was not already pregnant prior to the assault. Emergency contraception or morning-after pills are contraceptives that do not cause abortion. They act on follicular development and inhibit ovulation (Gemzell-Danielsson, 2010). If there is no egg available to the sperm, then pregnancy cannot occur.

Assessment data are carefully documented, including verbatim statements by the patient, detailed observations of emotional and physical status, and all results of the physical examination. All laboratory tests performed are noted and findings recorded as soon as they are available. One of the greatest concerns is that crucial evidence may be lost or overlooked.

Self-Assessment

Nurses' attitudes influence the physical and psychological care received by rape survivors. Knowing the myths and facts surrounding sexual assault can increase your awareness of your personal beliefs and feelings regarding rape. If you examine personal feelings and reactions *before* encountering a patient who has been sexually assaulted, you will be better prepared to give empathetic and effective care. Examining your feelings about abortion is also important because a patient might choose an abortion if a pregnancy results from rape. Table 29-2 compares rape myths and facts.

DIAGNOSIS

Several domains of functioning are impacted by sexual assault and rape. Specific to rape, the NANDA International coping/stress tolerance domain is the most relevant. Within this domain, the nursing diagnosis of *rape-trauma syndrome* applies to the physical and psychological effects of rape. **Rape-trauma syndrome** is defined as "sustained and maladaptive response to

TABLE 29-2 MYTH VERSUS FACT: RAPE

MYTH	FACT
Many women really want to be raped.	Women do not ask to be raped—no matter how they are dressed, what their behavior is, or where they are at any given time. Studies show that violence toward women in the media leads to attitudes that foster tolerance of rape.
Most rapists are oversexed.	Sex is used as an instrument of violence in rape. Rape is an act of aggression, anger, or power.
Most women are raped by strangers.	The majority (69%) of rape victims are raped by someone they knew.
No healthy adult female who resists vigorously can be raped by an unarmed man.	Most men can overpower most women because of differences in body build. Also, the victim may panic, which makes her actions less effective than usual.
Most charges of rape are unfounded.	There is no evidence to show that there are more false reports for rape than for other crimes. Most rape victims do not even report the rape.
Rapes usually occur in dark alleys.	Over 50% of all rapes occur in the home.
Rape is usually an impulsive act.	Most rapes are planned; over 50% involve a weapon.
Nice girls don't get raped.	Any woman is a potential rape victim. Victims range in age from 6 months to 90 years.
There was not enough time for a rape to occur.	There is no minimal time limit that characterizes rape. It can happen very quickly.
Do not fight or try to get away, because you will just get hurt.	There are no verifiable data to substantiate the theory that a victim will be injured if he or she tries to get away.
Only females are raped.	There are a growing number of male rape victims.
Rape is a sexual act.	Rape is a violent expression of aggression, anger, and need for power.

ASSESSMENT GUIDELINES

Sexual Assault

1. Assess psychological trauma, and document the patient's verbatim statements.
2. Assess level of anxiety. If in a severe-to-panic level of anxiety, the patient will not be able to problem solve or process information.
3. Assess physical trauma. Use a preprinted body map, and ask permission to take photographs.
4. Assess available support system. Often partners or family members do not understand the trauma of rape, and they may not be the best supports to draw on at this time.
5. Identify community supports (e.g., attorneys, support groups, therapists) that work in the area of sexual assault.
6. Encourage the patient to talk about the experience, but do not press the patient to tell.

a forced, violent sexual penetration against the victim's will and consent" (Herdman, 2012, p. 337). Defining characteristics of rape-trauma syndrome are listed in Box 29-1.

A variety of diagnoses would also apply to the victim of sexual assault. They include, but are not limited to, the following:

- Disturbed personal identity
- Situational low self-esteem
- Interrupted family processes
- Ineffective relationship
- Sexual identity
- Sexual dysfunction
- Anxiety
- Fear
- Social isolation

BOX 29-1 DEFINING CHARACTERISTICS OF RAPE-TRAUMA SYNDROME

Shame	Mood swings	Anxiety	Dissociation
Guilt	Aggression	Fear	Disorganization
Helplessness	Anger	Disturbed sleep	Shock
Powerlessness	Agitation	Nightmares	Confusion
Dependence	Revenge	Sexual dysfunction	Phobias
Low self-esteem	Substance abuse	Muscle tension	Paranoia
Depression	Suicide attempts	Hyperalertness	

OUTCOMES IDENTIFICATION

The long-term outcome includes the absence of any residual symptoms after the trauma. S*exual abuse recovery* is specifically linked to sexual assault. It is defined as "extent of healing of physical and psychological injuries due to sexual abuse or exploitation" (Moorhead et al., 2013, p. 76). Indicators for improvement include the following:

- Expressions of the right to have been protected from abuse
- Healing of physical injuries
- Relief of anger in nondestructive ways
- Feelings of empowerment and expressions of hope
- Evidence of comfort in relationships

PLANNING

Unless the patient has sustained serious physical or psychological injury, treatment is offered, and the patient is released. Because the ramifications of rape are experienced for an extended time after the acute phase, the plan of care includes information for follow-up care. The patient needs information about available community supports and how to access them. Nurses may also encounter rape survivors in other settings when they are no longer in acute distress but still dealing with the aftermath of rape. Such settings include inpatient facilities, the community, and the home. A comprehensive plan of care addresses the continuing needs of the rape survivor in any setting.

IMPLEMENTATION

Timely intervention can reduce the aftermath of rape. The occurrence of rape can be the most devastating experience in a person's life and constitutes an acute adventitious (unexpected) crisis. Typical crisis reactions reflect cognitive, affective, and behavioral disruptions. For survivors to return to their previous level of functioning, it is necessary for them to fully mourn their losses, experience anger, and work through their fears. Box 29-2 identifies interventions for rape-trauma syndrome.

Counseling

The sexual assault patient may be too traumatized, ashamed, or afraid to go to the hospital. Cultural definitions of what constitutes rape may also affect the decision to seek treatment. For these reasons, 24-hour telephone and online hotlines—such as the Rape, Abuse, and Incest National Network (RAINN)—are initiated through instant messaging and provide direct communication with volunteers trained in rape crisis support. These types of support services focus on helping the person through the period of acute distress by assessing what has happened and determining what kind of assistance is needed. Counselors provide empathetic listening, the survivor is encouraged to go to the emergency department, and the main focus is on the immediate steps the person may take.

The most effective approach for counseling in the emergency department or crisis center is to provide nonjudgmental care and optimal emotional support. Confidentiality is crucial. The most helpful things the nurse can do are to listen and to let the patient talk. A patient who feels listened to and understood is no longer alone and feels more in control of the situation.

It is especially important to help the survivor and significant others to separate issues of vulnerability from blame. Although the person may have made choices that made her more vulnerable, she is not to blame for the rape. She may, however, decide to avoid some of those choices in the future (e.g., walking alone late at night or excessive use of alcohol). Focusing on one's behavior (which is controllable) allows the survivor to believe that similar experiences can be avoided in the future.

BOX 29-2 INTERVENTIONS FOR RAPE-TRAUMA SYNDROME

Definition: Provision of emotional and physical support immediately following a reported rape

Activities:

- Provide support person to stay with patient.
- Explain legal proceedings available to patient.
- Explain rape protocol and obtain consent to proceed through protocol.
- Document whether patient has showered, douched, or bathed since incident.
- Document mental state, physical state (clothing, dirt, and debris), history of incident, evidence of violence, and prior gynecological history.
- Determine presence of cuts, bruises, bleeding, lacerations, or other signs of physical injury.
- Implement rape protocol (e.g., label and save soiled clothing, vaginal secretions, and vaginal hair combings).
- Secure samples for legal evidence.
- Implement crisis intervention counseling.
- Offer medication to prevent pregnancy, as appropriate.
- Offer prophylactic antibiotic medication against sexually transmitted disease.
- Inform patient of availability of human immunodeficiency virus testing, as appropriate.
- Give clear, written instructions about medication use, crisis support services, and legal support.
- Refer patient to rape advocacy program.
- Document according to agency policy.

From Bulechek, G. M., Butcher, H. K., Dochterman, J. M., & Wagner, C. (2013). *Nursing interventions classification (NIC)* (6th ed.). St. Louis, MO: Mosby.

VIGNETTE

Ms. Smith comes to see that it was not her fault that she was raped and feels comfortable that she is "believed." Ms. Smith is now verbal and able to recall the events of the sexual assault to the health care providers and SANE prior to discharge.

If the patient consents, involve her support system (e.g., family or friends, also group home providers as in this case with Ms. Smith) and discuss with them the nature and trauma of sexual assault and possible delayed reactions that may occur. One survivor expressed the aftermath of her assault as follows:

"It takes a few days to hit you. It was bad. It was really rough for my husband. I needed to be reassured. I needed to be told that there was nothing I could do to prevent it. Understanding helps." (Anonymous)

Social support effectively moderates somatic symptoms and subjective health ratings. The survivor who is able to confide comfortably in one or two friends or family members, especially immediately after the assault, is likely to experience fewer somatic manifestations of stress. In many cases, family and friends need support and reassurance as much as the survivor does. This is especially true for those from traditional cultures, particularly those cultures who believe that sexual assault brings shame to the entire family. The longstanding cultural myth that women are the property of men still prevents some people from empathizing with the woman's severe psychic injury and from being supportive. Instead, in these cases, the woman is devalued.

29-1 CASE STUDY AND NURSING CARE PLAN

Rape

Latisha Smith, a 36-year-old single mother of two, goes out one evening with some friends. Her children are at a slumber party, and she "needs to get away and have a little rest and relaxation." She and her friends go bowling. Later in the evening, Latisha is tired and ready to go home. A man who has joined the group offers to take her home. She has seen the man at the bowling alley before but does not know much about him. Not in the habit of going home alone with men she does not know, she hesitates. A friend whom she trusts encourages her to go with James because he is a "nice man."

James drives Latisha home. He then asks if he can come into her house to use the bathroom before driving the long distance to his house. She reluctantly agrees and sits on the living room couch. After using the bathroom, James sits next to Latisha and begins to kiss her and fondle her breasts. As she protests, James becomes more forceful in his advances. Latisha is confused and frightened. She manages to get away from him briefly, but he begins grabbing, squeezing, and biting her. He tells her gruffly, "If you don't do what I say, I'll break your neck." She screams, but he proceeds to rape her. James becomes nervous that the noise will alert the neighbors and races out of the house. A neighbor does in fact arrive just after James flees. The neighbor calls the police and then brings Latisha to the local hospital emergency department for a physical examination, crisis intervention, and support.

In the emergency department, Latisha is visibly shaken. She keeps saying, over and over, "I shouldn't have let him take me home. I should have fought harder; I shouldn't have let him do this."

The nurse takes Latisha to a quiet cubicle. She does not want Latisha to stay alone and asks the neighbor to stay with her. The nurse then notifies the doctor and the rape-victim advocate. When the nurse comes back, she tells Latisha that she would like to talk to her before the doctor comes. Latisha looks at her neighbor and then down. The nurse asks the neighbor to wait outside for a while and says she will call her later.

Latisha: *It was horrible. I feel so dirty.*

Nurse: *You have had a traumatic experience. Do you want to talk about it?*

Latisha: *I feel so ashamed. I never should have let that man take me home.*

Nurse: *You think that if you hadn't gone home with a stranger, this wouldn't have happened?*

Latisha: *Yes . . . . I shouldn't have let him do it to me anyway; I shouldn't have let him rape me.*

Nurse: *You mentioned that he said he would break your neck if you didn't do as he said.*

Latisha: *Yes, he said that . . . he was going to kill me; it was awful.*

Nurse: It seems you did the right thing in order to stay alive.

As the nurse continues to talk with Latisha, Latisha's anxiety level seems to lessen. The nurse talks to Latisha about the kinds of experiences rape victims often have after the rape and explains that the reactions she might have 2 or 3 weeks from now are normal in these circumstances. The nurse continues to collect the necessary information. She says that the doctor will want to examine Latisha and explains the procedure to her. She then asks Latisha to sign a consent form. While preparing Latisha for examination, the nurse notices bite marks and bruises on both breasts. She also notes Latisha's lower lip, which is cut and bleeding. The nurse keeps detailed notes on her observations and draws a body map of the injuries. After the examination, Latisha is given clean clothes and a place to shower.

Self-Assessment

The nurse has worked with rape survivors before and has helped develop the hospital protocol. It took a while for her to be able to remain both neutral and responsive because her own anger at rapists had initially interfered. She also remembers a time when a woman came in stating that she was raped but was so calm, smiling, and polite that the nurse initially did not believe her story. She had not at that point examined her own feelings or dealt with the popular societal myths regarding rape. It was only later, when she had talked to more experienced health care personnel, that she learned that crisis reactions can seem bizarre, confusing, and contradictory.

The nurse learned that staying with the patient, encouraging her to express her reactions and feelings, and listening are effective methods of reducing feelings of anxiety. Once the nurse learned through supervision and peer discussion to let go of her personal anger at the attacker and her ambivalence toward the survivor, her care and effectiveness improved greatly. All of this growth took time and support from more experienced nurses and other members of the health care team.

Assessment

Objective Data

- Crying and sobbing
- Bruises and bite marks on each breast
- Lip cut and bleeding
- Rape reported to the police

Subjective Data

- "He was going to kill me."
- "It was horrible. I feel so dirty."
- "I shouldn't have let him rape me."

Diagnosis

The nurse formulates the following diagnosis:
Rape-trauma syndrome

Supporting Data

- "I shouldn't have let him rape me."
- "He was going to kill me."
- Crying and sobbing
- Bruises and bite marks on both breasts
- Rape reported to the police
- "It was horrible. I feel so dirty."

Outcomes Identification

Overall outcome: Abuse Recovery: Emotional

Short-term indicator: Latisha will demonstrate appropriate affect for the situation.

Intermediate indicator: Latisha will demonstrate confidence.

Short-term and intermediate outcome indicators are measured on a 5-point Likert scale from 1 (none) to 5 (extensive).

Planning

The nurse plans to provide emotional and physical support to Latisha while she receives care in the emergency setting and to make sure that Latisha is aware of the importance of follow-up care.

Implementation

Latisha's plan of care is personalized as follows.

29-1 CASE STUDY AND NURSING CARE PLAN—cont'd

Rape

SHORT-TERM GOAL	INTERVENTION	RATIONALE
1. Latisha will demonstrate appropriate affect by discharge from the emergency department.	1a. Remain neutral and nonjudgmental and assure patient of confidentiality.	1a. Lessens feelings of shame and guilt and encourages sharing of painful feelings.
	1b. Do not leave patient alone.	1b. Deters feelings of isolation and escalation of anxiety.
	1c. Allow the patient negative expressions and behavioral self-blame while using reflective techniques.	1c. Fosters feelings of control.
	1d. Assure patient she did the right thing to save her life.	1d. Decreases burden of guilt and shame.
	1e. When anxiety level is down to moderate, encourage problem solving.	1e. Increases survivor's feeling of control in her own life. (When in severe anxiety, a person cannot problem solve.)
	1f. Tell survivor of common reactions experienced by people in long-term reorganization phase (e.g., phobias, flashbacks, insomnia, increased motor activity).	1f. Helps survivor anticipate reactions and understand them as part of recovery process.
	1g. Explain emergency department procedure to patient.	1g. Lowers anticipatory anxiety.
	1h. Explain physical examination.	1h. Allows for questions and concerns; victim may be too traumatized and may refuse.
	1i. Nurse/female rape advocate should stay with patient during physical examination.	1i. Physical examination may be experienced as a second assault. Nurse provides comfort and support.

Evaluation

Latisha is able to express her feelings in the emergency department and talk about the possible reactions she might experience as she moves through the reorganization phase. Her anxiety level is reduced to moderate.

Promotion of Self-Care Activities

When preparing the patient for discharge, the nurse provides all referral information and printed follow-up instructions, detailing potential physical concerns and emotional reactions, legal matters, victim compensation (state financial assistance paid through perpetrators' fines and fees), and ways that family and friends, advocates, and other health care providers can help. This is important because the amount of verbal information the patient can retain likely will be limited due to high levels of anxiety. Written material can be referred to repeatedly over time. Health care referrals are provided for continuity of care, and victim assistance program information can also be given. A list of printed online resources can be helpful as well.

Case Management

The emotional state and other psychological needs of the patient should be reassessed by telephone or personal contact within 24 to 48 hours of discharge from the hospital. Make sure you discuss this with the patient prior to discharge. Also, the most up-to-date contact information should be correctly on file in the medical record. Repeat referrals should be made for resources or support services. Effective crisis intervention and continuity of care require outreach activities and services beyond the emergency medical setting.

Survivors may avoid seeking treatment from psychiatric mental health care providers because medical treatment is more socially sanctioned, and they are likely to be experiencing physical symptoms of stress. Thus the outpatient nurse can make a more focused assessment of stress-related symptoms and/or depression and ascertain the need for mental health referral. Reporting symptoms and seeking medical treatment are adaptive coping behaviors and can be reinforced as such.

Follow-up visits should occur at least 2, 4, and 6 weeks after the initial evaluation. At each visit, the patient should be assessed for psychological progress, the presence of sexually transmitted diseases, and pregnancy. Follow-up examinations provide an opportunity to (1) detect new infections acquired during or after the assault; (2) complete hepatitis B vaccination, if indicated; (3) complete counseling and treatment for other STDs; and (4) monitor side effects and adherence to postexposure prophylactic medication, if prescribed (CDC, 2010).

Advanced Practice Interventions

Psychotherapy

The advanced practice nurse may offer individual or group psychotherapy for either the rape survivor or the perpetrator.

Survivors. Most of those who have been raped are eventually able to resume their previous lifestyle and level of functioning after supportive services and crisis counseling; however, many continue to experience emotional trauma, including flashbacks, nightmares, fear, phobias, and other symptoms associated with PTSD (refer to Chapter 16). Some people who survive rape may be susceptible to a psychotic episode or an emotional disturbance so severe that hospitalization is required. Others whose emotional lives may be overburdened with multiple internal and external pressures may require individual psychotherapy.

Depression and suicidal ideation too frequently follow rape. Depression is more common in those who do not disclose the assault to significant others because they have concerns about being stigmatized, have children living at home, or have a pending civil lawsuit. Any exposure to stimuli related to the traumatic event may activate a reliving of the traumatic state.

People who have been raped are likely to benefit from group therapy or support groups. These modalities may be particularly beneficial for survivors from cultures that are group oriented rather than individualistic and for women who derive much of their self-definition from cultural norms. Group therapy can make the difference between a person's coming out of the crisis at a lower level of functioning or gradually adapting to the experience with an increase in coping skills.

Perpetrators. Psychotherapy is essential for perpetrators of sexual assault if behavioral change is to occur. Unfortunately, most perpetrators do not acknowledge the need for behavioral change, and no single method or program of treatment has been found to be totally effective. The nurse's awareness of his or her own feelings and reactions will be crucial to avoid interference with the therapeutic process.

EVALUATION

We consider **sexual assault** survivors to be in recovery if they are relatively free of any signs or symptoms of acute stress disorder and PTSD. Signs of recovery include the following:

- Sleeping well with few instances of episodic nightmares or broken sleep
- Eating as they did before the rape
- Being calm and relaxed or only mildly suspicious, fearful, or restless
- Getting support from family and friends
- Generally positive self-regard about themselves
- The absence or only mild instances of somatic reactions
- Returning to pre-rape sexual functioning and interest

In general, the closer the survivor's lifestyle is to the pattern that was present before the rape, the more complete the recovery has been.

CONCLUSION

Nurses need to review hospital-based policy and procedures manuals to determine if protocols have been established in how to care for a sexual assault patient. If your facility does not have a policy, consider establishing one for your area. The International Association of Forensic Nurses (IAFN, 2008) provides SANE Education Guidelines for the evaluation of Adult/Adolescent and Pediatric patients. Certification is provided by the IAFN for nurse providers (i.e., SANE-A, SANE-P) and information regarding certification can be found at www.iafn.org.

KEY POINTS TO REMEMBER

- Sexual assault is a common and often underreported crime of violence in the United States.
- Females are far more likely to be victims of sexual assault and tend to know their perpetrators. Sexual assault of males tends to be underreported, owing to the humiliation and stigma attached to such victimization.
- Psychoactive substances play a major role in sexual assault, and alcohol is the most commonly used date-rape drug. Other disinhibiting and amnestic substances play a role in forcible sex acts.
- A rape survivor experiences a wide range of feelings, which may or may not be exhibited to others.
- Feelings of fear, degradation, anger and rage, helplessness, and nervousness; sleep disturbances; disturbed relationships; flashbacks; depression; and somatic complaints are all common following sexual assault.
- The circumstances of the initial medical evaluation may be frightening and stressful. A police interview, repeated questioning by health professionals, and the physical examination itself all have the potential to add to the trauma of the sexual assault.
- Nurses, in their role as case managers, can serve to minimize repetition of questions and support the patient as she goes through the medical and legal evaluation.
- Survivors require long-term health care that can include counseling to minimize long-term effects of the rape and assist in early return to a normal living pattern.
- Telephone and online resources are available to assist sexual assault and rape survivors.

CRITICAL THINKING

- Jonah, 18 years of age, is brutally beaten and sexually assaulted by an unidentified male as he makes his way home from a party in an unfamiliar part of town. He is found semiconscious by a passerby and taken to the emergency department. Isaac has bite marks on his neck, extensive bruises around his head, chest, and buttocks and has sustained a cracked rib and anal tears. Ms. Santinez, a nurse and rape counselor in the emergency department, works with Jonah using the hospital's sexual assault protocol and evidence collection kit. Jonah appears stunned and confused and has difficulty focusing on what the nurse says. He states repeatedly, "This is crazy, this can't be happening . . . . I can't believe this has happened to me . . . . Oh, my God, I can't believe this. Does this mean I am gay?"
  - **a.** What areas of Jonah's assessment should be given highest priority by Ms. Santinez and her staff while he is in the emergency department?
  - **b.** Chart the signs and symptoms of Jonah's physical and emotional trauma and verbatim statements in as much detail as you can.
  - **c.** What are some of the pivotal issues that need to be addressed in terms of assessing Jonah's signs and symptoms of physical trauma? Although the risk of pregnancy is not present, what other real physical health risks need to be assessed?
  - **d.** What are some of the signs and symptoms of rape-trauma syndrome?

e. Identify the short-term outcome criteria for Jonah that ideally would be met before he leaves the emergency department.
f. What information does Jonah need to have regarding potential signs and symptoms that may occur in the near future? Why is this important for him to understand at present?
g. Identify specific indicators that will be met if Jonah recovers with minimal trauma from the event. How would you evaluate these criteria?
h. If Jonah wishes not to report the sexual assault to police, would you still complete the examination?

CHAPTER REVIEW

1. Tara, a 19-year-old freshmen college student, arrives for a follow-up appointment at the mental health clinic where you work. She had previously been seen in the clinic for crisis intervention three weeks ago after being raped. Tara states, "My mom says I was asking for trouble because of the way I was dressed at the party. She says when girls dress so sexy, men can't help themselves." Your response is guided by the knowledge that:
   a. Statistics show that women who dress provocatively are more likely to be raped.
   b. The party setting is more a factor in rape occurrences than what the victim is wearing.
   c. Rape is an act of violence, aggression, and power, not an expression of sexual needs.
   d. Tara is exhibiting symptoms of an acute phase of rape-trauma syndrome and will need further counseling sessions.
2. You are working in the emergency department caring for 21-year-old Larissa, who has just been raped. Which is your best *initial* nursing response?
   a. "We need to examine you for injuries and collect evidence for the police."
   b. "May I get your consent to test you for pregnancy and HIV?"
   c. "You are safe here."
   d. "I will get you the number for the crisis intervention specialist."
3. Mindy is the nurse caring for Caitlin, who was raped the night before. Caitlin is considering the morning-after pill to prevent a possible pregnancy that may have resulted from the rape. Caitlin is concerned and states that she does not believe in abortion. Which of the following is the most appropriate action Mindy could take in this situation?
   a. Examine her own feelings about abortion before discussing this with Caitlin.
   b. Encourage Caitlin to take more time to consider her options.
   c. Provide Caitlin with the number to Planned Parenthood.
   d. Provide Caitlin with medication education.
4. You are working at a telephone hotline center when Abby, a rape victim, calls. Abby states she is afraid to go to the hospital. What is your best response?
   a. "I'm here to listen, and we can talk about your feelings."
   b. "You don't need to go to the hospital if you don't want to."
   c. "If you don't go to the hospital, we can't collect evidence to help convict your rapist."
   d. "Why are you afraid to seek medical attention?"
5. Josefina was raped 6 months ago. Which symptom(s) should you anticipate for long-term successful outcomes? *Select all that apply.*
   a. Evidence of comfort in relationships
   b. Numbness, shock, and disbelief
   c. Recognition of the right to be protected from abuse
   d. Fear of sexual encounters
   e. Dreams with violent content
   f. Anxiety being replaced by calmness
   g. Absence of phobia of being alone

Answers to Chapter Review
1. c; 2. c; 3. d; 4. a; 5. a, c, f, g.

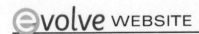

WEBSITE

Visit the Evolve website for a posttest on the content in this chapter: http://evolve.elsevier.com/Varcarolis

Post-Test interactive review

REFERENCES

Ackley, B., & Ladwig, G. (2011). *Nursing diagnosis handbook: An evidence-based guide to planning care.* St. Louis, MO: Mosby Elsevier.

Black, M. C., Basile, K. C., Breiding, M. J., Smith, S. G., Walters, M. L., Merrick, M. T., et al. (2011). *The National Intimate Partner and Sexual Violence Survey (NISVS): 2010 summary report.* Atlanta, GA: National Center for Injury Prevention and Control; Centers for Disease Control and Prevention.

Bulechek, G. M., Butcher, H. K., Dochterman, J. M., & Wagner, C. (2013). *Nursing interventions classification (NIC)* (6th ed.). St. Louis, MO: Mosby.

Centers for Disease Control and Prevention. (2010). *Sexually transmitted diseases treatment guidelines.* Retrieved from http://www.cdc.gov/std/treatment/2010/sexual-assault.htm.

Centers for Disease Control and Prevention. (2011). *Understanding intimate partner violence.* Retrieved from http://www.cdc.gov/violenceprevention/pdf/IPV_factsheet-a.pdf.

Drug-Induced Rape Prevention and Punishment. Drug-Induced Rape Prevention and Punishment Act, 21 U.S.C. 1996 § 841(b)(7).

Emergency Nurses Association. (2010). *Emergency Nurses Association position statements: Forensic evidence collection.* Retrieved from http://www.ena.org/SiteCollectionDocuments/Position%20Statements/Forensic%20Evidence.pdffrom http://www.ena.org/ about/position/forensicevidence.asp.

Emergency Nurses Association. (2010). *Emergency Nurses Association position statements: Care of sexual assault victims.* Retrieved from http://www.ena.org/SiteCollectionDocuments/Position%20Statements/SexualAssaultRapeVictims.pdf.

Federal Bureau of Investigation. (2011). *Preliminary crime stats for the first half of 2011.* Retrieved from http://www.fbi.gov/news/stories/2011/december/crime-stats_121911/crime-stats_121911.

Federal Bureau of Investigation. (2008). *Forcible rape: Crime in the United States.* Retrieved from http://www.fbi.gov/ucr/cius2007/offenses/violent_crime/forcible_rape.html.

Federal Bureau of Investigation. (2012). *Attorney General Eric Holder announces revisions to the Uniform Crime Report's definition of rape: Data reported on* rape will better reflect state criminal codes, victim experiences*. Retrieved from http://www.fbi.gov/news/pressrel/press-releases/attorney-general-eric-holder-announces-revisions-to-the-uniform-crime-reports-definition-of-rape.

Gaffney, D. (2011). The psychobiology of traumatic stress responses after sexual assault. In L. Ledray, A. Burgess, & A. Giardina (Eds.), *Medical response to adult sexual assault: A resource for clinicians and related professionals* (pp. 225–228). St. Louis, MO: STM Learning.

Gemzell-Danielsson, K. (2010). Mechanism of action of emergency contraception. *Contraception, 82*(5), 404–409.

Herdman, T. H. (Ed.), (2012). *NANDA international nursing diagnoses: Definitions and classification 2012–2014*. Oxford, UK: Wiley-Blackwell.

Marchetti, C. (2012). Regret and policy reporting among individuals who have experienced sexual assault. *Journal of the American Psychiatric Nurses Association, 18*(1), 32–39.

Moorhead, S., Johnson, M., Maas, M. L., & Swanson, E. (2013). *Nursing outcomes classification (NOC)* (5th ed.). St. Louis, MO: Mosby.

National Institute of Mental Health. (2009). *Post-traumatic stress disorder*. Retrieved from http://www.nimh.nih.gov/health/publications/post-traumatic-stress-disorder-ptsd/what-are-the-symptoms-of-ptsd.shtml.

Patel, A., Patel, D., Piotrowski, Z. H., & Panchal, H. (2008). Comprehensive medical care for victims of sexual assault: A survey of Illinois hospital emergency departments. *Contraception, 77*, 426–430.

Rape, Abuse and Incest National Network. (2008). *Who are the victims?* Retrieved from http://www.rainn.org/get-information/statistics/sexual-assault-victims.

Read, J., Hammersley, P., & Rudegeair, T. (2007). Why, when and how to ask about childhood abuse. *Advances in Psychiatric Treatment, 13*, 101–110.

The Library of Congress Thomas. (2005). *H. R. 3402*. Retrieved from http://thomas.loc.gov/cgi-bin/bdquery/z?d109:H.R.3402.

Tjaden, P., & Thonnes, N. (2008). *Prevalence, incidence, and consequences of violence against women: Findings from the National Violence Against Women Survey*. Washington, DC: U.S. Department of Justice. Report No. NCJ 172837.

Truman, J. L., & Rand, M. R. (2010). *Bureau of Justice statistics bulletin: National Crime Victimization Survey, criminal victimization, 2009*. Retrieved from http://bjs.ojp.usdoj.gov/content/pub/pdf/cv09.pdf.

U.S. Department of Justice. (2004). *A national protocol for sexual assault medical forensic examinations: Adults/adolescents (No. NCJ 206554.)*. Washington, DC: Office on Violence Against Women. Retrieved from https://www.ncjrs.gov/pdffiles1/nij/206554.pdf.

U.S. Department of Justice; Office of the Attorney General. (1997). *September 23 memorandum for all United States attorneys*. Retrieved from http://www.usdoj.gov/ag/readingroom/drugcrime.htm.

CHAPTER

30

Psychosocial Needs of the Older Adult

Leslie A. Briscoe

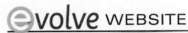

Visit the Evolve website for a pretest on the content in this chapter: http://evolve.elsevier.com/Varcarolis

Pre-Test interactive review

OBJECTIVES

1. Describe mental health disorders that may occur in older adults.
2. Discuss the importance of pain assessment, and identify three tools used to assess pain in older adults.
3. Explain the importance of a comprehensive geriatric assessment.
4. Recognize the significance of health care costs for older adults.
5. Discuss facts and myths about aging.
6. Analyze how ageism may affect attitudes and willingness to care for older adults.
7. Identify the requirements for the use of physical and chemical restraints.
8. Identify legislation and legal documents that protect the rights of older patients, and describe their impact on nursing care.
9. Describe the role of the nurse in various geriatric care settings.

KEY TERMS AND CONCEPTS

adult day care
advance directives
adverse drug reactions
ageism
late-life mental illness
Omnibus Budget Reconciliation Act (OBRA)
Patient Self-Determination Act (PSDA)
polypharmacy
prescribing cascade

The aging of the population is a global phenomenon occurring at a record-breaking rate, especially in developing countries around the world. The United States' economy, as well as its health and social services, is affected by this marked increase in the proportion of the older adults. According to the Administration on Aging 2012 estimates, the number of individuals over the age of 65 years has grown exponentially since 1900. At that point there were about 3 million, and in the year 2000 there were 35 million. Estimates for 2030 and 2050 are 72 million and 89 million, respectively. Among this group of older adults, the fastest-growing subgroups are minorities, the poor, and those aged 85 years and older.

As people live longer, they are more likely to deal with chronic illness and disability. At least 80% of individuals older than age 65 have one chronic condition, and many older persons have more than one. The likelihood of developing these chronic illnesses notably increases with age; individuals 75 years of age and older are the most prone to chronic illnesses and functional disabilities. After age 85, there is a 1-in-3 chance of developing dementia, immobility, incontinence, or another age-related disability.

Statistics indicate that women generally outlive men. This has significant ramifications for society at large and for the health care system in particular. Not only do women constitute the largest proportion of older adults, they also use health care services more frequently than men and seek services earlier, even for minor conditions.

Chronological age is considered an arbitrary indicator of function because there are significant variables that contribute to the capabilities of older adults. The National Council on Aging (2002) conducted surveys focusing on how older adults see themselves, revealing that nearly half of people 65 years and older consider themselves to be middle-aged or young. Only 15% of people aged 75 years and older consider themselves "very old."

Touhy (2012) provides a common classification for people 65 and older:

- **Young-old:** 65 to 74 years
- **Middle-old:** 75 to 84 years
- **Old-old:** 85 to 100 years
- **Elite-old (centenarians):** 100+ years of age

Aging is accompanied by increased medical and psychiatric illness. This increase is brought about in part by increasingly stressful life events (e.g., the loss of a spouse, family members, and independence) and comorbid illness. Polypharmacy also contributes to health problems and death in the elderly. Adverse drug reactions occur since there is a gradual reduction in renal, hepatic, and gastric function. Drug reactions can cause conditions such as delirium, dizziness, and confusion leading to serious complications and hospitalization.

MENTAL HEALTH ISSUES RELATED TO AGING

Late-Life Mental Illness

Older adults who develop late-life mental illness are less likely than young adults to be accurately diagnosed and receive mental health treatment. Psychiatric issues such as depression, cognitive deficits, and prolonged grieving are not a normal part of aging. Diagnosing and treating psychiatric disorders prolongs the individual's ability to remain independent and increases the ability to take the lead in personal decision making.

Depression

Depression is not a normal part of aging and is often underidentified because of comorbid medical conditions. Depression can be confused with dementia or delirium. A careful, systematic assessment is necessary to properly distinguish among the three. The cardinal differences include the following:

- Onset of mental-status change and course of illness
- Level of consciousness
- Attention span

Depression and Suicide Risk

Depression accounts for up to 70% of late-life suicides. The risk of suicide for men increases with age, particularly for white men ages 65 and older whose risk is 7 times that of females of the same age. The highest rate of suicide is in males 75 and older at 36 per 100,000; the rate of suicide for males and females aged 75 and older is about 16 per 100,000 (Centers for Disease Control and Prevention, 2012).

Even though the suicide rate among older adults is high, especially among white, non-Hispanic males (Figure 30-1), suicide in this group is probably underreported. The numbers also do not reflect those who passively or indirectly commit suicide by abusing alcohol, starving themselves, overdosing or mixing medications, stopping life-sustaining drugs, driving into bridge abutments, or simply losing the will to live. There is an ongoing effort to educate primary care providers to better recognize, treat, and refer older adults to mental health care providers. There is clear evidence that treating depression is cost effective and decreases health care expenditures (NIMH, 2004). Chapter 25 provides an in-depth discussion of suicide.

Early identification and treatment for depression are key measures for suicide prevention. Risks for suicide include demographics, diagnosable psychiatric illness (psychosis, anxiety, substance abuse, previous suicide attempts), psychological well-being (personality, emotional reactivity, impulsiveness), biological status (dysfunction of neurotransmitters), and stressful life events (Nock et al., 2008). Other risk factors include access to weapons, access to large doses of medications, and chronic or terminal illness. Protective factors include religious beliefs and practices, spirituality, perception of social/family support, and having children.

Selective serotonin reuptake inhibitors (SSRIs) are the first-line treatment for depression; this category is often helpful if anxiety, worry, or rumination is problematic. If pain or diabetic neuropathy is a comorbid condition, serotonin norepinephrine reuptake inhibitors (SNRIs) are often prescribed. Tricyclic antidepressants (TCAs) are effective, but they are utilized judiciously for those with chronic pain due to side effects and lethality in overdose. Treatment-resistant depression can be treated with psychostimulants such as methylphenidate or with

CONSIDERING CULTURE

Older African Americans' View of Depression

Older African Americans are underrepresented in all treatment settings but especially in psychiatric care settings. In regard to depression, understanding their beliefs and perceptions about depression would assist mental health care providers in developing interventions to overcoming barriers. In a recent qualitative study, 51 older African Americans responded to questions about depression, and four major themes were identified:

- "Keeping the Bully Out"—The belief that depression is something bad and can be kept out or avoided.
- "God Will Provide"—The role of God, faith, and prayer is vital to preventing depression.
- "Losing Control"—The experience of depression is a physical manifestation, which takes control.
- "That's Not Me"—Participants were clear that being depressed did not pertain to them.

These responses indicate that stigma remains a dominant response to depression in this population. There are clear beliefs that people who have depression are weak, choose to be depressed, or perhaps do not have enough faith. In this population, physical manifestations of depression may also be more prominent and a more acceptable way of expressing symptoms. This may lead to misdiagnosis and lack of treatment. Health care providers need to be keenly aware of the mind-body-spirit connection when assessing and treating older African American patients.

Shellman, J., Mokel, M., & Wright, B. (2007). Keeping the bully out: Understanding older African Americans' beliefs and attitudes toward depression. *Journal of the American Psychiatric Nurses Association, 13*(4), 230–236.

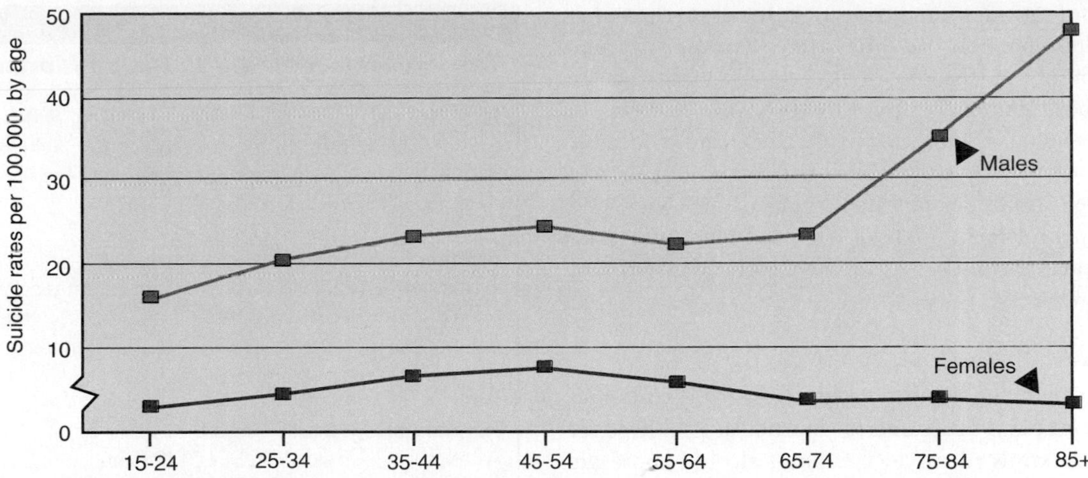

FIG 30-1 Suicide rates among persons 65 and older by race/ethnicity and sex, United States, 2005-2009. (From Centers for Disease Control. [2009]. Retrieved from http://www.cdc.gov/ViolencePrevention/suicide/statistics/rates05.html.)

monoamine oxidase inhibitors. Electroconvulsive therapy is a good alternative in care for depression, particularly in the elderly who may not tolerate medication or fail to improve.

Anxiety Disorders

Specific anxiety disorders peak at various ages (Lenze & Wetherell, 2011). This may be related to changes in brain structure or function. In older adults, anxiety disorders are even harder to diagnose, and prevalence estimates vary greatly. One unique anxiety in the elderly is the fear of falling; its impact on keeping the elderly at home is similar to agoraphobia. Psychosocial risk factors for anxiety include being childless, low socioeconomic status, and having experienced trauma. Protective factors may include social support, spiritual beliefs, physical activity, cognitive stimulation, and having acquired effective coping strategies.

Cassidy and Rector (2008) identify anxiety disorders in late life as "The Silent Geriatric Giant." Older adults often have multiple physical complaints, medication problems, pain, sleep disturbances, and psychiatric illness. Anxiety is twice as prevalent as dementia and four to eight times as common as major depressive disorders.

Treatment for anxiety disorders typically includes an SSRI along with cognitive behavioral therapy. Roy-Byrne and colleagues (2010) showed that relaxation training was an effective intervention for older adults. Antianxiety (benzodiazepines) agents are also used and frequently overprescribed. They should be used cautiously, as side effects can result in confusion, oversedation, increased risk of falls, and paradoxical agitation. Anxiety disorders are discussed in greater detail in Chapter 15.

Delirium

Delirium is a medical condition caused by physiological changes due to underlying pathology. It causes fluctuations in consciousness and changes in cognition that develop over a short period of time (hours to days). There is usually evidence from history, examination, or diagnostic testing that will help identify the cause (Caplan et al., 2010). Patients may be disoriented and often assumed to be demented because of their age; therefore, it is crucial to obtain data from family or caregivers about a baseline level of functioning. A patient who is newly confused, falling, disrobing, and fighting with staff should be assessed for delirium. Asking questions such as "Has your mother been shopping and cooking for herself?" or "Does she pay her own bills?" or "Does she ever get lost when driving?" may give subtle clues about whether changes are acute or have been coming on slowly. Other questions that can be revealing include "Has your father been started on any new medication?" or "Has your father fallen or hit his head recently?"

Treatment of delirium begins with identifying the cause. Adverse drug reactions, infections, electrolyte imbalances, anemia, thyroid dysfunction, vitamin deficiencies, and a multitude of other problems must be ruled out. A multidisciplinary approach is often helpful to identify causation: doctors of clinical pharmacology are helpful in identifying possible drug-related effects; geriatricians provide a comprehensive approach to physical assessment; and psychiatric consultation can provide mental status evaluation and recommendations for treatment of behaviors. If agitation or combative behaviors are present, it is common to provide short-term use of antipsychotic medications. Benzodiazepines should be avoided due to side effects and possible worsening of delirium.

Dementia

Dementia is usually of the Alzheimer's or vascular type. Both are characterized by aphasia (difficulty finding words), apraxia (difficulty carrying out motor functions despite intact functioning), agnosia (failure to recognize objects), and disturbances in executive functioning (organizing, planning, abstracting, insight, judgment) (Falk & Wiechers, 2010). Changes in executive functioning may include forgetting how to make old family recipes, the inability to manage bill paying, and limited insight and judgment, leading to increased vulnerability to exploitation.

Another symptom that often is not discussed is sexual disinhibition. Older patients may be overly flirtatious, grope caregivers or family during care, make sexually inappropriate comments, expose genitalia, or masturbate openly. These types of behaviors can cause staff and family to be uncomfortable and confused about how to respond. It is important for the nurse to be open and understanding about such behaviors and to recognize them as symptoms of a frontal lobe brain dysfunction. Chapter 23 presents a more complete description of delirium and dementia.

Alcohol Abuse

Although heavy drinking tends to decline with age, it continues to be a serious problem that can create particular problems for older adults. The antecedents to late-onset alcohol abuse are often related to environmental conditions and may include retirement, widowhood, and loneliness. Previous work and family responsibilities may help keep a person with vulnerabilities from drinking too much. Once these demands are gone and the structure of daily life is removed, for some there is little impetus to remain sober.

The risk factors for heavy drinking in older adults are being male and single, having less than a high school education, low income, and smoking (Karlamangla et al., 2006). Additionally, depression often plays a role in increased alcohol consumption in the elderly (National Institute on Aging, 2012). Identifying alcohol and substance abuse is often difficult because the accompanying personality and behavioral changes associated with alcohol abuse frequently go unrecognized in older adults.

Caution is required when medicating the older adult who abuses alcohol. Central nervous system toxicity from psychoactive drugs increases with aging. Ingestion of antidepressants or tranquilizers can be particularly harmful because their effect is further potentiated by alcohol. Whenever there is a suspicion or indication that an older adult is abusing alcohol, the health care provider should conduct a screening test. The MAST-G (Box 30-1) is an instrument commonly used to assess older adults' alcohol use.

The older person who misuses alcohol displays symptoms of confusion, malnutrition, self-neglect, weight loss, depression, and falls. Diarrhea, urinary incontinence, decreased functional status, failure to thrive, and dementia may also be present. Alcohol-induced dementia is caused by long-term excessive alcohol abuse. It typically presents with impaired executive function and significant lack of insight. This is in contrast to the memory or language problems of dementia.

Moos and colleagues (2010) conducted a study where participants were followed over a 20-year span. Drinking excessively late in life was found in about 33% of participants. Indicators of excessive use were past drinking history, reliance on substances for stress reduction, and support of peers in drinking behavior. There is evidence that older adults respond to treatment as well as, if not better than, younger adults. Intentional brief intervention by a health care provider or participation in a group setting can impact older adults to decrease alcohol consumption. Group therapy along with self-help groups like Alcoholics Anonymous can be effective. It is important that health care providers recognize this recovery potential.

EVIDENCE-BASED PRACTICE

The Impact of Wishing to Die on Mortality

Raue, P. J., Morales, K. H., Post, E. P., Bogner, H. R., Have, T. T., & Bruce, M. L. (2010). The wish-to-die and five-year mortality in elderly primary care patients. *American Journal of Geriatric Psychiatry, 18*(4), 341–350.

Problem

We know that suicide rates increase dramatically in the white male geriatric population. There is also concern that the wish-to-die, or passive suicidal ideation, may influence mortality rate for those who die of natural causes.

Purpose of the Study

A national study called PROSPECT (Prevention of Suicide in Primary Care Elderly: Collaborative Trial) provided longitudinal data to explore the correlation of natural cause deaths for those with a prior death wish, regardless of baseline depressive status. The researchers also compared mortality rates for those receiving usual care and for those receiving the specialized PROSPECT intervention.

Methods

Study data were collected from 20 primary care practices in New York City, Philadelphia, and Pittsburgh over a 5-year period. The sample of 1202 were given tests to evaluate mood and cognition, slong with a structured clinical interview.

Key Findings

- Rates of wish-to-die were 40% among depressed patients and 7% among nondepressed patients.
- Having a wish-to-die was linked with an increased mortality rate, regardless of whether depression was present or not.

Implications for Nursing Practice

Although elderly patients may not be depressed, assessing for a wish-to-die is an important intervention. This study also demonstrated that a targeted intervention for elderly individuals with depression is beneficial in increasing quality of life and reducing mortality.

Pain

Pain is common among older adults and affects their sense of well-being and quality of life. Up to 85% of the older population is thought to have conditions that predispose them to pain. These conditions include arthritis, peripheral vascular disease, and diabetic neuropathy. Pain is also associated with depression. Jann and Slade (2007) describe three categories of depressive symptoms: emotional (mood, motivation, apathy, anxiety), cognitive (concentration, memory), and physical (insomnia, fatigue, headache, and stomach, back, and neck pain).

The older adult's functioning and ability to perform activities of daily living such as walking, toileting, and bathing can be affected by pain, especially pain from musculoskeletal disease. Pain can lead to increased stress, delayed healing, decreased mobility, disturbances in sleep, decreased appetite, and agitation

BOX 30-1 MICHIGAN ALCOHOLISM SCREENING TEST—GERIATRIC VERSION (MAST-G)

Please answer "Yes" or "No" to each question by marking the line next to the question. When you finish answering the questions, please add up how many "Yes" responses you checked and put that number in the space provided at the end.

1. After drinking, have you ever noticed an increase in your heart rate or beating in your chest? _____ Yes _____ No
2. When talking to others, do you ever underestimate how much you actually drank? _____ Yes _____ No
3. Does alcohol make you sleepy so that you often fall asleep in your chair? _____ Yes _____ No
4. After a few drinks, have you sometimes not eaten or been able to skip a meal because you didn't feel hungry? _____ Yes _____ No
5. Does having a few drinks help you decrease your shakiness or tremors? _____ Yes _____ No
6. Does alcohol sometimes make it hard for you to remember parts of the day or night? _____ Yes _____ No
7. Do you have rules for yourself that you won't drink before a certain time of the day? _____ Yes _____ No
8. Have you lost interest in hobbies or activities you used to enjoy? _____ Yes _____ No
9. When you wake up in the morning, do you ever have trouble remembering part of the night before? _____ Yes _____ No
10. Does having a drink help you sleep? _____ Yes _____ No
11. Do you hide your alcohol bottles from family members? _____ Yes _____ No
12. After a social gathering, have you ever felt embarrassed because you drank too much? _____ Yes _____ No
13. Have you ever been concerned that drinking might be harmful to your health? _____ Yes _____ No
14. Do you like to end an evening with a nightcap? _____ Yes _____ No
15. Did you find your drinking increased after someone close to you died? _____ Yes _____ No
16. In general, would you prefer to have a few drinks at home rather than go out to social events? _____ Yes _____ No
17. Are you drinking more now than in the past? _____ Yes _____ No
18. Do you usually take a drink to relax or calm your nerves? _____ Yes _____ No
19. Do you drink to take your mind off your problems? _____ Yes _____ No
20. Have you ever increased your drinking after experiencing a loss in your life? _____ Yes _____ No
21. Do you sometimes drive when you have had too much to drink? _____ Yes _____ No
22. Has a doctor or nurse ever said he or she was worried or concerned about your drinking? _____ Yes _____ No
23. Have you ever made rules to manage your drinking? _____ Yes _____ No
24. When you feel lonely, does having a drink help? _____ Yes _____ No

TOTALS: _____ Yes _____ No

Scoring: A score of 3 points or less is considered to indicate no alcoholism; a score of 4 points is suggestive of alcoholism; a score of 5 points or more indicates alcoholism.

From Menninger, J. (2004). Assessment and treatment of alcoholism and substance-related disorders in the elderly. *Bulletin of the Menninger Clinic, 66*(2), 166–183.

with accompanying aggressive behaviors. Chronic pain can cause depression, low self-esteem, social isolation, and feelings of hopelessness (Wynne et al., 2000). There is mounting evidence that treatment of pain improves mood and treatment of mood improves pain.

Barriers to Accurate Pain Assessment

The appropriate assessment and treatment of pain in older adults may have complications. They may believe that pain is a punishment for past behaviors, an inevitable part of aging, indicative of pending death, related to serious illness, expensive to test and diagnose, or a sign of weakness. External obstacles include inadequate assessment by health professionals, complicated clinical presentation, assumptions by health care professionals that pain is part of aging, and communication deficits due to cognitive impairment.

McDonald and colleagues (2009) demonstrated that the phrasing of pain-related questions with older adults influenced their report. The use of open-ended questions such as "Tell me about your pain, aches, soreness, or discomfort" yielded significantly more information than use of a pain scale alone.

Changes in behavior may indicate pain and should be assessed, especially in patients who have language impairment (e.g., dementia, stroke). Unlike younger adults, older adults may understate pain using milder words such as *discomfort, hurting*, or *aching*. Multiple painful problems may occur together, making differentiation of new pain from preexisting pain difficult. Sensory impairments, memory loss, dementia, and depression can add to the difficulty of obtaining an accurate pain assessment. Interviews with family members, caregivers, or friends may be helpful.

Assessment Tools

When pain is suspected, the nurse begins with a physical assessment for medical origins of the pain and assesses the level of pain. The **Wong-Baker FACES Pain Rating Scale** (Hockenberry & Wilson, 2012) (Figure 30-2) is an active assessment instrument. The FACES scale shows facial expressions on a scale from 0 (a smile) to 5 (crying grimace). Respondents are asked to choose the face that depicts the pain they feel.

The present pain intensity (PPI) rating from the **McGill Pain Questionnaire (MPQ)** (Davis & Srivastana, 2003) is another tool accepted for use with older patients. Patients are asked to respond by selecting the description (from "no pain" [0] to "excruciating pain" [5]) that they believe identifies the pain they feel.

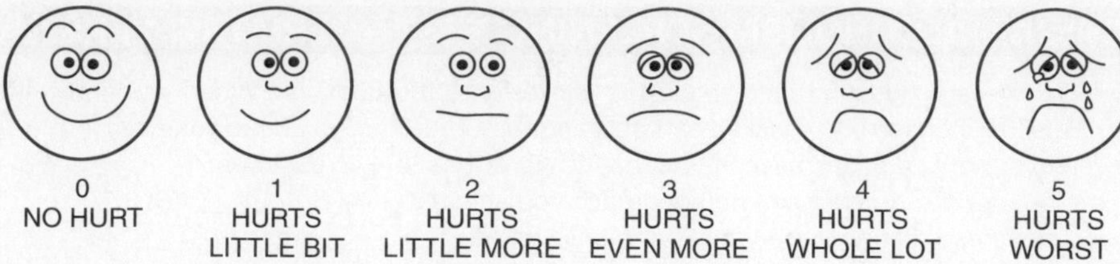
0
NO HURT
1
HURTS
LITTLE BIT
2
HURTS
LITTLE MORE
3
HURTS
EVEN MORE
4
HURTS
WHOLE LOT
5
HURTS
WORST

FIG 30-2 Wong-Baker FACES Pain Rating Scale. (From Hockenberry, M., & Wilson, D. [2013]. Wong's essentials of pediatric nursing [9th ed.]. St. Louis, MO: Mosby.)

	0	1	2	Score
Breathing Independent of vocalization	Normal	Occasional labored breathing; short period of hyperventilation	Noisy, labored breathing; long period of hyperventilation; Cheyne-Stokes respirations	
Negative Vocalization	None	Occasional moan or groan; low-level speech with a negative or disapproving quality	Repeated troubled calling out; loud moaning or groaning; crying	
Facial Expression	Smiling or inexpressive	Sad; frightened; frown	Facial grimacing	
Body Language	Relaxed	Tense; distressed pacing; fidgeting	Rigid; fists clenched; knees pulled up; pulling or pushing away; striking out	
Consolability	No need to console	Distracted or reassured by voice or touch	Unable to console, distract, or reassure	
			TOTAL	

FIG 30-3 Pain Assessment in Advanced Dementia (PAINAD) scale. (From Warden, V., Hurley, A. C., & Volicer, L. [2003]. Development and psychometric evaluation of the Pain Assessment in Advanced Dementia [PAINAD] scale. *Journal of the American Medical Directors Association, 4*[1], 9–15.)

The **Pain Assessment in Advanced Dementia (PAINAD) scale** is used to evaluate the presence and severity of pain in patients with advanced dementia who no longer have the ability to communicate verbally (Figure 30-3). The scale evaluates five domains: breathing, negative vocalization, facial expression, body language, and consolability (Box 30-2). The score guides the caregiver in the appropriate pain intervention.

Pain Management

Pharmacological Pain Treatments. Pain can be managed with pharmacological and/or alternative measures. Pharmacological pain management relies on the use of prescriptive and nonprescriptive medications, frequently based on the recommendation of the health care provider.

The treatment of acute pain is different from the approach for chronic pain. Acute pain can be helped with analgesics, such as opioids, nonsteroidal antiinflammatory drugs (NSAIDs), COX-2 inhibitors, and non-narcotic agents, such as tramadol. Chronic pain is treated with pain modulators such as gabapentin, pregablin, SNRIs, and TCAs. Consultation with a pain-management specialist is often helpful with chronic pain syndromes. Some considerations in pharmacological pain management in older adults are listed in Box 30-3. The current trend is to not utilize opioids for non–cancer-related chronic pain due to strong evidence that the risks are significant, including increased risk of fractures, hospitalization, and mortality. Prescribers also reported concern about abuse of opioids by family and friends.

A qualitative study by Teh and colleagues (2009) shows that older adults' successful response to pain treatment was the result of active participation in treatment decisions and a trusting and mutually respectful relationship with their providers. The concept of "being understood" was an important theme and underscores the importance of patient-centered care.

Nonpharmacological Pain Treatments. Nonpharmacological treatments for pain include physical therapy, vagal nerve stimulation, exercise, hydrotherapy, heat and cold packs, chiropractic,

BOX 30-2 THE FIVE ELEMENTS OF THE PAIN ASSESSMENT IN ADVANCED DEMENTIA (PAINAD) SCALE

1. Breathing
   Normal breathing is effortless breathing characterized by quiet, rhythmic respirations.
   Occasional labored breathing is characterized by episodic bursts of harsh, difficult, or wearing respirations.
   Short period of hyperventilation is characterized by intervals of rapid, deep breaths lasting a short period of time.
   Long period of hyperventilation is characterized by excessive rate and depth of respirations lasting a considerable time.
   Cheyne-Stokes respirations are characterized by rhythmic waxing and waning of breathing from very deep to shallow respirations with periods of apnea.
2. Negative Vocalization
   None is characterized by speech or vocalization that has a neutral or pleasant quality.
   Occasional moan or groan: *Occasional moaning* is characterized by mournful or murmuring sounds, wails, or laments. *Occasional groaning* is characterized by louder than usual inarticulate involuntary sounds, often abruptly beginning and ending.
   Low-level speech with negative or disapproving quality is characterized by muttering, mumbling, whining, grumbling, or swearing in a low volume with a complaining, sarcastic, or caustic tone.
   Repeated, troubled calling out is characterized by phrases or words being used over and over in a tone that suggests anxiety, uneasiness, or distress.
   Loud moaning or groaning: *Loud moaning* is characterized by mournful or murmuring sounds, wails, or laments in a much-louder-than-usual volume. Loud groaning is characterized by louder-than-usual inarticulate involuntary sounds, often abruptly beginning and ending.
   Crying is characterized by an utterance of emotion accompanied by tears. There may be sobbing or quiet weeping.
3. Facial Expression
   Smiling or inexpressiveness: Smiling is characterized by upturned corners of the mouth, brightening of the eyes, and a look of pleasure or contentment. *Inexpressive* refers to a neutral, at ease, relaxed, or blank look.
   Sad is characterized by an unhappy, lonesome, sorrowful, or dejected look. Eyes may be teary.
   Frightened is characterized by a look of fear, alarm, or heightened anxiety. Eyes may appear wide open.
   Frown is characterized by a downward turn of the corners of the mouth. Increased facial wrinkling in the forehead and around the corners of the mouth may appear.
   Facial grimacing is characterized by a distorted, distressed look. The brow is more wrinkled, as is the area around the mouth. Eyes may be squeezed shut.
4. Body Language
   Relaxed is characterized by a calm, restful, mellow appearance. The person seems to be taking it easy.
   Tense is characterized by a strained, apprehensive, or worried appearance. The jaw may be clenched.
   Distressed pacing is characterized by activity that seems unsettled. There may be a fearful, worried, or disturbed element present. The rate may be faster or slower.
   Fidgeting is characterized by restless movement. Squirming about or wiggling in the chair may occur. The person might be hitching a chair across the room. Repetitive touching, tugging, or rubbing body parts can also be observed.
   Rigid is characterized by stiffening of the body. The arms and/or legs are tight and inflexible. The trunk may appear straight and unyielding (exclude contractures).
   Fists clenched are characterized by tightly closed hands. They may be opened and closed repeatedly or held tightly shut.
   Knees pulled up is characterized by flexing the legs and drawing the knees upward toward the chest (exclude contractures).
   Pulling or pushing away is characterized by resistiveness upon approach or to care. The person is trying to escape by yanking or wrenching himself or herself free or by shoving you away.
   Striking out is characterized by hitting, kicking, grabbing, punching, biting, or other forms of personal assault.
5. Consolability
   No need to console is characterized by a sense of well-being. The person appears content.
   Distracted or reassured by voice or touch is characterized by a disruption in the behavior when the person is spoken to or touched. The behavior stops during the period of interaction, with no indication that the person is at all distressed.
   Unable to console, distract, or reassure is characterized by the inability to soothe the person or stop a behavior with words or actions. No amount of verbal or physical comforting will alleviate the behavior.

Scoring: (See Figure 30-5 on p. 577 for point allocation.)
0-1 = No significant pain
2-3 = Mild to moderate pain
4-6 = Moderate to severe pain
7-10 = Severe to very severe pain

From Lane, P., Kuntupis, M., MacDonald, S., McCarthy, P., Panke, J., Warden, V., & Volicer, L. (2003). A pain assessment tool for people with advanced Alzheimer's and other progressive dementias. *Home Healthcare Nurse, 21*(1), 36.

and transcutaneous electrical nerve stimulation (TENS). Yoga, biofeedback, hypnosis, acupuncture, massage, Reiki, guided imagery, reflexology, and therapeutic touch are integrative therapies for managing pain. Herbal remedies include cayenne, capsaicin, ginger extract, echinacea, kava, and willow bark. It is important to ask older adults if they are utilizing any alternative treatments for pain relief. Pain-management education is important for both the patient and caregivers. Refer to Chapter 35 for a full discussion of integrative therapies.

It is critical for nurses to evaluate the effectiveness of pain interventions at regular intervals and to be attentive to behavioral changes or verbal responses that indicate that the patient is experiencing pain. It is a common misconception to assume that the ability to perceive pain decreases with aging. No physiological changes in pain perception in older adults have been demonstrated. Careful and continuing assessments and an understanding of pain physiology are necessary for effective pain management of older adults.

BOX 30-3 TIPS FOR PHARMACOLOGICAL PAIN MANAGEMENT IN OLDER ADULTS

- Remember that older adults often receive pain medication less often than younger adults, which results in inadequate pain relief. Compensate for this.
- Safe administration of analgesics is complicated because of possible interactions with drugs used to treat multiple chronic disorders, nutritional alterations, and altered pharmacokinetics in older adults.
- Analgesics reach a higher peak and have a longer duration of action in older adults than in younger individuals. Start with one fourth to one half the adult dose and titrate up carefully.
- Give oral analgesics around the clock when initiating pain management. Administer on an as-needed basis later on, as indicated by the patient's pain status.
- If acute confusion occurs, assess for other contributing factors before changing the medication or stopping analgesic use. Confusion in postoperative patients has been found to be associated with unrelieved pain rather than with opiate use.
- **Acetaminophen** is an effective analgesic in older adults. Although there is an increased risk of end-stage renal disease with long-term use, it does not produce the gastrointestinal bleeding seen with **nonsteroidal antiinflammatory drugs (NSAIDs).**
- Analgesics and adjuvants, such as **anticholinergics** and **pentazocine**, may produce increased confusion in older adults. **NSAIDs** can have the same effect during their initial period of administration.
- **Opiates** have a greater analgesic effect and longer duration of action than nonopioid analgesics. Avoid the use of **meperidine**, whose active metabolite may stimulate the central nervous system and lead to confusion, seizures, and mood alterations. If this drug is selected, do not use it for more than 48 hours. Avoid intramuscular administration because of tissue irritation and poor absorption. **Morphine** is a safer choice than meperidine because its duration of action is longer, so a smaller overall dose is required.
- Assess bowel function daily because constipation can be a frequent side effect of opiates.

From Davis, M., & Srivastava, M. (2003). Demographics, assessment and management of pain in the elderly. *Drugs and Aging, 20*(1), 23–35.

HEALTH CARE CONCERNS OF OLDER ADULTS

Financial Burden

Health care expenses for older adults are nearly four times higher than the expenses for the rest of the population, and with the predicted growth in this population, illness prevention and maintenance of functional ability must be a priority in nursing care. To prepare for the future the average 65-year-old couple will need an estimated $215,000 to cover anticipated out-of-pocket expenses (Purcell, 2006). Many older adults on fixed incomes have to make a choice between buying medication or food.

The implementation of Medicare Part D has shifted some of the costs from seniors, but many continue to struggle. Medicare Part D pays 75% of total drug costs, after a $275 deductible, up to the initial limit of $2510. Once expenses exceed this $2510, there is no coverage until drug costs exceed $5726, at which time 95% of cost is covered. This "donut hole," or coverage gap, affects many seniors. There is a low-income subsidy, which allows for full or partial waivers for out-of-pocket costs, but to be eligible requires income no greater than 150% of the federal poverty level. A survey of 10,000 households revealed that older families spent 43.9% of their flexible spending on health care (Briesacher et al., 2010). This study also confirmed that, despite the implementation of Medicare Part D, the sickest population still has the highest level of cost-related medication nonadherence.

Caregiver Burden

Another phenomenon with the aging population is the increase in caregiver burden. Caregiver burden is defined as the amount of physical, emotional, financial, and psychosocial support provided to a loved one with a chronic illness. A common scenario is a two-income family, in the middle of raising children and planning for their future retirement, faced with aging parents in need of help. Another is one elderly spouse taking care of the other. Dwindling health care benefits, shorter hospital stays, limited home-care options, greater life expectancy, and complicated procedures to access care have increased the need for adult children and aging spouses to provide enormous amounts of care to loved ones. Resources for caregivers include the following:

- Books
  - Mace and Rabins, *The 36-Hour Day*
  - Lustbader, *Taking Care of Aging Family Members*
- Agencies & Associations
  - AARP: www.aarp.org/family/caregiving
  - Alzheimer's Association: www.alz.org & 24/7 helpline – 800-272-3900
  - U.S. National Library of Medicine: www.nlm.nig.gov/medlineplus
  - Family Caregiver Alliance: www.caregiver.org and 800-445-8106
  - U.S. Department of Veterans Affairs: www.va.gov and 800-827-1000
  - Caregiver Action Network: 800-896-3650
  - National Institute on Aging: www.nia.nih.gov
  - Administration on Aging: www.aoa.gov

Unfortunately, having family caregivers is not common for older adults who have lived with a chronic mental illness. Schizophrenia and bipolar disorders often take a toll on family members and intimate relationships, and it is not uncommon for those with severe mental illness to have no family available for support as they age. Grown children may be estranged because of a parent's frequent hospitalization, poor parenting ability, or paranoid symptoms. The support system of those aging with chronic mental illness often becomes case managers, community nurses, and mental health providers.

Ageism

In Western cultures, growing older is not usually viewed as a privilege, and old age does not tend to confer a revered social status upon those who have attained it. **Ageism** has been defined as a bias against older people based on advanced age.

Ageism differs from other forms of discrimination in that it cuts across gender, race, religion, and socioeconomic status to reach the majority of those over age 65.

Ageism and Public Policy

The results of ageism can be observed in every level of society. Financial and political support for programs for older adults is difficult to obtain; however, the Gray Panthers and the American Association of Retired Persons (AARP) are powerful lobbying groups that are fighting to change this trend. As listed previously, there are numerous federal, state, and local agencies dedicated to the interests of older adults.

Ageism and Research

In 1999 the U.S. Food and Drug Administration (FDA) began to require research specific to those over the age of 65. Barriers to inclusion in clinical trials are linked to older adults, being on multiple medications or to their already having an existing chronic illness. Information about medications for a younger, healthier general population often has to be generalized for older, sicker adults, and recommended (generally lower) doses of medication may not have ever been tested (Rochon, 2012). Other nonpharmacological intervention studies also struggle with obtaining subjects, so the knowledge base on older adults is frequently inadequate.

HEALTH CARE DECISION MAKING

Advance Directives

Since the 1960s, the public's desire to participate in decision making about health care has increased. This interest in patient advocacy was recognized when Congress passed the Patient Self-Determination Act (PSDA) in 1990, requiring that health care facilities provide clearly written information for every patient regarding his or her legal rights to make health care decisions, including the right to accept or refuse treatment. It also establishes the right of a person to provide directions (advance directives) for clinicians to follow in the event of a serious illness. Such a directive indicates preferences for the types and amount of medical care desired. The directive comes into effect should physical or mental incapacitation prevent the patient from making health care decisions. These wishes can be communicated through one or more of the following instruments: (1) a living will, (2) a directive to physician, and (3) a durable power of attorney for health care. These documents must be in writing, and the patient's signature must be witnessed; depending on state and institutional provisions, notarization of the documents may be required.

The American Nurses Association (1992) recommends that specific questions about advance directives be part of every nurse's admission assessment. Box 30-4 reproduces these questions and describes the responsibilities of health care workers under the Patient Self-Determination Act.

By signing a **psychiatric advance directive**, those with serious mental illness can designate a health care agent to make treatment decisions during an illness relapse (Elbogen et al., 2006). The National Resource Center on Psychiatric Advance Directives provides information about this method of treatment planning for those with serious mental illnesses such as schizophrenia and bipolar disorder. Both disorders characteristically have patterns of relapse, often combined with poor insight for needed intervention.

BOX 30-4 NURSES' RESPONSIBILITIES AND THE PATIENT SELF-DETERMINATION ACT OF 1990

Part of Nursing Admission Assessment

- Nurses should know the laws of the state in which [they] practice . . . and should be familiar with the strengths and limitations of the various forms of advance directive.
- The ANA recommends that the following questions be part of the nursing admission assessment:
  1. Do you have basic information about advance care directives, including living wills and durable power of attorney?
  2. Do you wish to initiate an advance care directive?
  3. If you have already prepared an advance care directive, can you provide it now?
  4. Have you discussed your end-of-life choices with your family or designated surrogate and health care workers?

Responsibilities of Health Care Workers Under the Patient Self-Determination Act of 1990

- Hospitals, skilled nursing facilities, home health agencies, hospice organizations, and health maintenance organizations serving Medicare and Medicaid patients must:
  1. Maintain written policies and procedures for providing information to their patients for whom they provide care.
  2. Give written material to patients concerning their rights under state law to make decisions about medical care, including the right to accept or refuse surgical or medical care and to formulate advance directives and provide written policies and procedures for the realization of these rights.
  3. Document in patients' records whether they have advance directives.
  4. Not discriminate in care or in other ways against patients who have or have not prepared advance directives.
  5. Make sure that policies are in place to ensure compliance with state laws governing advance directives.

From Schlossberg, C., & Hart, M. A. (1992). Legal perspectives. In M. Burke & M. Walsh (Eds.), *Gerontologic nursing care of the frail elderly* (p. 469). St. Louis, MO: Mosby; American Nurses Association. (1992). *Position statement on nursing and the patient self-determination act.* Washington, DC: Author.

Living Will

A **living will** is a personal statement of how and where one wishes to die. It is activated only when the person is terminally ill and incapacitated, and a competent patient may alter a living will at any time. The question of whether an incompetent person can change a living will is addressed on a state-by-state basis. Executing a living will does not always guarantee its application.

Directive to Physician

In a **directive to physician**, a physician is appointed to serve as a surrogate medical decision maker, particularly in cases of terminal illness when an individual has no family. There needs to be verification of terminal illness by the physician, and the patient must be competent at the time of signing. The physician must agree in writing to be the patient's agent and must also be one of the two physicians who made the original determination that the patient is terminally ill. Unlike the living will, the directive to physician can be revoked orally at any time without regard to patient competency.

Durable Power of Attorney for Health Care

The **durable power of attorney for health care** is the designation of a person to act as the patient's medical decision maker. The patient must be competent when making the appointment and must also be competent in order to revoke the power. Individuals do not have to be terminally ill or incompetent to allow the empowered individual to act on their behalf.

Guardianship

A **guardianship** is a court-ordered relationship in which one party, the guardian, acts on behalf of an individual, the ward. The law regards the ward as lacking capacity to manage his or her personal and/or financial affairs. After an evaluation, usually by a physician or psychologist, probate court determines if guardianship is warranted. Many people with mental illness, mental retardation, traumatic brain injuries, and organic brain disorders such as dementia have guardians. It is important that health care workers identify patients who have guardians and communicate with the guardians when health care decisions are being made.

The Nurse's Role in Decision Making

The nurse is often responsible for explaining the legal policies of the institution to both the patient and family and can help them understand advance directives. There are usually three common approaches to care:

1. **Full code:** All life-saving measures are initiated.
2. **Do not resuscitate–comfort care arrest (DNR–CCA):** All life-saving measures are initiated, except in the case of a full cardiac arrest and intubation.
3. **Do not resuscitate–comfort care only (DNR–CCO):** Medical care is focused on providing pain-free quality of life and comfort free of invasive procedures and intubation.

Ethical dilemmas can occur; for example, when a patient has a feeding tube and a DNR–CCO status is initiated later. There are many situations that can be called into question; there is usually a bioethics committee in hospital settings that can assist by looking at the situation objectively. The patient is encouraged to verbalize thoughts and feelings during this sensitive time of decision-making. Every health care facility receiving federal funds is required to have written policies, procedures, and protocols in compliance with the Patient Self-Determination Act. The law does not specify who talks with patients about treatment decisions, but nurses are often asked to discuss this issue with patients. If the advance directive of a patient is not being followed, the nurse intervenes on the patient's behalf. Although nurses may discuss options with their patients, they may not assist patients in writing advance directives, because this is considered a conflict of interest.

NURSING CARE OF OLDER ADULTS

Nurses encounter older adults in a variety of settings, and in each of these settings, the nurse is responsible for application of the nursing process to the individual patient's situation. Studies suggest that because nursing students are not given adequate information about nor exposure to older patients, they may hold ageist views when beginning their nursing careers (Williams et al., 2007). It is important for all nurses to gain a better understanding of the aging process and to recognize that with the aging of America this will be a population nurses will increasingly serve.

Evidenced-based practice recommendations are increasingly available to guide safe and excellent nursing care for older adults. The Hartford Institute for Geriatric Nursing was founded in 1996 and now provides priceless resources via the Internet. Nurses can access evidence-based information at ConsultGeriRN.org, which is supported by the Hartford Institute. Likewise, the American Psychiatric Nurses Association has recognized the need for specialized education and has competency recommendations for geropsychiatric nursing at its website, www.apna.org.

Positive attitudes toward older adults and their care need to be instilled during basic nursing education. It is vital for nurses to provide respect to older patients and appreciate their wisdom and life experience. Nursing educators need to teach the importance of using excellent communication skills with older adults. By utilizing role play, students may gain insight and empathy for those dependent on others for basic activities of daily living.

There are many theories about the process of aging from biological, genetic, psychological, and psychosocial perspectives (Box 30-5). Substantial literature is written on what shortens the life expectancy and on behaviors that predispose humans to disease. Current trends lean toward the concept of "aging well" and how this is accomplished. Nursing is about maintenance of health, prevention of illness, and helping individuals with their response to disease. There is a growing focus on healthy eating, exercise, socialization, spirituality, effective coping skills, avoiding alcohol/tobacco, and healthy relationships as a basis for "aging well." Nurses can play a vital role in this movement as educators and advocates for health.

Box 30-6 provides some facts and myths about aging that influence how society perceives the older adult.

Assessment Strategies

Nurses who work with older adults need specific knowledge about normal aging, drug interactions, and chronic disease. Those who work with older patients who have mental health problems or cognitive deficits need to have additional skills in effective communication, behavioral intervention, and recognition of how the care setting affects the older individual. The National Institutes of Health recommends a comprehensive geriatric assessment, which includes a focus on physical and mental health; functional, economic, and social status; and environmental factors that might

BOX 30-5 MAJOR THEORIES OF AGING

Biological

- **Cellular functioning:** Cells accumulate damage resulting in errors of replication
- **Error theory:** Error in protein synthesis results in impaired cellular function.
- **Oxidative stress theory:** Production of free radicals increases and the body's ability to remove them decreases, resulting in DNA damage
- **Wear-and-tear theory:** Internal and external stressors harm cells.
- **Programmed aging theory:** Biological or genetic clock plays out on genes.
- **Neuroendocrine theory:** A programmed decline in the functioning of the nervous, endocrine, and immune systems where cells lose their ability to reproduce.
- **Immunity theory:** An accumulation of damage and decline in the immune system.

Developmental

- **Jung's theory of personality:** Individuals move from outward achievement to self-acceptance.
- **Erikson:** Integrity is built on morality and ethics.
- **Peck:** Successful aging is accompanied by redefining self, letting go of occupational identity, rising above body discomforts, and establishing meaning.
- **Maslow:** Self-actualization and the evolution of developmental needs occur as the individual ages.
- **Tornstam:** Disengagement with the world can be a time of introspection leading to wisdom.

Psychosocial

- **Role theory:** The ability of an individual to adapt to changing roles predicts adjustment to aging.
- **Activity theory:** Actions, roles, and social pursuits are important for satisfactory aging.
- **Disengagement theory:** Mutual withdrawal occurs between the aging person and others.
- **Continuity theory:** Life satisfaction and activity are expressions of enduring personality traits.
- **Age-stratification theory:** Individuals are viewed as members of an age group (e.g., young, middle-age, old) with similarities to others in the group
- **Modernization theory:** Modern society devalues the contributions of elders and elders themselves.

From Jett, K. (2012). Theories of aging. In E. A. Touhy & K. Jett (Eds.), *Ebersole & Hess' toward healthy aging: Human needs and nursing response* (8th ed.). St. Louis, MO: Elsevier.

BOX 30-6 FACTS AND MYTHS ABOUT AGING

Facts

- The senses of vision, hearing, touch, taste, and smell decline with age.
- Muscular strength decreases with age. Muscle fibers atrophy and decrease in number.
- Regular sexual expressions are important to maintain sexual capacity and effective sexual performance.
- At least 50% of restorative sleep is lost as a result of the aging process.
- Older adults are major consumers of prescription drugs because of the high incidence of chronic diseases in this population.
- Older adults have a high incidence of depression.
- Many individuals experience difficulty when they retire.
- Older adults are prone to become victims of crime.
- Older widows appear to adjust better than younger ones.

Myths

- Most adults past the age of 65 are demented.
- Sexual interest declines with age.
- Older adults are unable to learn new tasks.
- As individuals age, they become more rigid in their thinking and set in their ways.
- The aged are well off and no longer impoverished.
- Most older adults are infirm and require help with daily activities.
- Most older adults are socially isolated and lonely.

impinge on the person's well-being. Figure 30-4 provides an example of a comprehensive geriatric assessment.

A thorough assessment, including a physical assessment and diagnostic testing, must precede any treatment and/or diagnosis of a mental illness in older adults. Common tests include thyroid, kidney, and liver function; complete blood count; comprehensive metabolic panel; vitamin B_{12}, folic acid, and therapeutic drug levels; urinalysis; serology (RPR); β-type natriuretic peptide (BNP); HIV testing; and computed tomography (CT) of the head when indicated.

A systematic review of current medication use must also occur (Rochon, 2012). **Adverse drug reactions**, or negative responses to drugs, are common among the elderly. Older adults are at special risk for these events due to multiple medical problems, memory issues that may result in taking too little or too much medication, and the use of multiple prescribed and nonprescribed medications. Renal impairment is a major problem associated with dose-related adverse reactions, and serum creatinine levels may not accurately reflect the actual efficiency of kidney function in older adults.

Assessing the use of multiple medications by patients, or **polypharmacy**, including prescription or over-the-counter drugs, is also essential. The presence of chronic conditions in the older population results in increased medication use that is associated with an increased risk for adverse drug events. Metabolic changes and decreased drug clearance compound the risk of drug-drug interactions. The risk of adverse drug reactions doubles for persons taking five to seven medications as compared to those taking fewer than five medications (Onder et al., 2010). For persons taking eight or more medications,

COMPREHENSIVE GERIATRIC ASSESSMENT					
Name:		Date of birth:		Gender:	
Physical Health					
Chronic disorder					
Vision	Adequate	Inadequate	Eyeglasses: Y N		Needs evaluation
Hearing	Adequate	Inadequate	Hearing aids: Y N		
Mobility	Ambulatory: Y N		Assistive device:		
	Falls: Y N				Needs evaluation
Nutrition	Albumin:	TLC:	HCT:		
	Weight:	Weight loss or gain: Y N			Needs evaluation
Incontinence	Y N	Treatment:	Y N		Needs evaluation
Medications	Total number:	Reviewed & revised:	Y N		
	Adverse effects/allergy:				
Screening	Cholesterol:	TSH:	B12:		Folate:
	Colonoscopy: Date:		N/A		
	Mammogram: Date:		N/A		
	Osteoporosis: Date:		N/A		
	Pap smear: Date:		N/A		
	PSA: Date:		N/A		
Immunization	Influenza: Date:				
	Pneumonia: Date:				
	Tetanus: Date:		Booster:		
Counseling	Diet	Exercise	Calcium	Vitamin D	
	Smoking	Alcohol	Driving	Injury prevention	
Mental Health					
Dementia	Y N	MMSE score:	Date:	Cause (if known):	
Depression	Y N	GDS score:	Date:	Treatment:	Y N
Functional Status					
ADL	Bathing: I D		Dressing: I D		Toileting: I D
	Transferring: I D		Feeding: I D		Continence: Y N

FIG 30-4 Comprehensive geriatric assessment. *ADL*, Activities of daily living; *B_{12}*, vitamin B12; *D*, dependent; *GDS*, Geriatric Depression Scale; *HCT*, hematocrit; *I*, independent; *MMSE*, Mini-Mental State Examination; *N*, no; *PSA*, prostate-specific antigen; *TLC*, total lymphocyte count; *TSH*, thyroid-stimulating hormone; *Y*, yes.

the risk of adverse drug reactions increases by four times. One screening tool, the Screening Tool of Older Person's Prescriptions (STOPP) (Gallagher et al., 2008), provides 65 criteria that measure potentially inappropriate prescribing.

Prescribing cascades happen when drug-induced symptoms are treated with another drug. The symptoms of the first drug (e.g., agitation) may be evaluated as part of the medical problem. Prescribing cascades are particularly problematic and complicated. One of the most common examples is when anti-Parkinson therapy is initiated for symptoms brought about by antipsychotics (Rochon, 2012). Anti-Parkinson drugs may bring about new and dangerous symptoms such as delirium

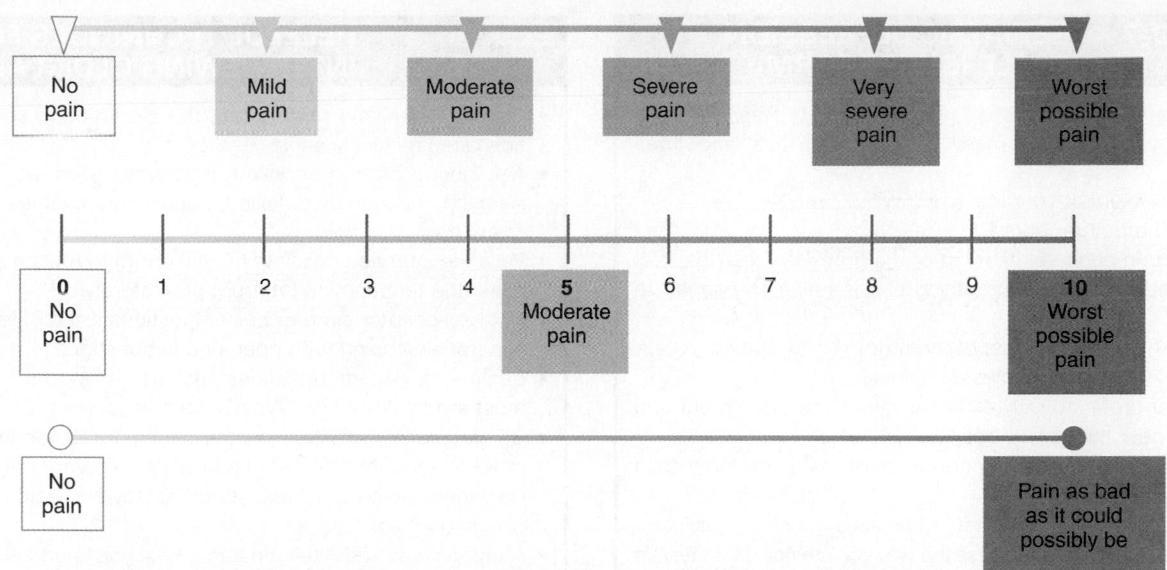

FIG 30-5 Visual analogue scales used in the management of cancer pain. (From Jacox, A., et al. [1994]. Management of cancer pain [Clinical Practice Guideline No. 9, AHCPR Publication No. 94-0952]. Rockville, MD: U.S. Department of Health and Human Services, Public Health Service, Agency for Health Care Policy and Research.)

and orthostatic hypotension. Anticholinesterase inhibitor drugs used to treat dementia (e.g., donepezil, rivastigmine, and galantamine) may cause urinary incontinence and diarrhea. These symptoms may result in a prescribing cascade when they are treated with an anticholinergic such as oxybutynin.

Common problems associated with medication include confusion, which can be caused by anticholinergics, antihistamines, and benzodiazepines. Psychosis has been linked to steroids and even cholesterol-lowering medications. Depression has been linked with beta-blockers, alpha adrenergics, and opiates. Serious medical conditions such as cancer, stroke, anemia, diabetes, infections, electrolyte imbalance, malnutrition, dehydration, and cardiac disease can manifest in mental status changes before more specific physical symptoms occur. Nurses are in a unique position to advocate for and coordinate appropriate medical evaluation for older adults.

An examination and interview of an older adult conducted in unfamiliar surroundings can produce anxiety. Unlike younger patients, who may be comfortable discussing personal issues—family conflicts, feelings of sadness, sexual practices, finances, and bodily functions—older adults may view these topics as private or taboo. As a result, they may be uncomfortable discussing them. It is important to respect these feelings while reviewing essential history by:

- Conducting the interview in a private area
- Introducing oneself and asking the patient what he or she would like to be called (use of the first name is rarely appropriate unless one is invited to do so)
- Establishing rapport and putting the patient at ease by sitting or standing at the same level as the patient
- Ensuring that lighting is adequate and noise level is low in recognition of the fact that hearing and vision may be impaired
- Using touch (with permission) to convey warmth while at the same time respecting the patient's comfort level with personal touch
- Summarizing the interaction, inviting feedback and questions, and thanking patients for giving their time and information

Assessment of the cognitive, behavioral, and emotional status of the older adult is important in managing the nursing care of the patient. The periodic repetition of these screening tools serves to evaluate the effectiveness of intervention. The Geriatric Depression Scale (Short Form) (Box 30-7) is a subjective yes/no questionnaire (Sheikh & Yesavage, 1986), and the Cornell Scale for Depression in Dementia is an objective behavioral checklist for caregivers to help identify the presence of depressive symptoms (Alexopoulos, 1988).

It is also essential to assess for suicidal thoughts and intent by asking specific questions such as:

- Have you ever thought about killing yourself?
- Have you ever felt that life is not worth living?
- Have you ever tried to hurt yourself in the past?
- Are you looking for ways to harm yourself?
- Do you have thoughts of harming others?
- Do you have any means to harm yourself or others? Weapons? Large amounts of medication? (This may need to be asked to family members as well.)

At times, when individuals, older adults included, are sick or are in significant pain, they may verbalize a death wish by saying "I just wish I would die" or "If I had a gun, I'd shoot myself." This should never be ignored; rather it needs to be explored. Often people just feel frustrated, desperate, ignored, unheard, or disrespected, but they aren't able to articulate these emotions. Encourage the individual to say more about what he or she is experiencing, get more information, provide active listening, and offer support. These types of statements and data need to be documented and reported to the care provider. If there are active suicidal thoughts and intent, the individual should not be left alone. Elicit help from other staff and the mental health team.

Interventions for the prevention of suicide in older adults are discussed in greater depth later in this chapter. Also refer to

BOX 30-7 GERIATRIC DEPRESSION SCALE (SHORT FORM)

1. Are you basically satisfied with your life? Yes/No
2. Have you dropped many of your activities and interests? Yes/No
3. Do you feel that your life is empty? Yes/No
4. Do you often get bored? Yes/No
5. Are you in good spirits most of the time? Yes/No
6. Are you afraid that something bad is going to happen to you? Yes/No
7. Do you feel happy most of the time? Yes/No
8. Do you often feel helpless? Yes/No
9. Do you prefer to stay at home rather than going out and doing new things? Yes/No
10. Do you feel you have more problems with memory than most? Yes/No
11. Do you think it is wonderful to be alive now? Yes/No
12. Do you feel pretty worthless the way you are now? Yes/No
13. Do you feel full of energy? Yes/No
14. Do you feel that your situation is hopeless? Yes/No
15. Do you think that most people are better off than you are? Yes/No

From Sheikh, J. I., & Yesavage, J. A. (1986). Geriatric Depression Scale (GDS): Recent evidence and development of a shorter version. In T. L. Brink (Ed.), *Clinical gerontology: A guide to assessment and intervention* (pp. 165–173). New York, NY: Hawthorn Press.

BOX 30-8 HELPFUL TECHNIQUES FOR INTERVIEWING OLDER ADULTS

- Gather preliminary data before the session and keep questionnaires relatively short.
- Ask about often-overlooked problems, such as difficulty sleeping, incontinence, falling, depression, dizziness, or loss of energy.
- Pace the interview to allow the patient to formulate answers; resist the tendency to interrupt prematurely.
- Use yes-or-no or simple-choice questions if the older patient has trouble coping with open-ended questions.
- Begin with general questions such as, "How can I help you most at this visit?" or "What's been happening?"
- Be alert for information on the patient's relationships with others, thoughts about families or co-workers, typical responses to stress, and attitudes toward aging, illness, occupation, and death.
- A request such as, "Tell me about how you spend your days" often provides important information.
- Assess mental status for deficits in recent or remote memory and determine if confusion exists.
- Be aware of all medications the patient is taking, and assess for side effects, efficacy, and possible drug interactions.
- Determine how fast the condition of the patient has been changing to assess the extent of the patient's concerns.
- Include the family or significant other in the interview process for added input, clarification, support, and reinforcement.

From National Institute on Aging. (2012). *Talking with your older patient: A clinician's handbook.* Retrieved from http://www.nia.nih.gov/health/publication/talking-your-older-patient-clinicians-handbook.

Chapter 25 for a more detailed discussion of suicide assessment and intervention.

Older adult abuse is another area to explore during a nursing assessment and is discussed in depth in Chapter 28. Questions about being hit, pushed, kicked, and slapped are important, but it is also imperative to inquire about care being withheld. Not being fed, cleaned, helped, or cared for is abuse also. Asking "How are you being treated at home?" or "Are you afraid of anyone?" may encourage further exploration. Financial exploitation is another issue that is difficult to uncover. Older adults may feel ashamed or embarrassed to admit they have been taken advantage of by family, friends, or strangers (Spangler & Brandl, 2007). Box 30-8 provides helpful interview techniques to use with older adults.

Intervention Strategies

The growing trends for patient-centered care, relationship-based care, and the patient as a participant in care are foreign concepts to the older adult. Most have experienced medical care as "listening to the doctor" regardless of whether they agree or not. This shift in care approach may need much reinforcement with the older adult, who has been socialized as a passive recipient of health care.

Certain psychotherapeutic methods are especially useful for older adults:

- Providing empathetic understanding and active listening
- Encouraging ventilation of feelings and normalizing emotional responses
- Reestablishing emotional equilibrium when anxiety is moderate to severe
- Providing health education, discussing alternative solutions, and encouraging questions
- Assisting in the use of problem-solving approaches
- Allowing adequate time to process information
- Ensuring hearing aids are working or using an amplifier to facilitate good communication
- Providing written information in large print

Environmental Interventions

An older adult may require acute inpatient mental health care for signs and symptoms of severe psychiatric conditions, such as nondementia psychiatric illnesses, major depression with suicidal thoughts, bipolar disorder, and schizophrenia (Hoover et al., 2008). Inpatient treatment is still recommended when the patient is at high risk of self-harm (whether intentional or unintentional) or poses a risk of harm to other people. The nurse also assesses for underlying medical problems. Often patients with chronic persistent mental illnesses (such as schizophrenia), as well as chronic medical conditions, do not report or misinterpret visceral cues, pain, and significant symptoms of illness (Reeves & Torres, 2003). One true-life example of this phenomenon follows:

A 65-year-old white female with schizophrenia was admitted to an acute psychiatry unit due to an exacerbation of psychosis. For several days she refused to get out of bed or leave the room.

She claimed there were "Japanese torture devices" hurting her legs when she got out of bed. Upon further exploration of her pain the nurse evaluated the lower legs. The assessment revealed marked redness, tenderness, and bilateral edema, with multiple small abrasions scattered over the skin. The patient described the pain as worsening upon standing up. This finding was brought to the attention of the medical provider, and the diagnosis of cellulitis was given. The patient was treated with antibiotics, the pain subsided, and she was able to exit the bed and room.

Hospitalization may be an opportunity for the patient to receive much-needed assessment of the skin, feet, hair, mouth, and perineal areas. These assessments often can uncover hidden infections, unhealed wounds, and growths that may otherwise have been missed and can lead to needed medical attention.

Specialized geropsychiatric units provide a comprehensive and specialized approach to care. These units utilize a multidisciplinary approach to assessment, treatment planning, implementation, and evaluation of care. Ideally, the team consists of a geriatric psychiatrist, geriatrician, social worker, nurses, a pharmacist, psychologist, dietitian, occupational therapist, physical therapist, and other specialists as indicated. Nurses play the major role in providing continuous care from admission to discharge.

Psychosocial Interventions

The nurse uses counseling skills to assist the patient with examining his or her present situation, looking at alternatives, and planning for the future. Sometimes counseling is provided in a group setting, as this approach helps build relationships, provides focus on the here and now, and reduces feelings of isolation. Psychoeducation is the goal of the nurse, including symptom identification, coping skills, stress management, self-care, healthy living, resources that will support recovery, medication education, and relapse prevention.

There is a growing interest in activities and mental exercises that maintain and improve cognitive function. An exercise that nurse generalists can use with those aims is cognitive stimulation therapy, which may be conducted individually or in groups of five to eight people (Woods et al., 2010). This evidence-based approach may result in significant improvement in language skills; that includes word finding, comprehension, and naming.

The advanced practice nurse may provide individual and/or group psychotherapy to older adults with mental illness. The group process focuses on instilling hope by diminishing social isolation and loneliness and helping members recognize they are not alone in their situation. Group members can learn creative ways to improve mood and increase quality of life (Yalom, 2005). Individual therapies such as cognitive-behavioral, motivational, interpersonal, and psychodynamic therapy are just a few commonly used. The recommended treatment for depression is the combination of therapy with medication. Because older adults often are reluctant to seek mental health care, primary care providers must have the skills to provide sensitive assessment for depression and suicide risk and be knowledgeable about methods of intervention. Collaboration with mental health providers is best practice. Table 30-1 describes three different group therapy methods for older adults.

Pharmacological Interventions

Evidence about the biology of mental illness and the discovery of new psychotropic medications has expanded the role of the geropsychiatric nurse. Nurses play a vital role in monitoring, reporting, and managing medication side effects such as acute dystonia, akathesia, pseudo-parkinsonism, neuroleptic malignant syndrome (NMS), serotonin syndrome, and anticholinergic effects. Physical assessment of response to medication is also important; this includes monitoring vital signs, pain, lab work, elimination (bowel and bladder), changes in gait, prevention of falls, and neurological checks when appropriate. Teaching patients and/or family about management of medications is a vital part of nursing care (Box 30-9).

Promotion of Self-Care Activities

Hospitalization may result in regression that ranges from needing assistance to requiring total care in accomplishing the activities of daily living. A goal for nurses is to encourage the patient to regain independence in the realm of personal care.

Teamwork and Safety

The major roles of the nurse in terms of milieu management are to assist the patient in adjusting to the environment, to keep the patient safe at all times (e.g., make sure roommates are compatible, call lights are within reach, patients at risk for falling are placed close to the nurses' station), to minimize the adverse effects of hospitalization on functional capacity (e.g., encourage patients to walk and to do so as independently as possible), to provide reality orientation, and to engage in therapeutic communication. It's important to realize that re-orienting a patient is NOT always therapeutic, especially if the patient has dementia and reorientation causes distress or agitation. Using distraction techniques in these cases is often the intervention of choice.

Another vital aspect of teamwork is the prevention and reduction of agitation by maintaining a visible presence on the unit and anticipating the patient's needs (Johnson & Delaney, 2007). Crisis intervention techniques may be utilized if an agitated patient does not respond to redirection or verbal attempts to deescalate agitation. As a crisis situation unfolds, staff response will largely determine the outcome, and a well-trained crisis team improves these outcomes. The crisis team leader is usually a nurse for several reasons:

1. Nurses provide professional care 24 hours a day, 7 days a week and have detailed knowledge of patients and the milieu.
2. The nurse is aware of the patient's medical condition.
3. The nurse is able to guide the team and help prevent injury to patients who may need physical restraint

After the crisis has been deescalated, the team leader, the team, and other patients (as indicated) need to discuss the situation; this will help restore a sense of safety and calm. As the agitated patient gains control, it is important to help the individual ease back into the milieu with dignity.

TABLE 30-1 USEFUL GROUP THERAPY MODALITIES FOR OLDER ADULTS

REMOTIVATION THERAPY	REMINISCENCE THERAPY (LIFE REVIEW)	PSYCHOTHERAPY
Purpose of Group		
Resocialize regressed and apathetic patients Reawaken interest in the environment	Share memories of the past Increase self-esteem Increase socialization Increase awareness of the uniqueness of each participant	Alleviate psychiatric symptoms Increase ability to interact with others in a group Increase self-esteem Increase ability to make decisions and function more independently
Format		
Groups are made up of 10 to 15 people. Meetings are held once or twice a week. Meetings are highly structured in a classroom-like setting. Group uses props. Each session discusses a particular topic.	Groups are made up of six to eight people. Meetings are held once or twice weekly for 1 hour. Topics include holidays, major life events, birthdays, travel, and food.	Group size is 6 to 12 members. Group members should share similar: Problems Mental status Needs Sexual integration Group meets at regularly scheduled times (certain number of times a week, specific duration of session) and place.
Desired Outcomes		
Increases participants' sense of reality Offers practice of health roles Realizes more objective self-image	Alleviates depression in institutionalized older adults Through the process of reorganization and reintegration, provides avenue by which members: Achieve a new sense of identity Achieve a positive self-concept	Decreases sense of isolation Facilitates development of new roles and reestablishes former roles Provides information for other groups Provides group support for effecting changes and increasing self-esteem

From Matteson, M. A., & McConnell, E. S. (Eds.), (1988). *Gerontological nursing: Concepts and practice* (p. 80). Philadelphia, PA: Saunders.

BOX 30-9 PATIENT AND FAMILY TEACHING: DRUG SAFETY

- Learn about your medicines: Read medicine labels and package inserts and follow the directions.
- If you have questions, ask your nurse, pharmacist, or primary care provider.
- Talk to your team of health care professionals about your medical conditions, health concerns, and all the medicines you take (prescription and over-the-counter medicines) as well as dietary supplements, vitamins, and herbal supplements. The more they know, the more they can help.
- Keep track of side effects or possible drug interactions, and let your doctor know right away about any unexpected symptoms or changes in the way you feel.
- Be sure to keep all care provider appointments.
- Use a calendar, pillbox, or something to help you remember what medications you need to take and when.
- Write down information your health care provider gives you about your medicines or your health condition.
- Take a friend or relative to your doctor's appointments if you think you need help to understand or remember what the doctor tells you.
- Have a "medicine check-up" at least once a year. Go through your medicine cabinet to get rid of old or expired medicines.
- Ask your health care provider or pharmacist to go over all the medicines you now take. Remember to tell them about all the over-the-counter medicines, vitamins, dietary supplements, and herbal supplements you take.

Care Settings

Skilled Nursing Facilities

As acute hospital care of older adults with nondementia psychiatric illnesses is decreasing, the use of long-term skilled nursing facilities is increasing (Hoover et al., 2008). The use of these facilities to treat older adults with severe mental illness is controversial, and opponents fear that "nursing homes" will become the mental institutions of the 21st century, providing little more than custodial care.

Whereas some long-term care settings provide specialized psychiatric mental health care, most do not. There may be little consistency in the education of nurses and nursing assistants in appropriate psychiatric assessment and intervention. Clinicians may believe that patients who refuse personal hygiene, medication, or wound care are exercising their rights to refuse care, rather than recognizing the negative symptoms of schizophrenia. Nurses who accept these refusals may inadvertently contribute to a patient's deterioration.

The skilled nursing facility setting can be a stabilizing environment for a person with severe mental illness who thrives within the structure of a therapeutic environment. Providing a documented plan of care and intervening when behavioral symptoms increase is as important as monitoring and intervening when a resident has signs of infection.

Legislation has had a significant impact on the treatment of older adults in extended-care facilities. The **Patient Self-Determination Act** of 1990 was an amendment to the **Omnibus Budget Reconciliation Act (OBRA)** that declared that nursing-home residents have the right to be free from unnecessary drugs and physical restraints. There now is much greater awareness and focus on the use of nonpharmacological interventions for the treatment of agitation, wandering, confusion, yelling, and aggression. Drugs deemed "unnecessary" are generally antipsychotics, antianxiety agents, and sedatives. Patients with a history of depression, schizophrenia, obsessive-compulsive disorder, generalized anxiety disorder, or bipolar disorder need ongoing treatment to prevent relapse and re-emergence of symptoms. Nurses can play an important role in advocating for psychiatric evaluation and intervention to assist with (1) medication management, (2) monitoring and documenting behavioral changes, (3) notifying the physician of behavioral changes, and (4) planning care for the needs of those residents with mental illness.

Due to past inappropriate use of restraints, which lead to injuries and deaths, federal legislation regarding their safe use was put into place. The requirements governing the use of restraints include the following:

1. Consultation with a physical and/or occupational therapist
2. The least restrictive measures must be considered and documented.
3. A physician's order is required.
4. Consent of the resident or family must be obtained.
5. Documentation must be provided that the restraint enables the resident to maintain maximum functional and psychological well-being.

Residential Care Settings

Nurses who work with older adults should be knowledgeable about residential care settings. This is especially important for older adults with chronic and persistent mental illness (e.g., schizophrenia), since placement becomes increasingly difficult. As discussed inChapters 4 the mental health system has increasingly become focused on the goal of community living rather than institutional living, but resources necessary to meet this goal have been chronically underfunded. Patients who would benefit from residential care are often moved from the most structured environment (inpatient care) to unstructured and unsupervised living situations in the community.

Partial Hospitalization

Partial hospitalization or day hospital programs are recommended for ambulatory patients who do not need 24-hour nursing care but require and would benefit from intensive, structured psychiatric treatment. A review of acute psychiatric day hospitals in the United Kingdom found that patients who received care in partial hospitalization programs showed a more rapid improvement in mental status than patients randomly assigned to inpatient care; this type of care also led to cost reductions ranging from 20.9% to 36.9%, compared with inpatient care (Marshall, 2003).

Day Treatment Programs

Multipurpose senior centers provide a broad range of services, including: (1) health promotion and wellness programs; (2) health screening; (3) social, educational, and recreational activities; (4) meals; and (5) information and referral services. For those in need of mostly custodial care services, **adult day care** is an appropriate choice. Older adults are cared for during the day and stay in a home environment at night. These programs are meant to provide a safe, supportive, and nonthreatening environment and fulfill a vital function for older adults and their families. The programs allow older adults to continue their present living arrangements and maintain their social ties to the community; they also relieve families of the burden of 24-hour-a-day care for older adult dependents. This is a great intervention to relieve caregiver burden.

Behavioral Health Home Care

Home-based behavioral health care is particularly recommended to assist the homebound older adult adjust to and manage illness and disability either before or after hospitalization. It is often the role of the behavioral health home-care nurse to help a person affected by a cognitive brain disorder or a severe and persistent mental illness to remain in the home. The National Association of Area Agencies on Aging assists with providing local home care services, such as housekeeping, meal preparation, and assistance with activities of daily living, to increase the older adult's ability to live independently. The target population for behavioral health home care includes older adults who need help with activities of daily living, have behavioral issues related to their physical illness, or have an enduring mental illness. Chapter 4 discusses home psychiatric mental health care in greater detail.

Community-Based Programs

Community-based programs are an alternative to promote the older adult's independent functioning and reduce the stress on the family system. These programs provide specialized case management services that assist older adults with coordination of care and with entitlements (such as Meals on Wheels and transportation). Federal funding has increased the accessibility to home-care options with the creation of the Administration on Aging, a part of the U.S. Department of Health and Human Services. Constant assessment of the changing needs of older adults requires frequent contact and rapid intervention when they become sick or need additional services. Hospitalization can be averted if aggressive and skilled case management is in place, and nurses are uniquely qualified to fulfill the role of case manager.

Driving and the Older Adult. Older adults living in the community may still be driving, which can become a safety concern for caregivers, family, and the public. If there is evidence an older adult can no longer safely drive a vehicle (e.g., failing visual acuity, hearing loss, cognitive deficits, impaired mobility, or movement disorders such as Parkinson's disease) or if there have been occurrences of frequent small collisions, it is appropriate to notify the state bureau of motor vehicles for a driving evaluation to determine capacity for safe operation of a vehicle.

KEY POINTS TO REMEMBER

- The older adult population continues to increase exponentially.
- The increase in the number of older adults poses a challenge not only to nurses but also to the entire health care system to be prepared to respond to the special needs of this population.
- Attitudes toward older adults are often negative, reflecting ageism—a bias against older adults based solely on age. Ageism is found at all levels of society and even among health care providers, which affects the way we render care to our older patients.
- Maintaining a positive regard that demonstrates respect will improve interactions with older adults.
- Nurses who care for older adults in various settings may function at different levels. All should be knowledgeable about the process of aging and be cognizant of the differences between normal and abnormal aging changes.
- The Omnibus Budget Reconciliation Act established guidelines and a philosophy of care that call for patients to be free from unnecessary use of drugs and physical restraints.
- Medication use in the older population is
- Adequate pain assessment is important, and the nurse must bear in mind that older adults tend to understate their pain. Sufficient pain medication should be administered and the drugs carefully titrated.
- Nurses working with elderly patients with concurrent mental health problems should be knowledgeable about psychotherapeutic approaches relevant for the older adult.
- When it comes to dying and death, older adults' wishes and those of their families are frequently ignored. The implementation of the Patient Self-Determination Act, passed in 1990, allows patients autonomy and dignity in death.

CRITICAL THINKING

1. Mr. Jackson is a 70-year-old African American who has been admitted to the intensive care unit with a diagnosis of alcohol withdrawal delirium. He is confused and combative and threatens to strike the nurse unless he is allowed to leave. After getting an order from the primary care provider, the nurse applies wrist restraints to keep Mr. Lopez from striking her and leaving the room.
   a. What are the mandates of OBRA (1990) regarding the use of restraints?
   b. Is the nurse working in accordance with the mandates of OBRA (1990) regarding the use of restraints? Explain your rationale.
2. Mr. Jackson has received treatment for alcohol withdrawal. He is quiet, refuses to eat, does not sleep at night, admits to thoughts of desperation, and wishes he could die. He also confides that he attempted suicide when his wife died 5 years earlier, and that is when he started drinking heavily.
   a. Culturally, what may be helpful to know about older African Americans' response to depression?
   b. Which depression assessment tool is appropriate to use in assessing the severity of Mr. Jackson's condition? Explain your answer.
3. Mrs. Duff is 75 years old and lives with her daughter's family. She has moderate-advanced Alzheimer's disease. Although Mrs. Duff's family wants to keep her at home for as long as possible, they are overwhelmed by her needs and being unable to leave her alone. What community placements might be best for Mrs. Duff? Explain your answer.

CHAPTER REVIEW

1. You are caring for Maggie, a 78-year-old with Alzheimer's disease and Stage III breast cancer who can no longer communicate verbally. What is the appropriate way to assess Maggie's pain?
   a. The Wong-Baker FACES Pain Rating Scale
   b. The McGill Pain Questionnaire
   c. Direct questioning with the use of a Likert 1-10 pain rating scale
   d. The Pain Assessment in Advanced Dementia scale
2. Carlton, age 85, is brought to the clinic by his daughter. She states that Carlton's wife and brother both recently passed away. He has been sad and crying frequently, not attending to hygiene, eating less, and sleeping much of the day. Your nursing assessment and intervention are guided by the knowledge that:
   a. Loss and depression are an expected part of the aging process, needing no specific intervention.
   b. Older male patients are more likely to be resilient and able to recover from life events.
   c. Electroconvulsive therapy (ECT) is the first-line treatment for those in this age group with depression.
   d. Older male patients have the highest rate of suicide.
3. You are caring for Miguel, age 76, who is experiencing delirium. Which nursing response is appropriate when the patient's daughter asks, "Will he ever stop acting like this?"
   a. "I'm sorry. I know this is hard for you, but your father will most likely be this way from now on."
   b. "Once we know the underlying medical cause of the delirium, we can begin treatment to attempt to reverse the process."
   c. "Delirium is caused by infections and electrolyte imbalances, and the damage is permanent."
   d. "A benzodiazepine will help alleviate the delirium."
4. Marco, age 83, has dementia and has difficulty feeding himself despite the fact that there is nothing wrong with his motor functions. Which term should the nurse use to document this finding?
   a. Aphasia
   b. Apraxia
   c. Agnosia
   d. Disinhibition anergia
5. You are caring for Ellie, age 91, whose provider has written a "DNR-CCO" order. Which nursing action would be appropriate if Ellie were to go into cardiac arrest?
   a. Immediately call for the code team
   b. Prepare for intubation by physician
   c. Administer prescribed medication morphine for pain control
   d. Initiate cardiopulmonary resuscitation

Answers to Chapter Review

1. d; 2. d; 3. b; 4. b; 5. c.

evolve WEBSITE

Visit the Evolve website for a posttest on the content in this chapter: http://evolve.elsevier.com/Varcarolis

Post-Test interactive review

REFERENCES

Alexopoulos, G .S. (1988). Cornell scale for depression in dementia. *Biological Psychiatry, 23*(3), 271–284.

American Nurses Association. (1992). *Position statement on nursing and the patient self-determination act.* Washington, DC: Author.

Briesacher, B. A., Ross-Degnan, D., Wagner, A. K., Fouayzi, H., Zhang, F., Gurwitz, J. H., et al. (2010). Out-of-pocket burden of health care spending and the adequacy of Medicare Part D low-income subsidy. *Medical Care, 48*(6), 503–509.

Caplan, J. P., Cassem, N. H., Murray, G. B., Park, J. M., & Stern, T. A. (2010). Delirious patients. In T. A. Stern, Fricchione, G. L., Cassem, N. H., Jellinek, M. S., & J. F. Rosenbaum, (Eds.), *Massachusetts General Hospital handbook of general hospital psychiatry* (6th ed., pp. 93–194). Philadelphia, PA: Saunders.

Cassidy, K., & Rector, N. (2008). The silent geriatric giant: Anxiety disorders in late life. *Geriatrics and Aging, 11*(3), 150–156.

Centers for Disease Control and Prevention. (2012). *Suicide: Facts at a glance.* Retrieved from www.cdc.gov/violenceprevention/pdf/suicide-datasheet-a.PDF.

Davis, M., & Srivastana, M. (2003). Demographics, assessment and management of pain in the elderly. *Drugs and Aging, 20*(1), 23–35.

Elbogen, E. B., Swartz, M. S., VanDorn, R., Swanson, M. K., & Scheyett, A. (2006). Clinical decision making and views about psychiatric advance directives. *Psychiatric Services, 57*, 350–355.

Falk, W. E., & Wiechers, I. R. (2010). Demented patients. In T. A. Stern, G. L. Fricchione, N. H. Cassem, M. S. Jellinek, & J. F. Rosenbaum (Eds.), *Massachusetts General Hospital handbook of general hospital psychiatry* (6th ed., pp. 105–118). Philadelphia, PA: Saunders.

Gallagher, P., Ryan, C., Byrne, S., Kennedy, J., & O'Mahony, D. (2008). STOPP (Screening Tool of Older Person's Prescriptions) and START (Screening Tool to Alert doctors to Right Treatment): Consensus validation. *International Journal of Clinical Pharmacological Therapy, 46*(2), 72–83.

Hockenberry, M., & Wilson, D. (2013). *Wong's essentials of pediatric nursing* (9th ed.). St. Louis, MO: Mosby.

Hoover, D. R., Akincigil, A., Prince, J. D., Kalay, E., Lucas, J. A., Walkup, J. T., et al. (2008). Medicare inpatient treatment of elderly non-dementia psychiatric illnesses 1992–2002: Length of stay and expenditures by facility type. *Administration and Policy in Mental Health, 35*, 231–240.

Ingersoll-Dayton, B., Campbell, R., & Jung-Hwa, H. (2009). Enhancing forgiveness: A group intervention for the elderly. *Journal of Gerontological Social Work, 52*(1), 2–16.

Institute of Medicine. (2008). *Retooling for an aging America: Building the healthcare workforce.* Retrieved from http://books.nap.edu/catalog.ph?record id=12089.

Jacox, A., Carr, D., Payne, R., & Berde, C. (1994). *Management of cancer pain (Clinical Practice Guideline No. 9, AHCPR Publication No. 94–0952).* Rockville, MD: U. S. Department of Health and Human Services, Public Health Service, Agency for Health Care Policy and Research.

Jann, M. W., & Slade, J. H. (2007). Antidepressant agents for the treatment of chronic pain and depression. *Pharmacotherapy, 27*, 1571–1587.

Johnson, M. E., & Delaney, K. R. (2007). Keeping the unit safe: The anatomy of escalation. *Journal of the American Psychiatric Nurses Association, 13*(1), 42–52.

Karlamangla, A., Zhou, K., Reuben, D., Greendale, G., & Moore, A. (2006). Longitudinal trajectories of heavy drinking in adults in the United States of America. *Addiction (Abingdon, England), 101*(1), 91–99.

Karsh, D. (2011). Sex differences in suicide incident characteristics and circumstances among older adults: Surveillance data from the national violent death reporting system–17 states, 2007 2009. *International Journal of Environmental Research in Public Health, 8*(8), 3479–3495.

Kolanowski, A., & Piven, M. (2006). Geropsychiatric nursing: The state of the science. *Journal of the American Psychiatric Nurses Association, 12*(2), 75–99.

Lenze, E., & Wetherell, J. (2011). A lifespan view of anxiety disorders. *Clinics of Neuroscience, 13*(4), 381–399.

Marshall, M. (2003). Adult psychiatric day hospital. *British Medical Journal, 327*(7407), 116–117.

McDonald, D. D., Shea, M., Rose, L., & Fedo, J. (2009). The effect of pain question phrasing on older adult pain information. *Journal of Pain Symptom Management, 37*(6), 1050–1060.

Menninger, J. (2004). Assessment and treatment of alcoholism and substance-related disorders in the elderly. *Bulletin of the Menninger Clinic, 66*(2), 166–183.

Moos, R. H., Schutte, K. K., Brennan, P. L., & Moos, B. S. (2010). Late-life and life history predictors of older adults of high-risk alcohol consumption and drinking problems. *Drug Alcohol Dependency, 108*(102), 13–20.

National Council on Aging. (2002). *American perceptions of aging in the 21st century.* Retrieved from www.brown.edu/Courses/BI_278/projects/.../perceptions.pdf.

National Institute on Aging. (2012). *Alcohol use in older adults.* Retrieved from http://www.nia.nih.gov/health/publication/alcohol-use-older-people.

Nock, M. K., Borges, G., Bromet, E. J., Cha, C. B., Kessler, R. C., & Lee, S. (2008). Suicide and suicidal behavior. *Epidemiology Review*, 1, 133–154.

Onder, G., Petrovic, M., Tangiisuran, B., Meinardi, M. C., Markito-Notenboom, W. P., Somers, A., et al. (2010). Development and validation of a score to assess risk of adverse drug reactions among in-hospital patients 65 years or older: The GerontoNet ADR risk score. *Archives of Internal Medicine, 170*(13), 1142–1148. doi:10.1001/archinternmed.2010.153.

Reeves, R. R., & Torres, R. A. (2003). Exacerbation of psychosis by misinterpretation of physical symptoms. *Southern Medical Journal, 96*(7). Retrieved from http://www.medscape.com/viewarticle/459197_print.

Rochon, P. A. (2012). *Drug prescribing for older adults.* Retrieved from http://www.uptodate.com/contents/drug-prescribing-for-older-adults.

Roy Byrne, P., Craske, M. G., Sullivan, G., Rose, R. D., Edlund, M. J., Lang, A. J. et al. (2010). Delivery of evidence-based treatment for multiple anxiety disorders in primary care: A randomized controlled trial. *Journal of the American Medical Association, 303*(19), 1921–1928.

Sheikh, J. I., & Yesavage, J. A. (1986). Geriatric Depression Scale (GDS): Recent evidence and development of a shorter version. In T. L. Brink (Ed.), *Clinical gerontology: A guide to assessment and intervention* (pp. 165–173). New York, NY: Haworth Press.

Spangler, D., & Brandl, B. (2007). Abuse in later life: Power and control dynamics and a victim-centered response. *Journal of the American Psychiatric Nurses Association, 12*, 322–331.

Teh, C. F., Karp, J. F., Kleinman, A., Reynolds, C. F., Weiner, D. K., & Cleary, P. D. (2009). Older people's experiences of patient-centered treatment for chronic pain: A qualitative study. *Pain Medicine, 10*(3), 521–530. doi:10.1111/j.1526–4637.2008.00556.x.

Touhy, T. A. (2012). Gerontological nursing and an aging society. In T. A. Touhy, T. A., & K. Jett (Eds.), *Ebersole & Hess' toward healthy aging: Human needs and nursing response* (pp. 1–20). St. Louis, MO: Elsevier.

United States Congress (1990). *Patient Self-Determination Act of* 1990. 42 U.S.C. 1395.

Warden, V., Hurley, A. C., & Volicer, L. (2003). Development and psychometric evaluation of the Pain Assessment in Advanced Dementia (PAINAD) scale. *Journal of the American Medical Directors Association, 4*(1), 9–15.

Williams, B., Anderson, M. C., & Day, R. (2007). Undergraduate nursing students' knowledge of and attitudes toward aging: Comparison of context-based learning and a traditional program *Journal of Nursing Education, 46*(3), 115–120.

Woods, B., Aquirre, E., Spector, A. E., & Orrell, M. (2012). Cognitive stimulation to improve cognitive functioning in people with dementia. *Cochrane Database System Review.* Retrieved from http://www.ncbi.nlm.nih.gov/pubmed/22336813.

Yalom, I. D. (2005). *The theory and practice of group psychotherapy* (5th ed.). Cambridge, MA: Basic Books.

CHAPTER

31

Serious Mental Illness

Edward A. Herzog

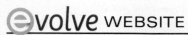

Visit the Evolve website for a pretest on the content in this chapter: http://evolve.elsevier.com/Varcarolis

Pre-Test interactive review

OBJECTIVES

1. Discuss the effects of serious mental illness on daily functioning, interpersonal relationships, and quality of life.
2. Describe three common problems associated with serious mental illness.
3. Discuss five evidence-based practices for the care of the person with serious mental illness.
4. Explain the role of the nurse in the care of the person with serious mental illness.
5. Develop a nursing care plan for a person with serious mental illness.
6. Discuss the causes of treatment nonadherence, and plan interventions to promote treatment adherence.

KEY TERMS AND CONCEPTS

anosognosia
assertive community treatment (ACT)
deinstitutionalization
National Alliance on Mental Illness (NAMI)
outpatient commitment
parity
psychoeducation
recovery model
rehabilitation
serious mental illness (SMI)
social skills training
stigma
supported employment
supportive psychotherapy
transinstitutionalization
vocational rehabilitation

Categorizing mental illness according to levels of severity has tremendous implications for setting mental health policy, establishing insurance reimbursement standards, and facilitating access to appropriate care. In the United States, each state determines how to classify mental illness for the purpose of insurance coverage. The definitions used by the states generally fall into one of three categories. "Broad-based mental illness" refers to any commonly accepted mental health diagnosis whereas "serious mental illness" and "biologically based mental illness" refer only to a limited number of brain-based disorders that have a significant impact on functioning.

The federal government's classifications of "severe and persistent mental illness (SPMI)" and "serious mental illness (SMI)" apply to those who are most deeply affected by psychiatric disorders. Disorders that fall into this category include severe forms of depression, panic disorder, and obsessive-compulsive disorder, as well as schizophrenia, schizoaffective disorder, and bipolar disorder. SPMI affects almost 3% of all adults (Substance Abuse and Mental Health Services Administration [SAMHSA], 2012), and overall, one third of the disabled are disabled due to a mental illness (Anderson et al., 2011).

This chapter focuses on the broader classification of **serious mental illness (SMI)**, which includes disorders in the SPMI group and affects more than 5% to 7% of the U.S. population (SAMHSA, 2012). Persons with SMI usually have difficulties in multiple areas, including activities of daily living (ADLs) (e.g., cooking, hygiene), relationships, social interaction, task completion, communication, leisure activities, remaining safe in the community, finances and budgeting, health maintenance, vocational and academic activities, coping with poverty, stigma, unemployment, and inadequate housing.

SMIs are chronic or recurrent. Some patients experience remissions interrupted by exacerbations of varying lengths; the remissions may be essentially symptom-free, but in most cases involve some degree of residual symptoms. For others, the illness follows a chronic and sometimes deteriorating course during which symptoms wax and wane but never remit.

People with serious mental illness are at risk for multiple physical, emotional, and social problems: they are more likely to be victims of crime, be medically ill, have undertreated or untreated physical illnesses, die prematurely, be homeless, be incarcerated, be unemployed or underemployed, engage in binge substance abuse, live in poverty, and report lower quality of life than persons without such illnesses.

Persons with SMI experience difficulties in a wide range of functions—from preparing meals to coping with everyday stressors. These impairments, along with related factors such as poverty, stigma, unemployment, and inadequate housing, can significantly impact quality of life and can cause persons with SMI to live in a "parallel universe" separate from "normals" (the name some use to describe people who do not have mental illnesses) (Fitch, 2007). Stigma, symptoms, or socially inappropriate behavior caused by SMIs can cause others to reject the patient and refuse friendship, housing, or employment.

VIGNETTE

During her adolescence and young adulthood, Marian was a resident at a facility that cared for people with SMI. On discharge, she moves to a community home, where she spends long periods sitting in front of the living room window. Marian does not ask to go out into the garden she watches for so many hours. Indeed, she rarely asks for anything, including snacks or recreational activities, instead waiting for others to approach her or provide for her. Her caregivers work for several months to help her to recognize and articulate or act on her needs. There is a major celebration the day she walks into the kitchen and makes a sandwich of her own volition. Some of the dependency caused by institutionalization is being positively altered.

VIGNETTE

After graduating from high school, Christopher enlists in the army and serves for 5 years. He settles on the West Coast and takes a job in the post office. In his first psychotic break, Christopher becomes paranoid and threatening at work and is hospitalized briefly. After discharge, Christopher refuses aftercare and will not take medication. He quits his job and moves to another city. For the next 15 years, Christopher works intermittently, is homeless off and on, and drinks heavily whenever he has money. His only treatment is when he is involuntarily hospitalized when his behavior is threatening to others. He consistently resists aftercare recommendations, showing no insight into his illness. One day Christopher simply disappears.

SERIOUS MENTAL ILLNESS ACROSS THE LIFESPAN

SMI occurs in persons of any gender, age, culture, or location; however, the population currently living with SMIs can be separated into two groups who have had different experiences with the mental health system: (1) those old enough to have experienced long-term institutionalization (common before approximately 1975), and (2) those young enough to have been hospitalized only for acute care during exacerbations of their disorders.

Older Adults

Before **deinstitutionalization**, the mass shift of patients with SMIs out of state hospitals and into the community that began in the 1960s and continued through the 1970s, many people lived long term in state psychiatric hospitals (refer to Chapter 4). Medical paternalism, in which the health care provider made all decisions for patients with SMIs, was pervasive at that time. Thus, patients became institutionalized. As a result, they became dependent on the services and structure of institutions and unable to function independently outside such institutions. It was difficult to distinguish whether behaviors such as regression were the result of the illness or institutionalization.

Younger Adults

People young enough never to have been institutionalized usually do not have problems of passivity and dependency; however, a series of short-term hospitalizations has given them limited experience with treatment and has contributed to a cycle of treatment, brief recovery, and relapse. Intermittent treatment can increase denial and puts young adults with SMI at particular risk for additional problems, including increased frequency of relapse, legal difficulties, homelessness, substance abuse, and unemployment.

DEVELOPMENT OF SERIOUS MENTAL ILLNESS

SMI has much in common with chronic physical illness: the original problem increasingly overwhelms and erodes basic coping mechanisms and increases the use of compensatory processes. As the disorder extends beyond the acute stage, more and more of the neighboring systems are involved. For example, in chronic congestive heart failure, the lungs and kidneys begin to deteriorate due to cardiac insufficiency. A person with schizophrenia may experience disturbed thought processes and social skills, which cause interactions with others to become increasingly awkward and anxiety provoking for both the patient and others. People begin to avoid interactions with the affected person, and in turn the person's self-esteem and social skills weaken.

REHABILITATION VERSUS RECOVERY: TWO MODELS OF CARE

For many years, the concept of **rehabilitation**, which focused on managing patients' deficits and helping them learn to live with their illnesses, dominated psychiatric care. Staff directed the treatment and focused on helping patients to function in their daily roles. Advocates and patients with SMI (many of whom prefer to call themselves "consumers" to emphasize the choices they have, or seek to have, over their treatment) have increasingly sought a different treatment approach. This **consumer movement** has criticized the rehabilitation model as being paternalistic and focused on living with disability rather than on quality of life and eventual cure.

The recovery model developed out of the consumer movement. It is supported by the National Alliance on Mental Illness (NAMI), perhaps the leading mental health consumer-advocacy organization, and the President's New Freedom Commission on Mental Health (2003) stresses it in its recommendations for the future of mental health care. The recovery model:

- Is patient/consumer-centered.
- Is hopeful and empowering.
- Emphasizes the person and the future rather than the illness and the present.
- Involves an active partnership between client and care providers.
- Focuses on strengths and abilities rather than dysfunction and disability.
- Emphasizes staff assisting the consumer in using strengths to achieve the highest quality of life possible.
- Encourages independence and self-determination.
- Focuses on achieving goals of the patient's choosing (not staff's).
- Aims for increasingly productive and meaningful lives for those with SMI.

A patient in recovery stated, "Slowly I accepted my illness but wanted to live a full life in spite of it. I was desperate to succeed in the real world, and I entered college. There I expanded my social ties, so I wouldn't have to be forced into the identity of schizophrenia. My teachers gave me courage and respect" (Group for the Advancement of Psychiatry [GAP], 2000, p. 22).

ISSUES CONFRONTING THOSE WITH SERIOUS MENTAL ILLNESS

Establishing a Meaningful Life

Finding meaning in life and establishing goals can be difficult for persons living with SMI, particularly if they also experience poor self-esteem or apathy. Patients may struggle with the possibility that they may never be the person they once expected to be. Finding a way to "reset" one's goals so that meaning can be found in new ways (e.g., helping others, volunteering, or simply surmounting a significant illness) is important to achieving a satisfactory quality of life and in avoiding despair.

If a person cannot work or attend school, there is a significant amount of free time to be filled. Unstructured free time and resulting boredom can be a significant problem. Options for constructive use of leisure time can be very limited if a person doesn't have transportation, lacks money for movies or other pastimes, doesn't live near parks or libraries, is afraid to go outside, or doesn't have enough confidence to join peers in social activities. Such issues can reduce access to potential support resources and can sometimes lead to maladaptive coping via substance abuse or petty theft.

Comorbid Conditions

Physical Disorders

Persons with SMI are at greater risk from co-occurring physical illnesses, particularly hypertension, obesity, cardiovascular disease, and diabetes. The risk of premature death is over three times greater than the general population, and on average, patients with SMI die more than 25 years prematurely (Daumit et al., 2010). Contributing factors include failing to provide for their own health needs (e.g., forgetting to take medicine), inability to access or pay for care, higher rates of smoking, poor diet, criminal victimization, and stigma.

Diagnostic overshadowing results when a mental illness distracts medical staff from the patient's real medical needs (Chadwick et al., 2010). For example, expressing health concerns in an eccentric or unclear manner can influence the quality of care received. One patient with schizophrenia experienced a priapism—a medically dangerous extended period of penile erection—as a medication side effect. Due to his psychosis, he described the resulting paresthesias to emergency department staff as "demons sticking needles in my [penis]." The ED resident did not assess for priapism partly because of the bizarre description and partly due to avoidance of this person. A response to this weighty problem has been a movement toward integrating mental and physical health care in a single setting to enhance access, improve coordination, and facilitate staff understanding and communication. While there are many models for this integration, one example is for mental health centers to partner with primary care providers so that their consumers can receive both forms of care in a single, coordinated delivery setting.

Depression and Suicide

Persons with SMIs may experience a profound sense of loss of their preillness life and potential. Consider a successful premed student who develops SMI, then 3 years later finds herself unemployed and living in a group home. There is a significant disconnect between her former life trajectory and her current living situation. This loss can lead to acute or chronic grief that, along with the chronicity of the illness and its demands and impact on daily life, can contribute to despair, depression, and risk of suicide, which occurs 12 times more frequently in persons with SMI (Dutta et al., 2010).

Substance Abuse

Comorbid substance abuse occurs in 60% of those with SMI (Kerfoot et al., 2011). It may be a form of self-medication, countering the dysphoria or other symptoms caused by illness or its treatment (e.g., the sedation caused by one's medications), or a maladaptive response to boredom. Nicotine use has always been higher in the population of those with SMI and is not declining as it has been in the general population. Substance abuse contributes to comorbid physical health problems, reduced quality of life, incarceration, relapse, and reduced effectiveness of medications.

Social Problems

Stigma

Stigma is the propensity to view and respond to others negatively based on a belief that they possess undesirable traits. Stigma about SMI stems from a lack of understanding and causes others to make assumptions about persons with SMI. For example, many people believe that SMI persons are violent, when in fact violence by SMI persons is unusual; nonetheless, the result of this stigmatizing belief is fear and avoidance of SMI persons. Stigma interferes with access to quality health care and related services, results in discrimination and isolation, and can cause shame and anger. The President's New Freedom Commission on Mental Health (2003) targeted stigma reduction as a focus for the next 25 years.

According to the Substance Abuse and Mental Health Services Administration (SAMHSA) (2008), only 25% of young adults believe that one can recover from mental illness; this belief is perpetuated by stereotypical images of mental illness in U.S. culture and limited corrective contact with persons with SMIs. Initiatives such as SAMHSA's "What a Difference a Friend Makes" program (2008) and NAMI's "Stigmabusters" campaign (2008) seek to improve understanding and acceptance through public education and reduction of stigma. As one patient explained, "We need to grieve the loss of normal lives, normal families, and normal places in society . . . we are placed at the very lowest rung on the ladder of society. We are believed by many to be axe-murdering fiends—all of us, even though statistics do not bear this notion out" (GAP, 2000, p. 9).

Isolation and Loneliness

Social isolation and loneliness are concerns of many people with chronic illnesses, not just those with SMIs. Stigma, poor self-image, passivity, impaired hygiene, and similar factors reduce interaction and interfere with relationships. Romantic relationships and opportunities for sexual expression, usually desired among persons with SMI just as in any population, are also affected by isolation (and by sexual dysfunction from medications). One response has been the creation of dating services specifically for persons with disabilities or mental illness.

Victimization

Stereotypes would have us believe that people with SMI are more likely to be violent than people who do not have mental illness, but the reverse is actually true: mentally ill people are more likely to be *victims* of violence than *perpetrators* (Hughes et al., 2012)). Sexual assault or coerced sexual activity also occurs in this vulnerable population. Impaired judgment, impaired interpersonal skills (e.g., unknowingly acting in ways that might provoke others, such as standing too close or not recognizing irritation in another's facial expression), passivity, poor self-esteem, dependency, living in high-crime neighborhoods, and appearing more vulnerable to criminals may contribute to this problem. Drug abuse and transient living conditions increase the risk of victimization and resulting worsening of one's mental health (Whitley, 2011).

Economic Challenges

Unemployment and Poverty

Most persons derive at least part of their identity and sense of value from the work they do. Many persons with SMI would like to work, but symptoms such as cognitive slowing or disorganization interfere with obtaining or succeeding at work. Eighty-five percent of persons with SMI are unemployed, and disability entitlements received by 50% of those with SMIs do not provide much income. Finding an employer open to hiring a person with SMI can be difficult, and antidiscrimination laws do not guarantee a job.

Newer antipsychotic medications can be extremely expensive (over $1000/month). Co-pays or Medicaid "spend-downs" (the monthly need to exhaust one's funds to reestablish Medicaid eligibility) are obstacles to treatment. Persons with insurance may find that their share of costs is prohibitively high or that their insurance provider limits mental health care coverage or does not cover it at all. Providing mental health care coverage equal to that for physical health care, or **parity**, has been legislated in many states (and somewhat at the national level), but "loopholes" reduce mental health care coverage for many. Changes in national health care policy may reduce these obstacles to needed physical and mental health care.

Housing Instability

Many persons with SMIs have limited funds, which equates to limited options for housing. Affordable housing may require living far from needed resources (e.g., stores, health care, and support persons) or in unsafe neighborhoods. Living with family can produce conflict about patient behavior (e.g., nonadherence, impaired self-care) that can lead to estrangement and disrupt housing with family.

An episode of inappropriate behavior could lead to eviction and a negative reputation among landlords, closing doors to future housing. Symptoms can cause behavior that leads to police arrest. One person asked a store clerk if he could pay him later for soda and, thinking concretely, mistook the clerk's sarcastic "Oh, sure" as genuine approval, only to leave with the soda and find himself charged with theft an hour later; this arrest could leave him ineligible for housing subsidies, public housing, and other entitlements. Even with a subsidy, waiting lists might be several years long. Finding and keeping good housing can be very challenging.

Caregiver Burden

Caregivers, particularly family members, have limits in terms of coping with the persistent and challenging needs of persons with SMI and may find themselves unable to shoulder the burden. They also age, become ill, and may require care themselves. For both the parent and child, living apart after 30 or 40 years can be a very difficult adjustment and can contribute to relapse (e.g., when a caregiver is hospitalized, leaving the patient alone for the first time in his life). Making the transition from home to alternate living arrangements before a crisis occurs and making arrangements for financial support (such as living trusts) when finances allow can preserve stability and avert relapse.

Treatment Issues

Nonadherence

At any point in time, nearly half of all persons with mental illness are not receiving treatment or are nonadherent to treatment; this can double the likelihood of relapse (Arango & Amador, 2010). Most health care providers address this problem with medication education, but patients faced with repetitive medication groups and exhortations to take medications often become more resistant rather than insightful. Other obstacles, such as side effects, drug costs, interruptions in treatment, and rotating treatment providers, increase the risk of nonadherence and threaten stability and prognosis. Box 31-1 describes nursing interventions that promote adherence.

BOX 31-1 INTERVENTIONS TO IMPROVE ADHERENCE TO TREATMENT

- Select medications that are most likely to be effective, well tolerated, and acceptable to the patient.
- Actively manage side effects to avert/minimize distress that could cause nonadherence.
- Carefully monitor medication decreases or changes to control side effects and maximize therapeutic effects.
- Simplify treatment regimens to make them more acceptable and understandable to the patient (e.g., once-a-day dosing instead of twice).
- Tie treatment adherence to achieving the *patient's* goals (not staff's or society's) to increase motivation. Reinforce improvements (e.g., such as living in the community without rehospitalization), connecting them to treatment adherence.
- Assign consistent, committed caregivers who are skilled at building trusting, therapeutic relationships and who will be able to work with the patient for extended periods of time.
- To improve patient insight and motivation, educate the patient and family about SMI and the role of treatment in recovery; however, education alone will not lead to adherence, particularly for persons with anosognosia (as described on this page).
- Minimize obstacles to treatment by providing assistance with treatment costs and access.
- Involve the patient and family in support groups with members who have greater insight and firsthand experience with illness and treatment—people whose viewpoints the patient may be more likely to appreciate and accept.
- Provide culturally sensitive care. Not attending to cultural beliefs and practices (e.g., mistrust of health care and authority figures, or valuing self-sufficiency or privacy above health care) can result in rejection of treatment.
- When other interventions have not been successful, use medication monitoring, long-acting forms of medication (depot injections or sustained-release forms) to increase the likelihood that needed medication will be in the patient's system. Note: mouth checks may not find pills hidden in the patient's mouth (engaging the patient in conversation for several minutes after he takes the pills is also helpful).
- Never reject, blame, or shame the patient when nonadherence occurs. Instead, label it as simply an issue for continuing focus, and accept that achieving adherence often requires numerous tries. Remind yourself that nonadherence is common and often is due to anosognosia from the illness itself.

Anosognosia

Many people assume that persons with mental illness who do not understand that they are mentally ill must be in denial, that is they know they are ill but cannot accept it. Although denial is a possibility, another is **anosognosia**, the inability to recognize one's deficits due to one's illness. In SMI, the brain—the organ one needs in order to have insight and make good decisions—is the organ that is diseased. An illness that makes one unable to recognize that he *has* an illness can understandably cause one to be resistant to treatment. It can take months or years for a person with SMI to recognize and acknowledge his mental illness.

Medication Side Effects

Psychotropic medications, especially antipsychotics, can produce a range of distressing side effects, from involuntary movements to increased risk of diabetes. Some side effects (e.g., dystonias) are treatable; others may diminish over time or can be compensated for via behavioral changes (e.g., changing position slowly to reduce dizziness from hypotension). Addressing side effects is essential to promoting adherence and maximizing quality of life. Refer to Chapter 3 for a detailed discussion of drugs used in the treatment of SMI.

Treatment Inadequacy

NAMI regularly evaluates services provided to those with SMI and finds most states lacking. The most recent such rating (in 2009) gave below-average ratings to 27 states, and the highest grade, a "B", to only 6 states; problems cited included fragmented and inadequately funded services, inadequate housing, and excessive institutionalization instead of treating persons in less restrictive settings (NAMI, 2010). Research has also suggested that racial, economic, and other nonmedical factors (e.g., uninsured persons being hospitalized less and blacks being more likely to be given antipsychotic medications) affect treatment decisions (Rost et al., 2011). Although standards of care now exist for most SMIs, they are not always followed; consumers must be informed and diligent in ensuring that they are receiving the most effective treatment, and agencies and staff must be diligent in updating their programs and practice.

Residual Symptoms

Residual symptoms are those that do not improve completely or consistently with treatment. This can be very frustrating, and patients may feel that these symptoms mean they will not get better or that treatments are not working. This leads to helplessness and hopelessness, and the patient may discontinue treatment in response, worsening the illness.

Relapse, Chronicity, and Loss

The majority of patients with an SMI face the possibility of relapse even when adhering to treatment, which may contribute to hopelessness and helplessness. Living with SMI paradoxically requires *more* effort and emotional resources from persons *less* able to cope with such demands. Each relapse can cause loss of relationships, employment, and housing, adding that much more loss to the patient's life and making discharge planning significantly more complicated.

RESOURCES FOR PERSONS WITH SERIOUS MENTAL ILLNESS

Comprehensive Community Treatment

Ideally, the community-based mental health care system provides comprehensive, coordinated, and cost-effective care for the consumer with mental illness; however, in 2003, the President's New Freedom Commission on Mental Health concluded that services—particularly for those with serious mental illness—were fragmented and inefficient, with blurring of responsibility among agencies, programs, and levels of government. Many consumers "fall through the cracks," and those who received treatment had difficulty achieving financial independence because of limited job opportunities and the fear of losing health insurance in the workplace (becoming employed and having an income may cause ineligibility for public health care coverage) (President's New Freedom Commission on Mental Health, 2003).

The overall goal of community psychiatric treatment is to improve the consumer's ability to function independently and achieve a satisfying quality of life. State hospitals and psychiatric units in general hospitals provide inpatient care. Community mental health centers (CMHCs), private providers (psychiatrists, psychologists, counselors, social workers, and advanced practice registered nurses [APRNs]), and other private, public, and governmental agencies provide outpatient care. Community services vary with local needs and resources; rural communities or those with limited finances may provide only mandated services (and limited access to them) whereas other communities may have a broad array of accessible services. Needed services may be unavailable or have long waiting lists, and consumers may have difficulty finding the services they need amid the maze of agencies and services.

Community Services and Programs

Psychiatric or **medical-somatic services** center on prescribing medications and related biological aspects of treatment (e.g., monitoring physical health status). Psychiatrists, advanced practice registered nurses, and sometimes physician assistants provide services, along with support from basic-level nurses.

Case management is usually provided by paraprofessional staff (people trained to assist professionals), who help patients with day-to-day needs, treatment coordination, and access to services. They work in their patient's home, school, and vocational settings and coordinate the patient's overall care, brokering and facilitating access to services while providing psychosocial education, guidance, and support. Case managers may also provide **medication monitoring**, observing and facilitating the patient's use of medications to promote adherence. One evidence-based model of case management for patients with SMIs is **assertive community treatment** (ACT), discussed later in this chapter.

Day programs provide structure and offer therapeutic activities to patients who come to the program 1 or more days per week. Social skills training, discussed later in this chapter, focuses on socialization, activities of daily living (ADLs), and prevocational training (the fundamentals needed before one can be successfully employed [e.g., interviewing, dressing for work, and interacting professionally with co-workers]). Day programs also provide social contact and peer support and allow staff to monitor the patient's status so that concerns can be detected and addressed quickly. A variety of staff, and some times consumers themselves, provide day program services.

Crisis intervention services focus on helping patients regain their ability to cope when facing overwhelming situations, such as psychological trauma or relapse. Impaired cognition and problem solving increase the risk of crisis in persons with SMI. Stressors, such as changes in routines at home or work, physical or financial problems, victimization, or anniversaries of traumatic events, may overwhelm coping and result in crises. A person with SMI and limited coping abilities may respond to a small stressor first by seeking hospitalization; crisis intervention seeks to help that person manage the stressor and avert a crisis and inpatient care.

Crisis intervention includes four steps: (1) clarify the reality of the situation; (2) build on the patient's strengths and support system; (3) identify realistic, step-by-step goals; and (4) promote problem solving. Direct interventions, such as finding new resources or calling on existing resources for additional support, are emphasized. Services range from staff on call to provide direct support 24 hours a day by phone or in person to support lines ("warm" lines) or hotlines providing phone-based screening, support, crisis intervention, and referral services. Crisis residential or stabilization programs in some communities help persons who are in crisis and/or facing impending relapse, typically providing a stay of several days to 2 weeks during which acuity is too great to remain in a community residence but not high enough to require hospitalization.

Emergency psychiatric services provide emergency assessments, crisis intervention, and sometimes emergency medications or adjustments. Persons with SMI may be unable to recognize that their illness is worsening or that they are becoming unsafe; therefore, most communities provide a 24-hour emergency psychiatric evaluation program that can initiate emergency inpatient admissions on an involuntary basis via a **mobile crisis team** (wherein mental health professionals respond to patient residences, jails, or even street corners) and/or specially trained personnel in a crisis center or emergency department setting. In some communities, law-enforcement officers are responsible for initiating involuntary psychiatric evaluations. Local probate courts can also order such evaluations upon petition by family members or other interested parties.

Group and individual psychotherapy includes counseling and therapy based on a variety of models, usually provided by independently licensed mental health professionals (e.g., licensed independent social workers or APRNs). Approaches appropriate for those with SMI include (1) family therapy (helping family members function more effectively and providing skills and knowledge necessary to support loved ones with mental illnesses), (2) **psychoeducation** groups (educating about mental health topics [e.g., psychotropic drugs] and building skills [e.g., conflict resolution]), and (3) support groups (providing support related to daily challenges of living with chronic illness). Three other approaches—cognitive therapy, cognitive-behavioral therapy (CBT), and supportive psychotherapy—are discussed later in this chapter.

Housing services include supervised or unsupervised group homes, "board-and-care" homes (wherein room, board, and limited supervision are provided by laypersons in their homes), independent community housing (apartments, houses), and programming for specialized populations, such as forensic patients (e.g., criminal offenders found "Not Guilty by Reason of Insanity," who no longer require inpatient care but require special or intensive monitoring and programming in the community). Housing services are designed to help the patient progress toward independent living, maintain stability, and avoid homelessness.

Partial hospital programs (PHPs) provide services similar to those received during inpatient psychiatric care on an outpatient basis. Often affiliated with inpatient programs, they typically include most of the services available to inpatients. Patients may be "stepped down" to PHP programs from inpatient units to further stabilize acute psychiatric conditions before being fully released to community-based services. **Intensive outpatient programs (IOPs)** are similar but typically community based and focused on services for high-need persons.

Guardianship involves the appointment of a person (guardian) to make decisions for the consumer during times when judgment is impaired. Guardians may be significant others or attorneys and typically are appointed during a court process addressing the issue of whether or not a patient is competent to provide for his own needs. Those with a guardian typically may not enter into contracts, consent to sexual activity, or authorize their own treatment; those actions require the guardian's approval. In some cases, the guardian's authority may be limited to the person's finances, as when a consumer is functional in most respects but unable to manage money, placing basic needs for food and shelter at risk; the guardian is responsible for using the consumer's funds to meet such needs. An alternative is the use of a **payee,** often a volunteer or staff member, whom the consumer agrees to allow to manage his finances, usually via a contract.

Community outreach programs, often focused on homeless persons, send professional or paraprofessional teams into the community to engage persons with mental illness in needed services, to foster self-care, and to provide patient advocacy. **Multiservice centers** collaborate with outreach programs to supply hot meals, laundry and shower facilities, clothing, social activities, transportation to and from services, and access to a telephone and a mailing address (often essential when seeking work or benefits) for persons who are homeless or living in drop-in shelters.

Substance Abuse Treatment

A variety of services exist for those who have a dual diagnosis of SMI and alcohol-related or drug-related problems (sometimes referred to as *substance abuse/mentally ill* [SAMI] patients). Substance abuse clinics provide therapeutic and rehabilitative services, including medical and psychosocial assessment, detoxification, and medication such as methadone. Help for families is also available. Most clinicians endorse SAMI treatment that is integrated (i.e., delivered by a single provider rather than split between a mental health agency and a drug/alcohol agency), using personnel with dual areas of expertise, but this standard has not yet been met in some settings (NAMI, 2010). Refer to Chapter 22 for a detailed discussion of treatment settings for patients with substance abuse issues.

> **VIGNETTE**
>
> After 3 years, Christopher returns home to his parents. A policeman tells him to leave a library where he is causing a disturbance, and he is arrested when he threatens the policeman. He is found "Guilty but Insane" on a charge of disorderly conduct and is released on the condition that he receive psychiatric treatment. He goes to a clinic and receives long-acting intramuscular antipsychotic medication due to his history of nonadherence. He also joins a day program and gets a case manager, who helps him apply for Supplemental Security Income. When his aging parents state that he can no longer live with them, he moves to a group home. Because he wants to work, he is referred to Goodwill Industries, where he gets job training and coaching, leading to a job unloading delivery trucks. He stays on that job for the next 5 years. When the requirements of his conditional release are completed, he continues in treatment and continues working nearly full time. Because he is stable, his medication is changed to an oral antipsychotic, and he continues to receive supervision in his group home.

EVIDENCE-BASED TREATMENT APPROACHES

Assertive Community Treatment

Assertive community treatment (ACT) involves consumers working with a multidisciplinary team that provides a comprehensive array of services; the consumer is cared for by the team rather than going to multiple departments or agencies to receive the needed range of services. ACT has been shown to improve the quality of life and reduce inpatient admissions, incarceration, and homelessness among persons with mental illness (Rice, 2011; Dixon et al., 2010). At least one member of the team is available 24 hours a day for crisis needs, and the emphasis is on treating the patient within his own environment. Although ACT programs cost more to operate, proponents believe those costs are offset by reduced care costs elsewhere.

Cognitive and Behavioral Therapy

Cognitive-behavioral therapy (CBT) has been shown to be effective in helping persons with SMI reduce and cope with symptoms such as delusions and impaired social functioning (Dixon et al., 2010). The cognitive component of CBT focuses on patterns of thinking and "self-talk" (i.e., what one says to oneself internally). It identifies distorted thinking and negative self-talk and guides patients to substitute more effective forms of thinking. The behavioral component of CBT uses natural consequences and positive reinforcers (rewards) to shape the

VIGNETTE

After 10 years of adherence, Christopher, now 50, decides to move out on his own. Although his nurse-therapist has noted the risks of a less-supervised setting, Christopher finds himself a room to rent. Over the next 2 months, his mental status remains stable; however, his medication nurse, who weighs him monthly, notices that he has lost 12 pounds. Christopher denies any change in his eating habits, and he is referred to his primary care provider for evaluation. He doesn't follow up with the primary care provider, and over the next 4 weeks, he loses another 10 pounds. His nurse therapist calls his work supervisor, who reports that Christopher is talking out loud to himself, is more isolated, and that one morning he smelled of alcohol; she is supportive of Christopher and hopes he'll get treatment. At his next appointment, the psychiatrist, nurse, and nurse-therapist discuss these changes and recommend that Christopher go into the partial hospital program for medication reevaluation. He reluctantly agrees, denying that he has any problem.

person's behavior in a more positive or adaptive manner. Refer to Chapter 2 for further information on CBT.

Cognitive Enhancement Therapy

Cognitive enhancement therapy (CET) is based on the principle that compromised neurological functions can be assumed by healthier areas of the brain. CET involves many hours (e.g., 60 or more) of structured computer-based drills and group exercises that incrementally challenge and strengthen functions, such as focusing attention, processing and recalling information, and interpreting social and emotional information (e.g., inferring a person's mood from his expression or tone of voice). Research has shown that CET leads to sustained improvement in cognition and improves social and vocational functioning (Hurford et al., 2011).

Family Support and Partnerships

Families and significant others can face significant stresses related to the mental illness of a loved one, and both may suffer from insufficiencies in empathy and understanding (Hasson-Ohayon et al., 2011). Sound **family support and partnerships** is one of the strongest predictors of recovery; response to treatment is enhanced and conflict is reduced when treatment providers work as empathic partners with patients and significant others. NAMI's Family-to-Family program focuses on understanding SMI, coping skills, and the recovery process; it has been found to enhance coping and empowerment (Dixon et al., 2011). NAMI meetings and support groups specific to various SMIs (e.g., the Depression and Bipolar Support Alliance) serve as excellent sources of support and practical guidance for primary consumers (patients) and secondary consumers (their significant others).

Social Skills Training

Social skills training focuses on teaching a wide variety of social and ADL skills. Persons with SMI often have social deficits that cause functional impairment; for example, persons unable to respond assertively may respond aggressively instead. Complex interpersonal skills, such as negotiating or resolving a conflict, are broken down into subcomponents that are then taught in a step-by step fashion. Role playing and group interaction are used to practice skills.

Supportive Psychotherapy

Supportive psychotherapy focuses on supporting the patient at the current stage of illness rather than confronting possible problems and pushing the patient toward change. It stresses empathic understanding, coping, and anxiety reduction. It is informal in style and can be used by any discipline alone or in combination with other modalities; it enhances the therapeutic alliance and improves long-term recovery in SMI (Douglas, 2008).

VIGNETTE

Christopher joins the partial hospital program, attending groups on medication, living with SMI, substance use, and healthy habits. In the first week, the nurse calls the therapist to report that he is severely paranoid; he will not eat or drink out of any open containers and is observed spitting out his pills. He admits that he has not taken any medication since he moved out of his group home His medication is changed to a quick-dissolving and long-acting injectable medication. He begins to eat normally, gaining 5 pounds in 2 weeks. Upon discharge 4 weeks later, he again attends the psychosocial program for structure, supportive group therapy, socialization, and case management to assist with finding a new home, medical care, and employment. His case manager finds him a room in a family care home with a supportive caregiver. Over the next 3 months, Christopher gradually returns to his baseline functioning. He returns to work 2 days per week and attends the day program 2 days per week. The nurse therapist now observes his physical status more closely and inquires specifically about his work, adherence, and social activities at each session.

Vocational Rehabilitation and Related Services

Consumers with SMI who are employed experience improved socialization, confidence, organizational abilities, socialization, income, and quality of life (Drake & Becker, 2011). Vocational services (**vocational rehabilitation**) can vary widely but can include vocational training, financial support for attaining employment, or supported-employment services (wherein the employer receives financial incentives to employ persons with SMI, and vocational staff monitor and guide the consumer to succeed as an employee).

Programs using a **clubhouse model** (in which consumers run their own business, such as a coffee shop or housekeeping service) teach all members to perform a job in order to run the business. Such programs have led to the **supported employment** model, which has been shown to be more effective in helping persons with SMI achieve employment. Elements of this approach include (Twamley et al., 2012):

1. Rapid placement in a competitive job preferred by the patient
2. Continuing, individualized support on the job (e.g., a coach at the worker's side, providing support, guidance, and training in coordination with supervisors)
3. Integration of mental health and employment services

EVIDENCE-BASED PRACTICE

Wellness Self-Management in Severe and Persistent Mental Illness

Salerno, A., Margolies, P., Cleek, A., Pollock, M., Gopalan, G., & Jackson, C. (2011). Wellness self-management: An adaptation of the Illness Management Program in New York state. *Psychiatric Services, 62*(5), 456–458. doi:10.1176/appi.ps.62.5.456.

Problem

The recovery model stresses client independence and ability; however, interventions that reflect this perspective tend to be more recently developed. Consequently, related research support tends to be less than for more-established treatments.

Purpose of Study

This study evaluated the implementation and effectiveness of a Wellness Self-Management treatment program designed to aid clients in enhancing their recovery by improving coping, understanding of illness, social supports, problem solving, and goal-focused activity.

Methods

Over 100 mental health agencies, from outpatient centers to prisons, implemented and evaluated the newly developed Wellness Self-Management group curriculum and client workbook. Program implementation fidelity and consumer achievement of personal goals were evaluated.

Key Findings

- The curriculum and groups were implemented as designed and continued to be provided after the study period ended.
- 75% of consumers reported significant achievement of their goals for the program.
- Inexpensive resources (e.g., client workbooks) contributed significantly to client goal achievement and program fidelity.

Implications for Nursing Practice

Well-designed, consumer-centered programming that is structured and includes useful and affordable resources is effectively implemented and sustained, resulting in enhanced consumer recovery outcomes.

OTHER POTENTIALLY BENEFICIAL SERVICES OR TREATMENT APPROACHES

Advance Directives

Advance directives are legal documents that allow the consumer whose disorder is in remission to direct how treatment needs should be managed if his judgment is later impaired during a relapse. For example, when well, a consumer can commit to accepting hospitalization or medications should he experience a relapse, maintaining control over his treatment and avoiding the need for involuntary admission and court involvement.

Consumer-Run Programs

Consumer-run programs range from informal "clubhouses," which offer socialization, recreation, and sometimes other services, to competitive businesses, such as snack bars or janitorial services, which provide needed services and consumer employment while encouraging independence and building vocational skills. NAMI and other programs offer training that enables consumers to assist peers effectively in the recovery process; often called Peer Specialists, such consumers may work in case management, hospitals, or day programs to support their peers, drawing on their firsthand experiences with SMI to enhance their effectiveness and achieve acceptance by their peers.

Wellness and Recovery Action Plans

Wellness and Recovery Action Plans (WRAPs) (Cook et al., 2011) and similar programs are psychoeducational programs that empower and train consumers in skills that promote recovery and prepare them to deal with stressors and crises. Training focuses on daily maintenance plans (actions and resources needed to maintain wellness, such as adequate rest and sleep), identifying and managing triggers that could provoke a relapse, early identification of impending relapse, and crisis plans (for managing crises or impending relapse). Typically, a wide variety of useful tools, templates, and techniques is provided, and the programs lead to developing practical and concrete action plans for promoting recovery.

Technology

Technology can reduce costs and improve treatment access and outcomes. Electronic records available in multiple locations can assist in assessments or service delivery anywhere in the community. Persons who cannot afford electronic access often have, or can be provided with, a cell phone, allowing for improved monitoring and faster response if, for example, a patient misses an appointment. Treatment adherence is being promoted through text reminders about medications or appointments. Personnel in remote locations are speaking with patients by telephone or Internet-based video when patients cannot otherwise access distant services or specialists.

Exercise

Exercise holds benefits for persons with SMI, including improved coping with symptoms, reduced anxiety and depression, enhanced self-esteem, weight control or loss (important for patients with weight-related comorbidities, such as diabetes and hypertension), and cost effectiveness. While SMI symptoms such as avolitionality can be obstacles to exercise, motivational and group interventions can improve exercise participation (Beebe et al., 2010).

NURSING CARE OF PATIENTS WITH SERIOUS MENTAL ILLNESS

Nurses encounter patients with SMI in a variety of inpatient and community settings. All roles and techniques used by psychiatric mental health nurses in inpatient psychiatric settings also apply in the community and other settings.

Assessment Strategies

Important aspects of assessment include the following:

- Signs of direct risk to self or others: suicidality or homicidality
- Signs of indirect risk to self or others: inadequate nutrition,

clothing inadequate for the weather, neglect of medical needs, or carelessness while driving, smoking, or cooking (e.g., leaving pots on the stove and becoming distracted or falling asleep)
- Depression or hopelessness
- Signs of impending relapse: especially decreased sleep, increased impulsivity or paranoia, diminished reality testing, increased delusional thinking, or command hallucinations (early detection and correction of relapse reduces its intensity and duration and prevents hospitalization, loss of housing, arrest, and loss of entitlements)
- Physical health problems, such as brain tumors or drug toxicity, which can cause psychiatric symptoms and be mistaken for mental illness or relapse
- Comorbid illnesses (ensuring that the patient provides appropriate self-care and receives adequate health care)
- Signs of treatment nonadherence such as worsening of symptoms, unused medications, missed appointments, or reluctance to discuss these issues.

Table 31-1 lists signs and symptoms of problems associated with SMI, potential nursing diagnoses that apply to the patient with SMI, and examples of specific nursing outcomes.

Intervention Strategies

Box 31-2 outlines two relevant *Nursing Interventions Classification (NIC)* interventions for the management of serious mental illness (Bulechek et al., 2013). Basic nursing interventions for patients with SMI include the following:

- Empowering the patient by involving him in goal setting and treatment planning; this increases the treatment adherence and improves treatment outcomes.
- Emphasizing quality of life rather than simply focusing on symptoms; this conveys an interest in the person rather than the illness and builds the therapeutic alliance.
- Developing and maintaining sustained therapeutic relationships; trust in providers is key to overcoming anosognosia and achieving treatment adherence. Persons with SMI often require extended periods to form these connections.
- Providing supportive psychotherapy, focusing on the here and now; this aids in maintaining rapport and positive self-esteem and reduces maladaptive coping.
- Aiding effective reality testing to enable consumers to recognize and counter hallucinations and delusional thinking. Training and encouraging the patient to validate whether experiences are real can help the patient distinguish symptoms from reality (e.g., if a person experiences frightening

TABLE 31-1 SIGNS AND SYMPTOMS, NURSING DIAGNOSES, AND OUTCOMES FOR PATIENTS WITH SERIOUS MENTAL ILLNESS

SIGNS AND SYMPTOMS	NURSING DIAGNOSES	OUTCOMES
Absence of eye contact, difficulty expressing thoughts, difficulty in comprehending usual communication pattern, inappropriate verbalization	*Impaired verbal communication*	Exchanges messages accurately with others, uncompromised spoken language, accurately interprets messages received
Withdrawal, inappropriate interpersonal behavior, social discomfort, lack of belonging	*Impaired social interaction*	Engages others, appears relaxed, cooperates with others, uses assertive behaviors as appropriate, exhibits sensitivity to others
Absence of supportive significant other(s), preoccupation with own thoughts, shows behaviors unaccepted by dominant cultural group, withdrawn, reports feeling alone, feels different from others, feels rejected	*Social isolation*	Interacts with others (e.g., family, friends, neighbors, mental health consumers), participates in community activities (e.g., church, volunteer work, clubs), participates in leisure activities with others
Failure to keep appointments, missing medication dosages, evidence of exacerbation of symptoms, failure to progress	*Nonadherence**	Discusses prescribed treatment regimen with health professional, performs treatment regimen as prescribed, keeps appointments with health professionals, monitors own treatment response
Self-negating verbalization, lacks success in life events, hesitant to try new situations, indecisive behavior, lack of eye contract, nonassertive behavior	*Chronic low self-esteem*	Describes feelings of self-worth, fulfills personally significant roles, maintains eye contact, accepts compliments from others
Apprehension about care receiver's care if caregiver unable to provide care, apprehension about possible institutionalization of care receiver, lack of time to meet personal needs, anger, stress, frustration, impatience, limited social life	*Caregiver role strain*	Caregiver receives adequate respite, social support, opportunities for leisure activities, supplemental services to assist with care; caregiver reports sense of control and certainty about future

*NANDA-I diagnosis is *noncompliance*.
From Herdman, T. H. (Ed.), (2013). *Nursing diagnoses—Definitions and classification 2012-2014.* Copyright © 2012, 1994-2012 by NANDA International. Used by arrangement with John Wiley & Sons Limited; Moorhead, S., Johnson, M., Maas, M., & Swanson, E. (2013). *Nursing outcomes classification (NOC)* (5th ed.). St. Louis, MO: Mosby.

BOX 31-2 *NIC* INTERVENTIONS FOR SERIOUS MENTAL ILLNESS

Self-Care Assistance: IADLs

Definition: Assisting and instructing a person to perform instrumental activities of daily living (IADLs) needed to function in the home or community

*Activities**:

- Instruct individual on appropriate and safe storage of medications.
- Assist the individual to understand how to use public transportation (e.g., buses and bus schedules, taxis, city or county transportation for disabled people).
- Assist individual in establishing safe methods and routines for cooking, cleaning, and shopping.

Family Support

Definition: Promotion of family values, interests, and goals

*Activities**:

- Listen to family concerns, feelings, and questions.
- Accept the family's values in a nonjudgmental manner.
- Identify congruence among patient, family, and health professional expectations.

*Partial list.

From Bulecheck, G. M., Butcher, H. K., & Dochterman, J. M. (2013). *Nursing interventions classification (NIC)* (6th ed.). St. Louis, MO: Mosby.

hallucinations while in public, he can learn to scan the room and determine if others seem frightened; if not, he can learn to attribute his experience to his illness and to ignore the hallucinations).

- Enabling consumers to recognize and respond to stigma. Stigma predisposes SMI persons to isolation and social discomfort; the resulting isolation contributes to loneliness and reduces access to support. Activities that increase social skills and comfort provide opportunities for socialization (especially with supportive persons and positive role models, such as other patients who are further along in recovery) and contribute to improved functioning and a higher quality of life.
- Involving consumers in support groups such as NAMI that expose them to members who "have been there." Such groups provide support, socialization opportunities, and practical suggestions for issues and problems facing patients and significant others. Involvement in support groups is often empowering for the patient.
- Educating consumers about their illness and recovery; since SMI may result in impaired judgment, isolation, or memory, and understanding one's illness enhances coping, treatment adherence, and quality of life, psychoeducation and reinforcement of this content are essential.
- Caring for the whole person. SMI patients have higher burdens of physical illness; poorer hygiene and health practices; less access to effective medical treatment; increased risk for victimization, STDs, and undesired pregnancies; and more premature mortality than the general population. Avoiding obesity through exercise and good nutritional practices can reduce the risk of comorbidities such as metabolic syndrome; sound physical health conserves energy and resources for use in coping with SMI.
- Involving persons with co-occurring substance abuse in AA/NA and other dual-diagnosis services. Substance abuse rates are high in SMI populations; they increase relapse and interfere with recovery. Achieving sobriety is most associated with AA and integrated treatment programs.

Evaluation

Identified outcomes serve as the basis for evaluation. Each *NOC* outcome has a built-in rating scale that helps the nurse to measure improvement.

CURRENT ISSUES

Mandatory Outpatient Treatment

Mandatory outpatient treatment is treatment mandated by a court and delivered without the patient's consent. Traditionally, this referred to involuntary inpatient care, but beginning in the 1980s, jurisdictions began to experiment with outpatient commitment, which provides mandatory treatment in a less restrictive setting. Typically ordered when a patient leaves the hospital or prison, it is intended for persons who would otherwise be unlikely to continue treatment and then come to represent a danger to self or society. Some consider outpatient commitment a form of assisted treatment in that it helps persons who do not realize they are mentally ill to maintain the best possible mental health status while others see it as a paternalistic approach at odds with the recovery model of care. Research on the effectiveness of outpatient commitment has been mixed. One difficulty is how to respond if the person does not follow the ordered treatment; rehospitalization or reincarceration are expensive consequences, and neither may cause the patient to relent and cooperate with treatment.

Criminal Offenses and Incarceration

People with SMIs may commit crimes due to desperation, impaired judgment, or impulsivity; most often they are nonviolent crimes, such as petty theft or disorderly conduct. Police may also become involved with persons who seem unable to care for themselves, have become a public nuisance, or cannot be persuaded to accept treatment but do not meet criteria for involuntary treatment (usually imminent danger to self or others). Consider a patient with impaired judgment who does not dress adequately for cold weather and spends time in libraries for warmth, causing disruption. When expelled, the individual is at risk of hypothermia. In such cases, the risk to self may not be "imminent," and hospitalization may not be possible. Loved ones or police may then seek the person's arrest simply for the patient's own safety.

Most advocates for the mentally ill believe that incarceration, even if "for the patient's own good," is harmful. Imprisonment can lead to victimization, despair, relapse due to stress or overstimulation, loss of housing or employment, inadequate treatment, and cessation of entitlements such as SSI or Medicaid. Felony convictions may make consumers ineligible for most housing or employment, trapping them in a cycle of release and reincarceration. Advocates instead support diversion from jail to clinical care. Interventions to achieve this include (1) **educating police** so that they can identify mental illness, distinguish it from criminal intent, and connect persons with SMI to help instead of jailing them, and (2) establishing special **mental health courts** designed to intercept persons whose crimes are secondary to mental illness and featuring specially trained officials with authority to order treatment in lieu of conviction (avoiding the stigma and other consequences of conviction and incarceration).

Transinstitutionalization

Transinstitutionalization is the shifting of a person or population from one kind of institution to another, such as from state hospitals to jails, prisons, nursing homes, or shelters. Although deinstitutionalization (the mass movement of SMI persons from state hospitals to outpatient care) has given the appearance of providing care in less restrictive settings, many who have left hospitals have ended up homeless or in trouble, such that there are now more persons with SMI in prisons than in hospitals (Sheth, 2009). Deinstitutionalization provided financial savings for the states, but those costs have been transferred to other payers (such as Departments of Corrections or the federal government). Nursing homes now house 125,000 persons with SMI and sometimes provide only limited mental health care at best; further, younger SMI patients may distress or endanger older, traditional nursing home residents (Meyer, 2009). Advocates believe that deinstitutionalization has often hurt the very people it intended to help and seek to have adequate, humane services alternatives available in the community.

BOX 31-3 WEB-BASED RESOURCES

Mental Health America (MHA, formerly the National Mental Health Association, www.mentalhealthamerica.net, founded in 1909, is a nonprofit organization of advocates, consumers, and significant others who are working to educate the nation about mental health issues and to strengthen mental health services. Its website provides a variety of resources pertaining to recovery, wellness, and severe mental illness.

The National Institute of Mental Health (NIMH, www.nimh.nih.gov), a division of the National Institute of Health, is a governmental agency charged with increasing the understanding and treatment of mental illnesses through basic and clinical research. Its website contains information about research findings, proposals and grants, as well as a variety of educational resources on mental illness.

The mission of the Substance Abuse and Mental Health Services Administration (SAMHSA, samhsa.gov) is to reduce the impact of substance abuse and mental illness. It works to move research findings into practice, and its website offers a wealth of useful information, including a mental health services locator to help consumers find local services.

BOX 31-4 VIDEO RESOURCES

PBS Frontline: The New Asylums (60 minutes, WGBH Boston; can be viewed free online at www.pbs.org/wgbh/pages/frontline/shows/asylums/view) details the societal factors that have led to the incarceration of hundreds of thousands of severely mentally ill persons in American jails and prisons and chronicles the financial and human consequences of this unintended and disastrous policy.

PBS Frontline: The Released (60 minutes, WGBH Boston; can be viewed free online at http://www.pbs.org/wgbh/pages/frontline/released/view/) is a companion video to The New Asylums that follows mentally ill inmates as they are released to the community. The inadequacies and strengths of the community mental health system become apparent as the inmates struggle to establish a life outside institutions.

Kings Park: Stories from an American Mental Institution (http://kingsparkmovie.com; Wildlight Productions, New York, NY). This documentary follows a group of former New York state hospital patients as they visit the now-closed state hospital where they spent months or years of their lives. Interviews chronicle the lives and experiences of those deinstitutionalized from the state hospital system, sometimes only to experience still sadder fates.

PBS: Minds on the Edge: Facing Mental Illness (can be viewed free online at http://www.mindsontheedge.org/watch/fullprogram/) features a fast-moving panel discussion of issues facing the severely mentally ill in our communities. Using hypothetical situations and featuring mental health professionals, advocates, policy makers, and consumers, the panel looks at the problems plaguing our mental health system and offers keen insights into ways that the mentally ill could be helped much more effectively.

KEY POINTS TO REMEMBER

- Patients with SMI suffer from multiple impairments in thinking, feeling, and interacting with others.
- The course of SMI involves exacerbations and remissions, as do many chronic medical illnesses.
- Persons with SMI often suffer complications due to insufficient housing, nonadherence to treatment, comorbid medical or substance use problems, and the stigma of mental illness.
- Coordinated, comprehensive community services help the SMI patient to function at an optimal level.
- The recovery model stresses hope, strengths, quality of life, patient involvement as an active partner in treatment, and eventual recovery.
- The family and support systems play a major part in the care of many persons with SMI and should be included as much as possible in planning, education, and treatment activities.

CRITICAL THINKING

1. John Yang, 42, dually diagnosed with schizophrenia and alcohol/marijuana abuse, is brought to the clinic by his mother, Mrs. Yang. During his assessment, Mrs. Yang reports that she has been caring for her son at home since he was 15; however, since recently moving to town, she is at a loss about what is available in the community. John takes haloperidol (Haldol), but Mrs. Yang says he often refuses it because of muscle rigidity and sexual side effects. They have tried many first-generation antipsychotic drugs without success.
   a. Given the problems faced by a person with a severe mental illness, what areas of John's life might you want to explore in your assessment? Consider relationships, employment history, cognitive abilities, social activity, and behavior. How would you use this information for long-term planning?
   b. As a patient advocate, how might you respond given John's medication history and his nonadherence to traditional antipsychotics? What obstacles to adherence exist for a dually diagnosed patient? What approach or change in treatment would offer the best chance of success?
   c. Which resources mentioned in this chapter might be appropriate for John?
   d. Identify three areas of psychoeducation you'd provide for John and his mother.
2. In your psychiatric rotation in a state hospital, many of the patients are diagnosed with schizophrenia. Although you had been apprehensive about this rotation, you are surprised that patients respond well to you, that you are fascinated by this specialty, and that you're considering it as a career. A fellow student remarks, "You must be crazy to want to work with these people."
   a. What social and other issues might be reflected in this student's remark?
   b. Identify other social prejudices that have been significant problems in the United States. What responses were effective in countering these and reducing their impact?

CHAPTER REVIEW

1. Sarah, a young woman with schizophrenia who has struggled with hygiene and other activities of daily living, has been on a 4-hour pass. She tearfully reports that on the bus back to the hospital, the woman she sat down next to immediately moved to another seat. Which response(s) would most likely be therapeutic? *Select all that apply.*
   a. Acknowledge Sarah's distress and remind her that dinner will be ready in 30 minutes so she has time to settle in before eating.
   b. State, "You sound discouraged. Sometimes persons who do not understand mental illness can be hurtful," and offer to talk with her.
   c. Advise Sarah that the woman's behavior was simply rude and should be ignored because it is something persons with mental illness have to get used to.
   d. Note that perhaps there was something about Sarah's hygiene or appearance that triggered the woman's prejudices about mental illness, and offer to help Sarah with this so that others will be less likely to reject her.
2. Christopher is a 25-year-old man who has been hospitalized three times for schizophrenia. Typically he is very disorganized, does not spend his money responsibly, loses his housing when he does not pay the rent, and in turn cannot be located by his case manager, leading to treatment nonadherence and relapse. Which response would be most therapeutic?
   a. Advise Christopher that if he does not pay his rent, he will be placed in a group home instead of independent housing.
   b. Discuss with Christopher the option of having a guardian who will assure that the rent is paid and assure that his money is managed to meet his basic needs.
   c. Suggest to Christopher's prescribing clinician that he be placed on a long-acting injectable form of antipsychotic medication to address the issue of treatment nonadherence.
   d. Encourage Christopher's case manager to hold him responsible for the outcomes of his poor decisions by allowing such periods of homelessness to serve as a natural consequence.
3. Elaine has experienced repeated episodes of severe depression and mania. These episodes and related hospitalizations have disrupted her employment and created discord within her marriage. She argues with the outpatient staff about medications, does not believe she has a mental illness, and, although she takes her medications while hospitalized, stops taking them after discharge. She will be discharged in 2 weeks. Which intervention is most likely to increase her medication adherence?
   a. Assign Elaine to new outpatient staff to reduce the conflicts she is experiencing with her current providers.
   b. Explain that the medications will help her and that all medications have side effects, but she can learn to live with these.
   c. Involve Elaine in a medication group that will teach her the types and names of psychotropic medications, their purpose, and possible side effects.
   d. Explore with Elaine her perceptions and experiences regarding medication and guide her to connect using medications with achieving her goals.
4. Which intervention(s) would be appropriate to promote recovery for persons with SMI who live in the community? *Select all that apply.*
   a. Meet regularly with the patients and encourage them to make steady progress toward independence.
   b. Introduce patients to others with similar illnesses, and encourage participation in social activities with peers.
   c. Support the development of advance directives and involvement in social and employment activities run by other consumers.
   d. Use public transportation to take patients to a museum and share a nutritious dinner with them at an inexpensive restaurant.
   e. Guide them to develop written plans that identify resources to maintain stability and steps to take when faced with unusual stressors.
   f. Over time, guide the patients to identify and switch to sources of support outside the family to reduce dependence on their loved ones as their primary support resource.

Answers to Chapter Review

1. b; 2. b; 3. d; 4. a, b, c, d, e, f.

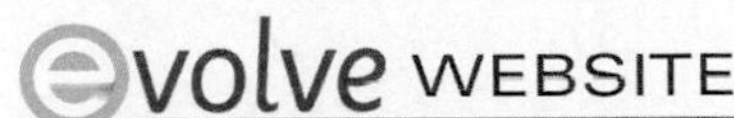

WEBSITE

Visit the Evolve website for a posttest on the content in this chapter: http://evolve.elsevier.com/Varcarolis

Post-Test interactive review

REFERENCES

Anderson, P., Jane-Llopis, E., & Hosman, C. (2011). Reducing the silent burden of impaired mental health. *Health Promotion International, 26*(Suppl 1), i4–i9.

Arango, C., & Amador, X. (2011). Lessons learned about poor insight. *Schizophrenia Bulletin, 37*(1), 27–28.

Beebe, L. H., Smith, K., Burk, R., Dessieux, O., Velligan, D., Tavakoli, A., et al. (2010). Effect of a motivational group intervention on exercise self-efficacy and outcome expectations for exercise in schizophrenia spectrum disorders. *Journal of the American Psychiatric Nurses Association, 16*(2), 105–113.

Bulechek, G. M., Butcher, H. K., Dochterman, J. M., & Wagner, C. (2013). *Nursing interventions classification (NIC)* (6th ed.). St. Louis, MO: Mosby.

Chadwick, A., Street, C., McAndrew, S., & Deacon, M. (2012). Minding our own bodies: Reviewing the literature regarding the perceptions of service users diagnosed with serious mental illness on barriers to accessing physical health care. *International Journal of Mental Health Nursing, 21*, 211–219.

Cook, J. A., Copeland, M. E., Jonikas, J. A., Hamilton, M. M., Razzano, L. A., Grey, D. D., et al. (2011). Results of a randomized controlled trial of mental illness self-management using wellness recovery action planning. *Schizophrenia Bulletin Advance Access.* Retrieved from http://schizophrenia bulletin.oxfordjournals.org/content/early/2011/03/14/schbul.sbr012.full.pdf.

Cook, J. A., Blyler, C. R., Burke-Miller, J. K., McFarlane, W. R., Leff, H. S., Mueser, K. T., et al. (2008). Effectiveness of supported employment for individuals with schizophrenia: Results of a multi-site, randomized trial. *Clinical Schizophrenia and Related Psychoses, 2*(1), 37–46.

Daumit, G. L., Anthony, C. B., Ford, D. E., Fahey, M., Skinner, E. A., Lehman, A. F., et al. (2010). Pattern of mortality in a sample of Maryland residents with severe mental illness. *Psychiatry Research, 176*(2010), 242–245.

Dixon, L. B., Dickerson, F., Bellack, A. S., Bennett, M., Dickinson, D., Goldberg, R. W., et al. (2010). The 2009 schizophrenia PORT psychosocial treatment recommendations and summary statements. *Schizophrenia Bulletin, 36*(1), 48–70.

Dixon, L. B., Lucksted, A., Medoff, D. R., Burland, J., Stewart, B., Lehman, A. F., et al. (2011). Outcomes of a randomized study of a peer-taught Family-to-Family education program for mental illness. *Psychiatric Services, 62*(6), 591–597.

Douglas, C. J. (2008). Teaching supportive psychotherapy to psychiatric residents. *American Journal of Psychiatry, 165*(4), 445–452.

Drake, R. E., & Becker, D. R. (2011). Why not implement supported employment? *Psychiatric Services, 62*(11). Retrieved from http://ps.psychiatryonline.org/article.aspx?articleID=179862.

Dutta, R., Murray, R. M., Hotopf, M., Allardyce, J., Jones, P. B., & Boydell, J. (2010). Reassessing the long-term risk of suicide after a first episode of psychosis. *Archives of General Psychiatry, 67*(12), 1230–1237.

Fitch, B. (2007). Growing through psychosis: The patient's journey toward mental health. Presentation at the Eighth Annual All-Ohio Institute on Community Psychiatry, Beachwood, OH.

Group for the Advancement of Psychiatry. (2000). *Now that we are listening.* Dallas, TX: Committee on Psychiatry and the Community Group for the Advancement of Psychiatry.

Hasson-Ohayon, I., Levy, I., Kravetz, S., Vollanski-Narkis, A., & Roe, D. (2011). Insight into mental illness, self-stigma, and the family burden of parents of persons with a severe mental illness. *Comprehensive Psychiatry, 52*(2011), 75–80.

Hughes, K., Bellis, M. A., Jones, L., Wood, S., Bates, G., Eckley, L., et al. (2012). Prevalence and risk of violence against adults with disabilities: A systematic review and meta-analysis of observational studies. *The Lancet Early Online Publication.* Retrieved from http://www.thelancet.com/journals/lancet/article/PIIS0140-6736%2811%2961851-5/abstract.

Hurford, I. M., Kalkstein, S., & Hurford, M. Cognitive rehabilitation in schizophrenia. *Psychiatric Times, 28*(3). Retrieved from http://psychiatrictimes.com/schizophrenia/content/article/10168/1822689.

Jans, L., Stoddard, S., & Kraus, L. (2004). *Chartbook on mental health and disability in the United States.* Washington, DC: U.S. Department of Education, National Institute on Disability and Rehabilitation Research. Retrieved from http://library.ncrtm.org/pdf/G926.0003.01.pdf.

Kerfoot, K. E., Rosenheck, R. A., Petrakis, I. L., Swartz, M. S., Keefe, R. S. E., McEvoy, J. P., et al. (2011). Substance use and schizophrenia: Adverse correlates in the CATIE study sample. *Schizophrenia Research, 132*(2011), 177–182.

Lawrence, D., & Kisely, S. (2010). Inequalities in healthcare provision for people with severe mental illness. *Journal of Psychopharmacology, 24*(11;Suppl 4), 61–68.

Mark, T. L., Levit, K. R., Coffey, R. M., McKusic, D. R., Harwood, H. J., & King, E. C. (2007). *National expenditures for mental health services and substance abuse treatment, 1993–2003.* SAMHSA Publication No. SMA 07-4227. Rockville, MD: Substance Abuse and Mental Health Services Administration. Retrieved from http://www.samhsa.gov/spendingestimates/SAMHSAFINAL9303.pdf.

Meyer, B. (2009). Nursing home patients endangered by mentally ill. *Cleveland Plain Dealer/Associated Press, March 22, 2009.* Retrieved from http://www.cleveland.com/nation/index.ssf/2009/03/nursing_home_patients_endanger.html.

Moorhead, S., Johnson, M., Maas, M., & Swanson, E. (2013). *Nursing outcomes classification (NOC)* (5th ed.). St. Louis, MO: Elsevier.

National Alliance on Mental Illness. (2008). *Stigma busters: Fight stigma.* Retrieved from http://www.nami.org/template.cfm?section = about stigmabusters2008.

National Alliance on Mental Illness. (2010). *Grading the states 2009.* Retrieved from http://www.nami.org/gtsTemplate09.cfm?section=Grading_the_States_2009&template=/ContentManagement/ContentDisplay.cfm&ContentID=75459.

President's New Freedom Commission on Mental Health. (2003). *Report of the president's new freedom commission on mental health.* Retrieved from http://govinfo.library.unt.edu/mentalhealthcommission/reports/FinalReport/downloads/FinalReport.pdf.

Rost, K., Hsieh, X-P., Xu, S., Menachemi, N., & Young, A. S. (2011). Potential disparities in the management of schizophrenia in the United States. *Psychiatric Services, 62*(6), 613–618.

Sheth, H. C. (2009). Deinstitutionalization or disowning responsibility. *The International Journal of Psychosocial Rehabilitation, 13*(2), 11–20.

Substance Abuse and Mental Health Services Administration (SAMHSA). (2012). *Results from the 2010 National Survey on Drug Use and Health: Mental health findings.* Retrieved from http://www.samhsa.gov/data/nsduh/2k10MH_Findings/2k10MHResults.htm

Substance Abuse and Mental Health Services Administration. (2008). *Campaign for mental health recovery.* Retrieved from www.whatadifference.org/docs/NASC_FactSheet.pdf2008.

Twamley, E. W., Vella, L., Burton, C. Z., Becker, D. R., Bell, M. D., & Jeste, D. V. (2012). The efficacy of supported employment for middle-aged and older people with schizophrenia. *Schizophrenia Research, 135*(2012), 100–104.

CHAPTER

32

Forensic Psychiatric Nursing

L. Kathleen Sekula and Alison M. Colbert

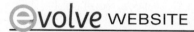

Visit the Evolve website for a pretest on the content in this chapter: http://evolve.elsevier.com/Varcarolis

Pre-Test interactive review

OBJECTIVES

1. Define forensic nursing, forensic psychiatric nursing, and correctional nursing.
2. Describe the educational preparation required for the forensic nurse generalist and the advanced practice forensic nurse.
3. Identify the functions of forensic nurses.
4. Discuss the specialized roles in forensic nursing.
5. Identify three roles of psychiatric nurses in the specialty of forensic nursing.
6. Discuss the roles of the forensic psychiatric nurse within the legal system.
7. Compare and contrast the roles of forensic psychiatric nurses and corrections nurses.

KEY TERMS AND CONCEPTS

advanced practice forensic nurse
competency evaluator
consultant
correctional nursing
criminal profiler
expert witness
fact witness
forensic nurse examiner
forensic nurse generalist
forensic nursing
forensic psychiatric nurse
hostage negotiator
legal sanity
nurse coroner/death investigator
sexual assault nurse examiner (SANE)

In the United States, crime accounts for more deaths, injuries, and loss of property than all natural disasters combined (Disaster Center, 2007). Approximately 13 million people (5% of the U.S. population) are victims of crime on a yearly basis, and of those crimes 1.5 million are violent. Violence has been targeted as a goal in *Healthy People 2020* to prevent injury and violence in the United States (U.S. Department of Health & Human Services [USDHHS], 2012) (Box 32-1).

Violence is often the focus in **forensics**. Forensics is an abbreviation derived from *forensic science* and refers to the application of a broad spectrum of sciences to answer questions of interest to the legal system. In recent years, nurses formalized a specialty of nursing called **forensic nursing**, which brings together traditional nursing practice and forensic knowledge to better serve victims and perpetrators of violence. In this chapter, we will explore a variety of roles that registered nurses assume within nursing that interface with the legal system.

FORENSIC NURSING

The International Association of Forensic Nurses (IAFN) (2006b) defines forensic nursing as:

- The application of nursing science to public or legal proceedings.
- The application of the forensic aspects of health care combined with the bio-psycho-social education of the registered

BOX 32-1 *HEALTHY PEOPLE 2020* GOALS: INJURY AND VIOLENCE PREVENTION (IVP) OBJECTIVES

IVP-29	Reduce homicides
IVP-30	Reduce firearm-related deaths
IVP-31	Reduce nonfatal firearm-related injuries
IVP-32	Reduce nonfatal physical assault injuries
IVP-33	Reduce physical assaults
IVP-34	Reduce physical fighting among adolescents
IVP-35	Reduce bullying among adolescents
IVP-36	Reduce weapon carrying by adolescents on school property
IVP-37	Reduce child maltreatment deaths
IVP-38	Reduce nonfatal child maltreatment
IVP-39	Reduce violence by current or former intimate partners
IVP-40	Reduce sexual violence
IVP-41	Reduce nonfatal intentional self-harm injuries
IVP-42	Reduce children's exposure to violence
IVP-43	Increase the number of states and the District of Columbia that link data on violent deaths from death certificates, law enforcement, and coroner and medical examiner reports to inform prevention efforts at the state and local levels

From U.S. Department of Health and Human Services. (2006). *Injury and violence prevention.* Retrieved from http://www.healthypeople.gov/Data/midcourse/html/focusareas/FA15Introduction.htm.

nurse in the scientific investigation and treatment of trauma and/or death of victims and perpetrators of abuse, violence, criminal activity, and traumatic accidents.

Forensic nurses provide direct services to crime victims and perpetrators of crime and consultation services to colleagues in nursing, medicine, social work, rehabilitation, and law, just to name a few. Forensic nurses can offer expert court testimony in cases related to their areas of practice and expertise, input on policy changes within the corrections settings, and evaluation services regarding specific medical and psychiatric diagnoses for inmates, among other services.

The IAFN was formed in 1992 when 74 nurses—most of whom were sexual assault nurse examiners (SANEs)—came together to create an organization to represent nurses whose practice overlapped with key areas of forensic science and law (IAFN, 2006a). The group currently represents nurses who are forensic nurse generalists, SANEs, forensic psychiatric nurses, death investigators, coroners, correctional nurse specialists, and those in other forensic nursing specialties that continue to evolve. A year after its creation, the organization had more than tripled in size, and by 2012, the IAFN's membership had grown to more than 3000 nurses (IAFN, 2006a). The ANA officially recognized forensic nursing as a specialty practice area in 1995 and combined efforts with the IAFN to develop the *Scope and Standards of Forensic Nursing* in 1997.

The goals of the IAFN (2006a) are to:

- Incorporate primary prevention strategies into our work at every level in an attempt to create a world without violence.
- Establish and improve standards of evidence-based forensic nursing practice.
- Promote and encourage the exchange of ideas and transmission of developing knowledge among its members and related disciplines.
- Establish standards of ethical conduct for forensic nurses.
- Create and facilitate educational opportunities for forensic nurses and related disciplines.

While there is no advanced practice certification at the master's level in forensic nursing, a portfolio recognition process has been established by the IAFN through the American Nurses Credentialing Center (ANCC). Various entry-level certifications, such as Sexual Assault Nurse Examiners (adult and pediatric) through the IAFN, Death Investigator through the American Board of Medicolegal Death Investigation, and the Legal Nurse Consultant through the American Association of Legal Nurse Consultants, are offered.

Education

Educational programs have been developed to prepare nurses for a career in forensic nursing. The IAFN calls for the incorporation of forensic content at all levels of nursing education. As students become more knowledgeable about forensic issues in the care of all patients, more graduate programs are offered that focus the nurse on forensic practice as a specialty area. Forensic education is offered at all academic levels.

Forensic Nurse Generalist

To be called a **forensic nurse generalist**, the nurse with a baccalaureate or associate degree or diploma may acquire additional knowledge and skills by completing a certificate program that comprises continuing education in an area of forensic nursing. Nurses can also gain expertise by taking secondary education electives and/or pursuing a minor in legal topics.

The role of the forensic nurse generalist may vary according to clinical setting, but consistent within this role is the need to be proficient in assessment and treatment of victims of violence, evidence collection and preservation, proper documentation, the legal system, and setting standards of care for victims and perpetrators. A forensic nurse generalist may work in a specialty area, such as on a trauma team or in an emergency department, critical care, or outpatient women's health clinic, or may serve as a general resource person for colleagues in the clinical setting. The forensic nurse generalist may also serve as a resource for the care provider who is working with a patient who has been a victim or perpetrator of violence. In addition to addressing patients' physical and psychological needs, forensic nurse generalists are prepared to identify and care for victims of violence and know when evidence should be collected and preserved.

Forensic Nurse in Advanced Practice

A forensic nurse in an advanced practice role (**advanced practice forensic nurse**) has completed graduate education with a broad focus in forensic nursing and may have obtained credentials as a clinical nurse specialist, certified nurse-midwife, or nurse practitioner. The education provides clinicians with nursing, medical, and legal content and focuses on the collaboration among disciplines in the care of victims and perpetrators. The advance practice registered nurse in forensics also has an educational background in psychiatric assessment and intervention skills, death investigation, forensic wound identification, evidence collection, family violence, sexual assault of all types and in varied populations, introductory law, and principles of criminal justice and forensic science.

Other advanced training takes place after the completion of a master's degree. Individuals who are prepared with a doctor of nursing practice (DNP) may evaluate and apply evidence-based forensic practice for the improvement of education, clinical practice, systems management, and nursing leadership. A doctor of philosophy (PhD) prepares nurses to initiate and conduct research in the area of forensics to ultimately enhance the practice of forensic nursing. Most forensic nursing researchers have completed a doctoral degree or have another advanced degree.

Postdoctoral education or fellowships are also available as additional coursework in the specialty of forensics and clinical experiences to enhance terminal nursing degrees.

Roles and Functions

Regardless of the preparation level of the nurse, the goal of forensic education is to provide nurses who are knowledgeable in the care of all victims and perpetrators of violence.

In forensic nursing, the nurse-patient relationship occurs based on the possibility that a crime has been committed, but it is not the role of the forensic nurse to make a decision as to guilt or innocence or whether a victim is being candid in reporting what happened. Basic roles of the forensic nurse include the following:

1. Identification of victims
2. Creation of appropriate treatment plans
3. Collection, documentation, and preservation of potential evidence.

The forensic nurse possesses expertise in assessment and treatment roles related to competency, risk, and danger. Forensic nurses are educated in theories of violence and victimology, legal issues, and nursing science that enable them to objectively assess the circumstances of the case.

An understanding of both the victim and the perpetrator enhances evidence collection. Forensic nurses may apply medical-surgical knowledge to the care of victims and perpetrators or may function in the legal role primarily as they collect evidence, testify in court, or collaborate with law practitioners with relationship to a victim or perpetrator.

Sexual Assault Nurse Examiner

The sexual assault nurse examiner (SANE) was the first specialized forensic role for nurses, and it represents the largest subspecialty in forensic nursing. SANEs are forensic nurse generalists who seek training in the care of adult and pediatric victims of sexual assault (SANE-A and SANE-P respectively). The IAFN has established clear guidelines for the preparation of SANEs and provides certification for nurses although not all nurses who work in this capacity have certification. A SANE training course is typically 5 days (40 contact hours) and is available online or in the classroom setting. Completion of the course is followed by a period in which the nurse is preceptored by an expert SANE until the nurse is deemed proficient in conducting the exam herself. At this point the nurse can then sit for the national certification exam through the IAFN. Chapter 29 addresses the role of the SANE nurse in more depth.

Nurse Coroner/Death Investigator

The nurse coroner/death investigator for nurses was first recognized in the mid-1990s. Traditionally, the coroner is a public official primarily charged with the duty of determining how and why people die. Increasingly, nurses are prepared as death investigators or deputy coroners. Nurses can practice as death investigators in medical examiners' or coroners' offices or independently in private offices. This expanding nursing role involves assessing the deceased through understanding, discovery, preservation, and use of evidence.

Nurses who work as nurse coroners/death investigators possess medical knowledge that allows them to make expert judgments regarding the circumstances of death based on observations of history, symptomatology, autopsy results, toxicology, other diagnostic studies, and evidence revealed in other aspects of the case. Their knowledge of anatomy and physiology, pathophysiology, pharmacology, grief and grieving, growth and development, interviewing, outcomes measurement, and many other areas of nursing practice bolsters the value of nurses serving in this capacity. Nurses are able to expand the role of the coroner and improve services provided to families, health care agencies, and communities by employing the basic principles of holistic nursing care.

FORENSIC PSYCHIATRIC NURSING

A forensic psychiatric nurse is one who is prepared as a generalist or at the advanced practice level. In the generalist role, nurses are prepared at the entry level as a college/university degree, associate degree, or diploma graduate, which prepares them to function as direct care providers and patient advocates. At this level a nurse who enters a forensic psychiatric setting is expected to advance her education through continuing education or certificate programs that provide education in caring for the forensic patient, usually in a corrections setting. At the advanced practice level, graduate education is required, which prepares nurses to function as psychiatric clinical nurse specialists or psychiatric nurse practitioners. Additional graduate work in forensics at the master's and post-master's levels provides the knowledge needed to practice with forensic populations. This specialty requires skills in psychiatric mental health nursing assessment, evaluation, and treatment of victims or perpetrators. Combining the skills of medical and psychiatric nursing with a thorough understanding of the criminal justice system is pertinent to expert practice (Lyons, 2009).

Evidence collection is central to the role of the forensic psychiatric nurse. For example, evidence is collected by a careful evaluation of intent or diminished capacity in the perpetrator's thinking at the time of the crime. This evaluation aids in determining the degree of crime and may later influence the sentence. Forensic psychiatric nurses who work as competency evaluators collect evidence by spending many hours with a defendant and carefully documenting the dialogue. In this capacity, the role of the forensic psychiatric nurse is not to determine guilt or innocence but to provide assessment data that can help make a final diagnosis within the multidisciplinary forensic team (Sekula & Burgess, 2006).

The forensic psychiatric nurse is highly skilled in interpersonal communications and able to develop collegial relationships with those in other disciplines. A prerequisite is the ability to listen and accept others' values and motivations in a nonjudgmental fashion. Forensic psychiatric nursing appeals to a particular type of nurse—one who thrives in a stimulating intellectual environment, seeks out opportunities to apply clinical skills to complex legal problems, and enjoys pushing the limits of traditional boundaries. Because of the value placed on tradition by the nursing profession, the forensic psychiatric nurse is sometimes viewed with skepticism and with caution in the legal system. These responses must be met with professionalism in practice, research, and education of future forensic psychiatric nurses, keeping in mind the tenets of evidence-based practice.

Roles and Functions of the Forensic Psychiatric Nurse

The forensic psychiatric nurse may function as a psychotherapist, forensic nurse examiner, competency evaluator, fact or expert witness, consultant to law enforcement agencies or the criminal justice system, hostage negotiator, or criminal profiler. These roles may involve providing therapy, witness testimony, services to a prosecutor or defense attorney, and criminal profile reports. Roles of the forensic psychiatric nurse may be examined in relationship to the outcomes for which the nurse is contracted to accomplish. These nurses may be contracted by the legal system to interface with the perpetrator for a variety of services. They may also be contracted by the correctional system or a private entity to offer direct services to the perpetrator. Or they may provide services to the victim in a variety of settings. A list of role functions of forensic psychiatric nurses is presented in Box 32-2.

Nurse Psychotherapist

In addition to the competencies possessed by the generalist, the forensic advanced practice registered nurse in psychiatric mental health (APRN-PMH) may function as a psychotherapist, providing individual, family, and group therapy. Depending on educational preparation and individual state statutes, an APRN-PMH may have prescriptive privileges and initiate psychopharmacology treatment along with psychotherapy. While this role is seriously limited within the corrections systems due to procedural and economic restrictions, the role is often filled in the private sector for perpetrators with the financial resources necessary.

BOX 32-2 FORENSIC PSYCHIATRIC NURSING FUNCTIONS

- Psychotherapist
- Forensic nurse examiner
- Competency evaluator
- Fact or expert witness
- Consultant to law enforcement agencies or the criminal justice system
- Hostage negotiator
- Criminal profiler

Forensic Nurse Examiner

Important functions of the forensic psychiatric nurse examiner are to conduct court-ordered evaluations regarding legal sanity or competency to proceed, to respond to specific medicolegal questions as requested by the court, and to render an expert opinion in a written report or courtroom testimony. The prosecution, the defense, or the judge may request an evaluation. Evaluations are usually based on the defendant's history, along with behavior at the scene of the crime, in jail, or in the courtroom. A comprehensive report is based on clinical data, observations of the defendant's behavior, any forensic evidence contained in crime-scene reports or laboratory reports, summary of any psychological testing, and a thorough psychosocial history. The forensic nurse examiner interviews the defendant and notes behavior, past diagnoses, personality traits, emotions, cognitive abilities, any symptoms of mental disorder, and the psychodynamics of interpersonal relationships.

The forensic psychiatric nurse examiner must be able to separate personal opinion from professional opinion. Personal opinion is based on one's background, upbringing, education, and value system. Professional opinion is based on scientific principle, advanced education in a specific field of endeavor, and the unbiased standards set by research in that area. Although other members of the treatment staff on a forensic unit strive to be supportive, accepting, and empathetic, the forensic nurse examiner strives to remain neutral, objective, and detached.

Legal sanity is defined as the individual's ability to distinguish right from wrong with reference to the act charged, capacity to understand the nature and quality of the act charged, and capacity to form the intent to commit the crime. Legal sanity is determined for the specific time of the act. The forensic nurse examiner must reconstruct the defendant's mental state by reviewing evidence left at the scene, any witness statements, the self-report of the defendant's symptoms, and the defendant's disclosed motivation. Some of the issues addressed in the forensic nurse examiner's determination are (1) whether or not the defendant was using drugs, (2) whether the defendant's reasoning ability was affected by any medical condition, and (3) what the social context of the crime was.

In most states, the presence of a major mental disorder (usually referring to those that cause psychoses—delusions, hallucinations, and disorganized thought—such as schizophrenia) is a prerequisite for a finding of *legal insanity*; however, a defendant who has a mental illness does not have to use this defense. It is the defendant's choice. The forensic nurse specialist must have a clear knowledge of which legal standard is being used and must be able to articulate it to the court and jury. Legal tests of sanity may include the McNaughton rules, irresistible impulse, and guilty but mentally ill.

The *McNaughton rules* derive from a trial in 1843 in which Daniel McNaughton was tried for the murder of a public official. McNaughton believed there was a conspiracy among the Tories of England to destroy him. In an attempt to assassinate the prime minister, who was the Tory leader, McNaughton mistakenly shot and killed the prime minister's secretary. McNaughton was judged to be criminally insane and acquitted of the murder (but institutionalized for the remainder of his life). There was a public outcry over the leniency of this verdict. The House of Lords convened a special session of the judges to give an advisory opinion regarding the law of England governing the insanity defense. The judges advised that to be considered legally insane, the accused person with a mental disorder either must not know the nature and quality of the act or must not know whether the act is right or wrong. Whether or not the individual is responsible for his or her action is the underlying issue in the McNaughton rules. *Irresistible impulse* was added to the McNaughton rules in 1929. This addition stipulates that even if the defendant knew the criminal act was wrong but could not control his or her behavior because of a psychiatric illness or a mental defect, the defendant is not guilty.

Guilty but mentally ill is another insanity defense. Those who plead guilty but mentally ill are remanded to the correctional system, where they receive treatment for their mental disorder. They are subject to the correctional system's parole decisions.

Whereas legal insanity is determined by the defendant's thinking in the past at the time of the offense, *competence to proceed* is determined by the defendant's present thinking at the time of the trial. It is defined as the capacity to assist one's attorney and understand the legal proceedings. Because competence to proceed is a determination of mental capacity in the present, the defendant's competency must be determined each time he or she goes to court. A prior finding of incompetence, even if due to a developmental disability or mental illness, does not preclude a subsequent finding of competency in a later, unrelated case.

Competency Evaluator

Under U.S. federal law, no person may be tried if deemed legally incompetent, and the defendant must be sent to a suitable facility (usually a locked unit in a psychiatric facility) for a specified time period for treatment to regain competency. Forensic psychiatric nurses working as competency evaluators have greatly enhanced the treatment of defendants deemed legally incompetent, which in the past usually meant only the prescribing of antipsychotic medications.

Roles of the **competency evaluator** include assessing mental health or illness, conducting a forensic interview, providing documentation, completing a formal report to the court, and testifying as an expert witness. Competency therapists work with the defendant in one-to-one and group activities, which should not be confused with psychotherapy. For competency therapists, the patient is the court, not the defendant, and the products of their work are a competent defendant and a completed report. Becoming an advocate for the defendant, rather than for the process, is a breach of professional boundaries (Jacobson, 2002).

Fact and Expert Witnesses

Three types of witnesses can be used in the courtroom trial: (1) the principals (plaintiffs and defendants), (2) fact witnesses, and (3) expert witnesses. Each witness has a specific role in the presentation of the case and in establishing the required burden of proof (Matthews, 2001). The **fact witness** is now used routinely in medical malpractice cases as an individual considered by the court to be capable and qualified to summarize and explain complex and voluminous medical records and medical terminology to the jury (Matthews, 2001).

The court can subpoena any nurse to testify as a fact witness. A fact witness testifies regarding what was *personally* seen or heard, performed, or documented regarding a patient's care and testifies as to first-hand experience only (Sekula & Burgess, 2006). An **expert witness** is recognized by the court as having a certain level of skill or expertise in a designated area and possesses superior knowledge because of education or specialized experience. A nurse may testify as a fact witness and an expert witness. For example, a SANE may testify regarding the facts of a case in which she examined the victim and collected evidence and may also testify in the case because of her expertise as a certified SANE-A. Refer to Chapter 29 for more discussion on sexual assault.

Forensic nurses with advanced degrees are more likely to be called upon as expert witnesses. To establish credibility as an expert witness and to have one's opinion given equal weight to that of other professionals in court, the forensic nurse specialist must have current and updated clinical expertise, trustworthiness, and a professional presentation style (Box 32-3). Professional credentials indicate clinical expertise, and trustworthiness is indicated by the degree of honesty in demeanor and opinion evidenced on the witness stand, as perceived by the judge or jury. The expert witness may be deemed an authority in a specialty area and trustworthy, but unless he or she has a professional presentation style (i.e., the ability to communicate in a concise and convincing fashion) the testimony given is of limited value. In addition if the expert has conducted research and published in the area, it is an added strength. Expert testimony is based on evidence-based practice.

Consultant

Over the last decades, deinstitutionalization has precipitated a need for interagency cooperation between mental health and law enforcement agencies. Although controversial, individuals who previously would have been institutionalized are now commonly homeless and often (intentionally or unintentionally) the focus of law enforcement. The forensic psychiatric

BOX 32-3 REQUIREMENTS FOR EXPERT WITNESS TESTIMONY

Establishment of Expertise

- Academic preparation
- Professional training
- Practical working experience in the field
- Involvement in professional organizations
- Research and publications in the area of expertise

Establishment of Trustworthiness and Objectivity

- Comfortable with self
- Good presentation style
- Successful communication to jury
- Dress, manner, and performance that communicate professionalism

nurse can provide consultation to mental health agencies regarding care of the patient with legal issues and to law enforcement agencies regarding the status and suggested treatment of mentally ill patients in the legal system. In this role, the nurse may also act as an advocate for families and patients. The bottom line for the nurse who serves in this capacity is the perpetrator's well-being, even if that results in civil detention and admission to a hospital.

A forensic psychiatric nurse may be used as a resource for education and information about mental illness by either side in a court case. In this **consultant** role, the nurse may be asked to listen to witness testimony for the purpose of guiding further cross-examination or to assist in the preparation for trial by giving information about mental illness, including personality disorders and paraphilias. The nurse may be asked to testify about mental health treatment options, medications, and community resources.

Hostage Negotiator

In the late 1970s, the Federal Bureau of Investigation (FBI) began expanding hostage-negotiation team structure by recommending the use of consultants who could address the mental state of the perpetrator and recommend appropriate negotiation strategies. In the 1980s, local police agencies began to develop specialized teams that included consultants. When the forensic psychiatric mental nurse functions as a **hostage negotiator**, the role may include the following:

- Being on call around the clock to assist law enforcement officers on the scene
- Providing suggestions regarding negotiation techniques
- Assessing the mental status of the perpetrator
- Providing a link to mental health agencies
- Participating in a critique of the hostage incident
- Assessing released hostages
- Assessing the stress level of the hostage negotiator
- Providing training in communication skills to law enforcement officers

The successful hostage negotiator thinks clearly under stress, is able to communicate with persons from all socioeconomic classes, and demonstrates common sense and "street smarts." Hostage negotiators need to cope with uncertainty, accept responsibility with no authority, and be committed to the negotiation process.

Criminal Profiler

A **criminal profiler** attempts to provide law enforcement officials with specific information about the type of individual who may have committed a certain crime. This service is usually requested when the crime scene indicates psychopathology or when serial crime is suspected. Historically, criminal profilers came from a variety of backgrounds, including law enforcement, psychology, psychiatry, and criminal justice. The criminal profiler collects all the available data, attempts to reconstruct the crime, formulates a hypothesis, develops a profile, and tests it against the known data.

This is familiar territory for the forensic psychiatric nurse, who is comfortable with the nursing processes of assessment, diagnosis (analysis), planning, implementation, and evaluation. Ann Burgess, one of the founders of the IAFN, was the first identified nurse criminal profiler with the FBI (Burgess et al., 2000). Skilled profilers have the ability to isolate their own emotions and reconstruct the crime using the criminal's reasoning process (Fintzy, 2000). Although this requires time and thoughtful consideration, the insights gained are usually critical for diagnosis and treatment. Psychiatric mental health nurses can serve as profilers of specific perpetrators because of their knowledge of psychiatry and human behavior.

CORRECTIONAL NURSING

Nursing care of patients who are incarcerated presents challenges to the way nurses think about the patient. There is debate as to the terminology used when referring to both correctional nurses and psychiatric mental health nurses within correctional settings. Education is key in determining the level of expertise and whether one merits the title *forensic nurse* (either psychiatric mental health or correctional). Working in a correctional setting does not qualify one as a forensic nurse; rather, it is the advanced education and clinical practice that qualify one as a forensic nurse (Sekula et al., 2001).

Currently, there are over 1.2 million incarcerated adults in the United Sates, and over 7 million adults under some kind of correctional supervision. The number of incarcerated individuals in the United States had been steadily increasing for both men and women over the last two decades. It now appears to have leveled off but at artificially high rates. Incarcerated men and women have higher rates of serious and chronic physical and mental illnesses than the general population, requiring enormous health care efforts (Maeve & Vaughn, 2001).

Prisoners are the only U.S. population group with a constitutional right to health care. Because most of their civil liberties are taken away from them when they are incarcerated, and their movements are (necessarily) severely restricted, prisoners are unable to seek and secure health care services on their own. Therefore, correctional facilities are required to provide "adequate" health services to inmates, either directly or through community health services organizations. This includes treatment for both mental and physical illness. **Correctional nursing** is defined by the location of the work or the legal status of the patient, rather than by the role functions being performed.

Treatment and services for inmates with chronic mental health diagnoses are a significant part of the job for correctional staff. According to the U.S. Department of Justice (2006), more than 1 in 3 state prisoners, 1 in 4 federal prisoners, and 1 in 6 jail inmates with a mental health problem received treatment during their incarceration, which amounts to hundreds of thousands of incarcerated adults. Additionally, nearly 25% of inmates with a mental health diagnosis have had three or more prior incarcerations. In general females have higher rates of mental health problems than males. In addition to those receiving care are the thousands of incarcerated adults known to have a mental health problem who are not receiving treatment. When compared to the rates in the general population (11% of whom have a mental health problem, with approximately 55,000 individuals hospitalized at an inpatient psychiatric hospital on any given day), it is clear that correctional facilities carry a disproportionate share of the burden for the provision of mental health services.

Correctional nurses provide care for many patients with serious mental illness who are caught in a cycle of homelessness, psychiatric hospitals, and jail. Frequently these individuals become incarcerated as a result of psychiatric emergencies that generally include threats made to others. Because psychiatric facilities for the management of such emergencies are scarce, often these patients end up in jail instead of in a hospital. Once they are in jail, their psychiatric condition often worsens without adequate psychiatric intervention. The fortunate patients end up in a secure treatment unit within the jail where they receive proper medication and psychiatric mental health nursing care.

Because of the long-term effects on recidivism (repeat offenders) and resource allocation, policy makers and legislators are beginning to recognize the importance of providing treatment for patients who are incarcerated. In a U.S. Department of Justice survey (2006), the most common mental health symptoms were insomnia and hypersomnia. Many of the commonly reported symptoms were related to major depression. Delusions and hallucinations were the most commonly identified psychotic symptoms, with 25% of state inmates, 15% of federal inmates, and 10% of jail inmates reporting at least one of the two symptoms. Especially critical within this population is treatment of those with a history of trauma or posttraumatic stress disorder (PTSD), owing to their long-term debilitating effects. The correctional setting, however, is not conducive to the intensive therapy required to adequately treat these issues; therefore, the needs of the vast majority of people with PTSD and/or trauma history in the correctional system are not appropriately addressed.

Substance use is another critical issue associated with incarceration. According to the National Institute on Drug Abuse (NIDA) (2012a), about half of all inmates at state and federal prisons meet the criteria for alcohol/drug dependence or abuse, but few receive treatment in jail or prison. There is still a great deal of controversy over how to respond to people with substance abuse problems who commit crimes: should we incarcerate or provide treatment? While much of this debate centers on whether incarceration should be punishment or rehabilitation, there is significant evidence to support the latter if the goal is improving safety in communities and reducing crime. Drug courts, mandatory drug treatment, and drug/alcohol treatment within correctional facilities have all been shown to decrease the likelihood of recidivism and increase the likelihood of abstinence from drugs and/or alcohol after release (NIDA, 2012b).

In addition to the needs of people living with mental illness while they are incarcerated, the needs of those same people when they are released and returning home must also be addressed. The reentry experience is more difficult for persons with mental illness due to factors such as physical health problems, housing difficulties, and poorer employment outcomes (Mallik-Kane & Visher, 2008). To be effective, services for this population must include comprehensive discharge planning. Nurses working in this setting are obligated to help try to facilitate ongoing care for people living with chronic mental illness. This may include advocating for alternatives to incarceration since the prison systems are often ill-equipped to deal with the needs of people with severe mental illness, nor is the purpose of incarceration that kind of care. The alarmingly high rates of mental illness in the offender population, often referred to as the "criminalization of mental illness," has spurred advocates to push for options other than jail or prison, such as treatment programs.

Correctional nurses working in facilities with comprehensive psychiatric services perform psychiatric mental health nursing role functions rather than forensic nursing role functions, including completing comprehensive mental status examinations and implementing psychiatric care plans. The following vignettes illustrate challenging situations facing correctional psychiatric nurses.

VIGNETTE

Suzanne is a 45-year-old woman incarcerated at a state facility in the general population. She was convicted of assault with a deadly weapon following a confrontation with a "friend." Her psychiatric diagnoses include major depression and PTSD (resulting from severe abuse in her childhood and from an intimate partner during her early 20s). Although she is not in a locked forensic unit, she is being treated with medication and is seen by the facility's psychiatric mental health nurse practitioner (NP) for medication management. While watching television in the common area one morning, Suzanne attacked a fellow inmate for no apparent reason, screaming and clawing at anyone who approached her. Staff were unable to control her physically. She was placed in solitary confinement with mechanical restraints; these actions did nothing to control her screaming. The NP on call, who reported that Suzanne was having a flashback related to her PTSD, saw her. The solitary confinement and mechanical restraints were only worsening her flashbacks. The staff and the NP were facing a common dilemma in correctional health care: custody versus caring. While the NP was focusing on the needs of the individual inmate, the correctional staff were focused on the goals of the correctional facility related to custody of violent offenders and protecting the environment. The successful correctional treatment team seeks to balance the two sides of this debate: creating an environment where possible rehabilitation of offenders is possible without compromising the compulsory "punitive" aspects of incarceration.

VIGNETTE

Susan Barnes is a 34-year-old woman recently incarcerated at the local jail after being arrested for public intoxication and retail theft; she has had multiple incarcerations over the past 10 years for drug use and minor property crimes. She is expected to be released from jail in 14 to 21 days. Previously diagnosed with bipolar I disorder, she has been on multiple medications. Past arrests were associated with discontinuing medications and self-medicating with crack cocaine and other drugs. At this time she reports being off her medications "for a while" and that "they don't really help much anyway." After 24 hours, the correctional staff notes that she is acting erratically, pacing the floor, and not sleeping. Her behavior is becoming more aggressive toward others, and the staff has threatened to put her in solitary confinement.

A psychiatric nurse practitioner is assigned to interview Ms. Barnes, who says she "feels great" and "the cops are just out to get me." Her speech is pressured, and she expresses significant hostility. She is diagnosed as being in an acute manic phase. Her plan of care focuses on stabilization, medications, patient education, and sleep hygiene. Safety is a key consideration.

The nurse practitioner orders Ms. Barnes to be housed in the infirmary until she can be stabilized, at which time she will be reevaluated for return to the general jail population. Discharge planning is especially critical in this case, as Ms. Barnes' involvement in the criminal justice system seems to coincide with stopping her medications. Ms. Barnes is to be assessed for Forensic Mental Health Court, which offers specialized services for offenders with severe mental illness. This program provides access to a variety of institutional and community-based services and allows the judge to require participation in treatment and follow-up as terms of release from jail. The treatment plan also includes intensive case management so that referrals are in place when Ms. Barnes is released for such critical needs as housing, health care, and food. While the NP is providing care in a correctional setting, she knows that her primary commitment is to high-quality patient care at the same level seen outside the facility. She also knows that Ms. Barnes' needs are complex and that the key outcomes for this patient include preventing a return to jail.

KEY POINTS TO REMEMBER

- Forensic nursing is an emerging specialty area of practice that combines elements of traditional nursing, forensic science, and criminal justice.
- Psychiatric forensic nursing requires that a nurse gain additional education in order to serve this unique population.
- The International Association of Forensic Nurses (IAFN) was established in 1992 as the professional association representing this specialty. Certification for the sexual assault nurse examiner is offered through the IAFN.
- Forensic psychiatric nurses can fulfill a variety of roles, including that of psychotherapist, forensic nurse examiner, competency evaluator, fact witness, expert witness, consultant, hostage negotiator, criminal profiler, and correctional nurse.
- The forensic psychiatric nurse must understand the roles of other forensic nurses in order to function on teams to provide quality care for all victims and perpetrators of violence.
- Forensic nursing brings together traditional nursing practice with forensic knowledge to better serve all persons within the health care system affected by violence in some way.
- The forensic nurse generalist must be proficient in assessment and treatment of victims of violence, evidence collection and preservation, proper documentation, the legal system, and setting standards of care for victims and perpetrators.
- In contrast to other members of the treatment staff on a forensic unit who can be supportive, accepting, and empathetic, the forensic nurse examiner must remain neutral, objective, and detached.

CRITICAL THINKING

1. Compare and contrast the roles of the forensic psychiatric nurse and the correctional nurse. How do their roles differ regarding their relationship with the patient?
2. Given the varied and complex roles within forensic psychiatric nursing, how does an advanced practice forensic psychiatric nurse prepare for these roles? What educational requirements should be considered?
3. The Institute of Medicine's report on the Future of Nursing: Leading Change, Advancing Health encourages all nurses to be full partners with physicians and other health care professionals in redesigning health care. How can a forensic psychiatric nurse prepare to be a part of that team?
4. As a forensic psychiatric nurse, describe circumstances in which you might be called to serve as a fact witness versus being called as an expert witness? What types of education and practice requirements are needed for each role?

CHAPTER REVIEW

1. Which role does a correctional nurse **not** fulfill within the corrections setting?
   a. Nursing assessment
   b. Maintain proper safety procedures
   c. Psychotherapist
   d. Document patient progress
2. Which statement regarding forensic nursing is accurate?
   a. Forensic nurses must all be prepared at the doctoral level.
   b. Forensic nurses focus on sexual assault examinations as this fits within the scope of practice.
   c. Forensic psychiatric nurse examiners are prepared to conduct court-ordered evaluations regarding sanity or competency.
   d. Forensic psychiatric mental health nurses are not permitted to act as hostage negotiators.
3. The psychiatric forensic nurse (PFN) has been asked to evaluate an incarcerated patient who has mental health problems for a competency hearing. As the patient is being considered for sentencing, what is the PFN's role? *Select all that apply.*
   a. Assess the patient for level of competency
   b. Determine whether the patient is guilty or innocent
   c. Assist in determining the length of the sentence
   d. Complete a formal report to the court
   e. Become an advocate for the incarcerated patient

4. In order to determine a patient's legal sanity or competency the psychiatric forensic nurse must assess all of the following, *except*:
   a. The patient's ability to distinguish right from wrong regarding the act
   b. The patient's capacity to understand the nature of the act committed
   c. The evidence with respect to the defendant's mental state at the time of the act
   d. The patient's social network

5. You are caring for Naomi, who has been arrested and is found to be at risk for alcohol and drug dependence/abuse. Which approach is thought to be most useful in treating Naomi?
   a. Recommend that the patient receive treatment when released from jail
   b. Provide immediate drug/alcohol treatment plan
   c. Immediately withdraw all medications
   d. Isolate the patient until withdrawal from drugs is complete

Answers to Chapter Review
1. c; 2. c; 3. a; 4. d; 5. b.

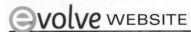

Visit the Evolve website for a posttest on the content in this chapter: http://evolve.elsevier.com/Varcarolis

Post-Test interactive review

REFERENCES

Burgess, A. W., Dowdell, E. B., & Brown, K. (2000). The elderly rape victim: Stereotypes, perpetrators, and implications for practice. *Journal of Emergency Nursing, 26*, 516–518.

Disaster Center. (2007). *United States: Uniform crime report: State statistics from 1960–2007*. Retrieved from http://www.disastercenter.com/crime/.

Fintzy, R. T. (2000). Criminal profiling: An introduction to behavioral evidence analysis. *American Journal of Psychiatry, 157*, 1532–1555.

International Association of Forensic Nurses. (2006). *About IAFN*. Retrieved from http://www.iafn.org/displaycommon.cfm?an=3.

International Association of Forensic Nurses. (2006). *What is forensic nursing*? Retrieved from http://www.iafn.org/displaycommon.cfm?an=1&subarticlenbr=137.

International Association of Forensic Nurses and American Nurses Association. (1997). *Scope and standards of forensic nursing practice*. Washington, DC: American Nurses Publishing.

Jacobson, G. (2002). Maintaining professional boundaries: Preparing nursing students for the challenge. *Journal of Nursing Education, 41*, 279–281.

James, D. J., & Glaze, L. E. (2006). *Bureau of Justice Statistics: Special report: Mental health problems of prison and jail inmates*. Washington, DC: U. S. Department of Justice, Office of Justice Programs.

Lyons, T. (2009). Role of the forensic psychiatric nurse. *Journal of Forensic Nursing, 5*(1), 53–57. doi:10.1111/j.1939-3938.2009.01033.x.

Maeve, M. K., & Vaughn, M. S. (2001). Nursing with prisoners: The practice of caring, forensic nursing or penal harm nursing? *Advances in Nursing Science, 24*(2), 47–64.

Mallik-Kane, K., & Visher, C. (2008). *Health and prisoner reentry: How physical, mental, and substance abuse conditions shape the process of reintegration*. Washington, DC: Urban Institute, Justice Policy Center. Retrieved from http://www.urban.org/UploadedPDF/411617_health_prisoner_reentry.pdf.

Matthews, M. D. (2001). *The nurse and the legal system*. Philadelphia, PA: Davis.

National Institute on Drug Abuse. (2012a). *Principles of drug addiction treatment: A research-based guide* (3rd ed.). Washington, DC: National Institute on Drug Abuse; National Institutes of Health; U.S. Department of Health and Human Services. Retrieved from http://www.drugabuse.gov/publications/principles-drug-addiction-treatment-research-based-guide-third-edition/frequently-asked-questions/what-role-can-criminal-justice-system-play.

National Institute on Drug Abuse. (2012b). *Program reduces recidivism among men with co-occurring disorders*. Retrieved from http://www.drugabuse.gov/news-events/nida-notes/2012/07/program-reduces-recidivism-among-men-co-occurring-disorders.

Sekula, L. K., & Burgess, A. W. (2006). *Forensic and legal nursing, vol. 1*. Boca Raton, FL: CRC.

Sekula, L. K., Holmes, D., Zoucha, R., DeSantis, J., & Olshansky, E. (2001). Forensic psychiatric nursing: Discursive practices and the emergence of a specialty. *Journal of Psychosocial Nursing & Mental Health Services, 39*(9), 51–57.

U.S. Department of Health and Human Services. Office of Disease Prevention and Health Promotion. *Healthy People 2020*. Retrieved from http://www.healthypeople.gov/2020/default.aspx.

U.S. Department of Justice. (2006). *Mental health problems of prison and jail inmates*. Retrieved from http://www.ojp.usdoj.gov/bjs/pub/pdf/mhppji.pdf.

U.S. Department of Justice-Federal Bureau of Investigation. (2006). *United States uniform crime report*. Washington, DC: Author.

Zhang, Z. (2004). *Drug and alcohol use and related matters among arrestees, 2003*. Washington, DC: U.S. Department of Justice.

CHAPTER

33

Therapeutic Groups

Donna Rolin-Kenny and Karyn I. Morgan

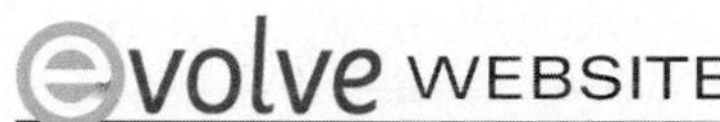

Visit the Evolve website for a pretest on the content in this chapter: http://evolve.elsevier.com/Varcarolis

Pre-Test interactive review

OBJECTIVES

1. Identify basic concepts related to group work.
2. Describe the phases of group development.
3. Define task and maintenance roles of group members.
4. Discuss the therapeutic factors that operate in all groups.
5. Discuss seven types of groups commonly led by basic-level registered nurses.
6. Describe a group intervention for (a) a member who is silent or (b) a member who is monopolizing the group.

KEY TERMS AND CONCEPTS

conflict
feedback
group content
group norms
group process
group psychotherapy
group themes
group work
maintenance roles
psychoeducational groups
self-help groups
support groups
task roles
therapeutic factors

We all live and interact among groups throughout our lives. Most of us are born into a family group and grow up with various peer groups, such as those at school, work, and places of worship and within our communities. As adults, we often establish our own family groups. A **group** consists of two or more people who come together for the purpose of pursuing common goals and/or interests. Each group has characteristics that influence its progress and outcomes, including the following:

- Size
- Defined purpose
- Degree of similarity among members
- Rules
- Boundaries
- Content (what is said in the group)
- Process (underlying dynamics among group members)

Box 33-1 defines terms related to types of groups and group work. **Group work** is a method whereby individuals with a common purpose come together and benefit by mutually giving and receiving feedback within the dynamic and unique group context. Bohm (1992) asserted the importance of dialogue within groups to form a coherent shared meaning, acting as the glue holding people and societies together. Group modalities are commonly used in the care of patients in psychiatric health care settings.

There are advantages and disadvantages of group approaches in the care of psychiatric patients. Advantages include the following:

- Engaging multiple patients in treatment at the same time, thereby saving resources.
- Participants benefiting not only from the feedback of the nurse leader but also from that of peers who may possess a unique understanding of the issues.

BOX 33-1 TERMS CENTRAL TO THERAPEUTIC GROUPS

Terms Describing Group Work

Group content: All that is said in the group (e.g., the group's topics)

Group process: The dynamics of interaction among the members (e.g., who talks to whom, facial expressions, body language, and progression of group work)

Group norms: Expectations for behavior in the group that develop over time and provide structure (e.g., rules about starting on time, not interrupting)

Group themes: Members' expressed ideas or feelings that recur and share a common thread. The leader may clarify a theme to help members recognize it more fully.

Feedback: Providing group members with awareness about how they affect each other

Conflict: Open disagreement among members. Positive conflict resolution within a group is key to successful outcomes.

Terms Describing Membership in Various Types of Groups

Heterogeneous group: A group in which a range of differences exists among members

Homogeneous group: A group in which all members share central traits (e.g., men's group, group of patients with bipolar disorder)

Closed group: A group in which membership is restricted; no new members are added when others leave

Open group: A group in which new members are added as others leave (e.g., inpatient group with transient membership)

Subgroup: An individual or a small group that is isolated within a larger group and functions separately. Members of a subgroup may have greater loyalty, more similar goals, or more perceived similarities to one another than they do to the larger group.

BOX 33-2 THERAPEUTIC FACTORS IN GROUPS

Instillation of hope: The leader shares optimism about successes of group treatment, and members share their improvements.

Universality: Members realize that they are not alone with their problems, feelings, or thoughts.

Imparting of information: Participants receive formal teaching by the leader or advice from peers.

Altruism: Members gain or profit from giving support to others, leading to improved self-value.

Corrective recapitulation of the primary family group: Members repeat patterns of behavior in the group that they learned in their families; with feedback from the leader and peers, they learn about their own behavior.

Development of socializing techniques: Members learn new social skills based on others' feedback and modeling.

Imitative behavior: Members may copy behavior from the leader or peers and can adopt healthier habits.

Interpersonal learning: Members gain insight into themselves based on the feedback from others during later group phases.

Group cohesiveness: This powerful factor arises in a mature group when each member feels connected to the other members, the leader, and the group as a whole; members can accept positive feedback and constructive criticism.

Catharsis: Through experiencing and expressing feelings, therapeutic discharge of emotions is shared.

Existential resolution: Members examine aspects of life (e.g., loneliness, mortality, responsibility) that affect everyone in constructing meaning.

From Yalom, I. D., & Leszcz, M. (2005). *The theory and practice of group psychotherapy* (5th ed.). New York, NY: Basic Books.

- Providing a relatively safe setting to try out new ways of relating to other people and practicing new communication skills.
- Promoting a feeling of belonging.

Disadvantages include the following:

- Time constraints in which an individual member may feel cheated for participation time, particularly in large groups.
- Concerns that private issues may be shared outside the group.
- Dealing with disruptive member behavior during an emotionally vulnerable point.

Not all patients benefit from group treatment. Until symptoms are stabilized, persons who are acutely psychotic, acutely manic, or intoxicated have difficulty interacting effectively in groups and may interfere with other members' ability to remain safely focused on group goals and progress.

THERAPEUTIC FACTORS COMMON TO ALL GROUPS

Irvin D. Yalom, one of the most noted researchers on group psychotherapy, is credited with identifying the factors that make groups therapeutic (Yalom & Leszcz, 2005). **Therapeutic factors** (Box 33-2) are aspects of the group experience that leaders and members have identified as curative and facilitative of therapeutic change. For example, as group members begin to share life experiences, feelings, and concerns, they may recognize for the first time that they are not "alone in the world," which allows them to genuinely connect with others. Yalom calls this factor *universality*—the patient's recognition that other persons feel the same way or have had the same experiences. Recognizing universality can provide a profound sense of relief. Different factors may overlap and operate at different phases of a group. The leader may role-model several therapeutic behaviors during the initial phase, such as *instilling hope* and *imparting information*. Just as with other types of treatment, each person's response to a group is highly individualized based on past experiences and level of participation.

PLANNING A GROUP

To develop a successful group, planning should include a description of specific characteristics, including the following:

- Name and objectives of the group
- Types of patients or diagnoses of members for inclusion
- Group schedule (frequency, times of meetings, etc.)
- Physical setting configuration
- Description of leader and member responsibilities
- Methods or means of evaluating outcomes of the group

Planning and structure are especially important when group leaders are likely to change (in inpatient settings where staffing patterns change) or when several groups are running concurrently with a common goal (in a research study), where consistency is most advantageous.

Thoughtful configuration of the physical space in which the group will meet is essential for promotion of comfort and function. Depending on the size of the group, the room and its physical boundaries should be organized with seats relatively close to each other in a nonhierarchical arrangement. Arranging chairs in a circle conveys equality among all present, whether a group member or leader, and allows for all members to see the whole group.

Basic comfort and sensory measures, such as room temperature, lighting, external noise, and privacy, should be optimized. Size of the room should be functional, as a huge room for a small group does not encourage intimacy, and an overcrowded room may contribute to discomfort and anxiety among members. It is also important to note that inpatient groups have significant differences from outpatient groups (Table 33-1), and the group planning must be adapted accordingly.

PHASES OF GROUP DEVELOPMENT

All groups go through developmental phases similar to those identified for individual therapeutic relationships (refer to Chapter 8). In each phase, the group leader has specific roles and challenges to address in support of positive interaction, growth, and change.

In the **orientation phase**, the group is forming. The group leader's role is to structure an atmosphere of respect, confidentiality, and trust. The purpose of the group is stated, and members are encouraged to get to know one another. Initially, members may be overly silent or overbearing because they have not yet established trust with one another. Therapeutic interaction is supported when the group leader points out similarities between members, encourages them to talk directly to each other rather than to the leader, and reminds members about ground rules for respectful, meaningful interaction.

In the **working phase**, the group leader's role is to encourage a focus on problem solving that is consistent with the purpose of the group. As group members begin to feel safe within the group, conflicts may be expressed, which should be viewed by the group leader as a positive opportunity for group growth. It is important for the leader to guide and support conflict resolution. Through successful resolution of conflicts, group members are empowered to develop confidence in their problem-solving abilities and better support one another in their individual efforts to grow and change. Tuckman (1965) outlined this working phase of groups with classic stages of "storming, norming, and performing." These collaborations generate group cohesion, followed by completion of group tasks, resulting in insight development.

In the **termination phase**, the group leader's role is to encourage members to reflect on progress they have made and identify post termination goals. Members may experience feelings of loss or anger about the group's ending; at times, these feelings can be directed toward other group members or the leader. It is important to openly address such feelings as part of the work toward successful group adjournment.

GROUP MEMBER ROLES

We each have a unique style of interacting with others, and we gravitate toward personal comfort zones within groups. Consider your own behaviors within groups. You may tend to sit back and mainly observe, giving your opinion only after careful consideration, or perhaps you feel it is important to keep everyone moving in a common direction or to help maintain order and actively urge people to continue working. The way we behave in groups is a function of our innate personalities (e.g., shy or outgoing),

TABLE 33-1 COMPARISON OF OUTPATIENT AND INPATIENT GROUPS

GROUP COMPONENT	OUTPATIENT GROUPS	INPATIENT GROUPS
Composition	The group has a stable composition.	The group is rarely the same for more than one or two meetings.
Membership selection	Patients are carefully selected and prepared.	Patients are admitted to the group with little prior selection or preparation.
Level of functioning	The group is homogeneous with regard to ego function.	The group has a heterogeneous level of ego function.
Motivation	Motivated, self-referred patients make up the group; therapy is growth oriented.	Patients are ambivalent, as therapy is often compulsory; therapy is relief oriented.
Length of group treatment	Treatment proceeds as long as required: may continue for 1 to 2 years.	Treatment is limited to the hospital period, with rapid patient turnover.
Boundary	The boundary of the group is well maintained, with few external influences.	Boundary diffuse; events in the milieu affect the group.
Cohesion	Group cohesion develops normally, given sufficient time in treatment.	There is no time for cohesion to develop spontaneously; group development and work progress are limited to the initial phases
Leadership	The leader allows the process to unfold; there is ample time to let group norms evolve.	The group leader structures time and is not passive.
Contact	Members convene only for scheduled meetings, are encouraged to avoid extra group contact.	Patients eat, sleep, and live together outside of the group, extra group contact is endorsed.

From Mackenzie, K. R. (1997). *Time-managed group psychotherapy: Effective clinical applications.* Washington, DC: American Psychiatric Press.

socialization (e.g., birth order, prior exposure to groups), and the specific context of the group (e.g., familiar and interesting topic or one outside of your comfort zone).

Studies of group dynamics have identified informal roles that group members often assume, which may or may not be helpful in the group's development. The classic descriptive categories for these roles are task, maintenance, and individual roles (Benne & Sheats, 1948). **Task roles** keep the group focused on its main purpose and get the work done. **Maintenance roles** keep the group together, help each person feel worthwhile and included, and create a sense of group cohesion. There are also *individual roles* that have nothing to do with helping the group but instead relate to specific personalities, personal agendas, and desires for having needs met by shifting the group's focus to them. Awareness of roles that individual members assume can assist the group leader in identifying behaviors that need to be reinforced or confronted. Members' self-awareness of their roles may encourage more deliberate and insightful group participation. Table 33-2 describes the informal roles of group members.

SELF-ASSESSMENT OF GROUP PARTICIPATION ROLES

You are automatically a part of several groups during nursing education: your large cohort and smaller course and clinical practicum groups. Review Table 33-2 and think about your position and ways you tend to participate in your current groups at school.

- Which task role do you assume in your groups? . . . based on what evidence?
- Which maintenance role do you assume? . . . based on what data?
- Which individual group role is yours? . . . based on what evidence?
- In your class groups in general, how would you characterize the group dynamics and why?

GROUP LEADERSHIP

Responsibilities

The group leader has multiple responsibilities in initiating, maintaining, and terminating a group. The leader is often most commanding during the orientation phase. Here, the structure, size, composition, purpose, and timing of the group are defined. Task and maintenance functions may be introduced and demonstrated. During the working phase, the leader facilitates communication, the flow of group processes, and group conduct. In the termination phase, the leader ensures that each member summarizes individual accomplishments and insights and gives positive and negative feedback regarding the group experience.

TABLE 33-2 **INFORMAL ROLES OF GROUP MEMBERS**

ROLE	FUNCTION	
Task roles	Coordinator	Tries to connect various ideas and suggestions.
	Elaborator	Gives examples and follows up meaning of ideas.
	Energizer	Encourages the group to make decisions or take action.
	Evaluator	Measures the group's work against objectives.
	Information giver	Provides facts or shares experience as an authority figure.
	Information seeker	Tries to clarify the group's values.
	Initiator-contributor	Offers new ideas or a fresh outlook on an issue.
	Opinion giver	Shares opinions, especially to influence group values.
	Orienter	Notes the progress of the group toward goals.
	Procedural technician	Supports group activity with physical tasks (e.g., distributing papers, arranging seating).
	Recorder	Keeps notes and acts as the group memory.
Maintenance roles	Compromiser	During conflict, yields to preserve group harmony.
	Encourager	Praises and seeks input from others.
	Follower	Agrees with the flow of the group.
	Gatekeeper	Monitors the participation of all members to keep communication open and equal.
	Group observer	Notes different aspects of group process and reports to the group.
	Harmonizer	Tries to mediate conflicts between members.
	Standard setter	Verbalizes standards for the group.
Individual roles	Aggressor	Criticizes and attacks others' ideas and feelings.
	Blocker	Disagrees with and halts group issues; oppositional.
	Dominator	Tries to control other members of the group with flattery or interruptions.
	Help seeker	Asks for sympathy of group excessively.
	Playboy	Acts disinterested in group process.
	Recognition seeker	Seeks attention by boasting and discussing achievements.
	Self-confessor	Verbalizes feelings or observations beyond the scope of the group topic.
	Special-interest pleader	Advocates for a special group, usually with own prejudice or bias.

From Benne, K., & Sheats, P. (1948). Functional roles of group members. *Journal of Social Issues, 4*(2), 41.

Sensitivity to cultural diversity and cultural needs of individual members is a key responsibility of the group leader. The leader initially sets a foundation for open communication by defining the importance of mutual respect and rules for group conduct. As group members begin to engage with one another, the leader's sensitivity to issues that may have a cultural basis can be pivotal in facilitating efforts to maintain open, respectful communication. Diversity exists in many forms, including racial, ethnic, economic, and sexual orientation. Encouraging members to share and explore their cultural foundations and beliefs promotes genuine, rich communication and provides the group with the opportunity to explore similarities and differences in a safe environment.

Consider the example of a woman who came to group after a significant suicide attempt. She remained silent and withdrawn until the leader encouraged her to explore her feelings about the group. The patient revealed that she "wasn't smart like everyone else" and that she was "basically just trailer trash." Other group members began to share their similarities and differences in backgrounds, with a focus on their common needs, fears, and insecurities. When this woman finished the group, she acknowledged having learned an important lesson: she could give and get help from persons she saw as different from her, and not everyone would treat her as if she were "unworthy."

Styles of Leadership

There are three main styles of group leadership, and a leader selects the style that is best suited to the therapeutic needs of a particular group. The **autocratic leader** exerts control over the group and does not encourage much interaction among members. For example, staff leading a community meeting with a fixed, time-limited agenda may tend to be more autocratic. In contrast, the **democratic leader** supports extensive group interaction in the process of problem solving. Psychotherapy groups most often employ this empowering leadership style. A **laissez-faire leader** allows the group members to behave in any way they choose and does not attempt to control the direction of the group. In a creative group, such as an art or horticulture group, the leader may choose a flexible laissez-faire style, directing minimally to allow for a variety of responses. In any group, the leader must be thoughtful about communication techniques since these can have a tremendous impact on group content and process. Table 33-3 describes communication techniques frequently used by group leaders.

Clinical Supervision

Clinical supervision is important for group leaders; it provides feedback about their performance and enhances their professional growth. Transference and countertransference issues occur in groups just as in therapeutic relationships within individual treatment (refer to Chapter 8), and more objective input supports a focus on therapeutic goals. Co-leadership of groups is a common practice and has several benefits, which include (1) providing training for less experienced staff, (2) allowing for immediate debriefing between leaders after sessions, and (3) offering two distinctive role models for teaching communication skills to members.

ASSESSMENT OF YOUR GROUP

While participating in your nursing education groups, you have surely taken note of the style and effectiveness of your groups' leaders or instructors. Review Table 33-3 and think about the communication you've been involved in.

- How would you characterize the dynamic of the group?
- Which overall leadership style have your instructors modeled?
- Were group members well prepared to participate in the class/group sessions? If not, how did this affect the dynamic of the group?
- How did the group leader handle group monopolization? . . . side conversations or distractions?

TABLE 33-3 GROUP LEADER COMMUNICATION TECHNIQUES

TECHNIQUE	EXAMPLE
Giving Information: Provides resources and information that support treatment goals	"Antidepressants may take as long as 4 weeks or more to show full therapeutic effects."
Clarification: Asks the group member to expand and clarify what he or she means	"What do you mean when you say 'I can't go back to work?'"
Confrontation: Encourages the group member to explore inconsistencies in his or her communication or behavior	"Jane, you're saying 'nothing's wrong,' but you're crying."
Reflection: Encourages the group member to explore and expand on feelings (rather than thoughts or events)	"I notice you're clenching your fists. What are you feeling right now?" "It sounds like that really upset you."
Summarization: Closes a discussion or group session by pointing out key issues and insights	"We've talked about different types of cognitive distortions, and everyone identified at least one irrational thought that has influenced his or her behavior in a negative way. In the next session, we'll explore some strategies for correcting negative thinking."
Support: Gives positive feedback and acknowledgement	"It took a lot of courage to explore those painful feelings. You're really working hard on resolving this problem."

NURSE AS GROUP LEADER

Psychiatric mental health nurses are involved in a variety of therapeutic groups in acute care and long-term treatment settings. For all group leaders, a clear theoretical framework is necessary to provide a foundation for analyzing the group dynamics and progress. Table 33-4 describes common theoretical frameworks underlying group work.

Registered nurses who are trained at the basic level (diploma, associate degree, or baccalaureate degree) have holistic training and an educational aptitude for providing leadership skills in a variety of group settings. Registered nurses with basic preparation may lead activity, educational, task, and support groups. Advanced practice registered nurses may lead these groups as well but are also qualified to facilitate other specialized group treatments, including psychotherapy, for which more complex skills are necessary. Potential focuses of group content for nurses as group leaders are further explored.

Basic-Level Registered Nurse

Psychoeducational Groups

Psychoeducational groups are groups set up to increase knowledge or skills about a specific psychological or somatic subject and to allow members to communicate emotional concerns. These groups may be time limited or may be supportive for long-term treatment. Generally, written handouts or audiovisual aids are used to focus on specific teaching points. Psychiatric mental health nurses, who are holistically trained, are well prepared to teach about a variety of health subjects.

Medication Education. The psychoeducational group for which the nurse most commonly assumes responsibility is the medication education group, as nurses hold the primary responsibility for teaching patients about their medications. These groups are designed to teach patients about their medications, answer all of their questions, and prepare them for self-management. The group setting facilitates discussion. When patients have concerns about taking medications, it is often the group members themselves who are in the position to most effectively respond to these questions. "Yes, I got a dry mouth when I first started taking that, but it got better. Hang in there." Box 33-3 outlines a template for a medication education group protocol, and Figure 33-1 shows a tool used to outline and evaluate a medication group.

Health Education. Nurses also frequently lead health education groups, including groups on medical conditions and general health topics, such as sex education. The majority of patients with

TABLE 33-4 THEORETICAL FOUNDATIONS FOR GROUP THERAPY

THEORY	CONCEPTS	ROLE OF THERAPIST
Psychodynamic/ psychoanalytic	Applies Freud's concepts of psychoanalysis to individual members and to the group itself; focus is on unconscious conflicts and transference; goal is insight	Helps members to recognize unconscious conflicts and encourages peer feedback, boundary management
Interpersonal	Applies Sullivan's theories about interpersonal learning; focus is on understanding how current relationships repeat early significant relationships; goal is to rebuild individual's personality	Agenda setting, role playing, helps to reduce anxiety and encourages members to validate feelings and thoughts with each other
Communication	Applies a systems model, holding that the whole (group) is greater than the sum of its parts (members); focus is on subgroups and communication, both verbal and nonverbal; goal is to learn clear, congruent communication skills	Helps point out confusing or contradictory messages; acts as a role model for clear communication, showing systemic effects of specific individual behaviors
Group process	Applies Tuckman's stages of group development, analyzes the group with a focus on individual roles and group patterns of behavior (phases, norms, etc.); goal is to resolve authority and intimacy issues	Helps develop a mature, cohesive group in which members trust each other and give supportive feedback
Existential/gestalt	Applies theories of Maslow, Yalom and Rogers to encourage individuals to develop to full potential; focus is on the here and now to increase members' awareness of feelings and meaning; goal is self-actualization in which individual takes full responsibility for choices	Helps focus members on here-and-now experiences to promote self-learning; promotes emphasis on "what" of behaviors, not "why," work with individual disperses as vicarious learning to benefit group
Cognitive-behavioral	Applies Beck's cognitive behavior therapy; focus is on behavior, linking symptom manifestations to thinking patterns, with the group used to reinforce adaptive behavior and minimize and reframe dysfunctional thought patterns; time limited; goal is to change behavior through shifting thinking patterns	Develops a structured group in which members give supportive feedback to identify thoughts and beliefs, reinforce healthier outlooks and behavior; may provide formal teaching, along with homework assignments and behavioral experiments

From Beck, J. S. (2011). *Cognitive behavior therapy: Basics and beyond* (2nd ed.). New York, NY: Guilford Press; Dies, R. (1992). Models of group psychotherapy: sifting through confusion. *International Journal of Group Psychotherapy, 42*, 1–16; Scheidlinger, S. (1997). Group dynamics and group psychotherapy revisited: Four decades later. *International Journal of Group Psychotherapy, 47*(2), 141–159; Tuckman, B. W. (1965). Developmental sequence in small groups. *Psychological Bulletin, 63*, 384–399.

BOX 33-3 TEMPLATE FOR MEDICATION EDUCATION GROUP PROTOCOL

Description of Group

A group for all patients that prepares patients for self-management of medication at home.

Criteria for Patient Selection

Open to all patients with stabilized acute symptoms except those who are displaying suicidal or homicidal behaviors or the potential for assault

Visual Aids

Projected slides, diagrams, films, patient medication education handouts

Purpose

1. To educate patients on the primary function of their medications, including specific symptom relief to expect
2. To provide information on side effects (also that benefits can outweigh risks)
3. To describe a mechanism to negotiate relationships with health care workers in obtaining medications and in discussing medication-related problems
4. To enhance a sense of self-control and mastery of treatment

Procedure

1. Orientation and introduction to the group
2. Brief description of major symptoms in a diagnosis
3. Overview of antipsychotics or antidepressants and their mechanism of action
4. Use of Albany Medical Center patient medication education sheets
5. Question-and-answer period

Behavioral Objectives

At the end of the 45-minute session, patients will be able to:

1. State one symptom they have that is treated by their medication.
2. Ask at least one question about their medication.
3. Identify one mechanism that helps in adhering to the medication regimen.

Theoretical Justification

Even people who think that they are adherent actually take only 80% of doses. Education and therapy are essential adjuncts to drug therapy.

From Ott, C. A. (2000). *Pediatric psychopharmacology.* South Easton, MD: American Healthcare Institute.

Criteria	Strongly Agree	Somewhat Agree	Agree	Disagree	Strongly Disagree
1. I know the name(s) of the medication(s) I am taking.					
2. I know what symptoms the medication(s) can help me with.					
3. I know the common side effects of my medication(s).					
4. I feel comfortable talking to my prescriber if I am having problems with my medication(s).					
5. It is important to take my medication(s) at the same time every day.					

FIG 33-1 Medication group evaluation tool.

a serious mental illness will have co-morbid chronic medical illnesses. Common topics for discussion may include the following:

- Diabetes
- Hypertension
- HIV/AIDS and other sexually transmitted infections
- Education on condom use and other forms of safer sex practices for harm reduction
- Nutrition and exercise

Dual-Diagnosis. Dual-diagnosis groups are designed to incorporate learning about coexisting mental illnesses and substance use disorders. Since treatment issues for patients with dual diagnoses can be complex, group leaders must have demonstrated competency in both mental health and chemical dependence treatment. The goals are to engage patients in treatment, decrease their use of substances in a step-by-step, meaningful process, and improve psychiatric symptoms. Research has shown that combined treatment for patients with serious mental illnesses and substance use disorders produces improvements in both psychiatric and substance use outcomes (Drake et al., 2001). Specific dual-diagnosis group treatment programs have been further developed, incorporating social learning, skills training, and motivational interviewing, yielding improved, longer-term outcomes in substance use, hospitalization, and quality of life (Bellack et al., 2006). Patients developing insights into both conditions will recognize early symptoms and be empowered with the tools needed for relapse prevention.

Symptom Management. For patients with common symptoms resulting from a disorder such as anger or anxiety, symptom management groups are ideal. The group focuses on sharing positive and negative experiences so that members learn coping skills from one another. A primary goal is to increase self-control by helping patients develop a plan for action at the first appearance of symptoms, establishing relapse prevention of psychiatric episodes.

Stress Management. Often time-limited, stress management groups teach members about various relaxation techniques, including deep breathing, exercise, music, and spirituality. One such technique that is increasingly demonstrating efficacy in stress management, as well as other distressing symptoms, is mindfulness (Chadwick et al., 2009). Mindfulness groups focus on developing awareness of the present moment with the intent to induce relaxation and promote insight into thoughts, emotions, and physical symptom responses. Although much of the research has focused on the use of this technique in outpatient settings, one recent study by Winship (2007) reports the benefits of this technique for acutely ill inpatients.

Therapeutic Community Meeting Groups

With the promotion of patient rights and advocacy, another common group consistently held on inpatient units is the therapeutic community meeting. As every interaction occurring on an inpatient milieu has the potential to be therapeutic, the community meeting is the essential venue at which unit happenings are processed and integrated into treatment. Group members adjust to authority, rules, and tolerance of peers. As described in Lego's seminal work, *The American Handbook of Psychiatric Nursing* (1984), group settings provide patients with the opportunity to develop social skills that are modeled on actual interactions Furthermore, behaviors are confronted and processed by the group. Patient governance and advocacy matters are managed during these groups, and nurses are ideally suited to lead these groups since they are in close daily contact with patients and make frequent individual and unit assessments.

Support and Self-Help Groups

Support groups and **self-help groups** are structured for the purpose of providing patients with the opportunity to maintain or enhance personal and social functioning through cooperation and shared understanding of life's challenges (Hayes et al., 2006; Yalom & Leszcz, 2005). Examples include support groups for survivors of cancer, bereavement support, or support groups for families who have lost a loved one to suicide. Hayes and colleagues (2006) present evidence of the benefits of supportive group therapy for severe mental illness as well. Their findings also indicated that adding structured cognitive exercises enhanced the overall improvement in this population over supportive group therapy alone.

The nurse may serve as a resource for patients and must be aware of the wide array of self-help groups available. The flagship example of self-help groups is Alcoholics Anonymous. One of the most important functions of such groups is to demonstrate universality to individuals, as they are not alone in having a particular problem. Thus, these groups provide members with support, and their members help one another by telling their stories and providing alternative ways to view and to resolve problems. Box 33-4 describes characteristics of support and self-help groups.

BOX 33-4 SUPPORT AND SELF-HELP GROUPS

Target Population
- Persons who have shared the experience of a common problem, issue, illness, crisis, or tragedy

Group Leader Activities
- May or may not be defined, often rotates among members
- Role is often more task oriented or facilitative

Examples of Support Groups
- Bereavement groups for those who have experienced the loss of a loved one
- Suicide survivor groups for those who have lost a loved one to suicide
- NAMI (National Alliance for the Mentally Ill) groups for patient/family support, education, and advocacy
- Cancer support groups for families and patients coping with the ramifications of this potentially terminal illness
- Internet support groups for a growing number of people, providing online, synchronous interaction and support, which may be perceived as more private or anonymous
- Veterans support groups

Examples of Self-Help Groups and Resources
- Twelve-step groups that use a common model for recovery: Alcoholics Anonymous (AA)—the prototype for other 12-step groups
- Gamblers Anonymous (GA)
- Overeaters Anonymous (OA)
- Narcotics Anonymous (NA)
- Co-Dependents Anonymous
- Adult Children of Alcoholics (ACOA) and Al-Anon (friends and families of alcoholics)
- Recovery International for persons who have had a mental illness; groups use prescribed model for managing illness and recovery
- National Mental Health Consumers Self-Help Clearinghouse, an information clearinghouse to guide consumers to the nearly 500 diverse types of self-help groups in operation (Yalom & Leszcz, 2005)

Goals
- To provide health education and networking for resources
- To reduce anxiety and decrease feelings of isolation through universality
- To provide support and encouragement of positive coping behaviors:
  - Decrease feelings of isolation
  - Provide mutual support
  - Provide psychoeducation and health education
  - Reduce stress
  - Help individuals cease self-destructive behaviors or come to terms with an overwhelming event or situation

Frequency and Duration
- Meets one or more times per week, some programs monthly, for an indefinite period of time
- Ongoing and open membership; membership may be transient and anonymous

Advanced Practice Nurse

Group Psychotherapy

Group psychotherapy is a specialized treatment intervention in which a trained leader (or co-leaders) establishes a group for the purpose of treating patients with psychiatric disorders. *Psychiatric-Mental Health Nursing: Scope and Standards of Practice* (American Nurses Association [ANA], 2007) defines group psychotherapy as a role of the advanced practice registered nurse in psychiatric mental health (APRN-PMH). Expertise is necessary since the group is used as a tool to bring about personality change (Sadock & Sadock, 2008). Often group psychotherapy is done in conjunction with individual psychotherapy as part of an ongoing plan of feedback in which intense one-to-one work is interspersed with opportunities to relive and work through early life experiences among a supportive group.

Recently, group psychotherapies have been implemented for gaining symptom improvements in both psychiatric disorders and in conjunction with standard treatments for serious medical illnesses. Belotto-Silva et al. (2012) found a cognitive behavioral group therapy intervention (33.3% with significant symptom improvement) to be similarly but even more effective in reducing symptoms of obsessive-compulsive disorder in an outpatient population (N=158) than the selective serotonin reuptake inhibitor medications (SSRIs) (27.7% with significant symptom improvement) prescribed to the comparison group. These results are meaningful because implementation of group therapy showed similar efficacy to the proven standard of care, SSRIs.

Herschbach and colleagues (2010) compared two different types of group therapy to treatment as usual for reducing "fear of disease progression" in a group of outpatients with cancer (N=174), with this variable a marker of distress during treatment. They compared cognitive behavioral group therapy to both supportive-experiential group therapy and to a control group receiving no therapy. Both groups receiving therapies showed significant decreases in fear of progression, which remained significant over time, where the control group improved only in the short term.

Psychodrama Groups. Psychodrama groups are specialized groups in which members are encouraged to act out life experiences or situations for the purpose of learning and insight. A psychodrama group is comprised of a director, a protagonist, and group members who play the cast (Scheidlinger, 1997). Psychodrama entails working in the present moment to process possible past encounters, leading to catharsis, insight, and the promotion of reality testing (Corey, 2007). Leaders should have graduate-level education and training specific to this approach.

Dialectical Behavior Treatment. Dialectical behavior treatment (DBT) groups are a type of group psychotherapy where patients are seen each week with the goal of improving interpersonal, behavioral, cognitive, and emotional skills and reducing self-destructive behaviors (Sadock & Sadock, 2008). Linehan originally developed DBT for the treatment of patients with borderline personality disorders and tenacious suicidal behaviors, but it has been extended to other illnesses. Unlike in other types of group therapy, DBT group members are discouraged from making observations about others in the group. Instead, the focus is on acceptance and mindfulness (Dimeff & Linehan, 2001). This treatment also requires specialized training and advanced education.

Dealing with Challenging Member Behaviors

Are you in a group? What are the most frustrating aspects of group work? Therapeutic groups are similar. Research into group dynamics has identified certain behaviors of individual members that are challenging to manage within a group. Many defensive behaviors used by patients interfere with their ability to function or achieve satisfaction in their lives. Group therapy is about working through problem behaviors and resistance, but some behaviors can be especially disruptive to the group process and difficult for the leader to manage. The patient who monopolizes the group, the patient who complains but continues to reject help, the demoralizing patient, and the silent patient are examples (Yalom & Leszcz, 2005), and specific group interventions may be beneficial.

In dealing with any problematic behaviors and issues in groups, members may appreciate help in disclosing their own feelings and responses. The leader encourages the use of statements that do not focus on what the other one did, but the "how" of expression, such as, "When you speak this way, I feel . . ." The leader helps by noting that feelings are not right or wrong but simply exist. People tend to feel less defensive when *I feel* statements rather than *you are* statements are used. This approach helps members feel like part of the group, not alienated from it or threatened.

Monopolizing Member

The compulsive speech of a person who monopolizes the group may be an attempt to deal with anxiety. As group tension grows, this patient's level of anxiety rises, and his or her tendency to speak increases even more. Some people are just extremely talkative or may exhibit pressured speech due to hypomania or mania. In any case, no one else gets a chance to be heard, and other group members eventually lose interest and begin to withdraw.

VIGNETTE

Mario is the most talkative member of the group until the nurse intervenes. Initially, Mario talks at length about his early experiences related to losing both of his parents and having to live with his grandparents. The other members of the group become bored with the same old story, and they drift off. They have heard these stories many times, not only in group therapy but also during other activities.

There are several useful strategies for dealing with an overly talkative group member. One subtle method is to address the entire group with a reminder that, during group work, everyone should have an equal chance to contribute and that members should consider whether or not they are dominating the group's time. Another strategy is to request a response from group members who have not had a chance to talk about the day's topic. If the behavior continues, it may be necessary to speak directly to the monopolizing group member, either privately or in the group setting. In private, you can share your observations and suggest that perhaps nervousness may be a factor causing the talkativeness. Asking for clarification of your observations may lead to a greater understanding of what the group member is experiencing. You may then ask him or her to limit contributions to a specific number of times (e.g., two or three). In the group setting, the leader may ask group members if they would like to share observations or feedback about other members, thereby offering a chance for redirecting growth. This strategy is probably the most challenging but potentially the most rewarding in that members feel empowered, and the real therapeutic forces of groups are realized.

Complaining Member Who Rejects Help

The patient who complains but continues to reject help continually brings environmental or somatic problems to the group and often describes the problems in a manner that makes them seem insurmountable. In fact, the patient appears to take pride in the insolubility of his or her problems. The patient comes across as entirely self-centered, and the group's attempts to help are continually rejected.

The person who uses these tactics generally has highly conflicting feelings about his or her own dependency or connection within the group; any notice from the leader temporarily increases the patient's self-esteem. On the other hand, the patient has a pervasive mistrust of all authority figures. Most patients who complain but continue to reject help have been subjected to severe emotional deprivation early in their lives and may have experienced emotional and/or physical abuse.

VIGNETTE

Julia is always complaining about how horrible her relationship with her boyfriend is, and she manages to get the entire group worked up over the situation. Members tell her to leave him, not to spend all her time with him, and not to spend all her money on him, but each week she reports a new incident or crisis. In every session, the group members become concerned and offer encouragement, advice, and solutions. Each time, the group becomes angry at her lack of change, and she is frustrated by her own inability to change. She asserts that the group is not helpful.

The leader should acknowledge the patient's pessimism but maintain a neutral affect. If the patient stays in the group long enough and the group develops a sense of cohesion, this individual can be helped to recognize reality-based relationship patterns. The leader should encourage the patient to look at the habitual "yes . . . but" behavior objectively.

Demoralizing Member

Some people whose behavior is self-centered, angry, or depressed may lack empathy, hope, or concern for other members of the group. They refuse to take any personal responsibility and can challenge the group leader and negatively affect the group process.

In this case, the group leader should listen to the comments objectively. Again, the leader may choose to speak to the group member in private and ask what is causing the anger. Sometimes this simple exchange can make the patient feel greater connection with the nurse and more important as a member of the group, which likely will decrease hostile behavior and increase the group's benefit. In the group setting, the leader can focus on positive group members whose comments may reduce the hostility of the negative group member.

VIGNETTE

Douglas comes to the support group on the inpatient psychiatric unit. He is very angry, stating, "I don't know why I come to these groups anyway! They don't help." Douglas is to be discharged the next day to a 28-day alcohol rehabilitation program. He has a previously scheduled dental appointment before the rehabilitation intake interview, and he is being strongly encouraged by his therapist to reschedule the appointment. The therapist fears that Douglas is at high risk for drinking again because he states that he has constant cravings to drink. When a group member who is an addictions therapist confronts Douglas about not being flexible and prioritizing his need for alcohol treatment, he explodes, "I thought this group was for support. This is outrageous!" Group members are obviously uncomfortable with his anger.

Remember that angry patients may be extremely vulnerable, and devaluing or demoralizing keeps others at a distance and maintains the patient's own precarious sense of safety. Leaders must empathize with the patient in a matter-of-fact manner, such as, "You seem angry that the group wants to support you in putting sobriety ahead of your dental needs."

Silent Member

Patients who are silent in the group may be observing intently until they decide the group is safe for them, or they may believe they are not so competent as other, more assertive group members. Silence does not mean that the member is not engaged or involved, but it should be addressed for several reasons. The person who does not speak cannot benefit from others' feedback, and other group members are deprived of this group member's valuable insights. Furthermore, a silent group member may make others uncomfortable and create a sense of mistrust.

Anyone who has led a group can attest to the challenges of a silent member. There are several techniques that may help, including allowing the person to have extra time to formulate his or her thoughts before responding. Saying, "I'll give you a moment to think about that," and waiting or coming back to the group member later is often helpful. Another tactic is to make an assignment that every person in the group respond

VIGNETTE

Anne has attended three group sessions for survivors of childhood sexual abuse. While she appears to be listening, she rarely makes eye contact with the leader or other group members. She will respond to yes or no questions, but when it comes to the open-ended type, such as "What do you think, Anne?" she tends to shrug her shoulders and respond with "I don't know." Other group members have tried to draw Anne out, as has the leader. Kathy, another group member, is beginning to exhibit frustration with Anne. "Look, I have shared some of the most private and painful memories of my childhood. I feel like you think you're too good to share what happened to you."

to a certain topic or question. For example, "Let's all think of a positive and assertive response to something that you generally feel helpless about. I'll give you a minute or so to think this over, and then I'm going to ask each of you to share."

Sometimes partnering with another group member will give the silent member the courage he or she needs to participate. You may break the group into pairs who are asked to discuss a certain topic and then each report back to the group what he or she heard the other one say. Follow-up privately with a silent member will safely identify the non participatory behavior as well as allow for personal discussion of what may be inhibiting his or her participation.

EXPECTED OUTCOMES

Expected outcomes of group participation will vary, depending on the type and purpose of the group. For educational groups, such as a medication education group, the expected outcome would be demonstration of precise knowledge such as the following:

- Patient identifies three significant side effects of his or her prescribed medication.
- Patient recognizes dangerous drug-drug and drug-food interactions for prescribed medications.
- Patient correctly identifies time of day and dose for each prescribed medication.

For therapy groups, the expected outcomes will focus more on insights, behavioral changes, and reduction in symptoms. For example, in an alcohol treatment group, an expected outcome might be that the patient develops insight into the connection between drinking and negative consequences. An expected behavioral outcome would be abstinence from alcohol use. In groups that focus primarily on emotional issues such as depression or anxiety, standardized symptom surveys can be used to measure symptom reduction as an outcome of group participation.

KEY POINTS TO REMEMBER

- When a new group is formed, similarities and differences in many dimensions, including diagnosis, age, gender, and culture, must be considered.
- A group format has advantages over individual therapy, including cost savings, increased feedback, an opportunity to practice new skills in a relatively safe environment, mutual learning, and instilling a sense of belonging.
- Research has identified 11 therapeutic factors that operate in groups and lead to therapeutic change for members. Yalom's therapeutic factors identify specific transformative aspects of groups, such as universality of experience and the instillation of hope.
- Groups develop through predictable phases over time.
- For a group to continue and be productive, members must fulfill specific functions known as *task or maintenance roles*. Individual roles are not productive and are based on individual personalities and needs, so the nurse leader should reinforce productive group roles and confront individual roles.
- Clinical supervision is important so that group leaders can objectively analyze group interactions and characteristics as well as leadership techniques.
- Nurses have many opportunities to lead or co-lead therapeutic groups, both in the hospital and community settings.
- Psychoeducational groups, health teaching groups, and support groups are often led by registered nurses and provide significant treatment.
- Advanced practice registered nurses may lead psychotherapy groups based on various theoretical models.
- Challenging member behaviors such as monopolizing, silence, complaining, or demoralizing can be especially difficult. A variety of interventions are recommended to minimize the disruption to the group and maximize the insight to the patient who is engaging in these behaviors.

CRITICAL THINKING

1. You are assigned to work with Mary, a 30-year-old who was admitted to the psychiatric unit with major depression and a suicide attempt. Her nurse has told her she needs to attend group therapy. While lying in bed and staring at the ceiling, Mary tells you that she is a private person and that listening to other people's problems won't help and will only make her more depressed.
   a. How would you describe the benefits of group therapy to Mary?
   b. What intervention(s) might make it easier for Mary to attend group therapy?
2. Construct an outline for a medication-teaching group that would cover information useful for your patients. If possible, co-lead this group with a staff member with guidelines from your instructor.
3. Ms. Rodriguez is a 22-year-old Puerto Rican–born nursing student admitted to the psychiatric unit after a nearly lethal overdose of acetaminophen. She admits to drinking excessively for the past 6 months. She is at risk of failing school. She complains of depressed mood, a loss of interest in her studies, decreased concentration, and social isolation. In the dual-diagnosis group, she has been silent for the past two sessions and sits staring at the floor.
   a. What is your evaluation of Ms. Rodriguez's situation?
   b. What might Ms. Rodriguez's nonverbal behavior mean?
   c. What approach would you use to involve her more in the group?
   d. What criteria could you use to evaluate the effectiveness of your intervention?
   e. What cultural implications should you consider?

CHAPTER REVIEW

1. The nurse is caring for four patients. Which patients would not be appropriate to consider for inpatient group therapy? *(Select all that apply.)* The patient who:
   a. Has limited financial and social resources
   b. Is acutely manic
   c. Has few friends on the unit
   d. Is preparing for discharge tomorrow
   e. Does not speak up often, yet listens to others

2. The nurse tells group members that they will be working on expressing conflicts during the current group session. Which phase of group development is represented?
   a. Formation phase
   b. Orientation phase
   c. Working phase
   d. Termination phase
3. Group members are having difficulty deciding what topic to cover in today's session. Which nurse leader response reflects autocratic leadership?
   a. "We are talking about fear of rejection today."
   b. "Let's go around the room and make suggestions for today's topic."
   c. "I will let you come to a conclusion together about what to talk about."
   d. "I'll work with you to find a suitable topic for today."
4. The nurse is planning care, which will include a dual-diagnosis group. Which patient would be appropriate for this group? The patient with:
   a. Depression and suicidal tendencies
   b. Anxiety and frequent migraine headaches
   c. Bipolar disorder and anorexia nervosa
   d. Schizophrenia and alcohol abuse
5. A patient continues to dominate the group conversation despite having been asked to allow others to speak. What is the most appropriate nursing response?
   a. "You are monopolizing the conversation."
   b. "When you talk constantly, it makes everyone feel angry."
   c. "You are supposed to allow others to talk also."
   d. "When you speak out of turn, I feel concerned that others cannot participate equally."

Answers to Chapter Review
1. b; 2. c; 3. a; 4. d; 5. d.

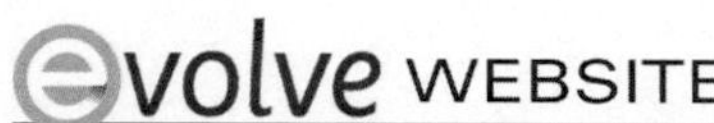

Visit the Evolve website for a posttest on the content in this chapter: http://evolve.elsevier.com/Varcarolis

Post-Test interactive review

REFERENCES

American Psychiatric Nurses Association, International Society of Psychiatric-Mental Health Nurses, & American Nurses Association. (2007). *Psychiatric-mental health nursing: Scope and standards of practice.* Silver Springs, MD: NurseBooks.org.

Beck, J. S. (2011). *Cognitive behavior therapy: Basics and beyond* (2nd ed.). New York, NY: Guilford Press.

Bellack, A. S., Bennett, M. E., Gearon, J. S., Brown, C. H., & Yang, Y. (2006). A randomized clinical trial of a new behavioral treatment for drug abuse in people with severe and persistent mental illness. *Archives of General Psychiatry, 63*, 426–432.

Belotto-Silva, C., Diniz, J. B., Malavazzi, D. M., Valerio, C., Fossaluza, V., Borcato, S., et al. (2012). Group cognitive-behavioral therapy versus selective serotonin reuptake inhibitors for obsessive-compulsive disorder: A practical clinical trial. *Journal of Anxiety Disorders, 26*(1), 25–31. doi:10.1016/j.janxdis.2011.08.008.

Benne, K. D., & Sheats, P. (1948). Functional roles of group members. *Journal of Social Issues, 4*(2), 41–49.

Bohm, D. (1992). On dialogue. *Noetic Sciences Review, 92*(23), 16–18.

Chadwick, P., Hughes, S., Russell, D., Russell, I., & Dagnan, D. (2009). Mindfulness groups for distressing voices and paranoia: A replication and randomized feasibility trial. *Behavioural and Cognitive Psychotherapy, 37*, 403–412. doi:10.1017/S1352465809990166.

Corey, G. (2007). *Theory and practice of group counseling* (8th ed.). Belmont, CA: Brooks/Cole Cengage Learning.

Dimeff, L., & Linehan, M. M. (2001). Dialectical behavior therapy in a nutshell. *The California Psychologist, 34*, 10–13.

Drake, R. E., Essock, S. M., Shaner, A., Carey, K. B., Minkoff, K., Kola, L., et al. (2001). Implementing dual-diagnosis services for clients with severe mental illness. *Psychiatric Services, 52*, 469–476. doi:10.1176/appi.ps.52.4.469.

Hayes, S. A., Hope, D. A., Terryberry-Spohr, L. S., Spaulding, W. D., Vandyke, M., Elting, D. T., et al. (2006). Discriminating between cognitive and supportive group therapies for chronic mental illness. *The Journal of Nervous and Mental Disease, 194*, 603–609. doi:10.1097/01.nmd.0000230635.03400.2d.

Herschbach, P., Book, K., Dinkel, A., Berg, P., Waadt, S., Duran, G., et al. (2010). Evaluation of two group therapies to reduce fear of progression in cancer patients. *Supportive Care in Cancer, 18*, 471–479. doi:10.1007/s00520-009-0696–1.

Leo, A. (1984). *The American handbook of psychiatric nursing.* Philadelphia, PA: Lippincott.

Sadock, B. J., & Sadock, V. A. (2008). *Kaplan & Sadock's concise textbook of clinical psychiatry* (3rd ed.). Philadelphia, PA: Lippincott Williams & Wilkins.

Tuckman, B. W. (1965). Developmental sequence in small groups. *Psychological Bulletin, 63*, 384–399.

Winship, G. (2007). A qualitative study into the experience of individuals involved in a mindfulness group within an acute inpatient mental health unit. *Journal of Psychiatric and Mental Health Nursing, 14*, 603–608.

Yalom, I. D., & Leszcz, M. (2005). *The theory and practice of group psychotherapy* (5th ed.). New York, NY: Basic Books.

CHAPTER

34

Family Interventions

Laura Cox Dzurec and Sylvia Stevens

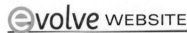

Visit the Evolve website for a pretest on the content in this chapter: http://evolve.elsevier.com/Varcarolis

Pre-Test interactive review

OBJECTIVES

1. Discuss the characteristics of a healthy family.
2. Differentiate between functional and dysfunctional family patterns of behavior as they relate to five universal family functions: management, boundaries, communication, emotional support, and socialization.
3. Compare and contrast insight-oriented family therapy and behavioral family therapy.
4. Identify five family theorists and their contributions to the family therapy movement.
5. Analyze the meaning and value of the family's sociocultural context when assessing and planning intervention strategies.
6. Construct a genogram using a three-generation approach.
7. Recognize the significance of self-assessment to successful work with families.
8. Formulate outcome criteria family might develop together.
9. Identify strategies for family intervention.
10. Distinguish between the nursing intervention strategies of a basic-level nurse and those of an advanced practice nurse with regard to counseling and psychotherapy.
11. Explain the importance of the nurse's role in psychoeducational family therapy.

KEY TERMS AND CONCEPTS

behavioral family therapy
boundaries
clear boundaries
diffuse or enmeshed boundaries
family systems theory
family triangle
genogram
insight-oriented family therapy
multigenerational issues
nuclear family
rigid or disengaged boundaries
sociocultural context

In Western culture, the uniqueness of the individual and the search for autonomy is celebrated, yet we are defined and sustained by interlocking systems of human relationships, including the relationships we develop with our own family members. Many of us struggle with these personal family relationships and wish they were better. When families are discussed, the tone ranges from a negative focus on differences and dissension to a positive focus on loyalty, tolerance, mutual aid, and assistance.

Political upheaval occurring around the world highlights the importance of family relationships to the well-being of individual family members. When children are deprived of family support—for instance, in cases of loss due to the ravages of war—they tend to respond with a range of adjustment difficulties and guilt reactions that can influence their well-being for years (Reeve, 2010). This sort of loss represents the most serious cases of fractured family dynamics.

In other cases, the family remains physically intact, yet family members are deprived of support. Emotional stress or trauma experienced by one family member, as well as complex life challenges faced by the family as a whole, can threaten interactions for the entire family. When individual deprivation occurs in intact families, and individual members exhibit behavioral, cognitive, or emotional dysfunction, the quality of family members' reciprocal and collective, day-to-day interactions may be impacted. For those families and for the members within them, family therapy may be recommended.

Family therapy focuses on changing the interactions among the people who make up the family and on changing the character of the interactions of the family unit as a whole. As a treatment approach, family therapy began to emerge in the 1920s, as social psychologists recognized that behaviors among group members mutually influenced the behaviors of individual members (Gilgulin, 2008). The aim of family therapy is to improve the skills of the individual members and to strengthen the functioning of the family as a whole, capitalizing on the notion that parts of a whole and the whole itself mutually influence each other. More specifically, family therapists concentrate on evaluating relationships and communication patterns, structure, and rules that govern the nature of family interactions.

Specific approaches to therapy vary according to the philosophical viewpoint, education, and training of individual therapists. It is fairly clear, though, that however it is practiced, family therapy is more effective for the mental health of individual family members than is treatment aimed at individuals separately (Baldwin et al., 2012).

OVERVIEW OF THE FAMILY

Families are defined by reciprocal relationships in which persons are committed to one another. Duvall (1957) was among early writers to describe the level of maturity of families as units. She addressed the quality of family functioning, noting that at one extreme some families function in immature or infantile ways, while at the other extreme, families may function in particularly healthy or adult-like ways.

The notion of family function refers to a range of characteristics. They include the family's:

- Ability to provide for the physical and emotional safety of individual members
- Quality of resources and support systems
- Underlying issues such as substance abuse, domestic violence, or chronic illnesses
- Cultural concerns
- Developmental needs
- Established patterns of behavior and interaction
- Responses to stressors
- Ability to interact with support services
- Parenting skill
- Relationships and interactions
- Overall flexibility or resilience

When Duvall described family functioning, she was referring to the "nuclear family"— mother, father, and children—that was prevalent in the 1950s. Today, family constellations are more complex. The National Health Interview Survey (Blackwell, 2010) identified the following types of families with children that exist in the United States:

- **Nuclear family:** One or more children who live with married parents who are the biological or adoptive parents to all the children.
- **Single-parent family:** One or more children who live with a single adult, male or female, related or unrelated to the children.
- **Unmarried biological or adoptive family:** One or more children who live with two parents who are not married to each other and are biological or adoptive parents to all children in the family.
- **Blended family:** One or more children living with a biological or adoptive parent and an unrelated stepparent who are married to each other.
- **Cohabitating family:** One or more children living with a biological or adoptive parent and an unrelated adult who are cohabitating together.
- **Extended family:** One or more children living with at least one biological or adoptive parent and a related adult who is not a parent (e.g., grandparent, adult sibling).
- **"Other" family:** One or more children living with related or unrelated adults who are not biological or adoptive parents. This includes children living with grandparents and foster families.

Still, Duvall's descriptions of family dynamics that describe family functioning on a maturity continuum remain useful in describing family dynamics, despite the increasing complexity of family makeup. The level of functioning of the family unit, regardless of its constellation, will influence the family's individual and collective abilities to deal with life events (Young, 2010).

The family is the primary system to which a person belongs, and in most cases, it is the most powerful system of which a person will ever be a member. The dynamics of the family subtly and significantly influence the beliefs and actions of individual members across the lifespan. Healthy families—those whose members communicate well, maintain fairly consistent expectations and roles, can support and nurture each other, and are adaptable in the face of change and stress—tend to deal better with developmental changes than do less healthy families. But the process of adaptation, even to "normal" changes such as the birth of a child, can test the strength of relationships even in the most resilient family. In those situations, family therapy can be beneficial to the overall functioning of the family and to the individual members as well. Family therapy provides an opportunity for emotional and social growth. In family therapy, a focus on family functions is aimed toward strengthening family interactions to foster family maturity.

As the notion of family has broadened to incorporate nontraditional family structures (Figure 34-1), family therapists and counselors have been challenged to recognize and incorporate similarly broad definitions of family in their work. Despite the increasing complexity of family definitions, family health still can be measured in terms of quality of communication, consistency of familial expectations and roles, support and nurturance of one another, and adaptability in the face of change and stress (Coulter & Mullin, 2012). The family provides an essential training ground for developing individuals' future skills for interacting in

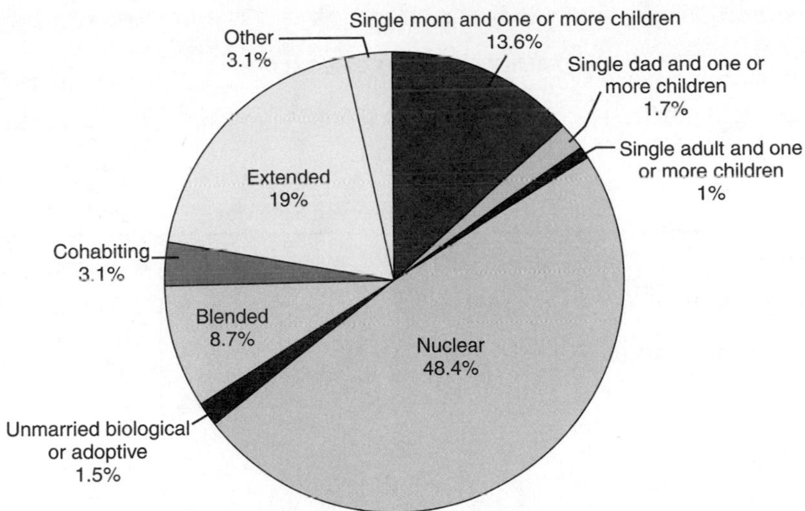

FIG 34-1 Percent distribution of family structure for children under age 18: United States 2001-2007. (From Blackwell, D. L. [2010]. Family structure and children's health in the United States: Findings from the national health interview survey, 2001-2007. *National Center for Health Statistics. Vital Health Statistics, 10*[246]. Retrieved from http://www.cdc.gov/nchs/data/series/sr_10/sr10_246.pdf.)

the greater community, and it is within the family that each of us initially learns sets of long-standing and fairly permanent social and emotional responses. Because family functioning represents behaviors that involve dynamics that extend beyond individuals to individuals-in-interaction, fully understanding the forces that influence family functioning is challenging. That is the challenge accepted by family therapists as they address family functioning.

Family Functions

A healthy family provides its members with tools to guide effective functioning within the family and extends to functioning in other intimate relationships, the workplace, culture, and society in general. These tools are acquired through the activities associated with family life and include management activities, boundary delineation, communication patterns, emotional support, and socialization (Nichols, 2009). Although family therapists may use various assessment strategies, these five areas are always included. Figure 34-2 presents an assessment overview developed by Roberts (1983) that can be used to examine and measure the effectiveness of family skills in these five areas.

Management

Every day in every family, decisions are made regarding issues of power, resource allocation (i.e. who gets what), rule making, and the provision of financial support. These decisions contribute to adaptive family functioning. In healthy families, it is usually the adults who mutually agree about how these management functions are to be performed. In families with a single parent, these management functions may sometimes become overwhelming, as the parent has no partner with whom to discuss management functions.

In more chaotic families, an inappropriate member, such as a teenager, may be the one who makes management decisions. Although children learn decision-making skills as they mature and increasingly make decisions and choices about their own lives, they should not be expected or forced to take on this responsibility for the family. A 12-year-old child, for example, should not be the one to decide whether to pay the gas bill or buy groceries.

Strong management supports the quality of day-to-day family operations. Assessing management functions contributes to a broad conceptualization of the quality of family functioning.

Boundaries

Boundaries serve to maintain distinctions between and among individuals in the family and between the family and individuals external to it. Establishment and maintenance of flexible and appropriate boundaries is essential to healthy family functioning. Boundary management is an important skill for families and often is a primary focus of family therapists. Minuchin (1974) identified three predominant types of boundaries within families: clear, diffuse, and rigid. **Clear boundaries** are adaptive and healthy. They are well understood by all members of the family and give family members a sense of "I-ness" and also "we-ness." They are firm, yet appropriately flexible, and provide a structure that responds and adapts to change. Clear boundaries allow family members to enact roles appropriately and to function without unnecessary or inappropriate interference from other members. They reflect structure and flexibility; at the same time, they support healthy family functioning and encourage growth in family members, often referred to as "differentiation" (Schnarch & Regas, 2011).

For example, a mother maintains her role as the parent by telling her 14-year-old son, "You don't need to worry whether your little brother eats his breakfast. Your father and I will handle that." This boundary, however, is not rigid and may be redefined from time to time, as in, "I want you to make sure that your little brother gets his homework done while your father and I are at the movies."

Diffuse or enmeshed boundaries are less supportive of family health and often are enacted in families in which members are

FAMILY FUNCTION CHECKLIST

Client Family ______________________ Date of Assessment ______________________

Family Functions	Observed Behavior	Assessed Need Level (I-IV)	Suggested Nursing Responses
I. *Management function* A. Use of power for all family members B. Rule making clear, accepted C. Fiscal support adequate D. Successful negotiations with extrafamilial systems E. Future planning present II. *Boundary function* A. Clear individual boundaries B. Clear generational boundaries C. Clear family boundaries III. *Communication function* A. Straight messages B. No manipulation C. Safe expression of positive and negative feelings IV. *Emotional-supportive function* A. Mutual positive regard B. Deals with conflict C. Uses resources for all family members D. Allows growth for all family members V. *Socialization function* A. Children growing and developing in a healthy pattern B. Mutual negotiation of roles by age and ability C. Parents feeling good about parenting D. Spouses happy with each other's role behavior			

FIG 34-2 Family Function Checklist. (From Roberts, F. B. [1983]. An interaction model for family assessment. In I. W. Clements & F. B. Roberts [Eds.], *Family health: A theoretical approach to nursing care* [p. 202]. New York, NY: Wiley. Copyright © 1983 by John Wiley & Sons. Reprinted by permission of John Wiley & Sons, Inc.)

overinvolved with one another. When boundaries are diffuse, individuals tend to become "enmeshed." As a consequence, it is not clear who is in charge, who is responsible for decisions, and who has permission to act or take charge. Diffuse boundaries are particularly problematic when parent/child role enactment becomes blurry. For example, when a parent is unemployed and one of the children takes responsibility for earning money to meet the family's basic needs, boundaries can be said to be diffuse.

In families with diffuse boundaries, individual family members are discouraged from expressing their own views or to differentiate. Thus, to an outsider, it may appear that family members are extremely close, and family members may believe that they are of one mind. That sense is typically false though, and deeper analysis often results in the discovery of suppressed frustrations, anger, and behaviors.

Because in enmeshed families any expression of separateness or independence is viewed as disloyalty to the family, members are prone to psychological or psychosomatic symptoms, probably as a function of the individuals' inability to actually say or even to recognize how they feel. During times of change or crisis, whether the crisis is one of normal development (such as when a new baby is born or an elderly grandparent dies) or is one that is unanticipated (such as the loss of a pregnancy, or serious, debilitating injury to a family member), adaptation of both individuals and of the family as a whole is extremely difficult.

When boundaries are diffuse, everyone, and thus no one, is in charge. Individuals expect other members of the family to know what they are thinking ("Why did you take that? You know I wanted it!"), believe they know what other family members are thinking ("I know exactly why you did that!"), and take comfort that everyone thinks the same way ("No one in our family likes seafood."). Assumptions at this basic level challenge the growth and maturation of the family over time, often serving to urge the family into family therapy.

Rigid or disengaged boundaries are characterized by the consistent adherence to rules and roles—some apparent and some less so—no matter what. Boundaries can be so closed that family members avoid each other, facilitating little sense of family loyalty. In that case, families are considered to be disengaged.

In families in which rigid boundaries predominate, communication is minimal, and thoughts and feelings rarely are shared. Isolation may be marked.

Disengaged family members lead highly separate and distinct lives, and no one is really involved with anyone else. Since intimacy is not learned in the family setting, individuals from disengaged families do not tend to develop insights into their own feelings and emotions. As a result, they may have a hard time bonding with others and participating in new family structures when they leave their families of origin and begin their lives as adults.

VIGNETTE

Lauren is a single, teenage mother living on public assistance; she has two preschool-aged children. Lauren is studying for a general equivalency degree and working part time as a seamstress. Her mother, Sandra, helps to watch the children, and the discipline of the children is an issue of contention between Lauren and Sandra. Sandra thinks that the children are allowed to run wild under Lauren's care. The lines of authority between Sandra as mother, Lauren as daughter, and Sandra as caregiver are blurred.

Sandra does not speak to Lauren about her concerns, but her nonverbal communications clearly express her feelings. Likewise, Lauren does not address her mother's attitude toward her parenting style. Instead, she complains about her mother's child-care skills to her friends and to her siblings. Neither Lauren nor Sandra is experiencing growth from this rigid set of expectations. Meanwhile, the children are learning poor communication skills.

When boundaries are functioning properly, family members work out arrangements in compromise based on understanding of appropriate roles and on open communication. Each generation within the family is made tacitly and explicitly aware of how decisions will be made. Individuals are clearly and appropriately involved in discussion so that they understand who is in charge and know when they are in charge. There is flexibility and room for discussion as family members work out difficult situations.

Alternatively, blurred boundaries, whether they are diffuse or rigid, result in family members interfering with each other's goals, in tension and anxiety between family members, and in intrapersonal anxiety. Children living within families with blurred boundaries become confused, tending to engage in manipulative and perhaps age-inappropriate behavior, and feel insecure and helpless as they mature.

Communication

Communication patterns are extremely important in family life. Healthy communication patterns are characterized by clear and comprehensible messages (e.g., "I would like to go now" or "I don't like it when you interrupt what I'm saying"). Healthy communication within the family encourages members to ask for what they want and need and to express their feelings appropriately. Thoughts and feelings can be openly, honestly, and assertively expressed in families where communication is healthy. Family members are able to ask for what they want and get the attention they need without resorting to manipulation. Alternatively, those in legitimate positions of power within the family, typically the parents, are able to make determinations about the appropriateness of requests.

In healthy families, there is a necessary and natural hierarchy, or power difference, for the protection and socialization of younger family members. Parents are the leaders in the family and children are the followers. Despite this arrangement, children can voice their opinions and have influence on family decisions. In dysfunctional families this seemingly simple equation goes off track. If the communication roles match speakers' functional roles—when, for example, parents communicate like parents—the communication remains clear; however, if a parent communicates like a child, refusing to enact communication expected of a parent, the child may need to take on a reciprocal parental communication role, significantly confusing both communication and boundary functions (Harris, 1967; Nichols, 2009).

When communication among family members is unclear, and when roles and the natural hierarchy become confused, communication cannot be used as a means to solve problems or to resolve conflict. The cardinal rule for effective and functional communication in families is "Be clear and direct in saying what you want and need," whether you are in a powerful or a subordinate position. As simple as this may seem, communication is one of the hardest skills to activate in a family system. To be direct, individuals must first have a sense that they are respected and loved and that it is safe to express personal thoughts and feelings. The consequences of being clear and direct may be unpleasant in a family system that will not tolerate openness.

The following vignette describes a spousal situation that shows how easily communication can be misunderstood when clear and direct messages are not sent, and Box 34-1 identifies some unhealthy communication patterns.

VIGNETTE

Liz would like to spend more time with her husband, Michael, on the weekends; however, Michael always seems to be busy doing projects around the house or talking with friends on the telephone. Liz believes that Michael does not notice her or maybe is not interested in her, so she spends a lot of time working out or playing tennis. Michael figures that Liz is doing what she wants to do and that it makes her happy, so he contents himself with finding things to do alone. The result is that Liz and Michael spend little time together.

Liz finally confronts Michael clearly, directly, and assertively, rather than angrily or aggressively, about her belief that he is "disinterested" in her and tells him what she wants and needs—to spend more time together on the weekends. Michael replies that he had no idea she felt that way. He had thought she enjoyed the way things were, and he would like to have more time together too.

BOX 34-1 EXAMPLES OF DYSFUNCTIONAL COMMUNICATION

Manipulating

Instead of asking directly for what is wanted, family members manipulate others to get what they want. For example, a child starts a fight with a sibling to get attention. Another example is a family member's making requests with strings attached so that the other person has a difficult time refusing the request: "If you do this for me, I won't tell Daddy you are getting poor grades in school."

Distracting

To avoid functional problem solving and resolving conflicts within the family, family members introduce irrelevant details into problematic issues.

Generalizing

When dealing with problematic family issues, members use global statements such as "always" and "never" instead of dealing with specific problems and areas of conflict. Family members may say "Harry is always angry" instead of "Harry, what is upsetting you?"

Blaming

Family members blame others for failures, errors, or negative consequences of an action to keep the focus away from themselves. This is a response to fear of being blamed by others.

Placating

Family members pretend to be inadequate but well meaning to keep peace in the family at any price: "Don't yell at the children, dear. *I* put the shoes on the stairs."

Emotional Support

All families, regardless of how healthy they are, encounter conflicts. In the most functionally healthy families, feelings of affection generally are uppermost, and family members realize that bursts of anger and conflict reflect a short-term response. Anger and conflict do not dominate the family's pattern of interaction.

Healthy families are concerned with one another's needs, and most of the family members' emotional and physical needs are met most of the time. When members' emotional needs are met, they feel support from those around them and are free to grow and explore new roles and facets of their personalities. A family that is dominated by conflict and anger alienates its members, leaving them isolated, fearful, and impaired emotionally.

Socialization

It is within families that individuals first learn social skills, such as how to interact in nonfamily venues, how to negotiate for personal needs, and how to plan. Children learn through role modeling and through behavioral reinforcement how to function effectively within the family and, when the system is successful, how to better develop an ability to apply those skills in society as adults. Parents are socialized into family roles as adult members as they address the growth and development and specific needs of each child throughout their developmental stages. Parents' roles change when the children mature and leave home; this may necessitate partners' renegotiation of the patterning of their lives together. As time goes on, the parents may need their adult children's help if they become less able to care for their own needs.

Each developmental phase for family members and for the family as a whole brings to bear new demands and requires new approaches to deal with changes. It is not surprising that families typically have difficulty negotiating role change. Change increases stress within families, sometimes for short periods if the family has in fact incorporated functioning that works well for them and their members, and sometimes for longer periods if the family functioning is not working well for all.

In response to the demands of change, healthy families demonstrate flexibility in adapting to new roles. Through well-organized management activities, firm but flexible boundary delineation, strong and appropriate communication patterns, ongoing provision of emotional support, and adept socialization, healthy families provide tools to their members to facilitate functioning for the present and into the future.

OVERVIEW OF FAMILY THERAPY

Family systems theory posits that interventions aimed especially toward addressing family dynamics will decrease emotional reactivity, encourage differentiation among individual family members (i.e., increase each member's sense of self), and/or improve patterns of family interaction. Interventions include encouraging family members to consider emotional patterns learned in their families of origin and to make use of family resources to engage in patterns of interaction that take them beyond the emotional responses of their pasts. Family members whose actions, perceptions, or beliefs are identified as problematic receive counseling and behavioral therapy encompassed in family work. The focus of family therapy is not on the problematic individual, however. Instead, it is on the ways the dynamics of the family system may contribute to the problems of individual family members.

By the 1960s and 1970s, therapists in clinical settings were beginning to notice the effects of the social milieu on their patients. At that point, the therapeutic community became established as a treatment modality, and group therapy and psychodrama were developed. All these changes were based on observations of patients and on an expanding belief that social systems played an integral role in psychological functioning and treatment. An **interactive** (interpersonal) rather than **indwelling** (intrapsychic Freudian) model of mental illness was becoming more widely accepted as family therapy took root in psychiatric care, paving the way for an interest in the family system as it related to psychiatric disorders.

Changing dynamics in families are difficult to recognize when they occur slowly over time. Thus, it is possible for the identified patient in a family to enact behaviors that get just a little bit worse every day or every week, sometimes for years before they become problematic. At the same time, before they are aware of the growing complexity of their dynamics and of changes in their patterns of interacting, family members can find themselves embroiled in situations they find intolerable. They may not recognize that their patterns of interrelationship have changed, finding only that the family no longer offers a sense of love, safety, value, and security. Thus, family members do not always welcome family therapy, as families adjust slowly to their new, if ultimately uncomfortable, ways of being together over time. Often the early sessions in family therapy are inadvertently threatening to family members because change is always difficult. The effective family therapist will demonstrate facility in recognizing and responding to family members' anxieties and concerns and will work to modify approaches accordingly to encourage the family to remain engaged.

Although there are a number of approaches useful in conducting family therapy, generally speaking, those approaches fall into one of two broad classifications or paradigms. One paradigm—**Insight-Oriented Family Therapy**—focuses on developing increased self-awareness, other-awareness, and family awareness among family members. The other paradigm—**behavioral family therapy**—focuses on changing behaviors of family members to influence overall patterns of family interactions. Table 34-1 lists specific therapies that can be classified within each paradigm, highlighting major concepts related to each individual therapy, and identifies some of the therapists who contributed to their development and use.

Alternatively, a family therapist might highlight the importance of relationship quality for family members rather than focusing on changing a specific pattern of behavior. At the same time, that therapist would likely emphasize the importance of flexibility in the family system that would allow for the changes inherent to normal growth and development.

Multiple-family group therapy often is used with families who are facing difficulties. These groups can help family members identify and gain insight into their own problems as they are reflected in the problems of other families (Deane et al., 2012) and develop skills for addressing the family member whose problems are foremost. In the case of multiple-family therapy, several families meet in one group with one or more therapists, usually once a week. The schedule of meetings can be tailored to meet the needs of the families involved.

TABLE 34-1 INSIGHT-ORIENTED AND BEHAVIORAL THERAPY

TYPE OF THERAPY	CONCEPTS	MAJOR THEORISTS
Insight-Oriented Family Therapy		
Psychodynamic therapy	Problems arise from developmental arrest,current interactions, projections, and current stresses Goal is to gain insight into problematic relationships originating in the past	Nathan Ackerman James Framo Ivan Boszormenyi-Nagy
Family-of-origin therapy	Emphasis is on the family of origin Family viewed as an emotional relationship system Triangulation Goal is to foster differentiation and decrease emotional reactivity	Murray Bowen
Experimental-existential therapy	Symptoms express family pain Family is responsible for its own solutions Therapist uses nurturing and identifies dysfunctional communication patterns Goal is to encourage growth of the family	Carl Whitaker Virginia Satir Leslie Greenberg Susan Johnson
Behavioral Family Therapy		
Structural therapy	Focus is on organizational patterns, boundaries, systems and subsystems, and use of scapegoating Enmeshment and disengagement Boundaries clarification Restructuring of dystunctional triangles	Salvador Minuchin
Strategic therapy	Identifies inequality of power, life-cycle perspectives, and use of double-bind messages Paradox Prescribes rituals Goal is to change repetitive and maladaptive interaction patterns	Jay Haley Chloe Madanes Milan group (Mara Palazzoli, Gianfranco Cecchin, Giuliana Prata)
Cognitive-behavioral therapy	Based on learning theory Focus is on changing cognition and behavior Skills training is emphasized	Gerald Patterson Richard Stuart Robert Liberman

VIGNETTE

Eight-year-old Tommy Gomez, who has recently become disruptive at school and at home, is brought to the community mental health clinic to be evaluated for attention deficit hyperactivity disorder (ADHD). The nurse clinician performs an assessment and finds that a great deal of turmoil exists within the Gomez family and that the parents do not talk about their stress openly. The family includes Tommy's married parents, their two other children, and a grandmother. Tommy's father has just lost his job, and his grandmother was recently diagnosed with bladder cancer. Tommy's mother is planning to file for separation because of constant, unresolved arguments with her husband. The nurse clinician who views this family from a strategic model would not focus solely on Tommy but would view Tommy's symptoms as a function of many difficult losses and transitions that are stressing the entire family's coping mechanisms.

The nurse identifies the multiple stressors in this family, believing that Tommy's symptoms of hyperactivity and acting out are related to the severe stresses in the family system. Once the issues within the family are addressed and plans are made to deal with these issues, perhaps Tommy's symptoms will subside. She refers the couple to a family therapist. In the meantime, she encourages the couple to focus more on their own issues and less on Tommy's behavior. An appointment is made to go to the clinic in 1 month, when Tommy will be reevaluated.

This vignette is an example of a family in which a pattern of communication, partly related to cultural norms, probably tends to exclude discussion with the children. For this family, decisions, whether or not they involve the children, are most likely made without informing them. Consequently, the children in this family often feel powerless, and Tommy has begun to engage in destructive behavior at school, which has precipitated a visit to a family therapist. The nurse seeing Tommy made astute and appropriate observations that supported the need for referral for family therapy. The family therapist will follow up to address Tommy's problem within the context of the family's dynamics.

Depending on personal beliefs, education, and training, a family therapist might work with the family to change their rigid pattern of communication to strengthen the decision-making process for the family as a whole. Family members, including Tommy, could comment and offer suggestions about how issues could be resolved. Tommy might be less anxious and less of a behavioral problem if given a sense of control over some aspects of his life; moreover, changing communication patterns could result in a systemic change in the way the Gomez family communicates overall.

In some cases, the focus of family therapy is psychoeducation. The primary goal of **psychoeducational family therapy** is the sharing of mental health care information. Family education groups help family members better understand their member's illness, prodromal symptoms (symptoms that may appear before a full relapse), medications needed to help reduce the symptoms, and more. Psychoeducational family meetings or multiple family meetings allow feelings to be shared and strategies for dealing with these feelings to be developed. Painful issues of anger or loss, feelings of stigmatization or sadness, and feelings of helplessness can be shared and put in a perspective that the family and individual members can deal with more satisfactorily. Psychoeducational family groups are extremely useful for people with all kinds of mental, as well as medical, disorders and for their families. In the case of the Gomez family, information and education about the pathophysiology and medical treatment plan for Tommy's ADHD symptoms would supplement information about family dynamics. This information collectively could help limit Tommy's disruptive behaviors as it provided insights for family members about ways to address and deal with Tommy's symptoms. The entire family would benefit as a result.

Psychoeducational family therapy has proven immensely effective, especially as a family treatment method combined with other modalities (e.g., psychopharmacology). An area in which psychoeducational family training has been applied successfully is in treatment of the patient with schizophrenia. Families are extremely valuable and positive resources for patients, and family work promotes and supports families in coping with a family member with a severe mental illness. Psychoeducational groups also have proven helpful in parent management training, such as teaching a parent to work with a child with a conduct disorder.

In summary, there is no single, universally accepted model for treating families. Presenting viewpoints that reflect differing theories and assumptions, family theorists and therapists have made substantial contributions to the knowledge and practice in the field of family therapy. All techniques are not applicable to all problems, and the experienced clinician must be discerning, as work with families is complex and challenging (Keeney & Keeney, 2012).

Concepts Central to Family Therapy

The "Identified Patient"

When a family comes for treatment, the first task of the therapist is to address the presenting problem. That problem often is one belonging to "the identified patient" whose symptoms might span a wide range, including specific psychiatric diagnoses (Monson et al., 2012). The identified patient is an individual in the family typically regarded by family members as "the problem," the family member whose beliefs, perceptions, actions, and responses demand an immediate fix. Sometimes known as the "family symptom-bearer," this family member serves generally as the focus of most of the family system's concern. From a therapeutic point of view, the identified patient probably serves to divert attention from the quality of life for the family; as noted previously, the slow decline that typically characterizes negative changes in family function is not always immediately recognizable to family members. As a result, families often tend to focus on the identified patient, or symptom bearer, when looking for an explanation for the difficulties they are facing.

The symptoms of the identified patient may actually serve as a stabilizing mechanism to bring about relatively cohesive behavior in a distressed family (Goldenberg & Goldenberg, 2008), at least in the short term, and the identified patient may be aware at some level—possibly at a level he or she is not even conscious of—of the role he serves in stabilizing the family. For example, adult children may sacrifice their autonomy by staying in the home to hold the parents together; this behavior demonstrates a violation of role boundaries.

The family member who is the identified patient may or may not be the one who initially seeks help from inpatient or outpatient services. The family may be referred by a clinician as noted in the example of the Gomez family previously. In some cases where criminal behavior is involved, family therapy may be court mandated. A family member other than the identified patient may initiate a request for therapy as well.

Family Triangles

A concept that is found in both the insight-oriented and behavioral paradigms categorizing approaches to family therapy is "family triangles" (Bowen, 1985; Minuchin, 1974, 1996; Young, 2012). Triangling describes an important and common relationship process that involves subsets of three family members. When the tension in a dyad (two people) builds, a third person (child, friend, and parent) may be brought in by one of the members. This third person of the dyad serves to help lower the tension by solving the crisis or offering understanding (Nichols, 2009). The **family triangle** (Figure 34-3) then serves to stabilize interpersonal relationships in the short term. For example, if parents are arguing about who "wears the pants" in the family, one parent may grant special favors to a child in the family, thereby using the child to establish personal superiority. The child becomes the means by which the parents communicate with each other about issues they cannot deal with directly and openly.

The intensity of the triangling process varies among families and within the same family over time (Young, 2012). Triangles are structurally stable; in other words, as family triangles are enacted, they tend to be maintained over time. At the same time, family triangles may create emotional instability in the long run. As family members demonstrate low levels of differentiation (Schnarch & Regas, 2011), that is, as they tend to hold similar beliefs without regard for their own personal thoughts and feelings in relation to those beliefs, they also tend to demonstrate more tension.

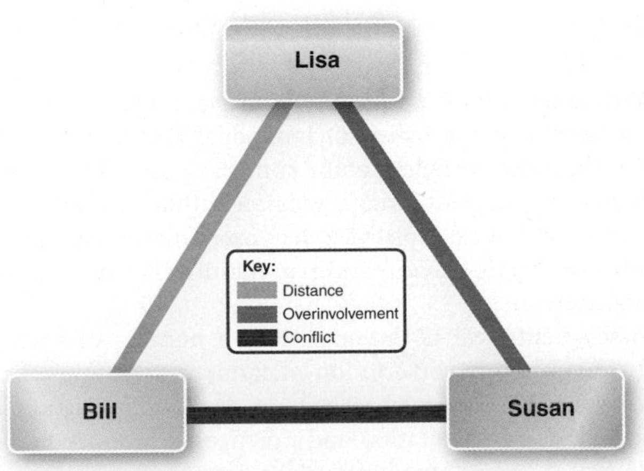

FIG 34-3 Example of a family triangle.

VIGNETTE

Six-year-old Mia is having trouble making friends. Her mother, Megan, has been feeling anxious and helpless as she tries to find ways to engage Mia with other youngsters. Megan develops an overprotectiveness that further inhibits Mia from venturing out to make friends. Megan believes that her husband, Shawn, is uncaring and disinterested because he thinks that she should be more relaxed about Mia's social life and let things develop naturally. Shawn's job requires that he travel most of the week, so he is not involved with Megan's daily experiences or in her struggles with Mia.

Megan and Shawn have been avoiding intimacy for almost a year. Megan is angry with Shawn for spending so much time with his parents, which further casts him in a peripheral role in their nuclear family. Shawn is angry with Megan, sensing her rejection of him. Both are feeling isolated and alienated and are consequently angry at each other. Neither Shawn nor Megan addresses this issue directly. Instead, they play out their anger in the parental arena as they battle over how to handle Mia's social isolation.

Triangling behavior is ubiquitous, occurring not only in families but among friends, in the workplace, and in social groups. Attention to its occurrence and efforts to ensure that it is not being used in a detrimental manner can strengthen relationships across many settings.

Box 34-2 provides an overview of terms used in regard to family therapy.

APPLICATION OF THE NURSING PROCESS

Nurses prepared at the basic level work to meet the needs of patients and families in inpatient and outpatient settings. Their work as part of the health care team can contribute significantly to the quality of intervention and patient outcomes. Advanced practice registered nurses (APRNs) who have graduate or postgraduate training in family therapy may conduct private family therapy sessions.

ASSESSMENT

Assessment typically is intermixed with treatment in family therapy, rather than constituting a distinct activity. As noted, families are inherently complex, and as a consequence, family assessment is complex as well, incorporating observations of the family both within and outside therapy sessions.

BOX 34-2 TERMS USED IN FAMILY THERAPY

Boundaries: Clear boundaries are those that maintain distinctions between individuals within the family and between the family and the outside world. Clear boundaries allow for balanced flow of energy between members. Roles of children and parent or parents are clearly defined. Diffuse or enmeshed boundaries are those in which there is a blending together of the roles, thoughts, and feelings of the individuals so that clear distinctions among family members fail to emerge. Rigid or disengaged boundaries are those in which the rules and roles are adhered to no matter what.

Differentiation: The ability to develop a strong identity and sense of self while at the same time maintaining an emotional connectedness with one's family of origin.

Double bind: A situation in which a positive command (often verbal) is followed by a negative command (often nonverbal), which leaves the recipient confused, trapped, and immobilized because there is no appropriate way to act. A double bind is a "no-win" situation in which you are "darned if you do, darned if you don't."

Family life cycle: The family's developmental process over time; refers to the family's past course, its present tasks, and its future course.

Hierarchy: The function of power and its structures in families, differentiating parental and sibling roles and generational boundaries.

Multigenerational issues: The continuation and persistence from generation to generation of certain emotional interactive family patterns (e.g., reenactment of fairly predictable and almost rituallike patterns; repetition of themes or toxic issues; and repetition of reciprocal patterns such as those of overfunctioner and underfunctioner).

Scapegoating: A form of displacement in which a family member (usually the least powerful) is blamed for another family member's distress. The purpose is to keep the focus off the painful issues and the problems of the blamers. In a family, the blamers are often the parents and the scapegoat a child.

Sociocultural context: The framework for viewing the family in terms of the influence of gender, race, ethnicity, religion, economic class, and sexual orientation.

Triangulation: The tendency, when two-person relationships are stressful and unstable, to draw in a third person to stabilize the system through formation of a coalition in which the two join the third.

VIGNETTE

The Jones family includes a single father, three adolescent children, and the paternal grandmother who is terminally ill with cancer. The eldest adolescent, Jocelyn, has just completed residential treatment for substance addiction. Her addiction brought the family to therapy initially 7 months ago.

Jocelyn is known to be close to her grandmother. She cries readily when others ask her about her grandmother's health status. She has spent increasingly less time at home and often skips meals or other situations in which she would be expected to talk with her father or siblings. Although she used to enjoy reading the evening newspaper with her grandmother, she has altogether stopped spending time with her. She has begun to refuse to attend therapy with the family although they continue to come weekly to the therapy center. Her interactions with the family have become increasingly limited. Often, she spends days away without contacting anyone at home.

During their sessions, family members demonstrate reluctance to admit that they are struggling with relationship issues. Mr. Jones has stated multiple times that life is hard. He has said, "Complaining is for whiny babies." The therapist has noted that boundaries between and among the family members appear rigid and that family members seem hard-pressed to provide evident support for one another, especially during this period of impending loss of the grandmother.

Because a pattern of addiction is already established in the family, the impending loss of an important family figure may be exacerbating Jocelyn's addiction. During therapy, the therapist may gently question family members to try to ascertain their recognition of the possibility that Jocelyn's drug use patterns will reoccur. An astute nurse will recognize that nonverbal messages often are more powerful than the spoken word in influencing behavior patterns (Patterson, 2012) and will address the ways that the family is dealing with the impending death. If the family has established a preferred pattern of dealing with grief and loss by using denial and discouraging the outward expression of painful feelings, the therapist may guide the family into learning about ways of dealing with grief that support family interactions and limit further symptomatic behaviors in other family members. Further, the nurse may help the family confront Jocelyn about her possible drug use and make referrals as appropriate.

Assessment begins with information that presents on the "face" of the family. This information includes appraisal of the family constellation and identification of individual family members as well as a description of family history. Family history would include past medical and mental illnesses experienced by family members across at least three generations—children, parent or parents, and grandparents. Through assessment of the intergenerational system, various patterns (such as a history of family members' suicides or diagnosed mental illnesses, established triangles, and family losses) become apparent. Often patterns of interaction passed down through the generations are notable among family members. In many cases, unspoken messages and legacies of the multigenerational family are observable as they influence the identified patient's presenting problem.

With a description of the family in place, the therapist can begin to address the beliefs of individual family members as well as the collective beliefs of the family as a unit. Sociocultural variables—country of origin, religious affiliation, education, and income, for example—all may exert direct influence on family members' behaviors and expectations (Priest et al., 2012; Roosa, 2009).

Assessments will be influenced by a number of variables that extend beyond description of family interactions. These variables—sociocultural background, including religious beliefs, and sexual orientation and practices— ground the constellation of family members' values, norms, traditions, roles, and acceptable rules for their day-to-day interactions

Cultural sensitivity, that is, acknowledging and nonjudgmentally addressing the sociocultural background of others, is increasingly important as our society becomes more global in nature. Cultural sensitivity involves recognition of personal history, not only of others but also of self. Personal histories are brought to bear on current interactions, influencing the expectations of all and shaping interaction. Religious beliefs, attitudes about the ways family members ought to interact, child-rearing practices, assumptions regarding appropriate jobs and how time and money should be allocated, and what constitutes beauty and art are all related to one's personal history, and all relate to the sociocultural context within which one was raised. As nurse and family work together, one was bring their own respective beliefs to the interaction. The interaction in turn will take shape within the context of those beliefs, as they are complementary or conflicting. Finding a common ground from which to address the family and provide appropriate and effective interventions requires provider openness to the expectations of the family.

For example, during Ramadan, the ninth month of the Islamic calendar, Muslims focus intently on the teachings of Islam. Ramadan is a time of spiritual reflection, personal improvement, and increased devotion and worship. It can involve periods of fasting and sexual abstinence. Understanding and valuing the context of family members' actions during Ramadan can help to strengthen the relationship between nurse and family. More broadly, recognizing the beliefs of families as they are influenced by religion will provide a strong base from which to plan interventions that are appropriate and acceptable to the family.

Because religious beliefs tend to be matters of faith rather than matters of "fact," they typically are not open to unbiased and rational discussion, nor are they readily amenable to change. The roles of nurse and therapist may be especially challenged if their religious beliefs conflict with those of the patient and family, yet it falls to them to build plans of care one that incorporate family members' beliefs and not to focus on changing them, except in instances that involve threat to family member safety.

Finally, assessment of sexual orientation and sexual history is essential to a thorough appraisal of family dynamics. This phase of assessment may prove challenging; despite training and practice in communication that is part of nursing curricula, direct questioning about the sexual practices and experiences of others approaches a level of intimacy that may be uncomfortable for the nurse or even the therapist, as well as for the patient and the family. Gentle questioning guided by an assessment template may assist the nurse to ask questions that will provide important information about the family and its members.

Assessment data collected by the nurse will help to focus more in-depth assessment of family interactions and communication styles. It is not likely that family members will be able to fully describe their patterns of interaction and communication directly, so building on assessment data, the therapist often will engage family members in conversation and brief role plays to facilitate identification and recognition of those behaviors. On the basis of these data, the therapist may begin to ascertain the developmental phase of the family and specific areas of stress as they influence family interactions.

Assessment Tools

Constructing a Genogram

Bowen (1985) provided much of the conceptual framework for the analysis of genogram patterns. He proposed that the family is organized according to generation, age, sex, roles, functions, and interests, and suggested that where each individual fits into the family structure influences the family functioning, relational patterns, and type of family formed in the next generation. He further contended that sex and birth order shape sibling relationships and characteristics, just as some patterns passed from one generation to the next result in persistent, interactive, emotional patterns and in triangling.

By creating a **genogram**, nurses and therapists are able to map the family structure and record family information that reflects both history and current functioning. The information included on a genogram should include demographic data such as geographic location of family members, their respective occupations, and educational levels. Functional information regarding medical, emotional, and behavioral status also is recorded. Finally, critical events, such as important transitions, moves, job changes, separations, illnesses, and deaths, are noted. Figure 34-4 provides an example of a genogram derived from the data from the family in the following vignette.

VIGNETTE

Hank and Catherine Schneider are both college educated, and each suffers from intermittent depression. Hank is an only child whose father died of a heart attack at age 55, Hank's present age. Hank's mother committed suicide at age 35. This is a toxic subject in Hank's family of origin. In Catherine's family of origin, she is the eldest, born after three miscarriages. Much pressure and many expectations were placed on her. Catherine's brother Mike was born 4 years after Catherine, and their mother died during Mike's birth. Mike never finished high school, has a serious alcohol addiction, and has had three marriages that ended in divorce. One can speculate about the level of guilt Mike may feel regarding the loss of his mother.

Hank and Catherine have two children, Keith and Jennifer. Keith, the identified patient, is 35 years old, has a college degree, and has not been able to hold down a job. He also has an addiction to alcohol. In 2004, Keith made a suicide attempt. In November 2006, Keith experienced a psychotic episode for which he was hospitalized, and he was diagnosed as having schizophrenia. His younger sister, Jennifer, has a college degree and works as a nurse. She married William in 2004, the year Keith attempted suicide. Jennifer and William have two young children 4 and 2 years of age.

Other Assessment Tools

A variety of assessment tools is available to help the nurse assess how the family functions as a unit and to identify individual members' perceptions of how the family communicates; how they deal with emotional issues such as anger, conflict, and

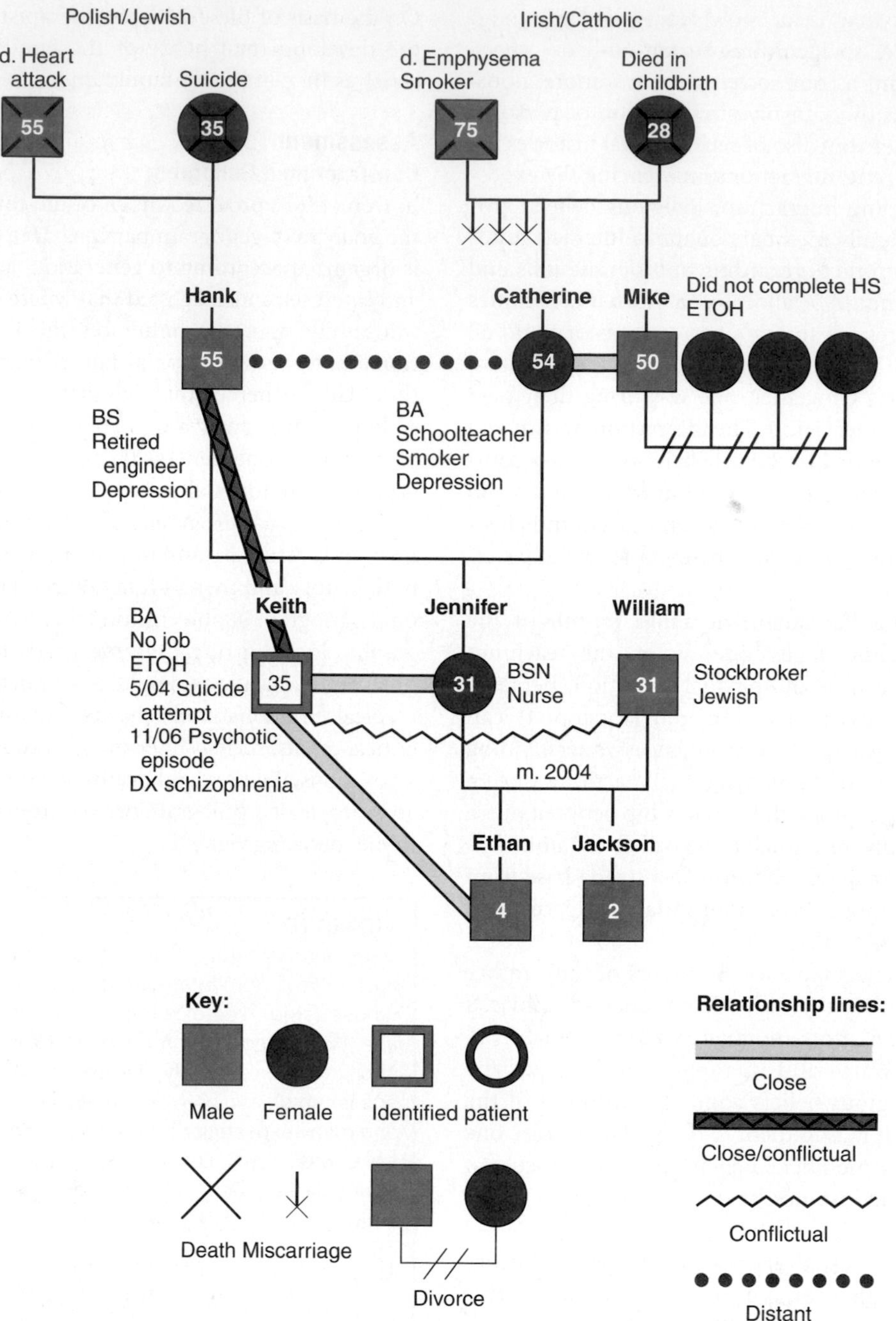

FIG 34-4 Genogram of the Schneider family. *DX,* Diagnosis; *ETOH,* alcohol; *HS,* high school; *m.,* married.

affection; how they work together as a unit to plan and solve problems; how they make the important decisions for the family; and how they function generally (Pritchett et al., 2011).

Self-Assessment

Assessment in psychiatric nursing in general and particularly in work with families begins with nurses' self-assessment. Although basic-level nurses do not provide family therapy, they do interact with patients and families, and they are not immune to the subtle messages that patients and family members convey, intentionally or unintentionally. Nurses should be aware that their personal histories and styles of interactions might affect their responses to patients and families as they express their feelings on the nursing unit. Unaware of triggers that subtly mimic and evoke past experiences, a nurse may become easily "triangled" into the family's system.

One could become triangled into a family system in any number of ways. Perhaps the nurse recently experienced the loss of a family member. The nurse may belong to an enmeshed family system in which the children are regularly drawn into spousal arguments, or perhaps stubbornness is an unresolved issue for the nurse. Any of these possibilities could allow the nurse to become triangled into a family system, which makes good therapeutic intervention difficult if not impossible. One indication that a nurse is being triangled is that his or her level of anxiety is greater than the situation warrants.

All nurses interact with families, whether in hospital acute care settings or in community-based settings. Most nurses come from a family, and because no family is perfect, all nurses are subject to becoming defensive when personal family anxieties are aroused or to experiencing role blurring or loosening of self-boundaries when sensitive personal issues and conflicts are triggered. Supervision can be conducted with peer professionals, in groups, or privately with a more experienced clinician.

DIAGNOSIS

Family needs vary over time and as a function of their situations over time. As discussed, families often find challenge in anticipated developmental change as well as in unanticipated change. Severe dysfunctional patterns such as marked relational conflict, sexual misconduct, abuse, violence, and suicide exist within many families, and these patterns can lead to physical or mental anguish among its members. As noted, nurses' understanding of family dynamics within a context of broader sociocultural and personal variables will foster appropriate planning and identification of diagnoses.

Numerous nursing diagnoses are useful in working with families. Box 34-3 identifies some of them.

OUTCOMES IDENTIFICATION

Although different therapists may adhere to different theories and use a wide variety of methods, the goals of family therapy (Nichols, 2009) are basically to:

- Reduce dysfunctional behavior of individual family members
- Resolve or reduce intrafamily relationship conflicts
- Mobilize family resources and encourage adaptive family problem-solving behaviors
- Improve family communication skills
- Heighten awareness and sensitivity to other family members' emotional needs and help family members meet their needs
- Strengthen the family's ability to cope with major life stressors and traumatic events, including chronic physical or psychiatric illness
- Improve integration of the family system into the societal system (e.g., school, medical facilities, workplace, and especially the extended family)
- Promote appropriate individual psychosocial development of each member of the family

Nurses often provide family psychoeducational treatment as part of their roles as team members to support consumers in understanding and better dealing with diagnoses. Through education, nurses reinforce patient and family strengths, help them to identify resources, and strengthen their coping skills. Family teaching may include helping them as they:

- Learn to accept the illness of a family member.
- Learn to deal effectively with an ill member's symptoms, such as hallucinations, delusions, poor hygiene, physical limitations, paranoia, and aggression.
- Develop understanding of what medications can and cannot do and when the family should seek medical advice.
- Learn what community resources are available and how to access them.
- Begin to feel less anxiety and regain or acquire a sense of control and balance in family life.

BOX 34-3 POSSIBLE NURSING DIAGNOSES FOR FAMILY PROBLEMS

- Risk for caregiver role strain
- Caregiver role strain
- Risk for impaired parenting
- Impaired parenting
- Readiness for enhanced parenting
- Risk for impaired attachment
- Dysfunctional family processes
- Interrupted family processes
- Readiness for enhanced family processes
- Parental role conflict
- Sexual dysfunction
- Risk for compromised resilience
- Ineffective denial
- Ineffective family therapeutic regimen management
- Deficient knowledge
- Defensive coping

From Herdman, T. H. (Ed.), (2012). *Nursing diagnoses—Definitions and classification 2012-2014.* Copyright © 2012, 1994-2012 by NANDA International. Used by arrangement with John Wiley & Sons Limited.

PLANNING

Planning nursing care for patients in the context of their families usually occurs within the context of individual care. You may be made aware of safety needs in the family. For example, is someone in the family at risk of a homicide or suicide? Is a member abusive or being abused? A determination of whether protective services or hospitalization is necessary to protect a suicidal or self-mutilating member must be made. A careful analysis of the data from a sound assessment helps the nurse and other members of the health care team to identify the most appropriate family interventions for troubled families.

Nurses are adept at helping family members learn about the illness of an afflicted family member (e.g., severe mental illness, dementia), understanding what medications can do (as well as side effects, etc.), and identifying support groups and community resources to help the family cope with crisis and improve the quality of life for all of its members. Identification of the extent of the family's knowledge deficit is equally important to organizing appropriate interventions.

IMPLEMENTATION

Counseling and Communication Techniques

Nurses prepared at the level of nurse generalist may provide counseling through the use of a problem-solving approach to address an immediate family difficulty related to health or well-being. Developing and practicing good listening skills and viewing family members in a positive, nonjudgmental way are critically important qualities for nurses at all levels, regardless of the practice setting.

An important function of basic-level nurses is to respond to cues from various family members that indicate the degree and amount of stress the family system is experiencing. These critical observations need to be readily reported so that appropriate interventions may be made in a timely manner. Some indicators of stress in a family system are the following:

- Inability of the family or a family member to understand and act on certain recommended treatment directives
- Various somatic complaints among family members
- High degree of anxiety
- Depression
- Problems in school
- Drug use

Promoting and monitoring a family's mental health can occur in virtually any setting and often requires making the most of an opportune moment. There does not have to be a formal meeting. Sometimes an informal conversation can have the greatest effect. Following a few general guidelines can help the nurse remain nonjudgmental in the information presented as well as in the tone of voice and questions asked. For example, the question "Don't you think you should at least try to comply with your medical regimen?" would probably cause the patient to tune the nurse out, whereas the invitation "Tell me what your medical regimen is like" could open the door to understanding and problem solving in a collaborative rather than a hierarchical way.

A nonjudgmental manner promotes open and flexible communication among all professionals and family members in the caregiving system. If other family members are involved in the conversation, whether in the hospital unit or a family therapy session, the nurse should consider each member's view, for example, by facilitating discussion about how an individual member's medical regimen affects the way the family functions and what the individual members consider a possible solution to the problem.

Information should be imparted in a clear and understandable manner to all family members so that they can decide what to do with the information. This is both a respectful and an empowering way to work with families, indicating to them that *they* are the ones who are accountable and responsible for how they choose to use the information.

The perspective of each family member must be elicited and heard. Often some family members hear another member's view for the first time in this democratic forum, and many times they are surprised ("I didn't know you felt that way"). The more family input there is, the more options usually exist for alternative ways of managing problematic situations. This approach defines the family as the central psychosocial unit of care. The following vignette provides an example of maintaining neutrality and hearing from all members.

As noted throughout this chapter, it is essential that the nurse keep track of his or her own feelings as these encounters evolve. For novice nurses especially, delving into family dynamics is challenging because it is, by nature, an intimate process. Over time, as nurses master their roles as helpers and facilitators, the process of encouraging discussion among family members becomes more natural.

VIGNETTE

Ms. Conway, the head nurse on the adolescent psychiatric unit, is concerned about all the negative comments the staff members are making regarding the fact that none of Aaron's family has been in to visit him for over a week. In fact, she is concerned that Aaron is picking up the staff's feelings as well. After many attempts, Ms. Conway finally reaches Aaron's mother by telephone and begins to assess the situation. She discovers that Aaron's mom is divorced and is working double shifts to meet the family's expenses. There is a 2-year-old at home and a set of twins in the fourth grade.

Aaron's mother had been planning to visit on the weekend, but the babysitter called to say she was sick. Once Ms. Conway is able to see the situation from another perspective, that this is a family with young children that is struggling to make ends meet, she calls a staff meeting to address the situation.

Further interventions in this situation would be to problem solve with Aaron and his mother concerning what is realistic for each of them regarding visiting. Perhaps an extended family member or a friend can visit when the mother cannot. Longer-range planning for supervision for Aaron when he is discharged should also be discussed as family supports are identified and assessed.

Unfortunately, negative comments about family members by staff occur all too often, probably as a function of nurses' own involvement in triangulation processes. This can present a difficult situation for the nursing student, who is entering the culture of the unit as an outsider and who realizes the negative effects this behavior has on family members. It is appropriate for the student to first seek supervision from the instructor so that the most effective approach can be planned out beforehand.

One useful technique for addressing a situation like this is for the student to ask questions of the supervising nurse and staff in such a manner that alternative ways of viewing the family in a broader perspective are embedded in the questions. An example of this is "Has anyone had a chance to contact Aaron's mother to see if there are any problems?" or "I wonder what it's like for Aaron's mother to have her son in a psychiatric unit." Consideration of the dynamics on the unit is as important as consideration of the dynamics of the family itself.

Pharmacological Interventions

The nurse often is the first to explain to the family the purpose of a prescribed medication, the desired effects, possible side effects, and adverse reactions. The following vignette describes a situation that occurred at the time of discharge.

VIGNETTE

David Gardiner, age 21 years, is leaving the hospital after experiencing his first psychotic episode while taking his final examinations before graduation from college. David is being discharged back to his family, which consists of his mother and father; his maternal grandfather, who has been recently bedridden; and a younger brother, Todd, who is 17 years of age. David's diagnosis is paranoid schizophrenia.

The nurse takes a psychoeducational approach with the family. The nurse addresses issues and needs during family meetings while David is still hospitalized and later in follow-up family therapy after discharge. Initial interventions involve imparting information about David's mental illness through reading materials and discussion. The nurse also gives the family information on and telephone numbers of psychosocial support groups and a local chapter of the National Alliance for the Mentally Ill (NAMI).

The nurse performs ongoing assessment of the family's strengths and weaknesses, including family supports and community support, identifying some of the areas that may need to be addressed during the next few meetings. Some of these areas include reorganizing family roles to accommodate a family member with a newly diagnosed serious mental illness; managing the bedridden grandfather; attending to Todd's probable fears that he too may have this illness; dealing with potential parental guilt feelings from a genetic point of view; planning how to mobilize should David experience another psychotic episode; managing medication and emphasizing the importance of adherence to the medication regimen; dealing with concerns about David's future and formulating realistic expectations; coping with feelings of loss for what was and what was hoped for; and finally, maintaining the integrity and functioning of the spousal subsystem.

The nurse discusses these and other issues with the family and identifies where and how these issues can best be addressed. For example, a visiting nurse is called in to evaluate the grandfather's situation and need for support in the home, and a multiple-family psychoeducation group is formed to increase the family's understanding of David's illness, help the family learn ways to cope with common problems that may arise, and provide a place for family members to share their feelings of loss and grief.

VIGNETTE

Susan Harris, a 45-year-old account executive and mother of three teenagers, has been referred by her physician to the mental health center for treatment of acute depression. The psychiatrist there has prescribed an antidepressant. Routinely, the nurse clinician reviews medications with new patients as part of the health teaching. Unfortunately, the nurse clinician is engaged with another patient in crisis at the time and misses meeting with Susan and her husband.

One week later, Susan makes an appointment with the advanced practice registered nurse (APRN), complaining of symptoms of insomnia and lack of sexual desire, which is a concern for both Susan and her husband. During the appointment, the nurse clinician reviews these side effects and adverse reactions associated with antidepressants. She informs Susan that the medication she is taking might not reach its full effects for 3 weeks or longer. She also explains that sleeplessness and lowered sexual drive are common side effects of the group of medications known as selective serotonin reuptake inhibitors (SSRIs), which includes the drug Susan is taking. They discuss ways to combat these side effects (refer to Chapter 14). The nurse urges Susan to continue taking the medication; however, if the side effects continue, the medication can be changed. Susan is due to visit the clinic 2 weeks later for follow-up. The nurse urges Susan to discuss the side effects of the medication with her husband and to encourage him to come with her to the clinic at her next appointment so that they can discuss Susan's response to the medication together.

In general, the more information family members have at their disposal, the less anxiety they will experience. Through follow-up visits, the APRN will closely monitor Susan to determine whether her symptoms represent an exacerbation of her depression or a reaction to the antidepressant medication.

Advanced Practice Interventions

Advanced practice registered nurses may be qualified to conduct family therapy. Family therapy has been applied to virtually every type of disorder among children, adolescents, and adults (Abbott, 2012), and its utility is not tied to any particular theoretical approach (Keeney & Keeney, 2012). Treating the whole family appears to be particularly effective in the treatment of substance abuse disorders, child behavioral problems, marital relationship distress, and as an element of the treatment plan for schizophrenia (Deane et al., 2012).

Family therapy may be not be helpful in some circumstances (Nichols, 2009):

- When the therapeutic environment is not safe and when someone will be harmed by information, uncontrolled anxiety, or hostility.
- When there is a lack of willingness to be honest.
- When there is an unwillingness to maintain confidentiality.
- When a parental conflict involves issues of sexuality that are not appropriate for the children.

In most other situations, however, family therapy is useful, especially when it is combined with psychopharmacology in the treatment of families who have a member with a mental illness such as bipolar disorder, depression, or schizophrenia. Other families may choose psychoeducational family therapy and/or self-help groups, which are good options that may be less costly and time consuming.

EVALUATION

In the treatment of families, evaluation focuses on the level of family members' individual and group functioning, whether conflicts reduced or resolved, communication skills improved, and coping strengthened, and whether family members have been better integrated into the broader societal system.

CASE MANAGEMENT

Employed commonly in psychiatric nursing, case management helps to assure successful outcomes for families once they are discharged from therapy. Case management focuses on client and family advocacy, identification of service resources, and service facilitation. As part of the therapeutic team, the case manager helps the family access a continuum of services that are both cost-effective and appropriate to the treatment needs of the family and its individual members. The goal of case management is to balance service quality and affordability, serving the objectives of providers, clients served, and the reimbursement source, typically an insurer. Case management is most successful when communication among the case manager, the family, and the treatment team is facilitated.

KEY POINTS TO REMEMBER

- Family therapy is based on a variety of theoretical concepts.
- The aim of family therapy is to decrease emotional reactivity, enhance awareness, strengthen communication among family members, and encourage personal differentiation.
- The primary characteristics essential to healthy family functioning are flexibility and clear boundaries.
- It is important to be aware of the phases in the changing family life cycle of a traditional family, a divorced family, and a remarried family.
- Family-oriented approaches that include helping a family gain insight and make behavioral changes are most successful.
- The genogram is an efficient clinical summary and format for providing information and defining relationships across at least three generations.
- The family's culture, ethnicity, socioeconomic status, and life-cycle phase, as well as its unique patterns and beliefs about illness, all affect the individual patient's progress and response to case management.
- Assessment of the family includes a focus on the phase of the family life cycle, multigenerational issues, the individual developmental stage of each member, and the family's sociocultural status.
- Nurses with basic training are frequently called upon to conduct psychoeducation with families.
- Advanced practice registered nurses who have specialized training may provide family therapy using a variety of theoretical approaches.

CRITICAL THINKING

1. Select a family with whom you've gotten to work during your clinical experience. Evaluate this family's status in terms of functionality/dysfunctionality with reference to the five family functions described in the text (i.e., management function, boundary function, communication function, emotional-supportive function, and socialization function).
2. Create your own personal genogram, including at least three generations. Be sure to include the following:
   a. Location, occupation, and educational level
   b. Critical events such as births, marriages, moves, job changes, separations, divorces, illnesses, and deaths
   c. Relationship patterns, if possible, such as cutoffs, distancing, overinvolvement, and conflict
3. A family has just found out that their young son is going to die. The parents have been fighting and blaming each other for ignoring the child's ongoing symptom of leg pain, which was eventually diagnosed as advanced cancer. There are two other siblings in the family.
   a. How would you apply family concepts to help this family?
   b. What would be your outcome criterion?

CHAPTER REVIEW

1. Just before you escort the Juarez family in for a meeting, their 17-year-old son confides to you that he is gay. He says he has not told any other adult, including his parents. What is your best response to him?
   a. "Your parents have a right to know about this."
   b. "How do you think your parents would react if you told them?"
   c. "That's your decision, but you need to be careful about risky sexual behavior."
   d. "Lots of famous people are gay. You don't need to worry."
2. When performing an intake assessment on a family who was referred for family counseling, you wish to map the family's structure and information that reflect both the family's history and current functioning. This assessment tool is called a __________.
3. While you are working with a family whose son was admitted due to a psychotic break, you observe the mother say to her son, "What, no hug for your mom?" As the son embraces his mother, she stiffens, which results in the young man backing away. She responds, "You only care about yourself." What behavior is this mother engaging in?
   a. Triangulation
   b. Scapegoating
   c. Double binding
   d. Differentiation
4. Which of the following family members should you refer to individual therapy rather than family therapy?
   a. A mother who has anxiety controlled by medication.
   b. A father who is questioning his sexuality.
   c. A son who is verbally abusive toward his parents.
   d. A daughter who has been treated for alcohol abuse.
5. You are evaluating the family therapy experience. Which behavior would indicate that further family therapy is needed?
   a. Wife talks to husband through the children.
   b. Son's grades have risen from a "D" average to a "C" average.
   c. Daughter's headaches have subsided.
   d. Mother has stopped using illicit substances.

Answers to Chapter Review

1. b; 2. genogram; 3. c; 4. b; 5. a.

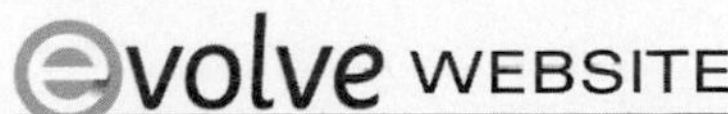

Visit the Evolve website for a posttest on the content in this chapter: http://evolve.elsevier.com/Varcarolis

Post-Test interactive review

REFERENCES

Abbott, D. A., Springer, P. R., & Hollist, C. S. (2012). Therapy with immigrant Muslim couples: Applying culturally appropriate interventions and strategies. *Journal of Couple and Relationship Therapy, 11*(3), 254–266.

Baldwin, S.A., Christian, S., Berkeljon, A., Shadish, W.R. (2012). The effects of family therapies for adolescent delinquency and substance abuse: A meta-analysis. *Journal of Marital & Family Therapy, 38*(1), 281–304.

Blackwell, D. L. (2010). Family structure and children's health in the United States: Findings from the national health interview survey, 2001–2007. *National Center for Health Statistics. Vital Health Statistics, 10*(246). Retrieved from http://www.cdc.gov/nchs/data/series/sr_10/sr10_246.pdf.

Bowen, M. (1985). *Family therapy in clinical practice*. New York, NY: Jason Aronson.

Bulechek, G. M., Butcher, H. K., Dochterman, J. M., & Wagner, C. (2012). *Nursing interventions classification (NIC)* (6th ed.). St. Louis, MO: Mosby.

Caporino, N. E., Morgan, J., Beckstead, J., Phares, V., Murphy, T. K., & Storch, E. A. (2012). A structural equation analysis of family accommodation in pediatric obsessive-compulsive disorder. *Journal of Abnormal Child Psychology, 40*(1), 133–143.

Coulter, S., & Mullin, A. (2012). Resilience and vulnerability in the midst of sociopolitical violence in Northern Ireland: One family's experience of a paramilitary style assault. *Journal of Family Issues, 33*(1), 99–111.

Deane, F. R., Mercer, J., Talyarkhan, A., Lambert, G., & Pickard, J. (2012). Group cohesion and homework adherence in multi-family group therapy for schizophrenia. *Australian & New Zealand Journal of Family Therapy, 33*(2), 128–141.

Duvall, E. M. (1957). *Family development*. Oxford, UK: J P Lippincott.

Garmezy, N., & Masten, A. S. (1994). Chronic adversities. In M. Rutter, E. Taylor, & L. Hersov (Eds.), *Child and adolescent psychiatry* (pp. 191–208). Cambridge, UK: Blackwell.

Gilgulin, A. S. (2008). *The history of family therapy*. Retrieved from http://socyberty.com/psychology/the-history-of-family-therapy/.

Goldenberg, H., & Goldenberg, I. (2008). *Family therapy: An overview* (7th ed.). Belmont, CA: Thomson.

Harris, T. (1967). *I'm OK, you're OK*. New York, NY: Avon.

Herdman, T. H. (Ed.), (2012). *NANDA international nursing diagnoses: Definitions and classification, 2012–2014*. Oxford, UK: Wiley-Blackwell.

Keeney, H., & Keeney, B. (2012). What is systemic about systemic therapy? Therapy models muddle embodied systemic practice. *Journal of Systemic Therapies, 31*(1), 22–37.

Minuchin, S. (1996). *Mastering family therapy*. New York, NY: John Wiley & Sons.

Minuchin, S. (1974). *Families and family therapy*. Cambridge, MA: Harvard University Press.

Monson, C. M., Macdonald, A., & Brown-Bowers, A. (2012). Couple/family therapy for posttraumatic stress disorder: Review to facilitate interpretation of VA/DOD Clinical Practice Guideline. *Journal of the Rehabilitation Research and Development Service, 49*(5), 717–728.

Moorhead, S., Johnson, M., Maas, M. L., & Swanson, E. (2013). *Nursing outcome classification (NOC)* (5th ed.) St. Louis, MO: Mosby.

Nichols, M. P. (2009). *Family therapy: Concepts and methods* (9th ed.). Upper Saddle River, NJ: Prentice Hall.

Patterson, J., Brandt, G., Burr, B., Hubler, D., & Roberts, K. (2012). Nonverbal behavioral indicators of negative affect in couple interaction. *Contemporary Family Therapy: An International Journal, 34*(1), 11–28. doi:10.1007/s10591-011-9170-6.

Priest, J. B., Edwards, A. B., Wetchler, J. J., Gillotti, C. M., Cobb, R. A., & Borst, C. W. (2012). An exploratory evaluation of the cognitive-active gener role identification continuum. *American Journal of Family Therapy, 40*(2), 152–168. doi:10.1080/01926187.2011.601196.

Pritchett, R., Kemp, J., Wilson, P., Minnis, H., Bryce, G., & Gillberg. C. (2011). Quick, simple measure of family relationships for use in clinical practice and research: A systematic review. *Family Practice, 28*(2), 172–187.

Reeve, J. T. (2010). Successfully living with the effects of posttraumatic stress disorder over the lifespan: Perceptions of combat veterans and their families, Ph.D. Dissertation, Texas A&M University. Corpus Christi, TX: ProQuest LLC.

Roberts, F. B. (1983). An interaction model for family assessment. In I. W. Clements, & F. B. Roberts (Ed.), *Family health: A theoretical approach to nursing care* (pp. 189–204). New York, NY: Wiley.

Roosa, M. W., Weaver, S. R., White, M. B. R., Tein, J-Y, Knight, G. P., Gonzales, N., et al. (2009). Family and neighborhood fit or misfit and the adaptation of Mexican Americans. *American Journal of Community Psychology, 44*(1–2), 15–27.

Schnarch, D., & Regas, S. (2011). The crucible differentiation scale: Assessing differentiation in human relationships. *Journal of Marital and Family Therapy, 38*(4), 639–652. doi:10.1111/j.1752–0606.2011.00259.x.

U. S. Department of Health and Human Services. *Administration for children and families: Child welfare information gateway*. Retrieved from http://www.childwelfare.gov/systemwide/assessment/family_assess/parental-needs/function.cfm.

Young, S. (2010). Two's company, three's a crowd: Revisiting triangles in family therapy. *Australian and New Zealand Journal of Family Therapy, 31*, 92–99.

CHAPTER

35

Integrative Care

Laura Cox Dzurec and Rothlyn P. Zahourek

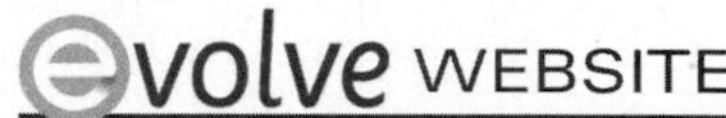

Visit the Evolve website for a pretest on the content in this chapter: http://evolve.elsevier.com/Varcarolis

Pre-Test interactive review

OBJECTIVES

1. Define the terms integrative care and complementary and alternative medicine.
2. Identify trends in the use of nonconventional health treatments and practices.
3. Explore the category of alternative medical systems along the domains of integrative care: natural products, mind and body approaches, manipulative and body-based practices, and other therapies.
4. Discuss the techniques used in major complementary therapies and potential applications to psychiatric mental health nursing practice.
5. Discuss how to educate the public in the safe use of integrative modalities and in the avoidance of false claims and fraud related to the use of alternative and complementary therapies.
6. Explore informational resources available through literature and online sources.

KEY TERMS AND CONCEPTS

acupuncture
aromatherapy
chiropractic medicine
complementary and alternative medicine (CAM)
conventional health care system
healing touch
herbal therapy
holism
homeopathy
integrative care
naturopathy
Reiki
therapeutic touch

This chapter considers *integrative care* as part of a holistic nursing philosophy. Integrative care is often referred to as *integrative medicine* or as **complementary and alternative medicine** (CAM). Since these terms are widely accepted, they are used interchangeably throughout this chapter.

Integrative care places the patient at the center of care, focuses on prevention and wellness, and attends to the patient's physical, mental, and spiritual needs (Institute of Medicine, 2009). Many of the philosophical underpinnings for the approaches presented in this chapter are derived from non-Western cultural traditions or from quantum physics and studies in the nature of energy and reality.

The trend toward adoption and use of integrative care modalities in Western health care is fairly recent and, over time, has been influenced by changes in dominant scientific theory and belief (Weldon, 2011). Across its individual therapies, integrative care is directed at healing, and its practitioners consider the whole person (mind, body, and spirit), along with the lifestyle of the person in their choice of treatment options. Establishing a therapeutic nurse/patient relationship is integral to integrative care, which includes both conventional and alternative therapies as required by the individual patient or client. Clinicians may choose to use integrative care as a substitute for, or combined with, conventional therapies or treatments.

INTEGRATIVE CARE IN THE UNITED STATES

The conventional health care system (also referred to as *allopathic, mainstream,* or *orthodox medicine; regular medicine;* and *biomedicine*) in the United States is based largely on highly controlled and federally regulated scientific research. One of the essential differences between conventional and integrative health care is that conventional medicine focuses on what is done to the patient whereas integrative practices are patient centered, meaning that the patient participates with the provider to heal the body and mind.

Due to the growing interest in and use of CAM in the United States, the National Institutes of Health (NIH) established the National Center for Complementary and Alternative Medicine (NCCAM) in 1998, making it one of 27 institutes and centers of the NIH. The NCCAM supports fair, evidence-based, scientific evaluation of integrative therapies and the dissemination of information to assist health care providers in making relatively informed choices regarding the safety and appropriateness of CAM. Since 2000, NCCAM has been awarded $2 billion for research, and as of 2011, NCCAM's annual budget was $134 million.

In 2011, NCCAM released a set of goals and objectives intended to benchmark its research priorities through 2015 in a document called Exploring the Science of Complementary and Alternative Medicine: Third Strategic Plan 2011–2015. Through this plan, NCCAM describes how it proposes to direct funding for research in complementary and alternative medicine for the next 5 years. The document addresses the conduct of research and the strengths and limitations of the scientific method for determining how CAM is used.

Study at this level—that is, study that questions research practices as well as the findings that those practices generate—is essential to optimal understanding of CAM modalities. Over the years since its establishment, NCCAM has been the subject of debate as questions of the efficacy of alternative therapies, and the appropriateness of allocating public funds for their study, continue to surface. The results of empirical studies have not convincingly established the efficacy of CAM modalities for improving the health of patients, nor have they ruled out the possibility of their worth.

What is clear in regard to CAM is that it is being used. The National Center for Health Statistics (NCHS) *National Health Interview Survey* included 31,000 people. They were surveyed regarding their use of 26 complementary and alternative treatments (Barnes et al., 2008). Below is a summary of the survey's findings:

- About 38% of adults (up from 36% in 2002) and almost 12% of children in the United States use some type of CAM.
- Use of CAM by adults is greater among women and those with higher levels of education and higher incomes.
- The most commonly used therapies are nonvitamin, nonmineral products such as fish oil/omega 3, glucosamine, echinacea, and flaxseed.
- Adults are most likely to use CAM for musculoskeletal problems such as back, neck, or joint pain.
- The use of CAM therapies for head or chest colds showed a substantial decrease from 2002 to 2007.

Despite debates surrounding its efficacy, CAM has been steadily integrated into Western health care practice since 2002. This increased use may be due to a greater availability of CAM-prepared practitioners and practice facilities, along with more public exposure to CAM through the media. Box 35-1 lists the

BOX 35-1 CAM THERAPIES INCLUDED IN THE 2007 NATIONAL HEALTH INTERVIEW SURVEY

- Acupuncture*
- Ayurveda*
- Biofeedback*
- Chelation therapy*
- Chiropractic or osteopathic manipulation*
- Deep breathing exercises
- Diet-based therapies
  - Atkins diet
  - Macrobiotic diet
  - Ornish diet
  - Pritikin diet
  - South Beach diet
  - Vegetarian diet
  - Zone diet
- Energy healing therapy/Reiki*
- Guided imagery
- Homeopathic treatment
- Hypnosis*
- Massage*
- Meditation
- Movement therapies
  - Alexander technique
  - Feldenkreis
  - Pilates
  - Trager psychophysical integration
- Natural products (nonvitamin and nonmineral)
- Naturopathy*
- Progressive relaxation
- Qigong
- Tai chi
- Traditional healers*
  - Botanica
  - Curandero
  - Espiritista
  - Hierbero or Yerbera
  - Native American healer/Medicine man
  - Shaman
  - Sobador
- Yoga

*Practitioner-based therapy.

From Barnes, P. M., Bloom, B., & Nahin, R. (2008). Complementary and alternative medicine use among adults and children: United States, 2007. *Centers for Disease Control and Prevention National Health Statistics Report #12.* Hyattsville, MD: National Center for Health Statistics. Retrieved from http://nccam.nih.gov/news/2008/nhsr12.pdf.

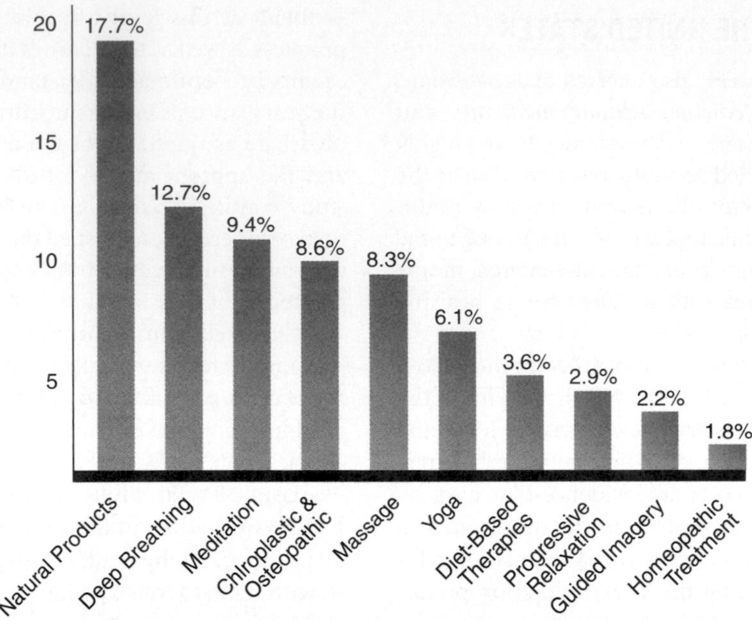

FIG 35-1 Ten most common CAM therapies used by adults in the United States. (The American Nurses Association and the American Holistic Nurses Association recognize holistic nursing as a specialty, which they describe in *Holistic Nursing: Scope and Standards of Practice* [2007].)

types of CAM included in the 2007 *National Health Interview Survey*, and Figure 35-1 is a graph comparing the 10 most commonly used therapies among adults surveyed.

The children of parents who use natural supplements, not surprisingly, were more likely to use them as well. The profile for a child who uses supplements is one who is white, non-Hispanic, adolescent, insured, lives in the western portion of the country, and has educated parents. Another factor that related to use of supplements was the presence of health conditions and frequent visits to the primary care provider.

In 2011, the AARP (formerly the American Association of Retired Persons) and the National Institutes of Public Health worked together to study conversations between people 50 and older and their health care providers regarding their use of CAM. They found that half of the people they surveyed used dietary supplements or herbal products and over 75% took one or more prescription medications. Study authors expressed concern that a significant number of respondents did not discuss their use of supplements and herbal products with their health care providers. Providers may not have a full picture of the ways people ages 50 and over seek to improve their health or of the implications of integration of CAM into traditional health care practices (AARP/NIH, 2011).

Research

As noted, although research on the efficacy of CAM is increasing, studies in the field are minimal and often controversial when compared to those of conventional medicine. At issue is not only the comparison of traditional and alternative therapies but also the question of what actually counts as evidence to support their use (Walach, 2009). Numerous explanations contribute to the current complexity of CAM research and knowledge, including (1) the relatively recent use of some of these therapies in the United States, (2) lack of financial incentive to support the research, (3) difficulties encountered by researchers when studying these modalities (Box 35-2), (4) the evolution of complementary science in the Western world (Weldon, 2011), and (5) the eagerness with which the public has begun to embrace these modalities.

Incorporation of CAM into Western health care practice has required a significant change in the way providers and researchers think about CAM. There has been a *paradigm shift*, or a major change, in the way that people think about things.

BOX 35-2 CAM RESEARCH CHALLENGES

- Individual, cultural, and environmental variables
- Lack of or limited funding sources
- Time as a variable to measure change
- Interpretation and meaning of an experience
- Impact of other intervening life experiences
- Effect and timing of a specific intervention or approach on a particular problem, specifically placebo and experimental effects
- Personality, belief systems, spiritual practices, and temperament of both the researcher and participants
- Difficulty in trying to standardize modalities; variations in methods, approach, and skill of the researcher
- Influence of studying a phenomenon or person within a naturalistic setting
- Interpretation of results
- The recognized value of both qualitative and quantitative results
- Acknowledging the importance of the relationship between the healer and the one being healed

This paradigm shift has instigated dramatic change in regard to perceptions of the legitimacy of nontraditional approaches to health care (van der Riet, 2011). CAM is being explored for such diverse and serious problems as neurocognitive disorders, substance abuse treatment, depression, traumatic life events, negative affect, trauma, pain, cancer, and diabetes (Edwards, 2012; Denneson, 2011). Reflexology, body work, prayer, visualization, breathing meditation, chiropractic, diet and/or megavitamin therapy, relaxation, massage, and poetry are among the CAM methods that are widely used.

Issues of finance also influence the use of integrative therapies. If a pharmaceutical company studies and patents a drug, it can reap considerable financial return; however, an herb cannot be patented and exclusively marketed, so there is little incentive to invest in researching its uses and effects. Governmental sources of funding such as the NCCAM and NIH, as well as nonprofit groups, are continuing to sponsor research that should contribute to further understanding of CAM. Nursing groups such as Healing Touch International and the American Holistic Nurses Association (AHNA) are emphasizing research and are beginning to catalogue findings and new interventions on their websites.

CAM is controversial, complex, and challenging. Full knowledge of integrative therapies of their effects, side effects, and interactions with dominant treatment modalities have yet to be determined. Both provider and consumer response to them continues to shift in response to available knowledge and understanding.

CONSUMERS AND INTEGRATIVE CARE

Consumers are attracted to integrative care for a variety of reasons, including the following:

- A desire to actively participate in their health care and engage in holistic practices that can promote health and healing
- A desire to find therapeutic approaches that seem to carry lower risks than traditionally used medications
- A desire to find less expensive alternatives to high-cost conventional care
- Positive experiences with holistic, integrative CAM practitioners, whose approach to patients is supportive and inclusive
- Dissatisfaction with the practice style of conventional medicine (e.g., rushed office visits, short hospital stays)
- A need to find modalities and remedies that provide comfort for chronic conditions for which no conventional medical cure exists, such as anxiety, chronic pain, and depression.

Because the demand for alternative medications is growing, the promise of financial gain is growing as well, and product marketing has become an industry. One marketer opens his website with the following comment: "FDA guidelines on supplement marketing have tightened in recent years. Supplement marketers now need more substantiation than ever" (Dougherty, 2011). Those companies selling supplements need to appeal to an increasingly well-informed audience. As a consequence, their marketing efforts need to reflect not only efforts to meet a growing public demand for CAM therapies and modalities, but also efforts to convince people of the legitimacy of the science surrounding their use and perceived efficacy.

Strong claims often are made on behalf of CAM therapies and modalities. One of the most common marketing angles is to use the term "natural" (Chiappedi, 2010). "Natural" emphasizes the notion that the chemicals in these medications are present in nature. Through its simplicity, the notion of "naturalness" suggests that alternative medications are harmless. However, even if they are naturally occurring, the chemicals contained in alternative medicines remain chemicals. The body does not distinguish between naturally occurring chemicals and those synthesized in a laboratory. Some natural substances are just not safe. Consider arsenic, for example, which is abundant in nature.

Knowledgeable consumers, relying on health information available through public libraries, popular bookstores, and the Internet, may question providers about aspects of conventional health care. Nurses' knowledge about CAM modalities and their commitment to ongoing evaluation of related evidence regarding the effectiveness of these modalities will provide information to patients and support general awareness of the efficacy of CAM in health care practice. For example, consumers are using herbal remedies to treat a variety of psychiatric conditions, including depression, which is among the most common complaints of all patients seeking medical treatment (Blues Busters, 2011). The wide range of herbs used without the guidance of a knowledgeable practitioner can result in serious side effects through their direct influence on the body and through interactions with other herbs and drugs.

Nurses' roles in collecting good assessment data about the integrative therapies their patients are using cannot be overemphasized; further, helping consumers actively evaluate the quality of information available to them is important. Information broadly available to consumers through sources such as the Internet and other readily accessible sources may not be especially useful or accurate (Evans et al., 2011).

Safety and Efficacy

As noted, people who use CAM therapies often do so without informing their conventional health care providers, which poses some risk. In the United States, there are no standards or regulations that guarantee the safety or efficacy of herbal products. Herbs and other food supplements do not have to undergo the same safety review as over-the-counter and prescription medications. Some consumers may believe that if they purchase a natural substance at a health food store, it must be safe and effective; however, as noted, "natural" does not mean "harmless." Herbal products and supplements may contain powerful active ingredients that can cause damage if taken inappropriately; furthermore, a consumer cannot be sure that the amount of the herb or other active ingredient listed on the label is actually the amount in the product. Consumers may waste a great deal of money and risk their health on unproven, fraudulently marketed, useless, or harmful products and treatments.

Another concern regarding CAM therapies is that diagnosis and treatment may be delayed while patients try alternative interventions, which is common with mental health symptoms such as major depression and anxiety. On the other hand, many CAM practitioners can recount stories of patients who have been injured by a noncaring conventional medical system or who have suffered terrible consequences from the use of conventional pharmaceuticals.

Cost

The growth in the use of CAM therapies is also linked to the rising cost of conventional medical care. There is mounting pressure to control health care spending in the United States and many other countries, and efforts are focused on the development of less expensive treatments. Before we can adopt alternative methods of treatment, however—even those that are relatively less expensive than traditional modalities—reliable information about the clinical effectiveness of these treatment methods is essential. Research on herbs such as St. John's wort, valerian, and ginkgo biloba and on mind-body interventions such as yoga and meditation is extensive, and results are available on the NCCAM website.

Reimbursement

Payment for CAM services comes from a wide array of sources, although third-party coverage is still the exception rather than the rule. Some health insurance companies include coverage for certain modalities, particularly chiropractic medicine, nutritional care, massage, mind-body approaches, and acupuncture. The covered benefits are quite narrowly defined, however. For instance, acupuncture can be used in some plans only as an alternative to anesthesia.

Placebo Effect

Some people make the claim that integrative therapies work through a mechanism known as the *placebo effect*. In fact, research indicates little difference between CAM to placebos. This lack of difference has fueled the debate about the efficacy of CAM modalities and spurred questions regarding the continuation of NCCAM funding. The placebo effect refers to a treatment that actually does nothing, even though the condition for which it is used improves in response to its use. Researchers and practitioners argue that improvements noted in response to placebo come about based on the power of suggestion and a belief that the treatment works. Research continues and is necessary to refute or support this claim; however, structuring research so that its outcomes accurately describe or predict reality is challenging.

The successes of integrative care may rely to a great degree on optimism. A positive approach and the use of positive suggestions, no matter what treatment modality is being implemented, typically yield a greater chance of success than do negative approaches and suggestions. The placebo effect can be most powerful when the need is greatest and a trusting relationship has been established between patient and caregiver. Saying "This will hurt" (more negative) may result in a *negative* placebo effect whereas saying "This may cause some brief discomfort, but I know it can make you better" (more positive) may result in a *positive* placebo effect. As a consequence of the complexities of the patient/caregiver relationship, the readiness of the patient to experience a positive result from CAM, and the actual efficacy of a given CAM intervention in itself, study of the effects of those modalities is challenged. The interrelationships of these factors make teasing out actual cause and effect difficult. A major report on the mechanism and value of the placebo as a mind-body response can be found in the *CAM at the NIH* newsletter (NCCAM, 2007b). It falls to the practitioner, and to the student learning about CAM, to determine whether or not use of CAM is optimal for a given patient.

INTEGRATIVE NURSING CARE

The American Nurses Association (ANA) recognizes holistic nursing as a specialty, publishing *Holistic Nursing: Scope and Standards of Practice* in 2007. Holistic nursing is defined as "all nursing that has healing the whole person as its goal" (AHNA, 1998). **Holism** is described as involving (1) the identification of the interrelationships of the bio-psycho-social-spiritual dimensions of the person, recognizing that the whole is greater than the sum of its parts, and (2) understanding of the individual as a unitary whole in mutual process with the environment (AHNA, 2004). Holistic nursing accepts both views and believes that the goals of nursing can be achieved within either framework.

Nurses in any setting should have a basic knowledge of treatments used in integrative care for several reasons. One is that they care for patients who increasingly are using a variety of unconventional modalities to meet their health needs. To fully understand the needs of patients, it is essential that nurses ask questions about the use of CAM as part of a holistic assessment. This practice is encouraged by NCCAM (2008f) and is emphasized in newer, published standards of nursing practice. Nursing education programs are including basic integrative modalities such as relaxation and imagery in nursing curricula, and some may include energy-based approaches such as therapeutic touch.

Holistic assessments include the traditional areas of inquiry such as history, present illness, family medical history, and history of surgeries as well as medications taken and response to these medications; however, the holistic-integrative assessment also includes areas such as the quality of social relationships, the meaning of work, the impact of major stressors in the person's life, strategies used to cope with stress (including relaxation, meditation, deep breathing, etc.), and the importance of spirituality and religion and cultural values in the person's life. Patients also are asked what they really love, how this is manifested in their lives, what their strengths are, and to identify the personal gifts they bring to the world (Maizes et al., 2003).

Credentials in Integrative Care

Graduate programs in the United States that prepare nurses with a specialty in holistic nursing are increasing in number. Doctor of nursing practice (DNP) programs with an emphasis in integrative health have been developed. Numerous post-master's certificate programs exist for advanced practice registered nurses.

The American Holistic Nurses' Credentialing Corporation (AHNCC) offers two levels of certification for registered nurses: the holistic nurse, board certified (HN-BC) for diploma or associate degree-prepared nurses, and the holistic baccalaureate nurse, board certified (HNB-BC) for baccalaureate-prepared nurses. AHNCC also offers two certificates for advanced practice nurses. Credentialing procedures are in place for many of the non-nursing modalities, such as acupuncture, chiropractic medicine, naturopathy, and massage therapy. Efforts are under way to regulate integrative care through credentialing of integrative physicians and non-physician practitioners, including nurses.

Integrative care is classified according to a general approach to care and is separated into these domains: (1) natural products, (2) mind and body approaches, (3) manipulative practices, (4) body-based practices, and (5) other CAM therapies (NCCAM, 2011). Some CAM therapies may fit into more than one domain.

Natural Products

Natural products include herbal medicine (botanicals) and also vitamins, minerals, and other "natural" products. With the proliferation of literature on herbal remedies and the accessibility of the products, increasing numbers of consumers are using these products to manage symptoms. Purchasing over-the-counter medications allows people to bypass a visit to a health care provider, thereby eliminating the cost and inconvenience of a visit as well as the real or perceived stigma on the part of the health care provider and others of a psychiatric label. As noted previously, however, use of these therapies may compromise treatment and/or health if they interact inappropriately or interfere with patient use of mainstream treatment approaches.

Diet and Nutrition

Because psychiatric illness affects the whole person, it is not surprising that patients with mental illnesses frequently have nutritional disturbances. Often their diets are deficient in the proper nutrients, or they may eat too much or too little. Obesity and diabetes coexist at a greater than average rate in persons with psychiatric disorders. Nutritional states may also cause psychiatric disturbances. Anemia, a common deficiency disease, is often accompanied by depression.

There is a good deal of study of the influence of diet and nutrition on health (Simpson et al., 2011). It is important that clinicians assess for patients' use of nutrients such as vitamins, protein supplements, herbal preparations, enzymes, and hormones that are considered dietary supplements. These dietary supplements are sold without the premarketing safety evaluations required of new food ingredients. Dietary supplements can be labeled with certain health claims if they meet published requirements of the U.S. Food and Drug Administration (FDA). They also may be labeled with a disclaimer saying that the supplement has not been evaluated by the FDA and is not intended to diagnose, treat, cure, or prevent any disease. Clinicians and consumers both should know, however, that the FDA does not regulate supplements and that claims offered on supplement labels may or may not be accurate.

Some nutritional supplements interact with medications. There are well-known interactions between prescription drugs and vitamins (e.g., vitamin E and anticoagulants), but drug interactions with other supplements are not so easily recognized or well understood. Nurses should specifically ask about patients' use of supplements during the assessment and should not expect patients to share this information without being asked. Nurses can review the use of the supplements and the potential interactions with foods, drugs, and other supplements to reduce risks. As an example, a serious hypertensive reaction can occur when a patient who is taking a monoamine oxidase inhibitor (MAOI) for depression ingests a food that contains tyramine, such as aged cheese, pickled or smoked fish, or red wine.

Megavitamin therapy, also called *orthomolecular therapy*, is a nutritional therapy that involves taking large amounts of vitamins, minerals, and amino acids. The theory is that the inability to absorb nutrients from a proper diet alone may lead to the development of illnesses. The earliest use of megavitamin therapy was for the treatment of schizophrenia, for which niacin was recommended.

Avoiding artificial food coloring became popular in the 1970s for treating children with attention deficit hyperactivity disorder (ADHD) and other developmental disorders. The Food and Drug Administration long ago determined that there is no definitive link between these disorders and food dyes; however, some clinicians and parents believe that children with attention deficit hyperactivity disorder are vulnerable to synthetic color additives (Food and Drug Administration, 2011).

Nutritional therapies are used to treat a variety of disorders, including depression, anxiety, ADHD, menopausal symptoms, dementia, and addictions. For instance, lower rates of anxiety and depression are reported among vegetarians than among non vegetarians. An analysis of the vegetarian diet found a higher antioxidant level compared with the non vegetarian diet, which suggests that antioxidants may play a role in the prevention of depression.

The efficacy of omega-3 fatty acids continues to be studied in the treatment of depression and bipolar depression. In a meta-analysis of studies of omega-3 supplements, Eisenberg and colleagues (2006) concluded that they could recommend them as adjuncts to standard treatment for depression and bipolar disorder. Chiu and colleagues (2008) reviewed epidemiological evidence, preclinical trials, and case-controlled studies on the use of omega-3 fatty acids and recommend that patients with depression and bipolar depression follow the same guidelines as for the American Heart Association. These stipulate that adults eat fish at least twice a week. Some authors (Chiu et al., 2008) argue that patients with mood disorders, impulse-control disorders, and psychotic disorders should consume 1 gram of omega-3 fatty acids a day.

Certain nutritional supplements, including *S*-adenosyl methionine (SAMe) and the B vitamins (especially vitamin B_6 and folic acid), also appear to improve depression (Lakhan & Vieira, 2008). Currently, B vitamins and folic acid are also being seen more favorably for the management of bipolar illness and schizophrenia. According to Lake (2006), these vitamins often augment conventional care with antipsychotic, antidepressant, and antimanic medications. The researchers recommend that combining such approaches with exercise and meditative practices such as yoga is helpful. In a recent random, controlled trial investigating vitamins B_{12} and B_6 and folic acid for the onset of depressive symptoms in older men (Ford et al., 2008), the vitamin supplements were found to be no more effective than placebo.

Herbal Therapy

A growing number of persons in the United States are using herbal therapy for preventive and therapeutic purposes and report good results; however, since manufacturers are not required to submit proof of safety or efficacy to the FDA, providers should be vigilant about their patients' use of herbal therapies. Food products also are supplemented with herbs, which may result in untoward reactions. For example, ginseng has anticoagulant effects. Drinking ginseng tea may increase the effects of prescription anticoagulants, and the consequences could seriously affect blood clotting.

St. John's wort has been used for centuries to improve mood and to alleviate pain. In ancient times, herbalists wrote of its efficacy as a sedative, antimalarial agent, and balm for burns and wounds (NCCAM, 2008d). Persons may use St. John's wort instead of traditional antidepressants to avoid the side effects (dry mouth, nausea, headache, diarrhea, and impaired sexual function). St. John's wort may be less costly (depending on insurance coverage), has fewer side effects (dry mouth, dizziness, gastrointestinal symptoms, photosensitivity, and fatigue), and does not require a prescription.

St. John's wort has been extensively researched and was generally found to be as effective as prescribed antidepressants in the treatment of mild to moderate depression (Randlov et al., 2006), but now its usefulness in treating severe depression has been established (Linde et al., 2008). The most recent studies suggest that St. John's wort has similar efficacy to standard antidepressants and causes fewer side effects. Because the FDA does not regulate St. John's wort, concentrations of the active ingredients may vary from preparation to preparation, which may account for some variation in research results.

Regulated preparations of St. John's wort are reasonably safe, but patients should be cautioned not to take it if they are already taking an SSRI antidepressant. St. John's wort is mildly serotonergic and may cause serotonin syndrome. St. John's wort also interacts negatively with other medications, including birth control pills, the antirejection transplant drug cyclosporine, Indivir and other anti-HIV medications, Irintocan and other cancer medications, and anticoagulants. Its safety has not been established for use during pregnancy or in children.

Ginkgo biloba has been used for the treatment of cerebral insufficiency, but this condition is broadly defined and ranges from memory loss to emotional instability. In a double-blind, random-controlled pilot study (Dodge et al., 2008) of 118 persons over 85 years of age, participants took 80 mg of ginkgo extract three times a day. Those who were medication adherent did better on memory tests and had fewer declines than did either the placebo group or the ginkgo group who did not take the medication as directed. According to NCCAM (2008b), however, other studies have failed to demonstrate that ginkgo was effective in improving memory. Ginkgo tends to be well tolerated, with rare, nonspecific side effects of gastrointestinal distress, headache, and allergic skin reactions. Ginkgo has anticoagulant effects and can cause bleeding in individuals who are using anticoagulants and antiplatelet agents or who are anticipating an invasive or operative procedure (NCCAM, 2008b). Ginkgo should be used with caution by patients who consume alcohol (which also thins the blood) or who have other risk factors for hemorrhagic stroke.

Black cohosh is an extract from a root that was used for centuries by Native Americans to ease pain associated with rheumatism, sore throat, and menstrual discomfort. It continues to be popular as a way of decreasing hot flashes and as an alternative to hormone replacement therapy for women in menopause. Research indicates, however, that it is probably no better than a placebo in reducing hot flashes and night sweats (Geller et al., 2009).

Kava is an herb from the South Pacific used in traditional ceremonial rites in Micronesian culture. Kava has also been used for anxiety and for its analgesic and anesthetic properties and was considered effective and safe until 2002, when at least 25 cases of liver toxicity, including hepatitis, cirrhosis, and liver failure were linked to its use. The FDA issued a consumer advisory based on this potential risk, and NCCAM discontinued its research (NCCAM, 2008c); however, according to Lake (2007), the cases of liver failure were associated with a processing error in the production of a single batch of Kava. This herbal medicine has been associated with dystonias (abnormal muscle movements) and scaly, yellow skin when taken long term.

Valerian is used as an antianxiety agent and has also been reported to have antidepressant and sedative properties (Lakhan & Vieira, 2010). Valerian is a root that when brewed as a tea has sedative, tranquilizing, and sleep-inducing effects. Valerian can also be made into a variety of extracts and tinctures, which may also include other ingredients. It is generally recognized as safe for the treatment of insomnia when taken at recommended dosages. Mild side effects at recommended dosages include headache, dizziness, tiredness, and upset stomach (NCCAM, 2008e). The major drug interactions are with other sedative-hypnotic agents, and the sedative effect of valerian may potentiate the effects of other central nervous system depressants.

Herbal teas have long been used for their sedative-hypnotic effects. Common ingredients in these teas, in addition to valerian, are hops, lemon balm, chamomile, and passionflower. The most studied of these is chamomile, a tea widely used as a folk remedy. Chamomile extract has been found to bind with gamma-aminobutyric acid (GABA) receptors. These teas, along with improved sleep hygiene, may be part of a set of interventions for insomnia; they are generally safely recommended but should be used with awareness of their potential effects, side effects, and interactions.

Figure 35-2 shows a comparison of the most commonly used natural products as reported by adults in the 2002 (A) and 2007 (B) *National Health Interview Survey* conducted by the NCHS.

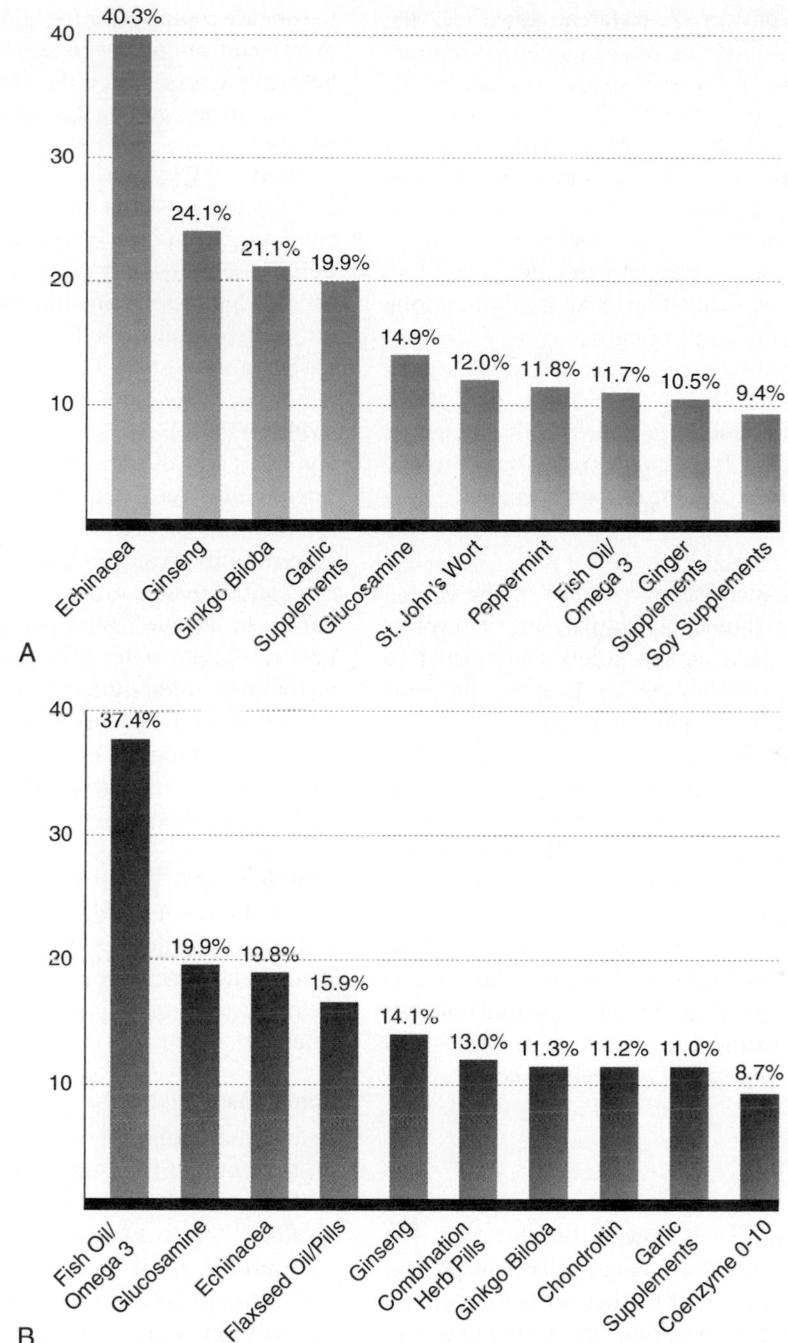

FIG 35-2 A, Ten most common natural products used by adults in the United States: 2002. **B,** Ten most common natural products used by adults in the United States: 2007. (**A,** From Barnes, P. M., Powel-Griner, E., McFann, K., & Nahin, R. [2004]. Complementary and alternative medicine use among adults: United States, 2002. In *Centers for Disease Control and Prevention Advance Data Report #343*. Hyattsville, MD: National Center for Health Statistics. **B,** From Barnes, P. M., Bloom, B., & Nahin, R. [2008]. Complementary and alternative medicine use among adults and children: United States, 2007. In *Centers for Disease Control and Prevention National Health Statistics Report #12*. Hyattsville, MD: National Center for Health Statistics.)

Mind and Body Approaches

Mind and body approaches are built on theories that regard continuous interaction between mind and body (Bedford, 2012). Most of these techniques emphasize facilitating the mind's capacity to affect bodily function and symptoms, but the reverse (the effects of bodily illness on mental health) is also part of the equation.

The significance of the mind-body relationship is well accepted in conventional medicine and to probably is the domain most familiar to psychiatric mental health nurses and nurses in general. Many of the mind-body interventions, such as cognitive-behavioral therapy, relaxation techniques, guided imagery, hypnosis, and support groups are now considered mainstream and have been the subject of considerable research (Anselmo, 2009; Schaub & Dossey, 2009).

Meditation

Meditation is an extremely popular method recommended to reduce physical and emotional stress and to promote wellness. It can be most simply accomplished by concentrating on slow, deep breathing and focusing on calming thoughts. Specific types of meditation include Benson's relaxation techniques (refer to Chapter 10) and mindfulness meditation by Kabat-Zinn, among others.

Yoga

Yoga is another popular method to both physically strengthen and emotionally relax people. It typically combines a variety of physical postures, meditation, and breathing techniques.

Acupuncture

Acupuncture is becoming increasingly popular in the United States. A skilled therapist should perform it, and it involves placing needles into the skin at key points (meridians) to modulate the flow of qi. According to Taoists, qi is a life force that circulates throughout the universe and in our bodies in precise channels called *meridians.*

Sometimes the needles are inserted and removed immediately; sometimes they are twirled and even attached to electrodes to stimulate; another method is to leave them in place for a certain period of time. Following needle placement, clients describe feeling sensations such as rushing, warmth, tingling, or occasionally pain. Acupuncture is believed to act by simulating and altering patients' physical responses, including those affecting cardiac, endocrine, neurological, and immune function. It is commonly used in the treatment of pain and in some blood disorders as well as for substance withdrawal and certain emotional disturbances.

Deep Breathing Exercises

Kitko (2007) described rhythmic breathing as an easy-to-learn-and-implement mind-body intervention for pain. The nurse helps the patient focus on an activity (purposeful breath) and in so doing usually breathes with the patient. This enhances the relaxation response in both nurse and patient and has implications for nurses working with agitated psychiatric patients. Maintaining a balance between inhalation and exhalation is important in order to avoid hyperventilation.

Guided Imagery

The use of **guided imagery** has been in the nursing literature for at least three decades. Different forms of imagery include (1) behavioral rehearsal imagery, (2) impromptu imagery, (3) biologically based imagery, and (4) symbolic and metaphoric imagery.

Imagery is used as a therapeutic tool for treating anxiety, pain, psychological trauma, and PTSD. Imagery may be combined with cognitive-behavioral therapy to help war veterans and people who have survived natural disasters. Imagery is used to enhance coping prior to childbirth or surgery, augment treatment, and minimize side effects of medications. It may help people cope with difficult times if they can imagine themselves as strong, coping, and eventually finding meaning in their experience.

Reed (2007) described several uses of imagery in clinical practice, as well as a successful hospital program and pilot study to evaluate the impact of imagery on pain and patients' opioid use. The study group that received the imagery intervention had significant improvements in pain relief and required fewer pain medications than did comparison study participants.

Hypnotherapy

Hypnosis is both a state of awareness (consciousness) and an intervention. As a state of consciousness, hypnosis is a natural focusing of attention that varies from mild to greater susceptibility to suggestion. In stress states, people are more susceptible to suggestion because their focus of attention is narrowed. People who dissociate in traumatic situations are in a trancelike state. When we use relaxation and imagery techniques, individuals frequently will enter a similarly altered state of awareness or trancelike state. Hypnosis is used to address a range of patient concerns, including weight loss, smoking cessation (Riegel & Tonnies, 2011), and depression (Schreiber, 2010).

Manipulative Practices

Manipulative, or body-based, practices relate to specific body systems and structures. These include joints and bones, circulation, and soft tissues. Two commonly used therapies—namely, spinal manipulation and massage—fall within this category.

Spinal Manipulation

Spinal manipulation is accomplished through chiropractic medicine, one of the most widely used integrative therapies. The term *chiropractic* comes from the Greek words *praxix* and *cheir*, meaning "practice" and "treatment by hand," respectively. Chiropractic medicine focuses on the relationship between structure and function and the way that relationship affects the preservation and restoration of health, using manipulative therapy as a treatment tool.

Daniel David Palmer, a grocery store owner, developed the method in the late 1800s in an effort to heal others without drugs. Palmer developed a series of manipulative procedures to bring health to muscles, nerves, and organs that had gotten out of alignment; he referred to these misalignments as *subluxations.* He believed that subluxations were metaphysical and that they interfered with the flow through the body of "innate intelligence" (spirit or life energy).

Contemporary chiropractic medicine continues to be based on the theory that energy flows from the brain to all parts of the body through the spinal cord and spinal nerves. Manipulation of the spinal column, called *adjustment*, returns the vertebrae to their normal positions. Back pain is the most common reason persons seek chiropractic treatment, but chiropractic manipulation is used to treat a variety of other conditions, including pain, allergies, and asthma (NCCAM, 2003). Manipulation is also helpful in reducing migraine, tension, or cervicogenic headache pain. Many chiropractors also treat patients with depression, anxiety, and chronic pain. Chiropractic treatment may be done in conjunction with herbs and supplements.

In randomized clinical trials investigating the treatment of tension headaches, one group of patients was treated with chiropractic manipulation, and another group received pain medication. Both groups experienced relief of pain, but there were fewer side effects from manipulation than from the use of medication (Freeman & Lawlis, 2004).

Massage Therapy

Massage therapy includes a broad group of medically valid therapies that involve rubbing or moving the skin. Massage therapists employ four basic techniques: effleurage (long, gliding strokes over the skin), pétrissage (kneading of the muscles to increase circulation), vibration and percussion (a series of fine or brisk movements that stimulate circulation and relaxation), and friction (which is decreased with the use of massage oils). Probably the best known massage technique in the United States is **Swedish massage**, which provides soothing relaxation and increases circulation. Japanese **Shiatsu massage** was strongly influenced by traditional Chinese medicine and developed from acupressure. It originated as a way to detect and treat problems in the flow of life energy (Japanese *ki).* The shiatsu practitioner uses fingers, thumbs, elbows, knees, or feet to apply pressure by massaging various parts of the body, known as *acupoints.*

Other Complementary Therapies

Homeopathy and Naturopathy

According to the National Center for Complementary and Alternative Medicine (2012), there is *little evidence* to support homeopathy as a complementary treatment. **Homeopathy** is an example of Western alternative medical systems. Homeopathy uses small doses (dilutions) of specially prepared plant extracts, herbs, minerals, and other materials to stimulate the body's defense mechanisms and healing processes. Infinitesimally small doses of diluted preparations that produce symptoms mimicking those of an illness are used to help the body heal itself. Homeopathy is based on the Law of Similars ("like cures like"), and dilutions are prescribed to match the patient's illness/symptom and personality profile. Healing occurs from the inside out, and symptoms disappear in the reverse order they appeared.

Adler and colleagues (2011) studied the use of homeopathy in depression and found no significant differences between response or remission rates in two groups of study participants, those using a conventional antidepressant and those using a homeopathic intervention. Homeopathy has been used in the treatment of short-term acute illnesses, migraine pain, allergies, chronic fatigue, otitis media, immune dysfunction, digestive disorders, and colic. It has also been used in the treatment of emotional disorders such as depression and anxiety. It is contraindicated as a treatment for advanced diseases, cancer, sexually transmitted diseases, conditions involving irreparable damage (e.g., defective heart valves), or brain damage due to stroke (Freeman & Lawlis, 2004).

Homeopathic remedies are available over the counter, but consumers should have a full evaluation by a homeopathic practitioner before using any treatments. Consumers who are given what is called a "constitutional remedy" to treat a specific symptom should be informed that occasionally the symptom will worsen before it gets better (e.g., a patient with anxiety should be warned not to fear a panic attack if anxiety worsens).

Naturopathy emphasizes health restoration rather than disease treatment and combines nutrition, homeopathy, herbal medicine, hydrotherapy, light therapy, therapeutic counseling, and other therapies. The underlying belief is that the individual assumes responsibility for his or her recovery. While psychiatric mental health nurses may not practice in these traditions, knowledge of the basic premises can be useful when assessing, treating, and referring patients. Such holistic concepts are also useful in considering the body-mind-spirit nature of mental health and illness

Aromatherapy

Aromatherapy, the use of essential oils for enhancing physical and mental well-being and healing, is a popular therapy in the mainstream market. Essential oils, often derived from herbs and plants, may be applied directly to the skin or an object such as cotton or diffused into the atmosphere through a diffuser. Essential oils are believed to stimulate the release of neurotransmitters in the brain. The sense of smell connects with the part of the brain that controls the autonomic (involuntary) nervous system. Depending on the essential oil used, the resulting effects are calming, pain reducing, stimulating, sedating, or euphoria producing.

Some nurses are trained in this art, and various oils have been introduced into hospitals, nursing homes, and hospice situations. Because these oils are believed to have unique energetic characteristics that facilitate changes in the human energy field, these interventions may also be seen as energy therapies (Smith & Kyle, 2008). Research evidence exists that combining aromatherapy with massage reduces anxiety and fosters mood elevation and stress reduction (Maddocks-Jennings & Wilkinson, 2004).

There are anecdotal reports that aromatherapy is useful for pain relief, memory improvement, and wound healing. Smith and Kyle (2008, p. 7) provide a convenient chart on how various classifications of oils affect people:

- Rooty oils such as patchouli and valerian affect calming, grounding, and stabilizing.
- Floral oils such as ylang-ylang and jasmine create mood uplifting, relaxation, and sensuality.
- Green herbaceous oils such as lavender and chamomile create balance, regulation, and clarification.

Some individuals, particularly those with pulmonary disease, may be sensitive or allergic to essential oils when they come into contact with the skin or are inhaled. Before massaging any essential oil into the skin, check for an allergic reaction by diluting the oil, administering a small amount and performing a 24-hour skin patch test.

Energy Therapies

Energy therapy includes therapies originating from many parts of the world. It is based on the belief that nonphysical bioenergy forces pervade the universe and people. Explanations vary as to the nature of this energy, the form of the therapies, and the rationale for how healing is believed to occur. Some cultures believe the energy comes from God. Those who practice shamanic healing rituals believe the energy comes from various spirits through a priest or shaman.

The NCCAM (2007a) coined the term *biofield energy.* Adherents believe that this energy takes a particular form in each person, called the *human energy field* or *aura*. This energy field is said to contain a number of layers, each with energy of different frequencies. Energy is transferred between layers and eventually into the physical body through *chakras*. Disturbances of the energy field are the cause of illness, and healing can occur only when the human energy field is balanced and energy is flowing freely.

More than 50 years ago, Russian researchers produced photographs of what they thought were human energy fields. The images captured by Kirlian photography show auras and streams of light emanating from people's hands and even from the leaves of plants. The conclusion was that the health of the person or organism could be evaluated by noting the intensity, shape, and color of these emanations. Unfortunately, the patterns on the Kirlian photographs have since been dismissed as explainable by variations in the techniques used in the photography.

Practitioners of energy medicine believe that they are able to increase their awareness of the human energy field and enhance healing through meditation and centering (finding the calm space within yourself) (Zahourek, 2005). Practitioners believe they can then detect problems in others' energy fields and adjust the quality or create balance. This is accomplished by placing one's hands in or through these fields to direct the energy through visualized or actual pressure and/or manipulation of the body. Therapeutic touch, healing touch, and Reiki are the most common energy therapies practiced by nurses.

Therapeutic Touch

Therapeutic touch is a modality developed in the 1970s by Dolores Krieger, a nursing professor at New York University, and Dora Kunz, a Canadian healer. The premise for therapeutic touch is that healing is promoted by balancing the body's energies. In preparation for a treatment session, practitioners focus completely on the person receiving the treatment without any other distraction. Practitioners then assess the energy field, clear and balance it through hand movements, and/or direct energy in a specific region of the body. The therapist never physically touches the patient. Ideally, after undergoing a session of therapeutic touch, patients report a sense of deep relaxation.

Practitioners of therapeutic touch believe that the therapy is useful in relieving pain, premenstrual syndrome, depression, complications in premature babies, and secondary infections associated with human immunodeficiency virus (HIV) infection; lowering blood pressure; decreasing edema; easing abdominal cramps and nausea; resolving fevers; and accelerating the healing of fractures, wounds, and infections.

Research in this area has generally been of medium quality and meets minimal standards for validity; there is a need for high-quality studies to repudiate or validate this therapy (Jain & Mills, 2010). Despite lack of absolute scientific support, therapeutic touch continues to occupy a place in mainstream health care. The American Cancer Society features an overview of therapeutic touch on its 2011 website "Find Support and Treatment—Therapeutic Touch" (http://www.cancer.org/Treatment/TreatmentsandSideEffects/ComplementaryandAlternativeMedicine/ManualHealingandPhysicalTouch/therapeutic-touch). The site overviews the history, research, and practice behind therapeutic touch as well as offering additional resources for patient use.

Healing Touch

Healing touch is a derivative of therapeutic touch developed by a registered nurse, Janet Mentgen, in the early 1980s. Healing touch combines several energy therapies and is based on the belief that the body is a complex energy system that can be influenced by another through that person's intention for healing and well-being. Healing touch is related to therapeutic touch in the belief that working energetically with persons to achieve their highest level of well-being, and not necessarily to relieve a specific symptom, is the goal.

A unified international program of study has evolved that teaches and certifies practitioners of healing touch. Healing touch involves gentle laying on of hands on a clothed body or moving over the body in the energy field. The practitioner may focus on a specific problem area or the full body. In a review of over 30 studies on healing touch, Wardel and Weymouth (2004) found that although the studies reported positive results in reducing stress, anxiety, and pain and in enhancing healing time and quality of life, the quality of the research was such that results could not be generalized to other settings and therapists.

Reiki

The Japanese spiritual practice of Reiki has become an increasingly popular modality for nurses to learn and practice. **Reiki** is an energy-based therapy in which the practitioner's energy is connected to a universal source (chi, qi, prana) and is transferred to a recipient for physical or spiritual healing (Miles & True, 2003). Numerous hospitals, hospices, cancer support groups, and clinics are now offering Reiki in complementary programs. Nursing research has been conducted on such topics as reducing anxiety and pain following abdominal hysterectomy, self-care for nurses, and orthopedic pain (Vitale & O'Conner, 2007; Brathovde, 2006*f*). LaTorre (2005) describes its use as an adjunct in psychotherapy. People may be hesitant about using Reiki because (1) there is little scientific support for Reiki and acceptance of its teaching about ki is a matter of faith; (2) the possibility exists that effects are due to a placebo effect; (3) it is incompatible with their religious beliefs; and (4) governmental regulation and licensing are controversial.

Thought Field Therapy and Emotional Freedom Technique

Thought field therapy (TFT) was first developed by Roger Callahan in the 1980s and then modified in the 1990s by

Gary Craig, who called his version the *emotional freedom technique* (EFT) (Borgatti, 2008). The basis for these interventions is the idea that negative emotions are the result of energy imbalances and blocks in the body. The goal is to release these blocks and view the problem with less distress by tapping specific acupuncture points and meridians and repeating a positive mantra. EFT is relatively easy to integrate into a psychotherapy or psychopharmacology practice and has some beginning research to support its practice (Wells et al., 2003).

Bioelectromagnetic-Based Therapies

Bioelectromagnetic-based therapies involve the unconventional use of electromagnetic fields, such as pulsed fields, magnetic fields, or alternating-current or direct-current fields. Transcranial magnetic therapy (TMS) and vagus nerve stimulus (VNS) treatments for depression are in this category. In TMS, pulsating magnetic fields are sent through a metal coil attached to the person's scalp. High-frequency pulses stimulate, and low-frequency pulses dampen neural impulses. A recent study indicates that when low-frequency TMS is used to "stun" parts of the brain of a person with schizophrenia, it tends to decrease auditory hallucinations (Aleman et al., 2007). TMS is approved by the FDA for the treatment of depression (refer to Chapter 14).

Prayer and Spirituality

Historically, there is a precedent for the inclusion of prayer and other spiritual practices as part of the care of the psychiatric patient. In England, a Quaker named William Tuke witnessed the failure of common practices of bleeding, purging, and ice baths that were used in the treatment of the mentally ill. He instituted compassionate psychological and spiritual treatments based on the idea that insanity was a disruption of both mind and spirit.

In the mid-1840s, the first form of psychiatric care in the United States was called "moral treatment." Religious superintendents ran the first mental institutions in Philadelphia, Hartford, and Worcester. A positive attitude toward prayer and spiritual practices continued in the United States until the influence of Sigmund Freud (1908 until 1939), who spoke and wrote about the emotionally destructive aspects of religion. These views subsequently influenced psychiatry's attitude toward religion for many years (Koenig, 2002).

The role of spirituality and religion in mental health has gained the attention of researchers (Meltzer et al., 2011; Koslander & Arvidsson, 2007). Patients with psychiatric disorders often have significant spiritual needs. Some feel angry with God for allowing them to suffer with disorders that affect every aspect of their lives. Some need to address issues of forgiveness, for example, for friends and family who have rejected them or been judgmental because of the psychiatric illness. Other patients may wish to seek forgiveness because of hurt they have caused others. Many patients rely on God as their source of strength and maintain a deep, abiding faith despite the circumstances of their illnesses (Carson & Koenig, 2004).

O'Reilly (2004) emphasizes the value of psychiatric mental health nurses who use spiritual assessment tools and interventions to support a patient's move toward wholeness and healing. One challenge in meeting the spiritual needs of psychiatric patients is in maintaining appropriate boundaries. Patients may experience difficulty in knowing where their own beliefs stop and those of the health care professional begin. The patient is in a vulnerable position of perhaps being unfairly influenced by someone with strong beliefs. In meeting the spiritual needs of psychiatric patients, it is imperative that nurses be continually aware and respectful of boundary issues and never impose beliefs on the patient.

To support the spiritual needs of psychiatric patients, we first assess the patient's beliefs and practices. The assessment itself is a powerful intervention. When we ask a patient about the importance of spiritual issues in his or her life, we are not only encouraging discussion, but also communicating that we are interested in and comfortable talking about an area of the patient's life. Asking about prayer, sources of hope and strength, and the patient's preferred spiritual practices allows us to know how we can provide spiritual support for the patient.

Historical Notes Regarding CAM

Traditional Chinese medicine (TCM) provides the basic theoretical framework for many CAM therapies, including acupuncture, acupressure, transcendental meditation, tai chi, and qigong. TCM is derived from the philosophy of Taoism and emphasizes the need to promote harmony (health) or to bring order out of chaos (illness). TCM is a vast medical system based on a constellation of concepts, theories, laws, and principles of energy movement within the body. Therapy is aimed at addressing the patient's illness in relation to the complex interaction of mind, body, and spirit.

Adherents of TCM say that it addresses not only physiological and psychological symptoms, but also "cosmologic" events that relate to the dynamics of the universe. These meridians become significant in the practice of acupuncture, touch therapy, and the more recent energy-based therapies used to treat emotional symptoms and promote mental health.

In TCM, health is the balance between yin and yang, and illness emanates from imbalances. The TCM practitioner uses the history and physical examination to understand the imbalances of mind, body, and spirit that have caused the patient's illness. Diagnosis involves both questioning and observing body structure, skin color, breath, body odors, nail condition, voice, gestures, mood, and pulse. Eastern goals, perspectives, and stages of healing are useful in treating mental illnesses, many of which are long term. The goals of healing in Eastern medicine include the following:

- Being in harmony with one's environment and with all of creation in mind, body, and spirit
- Reawakening the spirit to its possibilities
- Reconnecting with life's meaning

Also, active participation in TCM treatment is essential as healing progresses through a series of stages (Box 35-3).

Forms of movement such as qigong and tai chi demonstrate effects on a wide range of phenomena, including neuropsychiatric disorders, cognition, and neurodegeneration (Deslandes et al., 2009). Viewed as a stressor itself, movement seems to

BOX 35-3 STAGES OF HEALING IN TRADITIONAL CHINESE MEDICINE

- **Awakening:** Represents a time, often triggered by crisis or illness, in which the person is said to sense a need for change, a feeling of diminution in the quality of life.
- **Intentionality and focus:** Occurs when the person desires to change his or her consciousness from patterns of "disharmony" to patterns of healthy behaviors and seeks to ease the pain of spiritual discomfort and to obtain help.
- **Commitment:** Occurs when the person forges healing relationships and establishes goals for change.
- **Transformation:** Takes place when mutual, creative, active participation occurs between practitioner and patient directed toward ongoing change in mind, body, and spirit.
- **Attainment:** Occurs when the patient incorporates new, healthy behaviors, has a sense of well-being, and accepts new challenges for growth; he or she has a willingness to evaluate and change to move toward greater levels of wholeness.
- **Empowerment:** Occurs when the person feels a sense of stability and harmony.

mediate the effects of other stressors. Yoga is also based on the principles of TCM and can be helpful to people experiencing anxiety and depression to increase a sense of well-being and reduce symptoms of stress and depression.

Ayurvedic (pronounced "eye-yur-VEH-dik") medicine originated in India around 5000 BC and is one of the world's oldest medical systems. *Ayurveda* means "the science of life" and is a philosophy that emphasizes individual responsibility for health. It is holistic, promotes prevention, recognizes the uniqueness of the individual, and offers natural treatments (Pai et al., 2004).

The websites of both the NCCAM (http://nccam.nih.gov) and the NIH (http://nih.gov) provide detailed information and reviews about other complementary and alternative therapies.

KEY POINTS TO REMEMBER

- A philosophy of holism and promotion of therapeutic relationship are at the heart of psychiatric mental health nursing and are important no matter what modality is used, conventional or integrative.
- Complementary, alternative, and integrative therapies are in demand as consumers seek a broader range of therapies than those offered by traditional medicine.
- Integrative care is classified as: (1) natural products, (2) mind and body medicine, (3) manipulative practices, (4) body-based practices, and (5) other CAM therapies.
- With the availability of information on the Internet, consumers are more likely to have researched their symptoms or condition and identified potential CAM treatments.
- Utility of information from the Internet for informed patient decision making may be questionable.
- Nurses are ideally positioned to guide patients to reliable resources, such as the NCCAM, that provide up-to-date information for health care practitioners and consumers.
- Nurses' knowledge of current research about major CAM therapies will assist in purposeful promotion of holistic integrative care.
- As frontline health care providers, nurses help patients avoid wasting money on useless therapies and assist them in maximizing the benefits of CAM therapies.

CRITICAL THINKING

1. As a nurse, you may have patients who use integrative therapies in conjunction with the conventional therapies prescribed by the health care provider. Identify issues that are important to assess, and discuss how you would ask about the use of these nonconventional practices.
2. Discuss how herbal products sold in the United States can vary in quality. How does a patient determine the efficacy of the herb?
3. What can a patient do to guarantee the quality and dosage of an herbal product? What are resources for the patient and nurse to learn about the efficacy and safety of herbs and supplements?
4. By visiting their websites, determine how the NCCAM and other informational resources, such as the AHNA, provide information for the consumer and professionals.

CHAPTER REVIEW

1. Caitlin is being seen in the outpatient clinic for medication follow-up. She tells you that she is taking St. John's wort to help her symptoms of depression. Your response to make sure to let her primary care provider know that she is taking St. John's wort is guided by what knowledge?
   a. Many providers do not believe in herbal supplements.
   b. Taking St. John's wort along with an SSRI antidepressant may cause serotonin syndrome.
   c. The patient needs to increase her assertiveness with her provider.
   d. St. John's wort has not been shown to treat depression symptoms effectively.
2. You are caring for Georgia, who questions you about the safety of an herbal supplement. Which nursing response is true?
   a. "Herbal supplements are regulated by the FDA."
   b. "Natural ingredients in herbal supplements are harmless."
   c. "Your primary care provider needs to be aware of any supplements you take."
   d. "Marketing for herbal supplements demonstrates that all supplements are safe."

3. Which of the following patients may benefit from biofeedback? The one who:
   a. Is afraid of flying.
   b. Is about to give birth.
   c. Wants to quit smoking.
   d. Wants to relax and promote well-being.
4. Shelly is having menstrual problems and asks you which supplement might be helpful to her. Which supplement should you suggest for the patient to discuss with her primary care provider?
   a. Black cohosh
   b. St. John's wort
   c. Kava
   d. Ginkgo biloba
5. Which nursing question(s) should be included in a holistic assessment? *Select all that apply.*
   a. "Are you taking any herbal supplements or other natural remedies?"
   b. "Have you undergone any surgeries in the past?"
   c. "What gives you a sense of meaning and purpose in life?"
   d. "What methods do you use to cope with stress?"
   e. "Do you feel safe in your relationships?"
   f. "Do you have regular physical exams?"

Answers to Chapter Review

1. b; 2. c; 3. d; 4. a; 5. a, b, c, d, e, f.

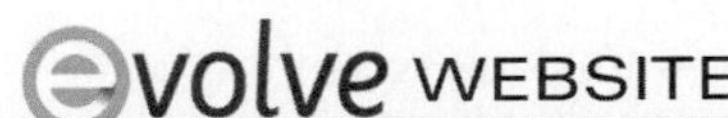

Visit the Evolve website for a posttest on the content in this chapter: http://evolve.elsevier.com/Varcarolis

Post-Test interactive review

REFERENCES

Adler, U. C., Krüger, S., Teut, M., Lüdtke, R., Bartsch, I., Schützler, L., et al. (2011). Homeopathy for depression–DEP-HOM: Study protocol for a randomized, partially double-blind, placebo controlled, four armed study. *Trials, 12*(1) 43–49.

Aleman, A., Summer, L., & Kahn, R. (2007). Efficacy of slow repetitive magnetic stimulation on auditory hallucinations. *Journal of Clinical Psychiatry, 68*, 416–421.

American Association of Retired People and National Center for Complementary and Alternative Medicine. (2011). *What people aged 50 and older discuss with their health care providers.* Washington, DC: USDHS, NIH.

American Holistic Nurses Association. (2004). *What is holistic nursing?* Retrieved from http://www.ahna.org.

American Holistic Nurses Association. (1998). *Description of holistic nursing.* Flagstaff, AZ: AHNA.

American Nurses Association & American Holistic Nurses Association. (2007). *Holistic nursing: Scope and standards of practice.* Silver Spring, MD: Author.

Anselmo, J. (2009). Relaxation. In B. Dossey, & L. Keegan (Eds.), *Holistic nursing: A handbook for practice* (pp. 259–285). Sudbury, MA: Jones and Bartlett.

Barnes, P. M., Bloom, B., & Nahin, R. (2008). Complementary and alternative medicine use among adults and children: United States, 2007. *Centers for Disease Control National Health Statistics Report #12.* Retrieved from http://nccam.nih.gov/news/2008/nhsr12.pdf.

Bedford, F. (2012). A perception theory in mind-body medicine: Guided imagery and mindful meditation as cross-modal adaptation. *Psychonomic Bulletin & Review, 19*(1), 24–45.

Block, D. R. (2008). Brain stimulation therapies for treatment-resistant depression: Evidence for the use of neurostimulating techniques. *Psychiatric Times, 25*(1), 37–38.

Blues Busters. (2011). 17 ways to fight depression naturally. *Better Nutrition, 73*(12), 34–37.

Borgatti, J. C. (2008). Tap your way to fast relief. *American Nurse Today, 3*(1), 32–33.

Brathovde, A. (2006). A pilot study of Reiki for self-care of nurses and healthcare providers. *Holistic Nursing Practice, 20*(2), 95–100.

Carson, B., & Koenig, H. G. (2004). *Spiritual caregiving: Healthcare as a ministry.* Philadelphia, PA: Templeton Foundation Press.

Chiappedi, H. G. (2010). Herbals and natural dietary supplements in psychiatric practice. *Recent Patents on CNS Drug Discovery, 5*(2), 164–171.

Chiu, C. C., Liu, J. P., & Su, K. P. (2008). The use of omega-3 fatty acids in the treatment of depression: The lights and shadows. *Psychiatric Times, 25*(9), 76–80.

Denneson, L. M., Corson, K., & Dobscha, S. K. (2011). Complementary and alternative medicine use among veterans with chronic noncancer pain. *Journal of Rehabilitation Research & Development, 48*(9), 1119–1127.

Deslandes, A., Moraes, H., Ferreira, C., Veiga, H., Silveira, H., Mouta, R., et al. (2009). Exercise and Mental health: Many reasons to move. *Neuropsychobiology, 59*(4), 191–198.

Dodge, H. H., Zitzelberger, T., Oken, B. S., Howieson, D., & Kaye, J. (2008). A randomized placebo controlled trial of gingko biloba for prevention of cognitive decline. *Neurology, 70*(19 Pt 2), 1809–1817.

Dougherty, P. J. S. (2009). *Substantiation and style.* Retrieved from http://naturalhealthwriter.com/

Edwards, E. (2012). The role of complementary, alternative, and integrative medicine in personalized health care. *Neuropsychopharmacology, 37*(1), 293–295.

Eisenberg, D. M., Kessler, R. C., Van Rompay, M. I., Kaptchuk, T. J., Wilkey, S. A., Apple, S., et al. (2006). Perceptions about complementary therapies relative to conventional therapies among adults who use both: Results from a national survey. *Annals of Internal Medicine, 135*, 344–351.

Evans, M., Perle, S., & Harrison, N. (2011). Chiropractic wellness on the web: The content and quality of information related to wellness and primary prevention on the Internet. *Chiropractic & Manual Therapies, 19*(1). Retrieved from http://www.chiromt.com/content/19/1/4.

Food and Drug Administration. (2011). *Background document for the food advisory committee.* Retrieved from http://www.fda.gov/downloads/AdvisoryCommittees/CommitteesMeetingMaterials/FoodAdvisoryCommittee/UCM248549.pdf.

Ford, A. H., Flicker, L., Thomas, J., Norman, P., Jamrozik, K., & Almedia, O. P. (2008). Vitamins B_{12}, B_6, and folic acid for onset of depressive symptoms in older men: Results from a 2-year placebo-controlled trial. *Journal Clinical Psychiatry, 69*, 1203–1209.

Freeman, L. W., & Lawlis, G. F. (2004). *Mosby's complementary and alternative medicine: A research based approach.* St. Louis, MO: Mosby.

Geller, S. E., Shulman, L. P., van Breemen, R. B., Banuvar, S., Zhou, Y., Epstein, G., et al. (2009). Safety and efficacy of black cohosh and red clover for the management of vasomotor symptoms: A randomized controlled trial. *Menopause, 16*(6), 1156–1166.

Institute of Medicine. (2009). *February summit on integrative medicine and the health of the public.* Retrieved from http://sev.prnewswire.com/health-care-hospitals/20090227/DC7670827022009–1.html#.

Jain, S., & Mills, P. J. (2010). Biofield therapies: Helpful or full of hype? A best evidence synthesis. *International Journal of Behavioral Medicine, 17*(1), 1–16. doi:10.1007/s12529-009-9062–4.

Kitko, J. (2007). Rhythmic breathing as a nursing intervention. *Holistic Nursing Practice, 21*(2), 85–88.

Koenig, H. G. (2002). *Spirituality in patient care: Why, how, when and what.* Philadelphia, PA: Templeton Foundation Press.

Koslander, A., & Tiburtius, B. (2007). Patients' conceptions of how the spiritual dimension is addressed in mental health care: A qualitative study. *Journal of Advanced Nursing, 57*(6), 597–604.

Lake, J. (2007). Integrative management of anxiety. *Psychiatric Times, 24*(12), 13–17.

Lake, J. (2006). Textbook of integrative mental health care. New York, NY: Thieme.

Lakhan, S. E., & Vieira, K. F. (2010). Nutritional and herbal supplements for anxiety and anxiety-related disorders: Systematic review. *Nutrition Journal, 9*(42). Retrieved from http://www.nutritionj.com/content/9/1/42.

Lakhan, S. E., & Vieira, K. F. (2008). Nutritional therapies for mental health disorders. *Nutrition Journal, 7*(2). doi:10.1186/1475-2891-7–2. Retrieved from http://www.nutritionj.com/content/7/1/2.

LaTorre, M. A. (2005). The use of Reiki in psychotherapy. *Perspectives in Psychiatric Care, 41*(4), 184–187.

Linde, K., Berner, M., & Kriston, L. (2008). St. John's wort for major depression. *Cochrane Database of Systematic Reviews* (Issue 4), Art No.: CD000448. doi:10.1002/14561858.CD000448.pub3.

Maddocks-Jennings, W., & Wilkinson, J. M. (2004). Aromatherapy practice in nursing: Literature review. *Journal of Advanced Nursing, 48*, 933–103.

Maizes, V., Koffler, K., & Fleishman, S. (2003). The integrative assessment. In D. Rakel (Ed.), *Integrative medicine* (pp. 11–16). Philadelphia, PA: Saunders.

Marglin, E. (2011). Energy medicine. *Natural Health, 41*(3), 88–90.

Mehl-Madrona, L. (2004). Integrative approach to psychiatry. In B. Kligler & R. Lee (Eds.), *Integrative medicine: principles for practice* (pp. 623–666). New York, NY: McGraw-Hill.

Meltzer, H. I., Dogra, N., Vostanis, P., & Ford, T. (2011). Religiosity and the mental health of adolescents in Great Britain. *Mental Health, Religion & Culture, 14*(7), 703–713.

Miles, P., & True, G. (2003). Reiki: Review of biofield therapy history, theory, practice, and research. *Alternative Therapies in Health and Medicine, 9*(2), 62–72.

Morris, D. (2006). Pilot study using reflexology. *Beginnings, 26*(5), 28–29.

National Center for Complementary and Alternative Medicine. (2003). *November research report: About chiropractic and its use in treating low-back pain.* Retrieved from http://nccam.nih.gov/health/chiropractic/.

National Center for Complementary and Alternative Medicine. (2007). *Energy medicine: An overview.* Retrieved from http://nccam.nih.gov/health/backgrounds/energymed.htm.

National Center for Complementary and Alternative Medicine. (2007b). Placebo: Sugar, shams, therapies or all of the above. *CAM at the NIH, 14*(3), 1–2, 4–5.

National Center for Complementary and Alternative Medicine. (2008a). *Herbs at a glance: Black cohosh.* Retrieved from http://nccam.nih.gov/health/blackcohosh.

National Center for Complementary and Alternative Medicine. (2008b). *Herbs at a glance: Ginkgo.* Retrieved from http://nccam.nih.gov.health/ginkgo.

National Center for Complementary and Alternative Medicine. (2008c). *Herbs at a glance: Kava.* Retrieved from http://nccam.nih.gov/health/kava.

National Center for Complementary and Alternative Medicine. (2008d). *Herbs at a glance: St. John's wort.* Retrieved from http://nccam.nih.gov/health/stjohnswort.

National Center for Complementary and Alternative Medicine. (2008e). *Herbs at a glance: Valerian.* Retrieved from http://nccam.nih.gov/health/valerian.

National Center for Complementary and Alternative Medicine. (2008f). New campaign encourages open communication about CAM. *CAM at the NIH, 15*(2), 1–2.

National Center for Complementary and Alternative Medicine. (2011). *What is complementary and alternative medicine?* Retrieved from http://nccam.nih.gov/health/whatiscam.

O'Reilly, M. L. (2004). Spirituality and mental health clients. *Journal of Psychosocial Nursing and Mental Health Services, 42*(7), 44–53.

Pai, S., Shanbhag, V., & Archarya, S. (2004). Ayurvedic medicine. In B. Kligler & R. Lee (Eds.), *Integrative medicine: Principles for practice* (pp. 219–240). New York, NY: McGraw-Hill.

Randlov, C., Mehlsen, J., Thomsen, C. F., Hedman, C., Von Fircks, H., & Winther, K. (2006). The efficacy of St. John's wort in patients with minor depressive symptoms or dysthymia—a double-blind placebo-controlled study. *Phytomedicine, 13*(4), 215–221.

Reed, T. (2007). Imagery in the clinical setting: A tool for healing. *Nursing Clinics of North America, 42*(2), 261–277.

Riegel, B., & Tonnies, S. (2011). Hypnosis in smoking cessation: The effectiveness of some basic principles of hypnotherapy without using formal trance–a case study. *Journal of Smoking Cessation, 6*(2), 83–84.

Schaub, B. G., & Dossey, B. M. (2009). Imagery. In B. M. Dossey & L. Kegan (Eds.), *Holistic nursing: A handbook for practice.* Sudbury, MA: Jones & Bartlett.

Schreiber, E. H. (2010). Use of hypnosis in psychotherapy with major depressive disorders. *Australian Journal of Clinical & Experimental Hypnosis, 38*(1), 44–51.

Selman, L. E., Williams, J., & Simms. V. (2012). A mixed-methods evaluation of complementary therapy services in palliative care: Yoga and dance therapy. *European Journal of Cancer Care, 21*(1), 87–97.

Simpson, J. S. A., Crawford, S. G., Goldstein, E. T., Field, C., Burgess, E., & Kaplan, B. J. (2011). Systematic review of safety and tolerability of a complex micronutrient formula used in mental health. *BMC Psychiatry, 11*(1), 62–68.

Smith, C., Hancock, H., Blake-Mortimer, J., &.Eckert, K. (2007). A randomised comparative trial of yoga and relaxation to reduce stress and anxiety. *Complementary Therapies in Medicine, 15*, 77–83.

Smith, M. C., & Kyle, L. (2008). Holistic foundations of aromatherapy for nursing. *Holistic Nursing Practice, 22*(1), 3–9.

Transcranial magnetic stimulation: The saga continues. (2008). *The Carlat Psychiatry Report, 6*(1), 1–3.

van der Riet, P. (2011). Complementary therapies in health care. *Nursing & Health Sciences, 13*(1), 4–8.

Vitale, A., & O'Conner, P. (2007). An integrative review of Reiki touch therapy research. *Holistic Nursing Practice, 21*(4), 167–179.

Walach, H. (2009). The campaign against CAM and the notion of "evidence-based." *Journal of Alternative & Complementary Medicine, 15*(10), 1139–1142.

Weldon, S. P. (Ed.), (2011). Current bibliography of the history of science and its cultural influences. *Isis, 102*(S1), i–327.

Wells, S., Polglase, K., Andrews, H. B., Carrington, P., & Baker, A. H. (2003). Evaluation of meridian based intervention: Emotional freedom technique (EFT) for reducing specific phobias for small animals. *Journal of Clinical Psychology, 59*, 943–966.

WNBC.com. (2004). *Complementary and alternative medicine undergoes new scrutiny: Americans spend $30 billion on alternative therapies.* Retrieved from http://www.wnbc.com/print/2815485/detail.html.

Zahourek, R. (2005). Intentionality: Evolutionary development in healing. *Journal of Holistic Nursing, 23*(1), 89–109.

A

DSM-5 Classification

Before each disorder name, ICD-9-CM codes are provided, followed by ICD-10-CM codes in parentheses. Blank lines indicate that either the ICD-9-CM or the ICD-10-CM code is not applicable. For some disorders, the code can be indicated only according to the subtype or specifier.

ICD-9-CM codes are to be used for coding purposes in the United States through September 30, 2014. ICD-10-CM codes are to be used starting October 1, 2014.

Following chapter titles and disorder names, page numbers for the corresponding text or criteria are included in parentheses.

Note for all mental disorders due to another medical condition: Indicate the name of the other medical condition in the name of the mental disorder due to [the medical condition]. The code and name for the other medical condition should be listed first immediately before the mental disorder due to the medical condition.

NEURODEVELOPMENTAL DISORDERS (31)

Intellectual Disabilities (33)

319	(—.—)	Intellectual Disability (Intellectual Developmental Disorder) (33)
		Specify current severity:
	(F70)	Mild
	(F71)	Moderate
	(F72)	Severe
	(F73)	Profound
315.8	**(F88)**	Global Developmental Delay (41)
319	**(F79)**	Unspecified Intellectual Disability (Intellectual Developmental Disorder) (41)

Communication Disorders (41)

315.39	**(F80.9)**	Language Disorder (42)
315.39	**(F80.0)**	Speech Sound Disorder (44)
315.35	**(F80.81)**	Childhood-Onset Fluency Disorder (Stuttering) (45)
		Note: Later-onset cases are diagnosed as 307.0 (F98.5) adult-onset fluency disorder.
315.39	**(F80.98)**	Social (Pragmatic) Communication Disorder (47)
307.9	**(F80.9)**	Unspecified Communication Disorder (49)

Autism Spectrum Disorder (50)

299.00	**(F84.0)**	Autism Spectrum Disorder (50)
		Specify if: Associated with a known medical or genetic condition or environmental factor; Associated with another neurodevelopmental, mental or behavioral disorder
		Specify current severity for Criterion A and Criterion B: Requiring very substantial support, Requiring substantial support, Requiring support
		Specify if: With or without accompanying intellectual impairment, With or without accompanying language impairment, With catatonia (use additional code 293.89 [F06.1])

Attention-Deficit/Hyperactivity Disorder (59)

—.—	(—.—)	Attention-Deficit/Hyperactivity Disorder (59)
		Specify whether:
314.01	**(F90.2)**	Combined presentation
314.00	**(F90.0)**	Predominantly inattentive presentation
314.01	**(F90.1)**	Predominantly hyperactive/impulsive presentation
		Specify if: In partial remission
		Specify current severity: Mild, Moderate, Severe
314.01	**(F90.8)**	Other Specified Attention-Deficit/Hyperactivity Disorder (65)
314.01	**(F90.9)**	Unspecified Attention-Deficit/Hyperactivity Disorder (66)

Specific Learning Disorder (66)

—.—	(—.—)	Specific Learning Disorder (66)
		Specify if:
315.00	**(F81.0)**	With impairment in reading (*specify* if with word reading accuracy, reading rate or fluency, reading comprehension)
315.2	**(F81.81)**	With impairment in written expression (*specify* if with spelling accuracy, grammar and punctuation accuracy, clarity or organization of written expression)

315.1 (F81.2) With impairment in mathematics (*specify* if with number sense, memorization or arithmetic facts, accurate or fluent calculation, accurate math reasoning)
Specify current severity: Mild, Moderate, Severe

Motor Disorders (74)

315.4 (F82) Developmental Coordination Disorder (74)
307.3 (F98.4) Stereotypic Movement Disorder (77)
Specify if: With self-injurious behavior, Without self-injurious behavior
Specify if: Associated with a known medical or genetic condition, neurodevelopmental disorder, or environmental factor
Specify current severity: Mild, Moderate, Severe

Tic Disorders

307.23 (F95.2) Tourette's Disorder (81)
307.22 (F95.1) Persistent (Chronic) Motor or Vocal Tic Disorder (81)
Specify if: With motor tics only, With vocal tics only
307.21 (F95.0) Provisional Tic Disorder (81)
307.20 (F95.8) Other Specified Tic Disorder (85)
307.20 (F95.9) Unspecified Tic Disorder (85)

Other Neurodevelopment Disorders (86)

315.8 (F88) Other Specified Neurodevelopmental Disorder (86)
315.9 (F89) Unspecified Neurodevelopmental Disorder (86)

SCHIZOPHRENIA SPECTRUM AND OTHER PSYCHOTIC DISORDERS (87)

The following specifiers apply to Schizophrenia Spectrum and Other Psychotic Disorders where indicated:

[a]*Specify* if: The following course specifiers are only to be used after a 1-year duration of the disorder: First episode, currently in acute episode; First episode, currently in partial remission; First episode, currently in full remission; Multiple episodes, currently in acute episode; Multiple episodes, currently in parital remission; Multiple episodes, currently in full remission; Continuous; Unspecified

[b]*Specify* if: With catatonia (use additional code 293.89 [F06.1])

[c]*Specify* current severity of delusions, hallucinations, disorganized speech, abnormal psychomotor behavior, negative symptoms, impaired cognition, depression, and mania symptoms

301.22 (F21) Schizotypal (Personality) Disorder (90)
297.1 (F22) Delusional Disorder[a,c] (90)
Specify whether: Erotomanic type, Grandiose type, Jealous type, Persecutory type, Somatic type, Mixed type, Unspecified type
Specify if : With bizarre content
298.8 (F23) Brief Psychotic Disorder[b,c] (94)
Specify if: With marked stressor(s), Without marked stressor(s), With postpartum onset
295.40 (F20.81) Schizophreniform Disorder[b,c] (96)
Specify if: With good prognostic features, Without good prognostic features
295.90 (F20.9) Schizophrenia[a,b,c] (99)
—.— (—.—) Schizoaffective Disorder[a,b,c] (105)
Specify whether:
295.70 (F25.0) Bipolar type
295.70 (F25.1) Depressive type
—.— (—.—) Substance/Medication-Induced Psychotic Disorder[c] (110)
Note: See the criteria set and corresponding recording procedures for substance-specific codes and ICD-9-CM and ICD-10-CM coding.
Specify if: With onset during intoxication, With onset during withdrawal
—.— (—.—) Psychotic Disorder Due to Another Medical Condition[c] (115)
Specify whether:
293.81 (F06.2) With delusions
293.82 (F06.0) With hallucinations
293.89 (F06.1) Catatonia Associated With Another Mental Disorder (Catatonia Specifier) (119)
293.89 (F06.1) Catatonic Disorder Due to Another Medical Condition (120)
293.89 (F06.1) Unspecified Catatonia (121)
Note: Code first 781.99 (R29.818) other symptoms involving nervous and musculoskeletal systems.
298.8 (F28) Other Specified Schizophrenia Spectrum and Other Psychotic Disorder (122)
298.9 (F29) Unspecified Schizophrenia Spectrum and Other Psychotic Disorder (122)

BIPOLAR AND RELATED DISORDERS (123)

The following specifiers apply to Bipolar and Related Disorders where indicated:

[a]*Specify:* With anxious distress (*specify* current severity: mild, moderate, moderate-severe, severe); With mixed features; With rapid cycling; With melancholic features; With atypical features; With mood-congruent psychotic features; With mood-incongruent psychotic features; With catatonia (use additional code 293.89 [F06.1]); With peripartum onset; With seasonal pattern

—.— (—.—) Bipolar I Disorder[a] (123)
—.— (—.—) Current or most recent episode manic
296.41 (F31.11) Mild

296.42 (F31.12) Moderate
296.43 (F31.13) Severe
296.44 (F31.2) With psychotic features
296.45 (F31.73) In partial remission
296.46 (F31.74) In full remission
296.40 (F31.9) Unspecified
296.40 (F31.0) Current or most recent episode hypomanic
296.45 (F31.73) In partial remission
296.46 (F31.74) In full remission
296.40 (F31.9) Unspecified
—.— (—.—) Current or most recent episode depressed
296.51 (F31.31) Mild
296.52 (F31.32) Moderate
296.53 (F31.4) Severe
296.54 (F31.5) With psychotic features
296.55 (F31.75) In partial remission
296.56 (F31.76) In full remission
296.50 (F31.9) Unspecified
296.7 (F31.9) Current or most recent episode unspecified
296.89 (F31.81) Bipolar II Disorder[a] (132)
Specify current or most recent episode: Hypomanic, Depressed
Specify course if full criteria for a mood episode are not currently met: In partial remission, In full remission
Specify severity if full criteria for a mood episode are not currently met: Mild, Moderate, Severe
301.13 (F34.0) Cyclothymic Disorder (139)
Specify if: With anxious distress
—.— (—.—) Substance/Medication-Induced Bipolar and Related Disorder (142)
Note: See the criteria set and corresponding recording procedures for substance-specific coded and ICD-9-CM and ICD-10-CM coding.
Specify if: With onset during intoxication, With onset during withdrawal
293.83 (—.—) Bipolar and Related Disorder Due to Another Medical Condition (145)
Specify if:
(F06.33) With manic features
(F06.33) With manic- or hypomanic-like episode
(F06.33) With mixed features
296.89 (F31.89) Other specified Bipolar and Related Disorder (148)
296.80 (F31.9) Unspecified Bipolar and Related Disorder (149)

DEPRESSIVE DISORDERS (155)

The following specifiers apply to Depressive Disorders where indicated:

[a]*Specify*: With anxious distress (*specify* current severity: mild, moderate, moderate-severe, severe); With mixed features; With melancholic features; With atypical features; With mood-congruent psychotic features; With mood-incongruent psychotic features; With catatonia (use additional code 293.89 [F06.1]); With peripartum onset; With seasonal pattern

296.99 (F34.8] Disruptive Mood Dysregulation Disorder (156)
—.— (—.—) Major Depressive Disorder[a] (160)
—.— (—.—) Single episode
296.21 (F32.0) Mild
296.22 (F32.1) Moderate
296.23 (F32.2) Severe
296.24 (F32.3) With psychotic features
296.25 (F32.4) In partial remission
296.26 (F32.5) In full remission
296.20 (F32.9) Unspecified
—.— (—.—) Recurrent episode
296.31 (F33.0) Mild
296.32 (F33.1) Moderate
296.33 (F33.2) Severe
296.34 (F33.3) With psychotic features
296.35 (F33.41) In partial remission
296.36 (F33.42) In full remission
296.30 (F33.9) Unspecified
300.4 (F34.1) Persistent Depressive Disorder (Dysthymia)[a] (168)
Specify if: In partial remission, In full remission
Specify if: Early onset, Late onset
Specify if: With pure dysthymic syndrome; With persistent major depressive episode; With intermittent major depressive episodes, with current episode; With intermittent major depressive episodes, without current episode
Specify current severity: Mild, Moderate, Severe
625.4 (N94.3) Premenstrual Dysphoric Disorder (171)
—.— (—.—) Substance/Medication-Induced Depressive Disorder (175)
Note: See the criteria set and corresponding recording procedures for substance-specific codes and ICD-9-CM and ICD-10-CM coding.
Specify if: With onset during intoxication, With onset during withdrawal
293.83 (—.—) Depressive Disorder Due to Another Medical Condition (180)
Specify if:
(F06.31) With depressive features
(F06.32) With major depressive-like episode
(F06.34) With mixed features
311 (F32.8) Other Specified Depressive Disorder (183)
311 (F32.9) Unspecified Depressive Disorder (184)

ANXIETY DISORDERS (189)

309.21 (F93.0) Separation Anxiety Disorder (190)
312.23 (F94.0) Selective Mutism (195)

300.29 (—.—) Specific Phobia (197)
Specify if:
(F40.218) Animal
(F40.228) Natural environmental
(—.—) Blood-injection-injury
(F40.230) Fear of blood
(F40.231) Fear of injections and transfusions
(F40.232) Fear of other medical care
(F40.233) Fear of injury
(F40.248) Situational
(F40.298) Other

300.23 **(F40.10)** Social Anxiety Disorder (Social Phobia) (202)
Specify if: Performance only

300.01 **(F41.0)** Panic Disorder (208)

—.— (—.—) Panic Attack Specifier (214)

300.22 **(F40.00)** Agoraphobia (217)

300.02 **(F41.1)** Generalized Anxiety Disorder (222)

—.— (—.—) Substance/Medication-Induced Anxiety Disorder (226)
Note: See the criteria set and corresponding recording procedures for substance-specific codes and ICD-9-CM and ICD-10-CM coding.
Specify if: With onset during intoxication, With onset during withdrawal, With onset after medication use

293.84 **(F06.4)** Anxiety Disorder Due to Another Medical Condition (230)

300.09 **(F41.8)** Other Specified Anxiety Disorder (233)

300.00 **(F41.9)** Unspecified Anxiety Disorder (233)

OBSESSIVE-COMPULSIVE AND RELATED DISORDERS (235)

The following specifiers apply to Obsessive-Compulsive and Related Disorders where indicated:
[a]*Specify* if: With good or fair insight, With poor insight, With absent insight/delusional beliefs

300.3 **(F42)** Obsessive-Compulsive Disorder[a] (237)
Specify if: Tic-related

300.7 **(F45.22)** Body Dysmorphic Disorder[a] (242)
Specify if: With muscle dysmorphia

300.3 **(F42)** Hoarding Disorder[a] (247)
Specify if: With excessive acquisition

312.39 **(F63.2)** Trichotillomania (Hair-Pulling Disorder) (251)

698.4 **(L98.1)** Excoriation (Skin-Picking) Disorder (254)

—.— (—.—) Substance/Medication-Induced Obsessive-Compulsive and Related Disorder (257)
Note: See the criteria set and corresponding recording procedures for substance-specific codes and ICD-9-CM and ICD-10-CM coding.
Specify if: With onset during intoxication, With onset during withdrawal, With onset after medication use

294.8 **(F06.8)** Obsessive-Compulsive and Related Disorder Due to Another Medical Condition (260)
Specify if: With obsessive-compulsive disorder-like symptoms, With appearance preoccupations, With hoarding symptoms, With hair-pulling symptoms, With skin-picking symptoms

300.3 **(F42)** Other Specified Obsessive-Compulsive and Related Disorder (263)

300.3 **(F42)** Unspecified Obsessive-Compulsive and Related Disorder (264)

TRAUMA- AND STRESSOR-RELATED DISORDERS (265)

313.89 **(F94.1)** Reactive Attachment Disorder (265)
Specify if: Persistent
Specify current severity: Severe

313.89 **(F94.2)** Disinhibited Social Engagement Disorder (268)
Specify if: Persistent
Specify current severity: Severe

309.81 **(F43.10)** Posttraumatic Stress Disorder (includes Posttraumatic Stress Disorder for Children 6 Years and Younger) (271)
Specify whether: With dissociative symptoms
Specify if: With delayed expression

308.3 **(F43.0)** Acute Stress Disorder (280)

—.— (—.—) Adjustment Disorder (286)
Specify whether:
309.0 **(F43.21)** With depressed mood
309.24 **(F43.22)** With anxiety
309.28 **(F43.23)** With mixed anxiety and depressed mood
309.3 **(F43.24)** With disturbance of conduct
309.4 **(F43.25)** With mixed disturbance of emotions and conduct
309.9 **(F43.20)** Unspecified

309.89 **(F43.8)** Other Specified Trauma- and Stressor-Related Disorder (289)

309.9 **(F43.9)** Unspecified Trauma- and Stressor-Related Disorder (290)

DISSOCIATIVE DISORDERS (291)

300.14 **(F44.81)** Dissociative Identity Disorder (292)

300.12 **(F44.0)** Dissociative Amnesia (298)
Specify if:
300.13 **(F44.1)** With dissociative fugue

300.6 **(F48.1)** Depersonalization/Derealization Disorder (302)

300.15 **(F44.89)** Other Specified Dissociative Disorder (306)

300.15 **(F44.9)** Unspecified Dissociative Disorder (307)

SOMATIC SYMPTOM AND RELATED DISORDERS (309)

300.82 **(F45.1)** Somatic Symptom Disorder (311)
Specify if: With predominant pain
Specify if: Persistent
Specify current severity: Mild, Moderate Severe

300.7 **(F45.21)** Illness Anxiety Disorder (315)
Specify whether: Care seeking type, Care avoidant type

300.11 **(—.—)** Conversion Disorder (Functional Neurological Symptom Disorder) (318)
Specify symptom type:
(F44.4) With weakness or paralysis
(F44.4) With abnormal movement
(F44.4) With swallowing symptoms
(F44.4) With speech symptom
(F44.5) With attacks or seizures
(F44.6) With anesthesia or sensory loss
(F44.6) With special sensory symptom
(F44.7) With mixed symptoms
Specify if: Acute episode, Persistent
Specify if: With psychological stressor (specify stressor), Without psychological stressor

316 **(F54)** Psychological Factors Affecting Other Medical Conditions (322)
Specify current severity: Mild, Moderate, Severe, Extreme

300.19 **(F68.10)** Factitious Disorder (includes Factitious Disorder Imposed on Self, Factitious Disorder Imposed on Another) (324)
Specify Single episode, Recurrent episodes

300.89 **(F45.8)** Other Specified Somatic Symptom and Related Disorder (327)

300.82 **(F45.9)** Unspecified Somatic Symptom and Related Disorder (327)

FEEDING AND EATING DISORDERS (329)

The following specifiers apply to Feeding and Eating Disorders where indicated:
[a]*Specify* if: In remission
[b]*Specify* if: In partial remission, In full remission
[c]*Specify* current severity: Mild, Moderate, Severe Extreme

307.52 **(—.—)** Pica[a] (329)
(F98.3) In children
(F50.8) In adults

307.53 **(F98.21)** Rumination Disorder[a] (332)

307.59 **(F50.8)** Avoidant/Restrictive Food Intake Disorder[a] (334)

307.1 **(—.—)** Anorexia Nervosa[b,c] (338)
Specify whether:
(F50.01) Restricting type
(F50.02) Binge-eating/purging type

307.51 **(F50.2)** Bulimia Nervosa[b,c] (345)

307.51 **(F50.8)** Binge-Eating Disorder[b,c] (350)

307.59 **(F50.8)** Other Specified Feeding or Eating Disorder (353)

307.50 **(F50.9)** Unspecified Feeding or Eating Disorder (354)

ELIMINATION DISORDERS (355)

307.6 **(F98.0)** Enuresis (355)
Specify whether: Nocturnal only, Diurnal only, Nocturnal and diurnal

307.7 **(F98.1)** Encopresis (357)
Specify whether: With constipation and overflow incontinence, Without constipation and overflow incontinence

—.— **(—.—)** Other Specified Elimination Disorder (359)
788.39 **(N39.498)** With urinary symptoms
787.60 **(R15.9)** With fecal symptoms

—.— **(—.—)** Unspecified Elimination Disorder (360)
788.30 **(R32)** With urinary symptoms
787.60 **(R15.9)** With fecal symptoms

SLEEP-WAKE DISORDERS (361)

The following specifiers apply to Sleep-Wake Disorders where indicated:
[a]*Specify* if: Episodic, Persistent, Recurrent
[b]*Specify* if: Acute, Subacute, Persistent
[c]*Specify* current severity: Mild, Moderate, Severe

780.52 **(G47.00)** Insomnia Disorder[a] (362)
Specify if: With non-sleep disorder mental comorbidity, With other medical comorbidity, With other sleep disorder

780.54 **(G47.10)** Hypersomnolence Disorder[b,c] (368)
Specify if: With mental disorder, With medical condition, With another sleep disorder

—.— **(—.—)** Narcolepsy[c] (372)
Specify whether:
347.00 **(G47.419)** Narcolepsy without cataplexy but with hypocretin deficiency
347.01 **(G47.411)** Narcolepsy with cataplexy but without hypocretin deficiency
347.00 **(G47.419)** Autosomal dominant cerebellar ataxia, deafness, and narcolepsy
347.00 **(G47.419)** Autosomal dominant narcolepsy, obesity, and type 2 diabetes
347.10 **(G47.429)** Narcolepsy secondary to another medical condition

Breathing-Related Sleep Disorders (378)

327.23 **(G47.33)** Obstructive Sleep Apnea Hypopnea[c] (378)

—.— **(—.—)** Central Sleep Apnea (383)
Specify whether:
327.21 **(G47.31)** Idiopathic central sleep apnea

786.04 **(R06.3)** Cheyne-Stokes breathing

780.57 **(G47.37)** Central sleep apnea comorbid with opioid use

Note: First code opioid use disorder, if present.

Specify current severity

—.— (—.—) Sleep-Related Hypoventilation (387)

Specify whether:

327.24 **(G473.34)** Idiopathic hypoventilation

327.25 **(G47.35)** Congenital central alveolar hypoventilation

327.26 **(G47.36)** Comorbid sleep-related hypoventilation

Specify current severity

—.— (—.—) Circadian Rhythm Sleep-Wake Disorders[a] (390)

Specify whether:

307.45 **(G47.21)** Delayed sleep phase type (391)

Specify if: Familial, Overlapping with non-24-hour sleep-wake type

307.45 **(G47.22)** Advanced sleep phase type (393)

Specify if: Familial

307.45 **(G47.23)** Irregular sleep-wake type (394)

307.45 **(G47.24)** Non-24-hour sleep-wake type (396)

307.45 **(G47.26)** Shift work type (397)

307.45 **(G47.20)** Unspecified type

Parasomnias (399)

—.— (—.—) Non–Rapid Eye Movement Sleep Arousal Disorders (399)

Specify whether:

307.46 **(F51.3)** Sleepwalking type

Specify if: With sleep-related eating, With sleep-related sexual behavior (sexsomnia)

307.46 **(F51.4)** Sleep terror type

307.47 **(F51.5)** Nightmare Disorder[b,c] (404)

Specify if: During sleep onset

Specify if: With associated non–sleep disorder, With associated other medical condition, With associated other sleep disorder

327.42 **(G473.52)** Rapid Eye Movement Sleep Behavior Disorder (407)

333.94 **(G25.81)** Restless Legs Syndrome (410)

—.— (—.—) Substance/Medication-Induced Sleep Disorder (413)

Note: See the criteria set and corresponding recording procedures for substance-specific codes and ICD-9-CM and ICD-10-CM coding.

Specify whether: Insomnia type, Daytime sleepiness type, Parasomnia type, Mixed type

Specify if: With onset during intoxication, With onset during discontinuation/withdrawal

780.52 **(G47.09)** Other Specified Insomnia Disorder (420)

780.52 **(G47.00)** Unspecified Insomnia Disorder (420)

780.54 **(G47.19)** Other Specified Hypersomnolence Disorder (421)

780.54 **(G47.10)** Unspecified Hypersomnolence Disorder (421)

780.59 **(G47.8)** Other Specified Sleep-Wake Disorder (421)

780.59 **(G47.9)** Unspecified Sleep-Wake Disorder (422)

SEXUAL DYSFUNCTIONS (423)

The following specifiers apply to Sexual Dysfunctions where indicated:

[a]*Specify* whether: Lifelong, Acquired

[b]*Specify* whether: Generalized, Situational

[c]*Specify* current severity: Mild, Moderate, Severe

302.74 **(F52.32)** Delayed Ejaculation[a,b,c] (424)

302.72 **(F52.21)** Erectile Disorder[a,b,c] (426)

302.73 **(F52.31)** Female Orgasmic Disorder[a,b,c] (429)

Specify if: Never experienced an orgasm under any situation

302.72 **(F52.22)** Female Sexual Interest/Arousal Disorder[a,b,c] (433)

302.76 **(F52.6)** Genito-Pelvic Pain/Penetration Disorder[a,c] (437)

302.71 **(F52.0)** Male Hypoactive Sexual Desire Disorder[a,b,c] (440)

302.75 **(F52.4)** Premature (Early) Ejaculation[a,b,c] (443)

—.— (—.—) Substance/Medication-Induced Sexual Dysfunction[c] (446)

Note: See the criteria and corresponding recording procedures for substance-specific codes and ICD-9-CM and ICD-10-CM coding.

Specify if: With onset during intoxication, With onset during withdrawal, With onset after medication use

302.79 **(F52.8)** Other Specified Sexual Dysfunction (450)

302.70 **(F52.9)** Unspecified Sexual Dysfunction (450)

GENDER DYSPHORIA (451)

—.— (—.—) Gender Dysphoria (452)

302.6 **(F64.2)** Gender Dysphoria in Children

Specify if: With a disorder of sex development

302.85 **(F64.1)** Gender Dysphoria in Adolescents and Adults

Specify if: With a disorder of sex development

Specify if: Posttransition

Note: Code the disorder of sex development if present, in addition to gender dysphoria.

302.6 **(F64.8)** Other Specified Gender Dysphoria (459)

302.6 **(F64.)** Unspecified Gender Dysphoria (459)

DISRUPTIVE, IMPULSE-CONTROL, AND CONDUCT DISORDERS (461)

313.81 **(F91.3)** Oppositional Defiant Disorder (462)
Specify current severity: Mild, Moderate, Severe
312.34 **(F63.81)** Intermittent Explosive Disorder (466)
—.— (—.—) Conduct Disorder (469)
Specify whether:
312.81 **(F91.1)** Childhood-onset type
312.32 **(F91.2)** Adolescent-onset type
312.89 **(F91.9)** Unspecified onset
Specify if: With limited prosocial emotions
Specify current severity: Mild, Moderate, Severe
301.7 **(F60.2)** Antisocial Personality Disorder (476)
312.33 **(F63.1)** Pyromania (476)
312.32 **(F63.3)** Kleptomania (478)
312.89 **(F91.8)** Other Specified Disruptive, Impulse-Control, and Conduct Disorder (479)
312.9 **(F91.9)** Unspecified Disruptive, Impulse-Control, and Conduct Disorder (480)

SUBSTANCE-RELATED AND ADDICTIVE DISORDERS (481)

The following specifiers and note apply to Substance-Related and Addictive Disorders where indicated:
[a]*Specify* if: In early remission, In sustained remission
[b]*Specify* if: In a controlled environment
[c]*Specify* if: With perceptual disturbances
[d]The ICD-10-CM code indicated the comorbid presence of a moderate or severe substance use disorder, which must be present in order to apply the code for substance withdrawal.

Substance-Related Disorders (483)

Alcohol-Related Disorders (490)

—.— (—.—) Alcohol Use Disorder[a,b] (490)
Specify current severity:
305.00 **(F10.10)** Mild
303.90 **(F10.20)** Moderate
303.90 **(F10.20)** Severe
303.00 (—.—) Alcohol Intoxication (497)
(F10.129) With use disorder, mild
(F10.229) With use disorder, moderate or severe
(F10.929) Without use disorder
291.81 (—.—) Alcohol Withdrawal[c,d] (499)
(F10.239) Without perceptual disturbances
(F10.232) With perceptual disturbances
—.— (—.—) Other Alcohol-Induced Disorder (502)
291.9 **(F10.99)** Unspecified Alcohol-Related Disorder (503)

Caffeine-Related Disorders (503)

305.90 **(F15.929)** Caffeine Intoxication (503)
292.0 **(F15.93)** Caffeine Withdrawal (506)
—.— (—.—) Other Caffeine-Induced Disorder (508)
292.9 **(F15.99)** Unspecified Caffeine-Related Disorder (509)

Cannabis-Related Disorders (509)

—.— (—.—) Cannabis Use Disorder[a,b] (509)
Specify current severity:
305.20 **(F12.10)** Mild
304.30 **(F12.20)** Moderate
304.30 **(F12.20)** Severe
292.89 (—.—) Cannabis Intoxication[c] (516)
Without perceptual disturbances
(F12.129) With use disorder, mild
(F12.229) With use disorder, moderate or severe
(F12.929) Without use disorder
With perceptual disturbances
(F12.122) With use disorder, mild
(F12.222) With use disorder, moderate or severe
(F12.922) Without use disorder
292.0 **(F12.288)** Cannabis Withdrawal[d] (517)
—.— (—.—) Other Cannabis-Induced disorders (519)
292.9 **(F12.99)** Unspecified Cannabis-Related Disorder (519)

Hallucinogen-Related Disorders (520)

—.— (—.—) Phencyclidine Use Disorder[a,b] (520)
Specify current severity:
305.90 **(F16.10)** Mild
304.60 **(F16.20)** Moderate
304.60 **(F16.20)** Severe
—.— (—.—) Other Hallucinogen Use Disorder[a,b] (523)
Specify the particular hallucinogen
Specify current severity:
305.30 **(F16.10)** Mild
304.50 **(F16.20)** Moderate
304.50 **(F16.20)** Severe
292.89 (—.—) Phencyclidine Intoxication (527)
(F16.129) With use disorder, mild
(F16.229) With use disorder, moderate or severe
(F16.292) Without use disorder
292.89 (—.—) Other Hallucinogen Intoxication (529)
(F16.129) With use disorder, mild
(F16.229) With use disorder, moderate or severe
(F16.929) Without use disorder
292.89 **(F16.983)** Hallucinogen Persisting Perception Disorder (531)
—.— (—.—) Other Phencyclidine-Induced Disorder (532)
—.— (—.—) Other Hallucinogen-Induced Disorder (532)
292.9 **(F16.99)** Unspecified Phencyclidine-Related Disorder (533)
292.9 **(F16.99)** Unspecified Hallucinogen-Related Disorder (533)

Inhalant-Related Disorder (533)

—.— (—.—) Inhalant Use Disorder[a,b] (533)
Specify the particular inhalant
Specify current severity:
305.90 **(F18.10)** Mild

ICD-9-CM	ICD-10-CM	
304.60	(F18.20)	Moderate
304.60	(F18.20)	Severe
292.89	(—.—)	Inhalant Intoxication (538)
	(F18.129)	With use disorder, mild
	(F18.229)	With use disorder, moderate or severe
	(F18.929)	Without use disorder
—.—	(—.—)	Other Inhalant-Induced Disorder (540)
292.9	(F18.99)	Unspecified Inhalant-Related Disorder (540)

Opioid-Related Disorders (540)

ICD-9-CM	ICD-10-CM	
—.—	(—.—)	Opioid Use Disorder[a] (541)
		Specify if: On maintenance therapy, In a controlled environment
		Specify current severity:
305.50	(F11.10)	Mild
304.00	(F11.20)	Moderate
304.00	(F11.20)	Severe
292.89	(—.—)	Opioid Intoxication[c] (546)
		Without perceptual disturbances
	(F11.129)	With use disorder, mild
	(F11.229)	With use disorder, moderate or severe
	(F11.929)	Without use disorder
		With perceptual disturbances
	(F11.122)	With use disorder, mild
	(F11.222)	With use disorder, moderate or severe
	(F11.922)	Without use disorder
292.0	(F11.23)	Opioid Withdrawal[d] (547)
—.—	(—.—)	Other Opioid-Induced Disorder (549)
292.9	(F11.99)	Unspecified Opioid-Related Disorder (550)

Sedative-, Hynotic-, or Anxiolytic-Related Disorders (550)

ICD-9-CM	ICD-10-CM	
—.—	(—.—)	Sedative, Hypnotic, or Anxiolytic Ue Disorder[a,b] (550)
		Specify current severity:
305.40	(F13.10)	Mild
304.10	(F13.20)	Moderate
304.10	(F13.20)	Severe
292.89	(—.—)	Sedative, Hypnotic, or Anxiolytic Intoxication (556)
	(F13.129)	With use disorder, mild
	(F13.229)	With use disorder, moderate or severe
	(F13.929)	Without use disorder
292.0	(—.—)	Sedative, Hypnotic, or Anxiolytic Withdrawal[c,d] (557)
	(F13.229)	Without perceptual disturbances
	(F13.232)	With perceptual disturbances
—.—	(—.—)	Other Sedative-, Hypnotic-, or Anxiolytic-Induced Disorder (560)
292.9	(F13.99)	Unspecified Sedative-, Hypnotic-, or Anxiolytic-Related Disorder (560)

Stimulant-Related Disorders (561)

ICD-9-CM	ICD-10-CM	
—.—	(—.—)	Stimulant Use Disorder[a,b] (561)
		Specify current severity:
—.—	(—.—)	Mild
305.70	(F15.10)	Amphetamine-type substance
305.60	(F14.10)	Cocaine
305.70	(F15.10)	Other or unspecified stimulant
—.—	(—.—)	Moderate
304.40	(F15.20)	Amphetamine-type substance
304.20	(F14.20)	Cocaine
304.40	(F15.20)	Other or unspecified stimulant
—.—	(—.—)	Severe
304.40	(F15.20)	Amphetamine-type substance
304.20	(F14.20)	Cocaine
304.40	(F15.20)	Other or unspecified stimulant
292.89	(—.—)	Stimulant Intoxication[c] (567)
		Specify the specific intoxicant
292.89	(—.—)	Amphetamine or other stimulant, Without perceptual disturbances
	(F15.129)	With use disorder, mild
	(F15.229)	With use disorder, moderate or severe
	(F15.929)	Without use disorder
292.89	(—.—)	Cocaine, Without perceptual disturbances
	(F14.129)	With use disorder, mild
	(F14.229)	With use disorder, moderate or severe
	(F14.929)	Without use disorder
292.89	(—.—)	Amphetamine or other stimulant, With perceptual disturbances
	(F15.122)	With use disorder, mild
	(F15.222)	With use disorder, moderate or severe
	(F15.922)	Without use disorder
292.89	(—.—)	Cocaine, With perceptual disturbances
	(F14.122)	With use disorder, mild
	(F14.222)	Without use disorder, moderate or severe
	(F14.922)	Without use disorder
292.0	(—.—)	Stimulant Withdrawal[d] (569)
		Specify the specific substance causing the withdrawal syndrome
	(F15.23)	Amphetamine or other stimulant
	(F14.23)	Cocaine
—.—	(—.—)	Other Stimulant-Induced Disorder (570)
292.9	(—.—)	Unspecified Stimulant-Related Disorder (570)
	(F15.99)	Amphetamine or other stimulant
	(F14.99)	Cocaine

Tobacco-Related Disorders (571)

ICD-9-CM	ICD-10-CM	
—.—	(—.—)	Tobacco Use Disorder[a] (571)
		Specify if: On maintenance therapy, In a controlled environment
		Specify current severity:
305.1	(Z72.0)	Mild
305.1	(F17.200)	Moderate
305.1	(F17.200)	Severe
292.0	(F17.203)	Tobacco Withdrawal[d] (575)
—.—	(—.—)	Other Tobacco-Induced Disorder (576)
292.9	(F17.209)	Unspecified Tobacco-Related Disorder (577)

Other (or Unknown) Substance-Related Disorders (577)

—.— (—.—) Other (or Unknown) Substance Use Disorder[a,b] (577)
Specify current severity:
305.90 (F19.10) Mild
304.90 (F19.20) Moderate
304.90 (F19.20) Severe
292.89 (—.—) Other (or Unknown) Substance Intoxication (581)
(F19.129) With use disorder, mild
(F19.229) With use disorder, moderate or severe
(F19.229) Without use disorder
292.0 (F19.23) Other (or Unknown) Substance Withdrawal[d] (583)
—.— (—.—) Other (or Unknown) Substance–Induced Disorders (584)
292.2 (F19.99) Unspecified Other (or Unknown) Substance–Related Disorder (585)

Non-Substance-Related Disorders (585)

312.31 (F63.0) Gambling Disorder[a] (585)
Specify if: Episodic, Persistent
Specify current severity: Mild, Moderate, Severe

NEUROCOGNITIVE DISORDERS (591)

—.— (—.—) Delirium (596)
[a]**Note:** See the criteria set and corresponding recording procedures for substance-specific codes and ICD-9-CM and ICD-10-CM coding.
Specify whether:
—.— (—.—) Substance intoxication delirium[a]
—.— (—.—) Substance withdrawal delirium[a]
292.81 (—.—) Medication-induced delirium[a]
293.0 (F05) Delirium due to another medical condition
293.0 (F05) Delirium due to multiple etiologies
Specify if: Acute, Persistent
Specify if: Hyperactive, Hypoactive, Mixed level of activity
780.09 (R41.0) Other Specified Delirium (602)
780.09 (R41.0) Unspecified Delirium (602)

Major and Mild Neurocognitive Disorders (602)

Specify whether due to: Alzheimer's disease, Frontotemporal lobar degeneration, Lewy body disease, Vascular disease, Traumatic brain injury, Substance/medication use, HIV infection, Prion disease, Parkinson's disease, Huntington's disease, Another medical condition, Multiple etiologies, Unspecified

[a]*Specify* Without behavioral disturbance, With behavioral disturbance. *For possible major neurocognitive disorder and for mild neurocognitive disorder, behavioral disturbance cannot be coded but should still be indicated in writing.*

[b]*Specify* current severity: Mild, Moderate, Severe. *This specifier applies only to major neurocognitive disorder (including probable and possible).*

Note: As indicated for each subtype, an additional medical code is needed for probable major neurocognitive disorder or major neurocognitive disorder. An additional medical code should *not* be used for possible major neurocognitive disorder or mild neurocognitive disorder.

Major or Mild Neurocognitive Disorder Due to Alzheimer's Disease (611)

—.— (—.—) Probable Major Neurocognitive disorder Due to Alzheimer's Disease[b]
Note: Code first **331.0 (G30.9)** Alzheimer's disease
294.11 (F02.81) With behavioral disturbance
294.10 (F02.80) Without behavioral disturbance
331.9 (G31.9) Possible Major Neurocognitive Disorder Due to Alzheimer's Disease[a,b]
331.83 (G31.84) Mild Neurocognitive Disorder Due to Alzheimer's Disease[a]

Major or Mild Frontotemporal Neurocognitive Disorder (614)

—.— (—.—) Probable Major Neurocognitive Disorder Due to Frontotemporal Labor Degeneration[b]
Note: Code first **331.19 (G31.09)** frontotemporal disease.
294.11 (F02.81) With behavioral disturbance
294.10 (F02.80) Without behavioral disturbance
331.9 (G31.9) Possible Major Neurocognitive Disorder Due to Frontotemporal Labor Degeneration[a,b]
331.83 (G31.84) Mild Neurocognitive Disorder Due to Frontotemporal Labor Degeneration[a]

Major or Mild Neurocognitive Disorder with Lewy Bodies (618)

—.— (—.—) Probable Major Neurocognitive Disorder With Lewy Bodies[b]
Note: Code first **331.82 (G31.83)** Lewy body disease.
294.11 (F02.81) With behavioral disturbance
294.10 (F02.80) Without behavioral disturbance
331.9 (G31.9) Possible Major Neurocognitive Disorder With Lewy Bodies[a,b]
331.83 (G31.84) Mild Neurocognitive Disorder With Lewy Bodies[a]

Major or Mild Vascular Neurocognitive Disorder (621)

—.— (—.—) Probable Major Vascular Neurocognitive Disorder[b]
Note: No additional medical code for vascular disease.
290.40 (F01.51) With behavioral disturbance
290.40 (F01.50) Without behavioral disturbance

331.9 (G31.9) Possible Major Vascular Neurocognitive Disorder[a,b]
331.83 (G31.84) Mild Vascular Neurocognitive Disorder[a]

Major or Mild Neurocognitive Disorder Due to Traumatic Brain Injury (624)

—.— (—.—) Major Neurocognitive Disorder due to Traumatic Brain Injury[b]
Note: For ICD-9-CM, code first **907.0** late effect of intracranial injury without skull fracture. For ICD-10-CM, code first **S06.2X9S** diffuse traumatic brain injury with loss of consciousness of unspecified duration, sequela.
294.11 (**F02.81**) With behavioral disturbance
294.10 (**F02.80**) Without behavioral disturbance
331.83 (**G31.84**) Mild Neurocognitive Disorder Due to Traumatic Brain Injury[a]

Substance/Medication-Induced Major or Mild Neurocognitive Disorder[a] (627)

Note: No additional medical code. See the criteria set and corresponding recording procedures for substance-specific codes and ICD-9-CM and ICD-10-CM coding.
Specify if: Persistent

Major or Mild Neurocognitive Disorder Due to HIV Infection (632)

—.— (—.—) Major Neurocogntive Disorder Due to HIV Infection[b]
Note: Code first **042** (**B20**) HIV infection.
294.11 (**F02.81**) With behavioral disturbance
294.10 (**F02.80**) Without behavioral disturbance
331.83 (**G31.84**) Mild Neurocognitive Disorder Due to HIV Infection[a]

Major or Mild Neurocognitive Disorder Due to Prion Disease (634)

—.— (—.—) Major Neurocognitvie Disorder Due to Prion Disease[b]
Note: Code first **046.79** (**A81.9**) prion disease.
294.11 (**F02.81**) With behavioral disturbance
294.10 (**F02.80**) Without behavioral disturbance
331.83 (**G31.84**) Mild Neurocognitive Disorder Due to Prion Disease[a]

Major or Mild Neurocognitive Disorder Due to Parkinson's Disease (636)

—.— (—.—) Major Neurocognitive Disorder Probably Due to Parkinson's Disease[b]
Note: Code first **332.0** (**G20**) Parkinson's disease.
294.11 (**F02.81**) With behavioral disturbance
294.10 (**F02.80**) Without behavioral disturbance
331.9 (**G31.9**) Major Neurocognitive Disorder Possibly Due to Parkinson's Disease[a,b]
331.83 (**G31.84**) Mild Neurocognitive Disorder Due to Parkinson's Disease[a]

Major or Mild Neurocognitive Disorder Due to Huntington's Disease (638)

—.— (—.—) Major Neurocognitive Disorder Due to Huntington's Disease[b]
Note: Code first **333.4** (**G10**) Huntington's disease.
294.11 (**F02.81**) With behavioral disturbance
294.10 (**F02.80**) Without behavioral disturbance
331.83 (**G31.84**) Mild Neurocognitive Disorder Due to Huntington's Disease[a]

Major or Mild Neurocognitive Disorder Due to Another Medical Condition[a] (641)

—.— (—.—) Major Neurocognitive Disorder Due to Another Medical Condition[b]
Note: Code first the other medical condition.
294.11 (**F02.81**) With behavioral disturbance
294.10 (**F02.80**) Without behavioral disturbance
331.83 (**G31.84**) Mild Neurocognitive Disorder Due to Another Medical Condition[a]

Major or Mild Neurocognitive Disorder Due to Multiple Etiologies (642)

—.—. (—.—) Major Neurocognitive Disorder Due to Multiple Etiologies[b]
Note: Code first all the etiological medical conditions (with the exception of vascular disease).
294.11 (**F02.81**) With behavioral disturbance
294.10 (**F02.80**) Without behavioral disturbance
331.83 (**G31.84**) Mild Neurocognitive Disorder Due to Multiple Etiologies[a]

Unspecified Neurocognitive Disorder (643)

799.59 (**R41.9**) Unspecified Neurocognitive Disorder[a]

PERSONALITY DISORDERS (645)

Cluster A Personality Disorders

301.0 (**F60.0**) Paranoid Personality Disorder (649)
301.20 (**F60.1**) Schizoid Personality Disorder (652)
301.22 (**F21**) Schizotypal Personality Disorder (655)

Cluster B Personality Disorders

301.7 (**F60.2**) Antisocial Personality Disorder (659)
301.83 (**F60.3**) Borderline Personality Disorder (663)
301.50 (**F60.4**) Histrionic Personality Disorder (667)
301.81 (**F60.81**) Narcissistic Personality Disorder (669)

Cluster C Personality Disorders

301.82 (**F60.6**) Avoidant Personality Disorder (672)
301.6 (**F60.7**) Dependent Personality Disorder (675)
301.4 (**F60.5**) Obsessive-Compulsive Personality Disorder (678)

Other Personality Disorders

310.1 **(F07.0)** Personality Change Due to Another Medical Condition (682)
Specify whether: Labile type, Disinhibited type, Aggressive type, Apathetic type, Paranoid type, Other type, Combined type, Unspecified type

301.89 **(F60.89)** Other Specified Personality Disorder (684)

301.9 **(F60.9)** Unspecified Personality Disorder (684)

PARAPHILIC DISORDERS (685)

The following specifier applies to Paraphilic Disorders where indicated:
[a]*Specify* if: In a controlled environment, In full remission

302.82 **(F65.3)** Voyeuristic Disorder[a] (686)

302.4 **(F65.2)** Exhibitionistic Disorder[a] (689)
Specify whether: Sexuallly aroused by exposing genitals to prepubertal children, Sexually aroused by exposing genitals to physically mature individuals, Sexually aroused by exposing genitals to prepubertal children and to physically mature individuals

302.89 **(F65.81)** Frotteuristic Disorder[a] (691)

302.83 **(F65.51)** Sexual Masochism Disorder[a] (694)
Specify if: With asphyxiophilia

302.84 **(F65.52)** Sexual Sadism Disorder[a] (695)

302.2 **(F65.4)** Pedophilic Disorder (697)
Specify whether: Exclusive type, Nonexclusive type
Specify if: Sexually attracted to males, Sexually attracted to females, Sexually attracted to both
Specify if: Limited to incest

302.81 **(F65.0)** Fetishistic Disorder[a] (700)
Specify: Body part(s), Nonliving object(s), Other

302.3 **(F65.1)** Transvestic Disorder[a] (702)
Specify if: With fetishism, With autogynephilia

302.89 **(F65.89)** Other Specified Paraphilic Disorder (705)

302.9 **(F65.9)** Unspecified Paraphilic Disorder (705)

OTHER MENTAL DISORDERS (707)

294.8 **(F06.8)** Other Specified Mental Disorder Due to Another Medical Condition (707)

294.9 **(F09)** Unspecified Mental Disorder Due to Another Medical Condition (708)

300.9 **(F99)** Other Specified Mental Disorder (708)

300.9 **(F99)** Unspecified Mental Disorder (708)

MEDICATION-INDUCED MOVEMENT DISORDERS AND OTHER ADVERSE EFFECTS OF MEDICATION (709)

332.1 **(G21.11)** Neuroleptic-Induced Parkinsonism (709)

332.1 **(G21.19)** Other Medication-Induced Parkinsonism (709)

333.92 **(G21.0)** Neuroleptic Malignant Syndrome (709)

333.72 **(G24.02)** Medication-Induced Acute Dystonia (711)

333.99 **(G25.71)** Medication-Induced Acute Akathisia (711)

333.85 **(G24.01)** Tardive Dyskinesia (712)

333.72 **(G24.09)** Tardive Dystonia (712)

333.99 **(G25.71)** Tardive Akathisia (712)

333.1 **(G25.1)** Medication-Induced Postural Tremor (712)

333.99 **(G25.79)** Other Medication-Induced Movement Disorder (712)

—.— **(—.—)** Antidepressant Discontinuation Syndrome (712)
995.29 **(T43.205A)** Initial encounter
995.29 **(T43.205D)** Subsequent encounter
995.29 **(T43.205S)** Sequelae

—.— **(—.—)** Other Adverse Effect of Medication (714)
995.20 **(T50.905A)** Initial encounter
995.20 **(T50.905D)** Subsequent encounter
995.20 **(T50.905S)** Sequelae

OTHER CONDITIONS THAT MAY BE A FOCUS OF CLINICAL ATTENTION (715)

Relational Problems (715)

Problems Related to Family Upbringing (715)

V61.20 **(Z62.820)** Parent-Child Relational Problem (715)

V61.8 **(Z62.891)** Sibling Relational Problem (716)

V61.8 **(Z62.29)** Upbringing Away From Parents (716)

V61.29 **(Z62.898)** Child Affected by Parental Relationship Distress (716)

Other Problems Related to Primary Support Group (716)

V61.10 **(Z63.0)** Relationship Distress With Spouse or Intimate Partner (716)

V61.03 **(Z63.5)** Disruption of Family by Separation or Divorce (716)

V61.8 **(Z63.8)** High Expressed Emotion Level Within Family (716)

V62.82 **(Z63.4)** Uncomplicated Bereavement (716)

Abuse and Neglect (717)

Child Maltreatment and Neglect Problems (717)

Child Physical Abuse (717)

Child Physical Abuse, Confirmed (717)
995.54 **(T743.12XA)** Initial encounter
995.54 **(T74.12XD)** Subsequent encounter

Child Physical Abuse, Suspected (717)
995.54 **(T76.12XA)** Initial encounter
995.54 **(T76.12XD)** Subsequent encounter

Other Circumstances Related to Child Physical Abuse (718)

V61.21 **(Z69.010)** Encounter for mental health services for victim of child abuse by parent

V61.21 **(Z69.020)** Encounter for mental health services for victim of nonparental child abuse

V15.41 **(Z62.810)** Personal history (past history) of physical abuse in childhood

V61.22 **(Z69.011)** Encounter for mental health services for perpetrator of parental child abuse

V62.83 **(Z69.021)** Encounter for mental health services for perpetrator of nonparental child abuse

Child Sexual Abuse (718)

Child Sexual Abuse, Confirmed (718)

995.53 **(T74.22XA)** Initial encounter

995.53 **(T74.22XD)** Subsequent encounter

Child Sexual Abuse, Suspected (718)

995.53 **(T76.22XA)** Initial encounter

995.53 **(T76.22XD)** Subsequent encounter

Other Circumstances Related to Child Sexual Abuse (718)

V61.21 **(Z69.010)** Encounter for mental health services for victim of child sexual abuse by parent

V61.21 **(Z69.020)** Encounter for mental health services for victim of nonparental child sexual abuse

V15.21 **(Z62.810)** Personal history (past history) of sexual abuse in childhood

V61.22 **(Z69.011)** Encounter for mental health services for perpetrator of parental child sexual abuse

V62.83 **(Z69.021)** Encounter for mental health services for perpetrator of nonparental child sexual abuse

Child Neglect (718)

Child Neglect, Confirmed (718)

995.52 **(T74.02ZA)** Initial encounter

995.52 **(T74.02XD)** Subsequent encounter

Child Neglect, Suspected (719)

995.52 **(T76.02XA)** Initial encounter

995.52 **(T76.02XD)** Subsequent encounter

Other Circumstances Related to Child Neglect (719)

V61.21 **(Z69.010)** Encounter for mental health services for victim of child neglect by parent

V61.21 **(Z69.020)** Encounter for mental health services for victim of nonparental child neglect

V15.42 **(Z62.812)** Personal history (past history) of neglect in childhood

V61.22 **(Z69.011)** Encounter for mental health services for perpetrator of parental child neglect

V62.83 **(Z69.021)** Encounter for mental health services for perpetrator of nonparental child neglect

Child Psychological Abuse (719)

Child Psychological Abuse, Confirmed (719)

995.51 **(T74.32XA)** Initial encounter

995.51 **(T74.32XD)** Subsequent encounter

Child Psychological Abuse, Suspected (719)

995.51 **(T76.32XA)** Initial encounter

995.51 **(T76.32XD)** Subsequent encounter

Other Circumstances Related to Child Psychological Abuse (719)

V61.21 **(Z69.010)** Encounter for mental health services for victim of child psychological abuse by parent

V61.21 **(Z69.020)** Encounter for mental health services for victim of nonparental child psychological abuse

V15.42 **(Z62.811)** Personal history (past history) of psychological abuse in childhood

V61.22 **(Z69.011)** Encounter for mental health services for perpetrator of parental child psychological abuse

V62.83 **(Z69.021)** Encounter for mental health services for perpetrator of nonparental child psychological abuse

Adult Maltreatment and Neglect Problems (720)

Spouse or Partner Violence, Physical (720)

Spouse or Partner Violence, Physical, Confirmed (720)

995.81 **(T74.11XA)** Initial encounter

995.81 **(T74.11XD)** Subsequent encounter

Spouse or Partner Violence, Physical, Suspected (720)

995.81 **(T76.11XA)** Initial encounter

995.81 **(T76.11XD)** Subsequent encounter

Other Circumstances Related to Spouse or Partner Violence, Physical (720)

V61.11 **(Z96.11)** Encounter for mental health services for victim of spouse or partner violence, physical

V15.41 **(Z91.410)** Personal history (past history) of spouse or partner violence, physical

V61.12 **(Z69.12)** Encounter for mental health services for perpetrator of spouse or partner violence, physical

Spouse or Partner Violence, Sexual (720)

Spouse or Partner Violence, Sexual, Confirmed (720)

995.83 **(T74.21XA)** Initial encounter

995.83 **(T74.21XD)** Subsequent encounter

Spouse or Partner Violence, Sexual, Suspected (720)

995.83 **(T76.21XA)** Initial encounter

995.83 **(T76.21XD)** Subsequent encounter

Other Circumstances Related to Spouse or Partner Violence, Sexual (720)

V61.11 **(Z69.81)** Encounter for mental health services for victim of spouse or partner violence, sexual

V15.41 **(Z91.410)** Personal history (past history) of spouse or partner violence, sexual

V61.12 **(Z69.12)** Encounter for mental health services for perpetrator of spouse or partner violence, sexual

Spouse or Partner Neglect (721)

Spouse or Partner Neglect, Confirmed (721)

995.85 **(T47.01XA)** Initial encounter

995.85 **(T74.01XD)** Subsequent encounter

Spouse or Partner Neglect, Suspected (721)
995.85 **(T76.01XA)** Initial encounter
995.85 **(T76.01XD)** Subsequent encounter
Other Circumstances Related to Spouse or Partner Neglect (721)
V61.11 **(Z69.11)** Encounter for mental health services for victim of spouse or partner neglect
V15.42 **(Z91.412)** Personal history (past history) of spouse or partner neglect
V61.12 **(Z69.12)** Encounter for mental health services for perpetrator of spouse or partner neglect

Spouse or Partner Abuse, Psychological (721)
Spouse or Partner Abuse, Psychological, Confirmed (721)
995.82 **(T74.31XA)** Initial encounter
995.82 **(T74.31XD)** Subsequent encounter
Spouse or Partner Abuse, Psychological, Suspected (721)
995.82 **(T76.31XA)** Initial encounter
995.82 **(T76.31XD)** Subsequent encounter
Other Circumstances Related to Spouse or Partner Abuse, Psychological (721)
V61.11 **(Z69.11)** Encounter for mental health services for victim of spouse or partner psychological abuse
V15.42 **(Z91.411)** Personal history (past history) of spouse or partner psychological abuse
V61.12 **(Z69.12)** Encounter for mental health services for perpetrator of spouse or partner psychological abuse

Adult Abuse by Nonspouse or Nonpartner (722)
Adult Physical Abuse by Nonspouse or Nonpartner, Confirmed (722)
995.81 **(T74.11XA)** Initial encounter
995.81 **(T74.11XD)** Subsequent encounter
Adult Physical Abuse by Nonspouse or Nonpartner, Suspected (722)
995.81 **(T76.11XA)** Initial encounter
995.81 **(T76.11XD)** Subsequent encounter
Adult Sexual Abuse by Nonspouse or Nonpartner, Confirmed (722)
995.83 **(T74.21XA)** Initial encounter
995.83 **(T74.21XD)** Subsequent encounter
Adult Sexual Abuse by Nonspouse or Nonpartner, Suspected (722)
995.83 **(T76.21XA)** Initial encounter
995.83 **(T76.21XD)** Subsequent encounter
Adult Psychological Abuse by Nonspouse or Nonpartner, Confirmed (722)
995.82 **(T74.31XA)** Initial encounter
995.82 **(T74.31XD)** Subsequent encounter
Adult Psychological Abuse by Nonspouse or Nonpartner, Suspected (722)
995.82 **(T76.31XA)** Initial encounter
995.82 **(T76.31XD)** Subsequent encounter
Other Circumstances Related to Adult Abuse by Nonspouse or Nonpartner (722)
V65.49 **(Z69.81)** Encounter for mental health services for victim of nonspousal adult abuse
V62.83 **(Z69.82)** Encounter for mental health services for perpetrator of nonspousal adult abuse

Educational and Occupational Problems (723)

Educational Problems (723)

V62.3 **(Z55.9)** Academic or Educational Problem (723)

Occupational Problems (723)

V62.21 **(Z56.82)** Problem Related to Current Military Deployment Status (723)
V62.29 **(Z56.9)** Other Problem Related to Employment (723)

Housing and Economic Problems (723)

Housing Problems (723)

V60.0 **(Z59.0)** Homelessness (723)
V60.1 **(Z59.1)** Inadequate Housing (723)
V60.89 **(Z59.2)** Discord With Neighbor, Lodger, or Landlord (723)
V60.6 **(Z59.3)** Problem Related to Living in a Residential Institution (724)

Economic Problems (724)

V60.2 **(Z59.4)** Lack of Adequate Food or Safe Drinking Water (724)
V60.2 **(Z59.5)** Extreme Poverty (724)
V60.2 **(Z59.6)** Low Income (724)
V60.2 **(Z59.7)** Insufficient Social Insurance or Welfare Support (724)
V60.9 **(Z59.9)** Unspecified Housing or Economic Problem (724)

Other Problems Related to the Social Environment (724)

V62.89 **(Z60.0)** Phase of Life Problem (724)
V60.3 **(Z60.2)** Problem Related to Living Alone (724)
V62.4 **(Z60.3)** Acculturation Difficulty (724)
V62.4 **(Z60.4)** Social Exclusion or Rejection (724)
V62.4 **(Z60.5)** Target of (Perceived) Adverse Discrimination or Persecution (724)
V62.9 **(Z60.9)** Unspecified Problem Related to Social Environment (725)

Problems Related to Crime or Interaction With the Legal System (725)

V62.879 **(Z65.4)** Victim of Crime (725)
V62.5 **(Z65.0)** Conviction in Civil or Criminal Proceedings Without Imprisonment (725)
V62.5 **(Z65.1)** Imprisonment or Other Incarceration (725)
V62.5 **(Z65.2)** Problems Related to Release From Prison (725)
V62.5 **(Z65.3)** Problems Related to Other Legal Circumstances (725)

Other Health Service Encounters for Counseling and Medical Advice (725)

V65.4 **(Z70.9)** Sex Counseling (725)
V65.40 **(Z71.9)** Other Counseling or Consultation (725)

Problems Related to Other Psychosocial, Personal, and Environmental Circumstances (725)

V62.89 **(Z65.8)** Religious or Spiritual Problem (725)
V61.7 **(Z64.0)** Problems Related to Unwanted Pregnancy (725)
V61.5 **(Z64.1)** Problems Related to Multiparity (725)
V62.89 **(Z64.4)** Discord With Social Service Provider, Including Probation Officer, Case Manager, or Social Service Worker (725)
V62.89 **(Z65.4)** Victim of Terrorism or Torture (725)
V62.22 **(Z65.5)** Exposure to Disaster, War, or Other Hostilities (725)
V62.89 **(Z65.8)** Other Problem Related to Psychosocial Circumstances (725)
V62.9 **(Z65.9)** Unspecified Problem Related to Unspecified Psychosocial Circumstances (725)

Other Circumstances of Personal History (726)

V15.49 **(Z91.49)** Other Personal History of Psychological Trauma (726)
V15.59 **(Z91.5)** Personal History of Self-Harm (726)
V62.22 **(Z91.82)** Personal History of Military Deployment (726)
V15.89 **(Z91.89)** Other Personal Risk Factors (726)
V69.9 **(Z72.9)** Problem Related to Lifestyle (726)
V71.01 **(Z72.811)** Adult Antisocial Behavior (726)
V71.02 **(Z72.810)** Child or Adolescent Antisocial Behavior (726)

Problems Related to Access to Medical and Other Health Care (726)

V63.9 **(Z75.3)** Unavailability or Inaccessibility of Health Care Facilities (726)
V63.8 **(Z75.4)** Unavailability or Inaccessibility of Other Helping Agencies (726)

Nonadherence to Medical Treatment (726)

V15.81 **(Z91.19)** Nonadherence to Medical Treatment (726)
278.00 **(E66.9)** Overweight or Obesity (726)
V65.2 **(Z76.5)** Malingering (726)
V40.31 **(Z91.83)** Wandering Associated With a Mental Disorder (727)
V62.89 **(R41.83)** Borderline Intellectual Functioning (727)

APPENDIX B

NANDA-I Nursing Diagnoses 2012-2014

Domain 1: Health Promotion

Class 1: Health Awareness
- Deficient Diversional Activity (00097)
- Sedentary Lifestyle (00168)

Class 2: Health Management
- Deficient Community Health (00215)
- Risk-Prone Health Behavior (00188)
- Ineffective Health Maintenance (00099)
- Readiness for Enhanced Immunization Status (00186)
- Ineffective Protection (00043)
- Ineffective Self-Health Management (00078)
- Readiness for Enhanced Self-Health Management (00162)
- Ineffective Family Therapeutic Regimen Management (00080)

Domain 2: Nutrition

Class 1: Ingestion
- Insufficient Breast Milk (00216)
- Ineffective Infant Feeding Pattern (00107)
- Imbalanced Nutrition: Less Than Body Requirements (00002)
- Imbalanced Nutrition: More Than Body Requirements (00001)
- Readiness for Enhanced Nutrition (00163)
- Risk for Imbalanced Nutrition: More Than Body Requirements (00003)
- Impaired Swallowing (00103)

Class 2: Digestion

Class 3: Absorption

Class 4: Metabolism
- Risk for Unstable Blood Glucose Level (00179)
- Neonatal Jaundice (00194)
- Risk for Neonatal Jaundice (00230)
- Risk for Impaired Liver Function (00178)

Class 5: Hydration
- Risk for Electrolyte Imbalance (00195)
- Readiness for Enhanced Fluid Balance (00160)
- Deficient Fluid Volume (00027)
- Excess Fluid Volume (00026)
- Risk for Deficient Fluid Volume (00028)
- Risk for Imbalanced Fluid Volume (00025)

Domain 3: Elimination and Exchange

Class 1: Urinary Function
- Functional Urinary Incontinence (00020)
- Overflow Urinary Incontinence (00176)
- Reflex Urinary Incontinence (00018)
- Stress Urinary Incontinence (00017)
- Urge Urinary Incontinence (00019)
- Risk for Urge Urinary Incontinence (00022)
- Impaired Urinary Elimination (00016)
- Readiness for Enhanced Urinary Elimination (00166)
- Urinary Retention (00023)

Class 2: Gastrointestinal Function
- Constipation (00011)
- Perceived Constipation (00012)
- Risk for Constipation (00015)
- Diarrhea (00013)
- Dysfunctional Gastrointestinal Motility (00196)
- Risk For Dysfunctional Gastrointestinal Motility (00197)
- Bowel Incontinence (00014)

Class 3: Integumentary Function

Class 4: Respiratory Function
- Impaired Gas Exchange (00030)

Domain 4: Activity/Rest

Class 1: Sleep/Rest
- Insomnia (00095)
- Sleep Deprivation (00096)
- Readiness for Enhanced Sleep (00165)
- Disturbed Sleep Pattern (00198)

Class 2: Activity/Exercise
- Risk for Disuse Syndrome (00040)
- Impaired Bed Mobility (00091)
- Impaired Physical Mobility (00085)
- Impaired Wheelchair Mobility (00089)
- Impaired Transfer Ability (00090)
- Impaired Walking (00088)

Class 3: Energy Balance
- Disturbed Energy Field (00050)
- Fatigue (00093)
- Wandering (00154)

Class 4: Cardiovascular/Pulmonary Responses
- Activity Intolerance (00092)
- Risk for Activity Intolerance (00094)
- Ineffective Breathing Pattern (00032)
- Decreased Cardiac Output (00029)
- Risk for Ineffective Gastrointestinal Perfusion (00202)
- Risk for Ineffective Renal Perfusion (00203)
- Impaired Spontaneous Ventilation (00033)
- Ineffective Peripheral Tissue Perfusion (00204)
- Risk for Decreased Cardiac Tissue Perfusion (00200)
- Risk for Ineffective Cerebral Tissue Perfusion (00201)
- Risk for Ineffective Peripheral Tissue Perfusion (00228)
- Dysfunctional Ventilatory Weaning Response (00034)

Class 5: Self-Care
- Impaired Home Maintenance (00098)
- Readiness for Enhanced Self-Care (00182)
- Bathing Self-Care Deficit (00108)
- Dressing Self-Care Deficit (00109)
- Feeding Self-Care Deficit (00102)
- Toileting Self-Care Deficit (00110)
- Self-Neglect (00193)

Domain 5: Perception/Cognition

Class 1: Attention
- Unilateral Neglect (00123)

Class 2: Orientation
- Impaired Environmental Interpretation Syndrome (00127)

Class 3: Sensation/Perception

Class 4: Cognition
- Acute Confusion (00128)
- Chronic Confusion (00129)
- Risk for Acute Confusion (00173)
- Ineffective Impulse Control (00222)
- Deficient Knowledge (00126)
- Readiness for Enhanced Knowledge (00161)
- Impaired Memory (00131)

Class 5: Communication
- Readiness for Enhanced Communication (00157)
- Impaired Verbal Communication (00051)

Domain 6: Self-Perception

Class 1: Self-Concept
- Hopelessness (00124)
- Risk for Compromised Human Dignity (00174)
- Risk for Loneliness (00054)
- Disturbed Personal Identity (00121)
- Risk for Disturbed Personal Identity (00225)
- Readiness for Enhanced Self-Concept (00167)

Class 2: Self-Esteem
- Chronic Low Self-Esteem (00119)
- Situational Low Self-Esteem (00120)
- Risk for Chronic Low Self-Esteem (00224)
- Risk for Situational Low Self-Esteem (00153)

Class 3: Body Image
- Disturbed Body Image (00118)

Domain 7: Role Relationships

Class 1: Caregiving Roles
- Ineffective Breastfeeding (00104)
- Interrupted Breastfeeding (00105)
- Readiness for Enhanced Breastfeeding (00106)
- Caregiver Role Strain (00061)
- Risk for Caregiver Role Strain (00062)
- Impaired Parenting (00056)
- Readiness for Enhanced Parenting (00164)
- Risk for Impaired Parenting (00057)

Class 2: Family Relationships
- Risk for Impaired Attachment (00058)
- Dysfunctional Family Processes (00063)
- Interrupted Family Processes (00060)
- Readiness for Enhanced Family Processes (00159)

Class 3: Role Performance
- Ineffective Relationship (00223)
- Readiness for Enhanced Relationship (00207)
- Risk for Ineffective Relationship (00229)
- Parental Role Conflict (00064)
- Ineffective Role Performance (00055)
- Impaired Social Interaction (00052)

Domain 8: Sexuality

Class 1: Sexual Identity

Class 2: Sexual Function
- Sexual Dysfunction (00059)
- Ineffective Sexuality Pattern (00065)

Class 3: Reproduction
- Ineffective Childbearing Process (00221)
- Readiness for Enhanced Childbearing Process (00208)
- Risk for Ineffective Childbearing Process (00227)
- Risk for Disturbed Maternal-Fetal Dyad (00209)

Domain 9: Coping/Stress Tolerance

Class 1: Post-Trauma Responses
- Post-Trauma Syndrome (00141)
- Risk for Post-Trauma Syndrome (00145)
- Rape-Trauma Syndrome (00142)
- Relocation Stress Syndrome (00114)
- Risk for Relocation Stress Syndrome (00149)

Class 2: Coping Responses
- Ineffective Activity Planning (00199)
- Risk for Ineffective Activity Planning (00226)
- Anxiety (00146)
- Defensive Coping (00071)
- Ineffective Coping (00069)
- Readiness for Enhanced Coping (00158)
- Ineffective Community Coping (00077)
- Readiness for Enhanced Community Coping (00076)
- Compromised Family Coping (00074)
- Disabled Family Coping (00073)
- Readiness for Enhanced Family Coping (00075)
- Death Anxiety (00147)
- Ineffective Denial (00072)

Adult Failure to Thrive (00101)
Fear (00148)
Grieving (00136)
Complicated Grieving (00135)
Risk for Complicated Grieving (00172)
Readiness for Enhanced Power (00187)
Powerlessness (00125)
Risk for Powerlessness (00152)
Impaired Individual Resilience (00210)
Readiness for Enhanced Resilience (00212)
Risk for Compromised Resilience (00211)
Chronic Sorrow (00137)
Stress Overload (00177)

Class 3: Neurobehavioral Stress
Autonomic Dysreflexia (00009)
Risk for Autonomic Dysreflexia (00010)
Disorganized Infant Behavior (00116)
Readiness for Enhanced Organized Infant Behavior (00117)
Risk for Disorganized Infant Behavior (00115)
Decreased Intracranial Adaptive Capacity (00049)

Domain 10: Life Principles

Class 1: Values
Readiness for Enhanced Hope (00185)

Class 2: Beliefs
Readiness for Enhanced Spiritual Well-Being (00068)

Class 3: Value/Belief/Action Congruence
Readiness for Enhanced Decision-Making (00184)
Decisional Conflict (00083)
Moral Distress (00175)
Noncompliance (00079)
Impaired Religiosity (00169)
Readiness for Enhanced Religiosity (00171)
Risk for Impaired Religiosity (00170)
Spiritual Distress (00066)
Risk for Spiritual Distress (00067)

Domain 11: Safety/Protection

Class 1: Infection
Risk for Infection (00004)

Class 2: Physical Injury
Ineffective Airway Clearance (00031)
Risk for Aspiration (00039)
Risk for Bleeding (00206)
Impaired Dentition (00048)
Risk for Dry Eye (00219)
Risk for Falls (00155)
Risk for Injury (00035)
Impaired Oral Mucous Membrane (00045)
Risk for Perioperative Positioning Injury (00087)
Risk for Peripheral Neurovascular Dysfunction (00086)
Risk for Shock (00205)
Impaired Skin Integrity (00046)
Risk for Impaired Skin Integrity (00047)
Risk for Sudden Infant Death Syndrome (00156)
Risk for Suffocation (00036)
Delayed Surgical Recovery (00100)
Risk for Thermal Injury (00220)
Impaired Tissue Integrity (00044)
Risk for Trauma (00038)
Risk for Vascular Trauma (00213)

Class 3: Violence
Risk for Other-Directed Violence (00138)
Risk for Self-Directed Violence (00140)
Self-Mutilation (00151)
Risk for Self-Mutilation (00139)
Risk for Suicide (00150)

Class 4: Environmental Hazards
Contamination (00181)
Risk for Contamination (00180)
Risk for Poisoning (00037)

Class 5: Defensive Processes
Risk for Adverse Reaction to Iodinated Contrast Media (000218)
Latex Allergy Response (00041)
Risk for Allergy Response (00217)
Risk for Latex Allergy Response (00042)

Class 6: Thermoregulation
Risk for Imbalanced Body Temperature (00005)
Hyperthermia (00007)
Hypothermia (00006)
Ineffective Thermoregulation (00008)

Domain 12: Comfort

Class 1: Physical Comfort
Class 2: Environmental Comfort
Class 3: Social Comfort
Impaired Comfort (00214)
Readiness for Enhanced Comfort (00183)
Nausea (00134)
Acute Pain (00132)
Chronic Pain (00133)
Social Isolation (00053)

Domain 13: Growth/Development

Class 1: Growth
Risk for Disproportionate Growth (00113)

Class 2: Development
Delayed Growth and Development (00111)
Risk for Delayed Development (00112)

Nursing Diagnoses Retired from the NANDA-I Taxonomy 2009-2014:
Health-Seeking Behaviors (00084); retired 2009-2011
Disturbed Sensory Perception (Specify: Visual, Auditory, Kinesthetic, Gustatory, Tactile, Olfactory) (00122); retired 2012-2014

APPENDIX

C

Historical Evolution of Psychiatric Mental Health Nursing

Pre-1860

Nursing care for young, ill, and vulnerable people has existed as long as the human race. Care was given by family members, other relatives, servants, neighbors, members of religious orders or humanitarian societies, or convalescing patients or prisoners.

1860

Florence Nightingale. The founder of nursing established the Nightingale School at St. Thomas's Hospital in London after the Crimean War and worked with untrained women caring for soldiers.

1860-1880

Nightingale emphasized the maintenance of a healthful environment, personal hygiene, cleanliness, and healthful living habits, such as adequate nutrition, exercise, and sleep, so that nature could heal. She emphasized kindness toward patients along with custodial care.

Linda Richards. First graduate nurse and first psychiatric nurse in the United States. After study under Florence Nightingale, she organized nursing services and educational programs in Boston City Hospital and in several state mental hospitals in Illinois.

Dorothea Lynde Dix. Worked to reform psychiatric care in mental hospitals and to correct overcrowding and the problem of an insufficient number of physicians and attendants.

1882

First school to prepare nurses to care for patients with acute and chronic mental illness opened at McLean Hospital in Waverly, Massachusetts, through collaboration of Linda Richards and Dr. Edward Cowles.

1890-1930

Psychiatrists in state and private hospitals begin to recognize nurses for their specialized preparation, although the role was primarily to assist the physician or carry out procedures for physical care. There were few psychosocial nursing skills, and nurses were concerned with maintaining a kind, tolerant attitude and humane treatment.

1913

Euphemia "Effie" Jane Taylor. At Johns Hopkins Hospital, she developed the first nurse-organized psychiatric nursing training program within a general nursing program.

1920

Harriet Bailey. First nurse educator to write a psychiatric nursing text, *Nursing Mental Disease.* She wrote of the importance of a nurse's knowing mental illness and of teaching mental health nursing, and she worked for provision of student experiences in psychiatry. She argued for more holistic care of patients.

1937

National League for Nursing recommended that psychiatric nursing be included in the basic nursing curriculum.

1940

Publication of *Psychiatry for Nurses* by Louis Karnosh, a psychiatrist, and Edith Gage, a registered nurse. This 327-page textbook was followed by several subsequent editions.

1943

Laura Fitzsimmons, a nurse consultant, was hired by the American Psychiatric Association to survey mental hospitals. She recommended that every nursing student have an experience in a psychiatric facility.

1946

The National Mental Health Act identifies psychiatric nurses as core mental health providers. It authorizes the establishment of the National Institute of Mental Health, with funds and programs to train professional psychiatric personnel, conduct psychiatric research, and aid in the development of mental health programs at the state level.

1950-1960

A nurse's role included physical care, administration of medications, and maintenance of therapeutic milieu.

Ruth Matheney and **Mary Topalis.** Emphasized the importance of milieu therapy and the nurse's use of this intervention.

1952

Hildegard E. Peplau. Formulated first systematic theoretical framework in psychiatric nursing, presented in *Interpersonal Relations in Nursing* (1952). She emphasized nursing as an interpersonal process and believed that psychological techniques and theoretical concepts were essential to nursing practice. She also defined steps in the nurse-patient relationship.

1953

The Therapeutic Community by Maxwell Jones (from Great Britain) laid the basis for a movement in the United States toward milieu therapy and for a nurse's role in this therapy.

1954

The antipsychotic medication chlorpromazine (Thorazine) was first used in the United States. It was synthesized in France in 1950.

Hildegard Peplau develops the first graduate psychiatric nursing program at Rutgers University.

1956

The National Conference on Graduate Education in Psychiatric Nursing introduced the concept of the psychiatric clinical nurse specialist. Theorists begin to differentiate functions based on a master's level of preparation in nursing.

1957

June Mellow. Introduced second theoretical approach to psychiatric nursing, called "nursing therapy," which applied psychoanalytical theory in one-to-one interactions with patients who had schizophrenia. She emphasized the provision of corrective emotional experiences rather than investigation of pathological processes.

1958

The American Nurses Association (ANA) established the Conference Group on Psychiatric Nursing.

1959

The National League for Nursing requires accredited schools of nursing to include a psychiatric nursing curriculum.

1960-1970

Hildegard E. Peplau, Gertrude Ujhely, Joyce Travelbee, Shirley Burd, Loretta Bermosk, Joyce Hays, Catherine Norris, Gertrude Stokes, Anne Hargreaves, Dorothy Gregg, and **Sheila Rouslin.** Nursing leaders emphasized the importance of self-awareness and use of self, nurse-patient relationship therapy, therapeutic communication, and psychosocial aspects of general nursing. Peplau identified the manifestations of anxiety and formulated steps in anxiety intervention now used by all health care professions. All of these nursing leaders converted various psychological concepts into operational definitions for use in nursing.

1961

Anne Burgess and **Donna Aguilera.** Engaged in crisis work and short-term therapy as well as long-term therapy. They applied crisis theory to psychiatric nursing.

Ida Orlando. Initiated the term *nursing process* and began to delineate its components. She presented a general theoretical framework for all nurse-patient relationships that focused on the patient identifying the meaning of behavior and what the nurse could do to help. She also wrote the classic book *The Dynamic Nurse-Patient Relationship.*

Hildegard E. Peplau. Promoted the primary role of the nurse as a psychotherapist or counselor rather than a mother surrogate, socializer, or manager.

1963

President John F. Kennedy's Comprehensive Community Mental Health Act was passed, providing an impetus for nurses to move from hospital to community settings.

The *Journal of Psychiatric Nursing and Mental Health Services* was established. It was later renamed *Journal of Psychosocial Nursing*

1965

Suzanne Lego established one of the first private psychiatric nursing practices.

1967

The ANA presented a "Position Paper on Psychiatric Nursing" that endorsed the role of clinical specialist as therapist in individual, group, family, and milieu therapies.

The ANA's Division on Psychiatric and Mental Health Nursing Practice published the first *Statement on Psychiatric and Mental Health Nursing Practice.*

1970-1980

Sheila Rouslin. Because of her leadership, certification of clinical specialists in psychiatric nursing was begun by the Division of Psychiatric Mental Health Nursing, New Jersey State Nurses Association. Later, certification was developed by the ANA.

Shirley Smoyak. Defined the patient as an individual, group, family, or community and defined the nurse as a family therapist. She also defined the expanded role of the nurse.

Gwen Marram and **Irene Burnside.** Emphasized that nurses with graduate-level preparation could conduct group and family psychotherapy.

Carolyn Clark. Emphasized the usefulness of a systems framework for psychiatric nurses. She also emphasized the importance of nurses acting as change agents and researchers.

Bonnie Bullough. Emphasized legal and ethical aspects of psychiatric care.

Madeleine Leininger. Reemphasized care of the whole person and introduced implications of cultural diversity for mental health services and psychiatric treatment.

1971

The Association for Child and Adolescent Psychiatric Nursing was formed.

1972

A group of Hildegard Peplau's graduate students, including Shirley Smoyak, founded the Society of Clinical Specialists in Psychiatric Nursing (now called the Society of Advance Practice Psychiatric Nurses) and developed the first credentialing examination for this specialty.

1973

The ANA published *Standards of Psychiatric-Mental Health Nursing.* The ANA also established certification of psychiatric-mental health nurse generalists.

1976

The ANA's Division on Psychiatric and Mental Health Nursing Practice published a revised *Statement on Psychiatric and Mental Health Nursing Practice.*

1978

The Report of the President's Commission on Mental Health described stigma as the primary barrier to providing services. It concluded that deinstitutionalization and discharge of patients to community facilities had not worked as expected and that improved financial, social, medical, and nursing resources; research; and coordination of services were needed.

1979

The ANA established certification of psychiatric-mental health clinical nurse specialists. The 1972 certification was no longer recognized, and Peplau herself lost her credentials.

1980-1990

Anne Burgess. Formulated a theory of victimology based on extensive studies of adult and child victims of rape and abuse, child victims of neglect, and family violence involving incest and battering. She described rape-trauma syndrome, silent rape trauma, and compound reactions to rape.

Lee Ann Hoff. Expanded crisis theory to be used in nursing practice. She contributed to the theory of suicidology. She also described battering syndrome after performing research on battered women and battered elderly persons.

1982

The ANA Executive Committee and Standards Committee, Division on Psychiatric and Mental Health Nursing Practice, published *Standards of Psychiatric and Mental Health Nursing Practice.*

The Century Celebration of Psychiatric Nursing in Washington, DC, was attended by more than 500 nurses.

1987

The American Psychiatric Nurses Association (APNA) was founded by a charter group composed of **Karen Babich, Fernando Duran, Judith Maurin, Mary Reres, Grayce Sills,** and **Shirley Smoyak.** It was supported by Slack Incorporated and was associated with Slack's *Journal of Psychosocial Nursing and Mental Health Services.*

1987

Maxine E. Loomis, Anita O'Toole, Marie Scott Brown, Patricia Pothier, Patricia West, and **Holly S. Wilson.** Began the development of a classification system for psychiatric and mental health nursing, first published in the new journal *Archives of Psychiatric Nursing, 1*(1), 16-24, 1987.

1990

Suzanne Lego. Opened the first psychoanalytic training program for nurses at the Columbia University School of Nursing.

The Americans with Disabilities Act was passed by the U.S. Congress. President George H.W. Bush declared the 1990s to be the "Decade of the Brain."

1994

The APNA was under new management, losing the *Journal of Psychosocial Nursing and Mental Health Services* and founding its own publication, *Journal of the American Psychiatric Nurses Association.*

1999

U.S. Surgeon General David Satcher released the first ever *Surgeon General's Report on Mental Health*, a science-based report that emphasized mental illness as an urgent health concern.

2003

The President's New Freedom Commission report emphasized the importance of mental health to overall health; recommended the reduction of disparities and stigma; and promoted recovery, resilience, early mental health interventions, and expansion of research and technology for mental health care.

2007

The APNA, the International Society of Psychiatric-Mental Health Nurses, and the ANA revised *Psychiatric-Mental Health Nursing: Scope and Standards of Practice.*

2010

The Institute of Medicine's report *The Future of Nursing: Leading Change to Advance Health* emphasized the role of psychiatric mental health nurses as national and international policy and program development leaders.

2011

The APNA and the International Society of Psychiatric Nurses Boards of Directors approved recommendations for implementations of the *Consensus Model for APRN Regulation: Licensure, Accreditation, Certification & Education (LACE).* This model establishes a more uniform system to ease mobility of practice across state lines.

Partially adapted from Murray, R.B., & Huelskoetter, M.M.W. (1991). *Psychiatric/mental health nursing: Giving emotional care* (3rd ed., pp. 94-97). Englewood Cliffs, NJ: Appleton and Lange; Carter, E., Peplau, H.E., & Sills, G.M. (1997). The ins and outs of psychiatric mental health nursing and the American Nurses Association. *Journal of the American Psychiatric Nurses Association, 3*(1), 10-16.

GLOSSARY

acculturation Adapting to the beliefs, values, and practices of a new cultural setting.

acquaintance (or date) rape A rape in which the perpetrator is known to, and presumably trusted by, the person who is raped.

active listening Being aware of a patient's verbal and nonverbal communications while monitoring one's own verbal and nonverbal communications.

acupuncture An aspect of traditional Chinese medicine that involves placement of needles into the skin at meridian points to modulate the flow of *qi*.

acute dystonia Acute, often painful, sustained contraction of muscles, usually of the head and neck, which typically occurs from 2 to 5 days after the introduction of antipsychotic medications.

acute phase One of three phases in bipolar disorder in which individuals are at risk for injury due to alterations in self-control, sleep, hydration, and nutrition.

acute stress disorder Severe numbing, derealization, inability to remember stressful event, fear, helplessness, or horror that occurs within 1 month of exposure to extreme stress.

addiction Obsession, compulsion, or loss of control with respect to use of a drug (e.g., alcohol), with genetic, psychosocial, and environmental factors that influence its development. Use of the drug continues despite the presence of related problems and a tendency to relapse after stopping use.

adjustment disorder A psychological response to identifiable stressors, with symptoms developing within 3 months of the stressors.

admission criteria Reasons for admitting an individual to an inpatient psychiatric unit. There will be evidence of one or more of the following: (1) imminent danger of harming self, (2) imminent danger of harming others, or (3) inability to care for basic needs, placing the individual at imminent risk of harming self.

adult day care A nonresidential facility that provides services and activities to elderly or handicapped individuals.

advance directives Directions provided by a patient for clinicians to follow in the event of a serious illness.

advanced practice forensic nurse A nurse who has completed graduate education with a broad focus in forensic nursing and obtained credentials as a clinical nurse specialist, certified nurse-midwife, or nurse practitioner.

advanced practice registered nurse–psychiatric mental health (APRN-PMH) A nurse generalist who has obtained additional training to provide care as a clinical nurse specialist with advanced nursing expertise or as a nurse practitioner who diagnoses, prescribes, and treats psychiatric disorders.

adventitious crisis A crisis that is not part of everyday life but involves an event that is unplanned and accidental. Adventitious crises include natural disasters and crimes of violence such as rapes or muggings.

adverse drug reactions Negative responses to drugs; particularly problematic in older adults. Drug reactions can cause conditions such as delirium, dizziness, confusion leading to serious complications, and hospitalization.

affect The external manifestation of a feeling or emotion that is manifested in facial expression, tone of voice, and body language. For example, a patient may be said to have a *flat affect*, meaning that there is an absence or a near absence of facial expression. The term may be used loosely to describe a feeling, emotion, or mood.

affective symptoms Symptoms involving emotions and their expression.

ageism A system of destructive, erroneous beliefs about the elderly; a bias against older people based solely on their age.

aggression Any verbal or nonverbal, actual or attempted, conscious or unconscious, forceful means of harm or abuse of another person or object.

agnosia Literally meaning *loss of knowledge* and referring to a wide range of cognitive losses. For example, a person may be unable to identify familiar sounds, such as the ringing of a doorbell (auditory agnosia), or familiar objects, such as a toothbrush or keys (visual agnosia).

agoraphobia An anxiety disorder characterized by fear of being in places or situations in which escape might be difficult or embarrassing or in which help may not be available should an anxiety attack occur.

agraphia Loss of a previous ability to write, resulting from brain injury or brain disease.

akathisia Regular rhythmic movements, usually of the lower limbs, with constant pacing sometimes seen; often noticed in people taking antipsychotic medication.

alternate personality (alter) A distinct personality state that recurrently takes control of the behavior of a person with dissociative identity disorder.

Alzheimer's disease (AD) A primary cognitive impairment disorder characterized by progressive deterioration of cognitive functioning.

ambivalence The holding, at the same time, of two opposing emotions, attitudes, ideas, or wishes toward the same person, situation, or object.

anergia Lack of energy; passivity.

anger An emotional response to the perception of frustration of desires or threat to one's needs. It can be used as a motivator or as an aid in survival, but problems begin to occur when anger is expressed through aggression and violence.

anhedonia The inability to experience pleasure.

anorexia nervosa A medical term that signifies a loss of appetite. A person with anorexia nervosa, however, may not have any loss of appetite and often is preoccupied with food and eating. A person with this disorder may suppress the desire for food in order to control his or her eating.

anosognosia A patient's inability to realize that he or she is ill, which is caused by the illness itself.

antagonists Drugs that block or depress the normal response of a specific receptor by only partly fitting the receptor site.

antianxiety (anxiolytic) drugs Drugs that increase the effectiveness of gamma aminobutyric acid (GABA), a neurotransmitter that modulates excitability and anxiety. These drugs are generally prescribed to reduce anxiety, but on a short-term basis due to problems with addiction.

anticholinesterase inhibitors Drugs that inhibit acetylcholinesterase, the enzyme that breaks down acetylcholine. This permits the accumulation of acetylcholine and increases stimulation of cholinergic receptors in the parasympathetic nervous system. Increasing acetylcholine slows heart action, lowers blood pressure, increases secretion, and increases contraction of smooth muscles.

anticonvulsant drugs Drugs commonly used to treat epilepsy that suppress the rapid and excessive firing of neurons and are used as mood stabilizers.

antisocial personality disorder A syndrome in which a person lacks the capacity to relate to others, does not experience discomfort in inflicting or observing pain in others, and may manipulate others for personal gain.

anxiety A state of feeling apprehension, uneasiness, uncertainty, or dread; results from a real or perceived threat whose actual source is unknown or unrecognized.

aphasia Difficulty in the formulation of words, which may progress to the loss of language ability.

apraxia Loss of ability to perform purposeful movements; for example, a person may be unable to shave, dress, or perform other once-familiar and purposeful tasks.

aromatherapy The use of essential oils for enhancing physical and mental well-being and healing.

assault An intentional threat designed to make the victim fearful; produces reasonable apprehension of harm.

assertive community treatment (ACT) An intensive type of case management for people with serious, persistent psychiatric symptoms. Repeated hospitalizations are reduced through a multidisciplinary team that provides a comprehensive array of services.

assimilation The incorporation of new ideas, objects, and experiences into the framework of one's thoughts.

associative looseness A disturbance of thinking in which ideas shift from one subject to another in an oblique or unrelated manner.

attempted rape Physical attempts and verbal threats of rape.

attention The ability to focus on environmental cues without distraction and to select and register information so that immediate recall (short-term memory) is possible.

attention deficit hyperactivity disorder Individuals with this disorder show an inappropriate degree of inattention, impulsiveness, and hyperactivity before the age of 12. Some individuals can have attention deficit disorder without hyperactivity

atypical antipsychotics See *second-generation (atypical) antipsychotics.*

autism spectrum disorders Complex neurobiological and developmental disabilities that typically appear during a child's first 3 years of life.

automatic thoughts Rapid, unthinking responses based on unique assumptions about ourselves and the world. These assumptions may be realistic or distorted. Common distortions include focusing on negative details and catastrophizing, which is assuming the worst possible outcome.

avoidant personality disorder A personality disorder in which the central characteristics are an extreme sensitivity to rejection and robust avoidance of interpersonal situations.

basal sleep requirement The amount of sleep required to feel fully awake and able to sustain normal levels of performance during periods of wakefulness

basic level registered nurse A professional who has completed a nursing program, passed the state licensure examination, and is qualified to work in almost any general or specialty area.

battery The harmful or offensive touching of another person.

behavior therapy A treatment method that is concerned with patterns of behavior rather than inner motivations. Maladaptive responses are replaced with adaptive responses.

behavioral family therapy A treatment in which family members identify undesirable behaviors, how they can unlearn these behaviors, and how they can learn more desirable behaviors.

bereavement exclusion A stipulation in which people who have experienced the loss of a significant loved one would not be given the diagnosis of major depression within the first 2 months of the loss. This exclusion was removed from the *DSM-5*.

bibliotherapy The use of literature to assist an individual to express feelings, gain insight into feelings and behavior, and learn new ways to cope with difficult situations.

binge eating disorder A disorder in which individuals engage in repeated episodes of binge eating, after which they experience significant distress. These binges occur at least once a week for 3 months. A common side effect of binge eating disorder is obesity.

bioethics The study of specific ethical questions that arise in health care.

biofeedback A technique for gaining conscious control over unconscious body functions, such as blood pressure and heartbeat. Feedback obtained by sensitive instruments can provide information on body function, and individuals can learn to monitor and control responses.

bipolar I disorder A mood disorder that is characterized by at least one week-long manic episode that results in excessive activity and energy. Manic episodes may alternate with depression, hypomania, or a mixed state of agitation and depression.

bipolar II disorder A form of bipolar disorder in which hypomanic episodes alternate with major depression.

body dysmorphic disorder An obsessive-compulsive disorder that involves preoccupation with an imagined defective body part, resulting in obsessional thinking and compulsive behavior.

borderline personality disorder A disorder characterized by disordered images of self, impulsive and unpredictable behavior, marked shifts in mood, and instability in relationships with others.

boundaries Those functions that maintain a distinction among individuals within a family or group and between family members and the outside world. Boundaries may be clear, diffuse, rigid, or inconsistent.

bulimia nervosa Episodes of excessive and uncontrollable intake of large amounts of food (binges), usually alternating with compensatory activities such as self-induced vomiting, use of cathartics and/or diuretics, and self-starvation.

chiropractic medicine Based on the theory that energy flows from the brain to the body through the spinal cord and spinal nerves. Manipulation of the spinal column is thought to return the vertebrae to their normal positions, thereby reducing pain, depression, or anxiety.

circadian drive Functions as part of the circadian rhythm that comes into play during the day to promote wakefulness. The circadian drive is balanced by the homeostatic mechanism of sleep drives.

circadian rhythms A 24-hour biological rhythm that influences specific regulatory functions such as the sleep/wake cycle, body temperature, and hormonal and neurotransmitter secretions. A "pacemaker" in the brain that sends messages to various systems in the body (such as those mentioned) controls the 24-hour biological rhythm.

civil rights The rights of personal liberty guaranteed under two U.S. constitutional amendments. These rights are extended to people with mental illness and include the right to vote, enter into contractual agreements, press charges, and receive humane care.

clang association The meaningless rhyming of words, often in a forceful manner.

classical conditioning Bringing about involuntary behavior or reflexes through conditioned responses to stimuli.

clear boundaries Boundaries that are understood by all members of the family and give family members a sense of "I-ness" and also "we-ness."

clinical epidemiology A broad field that examines health and illness at the population level.

clinical pathway A written plan or "map" identifying predetermined times that specific nursing and medical interventions (e.g., diagnostic studies, treatments, activities, medications, teaching, discharge teaching) will be implemented (e.g., day 1 or day 2 for hospital settings, week 1 or month 2 for community-based settings).

clinical supervision A mentoring relationship characterized by evaluation and feedback and a gradual increase in autonomy and responsibility.

closed-ended questions Questions that elicit a "yes" or "no" response. These are useful for getting information efficiently, as in an assessment, but do little to encourage the sharing of feelings.

codependence A term used to describe coping behaviors that prevent individuals from taking care of their own needs and have as their core a preoccupation with the thoughts and feelings of another or others; usually refers to the dependence of one person on another person who is addicted in one form or another.

codes Psychiatric emergencies. Many general and psychiatric hospitals have special teams made up of nurses, psychiatric technicians, and other professionals who respond to these codes.

cognitive-behavioral therapy (CBT) An evidence-based therapeutic modality for children, adolescents, and adults that seeks to identify negative and irrational patterns of thought and challenge them based on rational evidence and thoughts.

cognitive distortions Inaccurate and irrational automatic thoughts or ideas that lead to false assumptions and misinterpretations.

cognitive reframing A process of changing an individual's perceptions of stress by reassessing a situation and replacing irrational beliefs.

cognitive symptoms Abnormalities in how a person thinks.

command hallucinations An individual hearing voices that direct the person to take action.

communication disorders Deficits in language skills acquisition that create impairments in academic achievement, socialization, or self-care. These include speech disorders in which people have problems in making sounds or may stutter. Language disorders result in difficulty understanding or in using words in context and appropriately.

community mental health centers Centers created for those who have no access to private mental health care. The range of services available at such centers varies, but generally they provide emergency services, adult services, and children's services.

comorbid condition A condition that occurs along with another disorder.

competency The capacity to understand the consequences of one's decisions.

competency evaluator A forensic nurse who assesses mental health or illness, conducts forensic interviews, provides documentation, completes a formal report to the court, and testifies as an expert witness regarding the competency of the defendant.

complementary and alternative medicine (CAM) Also known as *integrative care* or *integrative medicine*, this approach places the patient at the center of care. It focuses on prevention and wellness and attends to the patient's physical, mental, and spiritual needs through treatment methods generally outside of mainstream medicine.

completed suicides Suicide attempts that result in death.

concrete thinking Thinking grounded in immediate experience rather than abstraction. There is an overemphasis on specific detail as opposed to general and abstract concepts.

conditional release A release from an inpatient psychiatric facility that is contingent upon outpatient commitment.

conditioning Involves pairing a behavior with a condition that reinforces or diminishes the behavior's occurrence.

conduct disorder A psychiatric disorder characterized by a persistent pattern of behavior in which the rights of others are violated and age-appropriate societal norms or rules are disregarded.

confabulation The filling in of a memory gap with a story that is believed by the teller. The purpose is to maintain self-esteem, and it is seen in organic conditions such as dementia.

confidentiality The ethical responsibility of a health care professional that prohibits the disclosure of privileged information without the patient's informed consent.

conflict Open disagreement among members of a group.

conscious Denoting experiences that are within a person's awareness.

consultant An expert who gives advice.

continuation phase The continuation phase of substance treatment lasts for 4 to 9 months. Although the overall outcome of this phase is relapse prevention, many other outcomes must be accomplished to achieve relapse prevention.

continuum of psychiatric mental health care A conceptualization of psychiatric care along the line of need for least restrictive to most restrictive environment and based on a patient's needs.

contract A written or stated agreement between patient and caregiver that contains the place, time, date, and duration of meetings.

conventional antipsychotics See *first-generation (conventional, typical) antipsychotics.*

conventional health care system Also known as *allopathic, mainstream*, or *orthodox medicine; regular medicine*; *and biomedicine*; based largely on highly controlled, evidence-based scientific research.

conversion disorder A somatic symptom disorder characterized by the presence of deficits in voluntary motor or sensory functions; may include blindness, paralysis, movement disorder, gait disorder, numbness, paresthesia, loss of vision or hearing, or episodes resembling epilepsy.

co-occurring disorders Disorders that occur at the same time as the psychiatric disorder and may be associated with the disorder.

coping styles Discrete personal attributes that people have and can develop to help manage stress.

copycat suicide A suicide that follows a highly publicized suicide of a public figure, idol, or peer in the community.

correctional nursing Nursing that occurs in correctional facilities and is defined by the location of the work or the legal status of the patient, rather than by the role functions performed.

countertransference The tendency of the nurse (or therapist or social worker) to displace onto the patient feelings that are a response to people in the nurse's past. Strong positive or strong negative reactions to a patient may indicate countertransference.

criminal profiler A person who attempts to provide law enforcement officials with specific information about the type of individual who may have committed a certain crime.

crisis intervention A brief, active, and collaborative therapy that draws on an individual's personal coping abilities and resources within the family, health care setting, or community.

crisis situation A situation that puts stress on a family with a violent member.

critical incident stress debriefing (CISD) A seven-phase group meeting that offers individuals who have experienced a crisis the opportunity to share their thoughts and feelings in a safe and controlled environment.

cultural competence A nurse's act of adjusting his or her practices to meet a patient's cultural beliefs, practices, needs, and preferences.

cultural filters Filters through which each person interprets self, others, and the surrounding world.

culture Culture is comprised of the shared beliefs, values, and practices that guide a group's members in patterned ways of thinking and acting. Culture guides actions that impact care, health, and well-being. Culture includes ethnicity, social norms, religion, geography, socioeconomic status, occupational, and ability/disability-related and sexual orientation–related beliefs and behaviors.

culture-bound syndromes Sets of signs and symptoms common in a limited number of cultures but virtually nonexistent in most other cultural groups.

cyclothymic disorder A disorder characterized by symptoms of hypomania that alternate with symptoms of mild to moderate depression for at least 2 years in adults and 1 year in children. Neither set of symptoms constitutes an actual diagnosis of either disorder, yet the symptoms are disturbing enough to cause social and occupational impairment.

debriefing Reflecting on and discussing a stressful experience; occurs within 12 to 48 hours of a traumatic event and is often offered as a group intervention.

decompensation Deterioration of mental health and loss of control due to an inability to compensate for mental illness due to stress.

de-escalation techniques Intentional techniques used for reduction of the intensity of a conflict.

defense mechanisms Usually unconscious intrapsychic processes used to ward off anxiety by preventing conscious awareness of threatening feelings. Defense mechanisms can be used in a healthy or a not-so-healthy manner. Examples are repression, projection, sublimation, denial, and regression.

deinstitutionalization Legislation that resulted in the mass movement of severely mentally ill (SMI) persons from state hospitals to outpatient care.

delayed ejaculation A man achieving ejaculation during coitus only with great difficulty.

delirium An acute, usually reversible alteration in consciousness typically accompanied by disturbances in thinking, memory, attention, and perception; has multiple causes.

delusions A false belief held to be true even with evidence to the contrary (e.g., a false belief that one is being singled out for harm by others).

dementia A progressive and usually irreversible deterioration of cognitive and intellectual functions and memory without impairment in consciousness.

dependent personality disorder A disorder in which people have a high need to be taken care of; this can lead to patterns of submissiveness with fears of separation and abandonment by others.

depersonalization A phenomenon whereby a person experiences a sense of unreality of or estrangement from the self. For example, one may feel that limbs or extremities have changed, that one is seeing self and events from a distance, or that one is in a dream.

derealization The false perception by a person that his or her environment has changed. For example, everything may seem bigger or smaller, or familiar objects may appear strange and unfamiliar.

Diagnostic and Statistical Manual of Mental Disorders, fifth edition (DSM-5) A medical manual that was published in 2013 for the purpose of classifying mental disorders and that influences treatment recommendations and reimbursement.

dialectical behavior therapy (DBT) An evidenced-based cognitive behavioral therapy developed by Dr. Marsha Linehan. It has been shown to successfully treat chronically suicidal persons with borderline personality disorder, and it focuses on impulse control..

diathesis-stress model A general theory that explains psychopathology using a multi-causational systems approach.

diffuse or enmeshed boundaries A blending together of roles, thoughts, and feelings of individuals so that clear distinctions among family members (or others) fail to emerge.

disaster A sudden event, such as an accident or a natural catastrophe, that causes great damage or loss of life.

disinhibited social engagement disorder A condition in which children demonstrate no normal fear of strangers, seem unfazed in response to separation from a primary caregiver, and are usually willing to go off with people who are unknown to them.

dissociation An unconscious defense mechanism that allows blocking of overwhelming anxiety stemming from disintegration of functions of consciousness, memory, identity, or perception of environment.

dissociative amnesia A dissociative disorder marked by the inability to recall important personal information, often the result of a trauma or severe stress.

dissociative fugue A dissociative disorder characterized by sudden, unexpected travel away from the customary locale and an inability to recall one's identity and information about some or all of one's past.

dissociative identity disorder A dissociative disorder in which two or more distinct personality states recurrently take control of behavior.

distress A negative, draining energy that results in anxiety, depression, confusion, helplessness, hopelessness, and fatigue.

double messages Conflicting messages (also known as *mixed messages*).

double-bind messages Communication that contains two contradictory messages given by the same person at the same time, to which the receiver is expected to respond. Constant double-bind situations result in feelings of helplessness, fear, and anxiety in the recipient of such messages.

duty to protect Ethical and legal obligations of health care workers to protect patients from physically harming themselves or others.

duty to warn An obligation to warn third parties when they may be in danger from a patient.

dysphoric mania Also referred to as a *mixed state* or *agitated depression;* includes depressive symptoms along with mania. A person with dysphoric mania may be irritable, angry, suicidal, or hypersexual and may experience panic attacks, pressured speech, agitation, severe insomnia, and grandiosity, as well as persecutory delusions and confusion.

dysthymic disorder (DD) A mild to moderate mood disturbance characterized by a chronic depressive syndrome that is usually present for many years. The depressive mood disturbance is hard to distinguish from the person's usual pattern of functioning, and the person has minimal social or occupational impairment.

early intervention programs Children with autism spectrum disorders are referred to these programs once communication and behavioral symptoms are identified, typically in the second or third year of life.

Eastern tradition Views the family as the basis for one's identity, so that family interdependence and group decision-making are the norm. Body-mind-spirit are seen as a single entity; there is no sense of separation between a physical illness and a psychological one.

echolalia Repeating of the last words spoken by another; mimicry or imitation of the speech of another person.

echopraxia Mimicry or imitation of the movements of another person.

economic abuse The withholding of financial support or the illegal or improper exploitation of funds or other resources for one's personal gain.

ego One of three psychological processes that make up the Freudian system of personality (id, ego, superego). The ego is one's sense of self and provides for such functions as problem-solving, mobilization of defense mechanisms, reality testing, and the capability of functioning independently. The ego is said to be the mediator between one's primitive drives (the id) and internalized parental and social prohibitions (the superego).

electroconvulsive therapy (ECT) An effective treatment for depression in which a grand mal seizure is induced by passing an electrical current through electrodes that are applied to the temples. The administration of a muscle relaxant minimizes seizure activity and prevents damage to long bones and cervical vertebrae.

electronic health care The provision of health care through methods that are not face-to-face but rather through an electronic medium.

elopement Escape or leaving from a psychiatric treatment facility without medical authorization or recommendation.

emotional abuse Depriving an individual of a nurturing atmosphere in which he or she can thrive, learn, and develop. Emotional abuse takes many forms (e.g., terrorizing, demeaning, consistently belittling, withholding warmth).

emotional dysregulation A poorly modulated mood characterized by mood swings. Individuals with emotion regulation problems have ongoing difficulty managing painful emotions in ways that are healthy and effective.

emotional lability Rapidly moving from one emotional extreme to another. Typically, these emotional shifts include responding to situations with emotions that are out of proportion to the circumstances, pathological fear of separation, and intense sensitivity to perceived personal rejection.

empathy The ability of one person to get inside another's world, see things from the other person's perspective, and communicate this understanding to the other person.

encopresis A term that refers to children who resist having bowel movements, causing impacted stool to collect in the colon and rectum. Liquid stool can then leak around the impacted stool and out of the anus and stain the child's underwear.

enculturation The process in which a culture's worldview, beliefs, values, and practices are transmitted to its members.

enuresis Nocturnal and/or daytime involuntary discharge of urine.

epidemiology The quantitative study of the distribution of mental disorders in human populations.

erectile disorder Refers to failure to obtain and maintain an erection sufficient for sexual activity or decreased erectile turgidity on 75% of sexual occasions and lasting for at least 6 months.

ethical dilemma A situation in which there is a conflict between two or more courses of action, each carrying favorable and unfavorable consequences.

ethics The discipline concerned with standards of values, behaviors, or beliefs adhered to by individuals or groups.

ethnicity The common heritage and history shared by a specific ethnic group.

ethnocentrism The universal tendency of humans to believe that their way of thinking and behaving is the only correct and natural way.

euphoric mania Individuals experiencing mania in bipolar disorder may experience euphoric mania. In this condition, they initially feel wonderful; however, feelings turn scary and dark as the mania progresses toward loss of control and confusion.

eustress A positive type of stress that reflects a person's confidence in the ability to successfully master given demands or tasks.

evidence-based practice (EBP) A method of care that integrates the latest and best available research; it stipulates that interventions should be based on scientific evidence and principles when available.

excessive sleepiness A subjective report of difficulty staying awake that is serious enough to impact social and vocational functioning and increase the risk for accident or injury.

executive functioning The ability to set priorities or make decisions.

exhibitionism An illegal activity that involves the intentional display of the genitals in a public place.

expert witness A witness recognized by the court as having a certain level of skill or expertise in a designated area and possessing superior knowledge because of education or specialized experience.

expressed emotion Refers to the qualitative amount of emotion displayed, usually in the context of family interactions.

extinction In operant conditioning, extinction occurs when reinforcement no longer results in a given behavior or response; in classical conditioning, extinction occurs when the stimulus no longer produces a response.

extrapyramidal side effects (EPSs) A variety of signs and symptoms that are often side effects of the use of certain psychotropic drugs, particularly phenothiazines. Three reversible extrapyramidal side effects are acute dystonia, akathisia, and pseudoparkinsonism. A fourth, tardive dyskinesia, is the most serious and is not reversible.

eye movement desensitization and reprocessing A first line treatment for traumatized children that processes traumatic memories though a specific eight-phase protocol that allows the person to think about the traumatic event while attending to other stimulation, such as eye movements, audiotones, or tapping.

fact witness A witness who testifies in court regarding what was *personally* seen, heard, performed, or documented regarding a patient's care and testifies to his or her firsthand experience only.

factitious disorders Psychiatric disorders in which people consciously pretend to be ill to get emotional needs met and attain the status of "patient."

false imprisonment May be a misdemeanor or tort brought against health care workers who illegally hold people in confinement. Confinement includes restraint within a limited area and restraint within an institution.

family systems theory A theory of human behavior that views the family as an emotionally connected unit and describes their interactions through a systems perspective.

family triangle A dysfunctional phenomenon in which a third person is brought into a two-person relationship to help relieve anxiety or stress between two family members. Triangles are dysfunctional because the lowering of anxiety comes from diversion from the conflict rather than from resolution of the conflict between the two members.

family violence The intentional intimidation, abuse, or neglect of children, adults, or elders by a family member, intimate partner, or caretaker in order to gain power and control over the victim.

fear An unpleasant emotion related to a specific danger.

feedback Communication of one person's impressions of and reactions to another person's actions or verbalizations.

female orgasmic disorder Defined as the recurrent or persistent inhibition of female orgasm, as manifested by the recurrent delay in, or absence of, orgasm after a normal sexual excitement phase (achieved by masturbation or coitus).

female sexual interest/arousal disorder Characterized by emotional distress caused by absent or reduced interest in sexual fantasies, sexual activity, pleasure, and arousal.

fetishism A sexual disorder characterized by a sexual focus on objects that are intimately associated with the human body.

fight-or-flight response The body's physiological response to fear or rage that triggers the sympathetic branch of the autonomic nervous system as well as the endocrine system. This response is useful in emergencies; however, a sustained response can result in pathophysiological changes such as high blood pressure, ulcers, and cardiac problems.

first-generation (conventional, typical) antipsychotics This original classification of antipsychotic medications works by D_2 receptor antagonism. These medications are accompanied by a variety of side effects, including extrapyramidal symptoms. They are effective in the treatment of positive symptoms (e.g., delusions, hallucinations, disorganized thought) but not negative symptoms (e.g., depression, avolition, anhedonia).

flashbacks Dissociative experiences during which an event is relived and a person behaves as though he or she is experiencing the event at that time,

flight of ideas A continuous flow of speech in which the person jumps rapidly from one topic to another. Sometimes the listener can keep up with the changes; at other times, it is necessary to listen for themes in the incessant talking. Themes often include grandiose and fantasized evaluation of personal sexual prowess, business ability, artistic talents, and so forth.

forensic nurse examiner A forensic psychiatric nurse who conducts court-ordered evaluations regarding legal sanity or competency to proceed, responds to specific medicolegal questions as requested by the court, and renders an expert opinion in a written report or courtroom testimony.

forensic nurse generalist A nurse with a baccalaureate or associate degree or diploma who has acquired additional knowledge and skills by completing a certificate program in forensic nursing.

forensic nursing The application of nursing science and care to public or legal proceedings or the application of forensic aspects of health care combined with the biopsychosocial education of the registered nurse.

forensic psychiatric nurse A psychiatric nurse prepared at the generalist or advanced practice level who cares for patients and/or victims involved with the forensic system.

frotteurism A sexual disorder characterized by rubbing or touching a nonconsenting person.

functional neurological disorder Also known as *conversion disorder;* manifests itself as neurological symptoms in the absence of a neurological diagnosis

gender dysphoria A person's feelings of unease about his maleness or her femaleness.

gender identity The sense of maleness or femaleness.

general adaptation syndrome (GAS) The body's organized response to stress, as elucidated by Hans Selye. It progresses through three stages: (1) the stage of alarm, (2) the stage of resistance, and (3) the stage of exhaustion.

generalized anxiety disorder Anxiety disorder characterized by excessive anxiety or worry about numerous things.

genito-pelvic pain/penetration disorder Pelvic and/or vaginal pain during or after intercourse.

genogram A systematic diagram of the three-generational relationships within a family system.

genuineness Self-awareness of one's feelings as they arise within the nurse-patient relationship and the ability to communicate them when appropriate.

grandiosity Exaggerated belief in or claims about one's importance or identity.

group content All that is said in a group.

group norms Expectations for behavior in a group that develop over time and provide structure for members.

group process The interaction continually taking place among members of a group.

group psychotherapy Psychotherapy based on the examination of group interaction with a view toward understanding and eventually changing the ways in which patients interact with others.

group themes Members' expressed ideas or feelings that recur and have a common thread.

group work A method whereby individuals with common purpose come together and benefit by both giving and receiving feedback within the dynamic and unique context of group life.

guided imagery A process whereby a person is led to envision images that are both calming and health enhancing.

hair pulling disorder Also known as *trichotillomania;* a distressing problem in which individuals compulsively pull hair out (typically from the scalp), resulting in varying degrees of disability, social stigma, and altered appearance.

hallucinations A sense perception (seeing, hearing, tasting, smelling, or touching) for which no external stimulus exists (e.g., hearing voices when none are present).

healing touch A derivative of therapeutic touch that combines several energy therapies and is based on the belief that the body is a complex energy system that can be influenced by another through that person's intention for healing and well-being.

Health Insurance Portability and Accountability Act (HIPAA) A bill enacted in 1996 that established national standards for the protection of electronic medical records.

health teaching Identification of the health education needs of a patient and the teaching of basic physical and mental health principles.

herbal therapy The use of plants or plant products to improve health, prevent illness, and/or treat illness.

histrionic personality disorder This disorder is characterized by attention-seeking behaviors, self-centeredness, low tolerance of frustration, and excessive emotionality. The person is often impulsive and melodramatic and may be flirtatious or provocative.

hoarding disorder An obsessive accumulation of belongings that may have little or no value and that prevents people from leading normal lives.

holism Involves identification of the interrelationships of the bio-psycho-social-spiritual dimensions of a person, recognizing that the whole is greater than the sum of its parts

holistic approach An approach to nursing care that emphasizes the interplay of biological, psychological, and sociocultural needs

homeopathy A Western alternative medical system in which small doses (dilutions) of specially prepared plant extracts, herbs, minerals, and other materials are used to stimulate the body's defense mechanisms and healing processes.

hostage negotiator A consultant who addresses the mental state of the perpetrator and recommends appropriate negotiation strategies.

humor Intensity of stressful thoughts or situations can be dissipated by viewing the absurd or comical aspects.

hypermetamorphosis The desire to touch everything in sight.

hyperorality The desire to taste everything, chew everything, and put everything into one's mouth.

hypersomnia The spending of increased time in sleep, possibly to escape from painful feelings; however, the increased sleep is not experienced as restful or refreshing.

hypersomnolence A condition associated with excessive daytime sleepiness and excessive sleep that is not experienced as restful or refreshing.

hypervigilance A state of extraordinary alertness that results in an exaggerated startle response.

hypnotic A classification of drugs used to promote sleep.

hypomania An elevated mood with symptoms less severe than those of mania. A person in hypomania does not experience impairment in reality testing, nor do the symptoms markedly impair the person's social, occupational, or interpersonal functions.

id One of three psychological processes that make up the Freudian system of personality (id, ego, and superego). The id is the source of all primitive drives and instincts and is considered to be the reservoir of all psychic energy.

ideal body weight The weight that is believed to be healthy for a person, based on height but impacted by factors such as gender, age, build, and degree of muscular development.

ideas of reference The false impression that outside events have special meaning for oneself.

illness anxiety disorder A psychiatric disorder that results in the misinterpretation of physical sensations as evidence of a serious illness.

illusions Errors in the perception of a sensory stimulus. For example, a person may mistake polka dots on a pillow for hairy spiders.

implied consent A form of consent that is not expressly given but is assumed from circumstances of a person's particular situation or a person's actions, especially in life-threatening or serious situations.

incidence Refers to the number of new cases of mental disorders in a healthy population within a given period.

indigenous culture The people and culture that have inhabited a country for thousands of years (e.g., Maoris of New Zealand, Australian aborigines, native Hawaiians, natives of North and South America).

informal admission One type of voluntary admission in which there is no formal or written application.

informed consent A legal term that indicates that a person has been provided with a basic understanding of risks, benefits, and alternatives and is receiving treatment voluntarily.

insight-oriented family therapy A traditional therapeutic modality that emphasizes understanding the origins of problems in order to address them.

integrative care Care that places the patient at the center of care, focuses on prevention and wellness, and attends to the patient's physical, mental, and spiritual needs.

intellectual development disorder Previously called *mental retardation,* this is a disorder characterized by deficits in three areas: intellectual functioning, social functioning, and practical functioning. Impairments must be evidenced during childhood development, range from mild to severe, and include consideration of the person's level of dependence on others for ongoing care and support

intentional torts Willful and intentional acts that violate another person's rights or property.

intermittent explosive disorder A psychiatric disorder with a pattern of behavioral outbursts characterized by an inability to control aggressive impulses in adults 18 years and older.

interpersonal psychotherapy A therapeutic modality that emphasizes what goes on between people. The basis of the therapy is on building interpersonal skills and correcting faulty processes of interacting.

intoxication Maladaptive behavioral or psychological changes caused by excessive use of a drug or alcohol.

involuntary admission Admission to a psychiatric facility without a patient's consent.

involuntary outpatient commitment Court mandates for medication and other treatments as a condition for remaining in the community rather than in the hospital. These mandates are controversial and not used in all communities in the United States.

journaling Keeping a diary; may be informal or part of a treatment plan of daily events, activities, and feelings.

kleptomania A repeated failure to resist urges to steal objects not needed for personal use or monetary value.

la belle indifference Literally *beautifully indifferent;* refers to an affect or attitude of unconcern about symptoms that most people would find distressing.

late-life mental illness Psychiatric disorders not discovered earlier in life but evident in older years.

least restrictive alternative doctrine Mandates that the least restrictive and least disruptive means be used to achieve a specific purpose.

least restrictive environment The setting that places the least restrictions on choices and freedom.

legal sanity An individual's ability to distinguish right from wrong with reference to the act charged, capacity to understand the nature and quality of the act charged, and capacity to form the intent to commit the crime.

lethality The relative deadliness of a chosen suicide method. For example, superficial cuts have a low degree of lethality, and a shotgun has a high degree of lethality.

light therapy A first-line treatment of seasonal affective disorder (SAD) in which the patient is exposed for 30 to 45 minutes daily to a 10,000-lux light source.

limbic system The part of the brain that is related to emotions and is referred to by some as the "emotional brain." It is involved in the mediation of fear and anxiety; anger and aggression; love, joy, and hope; and sexuality and social behavior.

lithium A mood stabilizer used in the treatment of bipolar disorder. It is a positively charged ion similar to sodium, and it may stabilize electrical activity in the brain.

lithium carbonate Known as an antimanic drug because it can stabilize the manic phase of a bipolar disorder. When effective, it can modify future manic episodes and protect against future depressive episodes.

long-term involuntary admission Used for extended care and treatment of those with mental illness. Commitments are obtained through medical certification, judicial hearings, or administrative action.

long-term memory A system for permanently storing, managing, and retrieving information for later use.

maintenance phase Phase in which health care providers focus on prevention of relapse and limitation of the severity and duration of future episodes.

maintenance roles Roles that keep a group together, help each person feel worthwhile and included, and create a sense of group cohesion.

major depressive disorder A mood disorder in which a patient presents with a history of one or more major depressive episodes and no history of manic or hypomanic episodes.

major neurocognitive disorder A disorder characterized by substantial cognitive decline that results in curtailed independence and functioning among affected individuals.

male hypoactive sexual desire disorder The male version of low interest in sex is characterized by a deficiency or absence of sexual fantasies or desire for sexual activity.

malpractice An act or failure to act that breaches the duty of due care and results in or is responsible for a person's injuries.

mania An unstable elevated mood in which delusion, poor judgment, and other signs of impaired reality testing are evident. During a manic episode patients have marked impairment of social, occupational, and interpersonal functioning.

maturational crisis A normal state in growth and development in which a specific maturational task must be learned but old coping mechanisms are no longer adequate or acceptable.

meditation A discipline for training the mind to develop greater calm and then using that calm to bring penetrative insight into one's experience.

mental health A state of well-being in which each individual is able to realize his or her own potential, cope with the normal stresses of life, work productively and fruitfully, and make a contribution to the community.

mental health continuum A conceptual line used to represent levels of mental health and mental illness that vary from person to person and vary for a particular person over time.

mental illness A clinically significant behavioral or psychological syndrome marked by the patient's distress or disability or the risk of suffering disability or loss of freedom.

mental status examination (MSE) A formal assessment of cognitive functions such as intelligence, thought processes, and capacity for insight.

metabolic syndrome Weight gain, dyslipidemia, and altered glucose metabolism caused by atypical antipsychotic drugs.

mild anxiety This first level of anxiety occurs in the normal experience of everyday living and allows people to perceive reality in sharp focus.

mild neurocognitive disorder A disorder characterized by symptoms that place individuals in a zone between normal cognition and noticeably significant cognitive deterioration.

milieu The physical and social environment of an individual.

milieu therapy A psychiatric philosophy that involves a secure environment (including people, setting, structure, and emotional climate) to effect positive change. Milieu therapy takes naturally occurring events in the environment and uses them as rich learning opportunities for patients.

mindfulness A centuries-old form of meditation that emphasizes awareness of ourselves and our mental activity from moment to moment.

minority status Describes economic and social standing in society. Many cultural, racial, and ethnic minority groups are economically and socially disadvantaged groups.

mitigation An attempt to limit a disaster's impact on human health and community function.

moderate anxiety This second level of anxiety results in selective inattention and some diminished thinking, although learning and problem solving can still occur. Symptoms include tension, pounding heart, increased pulse and respiration rate, perspiration, gastric discomfort, headache, urinary urgency, voice tremors, and shaking.

monoamine oxidase inhibitors (MAOIs) A classification of antidepressants that inhibit monoamine oxidase, an enzyme that breaks down amines such as serotonin and norepinephrine. The use of an MAOI necessitates the adoption of a tyramine-free diet because of potentially fatal interactions.

mood disorders A category of disorders characterized by disturbances of mood that range from elation to depression and interfere with normal functioning.

mood stabilizers Classes of drugs used to treat mood disorders characterized by highs (mania and hypomania) and lows (depression, depressive symptoms). Lithium and anticonvulsants are included in this class.

motor disorders A key feature of childhood growth and development is the acquisition of gross and fine motor skills and coordination. The ability to practice, exposure to new tasks, experience, and environment are factors that play a role in motor development.

multigenerational issues Various family patterns passed down through the generations.

narcissistic personality disorder A disorder characterized by a pervasive pattern of grandiosity, need for admiration, and lack of empathy for others.

National Alliance on Mental Illness (NAMI) The leading mental health consumer-advocacy organization that advocates for access to services, treatment, supports, and research.

naturopathy Emphasizes health restoration rather than disease treatment and combines nutrition, homeopathy, herbal medicine, hydrotherapy, light therapy, therapeutic counseling, and other therapies.

negative reinforcement Increasing the probability of a behavior by removing unpleasant consequences. This concept is related to positive reinforcement, which rewards or gives in to a specific behavior. A mouse that learns to press a lever to stop a shock has undergone negative reinforcement.

negative symptoms The absence of something that should be present (e.g., apathy, lack of motivation, anhedonia, poor thought processes).

neglect A form of abuse that involves failure to provide for or attend to basic physical, emotional, educational, or medical needs of another.

negligence An act, or failure to act, that breaches the duty of due care and results in or is responsible for another person's injuries.

neologisms Words a person makes up that have meaning only for that person; often part of a delusional system.

neuroleptic malignant syndrome (NMS) A rare and sometimes fatal reaction to high-potency neuroleptic drugs. Symptoms include muscle rigidity, fever, and elevated white blood cell count. It is thought to result from dopamine blockage at the basal ganglia and hypothalamus.

neurons Specialized cells in the central nervous system. Each neuron has a cell body, an axon, and dendrites.

neuroplasticity The state of malleability of the developing brain that can increase vulnerability to adverse life experiences.

neurotransmitter A chemical substance that functions as a neural messenger. Neurotransmitters are released from the axon terminal of the presynaptic neuron when stimulated by an electrical impulse.

non-suicidal self-injury Manifested by deliberate and direct attempts to cause bodily harm with no intent to cause death.

nontherapeutic communication techniques Any method of communication that detracts from the therapeutic relationship.

nonverbal behaviors Sending the "real" message through the tone or pitch of the voice.

nonverbal communication Communication without words, such as body language, eye contact, facial expressions, or gestures.

no-suicide contract A contract made between a nurse or counselor and a patient, outlined in clear and simple language, in which the patient states that he or she will not attempt self-harm and in which specific alternatives are given for the person instead.

nuclear family A family that includes a parent or parents and the children under the parents' care.

nurse coroner/death investigator A nurse who makes expert judgments of the circumstances of death based on observations of history, symptomatology, autopsy results, toxicology, other diagnostic studies, and evidence revealed in other areas of the case.

Nursing Interventions Classification (NIC) A listing of research-based nursing intervention labels that provides standardization of expected nursing interventions.

Nursing Outcomes Classification (NOC) A classification system that defines and describes patient outcomes to nursing interventions.

obsessive-compulsive disorder Obsessions are thoughts, impulses, or images that persist and recur. Compulsions are ritualistic behaviors an individual feels driven to perform to reduce anxiety. In obsessive-compulsive disorder, symptoms occur on a daily basis and may involve issues of sexuality, violence, contamination, illness, or death.

Omnibus Budget Reconciliation Act (OBRA) The 1990 act that declared that nursing home residents have the right to be free from unnecessary drugs and physical restraints.

open-ended questions Questions that encourage lengthy responses and information about experiences, perceptions, or responses to a situation and cannot be answered by a simple "yes" or "no" response.

operant conditioning A type of behavior modification in which voluntary behaviors are increased or decreased through positive reinforcement (reward), negative reinforcement (removal of objectionable event), or punishment.

oppositional defiant disorder Primarily a childhood disorder; characterized by a recurrent pattern of negativistic, disobedient, hostile, defiant behavior toward authority figures, without going so far as to seriously violate the basic rights of others.

orientation phase The phase of the nurse-patient relationship in which the nurse and patient meet and the nurse conducts the initial interview.

outcome criteria Hoped-for outcomes that reflect the maximal level of patient health that can realistically be achieved through nursing interventions.

outpatient commitment A form of mandatory treatment that requires persons to receive treatment in the community. Opponents of this care model view it as paternalistic and at odds with the patient-centered recovery model of care.

panic Panic is the fourth and most extreme level of anxiety and results in markedly disturbed behavior. Someone in a state of panic is unable to process what is going on in the environment and may lose touch with reality.

panic disorder An anxiety disorder in which panic attacks are the key feature.

paranoia A state characterized by the presence of intense and strongly defended irrational suspicions. These ideas cannot be corrected by experience and cannot be modified by facts or reality.

paraphilic disorder Refers to acts or sexual stimuli that are outside of what society considers normal but that are required for some individuals to experience desire, arousal, and orgasm.

parasuicide Self-injury with clear intent to cause bodily harm or death. Most people who eventually commit suicide have engaged in parasuicidal behaviors in the past.

parity Providing mental health care coverage equal to that for physical health care

patient-centered Refers to care that considers the patient a full partner whose values, preferences, and needs are respected.

patient-centered medical (health) home A facility that integrates primary care and behavioral health while emphasizing prevention and wellness. Care is provided by a diverse team, including advanced practice nurses, physicians, physician assistants, nurses, social workers, pharmacists, dieticians, care coordinators, and educators.

Patient Self-Determination Act (PSDA) The 1990 act that requires health care facilities to provide clear written information for every patient regarding his or her legal right to make health care decisions, including the right to accept or refuse treatment.

patient-centered care Care consisting of (1) dignity and respect, (2) information sharing, (3) patient and family participation, and (4) collaboration in policy and program development.

pedophilia A sexual disorder that involves sexual activity with a prepubescent child.

perpetrators Those who initiate violence.

perseveration The involuntary repetition of the same thought, phrase, or motor response (e.g., brushing teeth, walking); associated with brain damage.

personality Deeply ingrained personal patterns of behavior, traits, and thoughts that evolve, both consciously and unconsciously, as a person's style and way of adapting to the environment.

personality disorder An enduring pattern of experience and behavior that deviates significantly from the expectations within the individual's culture.

pharmacodynamics The physiological actions and effects of drugs in the body; includes receptor binding, postreceptor effects, and chemical interactions.

pharmacogenetics A field that focuses on how genes affect individual responses to medicines.

pharmacokinetics The physiological actions, effects, and responses of the body to drugs; includes absorption, distribution, excretion, onset of action, duration of effect, and the influence of substances such as enzymes.

phases of crisis The four phases of crisis are: (1) A crisis occurs and anxiety ensues; problem-solving techniques and defense mechanisms are used to cope with anxiety. (2) If usual defenses fail and a threat persists, anxiety rises, resulting in disorganization and discomfort. Trial-and-error is attempted for solutions. (3) If trial-and-error fails, anxiety may reach severe and panic levels, resulting in withdrawal or flight. Resolution in the form of compromising needs or redefining the situation may be made. (4) If the problem is not solved and new coping skills are ineffective, anxiety can overwhelm the person and lead to serious personality disorganization, depression, confusion, violence against others, or suicidal behavior.

phenomena of concern The central interests of a particular discipline. In nursing, these are commonly considered to be person, health, environment, and nursing.

physical abuse The infliction of physical pain or bodily harm on another.

physical restraint Any manual method or mechanical device, material, or equipment that inhibits free movement.

physical stressors Environmental and physical conditions that elicit the stress response.

pica Eating nonfood items after maturing past toddlerhood.

play therapy An intervention that allows a child to symbolically express feelings such as aggression, self-doubt, anxiety, and sadness through the medium of play.

polypharmacy The use of multiple medications by patients, including prescription and over-the-counter drugs. Individuals taking five to seven medications have twice the rate of adverse drug reactions as compared with those taking fewer than five medications.

positive reinforcement The presentation of a reward immediately following a behavior, making the behavior more likely to occur in the future.

positive symptoms The presence of something that is not normally present (e.g., hallucinations, delusions, bizarre behavior, paranoia).

posttraumatic stress disorder (PTSD) An anxiety disorder characterized by persistent reexperiencing of a highly traumatic event that involved actual or threatened death or serious injury to self or others, to which the individual responded with intense fear, helplessness, or horror.

postvention Therapeutic interventions with the significant others of an individual who has committed suicide.

preconscious Unconscious thoughts (including memory) that are available for retrieval by the conscious at any time.

premature ejaculation A sexual dysfunction in which a man persistently or recurrently achieves orgasm and ejaculation before he wishes to.

preparedness Enhancing efforts to develop greater resiliency at local community levels.

prescribing cascade Prescribing a new drug to treat the side effects of a previously prescribed drug; the symptoms of the first drug may be evaluated as part of the medical problem.

prevalence The total number of cases of a disease within a population at a given time.

prevention Reducing the incidence of health problems, stopping illnesses from progressing, and reducing disability, severity, and death.

primary care Care that promotes mental health and reduces mental illness.

primary intervention Interventions that include activities to provide support, information, and education to prevent or reduce the rate at which new cases of a disorder develop.

primary prevention Activities that provide support, information, and education, with the goal of prevention.

principle of least restrictive intervention Techniques are selected to ensure that the civil and legal rights of individuals are maintained.

progressive muscle relaxation (PMR) A method of decreasing anxiety in which the individual tenses groups of muscles as tightly as possible for 8 seconds and then suddenly releases them.

pseudoparkinsonism A medication-induced temporary constellation of symptoms associated with Parkinson's disease, including tremor, reduced accessory movements, impaired gait, and stiffening of muscles.

psychiatric case management A program that coordinates services for individual patient care.

psychiatric mental health nursing A specialty area in nursing and the core mental health profession that promotes mental health through use of the nursing process in the treatment of mental health problems and psychiatric disorders.

psychiatry's definition of mental health A definition of mental health that evolves over time and is shaped by the prevailing culture and societal values. It reflects changes in cultural norms, societal expectations, political climates, and even reimbursement criteria by third-party payers.

psychodynamic therapy A therapeutic modality based on classical psychoanalysis but with less focus on the early development of pathology. It uses free association, dream analysis, transference, and countertransference. The therapist is actively involved and interacts with the client in the here and now.

psychoeducation Educating about mental health topics (e.g., psychotropic drugs) and building skills (e.g., conflict resolution).

psychoeducational groups A group set up to increase knowledge or skills about a specific somatic or psychological subject and allow members to communicate emotional concerns.

psychological autopsies Retrospective review of a deceased person's life within several months of the death to establish likely diagnoses at the time of death.

psychological factors affecting medical condition A psychiatric classification that calls attention to how psychological factors may magnify and/or adversely affect medical conditions.

psychological stressors Stressors of the psyche, including divorce, loss of a job, unmanageable debt, death of a loved one, retirement, and fear of a terrorist attack, as well as changes one might consider positive, such as marriage, arrival of a new baby, or unexpected success.

psychomotor agitation Constant involvement in tension-relieving activities, such as pacing, biting one's nails, smoking, or tapping one's fingers on a tabletop.

psychomotor retardation Extreme slowness of and difficulty in physical and emotional reactions that in the extreme can entail complete inactivity and incontinence.

psychoneuroimmunology Study of the links among stress, the immune system, and disease.

psychosocial assessment Provides additional information from which to develop a plan of care.

psychosocial rehabilitation The development of the skills necessary for a person with chronic mental illness to live independently.

punishment Involves applying a stimulus after a behavior in order to reduce likelihood that the behavior will occur again in the future.

pyromania Repeated deliberate fire setting related to impulse control disorders.

race A group of humans within the population that share common heritable characteristics such as color of skin, eyes, and hair.

rape Defined in the context of nonconsensual activity and involving any penetration of the vagina or anus with any object or body part or the oral penetration by a sex organ of another person.

rape-trauma syndrome A syndrome characterized by an acute phase and a long-term reorganization process that occurs after an actual or attempted sexual assault. Each phase has separate symptoms.

rapid cycling Experiencing four or more mood episodes in a 12-month period.

rapport A relationship characterized by trust, support, and understanding.

reactive attachment disorder A disorder describing children who have a consistent pattern of inhibited, emotionally withdrawn behavior and who rarely direct attachment behaviors toward any adult caregivers.

reality testing A process by which a person is objectively able to evaluate the external world and adequately distinguish it from the internal world (the self).

receptors Protein molecules located within or on the outer membrane of cells of various tissues, such as neurons, muscles, and blood vessels. A receptor receives chemical stimulation that causes a chemical reaction, resulting in either stimulation or inhibition of the activity of the cell.

recovery Actions focusing on stabilizing the community and returning it to its normal status.

recovery model A model that is patient/consumer-centered, is hopeful and empowering, and emphasizes the person and the future rather than the illness and the present.

recovery-oriented systems of care (ROSC) Networks composed of formal and informal services that have been organized to support individuals and their families for long-term recovery in the face of substance use and addictive disorders.

refugee An immigrant who has left his or her native country to escape intolerable conditions and who would have preferred to stay in the original culture.

registered nurse–psychiatric mental health (RN-PMH) A registered nurse with experience as a psychiatric mental health nurse who may be employed as a staff nurse, case manager, or home care nurse.

rehabilitation A concept focused on managing patients' deficits and helping them learn to live with their illnesses; criticized by the consumer movement as being paternalistic and focused on living with disability rather than on quality of life and eventual cure.

Reiki An energy-based therapy in which a practitioner's energy is connected to a universal source (*chi, qi, prana*) and is transferred to a recipient for physical or spiritual healing.

reinforcement Responses from the environment that increase the probability that a behavior will be repeated.

relaxation response A set of physiological changes that result in decreased activity of the sympathetic part of the autonomic nervous system and a shift to the parasympathetic mode, which induces a state of relaxation. It is the opposite of the fight-or-flight response and has a stabilizing effect on the nervous system.

resilience The ability to adapt and cope that helps people to face tragedies, loss, trauma, and severe stress.

response Actual implementation of a disaster plan.

restraint See *physical restraint* and *chemical restraint.*

reticular activating system (RAS) The part of the brain stem that mediates alertness, arousal, and motivation and serves to filter out repetitive stimuli to prevent overload.

reuptake The reabsorption of neurotransmitters to the presynaptic cell that originally produced and secreted them after communication with receptors on the postsynaptic cell. Serotonin is most commonly associated with this process.

right to privacy The legal expectation of privacy concerning the sharing of medical information.

right to refuse treatment The right to reject forced treatment. This right takes into consideration a person's right for choice, or autonomy, and beneficence, actions that benefit others.

right to treatment The right to expect appropriate and adequate treatment.

rigid or disengaged boundaries Adherence to the "rules and roles" within a family, no matter what the situation. Rigid boundaries prevent family members from trying out new roles or taking on more mature functions.

rumination Regurgitation with rechewing, reswallowing, or spitting.

SAD PERSONS scale A simple and practical assessment tool to evaluate potentially suicidal patients.

safety plan A plan for rapid escape when abuse recurs.

schizoid personality disorder A disorder characterized by extreme emotional detachment and lack of relationships. Depersonalization, or feelings of detachment from oneself and the world, may be present.

schizotypal personality disorder A disorder characterized by lack of warmth, aloofness, and indifference to the feelings of others. Contributions to conversations tend to ramble and are lengthy, unclear, and overly detailed. Paranoia and mild, transient hallucinations and delusions distinguish this disorder from schizoid personality disorder.

Screening, Brief Intervention, Referral to Treatment (SBIRT) A public health approach that seeks to intervene early and provide treatment for people with substance use disorders and for those at risk of developing these disorders.

seclusion The last step in a process to maximize the safety of a patient and others, in which the patient is placed alone in a specially designed room for protection and close observation.

seclusion protocol The standardized procedure by which seclusion is used.

secondary care Establishes intervention during an acute crisis to prevent prolonged anxiety that may diminish personal effectiveness and personality organization.

secondary gain The benefits a person realizes from symptoms or relief behaviors he or she employs, including increased attention from others, avoidance of expected responsibilities, financial gain, and the ability to manipulate others in the environment.

secondary intervention Providing immediate intervention in times of crisis or acute illness.

secondary prevention Involves early detection and intervention in acute illness or situations to minimize disabling or long-term effects.

second-generation (atypical) antipsychotics A newer classification of drugs (compared to first-generation antipsychotics) that produces fewer extrapyramidal side effects (EPS) and targets both the negative and positive symptoms of schizophrenia.

selective serotonin reuptake inhibitors (SSRIs) First-line antidepressants that block the reuptake of serotonin, permitting serotonin to act for an extended period at the synaptic binding sites in the brain.

self-care activities The activities such as eating, attending to hygiene, and toileting that are necessary to live independently as an adult.

self-help groups Groups of people with similar problems or concerns who meet to receive peer support and encouragement and work together to use their strengths to gain control over their lives.

separation anxiety disorder Exhibiting developmentally inappropriate levels of concern over being away from a significant other.

separation-individuation A psychological process in which a child separates from the mother (or significant parent) into a physically and psychologically differentiated person. This process may be disrupted and result in a disturbance in maintaining a reliable feeling of individual identity.

serious mental illness (SMI) Persons with SMI usually have difficulties in multiple areas, including activities of daily living (ADLs; e.g., cooking, hygiene), relationships, social interaction, task completion, communication, leisure activities, remaining safe in the community, finances and budgeting, health maintenance, vocational and academic activities, coping with poverty, stigma, unemployment, and inadequate housing.

severe anxiety This third level of anxiety is debilitating and causes a person to focus on one particular detail or many scattered details. Learning cannot occur, and other aspects of the environment go unnoticed, even when another points them out.

sex reassignment surgery A surgical procedure that reshapes sexual organs from one gender to another.

sexual abuse Any form of sexual contact or exposure without consent or in circumstances in which the victim is incapable of giving consent.

sexual assault nurse examiner (SANE) The first specialized forensic role for nurses, SANEs are forensic nurse generalists who receive training in the care of adult and pediatric victims of sexual assault.

sexual assault Forced and violent vaginal, anal, or oral penetration against an adult victim's will and without the victim's consent. Legal definitions vary from state to state.

sexual disorders Psychiatric disorders in which sexual problems are considered to be socially atypical, have the potential to disrupt meaningful relationships, and may result in insult or even significant injury to other people.

sexual dysfunction A disturbance in the desire, excitement, or orgasm phases of the sexual response cycle, or pain during sexual intercourse.

sexual violence Includes sexual harassment, stranger rape, marital rape, date rape, and drug-facilitated sexual assault. Sexual violence also includes denying emergency contraception or measures to prevent sexually transmitted infections, organized rape during conflict or war, and sexual homicide.

shelters or safe houses Temporary residences that serve as refuges for abused spouses.

short-term memory Immediate recall of a small amount of information.

situational crisis A crisis arising from an external as opposed to an internal source. Most people experience situational crises to some extent during the course of their lives (e.g., death of a loved one, marriage, divorce, change in health status).

skin picking disorder Also known as *dermotillomania;* an anxiety-relieving activity in which individuals consciously pick at their skin. It is a distressing problem that may result in varying degrees of disability, social stigma, and altered appearance.

sleep architecture A term that refers to the structure and pattern of sleep.

sleep continuity The distribution of sleep and wakefulness across the sleep period.

sleep deprivation A state that occurs from a discrepancy between hours of sleep obtained and hours of sleep required for optimal functioning.

sleep drive Promotes sleep and is known as the *homeostatic process.* The longer the period of wakefulness, the stronger the sleep drive.

sleep efficiency Ratio of sleep duration to time spent in bed.

sleep fragmentation Disruption of sleep stages as indicated by excessive amounts of stage 1 sleep, multiple brief arousals, and frequent shifts in sleep staging.

sleep hygiene Conditions and practices that promote continuous and effective sleep.

sleep latency The time it takes to go to sleep.

sleep restriction Limiting the total sleep time, which creates a temporary, mild state of sleep deprivation and strengthens the sleep homeostatic drive.

social anxiety disorder Also called *social phobia*; characterized by severe anxiety or fear provoked by exposure to a social or performance situation that will be evaluated negatively by others.

social cognition The ability to "read" social situations in relation to how others might be feeling and determine what is appropriate for the environmental context.

social relationship A relationship that is primarily initiated for the purpose of friendship, socialization, enjoyment, or accomplishment of a task.

social skills training Focuses on socialization, activities of daily living (ADLs), and prevocational training (the fundamentals needed before one can be successfully employed [e.g., interviewing, dressing for work, interacting professionally with co-workers]).

sociocultural context The culture that a person lives in, which includes the people and environment with whom the person interacts.

somatic symptom disorder A psychiatric disorder characterized by a combination of distressing symptoms and an excessive or maladaptive response or associated health concerns without significant physical findings and medical diagnosis.

somatization The expression of psychological stress through physical symptoms.

specific learning disorders Identified during the school years. A learning disorder is diagnosed when a child demonstrates persistent difficulty in the acquisition of reading (dyslexia), mathematics (dyscalculia), and/or written expression (dysgraphia), and his or her performance is well below the expected performance of peers.

specific phobias Fear and avoidance of a single object, situation, or activity; common in the general population.

splitting A primitive defense mechanism in which the person sees self or others as all good or all bad, failing to integrate the positive and negative qualities of the self and others into a cohesive whole.

spousal (or marital) rape A rape in which the perpetrator (nearly always the male) is married to the person raped.

stabilization A treatment strategy aimed at support and preventing further decline in psychiatric functioning.

stereotyped behaviors A motor pattern that originally had meaning to the person (e.g., sweeping the floor, washing windows) but has become mechanical and lacks purpose.

stereotyping The assumption that all people in a similar cultural, racial, or ethnic group think and act alike.

stigma Negative attitudes or behaviors toward a person or group, based on a belief that they possess negative traits.

stimulus control A behavioral intervention that involves adherence to five basic principles that decrease the negative associations between the bed and bedroom and strengthen the stimulus for sleep.

stressors Psychological or physical stimuli that are incompatible with current functioning and require adaptation.

substance use disorder Complex diseases of the brain represented by drug use, craving, and seeking regardless of consequences.

suicidal ideation Thoughts a person has regarding killing himself or herself.

suicide The ultimate act of self-destruction in which a person purposefully ends his or her own life.

suicide attempt Any willful, self-inflicted, life-threatening attempt at suicide that did not lead to death.

sundowning Increasing destabilization of cognitive abilities (e.g., confusion) and lability of mood during the late afternoon, early evening, or night; seen in people with cognitive disorders.

superego One of three psychological processes that make up the Freudian system of personality (id, ego, and superego). The superego is the internal representative of the values, ideals, and moral standards of society. The superego is said to be the moral arm of the personality.

support groups Groups that use a variety of modalities to help people cope with overwhelming situations or alter unwanted behaviors during stressful periods.

supported employment Work and training in supportive settings for people with disabilities that helps them to become active workforce members.

supportive psychotherapy Therapy focused on supporting the patient at the current stage of illness rather than confronting possible problems and pushing the patient toward change.

survivor A term often used instead of *victim* because of its positive and assertive associations with recovery and healing.

synapse The gap between the membrane of one neuron and the membrane of another neuron. The synapse is the point at which the transmission of the nerve impulse occurs.

systematic desensitization A form of behavior modification therapy that involves the development of behavior tasks customized to a patient's specific fears. The patient is gradually exposed to his or her fears while using relaxation techniques.

tardive dyskinesia (TD or TDK) A serious and irreversible side effect of phenothiazines and related drugs; consists of involuntary tonic muscle spasms typically involving the tongue, fingers, toes, neck, trunk, or pelvis.

task roles Roles within a group that keep a group focused on its main purpose and get the work done.

temperament The style of behavior a child habitually uses to cope with the demands and expectations of the environment.

temporary admission Admitting patients with acute psychiatric symptoms on an emergency basis upon written order of a primary care provider for a limited amount of time.

termination phase The final, integral phase of the nurse-patient relationship.

tertiary care Provides support for those who have experienced a crisis or illness and are now recovering from a disabling mental state.

tertiary intervention Also known as *postvention.* Refers to interventions with the circle of survivors of a person who has completed suicide. This is done to both reduce the traumatic aftereffects and explore effective means of addressing survivor problems using primary and secondary interventions.

tertiary prevention Involves the facilitation of healing and rehabilitation to reduce the severity, impairment, or disability resulting from an illness or a situation.

therapeutic communication techniques Responses that maximize nurse-patient interactions.

therapeutic encounter A brief, informal meeting between nurse and patient in which the relationship is useful and important for the patient.

therapeutic factors Aspects of the group experience that leaders and members have identified as facilitating therapeutic change.

therapeutic games Games the nurse can play with a child to facilitate the development of a therapeutic relationship and provide an opportunity for conversation.

therapeutic index The ratio of the therapeutic dose of a drug and the toxic dose of a drug.

therapeutic milieu See *milieu.*

therapeutic relationship A relationship requiring that the nurse maximize his or her communication skills, understanding of human behaviors, and personal strengths in order to enhance personal growth in the patient. This relationship occurs in all clinical settings, not just those on a psychiatric unit.

therapeutic touch An energy therapy in which the practitioner focuses completely on the person receiving the treatment, assesses the energy field, clears and balances the energy field through hand movements, and/or directs energy in a specific region of the body.

therapeutic use of self Creative use of unique personality traits and talents to form positive bonds with others.

third-generation antipsychotics A newer classification of antipsychotics includes aripiprazole (Abilify), a unique antipsychotic known for dopamine system stabilization. In areas of the brain with excess dopamine, it lowers the dopamine level by acting as a receptor antagonist; however, in regions with low dopamine, it stimulates receptors to raise the dopamine level. Side effects include insomnia and akathisia.

tolerance Needing increased amounts of a substance in order to receive the desired result to become intoxicated or finding that using the same amount over time results in a much-diminished effect.

tort A civil wrong for which money damages (or other relief) may be obtained by the injured party (plaintiff) from the wrongdoer (defendant).

transcranial magnetic stimulation (TMS) A noninvasive treatment modality that uses MRI-strength magnetic pulses to stimulate focal areas of the cerebral cortex.

transference The experiencing of thoughts and feelings toward a person (often the therapist) that were originally held toward a significant person in one's past. Transference is a valuable tool used by therapists in psychoanalytical psychotherapy.

transinstitutionalization The shifting of a person or population from one kind of institution to another, such as from state hospitals to jails, prisons, nursing homes, or shelters.

transtheoretical model of care A model that describes the stages people go through when they change behaviors. The stages include precontemplation, contemplation, preparation, action, and maintenance.

trauma-informed care Based on an understanding of the vulnerabilities and triggers in psychiatric patients who have histories that include violence and victimization.

triage The process of sorting people based on their need for immediate treatment as compared to their chance of benefiting from such care.

tricyclic antidepressants (TCAs) Drugs that inhibit the reuptake of norepinephrine and serotonin by the presynaptic neurons in the central nervous system, increasing the amount of time they are available to the postsynaptic receptors. Muscarinic blockage leads to anticholinergic effects such as blurred vision, dry mouth, tachycardia, urinary retention, and constipation.

unconditional release Termination of a patient-institutional relationship.

unconscious Repressed memories, feelings, thoughts, or wishes that are not available to the conscious mind. Usually, these unconscious memories, feelings, thoughts, or wishes are associated with intense anxiety and can greatly affect an individual's behavior.

unintentional torts Unintended acts against another person that produce injury or harm.

vagus nerve stimulation (VNS) A pacemaker-like device is implanted surgically into the left chest wall; from this device, a thin, flexible wire is threaded up and wrapped around the vagus nerve on the left side of the neck. Electrical stimulation of the vagus nerve is thought to boost the level of neurotransmitters, improving mood and the action of antidepressants.

validation therapy A therapeutic modality that is typically used for older adults and focuses on emotional themes rather than content.

values Abstract standards that represent an ideal, either positive or negative.

vegetative signs of depression Significant changes from normal functioning in those activities necessary to support life and growth (such as eating, sleeping, elimination, and sex), occuring during a depressive episode.

verbal communication All of the words a person speaks.

violence An objectionable act that involves intentional use of force that results in, or has the potential to result in, injury to another person.

vocational rehabilitation State agencies that emphasized extensive prevocational training and employment in sheltered workshops before placement in competitive jobs. Success of this type of program was low.

voluntary admission Inpatient care sought by a patient or patient's guardian through a written application to the facility.

voyeurism An illegal activity that involves seeking sexual arousal through viewing, usually secretly, of other people in intimate situations.

vulnerable person A family member upon whom abuse is perpetrated.

Western tradition A worldview in which one's identity is found in individuality, which inspires the valuing of autonomy, independence, and self-reliance. Mind and body are seen as two separate entities, and different practitioners treat disorders of the body and the mind.

window of tolerance A term that refers to a balance between sympathetic and parasympathetic arousal.

withdrawal The negative physiological and psychological reactions that occur when a drug taken for a long period is reduced in dosage or no longer taken.

word salad A mixture of words meaningless to the listener and to the speaker as well.

working phase The phase of the nurse-patient relationship during which the nurse and patient identify and explore areas that are causing problems in the patient's life.

worldview A system for thinking about how the world works and how people should behave in it and in relationships with one another.

writ of habeas corpus A "formal written order" to "free the person."

INDEX

A

Page numbers followed by *f*, *t*, and *b* indicate figures, tables, and boxes, respectively.

B

C

D

E

F

G

Q

T